DIAGNOSTIC ULTRASOUND OF FETAL ANOMALIES: TEXT AND ATLAS

Diagnostic Ultrasound of Fetal Anomalies: Text and Atlas

DAVID A. NYBERG, M.D.
*Associate Clinical Professor of Radiology and Obstetrics
and Gynecology
University of Washington Hospital
Co-Director of Obstetric Ultrasound
Swedish Hospital Medical Center
Seattle, Washington*

BARRY S. MAHONY, M.D.
*Co-Director of Obstetric Ultrasound
Swedish Hospital Medical Center
Seattle, Washington*

DOLORES H. PRETORIUS, M.D.
*Associate Professor of Radiology
Department of Radiology
University of California at San Diego
San Diego, California*

YEAR BOOK MEDICAL PUBLISHERS, INC.
CHICAGO • LONDON • BOCA RATON • LITTLETON, MASS.

1 2 3 4 5 6 7 8 9 0 C Y 94 93 92 91 90

Library of Congress Cataloging-in-Publication Data

Nyberg, David A., 1952–
    Diagnostic ultrasound of fetal anomalies : text and atlas /
David A. Nyberg, Barry S. Mahony, Dolores H. Pretorius.
        p.   cm.
    Includes bibliographical references.
    ISBN 0-8151-6439-4
    1. Fetus—Abnormalities—Diagnosis.   2. Fetus—Diseases—
Diagnosis.   3. Diagnosis, Ultrasonic.   I. Mahony, Barry S.
II. Pretorius, Dolores.   III. Title.
    [DNLM: 1. Abnormalities—diagnosis.   2. Fetal Diseases—diagnosis.
3. Prenatal Diagnosis.   4. Ultrasonic Diagnosis.   WQ 211 N993d]
RG628.3.U58N93 1990
618.3'207543—dc20
DNLM/DLC   89–22409
for Library of Congress   CIP

Sponsoring Editor: James D. Ryan
Associate Director, Manuscript Services: Frances M. Perveiler
Production Project Coordinator: Karen Halm
Proofroom Supervisor: Barbara M. Kelly

To those who have cultivated our academic interest: Barbara, Brooke, Faye, George, Jim, Larry, Michael, Peter, and Roy.

CONTRIBUTORS

N. SCOTT ADZICK, M.D.
Assistant Professor of Surgery and Pediatrics
University of California at San Francisco
Attending Surgeon
Division of Pediatric Surgery
University of California at San Francisco Medical Center
San Francisco, California

JAMES P. CRANE, M.D.
Professor, Obstetrics-Gynecology and Radiology
Washington University School of Medicine
Director, Department of Obstetrics and Gynecology
Jewish Hospital at Washington University
St. Louis, Missouri

DONALD S. EMERSON, M.D.
Director of Ultrasound
Memphis Regional Medical Center
University of Tennessee
Memphis, Tennessee

HARRIS J. FINBERG, M.D.
Director of Diagnostic Ultrasound
Phoenix Perinatal Associates
Radiologist, Good Samaritan Medical Center
Phoenix, Arizona

PETER A. GRANNUM, M.D.
Associate Professor
Director of Medical Studies
Yale University School of Medicine
Director of Clinical High Risk Obstetrics
Yale New Haven Hospital
New Haven, Connecticut

FRANK P. HADLOCK, M.D.
Professor of Radiology
Baylor College of Medicine
Medical Director
Radiology Department
Lyndon B. Johnson General Hospital
Houston, Texas

FREDERICK N. HEGGE, M.D.
Director of Ultrasound
Emanuel Hospital
Portland, Oregon

LYNDON M. HILL, M.D.
Associate Professor of Obstetrics and Gynecology
Division of Maternal-Fetal Medicine
Director of Ultrasound

Magee-Women's Hospital
Pittsburgh, Pennsylvania

PAMELA L. HILPERT, M.D., PH.D.
Assistant Professor of Radiology
Thomas Jefferson University Hospital
Philadelphia, Pennsylvania

JACOB C. LANGER, M.D.
Assistant Professor of Surgery and Pediatrics
McMaster University
Hamilton, Ontario, Canada

GEORGE R. LEOPOLD, M.D.
Professor of Radiology
University of California at San Diego
Chairman, Department of Radiology
University of California at San Diego Medical Center
San Diego, California

DAVID A. NYBERG, M.D.
Associate Clinical Professor of Radiology and Obstetrics and
  Gynecology
University of Washington Hospital
Co–Director of Obstetric Ultrasound
Swedish Hospital Medical Center
Seattle, Washington

LAURENCE A. MACK, M.D.
Professor of Radiology
Adjunct Professor of Obstetrics-Gynecology and Orthopedics
University of Washington Medical Center
Director of Diagnostic Ultrasound
Seattle, Washington

BARRY S. MAHONY, M.D.
Co–Director of Obstetric Ultrasound
Swedish Hospital Medical Center
Seattle, Washington

DOLORES H. PRETORIUS, M.D.
Associate Professor of Radiology
Department of Radiology
University of California at San Diego
San Diego, California

YOGESH P. SHAH, M.D.
Assistant Clinical Professor of Radiology
Baylor College of Medicine
Houston, Texas

PREFACE

It would be a gross understatement to say that obstetric ultrasound has developed an essential role in the prenatal detection and diagnosis of congenital anomalies. Even when anomalies are not specifically sought, it is a fact of nature that anyone who performs, interprets, or requests obstetric sonograms will occasionally encounter anomalous fetuses. Such anomalies are not limited by geography, race, or social class. Rather, they reflect the complexity of normal human development.

The impetus for this textbook began with a series of unending questions not easily answered from other sources. How certain are we that the sonographic findings are normal or abnormal? Which sonographic findings permit a reliable diagnosis of a specific anomaly? What other findings might be demonstrated? How often should these findings be visualized? When should they be visualized? What other diagnoses should be considered? What is the likelihood we missed something? What sonographic findings are predictive of the eventual outcome for this pregnancy and fetus? What is the implication for future pregnancies? How do the sonographic findings compare with the pathologic findings?

This textbook is an attempt to answer some of these questions. It is primarily intended for those who perform and interpret obstetric sonograms, whether or not they are experienced in diagnosing fetal anomalies. Obstetricians and other health care providers should find it of interest, especially when one of their patients is diagnosed with a fetal anomaly. It is hoped that geneticists, neonatologists, pediatricians, surgeons and other members of the health care team involved in the care of the patient and anomalous fetus will also find it useful.

The ultimate goal of this textbook is to promote improved prenatal and perinatal management of pregnancies affected by an anomalous fetus. More immediate goals include improved *detection, diagnosis,* and *understanding* of congenital anomalies.

Detection of congenital anomalies assumes that an effective screening examination of the fetus is performed; Chapter 1 discusses the current guidelines recommended by various governing bodies regarding screening obstetric sonograms for congenital anomalies. Familiarity with these guidelines is strongly encouraged for improved detection of congenital anomalies during "routine" obstetric sonographic examinations. Detection of congenital anomalies also requires that the sonologist/sonographer be familiar with normal fetal anatomy and be able to recognize deviations from normal. The introductory sections of Chapters 5 through 15 discuss normal embryologic development, normal sonographic findings, and potential pitfalls related to detection of specific fetal anomalies. Because it is assumed that the anatomic area of interest is known even if the specific anomaly is uncertain, the chapters are arranged primarily on the basis of anatomic regions.

Correct *diagnosis* of congenital anomalies requires an appreciation of both typical and atypical sonographic findings that permits a reliable diagnosis of specific anomalies. Recognizing that the primary suspected diagnosis may be in error, differential diagnoses and potential pitfalls of specific anomalies are presented throughout the textbook to encourage consideration of alternative diagnoses. Correlation of sonographic and pathologic findings are emphasized to give the reader a full appreciation of the suspected anomaly. A large number of images and illustrations are included to compare images of the suspected anomaly with similar cases. Because the accumulative experience is greater than any individual experience in describing the spectrum of sonographic findings related to specific anomalies, we have freely borrowed illustrative cases from the literature.

Improved *understanding* of congenital anomalies requires a basic knowledge of the underlying pathophysiology. The more the sonologist/sonographer knows about the underlying condition, the better able he/she can contribute to the management of that pregnancy. Chapters 5 through 15 emphasize the significance and natural history of common anomalies. Frequently associated anomalies, chromosome abnormalities, and other predictors of outcome are described for each condition. Information derived from the prenatal literature is emphasized since it is often quite different than the postnatal experience. A large number of references are provided, arranged by the type of anomaly, to promote further reading and research.

In addition to chapters that address specific individual anomalies and disorders (Chapters 5 through 15), we have included chapters intended to promote a greater understanding of congenital anomalies as they relate to prenatal ultrasound. Chapter 2 presents an overview of congenital anomalies and compares the prenatal sonographic experience with postnatal data. Because oligohydramnios or polyhydramnios may be the first and foremost clue to many congenital anomalies, Chapter 3 discusses abnormalities of amniotic fluid volume and their relationship with anomalous fetuses.

Screening maternal serum alpha-fetoprotein is invaluable for identifying many anomalies; Chapter 4 is dedicated to this subject as it relates to obstetric sonography.

Chapter 16 discusses abnormalities of the placenta, placental membranes, and umbilical cord and their relation to fetal mortality. Prenatal sonographic findings that may increase the risk of an underlying chromosome abnormality have become a topic of great interest in recent years; Chapter 17 takes an in-depth look at common chromosome abnormalities and discusses sonographic findings that may indicate the need for chromosome analysis. Finally, awareness of corrective surgery provides hope for the newborn with congenital anomalies. Chapter 18 presents a surgical perspective for selected anomalies that are frequently detected on prenatal sonography.

DAVID A. NYBERG, M.D.
BARRY S. MAHONY, M.D.
DOLORES H. PRETORIUS, M.D.

ACKNOWLEDGMENTS

We greatly acknowledge the generosity of the many scientists in the United States and Europe who have contributed photographs and illustrations, or who permitted their data to be shared in this forum. Greater understanding of congenital anomalies is a collaborative effort by many individuals from various disciplines; we express our sincere appreciation to our many colleagues in the fields of radiology, obstetrics, surgery, pediatrics, pathology, and genetics, and especially to our perinatal colleagues. We also thank our colleagues who have trusted their patients to our observations, the sonographers who were largely responsible for the quality of images, and the patients for their patience in our endeavors. Special mention is given to Renee Durnell for tireless preparation of manuscript revisions, Lisa Ireland for data management, Swedish Medical Center photography department and Jeff Larsen for photography, Thomas Shepard and the Central Laboratory for Human Embryology for contributing pathologic photographs, Rob Schaller for his enthusiasm and insightful comments, and Cheryl Herndon and Dinah Wilson for original art work. We also thank the staff at Year Book Medical Publishers, especially Jim Ryan, whose assistance made this textbook possible.

Most importantly, we express our deep gratitude to our spouses and families for their quiet forebearance, unselfish devotion, and constant encouragement.

DAVID A. NYBERG, M.D.
BARRY S. MAHONY, M.D.
DOLORES H. PRETORIUS, M.D.

CONTENTS

The Role of Obstetrical Ultrasonography

Dolores H. Pretorius, M.D.

Barry S. Mahony, M.D.

Ultrasonography provides a window of unsurpassed clarity into the gravid uterus. Over the past 10 years, high-resolution real-time ultrasound has undeniably become the most prevalent and accurate means of obstetrical imaging, capable of providing exquisite detail regarding the fetus and the intrauterine environment. Information provided by prenatal sonography has been found to be indispensable for evaluating and managing a variety of common obstetric problems, including growth disturbances, vaginal bleeding, multiple gestations, and congenital anomalies.

INDICATIONS

The indications for obstetric sonography remain controversial. Some investigators advocate the use of ultrasonography as a routine screening modality in all pregnancies; others confine its use to pregnancies with a well-defined clinical indication.

To help define the clinical indications of obstetrical ultrasonography, the National Institutes of Health Consensus Development Conference (NIHCDC) evaluated available evidence regarding its bioeffects and clinical efficacy in 1984.[20] As a result of this conference, the NIHCDC listed clinical indications in which ultrasound imaging, although not mandatory, may be of benefit during pregnancy (Table 1–1). It concluded that the available data did not allow a recommendation of screening obstetrical ultrasonography at that time.[12]

The efficacy of routine obstetric sonography was also addressed earlier by several randomized, controlled clinical trials in Europe. Although each trial reached somewhat different conclusions, pooled data and review of the technical aspects of these trials supported the conclusion that routine scanning of all pregnancies was not justified at that time.[5, 8, 11, 13, 14, 15, 21]

Conclusions from these earlier studies do not necessarily remain applicable to contemporary ultrasonography, however, since dramatic interim advances have occurred in instrumentation, data analysis, and operator expertise since the original studies. For example, data analysis for intrauterine growth retardation now involves assessment of multiple parameters, whereas two of the European trials used biparietal diameter measurements as the sole criterion.

Some authors advocate the use of routine obstetrical sonography purely on the basis of improved detection and management of twin gestations. Screening sonography detected 95% of twin gestations prior to 20 weeks of gestation in one study, whereas a program which did not utilize screening ultrasonography detected only 47% of twins before 24 weeks.[16, 22, 23] Routine use of prenatal sonography might also be justified for its increasingly important role in the detection and management of congenital malformations (discussed below).

Arguments against routine obstetric scanning include its financial cost, concerns for safety to the developing fetus, and the potential to adversely affect the management of the pregnancy due to misuse or misinterpretation of sonographic findings. Of these, its financial cost is probably the most important obstacle to routine scanning. In the United States alone, the cost for one ultrasound examination for each of the 3 million babies born each year would total $450 million,

TABLE 1-1.

Conditions in Which, According to the National Institutes of Health Consensus Development Panel, Diagnostic Ultrasonography May Be Helpful During Pregnancy*

1. Estimation of gestational age for patients with uncertain clinical dates or verification of dates for patients who are to undergo scheduled elective repeated cesarean delivery, indicated induction of labor, or other elective termination of pregnancy.
2. Evaluation of fetal growth (e.g., when the patient has an identified cause for uteroplacental insufficiency, such as severe preeclampsia, chronic hypertension, chronic renal disease, severe diabetes mellitus), or for other medical complications of pregnancy where fetal malnutrition, i.e., intrauterine growth retardation or macrosomia, is suspected.
3. Vaginal bleeding of undetermined etiology.
4. Determination of fetal presentation when the presenting part cannot be adequately determined in labor or the fetal presentation is variable in late pregnancy.
5. Suspected multiple gestation based on detection of more than one fetal heartbeat pattern or fundal height larger than expected for dates and/or prior use of fertility drugs.
6. Adjunct to amniocentesis.
7. Significant discrepancy in uterine size compared with clinical dates.
8. Pelvic mass detected clinically.
9. Suspected hydatidiform mole on the basis of clinical signs of hypertension, proteinuria, and/or the presence of ovarian cysts felt on pelvic examination or failure to detect fetal heart tones with a Doppler ultrasound device after 12 weeks' gestation.
10. Adjunct to cervical cerclage placement.
11. Suspected ectopic pregnancy or pregnancy occurring after tuboplasty or prior ectopic gestation.
12. Follow-up evaluation of placental location for identified placenta previa.
13. Adjunct to special procedures, such as fetoscopy, intrauterine transfusion, shunt placement, in vitro fertilization, embryo transfer, or chorionic villi sampling.
14. Suspected fetal death.
15. Suspected uterine abnormality (e.g., clinically significant leiomyoma or congenital structural abnormalities, such as uterus bicornis or uterus didelphus.
16. Intrauterine (contraceptive) device (IUD) localization.
17. Ovarian follicle development surveillance.
18. Biophysical evaluation for fetal well-being after 28 weeks of gestation.
19. Observation of intrapartum events (e.g., version or extraction of second twin, manual removal of placenta).
20. Suspected polyhydramnios or oligohydramnios.
21. Suspected abruptio placentae.
22. Adjunct to external version from breech to vertex presentation.
23. Estimation of fetal weight and/or presentation in premature rupture of membranes and/or premature labor.
24. Abnormal serum alpha-fetoprotein (AFP) value for clinical gestational age.
25. Follow-up observation of identified fetal anomaly.
26. History of previous congenital anomaly.
27. Serial evaluation of fetal growth in multiple gestation.
28. Evaluation of fetal condition in late registrants for prenatal care.

*From Consensus Conference. The use of diagnostic ultrasound imaging during pregnancy. JAMA 1984; 252:669-672. Used by permission.

assuming a cost of $150 per examination. The potential cost of scanning each pregnancy twice approaches $1 billion per year.

Several European countries have accepted the cost of routine obstetric ultrasound examinations as a part of modern obstetric care. Indeed, the Republic of Germany recommends that every pregnant woman undergo two ultrasounds during the course of each pregnancy.[12] Increasing use of routine obstetric sonography is also apparent in the United States. In 1984, it was estimated that 50% of pregnant women underwent at least one prenatal sonographic examination.[30] The number of women undergoing prenatal sonography is probably much higher today, although the precise number is unknown. These trends indicate that obstetric sonography is increasingly being utilized for routine clinical indications.

ROLE IN DETECTION OF CONGENITAL ANOMALIES

Since only a small minority of women who carry a malformed fetus have a family history of congenital anomalies, other clinical risk factors are of great potential value for identifying anomalous fetuses. For example, advanced maternal age is strongly associated with chromosome abnormalities (see Chapter 17). Screening for either high or low levels of maternal serum alpha-fetoprotein (MS-AFP) can also help identify fetuses at risk for a neural tube defect or chromosome abnormality, respectively (see Chapter 3). Other clinical indications that may help to identify a high-risk pregnancy include small uterine fundal size for dates (due to intrauterine growth retardation or oligohydramnios); large fundal size for dates (due to polyhydram-

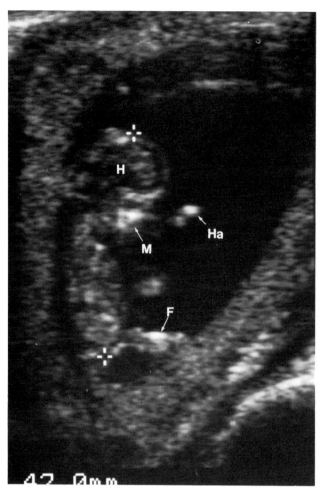

FIG 1–1.
Crown rump length. The crown rump length of this fetus measures 47 mm, which corresponds with a menstrual age of approximately 11.4 weeks. Measurement of the crown rump length during the first trimester of pregnancy provides accurate assessment of gestational age to within ± 0.6 - 1 week. *Graticules* = crown rump length; *H* = head; *M* = mandible; *F* = femur; *Ha* = hand.

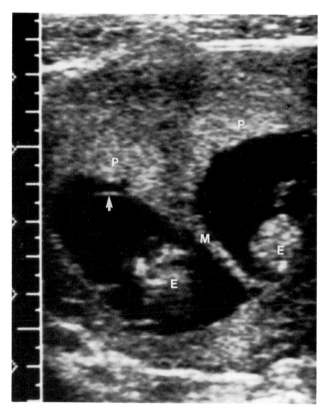

FIG 1–2.
Multiple pregnancy (see Chapter 15). Transverse scan of the gravid uterus at 9–10 weeks gestation shows two living embryos with a thick separating membrane. The separating membrane indicates diamnionicity. A thick separating membrane implies probable dichorionicity. *E* = twin embryos; *M* = thick dichorionic membrane; *arrow* = small portion of amnion; *P* = developing placentas.

nios or intrauterine mass); or irregular fetal heart rate, especially bradycardia.

Sonographic evaluation of patients considered to be at risk for carrying a fetus with a congenital anomaly has been found to be highly reliable and accurate. Most major congenital anomalies and even some minor anomalies have been successfully identified, particularly when the sonographic examination is performed by ultrasound specialists at referral centers for high-risk obstetrics. Factors that contribute to high detection rates of congenital anomalies, in addition to the expertise and training of the sonographer, include the high prevalence of anomalies in a referral population, use of sophisticated equipment, and the thoroughness of the examination.

Unfortunately, a large number of patients carrying

a fetus with a major congenital anomaly have no known risk factor. These anomalies usually remain unsuspected until the time of delivery or until an obstetric sonogram is performed for "routine" indications. This places responsibility for detection of major congenital anomalies on all those who perform obstetric sonography, not just the specialists at referral centers. Indeed, prospective parents often seek reassurance from a "normal" ultrasound examination to indicate that their baby is, in fact, normal. Because of the potential value of routine sonography, many authorities have suggested two scans for each pregnancy, one at 20 weeks to detect major fetal anomalies and the second examination at 32 to 34 weeks to detect additional anomalies and fetal growth disturbances.

Not surprisingly, the vast majority of "low-risk" obstetric sonograms are performed or supervised by physicians who actually devote a minority of their time to ultrasound and who have relatively little experience in the prenatal diagnosis of congenital malformations. When such examinations are also limited to one or

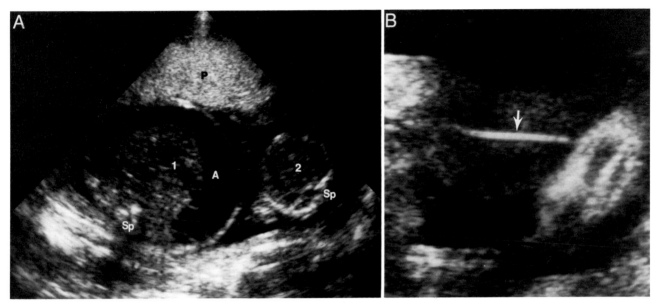

FIG 1–3.
Twins with discordant growth and the twin-twin transfusion syndrome (see chapters 14 and 15). **A,** sector scan through the abdomen of both twins at 21 weeks shows marked discrepancy in abdominal size with a large amount of ascites in the abdomen of one twin. A single placental site is noted anteriorly. Additional scans showed scalp and chest wall edema as well as pericardial effusion of the larger twin compatible with hydrops fetalis. **B,** linear scan demonstrates a thin membrane separating the twins indicative of diamnionicity. This diamniotic, monochorionic twin gestation has the twin-twin transfusion syndrome. *1* = hydropic twin; *2* = growth-retarded twin; *A* = ascites; *Sp* = spine; *P* = placenta; *arrow* = diamniotic separating membrane.

more biometric measurements without a survey of fetal anatomy, many major malformations will be missed. Despite these problems, physicians who perform or supervise routine obstetric sonograms need not be highly sophisticated in the prenatal diagnosis of congenital anomalies; rather, they need only to be thoroughly familiar with normal fetal appearances and to be able to recognize deviations from normal. Fetuses with suspected abnormalities can then be referred to centers where more sophisticated equipment and expertise is available. This screening approach emphasizes the need for minimum training requirements and the value of standard sonographic views that can help identify major fetal anomalies.

PROPOSED MINIMUM REQUIREMENTS

Increasingly common use of obstetric sonography has raised concerns regarding the wide variability in training and experience of the ultrasound examiner, expertise of the supervising physician, and comprehensiveness of the examination.[12, 20] Some physicians are trained in ultrasound for several years before applying it in clinical practice; others are trained in a few weeks or not at all. The NIHCDC recommended that all ultrasound examiners meet uniform credentialing standards

and minimum training requirements, and that all health care providers who utilize ultrasonography demonstrate knowledge of the basic physical principles of ultrasonography, equipment, recordkeeping requirements, indications, and safety.[12, 20] The American Institute of Ultrasound in Medicine recommends that all physicians who utilize ultrasonography but are not trained in its use receive at least (1) 1 month of supervised training; (2) 2 months of practical experience, including at least 200 ultrasound examinations; and (3) continuing education and self-assessment.[9]

In an effort to improve prenatal detection of fetal abnormalities and to standardize obstetric sonograms, the American Institute of Ultrasound in Medicine (AIUM), the American College of Radiology (ACR), and, more recently, the American College of Obstetricians and Gynecologists (ACOG) each adopted a set of recommendations which defines the minimum goals for an obstetrical ultrasound.[17, 27] Those performing obstetric sonograms in the United States should be familiar with these guidelines and are urged to implement them in their daily practice (Figs 1–1 to 1–16).

Most important in regard to detection of fetal anomalies are standard ultrasound planes and anatomic landmarks that are recommended during the second and third trimesters (AIUM recommendation D.6). Incorporation of these standard views into routine ob-

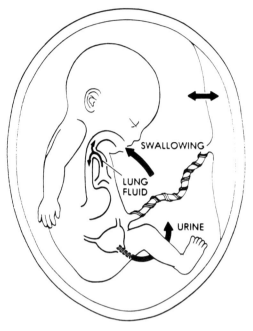

FIG 1–4.
Amniotic fluid (see Chapter 3). A variety of sites regulate the volume of amniotic fluid. Assessment of normal amniotic fluid volume, therefore, may provide an indicator of fetal well-being. (From Adzick NS, Harrison MR, Glick PL, et al: Experimental pulmonary hypoplasia and oligohydramnios. J Pediatr Surg 1984; 19:658–665. Used by permission.)

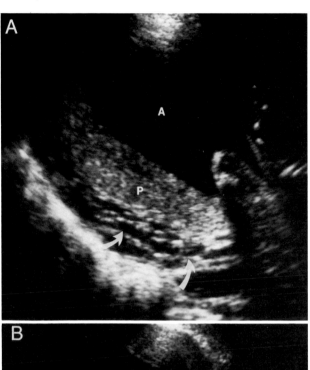

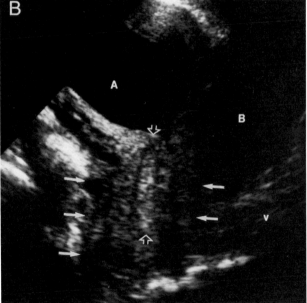

FIG 1–5.
Normal placenta (see Chapter 16). **A,** sagittal scan of the uterus shows the normal placenta. In this case, the posterior placenta extends to the fundus. The normal retroplacental venous complex and myometrium are hypoechoic and should not be confused with an abruption.[9] **B,** midline sagittal scan shows the cervix and cervical canal without overlying placenta. Typically, the cervix orients at a nearly antero-posterior angle with the maternal urinary bladder decompressed. *P* = placenta; *A* = amniotic fluid; *B* = maternal urinary bladder; *V* = maternal vagina; *curved arrows* = retroplacental venous complex; *solid straight arrows* = cervix; *open arrows* = cervical canal.

FIG 1–6.

Fetal growth. This graph illustrates the relationship between gestational age and fetal weight. *Shaded area* = 10th–90th percentiles; *dark shaded area* = 25th–75th percentiles; *light shaded areas* = less than 25th percentile and greater than 75th percentile. (From Brenner W, Edelman D, Hendricks C: A standard of fetal growth for the United States of America. Am J Obstet Gynecol 1976; 126:555–559. Used by permission.)

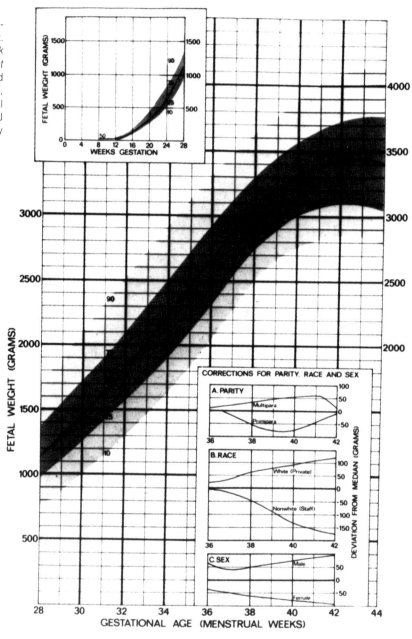

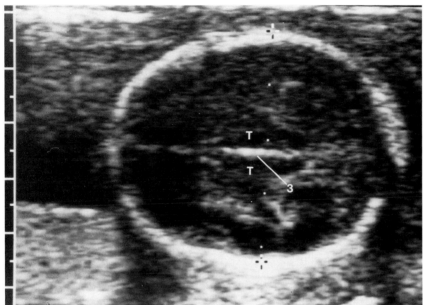

FIG 1–7.
Biparietal diameter. Axial scan of the head at the standardized level for biparietal diameter measurement shows the thalami and third ventricle at 18.5 weeks' gestation. Biparietal diameter measurements include only the calvarial diameter and exclude the soft tissues of the scalp. *Graticules* = biparietal diameter measurement; *3* = third ventricle; *T* = thalami.

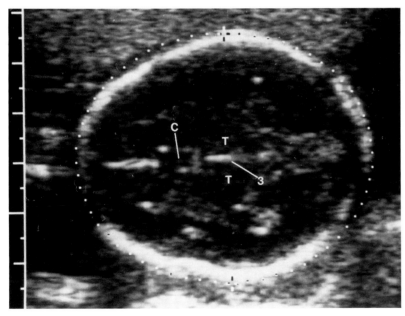

FIG 1–8.
Head circumference. The circumference of the head is measured at the same level as the biparietal diameter. The measurements of the head include the normal soft tissues of the scalp. *Graticules and dotted line* = head circumference; *3* = third ventricle; *T* = thalami; *C* = cavum septi pellucidi.

FIG 1–9.

Femur length. Measurement of the femur length includes only the ossified diaphysis and excludes the cartilaginous epiphyses. The specular echo from the edge of the *epiphyseal* cartilage at the knee should not be included in femur length measurement. *Graticules* = femur length measurement; *E* = hypoechoic non–ossified epiphyseal cartilage; *S* = specular echo from the edge of the epiphyseal cartilage.

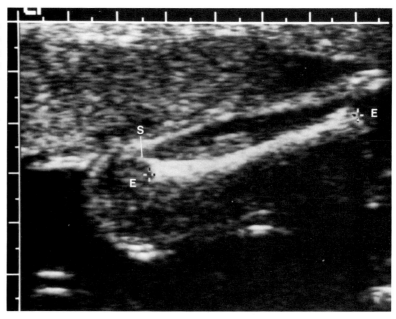

FIG 1–10.

Abdominal circumference. Transverse scan of the fetal abdomen at 27.5 weeks illustrates the standardized plane of section for measurement of the abdominal circumference. On this plane of section, the junction between the ascending left portal vein, pars transversus, and right portal vein form a "J," with the most anterior portion of the ascending left portal vein not extending to the anterior abdominal wall. The abdominal circumference measures the perimeter of the abdomen and includes the soft tissues. The stomach is documented to be left-sided. *Graticules* = perimeter of the abdomen; *A* = ascending left portal vein; *PT* = pars transversus; *R* = right portal vein; *S* = stomach; *Sp* = spine; *Rt* = right; *Lt* = left.

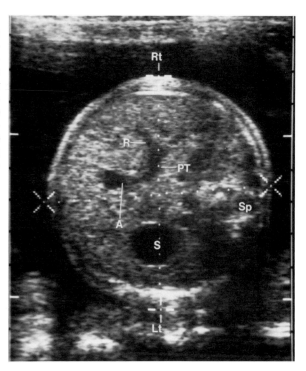

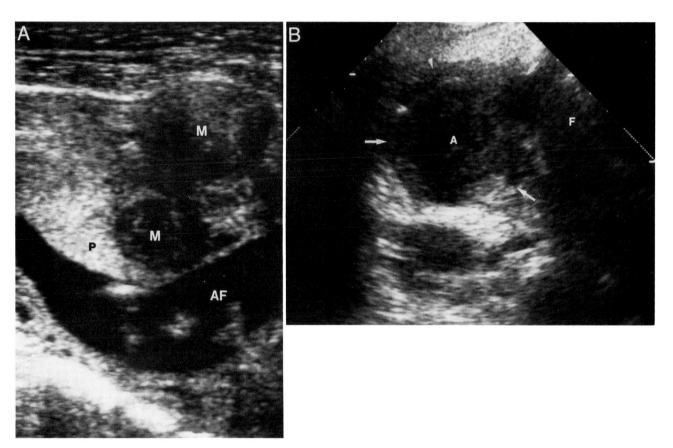

FIG 1–11.
The uterus and adnexae. **A,** sagittal scan of the uterus at 16 weeks shows two myomata, one of which is subjacent to the maternal surface of the placenta. This may be associated with an increased incidence of abruption later in gestation.[24] Myomata that measure greater than 3 cm in diameter may also signify an increased incidence of premature labor.[24] **B,** transverse scan of the maternal right lower quadrant at 36 weeks' gestation shows a complex 7 cm right adnexal mass confirmed to be an appendiceal abscess at surgery. *M* = myomata; *P* = placenta; *AF* = amniotic fluid; *A* = appendiceal abscess; *F* = right uterine fundus.

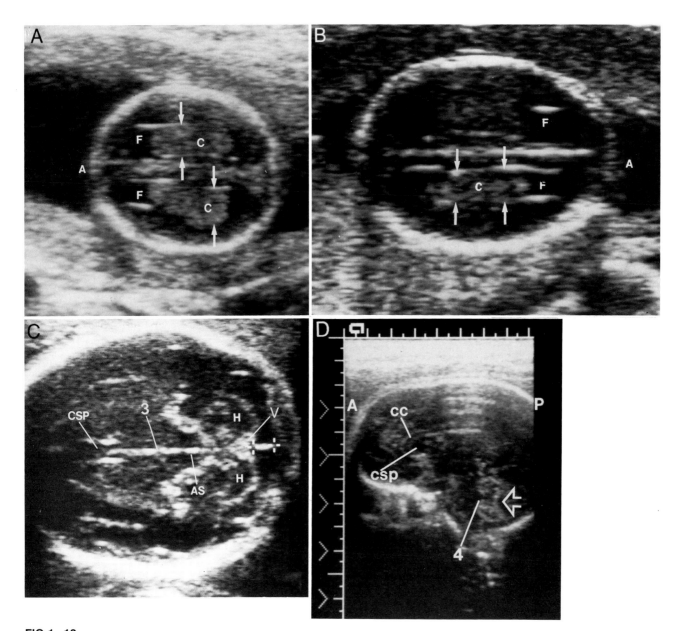

FIG 1–12.
Cerebral ventricles. **A** and **B,** axial scans of the head at 15.5 weeks **(A)** and 19 weeks **(B)** display the choroid plexus filling the bodies of the lateral ventricles but not extending into the frontal horns. Reverberation artifact from the skull obscures much of the lateral ventricle closest to the transducer on the 19-week scan **(B).** *C* = choroid plexus; *arrows* = medial and lateral walls of the bodies of the lateral ventricles; *F* = frontal horns; *A* = anterior. **C,** axial scan at 26 weeks obtained at approximately 10%–15% of transducer angulation from the canthomeatal line shows the cavum septi pellucidi, inferior portion of the third ventricle, aqueduct of Sylvius, cerebellar hemispheres, vermis, and cisterna magna. *CSP* = cavum septi pellucidi; *3* = inferior portion of the third ventricle; *AS* = aqueduct of Sylvius; *H* = cerebellar hemispheres; *V* = cerebellar vermis; *graticules* = cisterna magna. **D,** midsagittal scan of the head at 30 weeks displays portions of the corpus callosum, cerebellum, and fourth ventricle. Reverberation artifact from the ossified skull obscures a portion of the intracranial anatomy. This is not a routine plane of section. *CC* = corpus callosum; *CSP* = cavum septi pellucidi; *4* = fourth ventricle; *open arrow* = cerebellum; *A* = anterior, *P* = posterior.

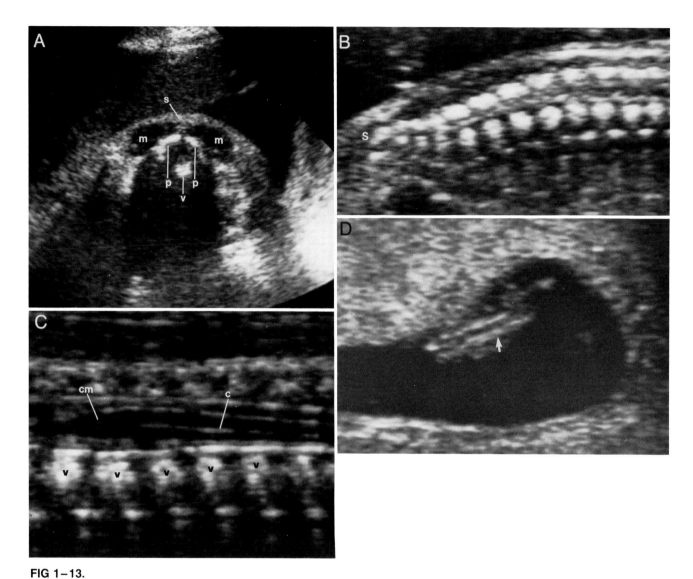

FIG 1–13.
Spine. **A,** transverse scan of a lumbosacral vertebra shows the normal posterior spinal elements converging posteriorly. Note the hypoechoic paraspinous musculature and intact skin overlying the spine. *P* = converging posterior elements; *V* = vertebral body; *M* = paraspinous muscles; *S* = skin. **B,** coronal image of the lumbosacral spine displays the gentle curvature of the spine extending to the inferior point of the sacrum. *S* = sacrum. **C,** midsagittal scan of the lumbar spine illustrates the spinal column within the vertebral canal. *V* = vertebral bodies; *CM* = conus medullaris; *C* = central canal. **D,** the spine begins to ossify during the first trimester, as this coronal scan of the spine at 8.4 weeks' gestation demonstrates. However, progressive ossification and size of the spine limits diagnostic accuracy in evaluation of the spine prior to 16–18 weeks' gestation. *Arrow* = spine.

FIG 1–14.
Urinary bladder. Transverse scan of the fetal pelvis at 19 weeks demonstrates the urinary bladder. In association with a normal amount of amniotic fluid, documentation of fluid within the urinary bladder after approximately 16 weeks' gestation confirms that the fetus is making urine. *B* = urinary bladder; *AF* = amniotic fluid; *IW* = iliac wing. *Arrows* = umbilical cord insertion site.

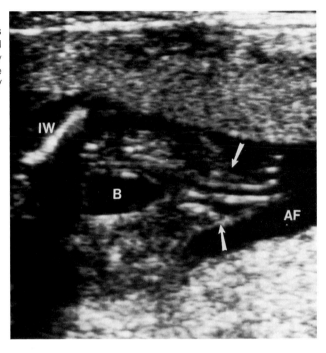

FIG 1–15.
Umbilical cord insertion site on the anterior abdominal wall. Transverse scan of the abdomen at 20 weeks displays the insertion site of the umbilical cord on the anterior abdominal wall. *Arrows* = umbilical cord insertion site; *B* = urinary bladder; *Sp* = spine.

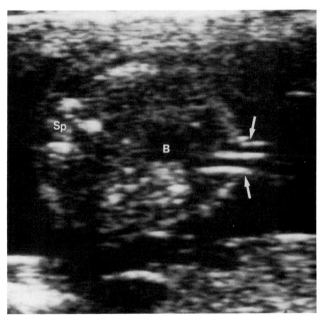

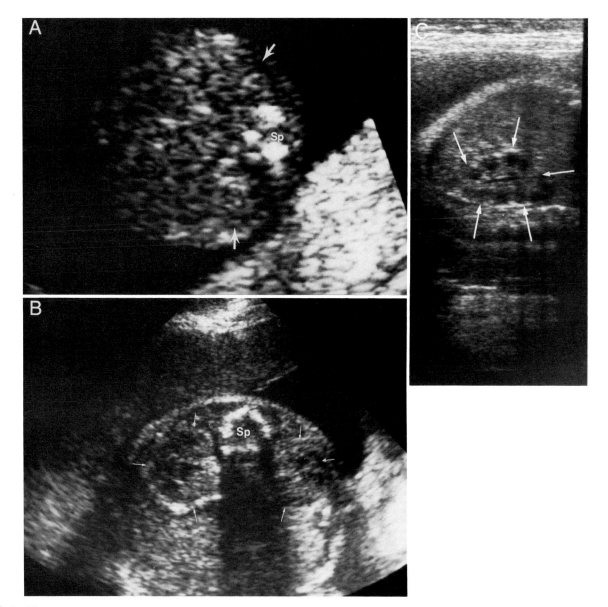

FIG 1–16.
Renal region. **A,** transverse scan of the renal region at 16 weeks shows the kidneys to have an echotexture similar to that of adjacent fetal tissues. **B** and **C,** Transverse **(B)** and parasagittal **(C)** scans during the third trimester, however, clearly show the kidneys with their hypo-echoic medullary pyramids and echogenic perinephric fat. *Arrows* = kidneys; *Sp* = spine.

FIG 1–17.
Four-chamber view of the heart. Scan through the thorax illustrates the normal cardiac axis and position as well as the four cardiac chambers. This view may provide a useful screen for many thoracic abnormalities (see Chapters 8 and 9). *Sp* = spine; *RA* = right atrium, *RV* = right ventricle; *LA* = left atrium; *LV* = left ventricle; *Ao* = aorta.

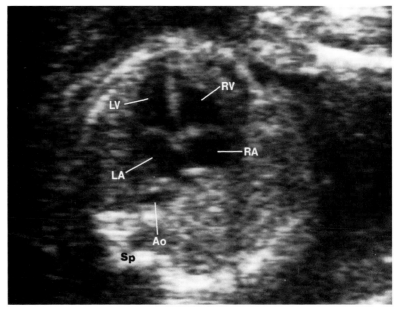

stetric scanning has the potential to detect or exclude the vast majority of major anomalies. Discussions of specific anomalies in subsequent chapters of this book reemphasize the importance of these standard views for recognition of a wide variety of anomalies.

Differences in standard sonographic views recommended by the AIUM and ACOG are minor. With regard to the heart, the AIUM guidelines suggest documentation of abnormal heart rate and/or rhythm, whereas the ACOG guidelines recommend that a four-chambered image of the heart be obtained, if possible (Fig 1–17). While neither the AIUM or ACOG guidelines mentions routine visualization of the cisterna magna, many authorities would also incorporate this view into a routine examination of the cranium. Undoubtedly, other modifications of a basic obstetric examination will be made in the future.

Because of the importance of such guidelines to the practicing sonographer, those adopted by the AIUM are reprinted in their entirety below. As a comparison, those guidelines adopted by ACOG are reproduced in Table 1–2.

AIUM GUIDELINES FOR ANTEPARTUM OBSTETRIC EXAMINATION*

A. Equipment

These studies should be conducted with real-time or a combination of real-time and static scanners, but

*This section from Leopold GR: Antepartum obstetrical ultrasound examination guidelines. J Ultrasound Med 1986; 5:241–242. Used by permission.

never solely with a static scanner. A transducer of appropriate frequency (3 to 5 MHz) should be used. *Comment:* Real-time is necessary to reliably confirm the presence of fetal life through observation of cardiac activity, respiration, and active movement. Real-time studies simplify evaluation of fetal anatomy as well as the task of obtaining fetal measurements.

The choice of frequency is a trade-off between beam penetration and resolution. With modern equipment, 3 to 5 MHz transducers allow sufficient penetration in nearly all patients while providing adequate resolution. During early pregnancy, a 5 MHz transducer may provide adequate penetration and produce superior resolution.

B. Documentation

Adequate documentation of the study is essential for high quality patient care. This should include a permanent record of the ultrasound images, incorporating whenever possible the measurement parameters and anatomical findings proposed in the following sections of this document. Images should be appropriately labeled with the examination date, patient identification, and image orientation. A written report of the ultrasound findings should be included in the patient's medical record, regardless of where the study is performed.

C. Guidelines for First Trimester Sonography

1. The location of the gestational sac should be documented. The embryo should be identified and the crown rump length recorded (see Fig 1–1). *Comment:*

The crown rump length is an accurate indicator of fetal age. Comparison should be made to standard tables. During the late first trimester, biparietal diameter and other fetal measurements may also be used to establish fetal age.

2. Presence or absence of fetal life should be reported. *Comment:* Real-time observation is critical in this diagnosis. It should be noted that fetal cardiac activity may not be visible prior to 7 weeks, as determined by crown rump length. Thus, confirmation of fetal life may require follow-up evaluation.

3. Fetal number should be documented. *Comment:* Multiple pregnancy should be reported only in those instances where multiple embryos are seen (see Fig 1–2). Due to variability in fusion between the amnion and chorion, the appearance of more than one sac-like structure in early pregnancy is often noted and may be confused with multiple gestation or amniotic bands.

4. Evaluation of the uterus (including cervix) and adnexal structures should be performed (see Fig 1–11). *Comment:* This will allow recognition of incidental findings of potential clinical significance. The presence, location, and size of myomas and adnexal masses should be recorded.

D. Guidelines for Second and Third Trimester Sonography

1. Fetal life, number, and presentation should be documented. *Comment:* Abnormal heart rate and/or rhythm should be reported. Multiple pregnancies require the reporting of additional information: placental number, sac number, and comparison of fetal size (see Fig 1–3).

2. An estimate of the amount of amniotic fluid (increased, decreased, normal) should be reported (see Fig 1–4). *Comment:* While this evaluation is subjective, there is little difficulty in recognizing the extremes of amniotic fluid volume. Physiologic variation with stage of pregnancy must be taken into account.

3. The placental location should be recorded and its relationship to the internal cervical os determined (see Fig 1–5). *Comment:* It is recognized that placental position early in pregnancy may not correlate well with its location at the time of delivery.

4. Assessment of gestational age in the second and third trimester should be accomplished using a combination of biparietal diameter (or head circumference) and femur length. Fetal growth assessment (as opposed to age) requires the addition of abdominal circumference measurements (see Fig 1–6). If previous studies have been done, an estimate of the appropriateness of

interval change should be given. *Comment:* Third trimester measurements may not accurately reflect gestational age. Initial determination of gestational age should be performed prior to 26 weeks whenever possible.

a. Biparietal diameter at a standard reference level (which should include the cavum septi pellucidi, the thalamus, or the cerebral peduncles) should be measured and recorded (see Fig 1–7). *Comment:* If the fetal head is dolichocephalic or brachycephalic, the biparietal diameter alone may be misleading. In such situations, the head circumference is required.

b. Head circumference is measured at the same level as the biparietal diameter (see Fig 1–8).

c. Femur length should be measured routinely and recorded after the 14th week of gestation (see Fig 1–9). *Comment:* As with biparietal diameter, considerable biological variation is present late in pregnancy.

d. Abdominal circumference should be determined at the level of the junction of the umbilical vein and portal sinus (see Fig 1–10). *Comment:* Abdominal circumference measurement may allow detection of asymmetric growth retardation—a condition of the late second and third trimester. Comparison of the abdominal circumference with the head circumference should be made. If the abdominal measurement is below that expected for a stated gestation, it is recommended that circumferences of the head and body be measured and the head circumference/abdominal circumference ratio be reported. The use of circumferences is also suggested in those instances where the shape of either the head or body is different from that normally encountered.

5. Evaluation of the uterus and adnexal structures should be performed (see Fig 1–11). *Comment:* This will allow recognition of incidental findings of potential clinical significance. The presence, location, and size of myomas and adnexal masses should be recorded.

6. The study should include, but not necessarily be limited to the following fetal anatomy: cerebral ventricles (see Fig 1–12), spine (see Fig 1–13), stomach (see Fig 1–10), urinary bladder (see Fig 1–14), umbilical cord insertion site on the anterior abdominal wall (see Fig 1–15), and renal region (see Fig 1–16). *Comment:* It is recognized that not all malformations of

these organ systems (such as the spine) can be detected using ultrasonography. Nevertheless, a careful anatomical survey may allow diagnosis of certain birth defects which would otherwise go unrecognized. Suspected abnormalities may require a specialized evaluation.

SPECIALIZED EXAMINATIONS

The AIUM, ACR, and ACOG also recognize that a comprehensive sonographic evaluation of the fetus, uterus, and adnexa may be necessary. These specialized examinations, termed "targeted" or "level II" sonograms, should be performed by an operator with special training and expertise in ultrasound scanning.[27] Common indications for a targeted sonogram include a family history of congenital anomalies, elevated MS-AFP, and anomalies suspected on a "routine" obstetric sonogram.

The following sections provide guidelines which, in conjunction with the minimal requirements set forth by the AIUM, ACR, and ACOG, may be useful in evaluation of targeted high-risk pregnancies. Subsequent chapters discuss each of these in greater detail.

CRANIOFACIAL REGION

Examination of the craniofacial region (see Chapters 5, 7) may include evaluation of:

1. Ossification, continuity, shape, and size of the cranium.
2. Identification of brain parenchymal structures such as the thalami, cerebral peduncles, cavum septi pellucidum, cerebral hemispheres, tentorium, cerebellar hemispheres, vermis, and cisterna magna.
3. Size and shape of the ventricles and choroid plexus and appearance of the ependyma.
4. The facial profile and assessment of the size, shape, and positioning of the eyes, nose, ears, and chin.
5. The size of the tongue and mouth and integrity of the upper lip and hard palate.
6. Positioning of the neck and identification of neck masses.

SPINE

Evaluation of the spine (see Chapter 6) may include assessment of:

1. Splaying of the posterior elements indicative of dysraphism at specific levels.
2. Ossification of the spine, including the three ossification centers at each level.
3. Configuration of the spine or vertebral body anomalies, best seen on longitudinal planes of section.

THORAX

Examination of the thorax (see Chapter 8) may include assessment of:

1. The size and configuration of the thoracic cage.
2. The size, shape, and echogenicity of thoracic masses or fluid collections.
3. The echogenicity of the lungs.
4. The presence or absence of extrathoracic compression and fetal respiratory movements.

HEART

The fetal echocardiographic examination is a very specialized study, often done by or in conjunction with a pediatric cardiologist and requiring as long as 60–90 minutes to perform (see Chapter 9). It may involve M-mode ultrasound for assessment of arrhythmias and extensive review of videotaped images of the parasternal long and short axis views, the four-chamber apical or subcostal view, and the oblique long axis views of the aortic arch and ductal arch. An abnormal echocardiographic study may include investigation with duplex Doppler or other sophisticated methods.

ABDOMEN

Examination of the abdomen (see Chapters 10, 11, and 12) may include evaluation of:

1. The size and location of the stomach.
2. The size and echogenicity of the bowel.
3. The location, size, and echogenicity of the gallbladder and liver.
4. The size, shape, location, and echogenicity of abnormal intraperitoneal fluid collections or masses.
5. The location, size, and contents of abdominal wall defects.
6. The location, size, and echogenicity of the kidneys as well as the presence of renal or perinephric cysts, pelvocaliectasis, ureterectasis,

and urinary bladder dilatation or thickening. Fetal gender assessment may be helpful in twin gestations and in fetuses at risk for a congenital anomaly associated with one sex.

EXTREMITIES

Examination of the extremities (see Chapter 13) may include evaluation of:

1. Lengths of the long bones as well as severity and distribution of shortening.
2. Extremity bowing, acute angulation, or focal absence of bone.

3. Presence or absence of polydactyly.
4. Presence or absence of contractures or postural deformities.
5. Extremity enlargement, masses, or abnormal echogenicity.

UMBILICAL CORD

Evaluation of the umbilical cord (see Chapter 16) may include documentation of:

1. Two arteries and one vein in the cord.
2. The size, position, and echogenicity of abnormal masses of the umbilical cord.

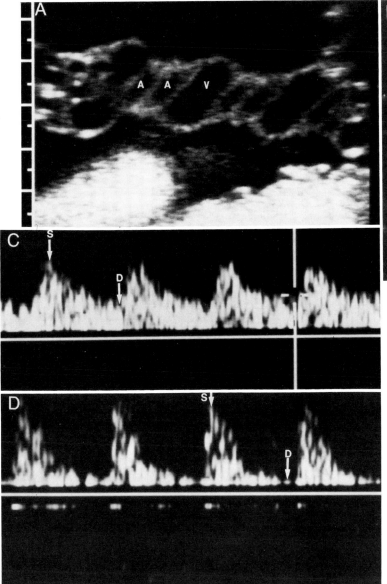

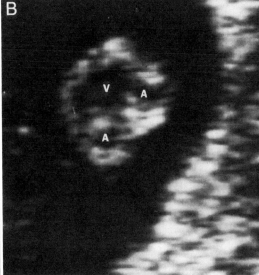

FIG 1–18.
Umbilical cord with umbilical artery and fetal internal cerebral artery Doppler wave form. **A** and **B,** longitudinal **(A)** and transverse **(B)** scans of the normal three-vessel umbilical cord display the two umbilical arteries and one umbilical vein. **C,** Doppler wave form from the free-floating portion of the umbilical artery documents a normal systolic to diastolic ratio of approximately 1.8. **D,** Doppler wave form from the fetal internal carotid artery at 33 weeks shows minimal, if any, diastolic flow. This infant was normal at delivery. *A* = umbilical arteries; *V* = umbilical vein; *S* = peak systole; *D* = end diastole.

TABLE 1–2.

American College of Obstetricians and Gynecologists
Components of a Basic Obstetrical Ultrasound Examination*

Components of a Basic Examination
Unless technically impossible, the following tasks should all be accomplished during a basic ultrasound examination of a pregnant patient:
- Fetal number.
- Fetal presentation (in second and third trimester).
- Documentation of fetal life.
- Placental localization.
- Amniotic fluid volume.
- Gestational dating.
- Detection and evaluation of maternal pelvic masses (best done in the first trimester).
- Survey of fetal anatomy for gross malformations (in second and third trimester).

Guidelines for Sonographic Screening
Although it is unrealistic to expect to detect anomalies with 100% accuracy, the following guidelines for a sonographic survey of fetal anatomy are designed to aid the practitioner in evaluating the fetus.

When the placental site is being localized in the second trimester, the term "placenta previa" should be avoided because of the potential for relative change secondary to lengthening of the lower uterine segment later in pregnancy.

The majority of obstetric ultrasound scans are performed to document gestational age when clinical dating is equivocal or when there is a discrepancy between uterine size and dates by last menstrual period. It is preferable for more than one parameter to be used in the second and third trimesters. The most commonly used fetal measurements are biparietal diameter, length of the femur or other long bones, and abdominal and head circumferences. Less frequently used biometric parameters include outer orbital diameter and transcerebellar diameter. In oligohydramnios, breech presentation, or multiple gestation, physiologic compression of the head may affect the biparietal diameter. This may be suspected if the head appears to be overly elliptical and confirmed when measurements of the cephalic index (biparietal diameter/occipital-frontal diameter) are below 0.75. In these cases, measurements of head circumference are more accurate than measurement of biparietal diameter alone in dating a pregnancy.

The biometric data are commonly averaged to determine a mean ultrasound age. This method, however, is affected by a single measurement that is out of synchrony with other measurements. In such situations, these "outlying" values can be discarded, and the clustered measurements should be averaged. It must be realized, however, that such values may also indicate an abnormality characterized by a large head or short limbs. Ultrasound dating is much less precise after 26 weeks of gestation, when biologic variation is greatest.

Early Pregnancy
An important component of a sonographic examination during pregnancy is a systematic survey of the maternal and fetal anatomy. The first trimester is the best time to examine the maternal uterus and ovaries for abnormalities. The following fetal characteristics should be visible at the indicated weeks of gestation. This timetable may be altered when a vaginal probe is used:

- Six weeks: Gestational sac.
- Seven weeks: Embryonic poles.
- Eight weeks: Fetal heart and crown-rump length (up to 12 weeks ± 4 days, crown-rump length is highly predictive of gestational age).
- Six to ten weeks: Yolk sac (this disappears by 12 weeks; a yolk sac without an embryo is highly suggestive of a missed abortion at this time of pregnancy).

Midpregnancy
At this time, it is possible to evaluate much of the fetal anatomy. More fetal anatomy can be observed at the end of this period.

Head: The head is normally elliptical in shape. In various types of abnormalities, the cranial configuration may provide valuable diagnostic information. For example, a cloverleaf-shaped cranium may accompany thanatophoric dysplasia or aneuploidy, and a lemon-shaped skull is frequently noted in spina bifida. Hydrocephaly is defined as enlargement of the ventricular system of the brain. Although dilation of the occipital horns occurs first in hydrocephaly, a common and useful screening practice is to estimate the ratio of the width of the lateral ventricle to that of the cerebral hemisphere. A measurement is made from the midline to the distal wall of the lateral ventricle and compared with a measurement made from the midline to the leading edge of the skull. This ratio varies with gestational age. The "midline" should be clearly identified as being midway between both skull outlines. Porencephaly, alobar or semilobar holoprosencephaly, and hydranencephaly can be suspected by abnormalities of the midline. Transcerebellar measurements may also be useful. Recent investigation indicates that in over 90% of cases of open spina bifida, the cerebellar structures are distorted by downward traction, resulting in an inability to identify the cerebellar bulbs or to obtain a transcerebellar measurement that is appropriate for gestation.

Spine: The spine is easier to study in the second trimester than in the third. A sagittal sonogram should reveal two parallel sets of echoes emanating from the spinal body and a spinal pedicle. In a coronal view, both pedicles produce a set of parallel echogenic tracts. With these views and a series of transverse sonograms, a spinal defect can be identified by observation of splaying of the lamina. It is also important to demonstrate the integrity of the skin overlying the spine, although approximately 10% of spinal defects are covered by intact skin.

Heart: An attempt should be made to obtain a four-chambered image of the fetal heart. Most major anomalies of the heart can be ruled out by demonstrating ventricles and atria of equal and appropriate sizes and an intact ventricular septum.

Abdomen: The fetal bladder and stomach can be visualized by 14 weeks of gestation. In most cases, gastrointestinal obstruction can be suspected by noting an enlarged stomach or dilated loops of bowel or both. Similarly, genitourinary obstruction can be suspected by noting an enlarged bladder or dilated renal pelvis. It is usually possible to visualize the kidneys after 16 weeks. Most ventral wall defects can be excluded by the demonstration of an intact abdomen in the area of the umbilical cord insertion.

Extremities: One should attempt to visualize the long bones of both lower extremities. In an active fetus, however, it is often difficult to identify all the bones of both upper extremities.

Genitalia: Although it is often possible to identify fetal genitalia late in the second trimester, determination of fetal gender should in no way be considered an essential part of a basic ultrasound scan.

Late Pregnancy

Often it is difficult to fully examine some fetal areas late in the third trimester. Difficulties may be posed by the relative paucity of amniotic fluid in the third trimester, the hyperflexed position of the fetus, engagement of the head, and compression of some fetal parts. An additional factor may be maternal obesity, which can make sonographic evaluation difficult at any time during pregnancy.

Evaluation of Fetal Behavior

In the third trimester, it is often useful to evaluate fetal behavior in addition to surveying the fetal anatomy. This would include a brief appraisal of the quantity and character of fetal movement, as well as a gross evaluation of fetal tone by noting the degree of flexion of the extremities and an assessment of amniotic fluid volume. The presence of fetal respiratory movements is a reassuring sign of fetal well-being. In high-risk patients, an assessment of fetal behavior may be useful. In these cases, a basic examination should also be performed.

*From ACOG Technical Bulletin, No. 116. Washington, DC, ACOG, May 1988. Used by permission.

PLACENTA/MEMBRANES

Evaluation of the placenta and intrauterine membranes (see Chapter 16) may include assessment of:

1. Placental echogenicity and grade and thickness.
2. Location, echotexture, and associated abnormalities of the placenta.
3. Size, thickness, and location of intrauterine membranes and the presence or absence of associated fetal entrapment or entanglement.

OBSTETRICAL DOPPLER EXAMINATION

The AIUM feels that sufficient data currently exist "to justify clinical use of continuous wave, pulsed, and color-flow Doppler ultrasound to evaluate blood flow in uterine, umbilical, and fetal vessels, the fetal cardiovascular system and to image flow in these structures using color-flow imaging technology."[2] Most commonly, Doppler evaluation involves interrogation of the umbilical arteries and/or the fetal internal carotid arteries in fetuses at risk for intrauterine growth retardation (Fig 1–18). Calculation of the ratio between velocities at peak end systole and peak end diastole and comparison of this ratio with normal values may provide useful information regarding placental resistance or fetal distress.[29, 32] Doppler evaluation includes several representative samples along the course of a vessel and several similar pulses on one tracing. Further discussion of obstetric Doppler can be found in Chapter 16.

SUMMARY

Obstetric sonography is increasingly utilized in the evaluation of a wide variety of both routine and specific obstetric indications. It is clear that detection of major congenital anomalies is an increasingly important role of obstetric sonography and that all obstetric sonograms share some responsibility for detection of major congenital anomalies. A systematic approach using standardized imaging planes, as recommended by the AIUM, ACR, and ACOG is necessary for improved detection of major anomalies. The utility of these specific views will be discussed in subsequent chapters on specific anomalies.

REFERENCES

1. Adzick NS, Harrison MR, Glick PL, et al: Experimental pulmonary hypoplasia: Relative contributions of lung fluid to development. J Pediatr Surg 1984; 19:658–665.
2. American Institute of Ultrasound in Medicine Newsletter. October 1988.
3. Bakketeig L, Eik-Nes S, Jacobsen G, et al: Randomized controlled trial of ultrasonographic screening in pregnancy. Lancet 1984; 2:207.
4. Belfrage P, Fernstrom I, Hallenberg G: Routine or selective ultrasound examinations in early pregnancy. Obstet Gynecol 1987; 69:747–750.
5. Bennett M, Little G, Dewhurst J, et al: Predictive value of ultrasound measurement in early pregnancy: A randomized controlled trial. Brit J Obstet Gynaecol 1982; 89:338–341.
6. Brenner W, Edelman D, Hendricks C: A standard of fetal growth for the United States of America. Am J Obstet Gynecol 1976; 126:555–559.
7. Bowerman RA: Using ultrasonography to diagnose fetal malformations. J Reprod Med 1982; 27:560–564.
8. Bracken M: Ultrasonography in antenatal management. Should it be a routine procedure? Fetal Ther 1987; 2:2–6.
9. Bundy AL, Jones TB: Guidelines for obstetrical scanning and reporting: The legal necessity. J Ultrasound Med 1985; 4:483–484.
10. Callen PW, Filly RA: The placental-subplacental complex: A specific indicator of placental position on ultrasound. J Clin Ultrasound 1980; 8:21–26.
11. Campbell SM, Pearch JM: The prenatal diagnosis of fetal structural anomalies by ultrasound. Clin Obstet Gynecol 1983; 10:475–506.
12. Consensus conference. The use of diagnostic ultrasound imaging during pregnancy. JAMA 1984; 252:669–672.
13. Cochlin DL: Effects of two ultrasound scanning regimes in the management of pregnancy. Br J Obstet Gynaecol 1984; 91:885–890.
14. Eik-Nes S, Okland O, Aure J, et al: Ultrasound screening

in pregnancy: A randomised controlled trial. Lancet 1984; 1:1347.

15. Grant A: Controlled trials of routine ultrasound in pregnancy. Birth 1986; 13:22–28.

16. Hawrylyshyn PA, Barkin M, Bernstein A, et al: Twin pregnancies—a continuing perinatal challenge. Obstet Gynecol 1982; 59:463–466.

17. Leopold GR: Antepartum obstetrical ultrasound examination guidelines. J Ultrasound Med 1986; 5:241–242.

18. Lacro R, Jones K, Benirschke K: The umbilical cord twist: Origin, direction, and relevance. Am J Obstet Gynecol 1987; 157:833–838.

19. Lilford R, Chard T: The routine use of ultrasound. Br J Obstet Gynaecol 1985; 92:434.

20. National Institutes of Health Consensus Development Conference. US Government Printing Office, Washington, 1984.

21. Neilson J, Munjanja S, Whitfield C: Screening for small for dates fetuses: A controlled trial. Br Med J 1984; 289:1179–1182.

22. Persson PH, Grennert L, Gennser G, et al: On improved outcome of twin pregnancies. Acta Obstet Gynecol Scand 1979; 58:3.

23. Persson PH, Kullander S: Long-term experience of general ultrasound screening in pregnancy. Am J Obstet Gynecol 1983; 146:942.

24. Rice JP, Kay HH, Mahony BS: The clinical significance of uterine leiomyomas in pregnancy. Am J Obstet Gynecol 1989; 160:1212–1216.

25. Shepard M, Filly RA: A standardized plane for biparietal diameter measurement. J Ultrasound Med 1982; 1:145–150.

26. Stark CR, Orleans M, Haverkamp AD, et al: Short- and long-term risks after exposure to diagnostic ultrasound in utero. Obstet Gynecol 1984; 63:194–200.

27. Technical Bulletin. American College of Obstetrics and Gynecology, No. 116. May 1988.

28. Thacker SB: Quality of controlled clinical trials. The case of imaging ultrasound in obstetrics: A review. Br J Obstet Gynaecol 1985; 92:437–444.

29. Trudinger BJ, Giles WB, Cook CM, et al: Fetal umbilical artery flow velocity wave forms and placental resistance: Clinical significance. Br J Obstet Gynaecol 1985; 92:23.

30. Wade RV, Smythe AR, Watt GW, et al: Reliability of gynecologic sonographic diagnoses, 1978–1984. Am J Obstet Gynecol 1985; 153:186–190.

31. Warsof SL, Cooper DJ, Little D, et al: Routine ultrasound screening for antenatal detection of intrauterine growth retardation. Obstet Gynecol 1986; 67:33–39.

32. Wladimiroff JW, Wijngaard JAGW, Degani S, et al: Cerebral and umbilical arterial blood flow velocity wave forms in normal and growth-retarded pregnancies. Obstet Gynecol 1987; 69:705–709.

An Overview of Congenital Malformations

Dolores H. Pretorius, M.D.

David A. Nyberg, M.D.

Congenital anomalies have become an increasingly common cause of human mortality and morbidity, parallel with improvements in medical and obstetrical care of other disorders. Major anomalies are present in 2%–5% of newborns and now account for 20%–30% of perinatal deaths.[5, 15, 28] Other malformations (for example, myelomeningocele) are not lethal themselves, yet cause significant physical or mental handicaps. Nearly half of institutionalized children carry a major chromosome abnormality (most commonly, trisomy 21), a single gene disease, or a severe developmental malformation syndrome.[15] The personal grief and suffering caused by the birth of a child with a major malformation are more difficult to quantify, but cannot be underestimated; birth of a child with a major anomaly commonly leads to domestic difficulties, feelings of guilt, alterations in lifestyle, and avoidance of future pregnancies.

For all these reasons, detection, prevention, and treatment of congenital anomalies are considered important goals in medicine. Intensified effort over the last 30 years has resulted in a virtual explosion in the prenatal detection and treatment of congenital anomalies. This chapter presents an overview of the pathogenesis, etiologies, prognosis, and management of congenital anomalies as a background for subsequent chapters regarding specific malformations. Both the benefits and limitations of prenatal sonographic diagnosis of congenital anomalies are emphasized.

INCIDENCE AND TERMINOLOGY OF CONGENITAL ANOMALIES

A congenital anomaly is defined as an anatomical or structural abnormality present at birth. Not all congenital anomalies are due to an embryologic defect *(malformation)*; other possible causes of congenital anomalies include abnormal intrauterine mechanical constraint *(deformation)*, disruption after normal embryologic development *(disruption)*, or abnormal organization of tissue in a specific tissue type *(dysplasia)*.[37, 38, 42, 43]

Independent of other classifications, congenital malformations are usually considered as single or multiple and of "minor" or "major" functional significance.[3, 19, 23, 31] In general, major anomalies are defined as those that produce significant long-term disability and/or death, whereas minor anomalies do not.[3] At least half of major anomalies will be detected at birth; other anomalies (for example, pyloric stenosis, inguinal hernia, Hirschsprung's disease, and some forms of congenital heart disease) may not be diagnosed until later in infancy or childhood. Other anomalies (for example, cystic fibrosis and polycystic kidney disease) are not fully manifested until adulthood.[15]

Table 2–1 shows the most common types of anomalies in live born and stillborn infants as reported by the Metropolitan Atlanta Congenital Defects Program. Cardiovascular and musculoskeletal malforma-

TABLE 2–1.

Selected Congenital Malformations in Live Born and Stillborn Infants in the Atlanta Metropolitan Area for All Races, 1982–1985*

Type of Malformation	Incidence per 10,000 Live Births	Percentage of Anomalies (%)
Central nervous system		**16.8%**
Anencephaly	6.0	3.3
Spina bifida	8.4	4.6
Hydrocephalus without spina bifida	9.3	5.1
Encephalocele	2.0	1.1
Microcephaly	4.9	2.7
Oro-facial		**12.8%**
Anopthalmia/microphthalmia	3.5	1.9
Congenital cataract	2.1	1.2
Coloboma	0.8	0.4
Aniridia/other anomalies of iris	0.5	0.3
Cleft palate	5.5	3.0
Cleft lip with and without cleft palate	11.0	6.0
Cardiovascular†		**34.4%**
Common truncus	0.9	0.5
Transposition of the great arteries	4.1	2.3
Tetralogy of Fallot	2.9	1.6
Ventricular septal defect	17.8	9.8
Atrial septal defect	10.5	5.8
Endocardial cushion defect	2.5	1.4
Pulmonic stenosis and atresia	2.6	1.4
Tricuspid valve stenosis and atresia	1.6	0.9
Aortic valve stenosis and atresia	2.4	1.3
Hypoplastic left heart	3.0	1.6
Coarctation of the aorta	3.5	1.9
Pulmonary artery anomaly	3.1	1.7
Conus arteriosus	7.7	4.2
Gastrointestinal		**3.6%**
Tracheoesophageal anomalies	2.3	1.3
Rectal and intestinal atresia	4.1	2.3
Genitourinary		**1.8%**
Renal agenesis	3.3	1.8
Abdominal wall defects		**2.8%**
Bladder exstrophy	0.4	0.2
Omphalocele	3.5	1.9
Gastroschisis	1.4	0.7
Musculoskeletal		**25.2%**
Clubfoot without CNS anomalies	36.6	20.0
Reduction deformity upper limbs	4.9	2.7
Reduction deformity lower limbs	2.2	1.2
Congenital arthrogryposis	2.3	1.3
Pulmonary		**2.5%**
Lung agenesis and hypoplasia	4.6	2.5

*Data from Metropolitan Atlanta Congenital Defects Program, in Congenital Malformations Surveillance. Centers for Disease Control Bulletin, March 1988.
†Excludes patent ductus arteriosus.

tions together comprise over half these anomalies. Other common malformations include cleft lip, cleft palate, and central nervous system (CNS) disorders. Other studies have reported the frequent occurrence of minor anomalies, such as polydactyly, syndactyly, hypospadias, skin tags, hemangioma, inguinal hernia, and hydrocele, which may be found in as many as 15% of newborns.[3, 23, 40] Although they are usually of little functional significance themselves, minor malformations may indicate the presence of a more serious underlying condition.[3]

It is well known that the presence of one congenital anomaly increases the probability of having additional anomalies.[9, 11] However, the presence of additional anomalies is not uniformly distributed, even among anomalous fetuses, since fetuses with multiple anomalies tend to have a large number of anomalies involving many organ systems. Although multiple anomalies coexist by chance in many cases, others are related. A *syndrome* is said to be present when two or more embryologically unrelated anomalies occur together at a higher than expected rate. The term *sequence* has been used to describe a pattern of multiple anomalies derived from a single known or presumed prior anomaly or mechanical factor (for example, the amniotic band sequence).[38] A number of excellent references can provide detailed descriptions of specific malformations and syndromes.[1, 8, 18, 24, 39, 40]

ETIOLOGY

A fundamental concept of teratology is that certain stages of embryogenesis are more vulnerable to development of malformations than are other stages, with the most critical stage being the period of organ development (fetal day 15 to day 60).[8, 27] As a corollary concept, the nature of the insult is less important than the time at which it occurs. Also, the fetus appears to be relatively limited in its ability to express errors in embryologic development. For example, the Dandy-Walker malformation may result from a wide range of causes, including inheritable syndromes (Meckel-Gruber syndrome), chromosome abnormalities (trisomies 13 and 18), teratogens, or idiopathic causes.[29]

Five major causes of malformations are generally recognized (Table 2–2).[16, 17, 26, 36] These include:

1. Chromosome abnormalities.
2. Single gene disorders.
3. Multifactorial inheritance (both genetic and environmental factors).

4. Teratogenic (environmental factors).
5. Unknown.

Although the etiology usually is not known at the time of the sonographic examination, this classification serves as a useful working system when counseling women who are suspected of carrying fetuses with congenital anomalies. It also emphasizes the importance of chromosome abnormalities and inheritable disorders as causes of congenital malformations. Each of these five types of etiologies is discussed in greater detail below.

Chromosome Abnormalities

Fetuses with abnormal karyotypes have a high frequency of anomalies, often multiple.[35, 41] Such fetuses often spontaneously abort or die in utero. For this reason, chromosome abnormalities are more frequently encountered in autopsy or stillborn series than in postnatal series. For example, major chromosome abnormalities are identified in 0.5% of live births compared to over 50% of first trimester abortuses.[27]

Chromosome abnormalities are also a more common cause of congenital malformations in prenatal sonographic series than in postnatal studies. For example, although neural tube defects are generally considered to result from multifactorial causes, prenatal series suggest that chromosome abnormalities are a relatively common cause. An underlying chromosome abnormality was found in 3 of 8 fetuses with cephaloceles in one prenatal series,[68] and in 6 of 26 fetuses with spina bifida in another series.[79] A similar experience has shown a high frequency of chromosome abnormalities for a wide range of other malformations, including cardiac defects, diaphragmatic hernia, abdominal wall defects, and intracranial anomalies.[46, 48, 54, 57] As chromosome banding techniques improve, the proportion of chromosome abnormalities as a recognized cause of malformations will undoubtedly increase.

Single Gene Disorders

Over 3,000 conditions with single gene inheritance (autosomal dominant, autosomal recessive, and X-linked recessive) have been identified.[24] It is estimated that single gene disorders occur in 1.3%–1.8% of all infants and account for 8% of congenital anomalies.[4, 31] However, these may be underestimates, since inheritable disorders may be misdiagnosed or go undetected until after the neonatal period. As perinatal mortality due to other causes has decreased with improvements in obstetrical care, genetic causes have become

TABLE 2–2.

Estimated Incidence of Causes of Major Congenital Anomalies*

Cause	Incidence
Chromosome abnormalities	6
Monogenic or single gene defects	8
Multifactorial	25
Teratogenic	7
Unknown	54

*Adapted from Connor JM, Ferguson-Smith MA: *Essential Medical Genetics*. Oxford, Blackwell Scientific Publications, 1984.

TABLE 2–3.

Potential Fetal Malformations Associated With Maternal Drug or Chemical Use*

Drug	Fetal Malformations
Acetaminophen overdose	Polyhydramnios
Acetazolamide	Sacrococcygeal teratoma
Acetylsalicylic acid	Intracranial hemorrhage, IUGR
Albuterol	Tachycardia
Alcohol (ethanol)	Microcephaly, micrognathia, cleft palate, short nose, hypoplastic philtrum, cardiac defects (VSD, ASD, double-outlet right ventricle, pulmonary atresia, dextrocardia, tetralogy of Fallot), IUGR, diaphragmatic hernia, pectus excavatum, radioulnar, synostosis, scoliosis, bifid xyphoid, NTDs
Amantadine	Cardiac defects (single ventricle with pulmonary atresia)
Aminopterin	NTDs, hydrocephalus, incomplete skull ossification, brachycephaly, micrognathia, clubfoot, syndactyly, hypoplasia of thumb and fibula, IUGR
Amitriptyline	Micrognathia, limb reduction, swelling of hands and feet, urinary retention
Amobarbital	NTDs, cardiac defects, severe limb deformities, congenital hip dislocation, polydactyly, clubfoot, cleft palate, ambiguous genitalia, soft tissue, deformity of neck
Antithyroid drugs	Goiter
Azathioprine	Cardiac defects (pulmonary valve stenosis), polydactyly
Betamethasone	Reduced head circumference
Bromides	Polydactyly, clubfoot, congenital hip dislocation
Busulfan	Pyloric stenosis, cleft palate, microphthalmia, IUGR
Caffeine	Musculoskeletal defects, hydronephrosis
Captopril	Leg reduction
Carbon monoxide	Cerebral atrophy, hydrocephalus, fetal demise
Carbamazepine	NTDs, cardiac defects (atrial septal defect), nose hypoplasia, hypertelorism, cleft lip, congenital hip dislocation
Chlordiazepoxide	Microcephaly, cardiac defects, duodenal atresia
Chloroquine	Hemihypertrophy
Chlorpheniramine	Hydrocephalus, polydactyly, congenital hip dislocation
Chlorpropamide	Microcephaly, dysmorphic hands and fingers
Clomiphene	NTDs, microcephaly, syndactyly, clubfoot, polydactyly, esophageal atresia
Cocaine	Spontaneous abortion, placental abruption, prematurity, IUGR, possible cardiac defects, skull defects, genitourinary anomalies
Codeine	Hydrocephalus, head defects, cleft palate, musculoskeletal defects, dislocated hip, pyloric stenosis, respiratory malformations
Cortisone	Hydrocephalus, cardiac defects (VSD, coarctation of aorta), clubfoot, cleft lip
Coumadin	NTDs, cardiac defects, scoliosis, skeletal deformities, nasal hypoplasia, stippled epiphyses, chondrodysplasia punctata, short phalanges, toe defects, incomplete rotation of gut, IUGR, bleeding
Cyclophosphamide	Cardiac defects, cleft palate, flattened nasal bridge, four toes on each foot, syndactyly, hypoplastic mid-phalanx
Cytarabine	NTDs, cardiac defects, lobster claw hand, missing digits of feet, syndactyly
Daunorubicin	NTDs, cardiac defects, syndactyly
Dextroamphetamine	NTDs, cardiac defects, IUGR
Diazepam	NTDs, cardiac defects, absence of arm, syndactyly, absence of thumbs, cleft lip/palate
Diphenhydramine	Clubfoot, cleft palate
Disulfiram	Vertebral fusion, clubfoot, radial aplasia, phocomelia, tracheoesophageal fistula
Diuretics	Respiratory malformations
Estrogens	Cardiac defects, limb reduction
Ethosuximide	Hydrocephalus, short neck, oral cleft
Fluorouracil	Radial aplasia, absent thumbs, aplasia of esophagus and duodenum, hypoplasia of lungs
Fluphenazine	Poor ossification of frontal bone, cleft palate
Haloperidol	Limb deformities
Heparin	Bleeding
Imipramine	NTDs, cleft palate, renal cysts, diaphragmatic hernia
Indomethacin	Fetal demise, hemorrhage
Isoniazid	NTDs
Lithium	NTDs, cardiac defects (VSD, Ebstein's anomaly, mitral atresia, dextrocardia)
Lysergic acid diethylamide (LSD)	NTDs, limb defects
Meclizine	Cardiac defects (hypoplastic left heart), respiratory defect
Meprobamate	Cardiac defects, limb defects

Methotrexate	Oxycephaly, absence of frontal bones, large fontanelles, micrognathia, long webbed fingers, low-set ears, IUGR, dextrocardia
Methyl mercury	Microcephaly, asymmetric head
Metronidazole	Midline facial defects
Nortriptyline	Limb reduction
Oral contraceptives	NTDs, cardiac defects, vertebral defects, limb reduction, IUGR, tracheoesophageal malformation
Paramethadione	Cardiac defects, IUGR
Phenobarbital	NTDs, digital anomalies, cleft palate, ileal atresia, IUGR, pulmonary hypoplasia
Phenothiazines	Microcephaly, syndactyly, clubfoot, omphalocele
Phenylephrine	Eye and ear abnormalities, syndactyly, clubfoot, hip dislocation, umbilical hernia
Phenylpropanolamine	Pectus excavatum, polydactyly, hip dislocation
Phenytoin (hydantoin)	Microcephaly, wide fontanelles, cardiac defects, IUGR, cleft lip/palate, hypertelorism, low-set ears, short neck, short nose, broad nasal bridge, hypoplastic distal phalanges, digital thumb, hip dislocation, rib-sternal abnormalities
Polychlorinated biphenyls	Spotted calcification in skull, fetal demise, IUGR
Primidone	Cardiac defects (VSD), webbed neck, small mandible
Procarbazine	Cerebral hemorrhage, oligodactyly
Progesterones	NTDs, hydrocephaly, cardiac defects (tetralogy of Fallot, truncus arteriosus, VSD), absent thumbs
Quinine	Hydrocephalus, cardiac defects, facial defects, vertebral anomalies, dysmelias
Retinoic acid (vitamin A)	Hydrocephalus, cerebral malformations, microcephaly, cardiac defects, limb deformities, fetal demise, cleft palate, rib abnormalities
Spermicides	Limb reduction
Sulfonamide	Limb hypoplasia, foot defects, urethral obstruction
Tetracycline	Limb hypoplasia, clubfoot
Thalidomide	Cardiac defects, spine defects, limb reduction (amelia), phocomelia, hypoplasia, duodenal stenosis or atresia, pyloric stenosis
Thioguanine	Missing digits
Tobacco	IUGR
Tolbutamide	Syndactyly, absent toes, accessory thumb
Toluene	IUGR, neonatal hyperchloremia acidosis, possible mental dysfunction, cardiac defects, dysmorphic facies
Trifluoperazine	Cardiac defects, phocomelia
Trimethadione	Microcephaly, low-set ears, broad nasal bridge, cardiac defects (ASD, VSD), IUGR, cleft lip and palate, esophageal atresia, malformed hands, clubfoot
Valproic acid	NTDs, microcephaly, wide fontanelle, cardiac defects, IUGR, cleft palate, hypoplastic nose, low-set ears, small mandible, depressed nasal bridge, polydactyly

*IUGR = Intrauterine growth retardation; ASD = atrial septal defect; VSD = ventricular septal defect; NTDs = neural tube defects.

---

relatively more important. In the United Kingdom, a threefold relative increase in death rate due to genetic causes was observed in the 1960s and 1970s compared to earlier data.[15]

Multifactorial Inheritance

Multifactorial inheritance is a combination of genetic and environmental factors. Multifactorial inheritance is responsible for many of the common isolated congenital anomalies, such as cleft lip/palate, neural tube defects, and congenital heart defects.[16, 17, 36] Some of these malformations may also occur as part of syndromes determined by chromosome abnormalities, single gene disorders, or an environmental teratogen.

Teratogens

A teratogen is any agent that can induce or increase the incidence of a congenital malformation. Possible teratogens include drugs or chemicals (Table 2–3), infectious agents (Table 2–4), radiation, or other toxic substances.[6, 10, 14, 30, 32, 34] Although commonly mentioned, drugs and chemicals are responsible for less than 2% of congenital malformations (see Table 2–3).[2, 20]

A variety of other maternal conditions leading to altered metabolism may be associated with fetal anomalies (Table 2–5).[5, 33] Maternal diabetes deserves special emphasis as a potential teratogen (Table 2–6). Women with maternal diabetes have a two- to threefold increased risk of congenital anomalies and a six times greater risk of fetal malformations.[5, 7, 11, 16–18] Although the cause for this relationship is uncertain, most evi-

TABLE 2-4.

Infectious Agents That May Produce Congenital Anomalies*

Cytomegalovirus	Spontaneous abortion
	IUGR†
	Microcephaly
	Periventricular calcification
	Chorioretinitis
	Mental retardation
	Deafness
	Dandy-Walker malformation
	Hepatosplenomegaly
Rubella	Stillbirth
	Microcephaly
	Cataract
	Cardiac malformation
	Deafness
	Dandy-Walker malformation
Herpes simplex	Microcephaly
	Hydranencephaly
	Microphthalmia
	Splenomegaly
	Liver necrosis
Varicella	Hypoplasia of limb
	Rudimentary digits
	Mental retardation, brain atrophy
Toxoplasma gondii	Microcephaly
	Hydrocephalus
	Periventricular calcification
	Dandy-Walker malformation
Treponema pallidum (syphilis)	Deafness
	Hydrocephalus
	Mental retardation
Human immunodeficiency virus (AIDS)	Congenital infection

*From Hutto et al,[14] Koren et al,[20] Naeye R et al,[30] and Reynolds DW et al.[32]
†IUGR = Intrauterine growth retardation.

TABLE 2-5.

Maternal Conditions Associated With Fetal Disorders

Maternal Condition	Fetal Disorder
Diabetes	See Table 2-6
Isoimmunization	Anemia
	Congestive heart failure
Connective tissue disease	Heart block
	Bradycardia
	Fetal loss
	Vascular lesions in placenta
	Skin lesions
	Hepatosplenomegaly
Graves' disease	Hyperthyroidism
	Hypothyroidism
	Stillborn
Thyroiditis	Hypothyroidism
Hypothyroidism	Hypothyroidism
	Ovarian cyst
	Fetal loss
	Fetal goiter
Hyperparathyroidism	Fetal demise
	Hypotonia
Phenylketonuria	Microcephaly
Cushing's syndrome	Fetal loss
Seizure disorders	Anomalies related to drug use
Myasthenia gravis	Fetal loss
	Myasthenia gravis
Heart disease	Fetal loss
	IUGR*
	Congenital malformation
Hypertension	Fetal loss
	IUGR*
	Abruptio placentae
Renal disease	Fetal loss
	Preterm delivery
	Low birth weight and IUGR*
Polycystic kidney disease	Polycystic kidney disease
Anemia	Fetal loss
	IUGR*
	Preterm delivery
Thalassemia	Hydrops
Hemophilia	AIDS
Advanced age (>35 yrs)	Chromosomal anomalies

*IUGR = Intrauterine growth retardation.

dence suggests that hyperglycemia or a related metabolite is the inciting agent.[5, 18]

Other Risk Factors

Multiple gestations are at increased risk for congenital anomalies and for other obstetric complications (see Chapter 15).[9] However, the risk of congenital anomalies appears to be increased only for monochorionic gestations. This additional burden is not unexpected, since monochorionic twinning is a type of malformation itself. By contrast, a dichorionic gestation results from simultaneous fertilization of multiple ova, and no increased risk of anomalies would be anticipated from this maternal predisposition.

AN OVERVIEW OF PRENATAL SONOGRAPHIC DETECTION OF FETAL MALFORMATIONS

Prenatal sonography has developed as a powerful tool for the detection and delineation of congenital anomalies. Optimal examination by experienced sonographers can diagnose the vast majority of major malformations, and even minor malformations have been correctly detected. Table 2-7 presents a partial list of malformations that have been successfully diagnosed on prenatal sonography and which are discussed

TABLE 2-6.

Congenital Anomalies Associated With Maternal Diabetes

Central nervous system	Anencephaly
	Encephalocele
	Meningomyelocele
	Spina bifida
Cardiac	Transposition of the great vessels
	Ventricular septal defect
	Atrial septal defect
	Tricuspid atresia
	Situs inversus
	Hypoplastic left ventricle
	Single ventricle
Skeletal	Caudal regression syndrome
	Arthrogryposis
Renal	Agenesis
	Multicystic dysplastic kidney
	Ureteral duplication
Gastrointestinal	Anorectal atresia
	Small left colon
	Situs inversus
Pulmonary	Hypoplasia

*From Cousins L,[5] Hollingsworth DR, Resnik R (eds),[11] and Koren G et al.[20]

in detail in subsequent chapters. In a clinical situation, however, it is useful to know the accuracy of sonographic diagnoses, including both false-negative and false-positive results. This information, as well as the limitations of prenatal sonography, are discussed below.

SONOGRAPHIC ACCURACY

The accuracy of prenatal sonography for diagnosing many major malformations has been assessed by various authors.[64, 66, 72, 83, 84, 91, 93] However, such reports invariably reflect the experience of high-risk centers that have considerable experience with prenatal diagnoses of fetal malformations. Also, many women seen at these centers are referred because of an abnormality suspected elsewhere or because of other high-risk factors (see Chapter 1 for a discussion of targeted and routine sonograms). The accuracy of sonography for diagnosing malformations in women referred for routine clinical indications or at institutions less experienced with fetal malformations is largely unknown.

In general, prenatal sonography is highly specific for the presence of major malformations when one or more anomalies are suspected. In one prenatal series, Manchester et al. reported that one or more anomalies were suspected in 215 fetuses and that 98.6% of these were confirmed to have a significant malformation

TABLE 2-7.

Fetal Malformations That Have Been Diagnosed by Prenatal Sonography

Cranial and intracranial
  Agenesis of the corpus callosum
  Anencephaly
  Aqueductal stenosis
  Arachnoid cyst
  Cephalocele
  Choroid plexus cysts
  Communicating hydrocephalus
  Dandy-Walker malformation
  Exencephaly
  Holoprosencephaly
  Iniencephaly
  Intracranial calcification
  Intracranial hemorrhage
  Intracranial neoplasm
  Microcephaly
  Porencephalic cyst
  Schizencephaly
  Unilateral hydrocephalus
  Vein of Galen aneurysm
Craniofacial
  Anophthalmia
  Cyclopia, ethmocephaly, cebocephaly
  Cystic hygroma
  Facial cleft
  Goiter
  Hypotelorism
  Hypertelorism
  Lacrimal duct cyst
  Micrognathia
  Microphthalmia
  Persistent choroidal artery
  Small ears
  Teratoma
Spine
  Hemivertebrae
  Lipomeningocele
  Sacral agenesis
  Sacrococcygeal teratoma
  Scoliosis
  Sirenomelia
  Spina bifida
Thoracic
  Absent lung
  Bronchial atresia
  Bronchogenic cyst
  Cystic adenomatoid malformation
  Diaphragmatic hernia
  Hydrothorax
  Pulmonary hypoplasia
  Pulmonary sequestration
Gastrointestinal
  Anorectal atresia
  Choledochal cyst
  Cholelithiasis
  Congenital chloridorrhea
  Duodenal atresia
  Enteric duplication cyst
  Hepatic cyst

(Continued.)

TABLE 2–7   (cont.).

Hepatic neoplasm
Hirschsprung's disease
Jejunoileal atresia
Meconium ileus
Meconium peritonitis
Mesenteric cyst
Persistent cloaca
Situs inversus
Tracheoesophageal fistula
Volvulus

Genitourinary
Ambiguous genitalia
Bladder outlet obstruction
Duplicated kidneys with ectopic ureterocele
Hydrometrocolpos
Megacystis microcolon intestinal
   hypoperistalsis syndrome
Multicystic dysplastic kidney
Ovarian cyst
Pelvic kidney
Renal agenesis
Tumors (mesoblastic nephroma,
   neuroblastoma)
Ureteropelvic junction obstruction
Ureterovesical obstruction

Cardiovascular
Arrhythmias
Atrioventricular septal defect (endocardial
   cushion defect)
Cardiomyopathy
Cardiosplenic syndromes
Coarctation of the aorta
Double outlet right ventricle
Ebstein's anomaly
Hypoplastic left ventricle
Hypoplastic right ventricle
Pericardial tumors (teratoma)
Rhabdomyoma
Tetralogy of Fallot
Total anomalous pulmonary venous return
Transposition of the great vessels
Valvular stenosis
Ventricular septal defect

Abdominal wall and trunk
Bladder exstrophy
Cloacal exstrophy
Ectopia cordis
Gastroschisis
Limb-body wall complex (body-stalk anomaly)
Lymphangioma
Omphalocele
Tumors (teratoma, melanoma, etc.)
Urachal cyst
Vascular malformation

Extremities
Arthrogryposis
Bone dysplasias
Clinodactyly
Clubfeet
Limb shortening
Polydactyly
Radial aplasia

postnatally.[72] There were only 4 "false-positive" diagnoses including 2 fetuses with suspected hydronephrosis, 1 with suspected intracranial cyst, and 1 fetus with intra-abdominal calcifications that could not be confirmed postnatally.

The sensitivity of prenatal sonography for detecting congenital anomalies is more difficult to determine, primarily because such analysis requires careful postnatal examinations of all fetuses who underwent obstetric sonography. Such a study ideally would include long-term clinical follow-up, since some malformations are not clinically apparent at birth. Nevertheless, such information is available for many major anomalies that are apparent at the time of delivery.

Table 2–8 shows the relative frequency and types of anomalies reported in several selected prenatal series.[63, 72, 84, 91] Major anomalies of the central nervous (see Chapters 5 and 6) and genitourinary systems (see Chapter 12) comprise a large share of reported anomalies in these and other prenatal studies, representing over 50% of detected malformations.[44, 45, 50, 51, 86] These data obviously differ from the frequency and types of anomalies encountered at birth, when musculoskeletal and cardiovascular anomalies are most common (see Table 2–1). Differences between prenatal and newborn studies can be explained by various factors, primarily by:

1. The relative insensitivity of prenatal ultrasound for detecting many minor anomalies.
2. Inclusion in prenatal series of more fetuses with severe and complex malformations who die before birth and who may be underreported in newborn studies.
3. Underrepresentation in newborn studies of anomalies that may be asymptomatic and not visible externally (for example, unilateral multicystic dysplastic kidney or unilateral renal obstruction).

As suggested by comparing Tables 2–1 and 2–8, cardiac anomalies are among the most commonly missed malformations prenatally. Manchester and associates detected 16 of 45 (36%) cardiac anomalies, and Hill et al. failed to detect a single cardiac defect (excluding arrhythmias) among 15 cardiac defects.[64, 72] The insensitivity of prenatal sonography for detecting many cardiac anomalies is in part due to various technical factors (rapid heart rate, fetal position, and limited resolution of real-time sonography) that make a thorough examination of the fetal heart a time-consuming procedure. Indeed, fetal echocardiography is generally considered a specialized examination that

TABLE 2–8.

Specific Congenital Malformations Detected in Selected Prenatal Series

Category of Anomaly	Grisoni (1986) (n=149)*	Manchester (1988) (n=211)†	Vandenberghe (1984) (n=186)‡	Sabbagha (1985) (n=79)§
CNS‖	54 (36%)	87 (41%)	65 (35%)	30 (38%)
Genitourinary	33 (22%)	38 (18%)	36 (19%)	12 (15%)
Gastrointestinal	16 (11%)	15 (7%)	19 (10%)	6 (8%)
Diaphragmatic hernia	6 (4%)	—	} 13 (7%)	—
Abdominal wall defects	11 (7%)	14 (7%)		10 (13%)
Hydrops fetalis	14 (9%)	21 (10%)	7 (4%)	3 (4%)
Cystic hygroma	3 (2%)	—	7 (4%)	6 (8%)
Cardiovascular	4 (3%)	16 (7%)	7 (4%)	—
Skeletal	4 (3%)	10 (5%)	7 (4%)	6 (8%)
Teratoma and tumors	3 (1%)	2 (1%)	6 (3%)	2 (2%)
Pulmonary	1 (1%)	—	4 (2%)	2 (2%)
Other		8 (4%)	15 (8%)	2 (2%)

*149 anomalies in 122 fetuses, excluding cardiac arrhythmia (n=2).
†From Table 2–2, excluding unspecified twins (n=16) or cardiac arrhythmia (n=7).
‡186 anomalies in 150 fetuses.
§Excluding fetuses wtih only detectable polyhydramnios (n=21) or oliogohydramnios (n=6).
‖ CNS = central nervous system anomalies, including cranial and spinal defects.

is performed separately from the remainder of the obstetric sonogram and that requires special expertise in cardiac imaging (see Chapter 9).[48, 58]

Although a few centers specializing in cardiac anomalies have reported a relatively high accuracy for detecting cardiac malformations,[48, 58] the majority of patients seen at such centers are first detected on outside sonograms. This emphasizes the value of routine evaluation of the fetal heart as a part of all routine obstetric sonograms. Incorporation of a four-chamber view and views of the great vessels should permit greater detection of many major cardiac anomalies which can then be referred to specialized centers for a more definitive diagnosis.

In addition to cardiac defects, other major anomalies that have been frequently missed in prenatal series include small myelomeningoceles, small abdominal wall defects, early hydrocephalus, bladder exstrophy, pulmonary hypoplasia, esophageal atresia, and sirenomelia.[56, 62, 67, 85, 91] Also, important "minor" abnormalities, such as facial clefts and skeletal abnormalities, are frequently missed.[64, 66, 83] Compiling a list of anomalies that are rarely or never seen with prenatal sonography is fraught with hazard, however, since improvements in detection of such anomalies are reported almost monthly. For example, recent observations of characteristic cranial findings associated with spina bifida (see Chapter 6) now make it possible to accurately detect nearly all cases of myelomeningoceles, even very small defects.[74, 78] Recognition of characteristic findings of bladder exstrophy and small abdominal wall defects (see Chapter 11) should also improve sonographic detection of these anomalies.

Detection of additional anomalies in fetuses with multiple malformations is of paramount importance for counseling patients and determining the optimal obstetric management. Hence, detection of one fetal anomaly demands a thorough search for other abnormalities. However, many associated anomalies can be overlooked. Manchester and associates reported that 25% of anomalous fetuses had multiple anomalies in their series, and 37% of associated anomalies were missed, even though the primary sonographic diagnosis was generally accurate.[72] Fortunately, individual fetuses with multiple anomalies can usually be identified, even if all the specific malformations are not. In the series of Manchester et al., 98% of fetuses with multiple anomalies were suspected by demonstrating more than one abnormality.[72] Therefore, detection of more than one anomaly should suggest the presence of additional non–detectable anomalies. Detection of multiple anomalies should also suggest the possibility of an underlying chromosome abnormality.[55, 57, 75, 92, 93]

An ideal screening test for fetal malformations would detect all major malformations prior to the time of fetal viability, thereby providing the prospective parents the choice of continuing the pregnancy or not. Indeed, certain types of malformations may be readily detected early in pregnancy (before 20 weeks). These include cystic hygromata, most CNS anomalies (including holoprosencephaly, anencephaly, spina bifida, and most cases of hydrocephaly), abdominal wall defects, many lethal bone dysplasias, and major genitourinary anomalies. On the other hand, some anomalies (for example, gastrointestinal obstruction) may not be

TABLE 2–9.

Fetal Anomalies That May Not Be Visualized by 24 Weeks' Gestation

Most gastrointestinal disorders (obstruction).
Some cases of infantile or adult-type polycystic kidney disease.
Heterozygous achondroplasia.
Some cases of microcephaly.
Some forms of hydrocephalus.
Some tumors.
Acquired disorders (for example, intracranial hemorrhage or arachnoid cyst).

detectable until after the time of fetal viability (Table 2–9).

LIMITATIONS OF PRENATAL SONOGRAPHY FOR DIAGNOSING FETAL MALFORMATIONS

It is important to recognize the limitations, as well as the benefits, of prenatal sonographic diagnoses of congenital anomalies. Some of these are within the control of the ultrasonographer, but many are not. These limitations may be secondary to various factors, categorized as follows:

1. Operator-dependence of ultrasound.
2. Technical limitations and artifacts.
3. Limitations due to embryologic development and physiology.
4. Limitations due to non–specificity of sonographic findings.

Each of these factors is discussed in greater detail below.

Operator-Dependence of Ultrasound

The operator-dependence of diagnostic ultrasound is widely recognized. Indeed, in few other areas of imaging are the experience and expertise of the operator so critical to the correct diagnosis. Fortunately, not all obstetric sonographers require special expertise in evaluation of fetal anomalies. Rather, most sonographers need only to distinguish normal from abnormal fetuses so that those fetuses with suspected abnormalities can be examined at a referral center for further evaluation. Nevertheless, the first step in this process requires recognition of a fetal abnormality. Since the vast majority of fetal malformations occur in women with no known risk factor, the responsibility for detection of major anomalies lies with all sonographers and physicians who perform obstetric sonograms. Many im-

portant anomalies will be missed if a systematic survey of fetal anatomy is not incorporated into "routine" examinations.[85]

Misinterpretation of a sonographically detectable abnormality continues to be problematic, even at referral centers for high-risk obstetrics. For example, Blane et al. reported nine fetuses who were thought to have obstructive hydronephrosis, but neonatal follow-up proved that some cases actually represented multicystic kidney, vesicoureteral reflux, Prune-Belly syndrome, cloacal abnormality, or ileal duplication.[49] Cranial malformations such as hydrocephaly, hydranencephaly, and holoprosencephaly may be mistaken for one another (see Chapter 5),[83] and abdominal wall defects such as omphalocele, gastroschisis, and cloacal exstrophy may be misinterpreted (see Chapter 11).[62, 83] Greater experience with prenatal sonographic findings of congenital anomalies can reduce the number of such misinterpretations, although some errors are partly attributable to the non–specificity of sonographic findings (see below). Correlation with postnatal clinical evaluation and thorough autopsy examinations are also essential in attempting to improve sonographic diagnoses.

Commonly encountered artifacts may result in either false-positive or false-negative diagnoses, particularly in the hands of less experienced sonographers.[87] For example, the normally sonolucent brain parenchyma may be mistaken for hydrocephalus, although this is a less common source of error currently than in previous years. In fetuses with true hydrocephalus, reverberation of the ultrasound beam often obscures the dilated ventricle in the near field and can lead to an erroneous diagnosis of unilateral hydrocephalus. An omphalocele may be falsely suspected by compression of the fetal abdomen.[83]

Technical Limitations

Technical limitations produced by fetal position, maternal obesity, and abnormal amniotic fluid volume may significantly limit sonographic evaluation of fetal anomalies.[66, 72, 83] Problems related to fetal position are easier to correct than other contributing factors. Changing the beam path by moving the transducer to various locations on the maternal abdomen may improve visualization of fetal parts. A change in maternal position, such as decubitus positions, may alter the fetal position and thus permit optimal imaging. We have also found that endovaginal scanning may be useful for examining fetal structures when the area of interest is low in the maternal pelvis. In some cases, a delayed study a few hours or days later may be necessary.

Although both oligohydramnios and polyhydramnios may be the initial clues to a significant underlying fetal malformation (see Chapter 3),[45] they may inhibit sonographic evaluation of fetal malformations in different ways. Since amniotic fluid normally provides an acoustic window to the fetus, oligohydramnios presents a major obstacle to visualization of fetal parts. Polyhydramnios permits the fetus to be unusually mobile so that specific images may be difficult to obtain. The fetus is also usually in the dependent portion of the uterus, increasing the distance from the fetus to the ultrasound transducer in the presence of polyhydramnios. The difficulties presented by abnormal amniotic fluid volume are emphasized by the study of Manchester and associates, who found that 43% of missed anomalies could be attributed to abnormalities of amniotic fluid volume.[72]

Embryologic Development and Physiology

As previously suggested, limitations inherent to fetal development and physiology may restrict detection of certain anomalies, particularly during the first trimester. For example, the bowel is normally eviscerated into the base of the umbilical cord between 8–12 weeks as part of normal gut migration.[58] Therefore, abdominal wall defects may not be reliably diagnosed before 12 weeks. As another example, fetal kidneys do not start producing urine until after 12 weeks and may not significantly contribute to amniotic fluid volume until after 16 weeks. Therefore, most renal malformations are usually not diagnosed until after 12–16 weeks.

Limitations of embryologic development and physiology may even restrict detection of certain anomalies until after the time of fetal viability (see Table 2–4). For example, the sonographic appearance of infantile or adult polycystic kidney disease may be entirely normal early in the second trimester, yet clearly abnormal by 25 weeks.[70, 81, 88] Also, gastrointestinal tract abnormalities (duodenal atresia, tracheoesophageal atresia) are usually not diagnosed until after 24 weeks, since fetal swallowing does not significantly contribute to amniotic fluid production until this time.[45] Prenatal diagnosis of esophageal atresia is particularly difficult, since this anomaly is usually associated with a tracheoesophageal fistula, thereby permitting amniotic fluid to accumulate in the stomach. Other malformations such as microcephaly and heterozygous achondroplasia may not become apparent until after 24 weeks, even with serial sonographic examinations.[69, 88]

Congenital anomalies may vary in their severity and hence in their likelihood of detection. For example, some cases of cerebral ventricular dilatation may progressively enlarge when due to obstructive hydrocephalus, whereas other cases of ventricular dilatation may resolve with advancing gestation, particularly when mild in severity.[71, 89] Other malformations that have been observed to spontaneously resolve include cystic adenomatoid malformation of the lung and cystic hygromata.

Non–Specificity of Sonographic Findings and Diagnostic Dilemmas

Prenatal sonography can permit a specific diagnosis for certain types of malformations such as alobar holoprosencephaly, myelomeningocele, and gastroschisis. Occasionally, however, the sonographic appearance suggests a list of diagnostic possibilities rather than a single, specific diagnosis. For example, a cystic structure in the lower fetal abdomen can represent an ovarian cyst, a duplication cyst, a meconium cyst, or some other unusual anomaly. Also, a hydroureter may be mistaken for dilated bowel.[67]

An even more difficult diagnostic problem is distinguishing suspected abnormalities from similar findings in normal fetuses. For example, the cystic mass in the pelvis should be distinguished from the unusually prominent colon found in some normal fetuses. Also, echogenic masses within the fetal abdomen have been reported as a sign of meconium ileus in some fetuses with cystic fibrosis, yet identical findings may occasionally be observed in normal fetuses.[59, 73] In both situations, the echogenic areas are thought to represent inspissated intraluminal meconium, with the inspissation being transient in normal fetuses but persistent and obstructive in fetuses with meconium ileus.

As another common dilemma, choroid plexus cysts are seen in 0.6%–2.5% of all fetuses during the second trimester; these usually resolve by 24 weeks (see Chapter 5).[52, 53] However, choroid cysts have also been associated with chromosome abnormalities, particularly trisomy 18.[53, 75] In determining the relative risk of a chromosome abnormality in a fetus who demonstrates choroid plexus cysts, other important factors include the size of the cysts and presence of associated abnormalities. Invariably, the likelihood of a chromosome abnormality must be weighed against the costs and potential risks of chromosome analysis (see Chapter 17).

In the quest to identify more fetuses with an underlying chromosome abnormality, especially fetuses with trisomy 21, two other sonographic findings that have been proposed as possibly useful are 1) increased nuchal thickening and 2) disproportionately short femur length.[47] The potential benefit of searching for such findings in all fetuses has not been clearly defined.[80] Nevertheless, such observations, based on prenatal sonographic findings, reflect the diagnostic dilemma in which both the ultrasonographer and obstetrician increasingly find themselves.

COUNSELING

As indicated by the previous discussion, a sonographic diagnosis of a fetal malformation raises a number of unexpected questions from the prospective parents. Although expressed in various ways, questions prospective parents commonly have include:

1. What is the sonographic accuracy for diagnosing this condition? (What is the chance that the ultrasound diagnosis could be in error?)
2. Assuming the diagnosis is correct, what is the likelihood of perinatal death, long-term handicaps, or mental retardation?
3. What can be done to correct the defect or improve the outcome?
4. What does this mean for this pregnancy in terms of the mode and time of delivery?
5. What is the recurrence risk of a similar abnormality affecting future pregnancies?

Although it is difficult and even hazardous to predict the outcome in any individual fetus with certainty, information based on a collective experience can provide the best possible answers. For this task, a multispecialty group of experts in ultrasound, obstetrics, pediatrics, genetics, and social work is most effective (see Chapter 18).[101, 102, 113] It is helpful for families to meet with pediatric specialists prior to the delivery of an abnormal baby, so that all parties concerned will know what to expect at the time of delivery. A reasonable estimate of prognosis can be discussed at that time, and the antenatal management may be planned. A physician should be available to explain the suspected abnormality to the prospective parents, who may require significant emotional support.

When counseling prospective parents about a particular malformation, it is important for the health care team to understand the differences in prognosis between fetal and neonatal studies of congenital anomalies. Since major anomalies are much more common in early abortuses and in stillborn infants (10%−15%) compared to live born infants,[8, 27] it is not surprising that prenatal series also generally include fetuses with more severe, lethal anomalies than neonatal studies.[46, 48, 54, 57] Hence, the prognosis for a malformed fetus detected prenatally is generally worse than the prognosis for a neonate with a similar malformation (for example, diaphragmatic hernia).[46, 54] In addition, some disorders are unique to fetal life, and thus little neonatal data are available regarding them. This includes entities such as oligohydramnios, amniotic bands, intrauterine growth retardation, placental pathology, umbilical cord pathology, and complications of multiple gestations (twin transfusion syndrome, acardiac twinning, conjoined twinning).

In a representative prenatal series reported by Manchester and associates, 59% of fetuses with a sonographically detectable anomaly died. Among survivors, 44% remained handicapped with disabilities ranging from limited use of limbs to ongoing hospitalization, while 56% of infants with structural abnormalities were functioning normally following treatment or repair of their birth defects.[72] A more meaningful estimate of the prognosis, however, depends on identification of the specific malformation or combination of malformations present. A common failing of many published series of congenital anomalies is grouping a variety of different malformations which may have very different outcomes under a single diagnosis, for example, aqueductal stenosis, Dandy-Walker malformation, holoprosencephaly, and hydranencephaly under the term "hydrocephalus." Whenever possible, therefore, the specific malformation should be identified and the outlook should be compared with prenatal experience for similar malformations.

The largest and most obvious malformations observed on sonography are often associated with the worst prognosis; however, this is not always the case. For example, cerebellar hypoplasia or the Dandy-Walker variant may appear relatively subtle, seen only as an enlarged cisterna magna, yet it is frequently associated with a chromosome abnormality (see Chapter 17).[76] On the other hand, the Dandy-Walker malformation (with ventricular dilatation) is a more obvious malformation that appears to be less frequently associated with chromosome abnormalities. As another example, small omphaloceles that contain only bowel might be expected to carry a better prognosis than large omphaloceles that also contain liver. While this may be true for surviving infants without additional malformations, there is evidence to suggest that for fetuses identified prenatally, an omphalocele that does not contain liver may carry a significantly greater risk of a chromosome abnormality (see Chapter 11).[77]

Rarely, anomalies seen in utero may actually have a better prognosis than suggested by neonatal studies.

One example is meconium peritonitis, a sterile chemical peritonitis caused by in utero bowel perforation. Postnatal studies suggest that in 15%−25% of cases, the meconium peritonitis results from meconium ileus and cystic fibrosis. By contrast, a prenatal study suggests that less than 10% of fetuses with meconium peritonitis prove to have cystic fibrosis.[60] The lower frequency of cystic fibrosis seen prenatally may reflect the greater detection rate of both asymptomatic fetuses who may not come to clinical attention after birth and fetuses who subsequently die before inclusion in neonatal studies.

MANAGEMENT OF FETAL MALFORMATIONS

The ultimate impact of prenatal sonographic diagnoses must be judged by its influence on patient management. Most importantly, detection of a malformation before the time of fetal viability permits the prospective parents to choose whether or not to continue the pregnancy. Even if the pregnancy is continued or if the malformation is not diagnosed until after the time of fetal viability, a diagnosis of a major fetal malformation will often influence obstetric decisions regarding the place, time, and mode of delivery. The parents, obstetrician, pediatrician, nursing staff, and pediatric surgeon can all be prepared for the birth of an anomalous infant, thereby providing the optimal management of such infants.

Certain malformations require surgical correction soon after birth (see Chapter 18). These include neural tube defects, diaphragmatic hernias, abdominal wall defects, intestinal atresias (including esophageal atresia and duodenal atresia), and some types of cardiac defects.[102, 107, 112] Optimal management of fetuses with such malformations includes delivery in a tertiary care center staffed by pediatric surgeons, thereby avoiding problems caused by delayed transport.

In reviewing the impact of prenatal diagnosis on surgically correctable defects, Grisoni et al. found that fetuses with abdominal wall defects and anomalies of the gastrointestinal tract who were detected prenatally had improved care and outcome and fetuses with genitourinary anomalies received earlier postnatal evaluation and treatment.[63] No difference in management was noted for central nervous system anomalies, however, since these malformations carry an inherently high mortality. Similarly, knowledge of cardiovascular malformations did not change postnatal treatment or the eventual outcome, with the exception of arrhythmias, which could be successfully treated in utero. Par-

adoxically, the mortality in neonates with congenital diaphragmatic hernia was increased compared to previous years, since management included newborns with more severe anomalies who previously would have died before transport to the primary care center.[63]

Rapid improvements in prenatal diagnosis and treatment have led to modes of treatment other than postnatal surgical management. The possible role of prenatal surgery for certain types of anomalies (diaphragmatic hernia and bladder outlet obstruction) has received much publicity.[85, 94, 103−105, 107, 110] Other surgical methods include catheter drainage of obstructed fluid collections, such as hydrocephalus and renal obstruction.[100, 104, 111] Pleuro-amniotic catheters have also been successfully utilized for drainage of hydrothorax which might otherwise contribute to breathing difficulties and pulmonary hypoplasia.[97, 114]

Equally dramatic progress has been made in less invasive methods for evaluating and treating fetal conditions. Development of percutaneous fetal umbilical vein sampling as an established technique now provides enormous potential opportunities for monitoring and treating fetal conditions such as thrombocytopenia, fetal hydrops due to anemia, infections, and genetic defects.[96, 99, 106, 108] Medical therapy has also been used successfully to treat fetal cardiac arrhythmias in utero. Indomethacin or other prostaglandin inhibitors have been used for treating polyhydramnios, and low-dose aspirin has been proposed for treating placental insufficiency.[115]

SUMMARY

In summary, prenatal ultrasound is remarkably accurate for detection of many major malformations. On the other hand, prenatal sonography is insensitive for detection of many minor anomalies present at birth. The potential benefits as well as the limitations of prenatal sonography should be recognized by health care providers who contribute to the management and counseling of women who are suspected of carrying an anomalous fetus. Differences in prognosis between prenatal series and postnatal series, the importance of associated anomalies to the eventual outcome, and possible options in management should also be recognized. Optimal management of fetal malformations requires a multidisciplinary approach of various specialties. Continued improvements in both invasive and non-invasive methods for treating fetal malformations can be anticipated in the near future.

REFERENCES

General Reference: Classification of Anomalies/ Risk Factors

1. Bergsma D: *Birth Defects Atlas and Compendium,* ed 2. New York, Alan R Liss Inc, 1979.
2. Brent RL: Radiation teratogenesis, in Sever JL, Brent RL (eds): *Teratogen Update: Environmentally Induced Birth Defect Risks.* New York, Alan R Liss Inc, 1986.
3. Chung CS, Myrianthopoulos C: Congenital anomalies: Mortality and morbidity, burden and classification. Am J Med Genet 1987; 27:505–523.
4. Connor JM, Ferguson-Smith MA: *Essential Medical Genetics.* Oxford, Blackwell Scientific Publications, 1984.
5. Cousins L: Congenital anomalies among infants of diabetic mothers: Etiology, prevention, prenatal diagnosis. Am J Obstet Gynecol 1983; 147:333–338.
6. Ernhart CB, Sokol RJ, Martier S, et al: Alcohol teratogenicity in the human: A detailed assessment of specificity, critical period, and threshold. Am J Obstet Gynecol 1987; 156:33–39.
7. Gomez KJ, Dowdy K, Allen G, et al: Evaluation of ultrasound diagnosis of fetal anomalies in women with pregestational diabetes: University of Florida experience. Am J Obstet Gynecol 1988; 159:584–586.
8. Gray SW, Skandalakis JE. *Embryology for Surgeons.* Philadelphia, Saunders, 1982.
9. Hay S, Wehrung D: Congenital malformations in twins. Amer J Genet 1970; 22:662–678.
10. Heinonen OP, Slone D, Shapiro S: *British Defects and Drugs in Pregnancy.* Littleton, MA, Publishing Sciences Group, 1977.
11. Hollingsworth DR and Resnik R (eds): *Medical Counseling Before Pregnancy.* New York, Churchill Livingstone, 1988.
12. Hook EB: Chromosome abnormalities and spontaneous fetal death following amniocentesis: Further data and associations with maternal age. Am J Hum Genet 1983; 35:110–116.
13. Hook EB: Spontaneous deaths of fetuses with chromosomal abnormalities diagnosed prenatally. N Engl J Med 1978; 299:1036–1038.
14. Hutto C, Arvin A, Jacobs R, et al: Intrauterine herpes simplex virus infections. J Pediat 1987; 110:97–101.
15. Kaback MM: The utility of prenatal diagnosis, in Rodeck CH, Nicolaides KH (eds): *Prenatal Diagnosis.* New York, John Wiley, 1984, pp 53–64.
16. Kalter H, Warkany J: Congenital malformations. Etiologic factors and their role in prevention, part 1. N Engl J Med 1983; 308:424–431.
17. Kalter H, Warkany J. Congenital malformations. Etiologic factors and their role in prevention, part 2. N Engl J Med 1983; 308:491–497.
18. Keeling JW: Examination of the fetus following prenatal suspicion of congenital abnormality, in Keeling JW (ed): *Fetal and Neonatal Pathology.* New York, Springer-Verlag, 1987, pp 99–122.
19. Kennedy WP: Epidemiologic aspects of the problem of congenital malformations. Birth Defects 1967; 3:1–18.
20. Koren G, Edwards M, Miskin M: Antenatal sonography of fetal malformations associated with drugs and chemicals: A guide. Am J Obstet Gynecol 1987; 156:79–85.
21. Kucera J: Rate and type of congenital anomalies among offspring of diabetic women. J Repro Med 1971; 7:73–82.
22. MacVicar J: Antenatal detection of fetal abnormality; physical methods. Br Med Bull 1976; 32:4.
23. Marden PM, Smith DW, McDonald MJ: Congenital anomalies in the newborn infant, including minor variations. J Pediatr 1964; 64:357–372.
24. McKusick VA: *Mendelian Inheritance in Man,* ed 6. Baltimore, Johns Hopkins University Press, 1983.
25. Miller E, Hare JW, Cloherty JP, et al: Elevated maternal hemoglobin A_{Ic} in early pregnancy and major congenital anomalies in infants of diabetic mothers. N Engl J Med 1981; 304:1331–1334.
26. Mills JL: Malformations in infants of diabetic mothers. Teratology 1982; 25:385–394.
27. Moore KL: *Essentials of Human Embryology.* Toronto, B.C. Decker, Inc, Philadelphia, 1988, p 54.
28. Morrison I: Perinatal mortality: Basic considerations. Semin Perinatol 1985; 9:144–150.
29. Murray JC, Johnson JA, Bird TD: Dandy-Walker malformation: Etiologic heterogeneity and empiric recurrence risks. Genetics 1985; 28:272.
30. Naeye R, Tafari N: *Risk Factors in Pregnancy and Diseases of the Fetus and Newborn.* Williams & Wilkins Co, Baltimore, 1983, pp 77–143.
31. Polani PE: Incidence of developmental and other genetic abnormalities. Proc R Soc Med 1973; 66:1118.
32. Reynolds DW, Stagno S, Alford CA: Congenital cytomegalovirus infection, in Sever JL, Brent RL (eds): *Teratogen Update: Environmentally Induced Birth Defect Risks.* New York, Alan R Liss, Inc 1986.
33. Rohr F, Doherty L, Waisbren S, et al. New England maternal PKU study of untreated and treated pregnancies and their outcomes. J Pediatr 1987; 110:391–398.
34. Scialli AR: A computerized consultation service in reproductive toxicology: Summary of the first five years. Obstet Gynecol 1988; 72:195–199.
35. Simpson JL, Golbus MS, Martin AO, et al: Autosomal chromosome abnormalities, in *Genetics in Obstetrics and Gynecology.* Philadephia, Grune & Stratton, 1982, pp 53–78.
36. Simpson JL, Golbus MS, Martin AO, et al: Single anatomical malformations usually inherited in polygenic/multifactorial fashion, in *Genetics in Obstetrics and Gynecology.* Philadelphia, Grune & Stratton, 1982, pp 79–94.
37. Smith DW: *Recognizable Patterns of Human Malformations,* ed 3. Philadelphia, WB Saunders Co, 1982, pp 10–19.
38. Spranger J, Benirschke K, Hall JG, et al: Errors of morphogenesis: Concepts and terms. J Pediatr 1982; 100:160–165.

39. Taybi H: *Radiology of Syndromes and Metabolic Disorders,* ed 2. Chicago, Year Book Medical Publishers, Inc, 1983.

40. Wacker MN: Congenital abnormalities. Am J Obstet Gynecol 1963; 86:310–320.

41. Warkany J: Syndromes of chromosomal abnormalities, in Warkany J (ed): *Congenital Malformations: Notes and Comments.* Chicago, Year Book Medical Publishers, 1971, pp 296-345.

42. Weaver DD: Classification of anomalies, in Sabbagha RE (ed): *Ultrasound Applied to Obstetrics and Gynecology,* ed 2. Philadelphia, JB Lippincott Co, 1987, pp 235–251.

43. Witt DR, Hall JG: Approach to multiple congenital anomaly syndromes. Semin Perinatol 1985; 9:219–231.

Prenatal Studies

44. Arger P, Coleman B, Mintz M, et al: Routine fetal genitourinary tract screening. Radiology 1985; 156:485–489.

45. Barkin SZ, Pretorius DH, Beckett MK, et al: Severe polyhydramnios: Incidence of anomalies. AJR 1987; 148:155–159.

46. Benacerraf BR, Adzick NS: Fetal diaphragmatic hernia: Ultrasound diagnosis and clinical outcome in 19 cases. Am J Obstet Gynecol 1987; 156:573–576.

47. Benacerraf BR, Gelman R, Frigoletto FD Jr: Sonographic identification of second-trimester fetuses with Down's syndrome. N Engl J Med 1987; 317:1371–1376.

48. Benacerraf BR, Pober BR, Sanders SP: Accuracy of fetal echocardiography. Radiology 1987; 165:847–849.

49. Blane C, Koff S, Bowerman R, et al: Nonobstructive fetal hydronephrosis: Sonographic recognition and therapeutic implications. Radiology 1983; 147:95–99.

50. Campbell S, Allan L, Griffin D, et al: Early diagnosis of fetal structural abnormalities, in *Prevention of Physical and Mental Congenital Defects, Part B: Epidemiology, Early Detection and Therapy, and Environmental Factors.* New York, Alan R Liss, Inc, 1985, pp 187–205.

51. Campbell S, Pearce JM: Ultrasound visualization of congenital malformations. Br Med Bull 1983; 3939:322–331.

52. Chan L, Hixson J, Laifer SA, et al: An ultrasound and karyotypic study of second trimester choroid plexus cysts. Presented to the Society of Perinatal Obstetricians, Las Vegas, NV, Feb 3–6, 1988.

53. Chitkara U, Cogswell C, Norton K, et al: Prenatal diagnosis of choroid plexus cysts: A benign anatomical variant or pathological entity? Report of 41 cases and review of the literature. Obstet Gynecol 1988; 72:185–189.

54. Comstock CH: The antenatal diagnosis of diaphragmatic anomalies. J Ultrasound Med 1986; 5:391–396.

55. Copel JA, Cullen M, Green JJ, et al: The frequency of aneuploidy in prenatally diagnosed congenital heart disease: An indication for fetal karyotyping. Am J Obstet Gynecol 1988; 158:409–413.

56. Corson VL, Sanders RC, Johnson JRB, et al: Midtrimester fetal ultrasound diagnostic dilemmas. Prenat Diagn 1983; 3:47–51.

57. Crawford DC, Chita SK, Allan LD: Prenatal detection of congenital heart disease: Factors affecting obstetric management and survival. Am J Obstet Gynecol 1988; 159:352–356.

58. Cyr D, Mack L, Schoenecker S, Patten R, et al: Bowel migration in the normal fetus: US detection. Radiology 1986; 161:119–121.

59. Fakhry J, Reiser M, Shapiro, et al: Increased echogenicity in the lower fetal abdomen: A common normal variant in the second trimester. J Ultrasound Med 1986; 5:489–492.

60. Foster MA, Nyberg DA, Mahony BS, et al: Meconium peritonitis: Prenatal sonographic findings and clinical significance. Radiology 1987; 165:661–665.

61. Gauderer MWL, Jassani MN, Izant RJ Jr: Ultrasonographic antenatal diagnosis: Will it change the spectrum of neonatal surgery? J Pediatr Surg 1984; 19:404–407.

62. Griffiths DM, Gough MH: Dilemmas after ultrasound diagnosis of fetal abnormality. Lancet 1985; 1:623–624.

63. Grisoni ER, Gauderer MWL, Wolfson RN, et al: Antenatal ultrasonography: The experience in a high risk perinatal center. J Pediatr Surg 1986; 21:358–361.

64. Hill LM, Breckle R, Gehrking WC: Prenatal detection of congenital malformations by ultrasonography. Am J Obstet Gynecol 1985; 151:44–50.

65. Hobbins JC, Grannum PAT, Berkowitz RL, et al: Ultrasound in the diagnosis of congenital anomalies. Am J Obstet Gynecol 1979; 134:331–344.

66. Horger EO III, Pai GS: Ultrasound in the diagnosis of fetal malformations. Implications for obstetric management. Am J Obstet Gynecol 1983; 147:163–170.

67. Hutson JM, McNay MB, MacKenzie JR, et al. Antenatal diagnosis of surgical disorders by ultrasonography. Lancet 1985; 621–624.

68. Jeanty P, Sacks G, Shah D, et al: In utero detection of fetal cephaloceles. Presented to the World Federation for Ultrasound in Medicine and Biology Meeting, Washington, DC, Oct 17–21, 1988.

69. Kurtz A, Filly R, Wapner J, et al: In utero analysis of heterozygous achondroplasia: Variable time of onset as detected by femur length measurements. J Ultrasound Med 1986; 5:137–140.

70. Mahony B, Callen P, Filly R, et al: Progression of infantile polycystic kidney disease in early pregnancy. J Ultrasound Med 1984; 3:277–279.

71. Mahony B, Nyberg DA, Hirsch JH, et al: Mild idiopathic lateral ventricular dilatation. Radiology 1988; 169:715–721.

72. Manchester D, Pretorius D, Avery C, et al: Accuracy of ultrasound diagnoses in pregnancies complicated by

suspected fetal anomalies. Prenat Diagn 1988; 8:109–117.

73. Muller F, Frot JC, Aubry J, et al: Meconium ileus in cystic fibrosis fetuses. Lancet 1984; 1:223.

74. Nicolaides KH, Campbell S, Gabbe SG: Ultrasound screening for spina bifida: Cranial and cerebellar signs. Lancet 1986; 2:72–74.

75. Nicolaides KH, Rodeck CH, Gosden CM: Rapid karyotyping in non–lethal fetal malformations. Lancet 1986; 1:283–287.

76. Nyberg DA, Cyr DR, Mack LA, et al: The Dandy-Walker malformation: Prenatal diagnosis and clinical significance. J Ultrasound Med 1988; 7:65–71.

77. Nyberg DA, Fitzsimmons J, Mack LA, et al: Chromosome abnormalities in fetuses with omphalocele: The significance of omphalocele contents. J Ultrasound Med, in press.

78. Nyberg DA, Mack LA, Hirsch J, et al: Abnormalities of fetal cranial contour in sonographic detection of spina bifida: Evaluation of the "lemon" sign. Radiology 1988; 167:387–392.

79. Nyberg D, Shepard T, Mack L, et al: Significance of a single umbilical artery in fetuses with central nervous system malformations. J Ultrasound Med 1988; 7:265–272.

80. Perrella R, Duerinckx AJ, Grant EG, et al: Second-trimester sonographic diagnosis of Down syndrome: Role of femur length shortening and nuchal-fold thickening. AJR 1988; 151:981–985.

81. Pretorius D, Lee M, Manco-Johnson M, et al: Diagnosis of autosomal dominant polycystic kidney disease in utero and the young infant. J Ultrasound Med 1987; 6:249–255.

82. Puri P, Gorman F: Lethal non–pulmonary anomalies associated with congenital diaphragmatic hernia: Implications for early intra-uterine surgery. J Pediatr Surg 1984; 19:29–32.

83. Rutledge JC, Weinberg AG, Friedman JM, et al: Anatomic correlates of ultrasonographic prenatal diagnosis. Prenat Diagn 1986; 6:51–61.

84. Sabbagha RE, Sheikh Z, Tamura RK, et al: Predictive value, sensitivity, and specificity of targeted imaging for fetal anomalies in gravid women at high risk for birth defects. Am J Obstet Gynecol 1985; 152:822–827.

85. Sack RA, Maharry JM: Misdiagnoses in obstetric and gynecologic ultrasound examinations: Causes and possible solutions. Am J Obstet Gynecol 1988; 158:1260–1266.

86. Sanders R, Graham D: Twelve cases of hydronephrosis in utero diagnosed by ultrasonography. J Ultrasound Med 1982; 1:341–348.

87. Schoenecker SA, Pretorius DH, Manco-Johnson ML: Artifacts seen commonly on ultrasonography of the fetal cranium. J Repro Med 1985; 30:541–544.

88. Simpson JL, Sabbagha RE, Elias S, et al: Failure to detect polycystic kidneys in utero by second trimester ultrasonography. Hum Genet 1982; 60:295.

89. Toi A: Spontaneous resolution of fetal ventriculomegaly in a diabetic patient. J Ultrasound Med 1987; 6:37–39.

90. Tolmie JL, McNay M, Stephenson JBP, et al: Microcephaly: Genetic counseling and antenatal diagnosis after the birth of an affected child. Am J Med Genet 1987; 27:583–594.

91. Vandenberghe K, De Wolf F, Fryns JP, et al: Antenatal ultrasound diagnosis of fetal malformations: Possibilities, limitations, and dilemmas. Eur J Obstet Gynecol Reprod Biol 1984; 18:279–297.

92. Williamson RA, Weiner CP, Patil S, et al: Abnormal pregnancy sonogram: Selective indication for fetal karyotype. Obstet Gynecol 1987; 69:15–20.

93. Wladimiroff JW, Sachs ES, Reuss A, et al: Prenatal diagnosis of chromosome abnormalities in the presence of fetal structural defects. Am J Med Genet 1988; 29:289–291.

Management

94. Adzick NS, Harrison MR, Glick PL, et al: Fetal urinary tract obstruction: Experimental pathophysiology. Semin Perinatol 1985; 9:79–90.

95. Appleman Z, Golbus MS: The management of fetal urinary tract obstruction. Clin Obstet Gynecol 1986; 29:483–489.

96. Benacerraf BR, Barss VA, Saltzman DH, et al: Fetal abnormalities: Diagnosis or treatment with percutaneous umbilical blood sampling under continuous US guidance. Radiology 1988; 166:105–107.

97. Blott M, Nicolaides KH, Greenough A: Pleuroamniotic shunting for decompression of fetal pleural effusions. Obstet Gynecol 1988; 71:798–800.

98. Bussel JB, Berkowitz RL, McFarland JG, et al: Antenatal treatment of neonatal alloimmune thrombocytopenia. N Engl J Med 1988; 319:1374–1378.

99. Daffos F, Capella-Pavlovsky M, Forstier F: Fetal blood sampling during pregnancy with use of a needle guided by ultrasound: A study of 606 consecutive cases. Am J Obstet Gynecol 1985; 153:665.

100. Flake AW, Harrison MR, Sauer L, et al: Ureteropelvic junction obstruction in the fetus. J Pediatr Surg 1986; 21:1058–1063.

101. Fletcher JC: Ethical considerations in and beyond experimental fetal therapy. Semin Perinatol 1985; 9:130–135.

102. Gauderer MWL, Jassani MN, Izant RJ Jr: Ultrasonographic diagnosis: Will it change the spectrum of neonatal surgery? J Pediatr Surg 1984; 19:404–407.

103. Glick PL, Harrison MR, Golbus MS, et al: Management of the fetus with congenital hydronephrosis. II: Prognostic criteria and selection for treatment. J Pediatr Surg 1985; 20:376–387.

104. Glick PL, Harrison MR, Adzick NS, et al: Correction of congenital hydronephrosis in utero IV: In utero decompression prevents renal dysplasia. J Pediatr Surg 1984; 19:649–657.

105. Golbus MS, Filly RA, Callen PW, et al: Fetal urinary tract obstruction: Management and selection for treatment. Semin Perinatol 1985; 9:91–97.

106. Gosden C, Rodeck CH, Nicolaides KH, et al: Fetal blood chromosome analysis: Some new indications for prenatal karyotyping. Br J Obstet Gynaecol 1985; 29:915–920.

107. Harrison MR, Adzick NS, Nakayama DK, et al: Fetal diaphragmatic hernia: Fatal but fixable. Semin Perinatol 1985; 9:103–112.

108. Hsieh F-J, Chang F-M, Ko T-M, et al: Percutaneous ultrasound-guided fetal blood sampling in the management of nonimmune hydrops fetalis. Am J Obstet Gynecol 1987; 157:44–49.

109. Machin GA, Nicholson SF, Nimrod GA: A multidisciplinary committee approach to prenatal diagnosis and management of fetuses with congenital anomalies. Birth Defects. 1987; 23:351–356.

110. Manning FA, Lange IR, Morrison I, et al: Treatment of the fetus in utero: Evolving concepts. Clin Obstet Gynecol 1984; 27:378–390.

111. Manning FA, Harrison MR, Rodeck C, et al: Catheter shunts for fetal hydronephrosis and hydrocephalus. Report of the International Fetal Surgery Registry. N Engl J Med 1986; 315:336–340.

112. Nakayama DK, Harrison MR, Gross BH, et al: Management of the fetus with an abdominal wall defect. J Pediatr Surg 1984; 19:408–413.

113. Porter KB, Wanger PC, Cabaniss ML: Fetal board: A multidisciplinary approach to management of the abnormal fetus. Obstet Gynecol 1988; 72:275–278.

114. Rodeck CH, Fisk NM, Fraser DI, et al: Long-term in utero drainage of fetal hydrothorax. N Engl J Med 1988; 319:1135–1138.

115. Trudinger BJ, Cook CM, Thompson RS, et al: Low-dose aspirin therapy improves fetal weight in umbilical placental insufficiency. Am J Obstet Gynecol 1988; 159:681–685.

3

Abnormalities of Amniotic Fluid

Lyndon M. Hill, M.D.

Abnormalities of amniotic fluid, whether deficient (oligohydramnios) or excessive (polyhydramnios), are frequently the first clues to an underlying fetal or maternal disorder. Even when not associated with a fetal malformation, abnormalities of amniotic fluid volume correlate strongly with increased rates of perinatal morbidity and mortality. For these reasons, the obstetric sonographer should have a basic understanding of the mechanisms responsible for normal amniotic fluid production and the potential effect of abnormal amniotic fluid volume on the fetus.

This chapter discusses current concepts in the derivation of both normal and abnormal amniotic fluid volume. Definitions and sonographic criteria for oligohydramnios and polyhydramnios, their possible causes, sequelae, and potential treatment are also discussed.

DERIVATION OF AMNIOTIC FLUID

The fetus and intrauterine environment have intrigued man for centuries. Hippocrates was the first to attribute the derivation of amniotic fluid to fetal urine.[79] However, prior to the 20th century, relatively little was known about the formation, maintenance, and volume of amniotic fluid. During the 1930s and 1940s, observations on experimental animal preparations added significantly to our knowledge of fetal physiology.[51] Isotope, as well as dye dilution techniques, have helped determine not only the volume of amniotic fluid at various gestational ages, but also some of the complex mechanisms involved in its formation.[38, 66]

Amniotic fluid volume normally increases until 34 weeks' gestation and then declines progressively (Fig 3–1). The amount of amniotic fluid present at any one time reflects a balance between amniotic fluid production and amniotic fluid removal (Figs 3–2 and 3–3). Hence, maintenance of amniotic fluid volume is a dynamic process, with different contributing factors at different stages of pregnancy.

During the early weeks of pregnancy, amniotic fluid is essentially an ultrafiltrate of maternal plasma.[81] Between 10 and 20 weeks' gestation, the composition of amniotic fluid more closely resembles fetal plasma, and its volume correlates directly with fetal weight (Fig 3–4).[79] This equilibration between fetal plasma and amniotic fluid probably is secondary to diffusion across the fetal skin, which at this stage of pregnancy is composed of only four cells. The presence of numerous microvilli within the fetal skin also suggests that it is a site of sodium transport during the second trimester. A correlation (R = 0.85) between $\log_e$ fetal weight and the rate of sodium transfer across the fetal skin has been noted (Fig 3–5).

In the second half of pregnancy, the skin becomes more closely bound at the desmosomes, and both stratification and cornification increase. Twenty years ago, this maturational process was felt initially to reduce, and finally to prevent, the diffusion of fetal extracellular fluid into the amniotic cavity.[81] However, because postnatal treatment of extremely premature infants requires three times the normal fluid intake of the term neonate due to transcutaneous fluid losses, the fetal skin may continue to play an important role in amniotic fluid volume regulation even in the second and early third trimester.[133]

As early as 12–14 weeks' gestation, the fetal kid-

38

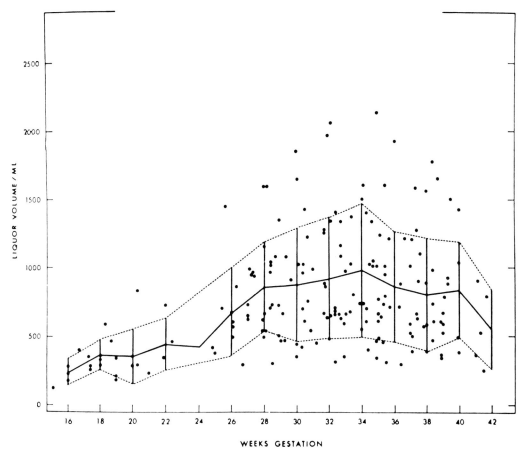

FIG 3–1.

Mean (± 1SD) amniotic fluid volume throughout gestation as determined by a dye dilution technique. (From Queenan JT, Thompson W, Whitfield CR, et al: Amniotic fluid volumes in normal pregnancies. Am J Obstet Gynecol 1972; 114:34–38. Used by permission.)

ney has the ability to remove sodium and concentrate urea, thereby altering the composition of amniotic fluid.[80] Simultaneously, fetal swallowing becomes established. Swallowed amniotic fluid is reabsorbed by the gastrointestinal tract and then recirculates through the kidneys. By 18 weeks, the fetus excretes an estimated urine volume of 7–14 ml/24 hr and swallows 4–11 ml/24 hr. However, the contribution of fetal urination and swallowing to the total amniotic fluid volume remains relatively small at this time (less than 10%).[1, 2]

During the latter stages of mid-pregnancy, the amniotic fluid volume increases by approximately 10 ml/day and reaches an average volume of 500 ml at 20 weeks.[1] Since the amount of amniotic fluid produced by fetal urination only slightly exceeds the amount removed by fetal swallowing at this time, more than 40% of the incremental increase in amnionic fluid probably originates from other sources. In addition to transdermal diffusion, the fetal surface of the placenta is a

source of fluid exchange that probably becomes quantitatively more important with advancing gestational age. The fetal gastrointestinal tract, respiratory system, and umbilical cord are other potential sources of amniotic fluid production (see Fig 3–2).[1, 39, 65, 92]

During the third trimester, fetal swallowing and urination strongly influence the constitution and volume of amniotic fluid. Near term, the fetus swallows approximately 200–450 ml/24 hr and voids approximately 600–800 ml/24 hr.[1, 134, 160] The amniotic fluid volume is approximately 700 ml at the beginning of the third trimester, 1000 cc in the mid-third trimester, and 800–900 cc at term. However, significant individual variation is observed. In some patients, the amniotic fluid volume was found to progressively increase until 40 weeks' gestation, while in others it either gradually declines or is maintained at a constant volume until term.[123]

The amniotic fluid at term has a constant sodium concentration of 120 mEq/liter. Since the sodium con-

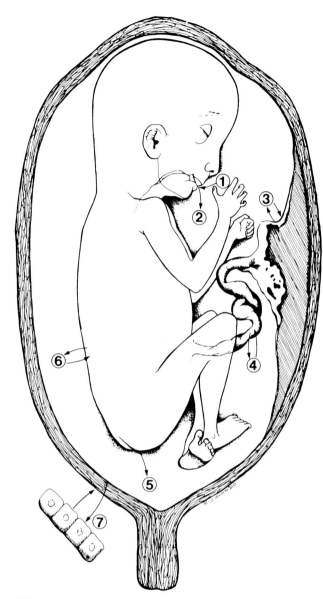

FIG 3–2.
Schematic diagram of amniotic fluid volume formation. *1*, respiratory tract; *2*, gastrointestinal tract; *3*, placenta; *4*, umbilical cord; *5*, urine; *6*, skin; *7*, extraplacental fetal membranes.

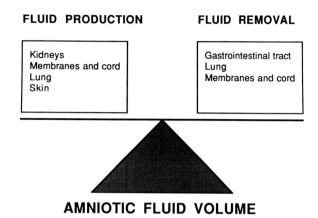

FIG 3–3.
Schematic diagram illustrating that amniotic fluid volume is a dynamic balance determined by formation and removal of amniotic fluid.

amniotic fluid circulates through the fetal lungs via respiratory movements each day with net reabsorption in the alveolar capillary bed.

A strong correlation exists between amniotic fluid volume and maternal plasma volume after 29 weeks' gestation, indicating that uterine perfusion may also contribute to amniotic fluid production and regulation.[47]

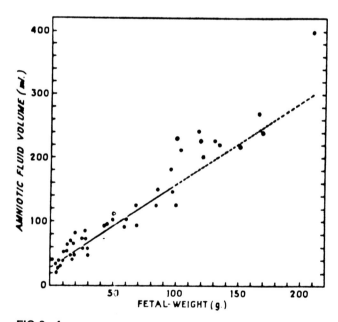

FIG 3–4.
Relationship between amniotic fluid volume and fetal weight in 46 cases up to 21 weeks' gestation, including five cases of uncertain gestation. The solid line is the regression calculated from 31 cases up to 15 weeks' gestation; the extrapolation *(dotted line)* indicates that the relationship may hold beyond 15 weeks. (From Lind T, Hytten FE: Lancet 1970; 1:1147–1149. Used by permission.)

centration of fetal urine is approximately 70 mEq/liter, there must be an additional source for amniotic fluid sodium. This discrepancy may be due, in part, to sodium transfer through the amnion and chorion, which behave as a simple semipermeable membrane.[80]

Reabsorption of hypotonic fluid by the fetal lungs is another mechanism for maintaining the sodium concentration in the amniotic fluid. This would also help to account for the difference between the volume of urine voided and the volume of fluid swallowed during the third trimester.[134] Approximately 600–800 ml of

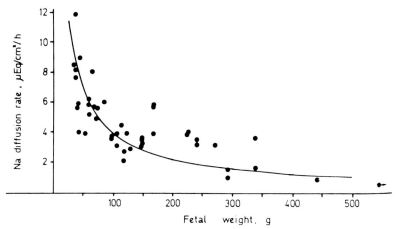

FIG 3–5.
Relationship of the rate of simple sodium diffusion across fetal skin to fetal weight in 44 fetuses. (From Lind T, et al: Br J Obstet Gynaecol 1972; 79:289. Used by permission.)

Hormonal factors may also play a role in amniotic fluid regulation. Josimovich et al., for example, reported a 50% decrease in amniotic fluid volume in all ten rhesus monkeys injected intra-amniotically with prolactin.[68] A decline in the maternal hematocrit and plasma protein concentration was further proof that prolactin stimulated fluid transport out of the amniotic cavity. This effect was not as evident with preterm membranes, implying that perhaps the number of prolactin receptors, as well as the significance of this pathway, increases with gestational age. Cortisol and ADH also influence the permeability of the amnion to water.[83]

Despite the multiple potential sources of amniotic fluid, its solute concentration is rigidly maintained. Lingwood and associates for example, replaced 20% to 30% of the amniotic fluid volume in 17 pregnant ewes with isotonic saline, mannitol, or dextrose.[83] As expected, the concentration of electrolytes was immediately reduced by 70%. Creatinine and urea returned to normal levels within 2–3 hours, and concentrations of sodium, potassium, and chloride returned to pre-infusion level by 6 hours. In each case, the amniotic fluid volume rose significantly ($p < 0.005$) above the control value by 1 hour, indicating that the composition of amniotic fluid is closely regulated (in sheep), even at the expense of fluid volume.

A similar rapid equilibration of total solute concentration occurs when the amniotic fluid of rhesus monkeys is replaced with distilled water.[132] Once again, the amniotic fluid volume is altered in order to attain a normal solute concentration. In humans, high or rising amniotic fluid osmolality is an indication of fetal compromise; reversal of rising osmolality can be accomplished by treatment of the underlying condition, for example, by intrauterine transfusion of Rh-sensitized fetuses.[19] Each of these examples indicates that multiple factors closely regulate and maintain the composition of amniotic fluid, even at the expense of amniotic fluid volume.

OLIGOHYDRAMNIOS

Definition and Sonographic Criteria

No universally accepted sonographic standard for assessing amniotic fluid volume exists. Since the amount of amniotic fluid varies with gestational age, an amniotic fluid volume more than 2 SD below or above the mean for a given gestational age would ideally define oligohydramnios and polyhydramnios, respectively. Unfortunately, the objective quantification of amniotic fluid volume requires amniocentesis and the instillation of a dye or isotope. This is impractical, and as a result one is left with various sonographic attempts to measure amniotic fluid volume.

Over 10 years ago, calculation of total intrauterine volume (TIUV)[82] was proposed as an objective means by which amniotic fluid volume could be assessed.[115] However, since the fetus and the placenta are included in the estimate of total intrauterine volume, it was relatively insensitive for diagnosing polyhydramnios and oligohydramnios. Also, this technique was tedious, requiring a static scanner to obtain the length, height, and transverse measurements of uterine volume. For these reasons, and because virtually all obstetrical ultrasound examinations are now performed with real-time units, calculation of TIUV is not currently employed.

Accepted sonographic methods for assessing amniotic fluid are subjective (visual criteria); semiquantitative (measuring one or more pockets of amniotic fluid); or a combination of the two. Whatever method is utilized, determination of amniotic fluid volume has

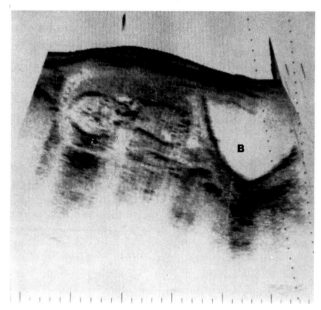

FIG 3–6.
Marked oligohydramnios. Longitudinal scan at 17 weeks' gestation (breech presentation) demonstrates no detectable amniotic fluid (anhydramnios) and crowding of fetal parts. *B* = maternal urinary bladder.

good to excellent intra-observer and inter-observer reliability.[45]

With regard to subjective visual criteria, the fetus normally occupies less of the amniotic fluid volume before 22 weeks and a progressively greater proportion of the amniotic volume as the pregnancy advances. During the third trimester, the fetal abdomen normally touches the anterior and posterior walls. Criteria for

oligohydramnios include visual evidence of fetal crowding, poor interface, and an obvious lack of fluid (Figs 3–6 and 3–7).[114]

Semiquantitative criteria with measurements of normal amniotic fluid pockets have been reported by various authors (see Fig 3–6). In measuring the largest single pocket of amniotic fluid, oligohydramnios has been variously defined as ≤ 3 cm (Halpern et al.),[48] ≤ than 1 cm, (Manning et al.,)[83] or ≤ 0.5 cm, (Mercer and colleagues).[91] More recently, Phelan and coworkers reported a four-quadrant technique for the assessment of amniotic fluid volume (Fig 3–8).[111, 113] In this latter schema, the largest pocket of amniotic fluid in each quadrant of the uterus is measured vertically, and the four measurements are then added together to obtain an amniotic fluid index (AFI). Normal amniotic fluid is defined as an AFI between 5 and 20; oligohydramnios as ≤ 5; and polyhydramnios as ≥ 20 (Fig 3–9).[113] Anhydramnios would indicate an absence of any detectable amniotic fluid within the intrauterine cavity (see Fig 3–6).

At the author's institution (University of Pittsburgh), oligohydramnios is defined by the 1 cm rule proposed by Manning et al.,[88] but gradations in the reduction of amniotic fluid volume from normal to oligohydramnios are also quantitated. A pocket of amniotic fluid ≥ 1.0 cm but ≤ 2.0 cm in vertical dimension is considered marginal (see Fig 3–7). Extensive antepartum assessment and consideration for delivery are undertaken when the amniotic fluid volume has fallen to this level without a history of premature rupture of the membranes.

FIG 3–7.
Oligohydramnios. This pocket of fluid measures 1.9 cm in vertical dimension, which is considered to be oligohydramnios by some semi-quantitative methods of amniotic fluid assessment but is marginally decreased by other criteria. *E* = extremity.

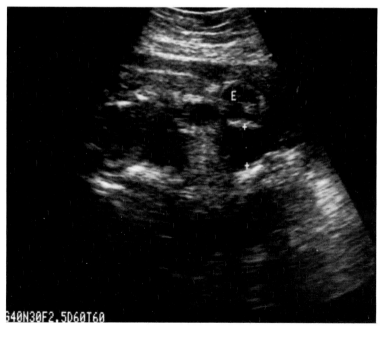

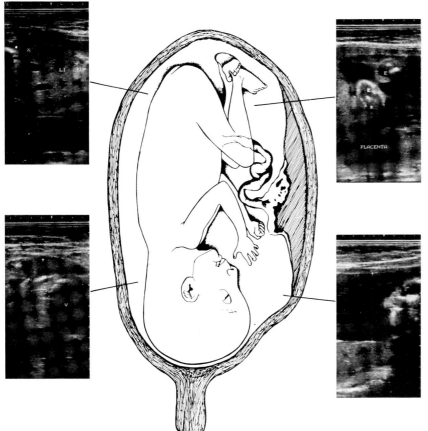

FIG 3–8.
Four-quadrant amniotic fluid index. The largest vertical pocket of amniotic fluid in each uterine quadrant is measured and then added together to obtain the amniotic fluid index *(AFI).*

Not infrequently, amniotic fluid volume appears subjectively decreased, even though the largest fluid pocket is greater than 2 cm. Although the perinatal mortality has not been found to be significantly increased for patients in this category, they are rescanned at frequent intervals in order to ensure that

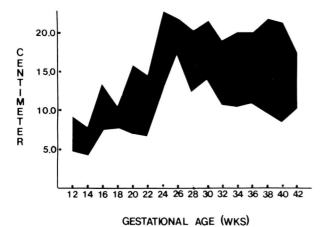

GESTATIONAL AGE (WKS)

FIG 3–9.
Amniotic fluid index compared with gestational age for 197 patients who underwent 262 ultrasound examinations (From Phelan JP, Ahn MO, Smith CV, et al: J Reprod Med 1987; 32:601–604. Used by permission.)

the amniotic fluid volume does not decline further.

Goldstein and Filly advocate a combination of the semiquantitative measurements of the largest amniotic fluid pocket and a subjective impression to identify abnormalities of amniotic fluid volume.[45] They define oliogohydramnios as an amniotic fluid volume that appears subjectively decreased, when the largest pocket of amniotic fluid measures < 3 cm in vertical dimension. Similarly, polyhydramnios is defined by a subjective impression and a pocket of amniotic fluid that measures greater than 7 cm. Good correlation was shown between subjective assessment and semiquantitative measurements (Fig 3–10); there was no discrepancy between the two methods among patients with normal amniotic fluid volume or unequivocally abnormal fluid volume.[45]

Pathophysiology

Significant oligohydramnios can usually be attributed to one of four causes:

1. fetal anomalies.
2. intrauterine growth retardation.
3. post-term pregnancies.
4. rupture of the membranes.

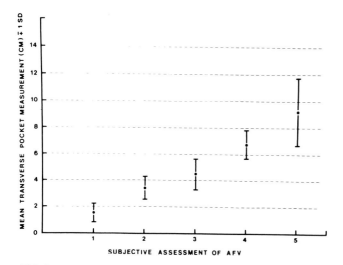

FIG 3–10.
Relationship between objective and subjective evidence of amniotic fluid volume. Subjective assessment of amniotic fluid was ranked from 1–5 and compared with mean transverse dimension of the largest pocket of amniotic fluid. (From Goldstein R, Filly RA: J Ultrasound Med 1988; 7:363–369. Used by permission.)

Less common causes of oligohydramnios include (5) presumed placental dysfunction, often in association with elevated maternal serum alpha-fetoprotein (MS-AFP) levels, and (6) drug therapy, particularly anti-prostaglandin therapy (e.g., indomethacin). Each of these will be discussed in following sections.

Fetal Anomalies

Fetal anomalies that result in oligohydramnios predictably involve obstruction or dysfunction of the urinary tract in the vast majority of cases (Table 3–1). Therefore, a diagnosis of oligohydramnios mandates a careful search of the urinary tract. Fortunately, sonography accurately detects the vast majority of significant renal anomalies resulting in oligohydramnios, including

renal obstruction, multicystic dysplastic kidneys, and infantile polycystic kidney disease.

Renal agenesis should be suspected when amniotic fluid is absent to markedly decreased and fetal kidneys are not reliably demonstrated (see Chapter 12). Because renal agenesis is uniformly fatal, accurate prenatal diagnosis is important. Paradoxically, although renal agenesis is frequently suspected when amniotic fluid is markedly decreased to absent, it is also one of the most difficult malformations to confirm. This difficulty can be attributed to poor visualization of fetal structures in the presence of marked oligohydramnios. Also, demonstrating the absence of normal structures is more difficult than showing the presence of a particular malformation. Finally, hypertrophied adrenal glands can be confused with normal kidneys.

Because of the difficulties outlined above, evaluation of the urinary bladder frequently provides as much information as evaluation of the kidneys themselves when amniotic fluid is markedly decreased. Demonstrating spontaneous filling and emptying of the urinary bladder virtually excludes a diagnosis of bilateral renal agenesis and should suggest alternative diagnoses, including less severe renal malformations (dysplasia, Fig 3–11), severe intrauterine growth retardation, or occult rupture of membranes. Conversely, non–visualization of the bladder, despite a careful search during intermittent observation for over an hour, is supportive evidence for renal agenesis.

Some authors have advocated maternal administration of furosemide as a means of distinguishing fetal causes of anhydramnios (renal agenesis/dysplasia) from fetuses with severe intrauterine growth retardation when a urinary bladder is not identified.[74] However, fetuses with severe intrauterine growth retardation may also be incapable of responding to furosemide, due to an impairment in glomerular filtration rate.[25, 44] Hence,

TABLE 3–1.

Outcome Data Utilizing the 1 cm Rule for the Detection of Intrauterine Growth Retardation (IUGR)

| Author | Population | | Prevalence | | | |
	Type	No.	Oligohydramnios (&)	Congenital Anomalies (%)	Corrected Perinatal Mortality (per 1,000 Live Births)	Prevalence IUGR (%)
Hill et al, 1983[56]	General	1408	0.43	33	0	83.3
Mercer et al, 1984[91]	General	8626	5.5	7	Same as general population	Same as general population
Manning et al, 1981[88]	Referred	120	25.8	9.7	8.3	89.6
Chamberlain et al, 1984[21]	High risk	7582	0.85	9.37	109.4	38.6
Bastide et al, 1986[10]	High risk	15,431	0.70	13.3	17.7	36.5

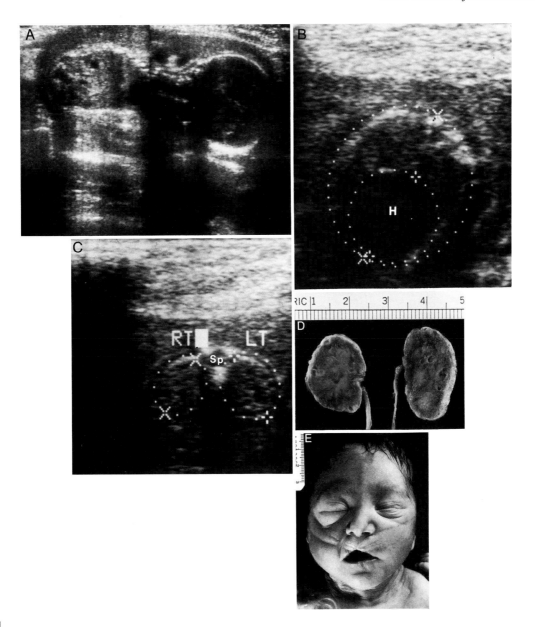

FIG 3–11.
Anhydramnios, renal dysplasia. **A,** longitudinal scan at 35 weeks' gestation shows absence of amniotic fluid. **B,** transverse scan of the fetal chest shows normal heart *(H)* circumference (inner graticules, 50th percentile for age) but small chest circumference (outer graticules, 2.5 percentile). These findings are consistent with pulmonary hypoplasia. **C,** transverse scan of the kidneys (outlined by graticules) shows echogenic parenchyma with numerous tiny cysts and absence of a definable renal pelvis. *Sp* = spine; *RT* = right kidney; *LT* = left kidney. **D,** postmortem section of kidneys in coronal plane shows small, multicystic dysplastic kidneys, absent renal pelvises, and thread-like ureters. **E,** Potter's facies. The nose is blunt; there is a prominent fold of skin covering the inner canthus; the depression below the lower lip is prominent; and the ears are pressed against the side of the head.

a false-positive diagnosis may occur after the furosemide test. Since this test provides no additional information to intermittent bladder observation, it has been abandoned by most centers.

In an attempt to identify fetal causes of severe oligohydramnios, a novel approach proposes instillation of warmed isotonic fluid into the amniotic cavity.[41] Gembruch et al. instilled 100 cc of fluid prior to 24 weeks' gestation and 150 cc after 24 weeks into the amniotic cavity.[41] Although this method does allow improved visualization of fetal anatomy, acute distention of the uterus may lead to premature rupture of the membranes. Also, because of the poor prognosis associated with severe oligohydramnios of any cause, this method is not widely employed.

Intrauterine Growth Retardation

Oligohydramnios is an accepted clinical marker for intrauterine growth retardation (IUGR). Indeed, the maximum vertical pocket of amniotic fluid is significantly related to growth (analysis of variance, p < 0.001) (Fig 3–12). Table 3–1 outlines the results from five studies utilizing ≤ 1 cm as a definition of oligohydramnios for the detection of IUGR. The prevalence of oligohydramnios in the population under study, the congenital anomaly and perinatal mortality rates, and the prevalence of IUGR all vary widely.

Severe IUGR might be considered a relative state of dehydration.[26] Hourly fetal urine production rates (HFUPR) can be assessed in normal and growth-retarded fetuses by measuring bladder volumes at 15-minute intervals over 1 to 2 hours.[160] Figure 3–13 illustrates the HFUPR regression line for a control group and a group of fetuses who, at delivery, were confirmed to have IUGR. With advancing gestational age, the HFUPR increases significantly less in patients with growth retardation. A reduction in the perfusion of the fetal kidney results in a decreased glomerular filtration rate and, hence, a reduction in HFUPR.[31] Fetal renal tubular function does not seem to be affected.[74]

Demonstration of early symmetric IUGR with marked oligohydramnios should suggest the possibility of an underlying chromosomal disorder, notably triploidy or trisomy 18 (Fig 3–14). Nicolaides et al. reported that two of six cases with early IUGR and oligohydramnios not caused by renal agenesis had chromosomal abnormalities, both with triploidy.[103]

Post-dates

Elliott and Inman have demonstrated a close relationship between declining amniotic fluid volume and diminishing placental function.[34] Consequently, the antepartum assessment of amniotic fluid volume has become an accepted practice in the evaluation of the post-dates pregnancy. Once again, however, the definition of oligohydramnios varies from author to author (subjective impression of amniotic fluid volume; ≤ 1 cm; and ≤ 3.0 cm).[28, 29, 97, 112]

Oligohydramnios has developed within 24 hours in both post-dates patients and in patients with chronic hypertension and superimposed preeclampsia.[24, 155] Although in the latter instance an acute reduction in fetal urinary output was postulated, there is nothing to suggest an impaired urinary output in post-date pregnancies. Reports of acute oligohydramnios suggest that weekly testing for conditions in which the fetus is at risk for oligohydramnios may be inadequate.

Spontaneous Rupture of Membranes

Oligohydramnios secondary to spontaneous rupture of the membranes is usually diagnosed by clinical means. However, the diagnosis may sometimes be uncertain, especially when the leak is chronic. Patients with oligohydramnios should be rescanned in 1 week in order to allow a sufficient amount of time for the amniotic fluid to reaccumulate. Persistent leakage and oligohydramnios carries a poor prognosis, particularly during the second trimester, and the patient should be counseled appropriately.

Prognosis and Sequelae of Oligohydramnios

Regardless of the cause, potential complications that may occur as a result of oligohydramnios include fetal demise, pulmonary hypoplasia, various skeletal and facial deformities, and intrauterine growth retardation (Figs 3–11 and 3–15).[106, 148, 149] Also, an association between second trimester oligohydramnios and increased MS-AFP has been noted.[6, 72, 137, 143] The latter association is possibly secondary to fetal renal hypoperfusion or placental hemorrhage and resultant diminution of water flow across the placental membranes.

A direct relationship has been noted between the objective measurement of amniotic fluid volume and perinatal outcome.[20] Severe oligohydramnios in the second trimester is a particularly poor prognostic sign secondary to development of pulmonary hypoplasia (see

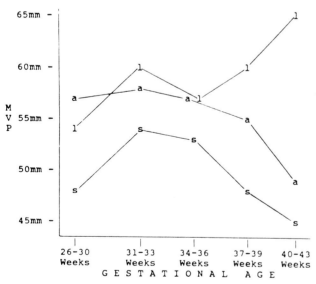

FIG 3–12.
Maximum vertical pocket (MVP) of amniotic fluid by gestational age and growth. Mean values for small *(S)*, appropriate *(A)*, and large *(L)* for gestational age infants are indicated. Small for gestational age fetuses tend to have smaller amounts of amniotic fluid, and large for gestational age fetuses tend to have greater amounts of amniotic fluid. (From Bottoms SF, et al: Am J Obstet Gynecol 1986; 155:154. Used by permission.)

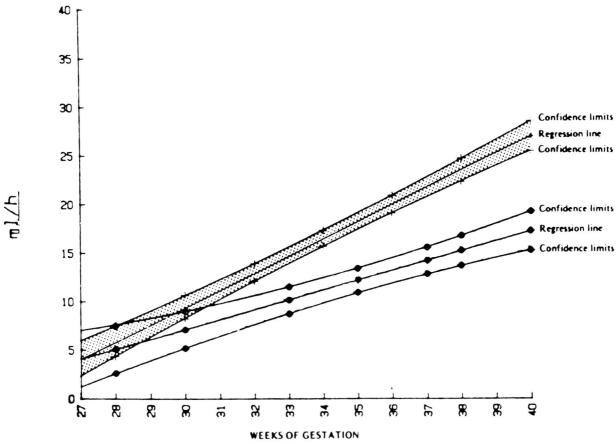

FIG 3-13.

Hourly fetal urine production rate (HFUPR) regression lines and 90% confidence limits for a control group *(shaded lines)* and a group with intrauterine growth retardation (IUGR). With advancing gestational age, the HFUPR increases significantly less in fetuses with IUGR due to decreased perfusion of the kidneys. (From Deutinger J, Bartl W, Pfersmann C, et al: J Perinat Med 1987; 15:307–315. Used by permission.)

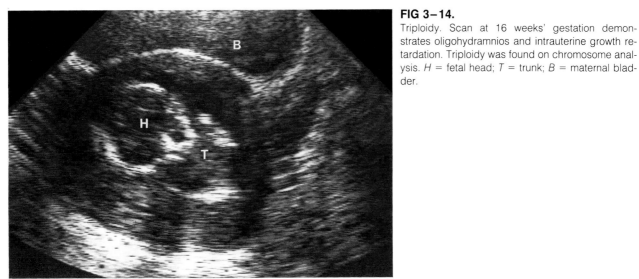

FIG 3-14.

Triploidy. Scan at 16 weeks' gestation demonstrates oligohydramnios and intrauterine growth retardation. Triploidy was found on chromosome analysis. *H* = fetal head; *T* = trunk; *B* = maternal bladder.

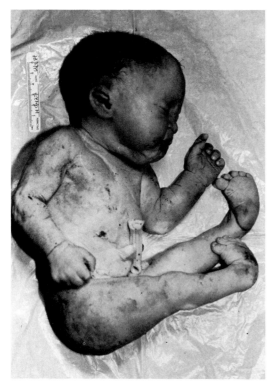

FIG 3–15.
Potter's syndrome. Postmortem photograph of an infant with renal agenesis detected prenatally shows Potter's facies and deformation of the feet and lower extremities secondary to oligohydramnios.

TABLE 3–2.
Second Trimester Oligohydramnios*

Diagnosis	Number
Renal agenesis	12
Urethral obstruction	2
Prune-belly syndrome	1
Skeletal dysplasia	1
Polycystic kidney	1
Multiple anomalies	1†
Triploidy	1
Intrauterine growth retardation	4†
Spontaneous miscarriage	2
Premature rupture of the membranes	1
Spontaneous labor 22 weeks	1
Intrauterine fetal demise	1
Therapeutic abortion	1
Neonatal death	1
Normal neonate	2†
Total	32

*From references [6, 9, 72, 137, 144].
†One surviving neonate from each of these categories.

Fig 3–5). Table 3–2 outlines the results of 32 published pregnancies with second trimester oligohydramnios. Only three of the 27 (11.1%) cases that were not terminated survived the neonatal period.[6, 9, 72, 143, 144] Oligohydramnios in the post-dates patient is also asso-

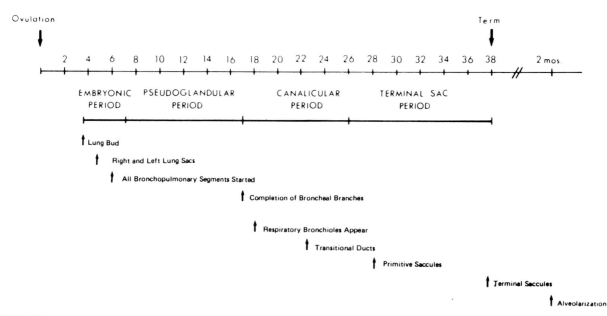

FIG 3–16.
Chronology of normal lung development. A general outline of the major events of normal human lung maturation is indicated against time in weeks following ovulation. Development of oligohydramnios after development of the terminal sac will not result in pulmonary hypoplasia. (From Beard RW, Nathanielz PW: *Fetal Physiology and Medicine,* ed 2. New York, Marcel Dekker, 1984, p 318. Used by permission.)

ciated with increased perinatal morbidity and mortality.[77]

Adzick et al. demonstrated that lung hypoplasia probably results from loss of the normal internal stenting force provided by pulmonary fluid.[3] At approximately 26 weeks' gestation (canalicular period), maturational development is extremely susceptible to extrathoracic compression.[145] Relieving thoracic compression will restore intrapulmonary fluid volume and allow respiratory maturational processes to continue.[102, 158] Also, development of oligohydramnios after sufficient lung development will not result in pulmonary hypoplasia (Fig 3–16).[60]

Nimrod and associates reported that eight of nine cases of pulmonary hypoplasia occurred in patients who experienced rupture of the membranes prior to 26 weeks.[106] Oligohydramnios was present in six cases; in one instance, the amniotic fluid volume was considered normal, and the information was not available in the final two patients. The prevalence of pulmonary hypoplasia with rupture of the membranes before 26

weeks' gestation and with a latent period of 5 weeks was 26.6% (8 of 30 cases). Other authors have found that pulmonary hypoplasia can result from premature rupture of the membranes associated with severe oligohydramnios in as little as 6 days.[148]

The eventual outcome in infants with bilateral pulmonary hypoplasia is dependent upon the severity of respiratory underdevelopment. When the lungs weigh ≤ 50% of normal, virtually all the infants will succumb to their lung disease.[146]

Fetal breathing movements were initially felt to preclude development of pulmonary hypoplasia in fetuses subjected to oligohydramnios.[13] More recently, however, Moessinger et al. reported observing fetal breathing activity in eight fetuses with oligohydramnios who had lung hypoplasia at necropsy.[94] Thus, diaphragmatic activity does not guarantee that anatomic maturation of the fetal respiratory system has occurred.

Several authors have suggested that ultrasonically measured fetal chest and heart circumference can predict pulmonary hypoplasia (Figs 3–11 and 3–17).[23, 104]

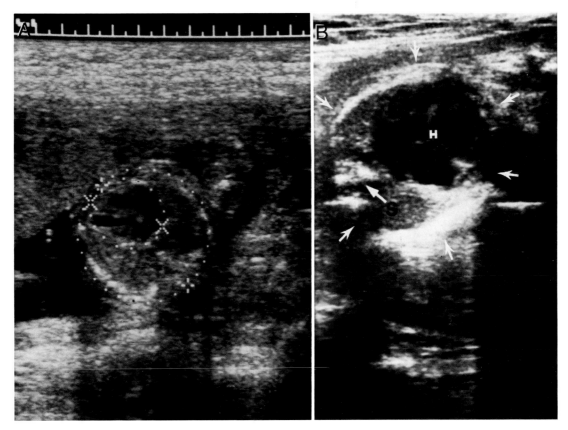

FIG 3–17.
Transverse scan of the fetal chest at the level of the four-chamber cardiac view. **A,** normal relationship. *Outer graticules* = chest circumference; *inner graticules* = heart circumference. **B,** pulmonary hypoplasia. The heart *(H)* appears to encompass most of the thorax. Actually, the heart circumference is normal, while the chest circumference *(arrows)* is at the third percentile. *S* = spine.

In one study of 45 patients at risk for developing pulmonary hypoplasia the sensitivity, specificity, positive predictive value, and negative predictive value of chest circumference measurements below the 5th percentile were 88%, 96%, 94%, and 93%, respectively.[105] Others, however, have shown difficulty in reproducing thoracic measurements. Nevertheless, it is the author's opinion that such measurements can help predict pulmonary hypoplasia and should be included in any complete sonographic evaluation of the fetus with oligohydramnios.

The incidence of skeletal deformities [i.e., talipes equinovarus and craniofacial deformities] (see Fig 3–15) is also significantly higher in fetuses with prolonged rupture of the membranes. As one would expect, there is an association between skeletal deformities and pulmonary hypoplasia. Neonates with deformities associated with oligohydramnios have a lower radial alveolar count (clinical evidence for pulmonary hypoplasia) than those without such deformities (Fig 3–18). In addition, those infants with skeletal deformities had more severe pulmonary hypoplasia, reflected by higher mortality, than those without skeletal deformities.[148]

In addition to pulmonary hypoplasia and skeletal deformities, oligohydramnios can result in intrauterine

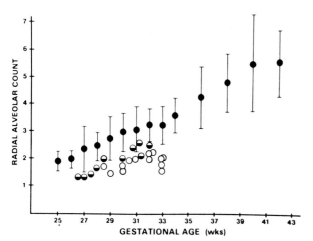

FIG 3–18.
Relationship of radial alveolar counts (determinate of lung development) to gestational age in three groups of infants *(solid dots)*. One hundred and eleven infants with premature rupture of the membranes < 24 hours who had RDS or asphyxia and required ventilatory support (control, ventilated infants); *hatched circles* = ten infants with PROM > 5 days requiring ventilator assistance and without skeletal deformities; *open circles* = 13 infants with PROM > 5 days and with skeletal deformities. These data indicate that infants with both oligohydramnios and skeletal deformities carry a higher frequency of pulmonary hypoplasia. (From Thibeault DW, Beatty EC, Hall RT, et al: J Pediatr 1985; 107:273–277. Used by permission.)

growth retardation (oligohydramnios tetrad).[149] Since amniotic fluid provides between 10% and 14% of the nutritional requirements of the normal fetus, this association is not unexpected.[99]

POLYHYDRAMNIOS
Criteria and Definition

By term, most authors consider an amniotic fluid volume > 2,000 ml as increased.[97, 121] This upper limit of normal is supported by Queenan's estimates of amniotic fluid volume in normal pregnancies utilizing a dye dilution technique.[123] Although the reported prevalence of polyhydramnios from ultrasound studies varies considerably, rates between 0.4% and 1.5% are most frequently quoted.[122, 154] The rate for a given institution will depend upon the clinical experience of the medical staff, the criteria for polyhydramnios, the proportion of high-risk obstetrical patients, and the frequency with which ultrasound examinations are ordered for low, as well as high-risk patients. Quite often, mild polyhydramnios will be diagnosed sonographically when it has not been suspected clinically.

Subjective, visual criteria for polyhydramnios include an obvious discrepancy between the size of the fetus and the amount of amniotic fluid, with the fetus appearing to swim freely within a sea of amniotic fluid. In severe polyhydramnios, the placenta also appears thin due to the marked distension of the amniotic cavity. While mild polyhydramnios can improve the sonographic resolution of fetal anatomy, severe polyhydramnios may actually hinder evaluation of fetal anatomy by increasing the distance between the patient's anterior abdominal wall and the fetus. In patients with severe polyhydramnios, development of hypotension in the supine position may require that the ultrasound examination be performed with the patient sitting or in a decubitus position.

Sonographic recognition of mild polyhydramnios shows more inter-observer variability than does recognition of moderate to marked polyhydramnios. Since the fetus usually lies in the dependent portion of a polyhydramniotic sac, attention should be directed to the amount of amniotic fluid overlying the fetal trunk. As noted previously, the fetal trunk normally comes into contact with the anterior uterine wall during the third trimester.

A false impression of polyhydramnios may be noted during the second trimester when the fetus comprises disproportionately less space than in the third trimester. One study reported that seven of 40 cases of

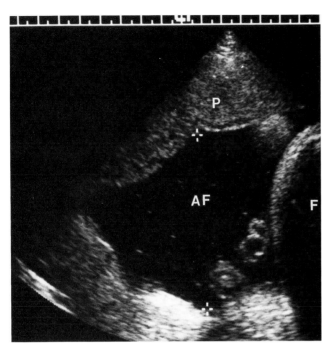

FIG 3–19.
Mild polyhydramnios. Largest pocket of amniotic fluid *(AF)* in a large-for-gestational age fetus measures 9 cm *(graticules)*. Mild polyhydramnios commonly accompanies a large-for-gestational age fetus, whether or not maternal diabetes is present. *F* = fetus; *P* = placenta.

sonographically documented polyhydramnios between 16 and 27 weeks' gestation had normal amniotic fluid volume when reexamined in the third trimester.[21] In equivocal cases, therefore, it would seem prudent to defer a diagnosis of abnormal amniotic fluid volume until the third trimester.

Using the four-quadrant approach, Phelan et al. consider polyhydramnios to be present when the AFI (see Figs 3–7 and 3–8) is ≥ 20.[113] Others, including the author, prefer to select the largest pocket of amniotic fluid free of fetal body parts and measure it vertically. Utilizing this technique, mild polyhydramnios is considered present when a vertical pocket of amniotic fluid measures 8–12 cm (Fig 3–19); moderate polyhydramnios is diagnosed when the pocket measures 12–16 cm; and severe polyhydramnios is diagnosed when the pocket is greater than 16 cm (Fig 3–20). Because mild polyhydramnios can subsequently become normal, a second study is performed in these patients in 1 month.

Polyhydramnios may develop acutely over a few days or chronically over weeks. The former usually occurs in the latter part of the second trimester, while chronic polyhydramnios is more prevalent in the third trimester. In one series, a diagnosis of acute polyhydramnios was made at an average gestational age of 23.4 weeks; delivery occurred within 2.6 weeks of the diagnosis.[122] Acute polyhydramnios is a frequent complication of monozygotic twin gestations (see Fig 3–20).[156] The recurrence of idiopathic acute polyhydramnios in subsequent pregnancies has been the subject of several case reports.[117, 124, 157]

Etiology

Polyhydramnios is associated with a wide variety of both maternal and fetal conditions (Table 3–3). Prior to the universal availability of ultrasound, Queenan and Gadow found the following diagnoses

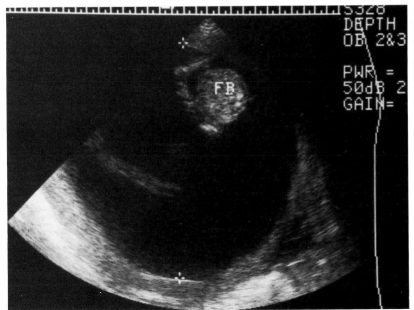

FIG 3–20.
Severe polyhydramnios and "stuck" twin. Severe polyhydramnios (marked by graticules) at 22 weeks' gestation in a monochorionic diamniotic twin gestation surrounding fetus A (not shown). Fetus B *(FB)* is actually in a oligohydramniotic scan and appears suspended (stuck) due to closely adherent membrane.

TABLE 3–3.

Congenital Anomalies Associated With Polyhydramnios*

	References
Gastrointestinal system	
Esophageal atresia/tracheoesophageal fistula	36, 67, 119, 151
Duodenal atresia	116, 151
Jejunoileal atresia	116
Gastroschisis	12
Omphalocele	67, 151
Diaphragmatic hernia	67
Meckel's diverticulum	67
Congenital megacolon	67
Meconium peritonitis	37, 135
Annular pancreas	135
Pancreatic cyst	63
Head and neck	
Cystic hygroma	135
Goiter	8
Cleft palate	64, 73
Epignathus	70
Respiratory system	
Cystic adenomatoid malformation	127
Congenital hydrothorax	67
Extralobar sequestration	69
Primary pulmonary hypoplasia	90
Congenital pulmonary lymphangiectasia	69
Pulmonary cyst	151
Asphyxiating thoracic dystrophy	63, 150
Cardiovascular system	
Arrhythmias	55
Coarctation of the aorta	67
Myxomas/hemangiomas	118
Ectopia cordis	135
Cardiac tumors	Chapter 9
Heart anomalies with hydrops	Chapter 9
Central nervous system	
Anencephaly	46, 67
Hydrocephaly	67
Microcephaly	135
Iniencephaly	67
Hydranencephaly	55
Holoprosencephaly	150
Encephalocele	135
Spina bifida	135
Dandy-Walker malformation	107
Genitourinary system	
Ureteropelvic junction obstruction	110, 126, 162
Posterior urethral valves	151
Urethral stenosis	110
Multicystic kidney disease	67, 151
Large ovarian cyst	108
Mesoblastic nephroma	76
Bartter's syndrome	140
Megacystis microcolon hypoperistalsis syndrome	Chapter 12
Skeletal system	
Thanatophoric dwarf	150, 161
Campomelic dwarf	161
Osteogenesis imperfecta	54, 151
Heterozygous achondroplasia	150, 161
Arthrogryposis multiplex	93
Klippel-Feil syndrome	73
Nager's acrofacial dysostosis	11
Achondrogenesis	150
Congenital infections	
Cytomegalovirus	120
Toxoplasmosis	62
Listeriosis	42
Congenital hepatitis	62
Miscellaneous	
Sacrococcygeal teratoma	27, 64
Cranial teratoma	64
Cervical teratoma	129
Congenital sarcoma	138
Placental chorioangioma	154
Cavernous hemangioma	67
Metastatic neuroblastoma	40
Myotonic dystrophy	33
Fetal acetaminophen toxicity	22
Retroperitoneal fibrosis	32
Multisystem anomalies	21, 141
Pena-Shokeir syndrome	5
Cutaneous vascular hemartosis	127
Twin reversed arterial perfusion (TRAP) sequence—acardiac anomaly	43

*Data from references 12, 36, 37, 63, 67, 116, 119, 135, 151.

among 358 cases of polyhydramnios: idiopathic (34%); diabetes mellitus (24.6%); congenital anomalies (20%); erythroblastosis fetalis (11.5%); multiple births (8.4%); and acute polyhydramnios (1.5%).[122] Polyhydramnios also frequently accompanies fetuses who are large for gestational age, whether or not maternal diabetes mellitus is present (see Fig 3–19).

Advances in maternal-fetal medicine over the past 15 to 20 years have significantly altered not only the overall prevalence, but also the types of cases seen with polyhydramnios. For example, Rh immune globulin has markedly reduced the incidence of erythroblastosis fetalis; rigidly maintaining euglycemia in the pregnant diabetic has significantly reduced the frequency with which hydramnios is seen with this disease entity; and the discovery of additional fetal and maternal conditions associated with polyhydramnios has resulted in fewer patients being placed in the idiopathic group.[58]

As the severity of polyhydramnios increases, so does the likelihood of determining an underlying etiology. In one study, 66 of 79 patients (83.5%) with mild polyhydramnios were categorized as idiopathic, while 21 of 23 patients (91.3%) with moderate or severe polyhydramnios had a maternal or fetal condition known to be associated with polyhydramnios.[58] However, in cases of mild polyhydramnios, patients were distributed within all of the common etiologic categories (Table 3–4).[58]

The prognostic significance of polyhydramnios is also directly related to its severity. Among 165 preg-

TABLE 3–4.

Severity of Polyhydramnios and Associated Maternal/Fetal Conditions*

Polyhydramnios	No. 102	(%) (100)	Mild 79	Moderate 19	Severe 4
Idiopathic	68	(66.7)	66	2	
Anomalies	13	(12.7)	2	9	2
Insulin-dependent diabetes	8	(7.8)	3	5	
Gestational diabetes	7	(6.9)	7		
Twins	5	(4.9)	1	2	2
Other maternal/fetal diseases	1	(1.0)	1		

*From Hill LM, Breckle R, Thomas M, et al: Polyhydramnios: Ultrasonically detected prevalence and neonatal outcome. Obstet Gynecol 1987; 69:23. Used by permission.

nancies with mild polyhydramnios combined from three series, 81% of neonates survived. In comparison, only 46% (39 of 85) of pregnancies with severe polyhydramnios survived the neonatal period.[7, 35, 58] Furthermore, 9% (9 of 104) of infants born from a mildly polyhydramniotic pregnancy had congenital anomalies compared to 66% (10 of 29) infants resulting from a severely polyhydramniotic pregnancy. An underlying chromosomal abnormality was found in six of 57 fetuses (10.5%) with severe polyhydramnios reported by Barkin et al. and three of 28 fetuses (11%) with marked polyhydramnios reported by Filly et al.[7, 35]

Fetal Anomalies

A wide variety of congenital malformations has been associated with polyhydramnios. However, it should be emphasized that association is not necessarily causation, and single case reports cannot be statistically evaluated with respect to prevalence. The fact that not all fetuses with any of the congenital anomalies mentioned will have polyhydramnios is in part due to the severity of the impairment in a given case, as well as the ability of the maternal-fetal unit to compensate by utilizing other pathways for fluid removal from the amniotic cavity. Finally, the role of deficiencies in amniochorionic membrane receptors (prolactin, antidiuretic hormone, etc.) as a possible final common pathway for the accumulation of an excess amount of amniotic fluid remains to be determined.[52, 53, 68, 87]

Despite the diversity of anomalies associated with polyhydramnios, certain types of malformations are so common that they should be specifically excluded. In fetuses with severe polyhydramnios reported by Barkin et al. (some of which had multiple anomalies), the organs most commonly involved included the central nervous system (52%), gastrointestinal tract (47%), cardiovascular system (30%), musculoskeletal system (19%), and genitourinary tract (16%).[7] In this series,

sonography also correctly identified 90%–95% of major fetal malformations.

The etiologic mechanism for polyhydramnios due to some malformations is usually self-evident: Central nervous system anomalies presumably cause neural depression of fetal swallowing; proximal bowel obstruction leads to decreased amniotic fluid reabsorption by the bowel; and cardiac malformations lead to congestive heart failure (hydrops). However, it is less certain why other types of anomalies, such as skeletal dysplasias or urinary malformations, may be associated with polyhydramnios.

In the following sections, major types of fetal anomalies that are most frequently associated with polyhydramnios will be considered as belonging to one of five major categories:

1. Central nervous system disorders.
2. Gastrointestinal disorders.
3. Hydrops fetalis.
4. Skeletal disorders.
5. Renal disorders.

Central Nervous System Disorders

A wide variety of primary central nervous system abnormalities may produce polyhydramnios, probably by depression of fetal swallowing (Fig 3–21). Hence, the onset of polyhydramnios may be related to menstrual age. Among anencephalics, Goldstein et al. reported that six of seven cases had polyhydramnios after 25 weeks' gestation, but only one of 13 cases had polyhydramnios before 25 weeks (Fig 3–22).[46]

Gastrointestinal Disorders

Polyhydramnios is a commonly associated finding of gastrointestinal disorders, most often resulting from atresia of the esophagus, duodenum, jejunum, or ileum (Fig 3–23); large bowel obstruction alone does not

FIG 3–21.
Dandy-Walker malformation and polyhy-dramnios. **A,** transverse scan of cranium at 35 weeks demonstrates posterior fossa cyst *(C)* and absence of cerebellar vermis *(arrow),* indicating Dandy-Walker malforma-tion. *H* = cerebellar hemispheres. **B,** mark-edly increased volume of amniotic fluid *(AF)* surrounds the fetus *(F).*

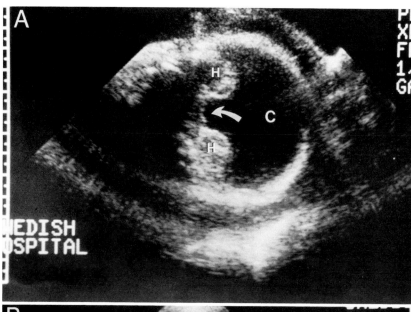

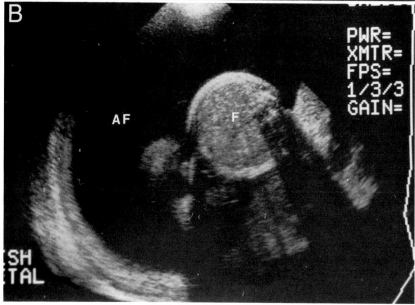

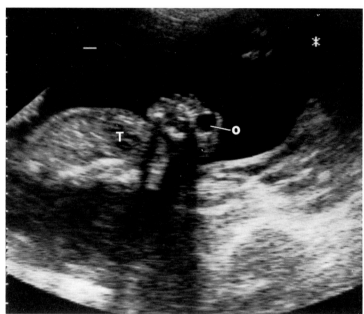

FIG 3–22.
Anencephaly and mild polyhydramnios. Longitudinal scan at 21 weeks shows characteristic findings of anencephaly with absence of cranium cephalad to orbits *(O)*. Mild polyhydramnios is present. *T* = thorax.

produce polyhydramnios. Other gastrointestinal disorders that may cause partial bowel obstruction include intestinal volvulus, meconium ileus, abdominal wall defects, and meconium peritonitis (see Fig 3–23).[37] In these cases, polyhydramnios presumably develops when the amount of swallowed amniotic fluid exceeds the absorptive capacity of the stomach and the bowel proximal to the site of obstruction. Similarly, polyhydramnios often accompanies diaphragmatic hernia (Fig 3–24) (see Chapter 8). Polyhydramnios also develops in 10% of cases of ovarian cysts (see Fig 3–23), presumably from compression on the adjacent bowel (see Chapter 9).

Facial clefts and neck masses, such as goiters and teratomas, have also been associated with polyhydramnios (see Chapter 7). Neck masses presumably cause mechanical obstruction to fetal swallowing, while facial clefts probably cause ineffective fetal swallowing.

A combination of congenital anomalies may result in an unpredictable amniotic fluid volume. For example, fetuses with both esophageal atresia and renal agenesis may have normal amniotic fluid volume.[149] Also, anorectal atresia, which is usually associated with a normal to decreased amount of amniotic fluid, may have increased fluid in conjunction with esophageal atresia (Fig 3–25).[50] It is also worthwhile to note that polyhydramnios does not universally accompany gastrointestinal obstruction, even when complete. For example, esophageal ligation in the sheep model or esophageal atresia in humans may not necessarily result in polyhydramnios.[119, 159, 162]

Fetal Hydrops

Approximately 50% of fetuses with hydrops fetalis have polyhydramnios (Fig 3–26). Given the diverse etiologies of hydrops fetalis, the underlying mechanism for polyhydramnios undoubtedly differs with the underlying disorder. In conditions associated with high output congestive heart failure (twin-twin transfusion, sacrococcygeal teratoma, chorioangioma, etc.), polyhydramnios may result predominantly from excess urine formation. By contrast, conditions associated with low output heart failure or other etiologies probably involve various mechanisms, including diminished swallowing, decreased lung reabsorption, or increased transudation of fluid secondary to fetal compromise.

Polyhydramnios may precede any other evidence of fetal hydrops. For example, fetuses with sacrococcygeal teratoma or chorioangioma may demonstrate polyhydramnios independent of hydrops. However, the etiology of arteriovenous shunting is presumably the same.

Skeletal Disorders

Polyhydramnios has been frequently associated with skeletal abnormalities (Fig 3–27), although the etiology for the polyhydramnios remains speculative. Thomas and associates reviewed 45 cases of skeletal dysplasias associated with polyhydramnios.[150] Skeletal dysplasias most frequently reported included thanatophoric dwarf (58%) and achondroplasia (27%).[150] They suggest that the presence of polyhydramnios is a poor prognostic finding since only five survivors

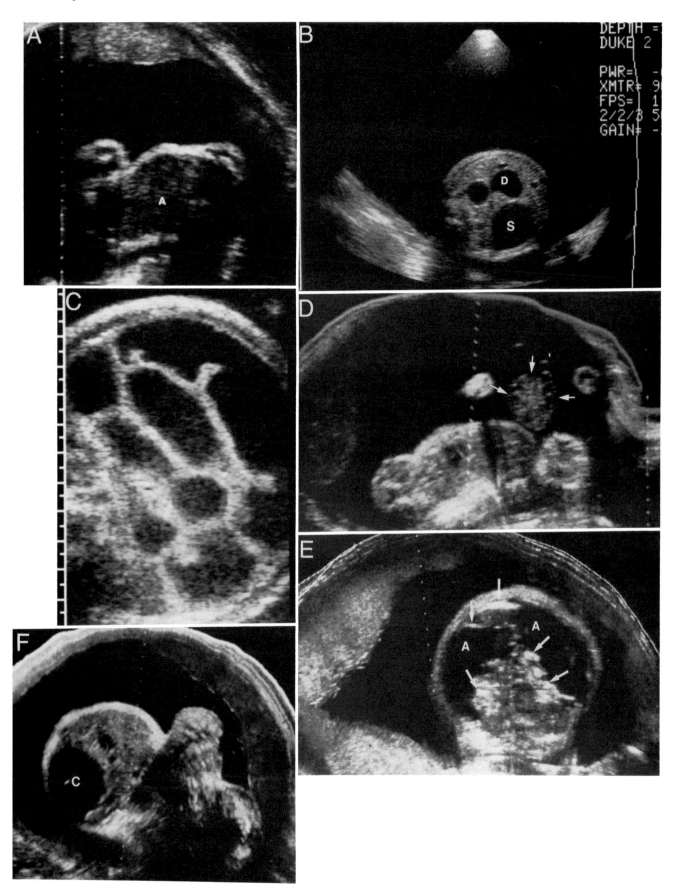

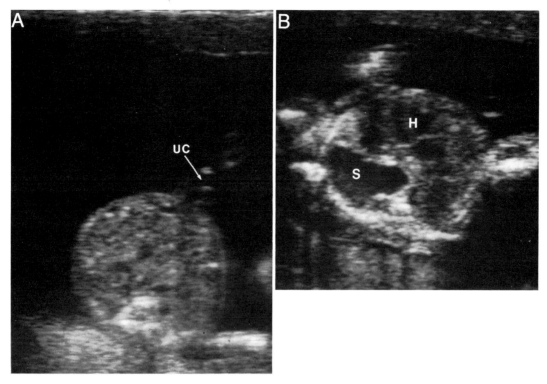

FIG 3–24.
Diaphragmatic hernia with multiple anomalies and polyhydramnios. **A,** transverse scan at 19 weeks' gestation in a twin pregnancy shows polyhydramnios and a single umbilical artery, seen as a two-vessel umbilical cord *(UC)*. **B,** transverse scan of the thorax demonstrates the fluid-filled stomach *(S)* in the right chest adjacent to the heart *(H)*. Also identified are cerebellar hypoplasia and a high thoracic myelomeningocele. Other abnormalities identified on postmortem examination included absent spleen, right clubfoot, hypoplastic left heart, and rib abnormalities. Chromosome analysis yielded a normal female karyotype.

(11%) were reported, and all of these were cases of heterozygous achondroplasia.

Renal Malformations

Paradoxically, various renal abnormalities have been associated with polyhydramnios (Fig 3–28). These usually involve unilateral renal disorders (ureteropelvic obstruction, multicystic dysplasia, and renal tumors), although occasional bilateral renal disorders have also been reported (bilateral ureteropelvic obstruction).[7, 71, 86] Approximately 25% of fetuses with ureteropelvic junction obstruction demonstrate polyhydramnios.[71]

The underlying mechanism leading to polyhydramnios from unilateral renal anomalies remains specula-

tive, but probably results either from glomerular hypertrophy or from hormonally induced polyuria. In cases of bilateral renal disorders, alternative mechanisms of polyhydramnios may include increased transudation of fluid into the amniotic cavity or decreased fetal swallowing.

Several studies have evaluated hourly fetal urinary production rates in various maternal-fetal disease entities. In the chronic ewe preparation, increased urinary output follows infusion of intravenous isotonic saline, if infusion rates are greater than the basal urinary flow rate (Fig 3–29). These data imply that if a normal fetus is overhydrated, an increase in the amniotic fluid volume will result from an increase in urinary output.[16] In human fetuses, correction of specific fetal disease states

FIG 3–23.
Gastrointestinal causes of polyhydramnios. **A,** esophageal atresia and trisomy 18. No stomach was visualized in the fetal abdomen *(A)*. **B,** duodenal atresia. Characteristic "double bubble" appearance with fluid-filled stomach *(S)* and duodenum *(D)*. **C,** ileal atresia. Multiple loops of dilated small bowel are demonstrated. **D,** omphalocele. A portion of liver *(arrows)* is seen external to the abdominal cavity. **E,** meconium peritonitis. Transverse scan demonstrates ascites *(A)* and multiple peritoneal calcifications *(arrows)* on the visceral and parietal peritoneum. **F,** ovarian cyst. Scan demonstrates large intra-abdominal cyst *(C)* representing an ovarian cyst. Polyhydramnios is associated with ovarian cysts in approximately 10% of cases, probably due to extrinsic compression on adjacent bowel.

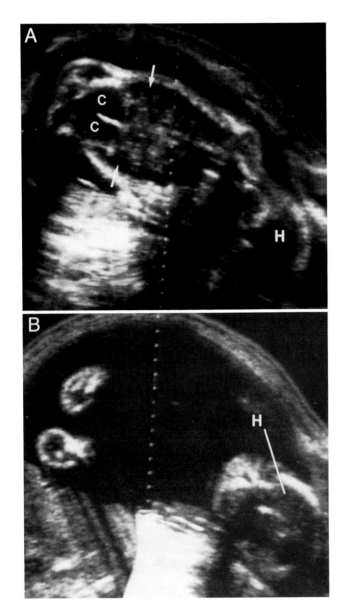

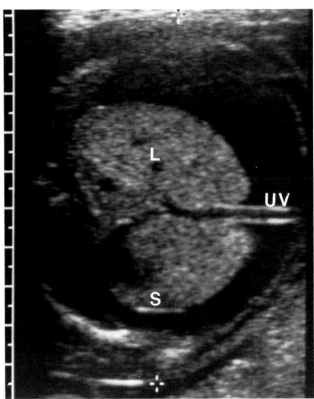

FIG 3–26.
Fetal hydrops from fetal tachycardia. Transverse scan of the abdomen in a fetus with supraventricular tachycardia demonstrates a large amount of ascites surrounding the liver *(L)* and spleen *(S)*. Mild polyhydramnios was also present. *UV* = umbilical vein.

FIG 3–25.
Multiple anomalies and polyhydramnios. **A,** longitudinal view demonstrates a bi-lobed cystic mass *(C)* in the lower pelvis that proved to represent dilated colon from anorectal atresia. A small amount of ascites *(arrows)* is also noted. *H* = head. **B,** marked polyhydramnios is identified on other views. Postmortem examination found multiple anomalies, including anorectal atresia and esophageal atresia with tracheoesophageal fistula. *H* = fetal head.

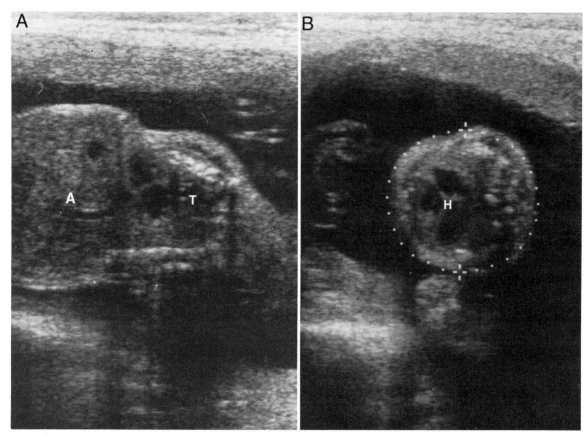

FIG 3–27.
Thanatophoric dwarf and polydramnios. **A,** sagittal scan demonstrates narrowed thorax *(T)* and normal size of abdomen *(A)*. Short extremities characteristic of thanatophoric dysplasia were also identified. **B,** transverse view of thorax demonstrates normal heart *(H)* size, but chest circumference is below the second percentile. Mild polyhydramnios is also identified.

FIG 3–28.
Renal causes of polyhydramnios. **A,** multicystic dysplastic kidney and mild polyhydramnios. Transverse scan demonstrates multiple cysts *(C)* of varying size due to unilateral multicystic dysplastic kidney and mild polyhydramnios. **B,** mildly increased amniotic fluid *(AF)* volume is identified in this fetus who demonstrated unilateral absence of one kidney on other views. Mild polyhydramnios is commonly observed in unilateral renal disorders, although the etiology is uncertain.

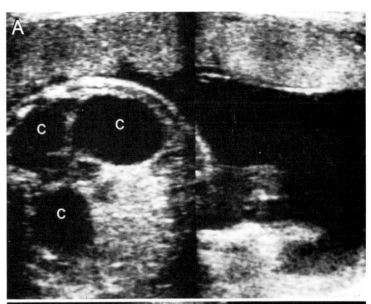

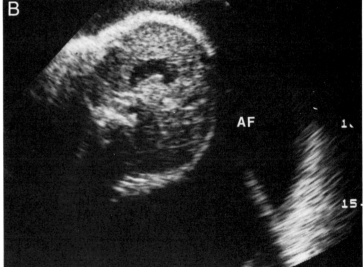

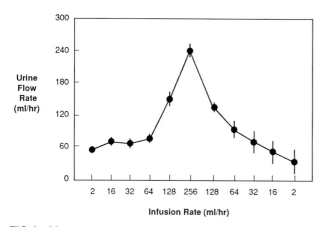

FIG 3–29.
Effects of intravenous saline infusions for 11 days on urinary output of fetal lambs (N = 3). Each infusion rate was maintained for 24 hours (From Brace RA: Amniotic fluid volume and its relationship to fetal fluid balance: Review of experimental data. Semin Perinatol 1986; 10:103–112. Used by permission.)

can also lead to a sudden change in the hourly fetal urinary output. For example, administration of intraperitoneal albumin in idiopathic non–immune hydrops has been shown to increase the hourly fetal urinary output, presumably because of the increase in the intravascular volume.[139] At least in some cases, therefore, increased urinary output probably contributes to development of polyhydramnios.

Treatment

Prenatal treatment of polyhydramnios is desirable to decrease the risk of potential complications of pre-term labor, rupture of membranes, and placental abruption. However, an effective treatment plan for polyhydramnios must take into consideration the underlying etiology. By correcting either a maternal cause (e.g., poor diabetic control) or fetal cause (e.g., anemia or arrhythmia), polyhydramnios can gradually improve.[59] On the other hand, removal of amniotic fluid by amniocentesis does not treat the underlying disease process, and the amniotic fluid volume predictably returns to preexisting levels within a few days. In addition, the potential complications of repeated amniocenteses—placental abruption after the precipitous removal of too much amniotic fluid, premature labor, and chorioamnionitis—must be considered.[154]

In patients with polyhydramnios, marked reduction in amniotic fluid volume has been observed within 1 week of maternal administration of indomethacin, a non–steroidal anti-inflammatory agent whose mechanism of action involves inhibition of prostaglandin synthesis.[17] In patients with normal amniotic fluid who are

treated for pre-term labor, reduction in fluid volume has also been observed within 4 to 56 days after initiation of indomethacin.[82] Amniotic fluid volume can return to normal within 2 days of discontinuing the medication in such patients. Possible mechanisms of action of indomethacin and other prostaglandin synthetase inhibitors for decreasing amniotic fluid volume include: decreasing fetal urinary output; increasing reabsorption of amniotic fluid via the lungs; and/or promoting water transport across fetal membranes.[17]

Unfortunately, Moise and coworkers have documented fetal ductal constriction by echocardiography in seven of 14 fetuses whose mothers received oral indomethacin for a maximum of 72 hours to inhibit labor.[95] Tricuspid regurgitation resulting from an increase in pressure in the right ventricular outflow tract led to mild endocardial ischemia and papillary muscle dysfunction. In this author's opinion, therefore, indomethacin should not be used in the treatment of idiopathic polyhydramnios without serial fetal echocardiographic surveillance of the ductus.

Treatment options for oligohydramnios are more limited than those for polyhydramnios. Correction of the underlying cause (for example, hypertension) is the most effective management. Other options include bed rest and fluid intake. Goodlin and coworkers, who suggest that amniotic fluid volume depends upon the degree of maternal plasma volume expansion after 29 weeks' gestation, treated 12 patients with hypovolemia and an admitting diagnosis of hypertension, intrauterine growth retardation, diabetes mellitus, or pre-term labor.[47] Plasma volume expansion was attempted by means of bed rest and forced oral fluid intake. If the hematocrit did not decline by 15%, acute intravenous volume expansion was performed with 25% albumin. Nine of the 12 patients studied increased their plasma volume; six of the nine had a sonographically documented increase in amniotic volume; and two patients ruptured membranes soon after volume expansion. The latter two cases are interesting in view of Gumbruch and Hansmann's cautionary note about the sudden over-distention of the uterine cavity leading to rupture of the membranes.[41]

CONCLUSION

Amniotic fluid is a major component of the intrauterine environment. Since its formation and maintenance is dependent upon intricate maternal and fetal interrelationships, an abnormal quantity of amniotic fluid (oligohydramnios or polyhydramnios) requires a careful evaluation of *both* patients. With treatment of the primary disease process, the amniotic fluid volume can return to normal. For conditions in which antenatal treatment is not yet available, the sonologist should direct attention toward evaluating the potential complications of abnormal amniotic fluid volume.

REFERENCES

1. Abramovich DR, Garden A, Jandial L, et al: Fetal swallowing and voiding in relation to hydramnios. Obstet Gynecol 1979; 54:15–20.
2. Abramovich DR: The volume of amniotic fluid and its regulating factors, in Fairweather DVE, Eskes TKAB (eds): *Amniotic Fluid-Research and Clinical Application* ed 2. Amsterdam, Excerpta Medica, 1978, pp 31–49.
3. Adzick NS, Harrison MJR, Glick PL, et al: Experimental pulmonary hypoplasia and oliogohydramnios: Relative contributions of lung fluid and fetal breathing movements. J Pediatr Surg 1984; 19:658–665.
4. Alexander ES, Spitz HB, Clark RA: Sonography of polyhydramnios. AJR 1982; 138:343–346.
5. Arienzo R, Ricco C, Romeo F: A very rare fetal malformation: The cutaneous widespread vascular hematomatosis. Am J Obstet Gynecol 1987; 157:1162–1163.
6. Balfour RP, Lawrence KM: Raised serum alpha-fetoprotein levels and fetal renal agenesis. Lancet 1980; 1:317.
7. Barkin SZ, Pretorius DH, Beckett MK, et al: Severe polyhydramnios: Incidence of anomalies. AJR 1987; 148:155–159.
8. Barone CM, Van Natta FC, Kourides IA, et al: Sonographic detection of fetal goiter, an unusual cause of hydramnios. J Ultrasound Med 1985; 4:625–627.
9. Barss VA, Benacerraf BR, Frigoletto FD: Second trimester oligohydramnios, a predictor of poor fetal outcome. Obstet Gynecol 1984; 64:608–610.
10. Bastide A, Manning F, Harman C, et al: Ultrasound evaluation of amniotic fluid: Outcome of pregnancies with severe oligohydramnios. Am J Obstet Gynecol 1986; 154:895–900.
11. Benson CB, Pober BR, Hirsch MP, et al: Sonography of Nager's acrofacial dysostosis syndrome in utero. J Ultrasound Med 1988; 7:163–167.
12. Bjornstahl H, Kullendorf C-M, Westgren M: Gastroschisis diagnosed in utero by ultrasound. Acta Obstet Gynecol Scand 1983; 62:683–684.
13. Blott M, Nicolaides KH, Gibb D, et al: Fetal breathing movements as predictor of favorable pregnancy outcome after oligohydramnios due to membrane rupture in second trimester. Lancet 1987; 2:129–131.
14. Bottoms SF, Welch RA, Zador IE, et al: Limitations of using maximum vertical pocket and other sonographic evaluations of amniotic fluid volume to predict fetal growth: Technical or physiologic? Am J Obstet Gynecol 1986; 155:154–158.
15. Boylan P, Paresi V: An overview of hydramnios. Semin Perinatol 1986; 10:136–141.
16. Brace RA: Amniotic fluid volume and its relationship to fetal fluid balance: Review of experimental data. Semin Perinatol 1986; 10:103–112.
17. Cabrol D, Landesman R, Muller J, et al: Treatment of polyhydramnios with prostaglandin synthetase inhibitor (indomethacin). Am J Obstet Gynecol 1987; 157:422–426.
18. Cardwell MS: Polyhydramnios: A review. Obstet Gynecol Survey 1987; 42:612–617.
19. Cassady G, Barnett R: Amniotic fluid electrolytes and perinatal outcome. Biol Neonate 1968; 13:155–174.
20. Chamberlain PF, Manning FA, Morrison I, et al: Ultrasound evaluation of amniotic fluid. I: The relationship of marginal and decreased amniotic fluid volumes to perinatal outcome. Am J Obstet Gynecol 1984; 150:245–249.
21. Chamberlain PF, Manning FA, Morrison I, et al: Ultrasound evaluation of amniotic fluid. II: The relationship of increased amniotic fluid volume to perinatal outcome. Am J Obstet Gynecol 1984; 150:250–254.
22. Char VC, Chandra R, Fletcher AB, et al: Polyhydramnios and neonatal renal failure—a possible association with maternal acetaminophen ingestion. J Pediatr 1975; 86:638.
23. Chitkara U, Rosenberg J, Chervenak FA, et al: Prenatal sonographic assessment of the fetal thorax: Normal values. Am J Obstet Gynecol 1987; 156:1069–1074.
24. Clement D, Schifrin BS, Kates RB: Acute oligohydramnios in post-date pregnancy. Am J Obstet Gynecol 1987; 157:884–886.
25. Cohn HE, Sacks EJ, Heymann MA, et al: Cardiovascular responses to hypoxemia and acidemia in fetal lambs. Am J Obstet Gynecol 1974; 120:817–824.
26. Cook CD, Brodie HR, Allen DW: Measurement of fetal hemoglobin in newborn infants. Correlation with gestational age and intrauterine hypoxia. Pediatrics 1957; 20:272–278.
27. Cousins L, Benirschke K, Porreco R, et al: Placentomegaly due to fetal congestive failure in a pregnancy with a sacrococcygeal teratoma. J Reprod Med 1980; 25:142–144.
28. Crowley P, O'Herlihy C, Boylan P: The value of ultrasound measurement of amniotic fluid volume in the management of prolonged pregnancies. Br J Obstet Gynaecol 1984; 91:444–448.
29. Crowley P: Non-quantitative estimation of amniotic fluid volume in suspected prolonged pregnancy. J Perinat Med 1980; 8:249–251.
30. Daniel SS, Yeh MN, Bowie ET, et al: Renal response of the lamb fetus to partial occlusion of the umbilical cord. J Pediatr 1975; 87:788–794.
31. Deutinger J, Bartl W, Pfersmann C, et al: Fetal kidney volume and urine production in cases of fetal growth retardation. J Perinat Med 1987; 15:307–315.
32. Duffy JL: Fetal retroperitoneal fibrosis associated with hydramnios. JAMA 1966; 198:993–996.

33. Dunn LJ, Dierker LJ: Recurrent hydramnios in association with myotonia dystrophica. Obstet Gynecol 1973; 42:104–106.

34. Elliot PM, Inman WHW: Volume of amniotic fluid in normal and abnormal pregnancy. Lancet 1961; 2:835–840.

35. Filly RA. Polyhydramnios, in Marguilis AR, Gooding CA (eds): *Diagnostic Radiology.* San Francisco, Radiology Research Foundation, 1987, pp 263–270.

36. Flowers WK: Hydramnios and gastrointestinal atresias. A review. Obstet Gynecol Surv 1983; 38:685–688.

37. Foster MA, Nyberg DA, Mahony BS, et al. Meconium peritonitis: Prenatal sonographic findings and clinical significance. Radiology 1987; 165:661–665.

38. Fuchs F: Volume of amniotic fluid at various stages of pregnancy. Clin Obstet Gynecol 1966; 9:449–460.

39. Fujiwara T, Adams FH, Scudder A: Fetal lamb amniotic fluid: Relationship of lipid composition to surface tension. J Pediatr 1964; 65:824–830.

40. Gadwood KA, Reynes CJ: Prenatal sonography of metastic neuroblastoma. J Clin Ultrasound 1983; 11:512–515.

41. Gembruch U, Hansmann M: Artificial instillation of amniotic fluid as a new technique for the diagnostic evaluation of cases of oligohydramnios. Prenat Diagn 1988; 8:33–45.

42. Gembruch U, Niesen M, Hansmann M, et al: Listeriosis: A case of non–immune hydrops fetalis. Prenat Diagn 1987; 7:277–282.

43. Gibson JY, D'Cruz CA, Patel RB, et al: Acardiac anomaly: Review of the subject with case report and emphasis on practical sonography. J Clin Ultrasound 1986; 14:541–545.

44. Goldenberg RL, Davis RO, Blumfield CG: Transient fetal anuria of unknown etiology: A case report. Am J Obstet Gynecol 1984; 149:87.

45. Goldstein RB, Filly RA: Sonographic estimation of amniotic fluid volume: Subjective assessment versus pocket measurements. J Ultrasound Med 1988; 7:363–369.

46. Goldstein RB, Filly RA: Prenatal diagnosis of anencephaly: Spectrum of sonographic appearances and distinction from the amniotic band syndrome. AJR 1988; 151:547–550.

47. Goodlin RC, Anderson JC, Gallagher TF: Relationship between amniotic fluid volume and maternal plasma volume expansion. Am J Obstet Gynecol 1983; 146:505–511.

48. Halpern ME, Fong KW, Zalev AH, et al: Reliability of amniotic fluid volume estimation from ultrasonograms: Intraobserver and interobserver variation before and after the establishment of criteria. Am J Obstet Gynecol 1985; 153:264–267.

49. Harman CR: Maternal furosemide may not provoke urine production in the compromised fetus. Am J Obstet Gynecol 1984; 150:322–323.

50. Harris RD, Nyberg DA, Mack LA, et al: Anorectal atresia: Prenatal sonographic diagnosis. AJR 1987; 15:469–474.

51. Harrison MR, Golbus MS, Filly RA: *The Unborn Patient. Prenatal Diagnosis and Treatment.* Philadelphia, Grune & Stratton Inc, 1984, pp 1–10.

52. Healy DL, Herington AC, O'Herlihy C: Chronic idiopathic polyhydramnios: Evidence for a defect in the chorion laeve receptor for lactogenic hormones. J Clin Endocrinol Metab 1983; 56:520–523.

53. Healy DL, Herington AC, O'Herlihy C: Chronic polyhydramnios is a syndrome with a lactogen receptor defect in the chorion laeve. Br J Obstet Gynaecol 1985; 92:461–467.

54. Heller RH, Winn KJ, Hell RM: The prenatal diagnosis of osteogenesis imperfecta congenita. Am J Obstet Gynecol 1975; 121:572–573.

55. Hill LM, Breckle R, Driscoll DJ: Sonographic evaluation of prenatal therapy for supraventricular tachycardia and congestive failure. A case report. J Reprod Med 1983; 28:671–676.

56. Hill LM, Breckle R, Wolkfgram KR, et al: Oligohydramnios: Ultrasonically detected incidence and subsequent fetal outcome. Am J Obstet Gynecol 1983; 147:407–410.

57. Hill LM, Breckle R: Vernix in amniotic fluid: Sonographic detection. Radiology 1986; 158:80.

58. Hill LM, Breckle R, Thomas M, et al: Polyhydramnios: Ultrasonically detected prevalence and neonatal outcome. Obstet Gynecol 1987; 69:21–25.

59. Hill LM: Resolving polyhydramnios: A sign of improved fetal status. Am J Perinatol 1988; 5:61–63.

60. Hislop A, Reid L: Persistent hypoplasia of the lung after repair of congenital diaphragmatic hernia. Thorax 1976; 31:450–455.

61. Hoddick WK, Callen PW, Filly RA, et al: Ultrasonographic determination of qualitative amniotic fluid volume in intrauterine growth retardation: Reassessment of the 1 cm rule. Am J Obstet Gynecol 1984; 149:758–762.

62. Holzgreve W, Curry CJR, Golbus MS, et al: Investigation of non–immune hydrops fetalis. Am J Obstet Gynecol 1984; 150:805–812.

63. Hooper MSC, Boultbee JE, Watson AR: Polyhydramnios associated with congenital pancreatic cysts and asphyxiating thoracic dysplasia. S Afr Med J 1979; 7:32–33.

64. Horger EO, Pai GS: Ultrasound in the diagnosis of fetal malformations. Implications for obstetric management. Am J Obstet Gynecol 1983; 147:163–170.

65. Hutchinson DL, Gray MJ, Plentl AA, et al: The role of the fetus in the water exchange of the amniotic fluid of normal and hydramniotic patients. J Clin Invest 1959; 38:971–980.

66. Hutchinson DL, Hunter CB, Neslen ED, et al: The exchange of water and electrolytes in the mechanism of amniotic fluid formation and the relationship to hydramnios. Surg Gynecol Obstet 1955; 100:391–396.

67. Jacoby HE, Charles D: Clinical conditions associated with hydramnios. Am J Obstet Gynecol 1966; 94:910–919.

68. Josimovich JB, Merisko K, Buccella L: Amniotic prolac-

tin control over amniotic and fetal extracellular fluid water and electrolytes in the rhesus monkey. Endocrinology 1977; 100:564–570.

69. Jouppila P, Kirkinen P, Herva R, et al: Prenatal diagnosis of pleural effusions by ultrasound. J Clin Ultrasound 1983; 11:316–319.

70. Kang KW, Hissong SL, Langer A: Prenatal ultrasonic diagnosis of epignathus. J Clin Ultrasound 1978; 6:330–331.

71. Kleiner B, Callen PW, Filly RA. Sonographic analysis of the fetus with ureteropelvic junction obstruction. AJR 1987; 148:359–363.

72. Koontz WL, Seeds JW, Adams NJ, et al: Elevated maternal serum alpha-fetoprotein, second-trimester oligohydramnios and pregnancy outcome. Obstet Gynecol 1983; 62:301–304.

73. Kramer EE: Hydramnios, oligohydramnios and fetal malformations. Clin Obstet Gynecol 1966; 9:508–519.

74. Kurjak A, Kirkinen P, Latin V, et al: Ultrasonic assessment of fetal kidney function in normal and complicated pregnancies. Am J Obstet Gynecol 1981; 141:266–270.

75. Landy HJ, Isada NB, Larsen JW. Genetic implications of idiopathic hydramnios. Am J Obstet Gynecol 1987; 157:114–117.

76. Lee KH: Hydramnios in the Chinese: A clinical study of 256 cases. Br J Obstet Gynaecol 1967; 74:868–874.

77. Leveno KJ: Amniotic fluid volume in prolonged pregnancy. Semin Perinatol 1986; 10:154–161.

78. Lind T, Billewicz WZ, Cheyne GA: Composition of amniotic fluid and maternal blood through pregnancy. Br J Obstet Gynaecol 1971; 78:505–512.

79. Lind T, Hytten FE: Relation of amniotic fluid volume to fetal weight in the first half of pregnancy. Lancet 1970; 1:1147–1149.

80. Lind T, Kendall A, Hytten FE: The role of the fetus in the formation of amniotic fluid. Br J Obstet Gynaecol 1972; 79:289–298.

81. Lind T, Parkin FM, Cheyne GA: Biochemical and cytological changes in liquor amnii with advancing gestation. Br J Obstet Gynaecol 1969; 76:673–680.

82. Lindenbaum C, Chhibber G, Cohen A: Oligohydramnios due to chronic indomethacin therapy in the treatment of premature labor. Presented at the eighth annual meeting of the Society of Perinatal Obstetricians, poster session, 1988.

83. Lingwood BE, Hardy KJ, Long JG, et al: Amniotic fluid volume and composition following experimental manipulations in sheep. Obstet Gynecol 1980; 56:451–458.

84. Lingwood BE, Wintour M: Amniotic fluid volume and in vivo permeability of ovine fetal membranes. Obstet Gynecol 1984; 64:368–372.

85. Lumbers ER, Stevens AD: Changes in fetal renal function in response to infusions of a hyperosmotic solution of mannitol to the ewe. J Physiol 1983; 343:429–436.

86. Mahony BS, Filly RA, Callen PW, et al: Severe nonimmune hydrops fetalis: Sonographic evaluation. Radiology 1984; 151:757–761.

87. Manku MS, Mtabaj, JP, Horrobin DF: Effect of cortisol, prolactin, and ADH on the amniotic membrane. Nature 1975; 258:78–82.

88. Manning FA, Hill LM, Platt LD: Qualitative amniotic fluid volume determination by ultrasound: Antepartum detection of intrauterine growth retardation. Am J Obstet Gynecol 1981; 139:254–258.

89. Mellor D, Slater JS: Daily changes in amniotic and allantoic fluid during the last three months of pregnancy in conscious, unstressed ewe with catheters in their foetal fluid sacs. J Physiol 1971; 217:573–604.

90. Mendelsohn G, Hutchins GM: Primary pulmonary hypoplasia. Report of a case with polyhydramnios. Am J Dis Child 1977; 131:1220–1223.

91. Mercer LJ, Brown LG, Petres RE, et al: A survey of pregnancies complicated by decreased amniotic fluid. Am J Obstet Gynecol 1984; 149:355–361.

92. Minei LJ, Suzuki K: Role of fetal deglutition and micturation in the production and turnover of amniotic fluid in the monkey. Obstet Gynecol 1976; 48:177–181.

93. Miskin M, Rudd NL, Benzie RJ, et al: Arthrogryposis multiplex congenita—Prenatal assessment with diagnostic ultrasound and fetoscopy. J Pediatr 1979; 95:463–464.

94. Moessinger AC, Higgins A, Fox HE, et al: Fetal breathing movements are not a reliable predictor of continued lung development in pregnancies complicated by oligohydramnios. Lancet 1987; 2:1297–1300.

95. Moise KL, Huhta JC, Sharif DS, et al: Indomethacin in the treatment of premature labor. Effect on the fetal ductus arteriosus. N Engl J Med 1988; 319:327–331.

96. Moya F, Apgar V, James LS: Hydramnios and congenital anomalies. JAMA 1960; 173:1552–1556.

97. Moya F, Grannum P, Pinto K, et al: Ultrasound assessment of the postmature pregnancy. Obstet Gynecol 1985; 65:319–322.

98. Moya F, Apgar V, James S, et al: Hydramnios and congenital anomalies: Study of series of 74 patients. JAMA 1960; 173:110–114.

99. Mulvihill SJ, Stone MM, Debas HT, et al: The role of amniotic fluid in fetal nutrition. J Pediatr Surg 1985; 20:668–672.

100. Murray SR: Hydramnios: A study of 846 cases. Am J Obstet Gynecol 1964; 88:65–67.

101. Naeye RL, Milic HMB, Blaanc W: Fetal endocrine and renal disorders: Clues to the origin of hydramnios. Am J Obstet Gynecol 1970; 108:1251–1256.

102. Nakayama DK, Glick PL, Harrison MR, et al: Experimental pulmonary hypoplasia due to oligohydramnios and its reversal by relieving thoracic compression. J Pediatr Surg 1983; 18:347–353.

103. Nicolaides KH, Rodeck CH, Gosden CM: Rapid karyotyping in non–lethal fetal malformations. Lancet 1986; 1:283–287.

104. Nimrod C, Davies D, Iwanieki S, et al: Ultrasound prediction of pulmonary hypoplasia. Obstet Gynecol 1986; 68:495–498.
105. Nimrod C, Nicholson S, Davies D, et al: Pulmonary hypoplasia testing in clinical obstetrics. Am J Obstet Gynecol 1988; 158:277–280.
106. Nimrod C, Varela-Gittings F, Machin G, et al: The effect of very prolonged membrane rupture on fetal development. Am J Obstet Gynecol 1984; 148:540–543.
107. Nyberg DA, Cyr DR, Mack LA, et al: The Dandy-Walker malformation. Prenatal sonographic diagnosis and its clinical significance. J Ultrasound Med 1988; 7:65–71.
108. Ott WJ: Acute polyhydramnios and a fetal ovarian cyst. J Reprod Med 1985; 30:887–889.
109. Perks AM, Cassin S: The effects of arginine vasopression and other factors on the production of lung fluid in fetal goats. Chest 1982; 81 (suppl):1–39.
110. Perlman M, Potashnik G, Wise S: Hydramnion and fetal renal anomalies. Am J Obstet Gynecol 1976; 125:966–968.
111. Phelan JP, Ahn MO, Smith CV, et al: Amniotic fluid index measurements during pregnancy. J Reprod Med 1987; 32:601–604.
112. Phelan JP, Platt LD, Yeh S, et al: The role of ultrasound assessment of amniotic fluid volume in the management of the post-date pregnancy. Am J Obstet Gynecol 1985; 151:304–308.
113. Phelan JP, Smith CV, Broussard P, et al: Amniotic fluid volume assessment with the four-quadrant technique at 36–42 weeks' gestation. J Reprod Med 1987; 32:540–542.
114. Philipson EH, Sokol RJ, Williams T: Oligohydramnios: Clinical associations and predictive value for intrauterine growth retardation. Am J Obstet Gynecol 1983; 146:271–278.
115. Phillips JF, Goodwin DW, Thomason SB, et al: The volume of the uterus in normal and abnormal pregnancy. J Clin Ultrasound 1977; 5:107–110.
116. Pierro A, Cozzi F, Colarossi G, et al: Does fetal gut obstruction cause hydramnios and growth retardation? J Pediatr Surg 1987; 22:454–457.
117. Pitkin RM: Acute polyhydramnios recurrent in successive pregnancies. Obstet Gynecol 1976; 48(suppl):42–43.
118. Platt LD, Geierman C, Turkel SB, et al: Atrial hemangioma and hydrops fetalis. Am J Obstet Gynecol 1981; 141:107–109.
119. Pretorius DH, Drose JA, Dennis MA, et al: Tracheoesophageal fistula in utero. J Ultrasound Med 1987; 6:509–513.
120. Price JM, Fisch AE, Jacobson J: Ultrasonic findings in fetal cytomegalovirus infection. J Clin Ultrasound 1978; 6:268.
121. Pritchard JA, MacDonald PC, Gant NF: *Williams Obstetrics,* ed 17. New York, Appleton-Century Crofts, Inc, 1985, pp 462–465.
122. Queenan JT, Gadow EC: Polyhydramnios: Chronic versus acute. Am J Obstet Gynecol 1970; 108:349–355.
123. Queenan JT, Thompson W, Whitfield CR, et al: Amniotic fluid volumes in normal pregnancy. Am J Obstet Gynecol 1972; 114:34–38.
124. Queenan JT: Recurrent acute polyhydramnios. Am J Obstet Gynecol 1970; 106:625–626.
125. Raghavendra BN, Young BK, Greco MA, et al: Use of furosemide in pregnancies complicated by oligohydramnios. Radiology 1987; 165:455–458.
126. Ray D, Berger N, Enson R: Hydramnios in association with unilateral fetal hydronephrosis. J Clin Ultrasound 1982; 10:82–84.
127. Reece EA, Lockwood CJ, Rizzo N, et al: Intrinsic intrathoracic malformations of the fetus: Sonographic detection and clinical presentation. Obstet Gynecol 1987; 70:627–632.
128. Rosenberg ER, Bowie JD: Failure of furosemide to induce diuresis in a growth-retarded fetus. AJR 1984; 142:485–486.
129. Rosenfeld CR, Coln CD, Duenhoelter JH: Fetal cervical teratoma as a cause of polyhydramnios. Pediatrics 1979; 64:176–179.
130. Rutherford SE, Smith CV, Phelan JP, et al: Four-quadrant assessment of amniotic fluid volume. Interobserver and intraobserver variation. J Reprod Med 1987; 32:587–589.
131. Schroder H, Gilbert RD, Power GG: Urinary and hemodynamic responses to blood volume changes in fetal sheep. J Dev Physiol 1984; 6:131–141.
132. Schruefer JJ, Seeds AE, Behrman RE, et al: Changes in amniotic fluid volume and total solute concentration in the rhesus monkey following replacement with distilled water. Am J Obstet Gynecol 1972; 112:807–815.
133. Sedin G, Hammarlund K, Nilsson GE, et al: Water transport through the skin of newborn infants. Ups J Med Sci 1981; 86:27–31.
134. Seeds AE: Current concepts of amniotic fluid dynamics. Am J Obstet Gynecol 1980; 138:575–586.
135. Seeds JW, Cefalo RC: Anomalies with hydramnios—Diagnostic role of ultrasound. Contrib Gynecol Obstet 1984; 23:32–43.
136. Seeds JW, Cefalo RC, Herbert WNP, et al: Hydramnios and maternal renal failure: Relief with fetal therapy. Obstet Gynecol 1984; 64:26s–29s.
137. Seller MJ, Child AH: Raised maternal serum alpha-fetoprotein, oligohydramnios and the fetus. Lancet 1980; 1:317–315.
138. Semchyshyn S, Mangurten H, Benawra R, et al: Fetal tumor, antenatal diagnosis and its implications. J Reprod Med 1982; 27:231–234.
139. Shimokawa H, Hara K, Fukuda A, et al: Idiopathic hydrops fetalis successfully treated in utero. Obstet Gynecol 1988; 71(suppl):984–986.
140. Sieck U, Ohlsson A: Fetal polyuria and hydramnios associated with Bartter's syndrome. Obstet Gynecol 1984; 63(suppl):22–24.

141. Sivit CJ, Hill MC, Larsen JW, et al: Second-trimester polyhydramnios: Evaluation with ultrasound. Radiology 1987; 165:467–469.

142. Sivit CJ, Hill MC, Larsen JW, et al: The sonographic evaluation of fetal anomalies in oligohydramnios between 16 and 30 weeks' gestation. AJR 1986; 146:1277–1281.

143. Sowers SG, Nelson LH, Burton BK: Raised maternal serum alpha-fetoprotein and severe oligohydramnios. Proceedings of March of Dimes Birth Defects Foundation Birth Defects Conference, Birmingham, Alabama, 1982, p 139.

144. Svigos JM: Early mid-trimester oligohydramnios: A sign of poor fetal prognosis. Aust N Z J Obstet Gynaecol 1987; 27:90–91.

145. Swischuk LE, Richardson CJ, Nichols MM, et al: Bilateral pulmonary hypoplasia in the neonate. AJR 1979; 133:1057–1063.

146. Swischuk LE, Richardson CJ, Nichols MM, et al: Primary pulmonary hypoplasia in the neonate. J Pediatr 1979; 95:573–577.

147. Taylor J, Garite TJ: Premature rupture of membranes before fetal viability. Obstet Gynecol 1984; 64:615–620.

148. Thibeault DW, Beatty EC, Hall RT, et al: Neonatal pulmonary hypoplasia with premature rupture of fetal membranes and oligohydramnios. J Pediatr 1985; 107:273–277.

149. Thomas IT, Smith DW: Oligohydramnios, cause of the nonrenal features of Potter's syndrome, including pulmonary hypoplasia. J Pediatr 1974; 84:811–814.

150. Thomas RL, Hess LW, Johnson TRB: Prepartum diagnosis of limb-shortening defects with associated hydramnios. Am J Perinatol 1987; 4:293–299.

151. Van Regemorter N, Vamos E, DeFleur V, et al: Pathological pregnancies. Results of amniotic fluid studies and fetal outcome. Acta Obstet Gynecol Scand 1986; 65:27–32.

152. Vintzileos AM, Campbell WA, Nochimson DJ, et al: Degree of oligohydramnios and pregnancy outcome in patients with premature rupture of membranes. Obstet Gynecol 1985; 66:162–167.

153. Vintzileos AM, Turner GW, Campbell WA, et al: Polyhydramnios and obstructive renal failure: A case report and review of the literature. Am J Obstet Gynecol 1985; 152:883–885.

154. Wallenburg HCS, Wladimiroff JW: The amniotic fluid. II: Polyhydramnios and oligohydramnios. J Perinat Med 1977; 5:233–243.

155. Weinbaum PJ, Vintzileos AM, Campbell WA, et al: Acute development of oligohydramnios in a pregnancy complicated by chronic hypertension and superimposed pre-eclampsia. Am J Perinatol 1986; 3:47–49.

156. Weir PE, Ratten GJ, Beischer NA: Acute polyhydramnios—A complication of monozygous twin pregnancy. Br J Obstet Gynaecol 1979; 86:849–853.

157. Weissman A, Zimmer EZ: Acute polyhydramnios recurrent in four pregnancies. A case report. J Reprod Med 1987; 32:65–66.

158. Wigglesworth JS, Desai R, Guerrini P: Fetal lung hypoplasia: Biochemical and structural variations and their possible significance. Arch Dis Child 1981; 56:606–615.

159. Wintour EM, Barnes A, Brown EH, et al: Regulation of amniotic fluid volume and composition in the ovine fetus. Obstet Gynecol 1978; 52:689–693.

160. Wladimiroff JW: Effect of furosemide on fetal urine production. Br J Obstet Gynaecol 1975; 82:221–224.

161. Wong WS, Filly RA: Polyhydramnios associated with fetal limb abnormalities. AJR 1983; 140:1001–1003.

162. Zamah NM, Gillieson MS, Walters JH, et al: Sonographic detection of polyhydramnios: A five-year experience. Am J Obstet Gynecol 1982; 143:523–527.

Maternal Serum AFP Screening

George R. Leopold, M.D.

Those practicing modern obstetrical sonography must recognize the value of combining their interpretations with other indicators of fetal well-being. Sonography does not exist in a vacuum, and to fathom the complexities of fetal life, a wise physician takes advantage of all possible clues. Nowhere is this statement more valid than in analysis of alpha-fetoprotein (AFP) values of amniotic fluid and maternal serum. Initially designed for prenatal identification of neural tube defects, AFP testing has also been found to be useful for detecting a variety of other abnormalities. Over the past 30 years, these have evolved into extremely useful adjunctive tests and are now the basis for screening programs in many countries of the world.

This chapter presents an overview of alpha-fetoprotein (AFP) and the role of sonography in interpreting both high and low levels. Related discussion may be found in chapters addressing the spine and neural tube defects (see Chapter 6), abdominal wall defects (see Chapter 11), placental abnormalities (see Chapter 16), and chromosome abnormalities (see Chapter 17).

BACKGROUND

Neural Tube Defects

Neural tube defects (NTDs) include anencephaly, encephalocele, and various forms of spinal dysraphism. These are second in incidence only to cardiac malformations as major congenital anomalies.[43] Although regional variations are marked (suggesting some yet unknown environmental factors), NTDs occur in approximately 1 in 1,000 live births. The vast majority of NTDs are sporadic; the recurrence risk for NTDs is generally quoted as 3%–5%.

Anencephaly is the most severe type of NTD and comprises 40%–50% of cases. Since the sonographic diagnosis of anencephaly is highly reliable and anencephaly is a uniformly lethal disorder, pregnancy termination may be offered at any age of gestation. Encephalocele (5% of NTDs) is also usually associated with a poor outcome, although it is not universally fatal. If the pregnancy is continued, counseling should be done in consultation with neurosurgeons who will help treat the child after birth.

Spinal dysraphism, which comprises 40%–50% of NTDs, presents the most difficult counseling problems, since most infants survive with their deformity. In 90% of cases the defect is "open," while in the remainder, skin covers the defect ("closed defect"). This is of great significance, since in the latter case, there will be no elevation of AFP values in either amniotic fluid or maternal serum, and sonography will be the sole means of detection. With either type, the prognosis for the fetus varies greatly, although, in general, a worse prognosis is associated with the more proximal location of the spinal defect.[43]

Alpha-fetoprotein

The presence of "fetospecific" substances was suspected for many years prior to their demonstration in the fetal calf by Pedersen.[37] In 1956, Bergstrand and Czar, performing protein electrophoresis on human amniotic fluid, were the first to report a new fraction migrating between albumin and alpha-1-globulin. Its proximity to the peak of albumin is probably at least partially responsible for early detection difficulties. Later, this substance was named alpha-fetoprotein (AFP) by Gitlin, and this designation was officially adopted by the International Agency for Research on Cancer in 1952.[37]

AFP is a glycoprotein with a molecular weight of approximately 70,000. In the human, production of this material is initially from the yolk sac for 4 to 8 weeks following conception. Subsequently, fetal liver is the major source of AFP, with trace amounts also produced by the mucosa of the stomach and small bowel. In lower species of life, the yolk sac is of lesser importance, and gastric mucosa is the principle source of AFP.

Although much is known about AFP, the precise function of this material remains uncertain. Before albumin becomes the major protein of the fetus, some believe it serves as the principle oncotic substance of the fetal vascular system. Others have postulated an anti-immune role, preventing the mother from rejecting the fetus as foreign protein. Those interested in a detailed treatise of the biochemistry of AFP are referred to the excellent review by Lau and Linkins.[37]

DISTRIBUTION OF AFP

Figure 4–1 shows the normal production, pathways, and compartments for AFP in humans.[27] Fetal serum concentration of AFP peaks at 12–13 weeks' gestation at a level of approximately 3,000 µg/ml before falling dramatically (Fig 4–2).[43] Production of AFP actually increases until about 32 weeks of gestation, but concentrations fall because of a dilution effect caused by rapid fetal growth.

AFP in the fetal serum passes through the glomeruli intact and is then reabsorbed in the renal tubules. Normally, only a small amount escapes and appears in the fetal urine and amniotic fluid. The concentration of amniotic fluid AFP (AF-AFP) is approximately 200 times less than that of the fetal serum in midpregnancy. Just as with fetal serum, concentrations peak at around 13 weeks' gestation (see Fig 4–2). Measurable quantities of AF-AFP exist prior to the onset of fetal renal function, presumably secondary to simple transdermal diffusion.

AFP normally appears in very low concentrations in the maternal serum. Unlike fetal serum and amniotic fluid AFP levels, maternal serum AFP (MS-AFP) peaks at 28 to 32 weeks' gestation, with the highest concentrations reaching 500 ng/ml (one nanogram = one billionth of a gram). Between 16 to 20 weeks' gestation, levels of AFP in the maternal serum are approximately

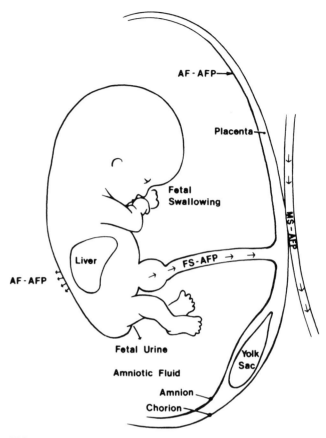

FIG 4–1.
Schematic drawing showing the production and distribution of AFP into its three compartments: Fetal tissues; amniotic fluid; and maternal serum. (From Glick P, Pohlson E, Resta R, et al: Maternal serum alpha-fetoprotein is a marker for fetal anomalies in pediatric surgery. J Ped Surg 1988; 23:16–20. Used by permission.)

100,000 times less than found in the fetal serum.[43] Radioimmunoassay techniques are necessary for quantitative determinations of such low MS-AFP.

The precise mechanism by which AFP enters maternal serum remains unclear. Comparisons of AF-AFP and MS-AFP in patients indicate that the relationship is non–linear, speaking against a simple diffusion gradient. Nevertheless, the concept of diffusion appears valid for fetal abnormalities associated with elevated levels of MS-AFP, since AF-AFP levels are substantially higher in these cases. In comparison, elevated MS-AFP resulting from placental hemorrhage or placental abnormalities usually has normal levels of AF-AFP. It is also worthwhile to note that prior amniocentesis may cause elevation in MS-AFP, probably secondary to fetal-maternal transfusion,[68] but chorionic villus sampling (CVS) generally does not.[63]

Although it would seem logical to report the results of AFP concentrations in the amniotic fluid and maternal serum as absolute levels, this turns out to be

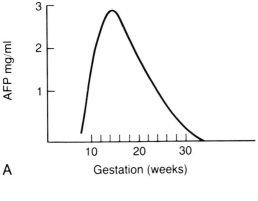

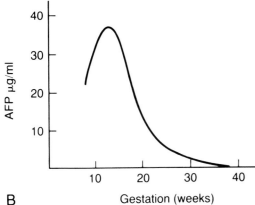

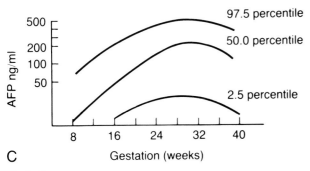

FIG 4–2.
Approximate relationship between alpha-fetoprotein values in *a)* fetal serum; *b)* amniotic fluid; and *c)* maternal serum. Note different units of measurement for each graph. (Habib A: Maternal serum alpha-fetoprotein: Its value in antenatal diagnosis of genetic disease and in obstetrical-gynecological care. Acta Obstet Gynecol Scand [Suppl] 1977; 61:1–72. Used by permission.)

impractical. Individual laboratories are often internally standardized, making direct comparisons difficult, if not impossible. It is therefore the custom to report AFP levels in terms of multiples of the median (MoMs). Since the median is the middle value in an array of values, it is not as sensitive as the mean to wide variations at either extreme of the measurement. However, this

method allows consistent reporting between institutions.

SIGNIFICANCE OF AFP TESTING

AF-AFP

In 1972, Brock and Sutcliffe were the first to report increased levels of AF-AFP in a patient bearing a fetus with neural tube defect,[8] a finding soon confirmed by others.[12, 42, 45, 71] The United Kingdom Collaborative Study found that using a series of cutoff levels that varied from 2.5 MoM at 13–15 weeks and 4.0 MoM at 22–24 weeks, elevated AF-AFP identified 98% of cases of anencephaly and 98% of cases of open spina bifida.[72] Only 0.5% of normal fetuses had AF-AFP levels above the cutoff level for a specificity of 99.5%.[72]

Despite the very high sensitivity and specificity of AF-AFP, less than one half of pregnancies with elevated AF-AFP actually result from those affected by an open NTD, because of the low prevalence of NTDs in the general population.[43] Since absolute levels of AFP are highly dependent on the age of gestation, poor obstetrical dating is by far the most common reason for "elevations" (the same is true for maternal serum screening). Abnormally high values of AFP also occur if the sample of amniotic fluid contains even small amounts of fetal blood, because of the high concentration gradient normally present between fetal blood and amniotic fluid. In this situation, Kleihauer testing can identify fetal contamination of blood in the sample. Other causes of elevated AF-AFP include previous fetal demise (presumably due to tissue autolysis) and other congenital anomalies, notably anterior wall defects.

The specificity of analyzing amniotic fluid for neural tube defects is significantly improved by also testing for acetylcholinesterase.[14, 46] This substance, normally present at synapses to facilitate impulse transmission, should be distinguished from the more abundant "pseudocholinesterases" found in many tissues. With the current technique that uses slab gel electrophoresis, acetylcholinesterase is a purely qualitative test, yielding either a positive or negative result. Occasionally, however, faint bands of activity may be identified, and this has been termed an inconclusive or indeterminate result. An inconclusive test is a more common, but less ominous finding early in gestation, but is frequently associated with congenital anomalies after 20 weeks.[22]

Large studies have found that 95.5% of fetuses with NTDs will have a positive acetylcholinesterase result,[4, 22, 72] and false-positive tests occur in less than 1% of cases.[38] In the presence of both elevated

AFP and acetylcholinesterase in the amniotic fluid, the chance of having a fetal neural tube defect is 99.5%.[14,71] Therefore, if this information is known prior to sonographic examination, the sonographer should have a very high suspicion of a NTD or other congenital anomaly. On the other hand, acetylcholinesterase is not an infallible test, and a normal ultrasound examination may alter the interpretation of a positive or indeterminate result.[22,38]

A positive acetylcholinesterase result does not significantly alter the differential diagnosis since, like AFP, acetylcholinesterase can become elevated from fetal blood admixture, abdominal wall defects, cystic hygroma, hydrops, or from transudation of plasma through the skin after fetal death.[22,43] However, other congenital anomalies are more likely to show a weakly positive result. A higher ratio of acetylcholinesterase to pseudocholinesterase has also been found to be useful for distinguishing NTDs from abdominal wall defects.[10]

MS-AFP

Although extremely valuable, measurements of AF-AFP are not suitable for mass screening surveys because of the invasive nature and expense of amniocentesis. As correctly predicted by Brock and Sutcliffe, analysis of MS-AFP would overcome this difficulty.[8] Initial series prior to 1970 showed AFP in the sera of very few patients, but it soon became apparent that this was secondary to the insensitivity of the gel diffusion technique. With the advent of radioimmunoassays, many authors quickly reported the ability to detect serum

levels as low as 10 ng/ml. These developments led to testing with AFP.

Those factors responsible for elevation of AF-AFP also cause similar changes in maternal serum. Typical MS-AFP curves for a population of normals, anencephaly, and open spina bifida are shown in Figure 4–3.[71] It is apparent that while there is reasonable separation between normals and those with neural tube defect, it is not perfect. Cutoff levels between 2.0 and 3.0 MoM have been utilized, with most centers using 2.5 MoM for a singleton gestation. The sensitivity of detecting NTDs could be improved by lowering this figure, but this would also increase the number of normal patients who would then require further extensive testing (Table 4–1). Similarly, raising the threshold level could avoid testing many normal patients, but would also overlook a greater number of fetuses with a NTD.

Optimal interpretation of MS-AFP levels also takes into account other contributing factors such as maternal weight, diabetes mellitus, and race. The prevalence of neural tube defects in the community should also be considered, since this affects the positive predictive value of an abnormal test.[1]

MS-AFP SCREENING

The benefits and risks of routine screening for MS-AFP have been debated. The American College of Obstetricians and Gynecologists has supported AFP screening in the United States, although it has not endorsed it for all women in all communities. Obstacles

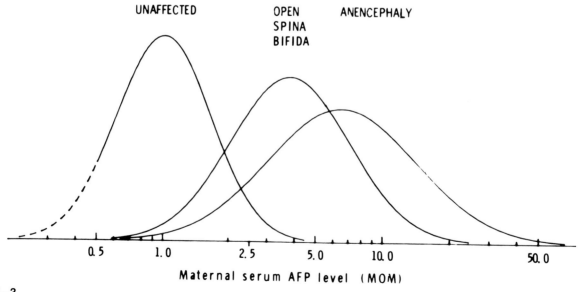

FIG 4–3.
Distribution of maternal serum alpha-fetoprotein (MS-AFP) values in a series of normal patients and in patients carrying a fetus with spina bifida or anencephaly. (Wald NJ, Cuckle HS: Neural tube defects: Screening and biochemical diagnosis. Prenat Diagn 1983; 3:219–241. Used by permission.)

TABLE 4–1.

Comparison of Normal and Abnormal Pregnancies for Various Cut-off Levels of Maternal Serum AFP Between 16 to 18 Weeks Gestation*

| Outcome | Cut-off Level Expressed as Multiple of the Normal Median | | |
	2.0 (%)	2.5 (%)	3.0 (%)
Anencephaly	90	88	84
Open spina bifida	91	79	70
All spina bifida	83	69	60
Normal singleton	7.2	3.3	1.4

*Adapted from UK Collaborative Study on alpha-fetoprotein in relation to neural-tube defects: Maternal-serum-alpha fetoprotein measurement in antenatal screening for anencephaly and spina bifida in early pregnancy. Lancet 1977; 1:1323–1332.

to routine screening include the economic costs involved; the lack of suitable or standardized laboratory testing, especially in remote areas; and the risks resulting from false-positive tests. Most of these obstacles have now been overcome, and the question appears to be not should we routinely screen MS-AFP, but rather how should we implement such programs.

A variety of different approaches has been adopted in the implementation of MS-AFP screening and in the evaluation of women found to have elevated levels.[23, 24, 58] In 1986, California began a statewide screening program with coordinated regional centers.[66] Participation in the program is voluntary, but non-participants must sign a statement of "informed consent/refusal." The fee to individual patients (now $49) is somewhat in excess of that required for the AFP test itself, but women found to have elevated AFP levels are then offered comprehensive evaluation (targeted sonogram and amniocentesis) at one of nine regional centers at no additional cost. In this way, all participating patients help to pay for those patients found to have elevated levels, and patients who may be unable to afford expensive tests are assured of equal access to AFP screening.

Despite some opposition,[36] the California State program appears to be successful, with over 500,000 women screened to date. In the first year of the program 176,000 women were screened. Of these, 122 neural tube defects were identified, including 71 cases of anencephaly, 40 cases of spina bifida, and 11 cases of encephalocele (R. Filly, personal communication). At the same time, 56 abdominal wall defects were identified.

Since sonography can never be 100% accurate in detecting congenital anomalies, some insist amniocentesis must follow every apparently normal ultrasound study.[23] Others, however, maintain that each case must be individualized and consider adequacy of visualiza-

tion, level of AFP, etc.[59] Presently, each center must make its own decision in this matter.

ROLE OF SONOGRAPHY IN EVALUATING HIGH MS-AFP VALUES

Commonly cited etiologies for elevated maternal serum alpha-fetoprotein (MS-AFP) are listed in Table 4–2. Prenatal sonography can help identify one or

TABLE 4–2.

Causes and Associations of Elevated Maternal Serum AFP

Incorrect dates
Multiple gestation
Neural tube defects
  Anencephaly
  Exencephaly
  Encephalocele
  Spina bifida
Abdominal wall defects
  Gastroschisis
  Omphalocele
  Cloacal exstrophy
  Bladder exstrophy
  Ectopia cordis
  Limb-body wall complex
Gastrointestinal obstruction
  Esophageal atresia
  Duodenal atresia
  Annular pancreas
Renal anomalies
  Congenital nephrosis
  Renal agenesis
  Urinary tract obstruction
  Polycystic kidney disease
Other
  Sacrococcygeal teratoma
  Epignathus
  Amniotic band syndrome
  Cystic hygroma
  Skin defects
  Pilonidal cyst
  Cystadenomatoid malformation
  Necrosis of fetal liver
  Liver tumor
  Chromosome abnormalities (trisomies 18, 13, Turner's syndrome, triploidy)
Placental/amniotic fluid abnormalities
  Placental or cord hematoma
  Chorioangioma
  Umbilical cord hemangioma
  Oliogohydramnios
Fetal demise
Maternal liver disease
  Hepatocellular carcinoma
  Hepatitis
Unexplained

more of these etiologies for many patients referred with elevated MS-AFP. A targeted sonogram performed by skilled ultrasonographers has been found to be of particular benefit in identifying fetal malformations associated with elevated MS-AFP.[31]

Incorrect Dates

Although MS-AFP screening was primarily designed to detect neural tube defects, less than 5% of patients initially reported as having an elevated test actually carry a fetus with a NTD.[43] Incorrect dating is a common reason for false-positive results; from 30% to 40% of patients with high AFP levels suffer only from incorrect dating. Since mean values are strongly dependent upon the actual age of the gestation, those in a more advanced state of pregnancy than suggested by their apparent menstrual dates may appear to be elevated. Recalculation following determination of correct gestational age eliminates the need for further study in this group.

Multiple Gestation

Multiple fetuses account for approximately 10% of high values in screening programs. If amniocentesis is performed and AF-AFP is examined, however, it is usually normal, since nearly all fetuses are contained within their own amniotic sac. In cases without a membrane (e.g., monoamniotic, monochorionic twinning), AF-AFP values may also be elevated.[67]

Sonographers should realize that an elevated MS-AFP in association with a multiple gestation should not automatically be ascribed to that process. In fact, the incidence of neural tube defects in twins is considerably higher (up to 20 times) than in singleton gestations, especially for monozygotic twins. Therefore, this diagnosis should prompt increased awareness and stimulate detailed sonographic search for these anomalies. If amniocentesis is performed in the presence of an anomalous twin, the AF-AFP concentration in the sac of the normal co-twin depends on placental anatomy and diffusion across the intervening membrane. In twins with discordant AF-AFP and acetylcholinesterase levels, Stiller and associates found that unaffected twins with a dichorionic, diamniotic membrane had normal AF-AFP levels, whereas unaffected twins with a monochorionic, diamniotic membrane had elevated AF-AFP and acetylcholinesterase levels.[67]

Fetal Demise

If fetal demise occurs before the maternal sample is drawn, markedly elevated MS-AFP levels result. This presumably is a reflection of autolysis of fetal tissue and liberation of AFP, but there is some indication that fetal distress itself causes elevated AF-AFP even prior to demise.[28] The role of real-time sonography in establishing fetal life is apparent in this situation.

Neural Tube Defects

AFP screening was originally designed to detect NTDs and, indeed, this remains its primary utility. As suggested by Brock and Sutcliffe, elevated MS-AFP apparently reflects high levels of AFP in the amniotic fluid, and this in turn results from transudation of AFP across exposed neural tissue.[8] As might be expected, the very highest AFP values occur with anencephaly and the lowest levels occur with closed spinal defects. Some authors have calculated the risk of having a neural tube defect based on the level of MoM. While, in general, the prognosis becomes worse with higher levels of AFP, in any individual case it is difficult to make assumptions based on this hypothesis.[49]

The potential for even experienced ultrasonographers to miss small spinal defects before 20 weeks has been emphasized.[23, 39, 69] Therefore, sonographic evaluation of patients with elevated MS-AFP requires a careful evaluation by trained sonographers to identify congenital defects such as small spinal defects (Fig 4–4) or small encephaloceles (Fig 4–5). Fortunately, sonographic recognition of cranial findings that have been associated with neural tube defects has been found to be of great value in conjunction with a MS-AFP screening program (see Chapter 6).[50, 51]

Other Congenital Abnormalities

A variety of other congenital anomalies has been associated with elevated MS-AFP levels. These can be categorized by their mechanism of elevating MS-AFP or into groups of anomalies, as follows: 1) abdominal wall defects, sacrococcygeal teratoma, cystic hygroma, skin defects, and other anomalies resulting in exposure of fetal tissue to amniotic fluid;[15, 32, 54] 2) proximal gastrointestinal obstructions;[43] 3) renal anomalies;[2, 43, 69] and 4) otherwise unexplained (for example, cystadenomatoid malformation).[33] Ordinarily, most such anomalies should be easily detected by sonography, although some (for example, skin defects) are not.

Following NTDs, abdominal wall defects are the second most common type of anomalies identified in most AFP screening programs. Early detection of such defects is an important secondary benefit of AFP screening. Figure 4–6 shows the normal distribution of MS-AFP in fetuses with gastroschisis, omphalocele, and normal controls. Fetuses with gastroschisis usually are

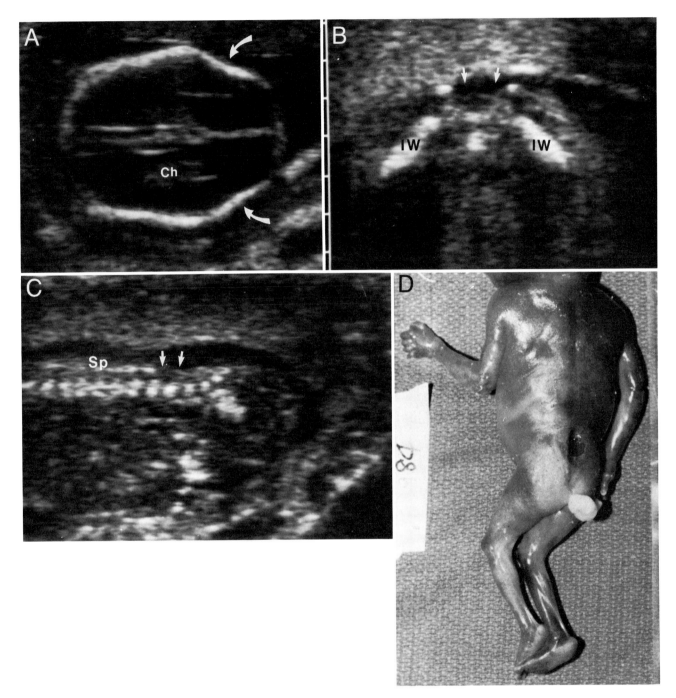

FIG 4–4.
Myelomeningocele. **A,** transverse scan of cranium at level of lateral ventricles demonstrates "lemon" deformity of frontal calvarium *(curved arrows)*. Note minimal separation of the choroid *(Ch)* from the medial ventricular wall. **B,** transverse scan demonstrates small dysraphic defect *(arrows)* without a surrounding sac at the lower lumbar spine. *IW* = iliac wing. **C,** longitudinal view of the spine *(Sp)* shows absence of overlying skin and dorsal ossification centers *(arrows)*. **D,** postmortem photogram confirms small open defect of lower lumbar spine.

FIG 4–5.
Encephalocele with Meckel-Gruber syndrome. Transverse scan in a woman with elevated MS-AFP demonstrates a small encephalocele *(arrows)* protruding through a posterior cranial defect *(open arrows)*. Oligohydramnios and cystic kidneys were also demonstrated. Meckel-Gruber syndrome was confirmed at postmortem examination. The woman had recurrence of Meckel-Gruber syndrome in subsequent pregnancies. *A* = anterior; *P* = posterior.

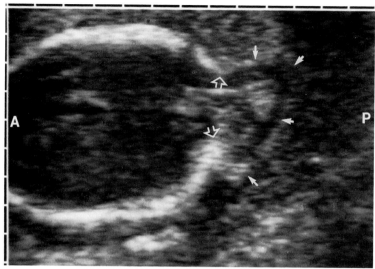

associated with high AFP levels, since eviscerated bowel comes into direct contact with the amniotic fluid (Fig 4–7). In comparison, the limiting membrane of omphalocele presents a relative barrier to amniotic fluid, and AFP levels are both generally lower and show a broader range than observed with gastroschisis (Fig 4–8).

It is currently unclear why renal and gastrointestinal abnormalities are sometimes associated with elevated levels of MS-AFP. Increased proteinuria has been postulated for some types of renal anomalies, such as congenital nephrosis. However, other renal abnormalities, such as renal agenesis or autosomal recessive polycystic kidney disease, are not associated with proteinuria after birth and do not affect the glomeruli.[2, 69] Secondary oligohydramnios may be an important contributing factor, since it has frequently been associated with elevated MS-AFP, even in the absence of renal anomalies (Fig 4–9).[34, 60, 62] However, in fetuses without renal abnormalities, oligohydramnios may simply reflect an underlying placental disorder that results in increased fetal-maternal transfer of AFP. The association of elevated MS-AFP with proximal bowel obstructions suggests that fetal swallowing and digestion are somehow important for AFP metabolism.

Chromosome abnormalities are probably associated with elevated MS-AFP because of coexistent malformations. For example, triploidy may be associated with elevated MS-AFP because of either the oligohydramnios or placental abnormalities that are characteristic of this disorder.[52] Similarly, neural tube defects, renal disorders, and bowel obstructions are commonly found in fetuses with other types of aneuploidy.

Some types of anomalies surprisingly are not associated with elevated AFP levels. For example, some facial clefts have been observed with normal levels of AFP, even within the amniotic fluid (Fig 4–10). This

FIG 4–6.
Distribution of MS-AFP values in patients carrying a fetus with gastroschisis or omphalocele compared to a control group. The lower values with omphalocele probably relate to the covering membrane usually present. (From Palomaki GE, Hill L, Knight G, et al: Obstet Gynecol 1988; 71:906–909. Used by permission.)

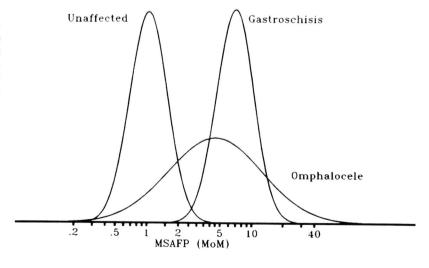

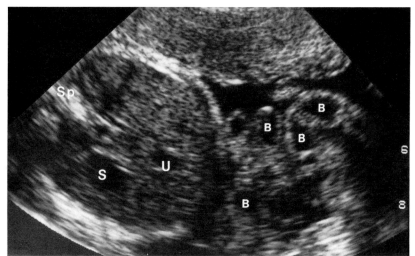

FIG 4–7.
Gastroschisis. Transverse scan at 24 weeks shows typical findings of gastroschisis with multiple segments of eviscerated bowel (*B*) that are not surrounded by a membrane. The absence of a surrounding membrane is associated with higher levels of AFP for gastroschisis than omphalocele. *Sp* = spine: *S* = stomach; *U* = umbilical vein.

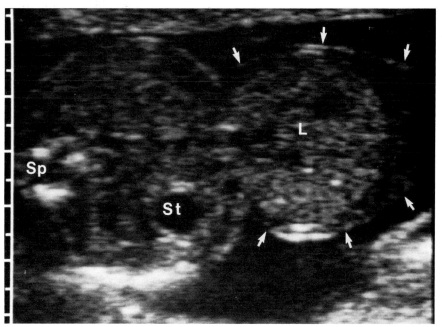

FIG 4–8.
Omphalocele. Scan at 22 weeks shows typical findings of omphalocele with liver (*L*) eviscerated through a central defect and surrounded by a membrane (*arrows*) representing the amnion. *Sp* = spine; *St* = stomach.

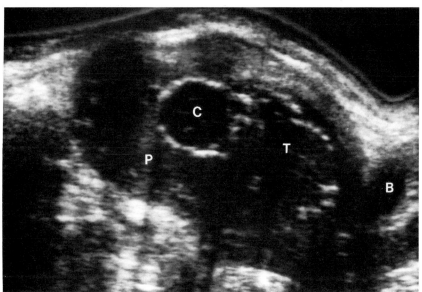

FIG 4–9.
Oligohydramnios and elevated MS-AFP. Longitudinal scan at 18 weeks in a woman referred with elevated MS-AFP (3.0 MoM) demonstrates marked oligohydramnios. There was no history of amniotic fluid leakage, and follow-up scans showed no change in oligohydramnios. Fetal kidneys and a urinary bladder were identified. Following voluntary termination of pregnancy at 22 weeks, postmortem examination confirmed normal fetal kidneys, and the oligohydramnios remained unexplained. *C* = cranium; *T* = trunk; *P* = placenta; *B* = maternal bladder.

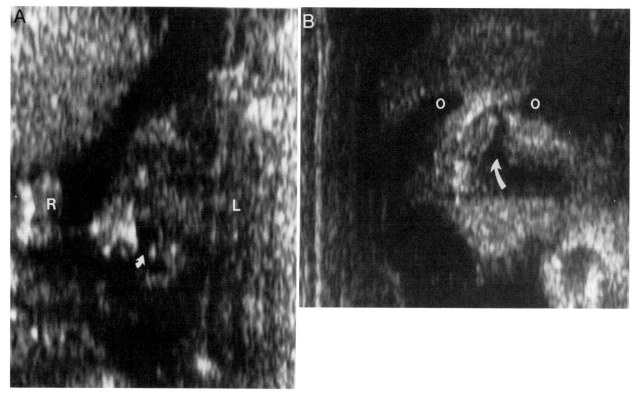

FIG 4–10.
Facial cleft and normal AFP. **A,** coronal scan at 17 weeks shows a facial cleft of the upper lip and palate (*curved arrow*). Amniotic fluid AFP and acetylcholinesterase were normal at the time of amniocentesis. *R* = right; *L* = left. **B,** follow-up sonogram at 30 weeks again demonstrates a facial cleft. *(curved arrow)*. This was confirmed on follow-up sonogram at 30 weeks and at the time of delivery. *O* = orbits.

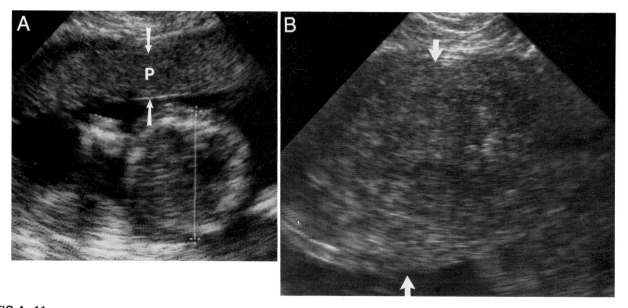

FIG 4–11.
Placental abruption. **A,** transverse scan at 18 weeks in a woman with elevated MS-AFP (2.5 MoM) demonstrates a normal-appearing placenta (*P*) with normal thickness. *F* = fetus. **B,** the patient returned 3 days later with acute onset of severe abdominal pain. Scan at this time demonstrates a markedly thickened placenta (*arrows*) representing an acute placental abruption and associated with fetal demise. Large abruption was confirmed at delivery.

suggests that such defects are not vascular and do not result in exposure of fetal blood to amniotic fluid.

Placental Hemorrhage/Dysfunction

Some observers have noted that patients with elevated MS-AFP may demonstrate increased numbers of lucent spaces within the placenta in excess of those seen in normal pregnancy.[7, 26, 55] Others report histopathologic changes of chronic villitis, infarction, and intervillous thrombosis in the placentas of some patients at delivery.[7, 61] One interesting theory suggests that these observations reflect an episode of fetal-maternal transfusion early in pregnancy. Since the concentration of AFP in the fetal serum is approximately 100,000 times greater than in the maternal serum during the mid trimester, it is easy to understand how a small amount of fetal blood may cause major elevations in MS-AFP.

If the pregnancy continues, the underlying placental abnormality may return to haunt the fetus in the form of placental insufficiency and increased perinatal loss (Fig 4–11).[11, 30, 42, 57, 68] Brumfield and her associates point out that the prediction of poor outcome from elevated MS-AFP does not apply to AF-AFP, adding some support to the theory that fetal-maternal transfusion is in some way responsible.[9] Vaginal bleeding has been shown to be an independent risk factor with elevated MS-AFP with risks being higher when both are present together.[29]

Vascular tumors of the placenta (chorioangioma) and umbilical cord (hemangioma) have also been associated with elevated MS-AFP levels (Fig 4–12). Indeed, markedly elevated AFP levels may result from these lesions. In these cases, elevated AFP is thought to be secondary to either hemorrhage in the tumor or increased transudation of fetal proteins to the amniotic fluid. Further discussion regarding placental abnormalities and elevated MS-AFP can be found in Chapter 16.

Unexplained

Even after thorough sonography and amniotic fluid analysis, there remains a large group of patients (>30%) for whom no explanation of elevated MS-AFP can be found. This unique subset of patients is regarded as high risk, since many studies document an increased risk of prematurity, low birth weight, fetal mortality (see Fig 4–11), and intrauterine growth retardation in this population.[11, 30, 42, 57, 68] These adverse outcomes can be explained by underlying placental dysfunction. A very rare cause of "unexplained" elevation of MS-AFP is maternal production of AFP, i.e., an AFP-secreting tumor (Fig 4–13).

LOW MS-AFP VALUES

In 1984, Merkatz et al. became the first to report the association of low MS-AFP values with chromosome abnormalities.[44] The index case was a fetus with trisomy 18. Following this report, many centers

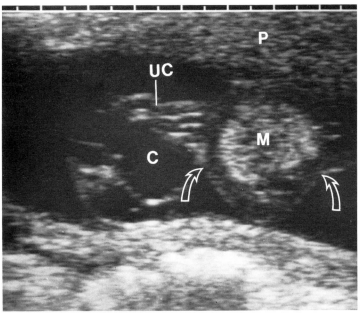

FIG 4–12.
Umbilical cord hemangioma. Scan in a woman with very high MS-AFP (31 MoM) demonstrates an echogenic mass, (*M*, demarcated by arrows) arising from the umbilical cord insertion site with the placenta (*P*). Also noted is a cystic component (*C*) which, when aspirated, yielded levels of AFP and acetylcholinesterase similar to those of serum. *UC* = umbilical cord. (Case reported by Resta et al.[58])

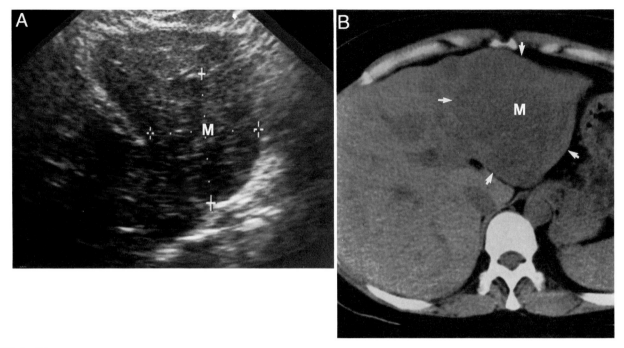

FIG 4–13.
Maternal hepatoma. **A,** transverse scan of the liver in a woman with elevated MS-AFP demonstrates a mass (*M*), demarcated by graticules, representing a hepatoma. **B,** non–contrast computed tomography scan confirms mass (*M*) in the left lobe of liver. AFP-secreting tumors are a very rare cause of elevated MS-AFP. (Courtesy of Harris Finberg, MD, Phoenix, AZ.)

confirmed an association of low MS-AFP with chromosome abnormalities, particularly with trisomy 21 and to a lesser extent with trisomy 18 and possibly 13.[4, 5, 18–20, 44, 65, 73] Some authors suggest that the low MS-AFP levels are of value only for detecting trisomy 21,[13] whereas others believe they are useful for identifying a variety of chromosome abnormalities, including triploidy and sex-chromosome abnormalities.[21]

While the reason for the association between low MS-AFP and chromosomal abnormalities has not yet been established, it cannot be explained by other factors such as maternal weight, birth weight, fetal sex, or diabetes mellitus. Wald et al. suggest that low AFP reflects immature placental function for gestational age.[73]

Screening patients for low levels of MS-AFP is of potential importance, since 75% to 80% of all infants with Down syndrome are born to mothers less than 35 years of age, and identification of all women with low MS-AFP levels (< 0.5 multiples of the median) could identify 20% to 30% of fetuses with Down syndrome. However, testing for low MS-AFP is still far from perfect for detecting Down syndrome, and it has not been universally accepted as a screening modality.[43, 56, 75] Figure 4–14 shows the distributions for a series of patients with Down syndrome and normal controls. Due to the overlap in AFP levels, screening for low MS-AFP levels would require testing 4%–8% of normal preg-

nancies.[19] The reliability of laboratory testing for low levels of MS-AFP is also of concern.[24, 34, 41]

Despite the potential problems involved, most centers that screen for elevated levels of MS-AFP now also screen for low levels of MS-AFP. Screening programs that utilize 0.4 and 2.5 MoMs as the lower and upper limits of normal will find they have approximately twice as many lows as highs to examine. Thus, programs which started as neural tube detection centers

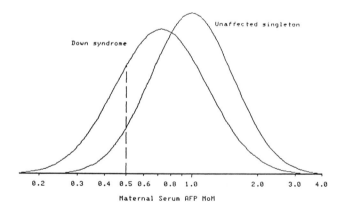

FIG 4–14.
Distribution of MS-AFP values in controls and a series of patients with Down syndrome. (From Wald NJ, Cuckle HS: Neural tube defects: Screening and biochemical diagnosis. Prenat Diagn 1983; 3:219–241. Used by permission.)

now find themselves with a considerably expanded task.

Some have suggested using age and MS-AFP concurrently to estimate more accurately the risk of Down syndrome.[17, 53] Since advanced maternal age and low MS-AFP are independent risk factors for trisomy 21, using both determinants together can detect more fetuses with trisomy 21 than can either alone (see Chapter 16).[53] Combining age and AFP can also provide a more precise estimate of risk for individual patients prior to choosing chromosome analysis.

ROLE OF SONOGRAPHY IN EVALUATING LOW MS-AFP VALUES

As with screening for high values of MS-AFP, there is a variety of reasons for results in the abnormally low range (Table 4-3). The role of sonography in evaluating these possibilities is described below.

Chromosomal Abnormalities

Sonography is not nearly as fruitful in identifying fetuses with chromosome abnormalities among patients with low values of MS-AFP as it is in identifying fetal anomalies associated with high levels of MS-AFP. Congenital anomalies that have been associated with trisomy 21 and that can be detected on prenatal sonography include cardiac anomalies, duodenal atresia, cystic hygroma, and hydrothorax. Although Benacerraf et al. have reported nuchal thickening in the early second trimester as a potentially useful indicator in Down syndrome,[5] others debate the utility of this finding. In short, sonographic examination of patients with low MS-AFP seldom yields definitive information about an underlying chromosomal abnormality.

Incorrect Dates

As with high levels of MS-AFP, interpretation of low levels is dramatically affected by calculation of ges-

TABLE 4-3.

Causes and Associations of Decreased Maternal Serum AFP

Chromosome abnormalities
Incorrect dates
Fetal death
Not pregnant
Hydatidiform mole
Unexplained

tational age from the last menstrual period. If a dating error is responsible, the patient usually believes she is further advanced in her pregnancy than is actually the case. Sonography performs a valuable function in eliminating concern for these patients by correcting dates.[48]

Fetal Demise

Since fetal function is necessary for continued production of AFP, fetal death some time before the blood sampling may be associated with low levels of MS-AFP.

Not Pregnant

Strangely, there are patients who enter screening who turn out not to be pregnant at all. In some cases the patient will actually have been pregnant, but fetal demise occurred much earlier in the gestation and values have now fallen to the normal non-pregnant level. Patients with any of the forms of molar pregnancy also present in this category, since high circulating levels of chorionic gonadotropin produce the side effects of pregnancy, but there is no fetus to produce AFP. In both of these situations, sonography provides a ready explanation of the findings.

Unexplained

The vast majority of patients with low MS-AFP levels remain unexplained following a thorough sonographic evaluation. Since sonography is usually unrewarding in this situation, amniocentesis is usually recommended for these patients. Unlike the situation with high values, unexplained lows do not appear to carry an adverse prognosis.[64]

FUTURE DEVELOPMENTS IN MATERNAL SERUM TESTING

Screening for low levels of MS-AFP in the first trimester has been shown to be feasible.[47] Detection of Down syndrome at an early age would be highly desirable. In another development, low levels of estriol and high levels of human chorionic gonadotropin (HCG) in the maternal serum have also been associated with chromosomally anomalous fetuses.[73] Like low AFP levels, low estriol and high HCG could be explained by placental function that is immature for gestational age.[73] In the future, maternal blood testing may include a battery of tests to define the specific risk of carrying a fetus with a chromosome abnormality.

REFERENCES

1. Adams MJ Jr, Windham GC, Greenberg JF, et al: Clinical interpretation of maternal serum alpha-fetoprotein concentrations. Am J Obstet Gynecol 1984; 148:241–254.
2. Balfour RP, Laurence KM: Raised serum AFP levels and fetal renal agenesis. Lancet 1980; i:317.
3. Barford D, Dickerman L, Johnson W: Alpha-fetoprotein: Relationship between maternal serum and amniotic fluid levels. Am J Obstet Gynecol 1985; 151:1038–1041.
4. Baumgarten A, Schoenfeld M, Mahoney MH, et al: Prospective screening for Down syndrome using maternal serum AFP. Lancet 1985; 1:1280–1281.
5. Benacerraf BR, Frigoletto FD Jr, Cramer DW: Down syndrome: Sonographic sign for diagnosis in the second trimester fetus. Radiology 1987; 163:811–813.
6. Bogart MH, Pandian MR, Jones OW: Abnormal maternal serum chorionic gonadotropin levels in pregnancies with fetal chromosomal abnormalities. Prenat Diagn 1987; 7:623–670.
7. Boyd PA, Keeling JW: Raised maternal serum alpha-fetoprotein in the absence of fetal abnormality—placental findings. A quantitative morphometric study. Prenat Diagn 1986; 6:369–373.
8. Brock DJH, Sutcliffe RG. Alpha-fetoprotein in the antenatal diagnosis of anencephaly and spina bifida. Lancet 1972; ii:197–199.
9. Brumfield C, Cloud G, Finley S, et al: Amniotic fluid alpha-fetoprotein levels and pregnancy outcome. Am J Obstet Gynecol 1987; 157:822–825.
10. Burton BK: Positive amniotic fluid acetylcholinesterase: Distinguishing between open defects of the neural tube and ventral wall defects. Am J Obstet Gynecol 1986; 155:984–986.
11. Burton BK, Dillard RG: Outcome in infants born to mothers with unexplained elevations of maternal serum alpha-fetoprotein. Pediatrics 1986; 77:582–586.
12. Burton BK, Sowers SG, Nelson LH: Maternal serum α-fetoprotein screening in North Carolina: Experience with more than twelve thousand pregnancies. Am J Obstet Gynecol 1983; 146:439–444.
13. Crandall BF, Matsumoto M, Perdue S: Amniotic fluid AFP in Down syndrome and other chromosome abnormalities. Prenat Diagn 1988; 8:255–262.
14. Crandall BF, Kasha W, Matsumoto M: Prenatal diagnosis of neural tube defects—experiences with acetylcholinesterase gel electrophoresis. Am J Med Genet 1982; 12:361–366.
15. Cruikshank SH, Granados JL: Increased amniotic acetylcholinesterase activity with a fetus papyraceus and aplasia cutis congenita. Obstet Gynecol 1988; 71:997–999.
16. Cuckle HS, Wald NJ, Lindenbaum RH: Maternal serum alpha-fetoprotein measurement: A screening test for Down's syndrome. Lancet 1984; 1:926–929.
17. Cuckle HS, Wald NJ, Thompson S: Estimating a woman's risk of having a pregnancy associated with Down's syndrome using her age and serum alpha-fetoprotein level. Br J Obstet Gynecol 1987; 94:387–402.
18. Davis RO, Cosper P, Huddleston JF, et al: Decreased levels of amniotic fluid alpha-fetoprotein associated with Down syndrome. Am J Obstet Gynecol 1985; 153:541–544.
19. DiMaio MS, Baumgarten A, Greenstein RM, et al: Screening for fetal Down's syndrome in pregnancy by measuring maternal serum alpha-fetoprotein levels. N Engl J Med 1987; 317:342–346.
20. Doran TA, Cadesky K, Wong PY, et al: Maternal serum alpha-fetoprotein and fetal autosomal trisomies. Am J Obstet Gynecol 1986; 154:277–281.
21. Drugan A, Dvorin E, Doppitch FC III, et al: Counseling for low maternal serum alpha-fetoprotein should emphasize all chromosome anomalies, not just Down syndrome! Obstet Gynecol 1989; 73:271–274.
22. Drugan A, Syner FN, Belsky R, et al: Amniotic fluid acetycholinesterase: Implications of an inconclusive result. Am J Obstet Gynecol 1988; 159:469–474.
23. Drugan A, Zador I, Syner F, et al: A normal ultrasound does not obviate the need for amniocentesis in patients with elevated serum alpha-fetoprotein. Obstet Gynecol 1988; 72:627–630.
24. Evans MI, Belsky RL, Clementino NA: Establishment of a collaborative university-commercial maternal serum α-fetoprotein screening program: A model for tertiary control. Am J Obstet Gynecol 1987; 156:1441–1449.
25. Farine D, Maidman J, Rubin S, et al: Elevated alpha-fetoprotein in pregnancy complicated by aplasia cutis after exposure to methamazole. Obstet Gynecol 1988; 71:996–997.
26. Fleischer AC, Kurtz AB, Wapner RJ, et al: Elevated alpha-fetoprotein and a normal fetal sonogram: Association with placental abnormalities. AJR 1988; 150:881–883.
27. Glick P, Pohlson E, Resta R, et al: Maternal serum alpha-fetoprotein is a marker for fetal anomalies in pediatric surgery. J Ped Surg 1988; 23:16–20.
28. Habib A: Maternal serum alpha-fetoprotein: Its value in antenatal diagnosis of genetic disease and in obstetrical-gynecological care. Acta Obstet Gynecol Scand [Suppl] 1977; 61:1–72.
29. Haddow JE, Knight GJ, Kloza EM, et al: Alpha-fetoprotein, vaginal bleeding and pregnancy risk. Br J Obstet Gynecol 1986; 93:589–593.
30. Hamilton MPR, Abdalla HI, Whitfield CR: Significance of raised maternal serum α-fetoprotein in singleton pregnancies with normally formed fetuses. Obstet Gynecol 1985; 65:465–470.
31. Hashimoto BE, Mahony BS, Filly RA, et al: Sonography, a complementary examination to alpha-fetoprotein testing for neural tube defects. J Ultrasound Med 1985; 4:307–310.
32. Hecht F, Hecht B, O'Keefe D: Sacrococcygeal teratoma: Prenatal diagnosis with elevated alpha-fetoprotein and acetylcholinesterase in amniotic fluid. Prenat Diagn 1982; 2:229–231.
33. Johnston RJ, McGahan JP, Hanson FW, et al: Type III congenital cystic adenomatoid malformation associated

with elevated maternal serum alpha-fetoprotein. J Perinatol 1987; 8:222–224.

33a. Kelly R, Nyberg DA, Mack LA, et al: Placental abnormalities and oligohydramnios in women with elevated alpha-fetoprotein: Comparison with normal controls. AJR, in press.

34. Knight GJ, Palomaki GE, Haddow GE: Maternal serum alpha-fetoprotein: A problem with a test kit. N Engl J Med 1986; 314:516.

35. Koontz WL, Seeds JW, Adams NJ, et al: Elevated maternal seum alpha-fetoprotein, second-trimester oligohydramnios, and pregnancy outcome. Obstet Gynecol 1983; 62:301–304.

36. Lasnover AL: Criticism of the California alpha-fetoprotein screening program. West J Med 1987; 146:100.

37. Lau L, Linkins S: Alpha-fetoprotein. Am J Obstet Gynecol 1976; 124:533–554.

38. Lee JES, Won WG, Falk RE, et al: False positive amniotic fluid acetylcholinesterase results: The need for a multifaceted approach to the prenatal diagnosis of neural tube defects. Obstet Gynecol 1985; 66:22s–24s.

39. Lindfors KK, McGahan JP, Tennant FP, et al: Midtrimester screening for open neural tube defects: Correlation of sonography with amniocentesis results. AJR 1987; 149:141–145.

40. Macri JN: Critical issue in prenatal maternal serum α-fetoprotein screening for genetic anomalies. Am J Obstet Gynecol 1986; 155:240.

41. Macri JN, Kasturi RV, Krantz DA, et al: Maternal serum alpha-fetoprotein screening. II: Potential pitfalls in low-volume decentralized laboratory performance. Am J Obstet Gynecol 1987; 156:533–535.

42. Macri JN, Weiss RR: Prenatal serum α-fetoprotein screening for neural tube defects. Higher perinatal loss with elevated levels. Obstet Gynecol 1982; 59:663–639.

43. Main DM, Mennuti MT: Neural tube defects: Issues in prenatal diagnosis and counselling. Obstet Gynecol 1986; 67:1–16.

44. Merkatz IR, Nitowsky HM, Macri JN, et al: An association between low maternal serum alpha-fetoprotein and fetal chromosome abnormalities. Am J Obstet Gynecol 1984; 148:886–894.

45. Milunsky A, Elliot A: Results and benefits of a maternal serum alpha-fetoprotein screening program. JAMA 1984; 252:1438–1442.

46. Milunsky A, Sapirstein V: Prenatal diagnosis of open neural tube defects using the amniotic fluid acetylcholinesterase assay. Obstet Gynecol 1981; 59:1–6.

47. Milunsky A, Wands J, Brambati B, et al: First-trimester maternal serum α-fetoprotein screening for chromosome defects. Am J Obstet Gynecol 1988; 159:1209–1213.

48. Nelson LH, Burton BK, Sowers SG: Ultrasonography in patients with low maternal serum alpha-fetoprotein. J Ultrasound Med 1987; 6:59–61.

49. Nelson LH, Bensen J, Burton BK: Outcomes in patients with unusually high maternal serum alpha-fetoprotein levels. Am J Obstet Gynecol 1987; 157:572–576.

50. Nicolaides KH, Campbell S, Gabbe SG: Ultrasound screening for spina bifida: Cranial and cerebellar signs. Lancet 1986; 2:72–74.

51. Nyberg DA, Mack LA, Hirsch J, et al: Abnormalities of fetal cranial contour in sonographic detection of spina bifida: Evaluation of the "lemon" sign. Radiology 1988; 167:387–392.

52. O'Brien WF, Knuppel RA, Kousseff B, et al: Elevated maternal serum alpha-fetoprotein in triploidy. Obstet Gynecol 1988; 71:994–995.

53. Palomaki GE, Haddow JE: Maternal serum α-fetoprotein, age, and Down syndrome risk. Am J Obstet Gynecol 1987; 156:460–463.

54. Palomaki GE, Hill L, Knight G, et al: Second trimester maternal serum alpha-fetoprotein levels in pregnancies associated with gastroschisis and omphalocele. Obstet Gynecol 1988; 71:906–909.

55. Perkes EA, Baim RS, Goodman KJ, et al: Second trimester placental changes associated with elevated maternal serum alpha-fetoprotein. Am J Obstet Gynecol 1982; 144:935–938.

56. Pueschel SM: Maternal alpha-fetoprotein screening for Down's syndrome. N Engl J Med 1987; 317:376–378.

57. Purdie DW, Young JL, Guthrie KA, et al: Fetal growth achievement and elevated maternal serum α-fetoprotein. Br J Obstet Gynaecol 1983; 90:433–436.

58. Resta RG, Luthy DA, Mahony BS: Umbilical cord hemangioma associated with extremely high alpha-fetoprotein levels. Obstet Gynecol 1988; 72:488–491.

59. Richards DS, Seeds JW, Katz VL, et al: Elevated maternal serum alpha-fetoprotein with normal ultrasound. Is amniocentesis always appropriate? A review of 26,069 screened patients. Obstet Gynecol 1988; 71:203–207.

60. Richards DS, Seeds JW, Katz VL, et al: Elevated maternal serum alpha-fetoprotein with oligohydramnios: Ultrasound evaluation and outcome. Obstet Gynecol 1988; 72:337–341.

61. Salafia CM, Silberman L, Herrera NE, et al: Placental pathology at term associated with elevated midtrimester maternal serum alpha-fetoprotein concentration. Am J Obstet Gynecol 1988; 158:1064–1066.

62. Seller MJ, Child AH: Raised maternal serum alpha-fetoprotein, oligohydramnios, and the fetus. Lancet 1980; i:317–318.

63. Sigler M, Colyer C, Rossiter J, et al: Maternal serum alpha-fetoprotein screening after chorionic villus sampling. Obstet Gynecol 1987; 70:875–877.

64. Simpson JL, Baum LD, Depp R, et al: Low maternal serum alpha-fetoprotein and perinatal outcome. Am J Obstet Gynecol 1987; 156:852–862.

65. Simpson JL, Baum LD, Marder R, et al: Maternal serum α-fetoprotein screening: Low and high values for detection of genetic abnormalities. Am J Obstet Gynecol 1986; 155:593–597.

66. Steinbrook R: In California, voluntary mass prenatal screening. Hastings Cent Rep 1986; 16:5–7.

67. Stiller RJ, Lockwood CJ, Belanger K, et al: Amniotic fluid α-fetoprotein concentration in twin gestation: Dependence on placental membrane anatomy. Am J Obstet Gynecol 1988; 158:1088–1092.

68. Thomsen S, Lennart I, Lange A, et al: Elevated maternal serum alpha-fetoprotein and perinatal outcome. Am J Obstet Gynecol 1983; 62:297–300.

69. Townsend RR, Goldstein RB, Filly RA, et al: Sonographic identification of autosomal recessive polycystic kidney disease associated with increased maternal serum/ amniotic fluid alpha-fetoprotein. Obstet Gynecol 1988; 71:1008–1012.

70. Tyrrell S, Howel D, Bark M, et al: Should maternal α-fetoprotein estimation be carried out in centers where ultrasound screening is routine? Am J Obstet Gynecol 1988; 158:1092–1099.

71. Wald NJ, Cuckle HS: Neural tube defects: Screening and biochemical diagnosis. Prenat Diagn 1983; 3:219–241.

72. Wald NJ, Cuckle HS, Brock DJH, et al: Maternal serum alpha-fetoprotein measurement in antenatal screening for anencephaly and spina bifida in early pregnancy. Report of U.K. Collaborative Study of alpha-fetoprotein in relation to neural tube defects. Lancet 1977; i:1323–1332.

73. Wald NJ, Cuckle HS, Densem JW, et al: Maternal serum screening for Down's syndrome in early pregnancy. Br Med J 1988; 297:883–887.

74. Willard DA, Moeschler JB. Placental chorioangioma: A rare cause of elevated amniotic fluid alpha-fetoprotein. J Ultrasound Med 1986; 5:221–222.

75. Wu LR: Maternal serum α-fetoprotein screening and Down's syndrome (letter). Am J Obstet Gynecol 1986; 155:1362.

Cerebral Malformations

David A. Nyberg, M.D.

Dolores H. Pretorius, M.D.

Cerebral malformations are some of the most common, yet most devastating of congenital anomalies. Because the vast majority of major cerebral disorders (holoprosencephaly, hydrocephalus, Dandy-Walker malformation) are well established early in embryologic development, they are potentially detectable on prenatal sonography before the time of fetal viability. Such malformations are often first discovered on "routine" obstetric sonograms, particularly when the sonogram is performed during the second trimester before polyhydramnios develops, or when the malformation is unassociated with spina bifida or other defects that might increase the maternal serum alpha-fetoprotein (MS-AFP). Importantly, prenatal sonography has proved to be exceedingly sensitive for detecting major cerebral malformations.

This chapter presents a systematic sonographic approach for imaging the fetal brain and for detecting major cerebral malformations. The pathogenesis, typical sonographic findings, prognosis, and options in management are discussed for each of the major cerebral malformations. Cerebral malformations related to neural tube defects are discussed separately (see Chapter 6), since they have a distinctive pathogenesis and are frequently referred for sonography in association with elevated MS-AFP.

EMBRYOGENESIS

The neural plate develops at approximately 18 to 20 days after conception (4.5 menstrual weeks) and subsequently forms the neural crest and neural tube.

The neural tube further differentiates into the brain and spinal cord. By the end of the fourth fetal week (sixth menstrual week), the brain segments into three primary vesicles: the forebrain (prosencephalon), midbrain (mesencephalon), and hindbrain (rhombencephalon) (Fig 5–1).[12]

At an early stage of development, the forebrain differentiates into the diencephalon and telencephalon. The telencephalic vesicles (future cerebral hemispheres) appear as outgrowths on either side of the diencephalon. The choroid plexus, which forms from an ependymal layer together with the overlying pia, invaginates into the lateral ventricles. The rapidly enlarging cerebral hemispheres grow and rotate over the dorsum of the diencephalon and mesencephalon (midbrain) to approach each other in the midline. Failure of this normal process of diverticularization and rotation results in holoprosencephaly.

By 8 to 10 menstrual weeks, the rhombencephalon can be demonstrated as a well-defined cystic area in the posterior aspect of the head.[3] This normal embryologic structure should not be mistaken for an abnormal cystic mass. The rhombencephalon differentiates into the metencephalon and myelencephalon with development of the pontine flexure. The metencephalon gives rise to the medulla, and the myelencephalon gives rise to the pons and cerebellum.[12] The ependyma and overlying pia form the tela choroidea of the fourth ventricle. The tela perforates in three places to form the foramina of Magendie and Luschka. Dysgenesis of the fourth ventricle results in the Dandy-Walker malformation.

The corpus callosum is a large bundle of white

FIG 5-1.

Normal brain development. **A,** diagramatic sketch of the brain vesicles, indicating the adult derivatives. **B,** diagram to illustrate normal brain development between 25 to 100 fetal days (6 to 18 menstrual weeks). (Part **A** from Moore KL: *The Developing Human.* Philadelphia, WB Saunders Co, 1988. Part **B** from Wigglesworth JS: *Perinatal Pathology.* Philadelphia, WB Saunders Co, 1984, pp 243-288.)

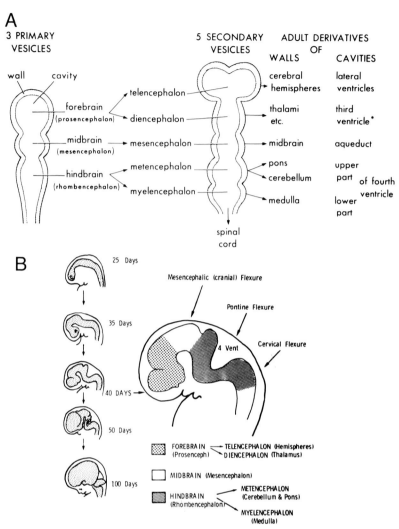

matter tracts that decussate between the cerebral hemispheres. Formation of the corpus callosum is a complex process that begins anteriorly at the genu and proceeds posteriorly to the splenium (Fig 5-2).[119] Unlike development of other major cerebral structures, this process does not begin until 8 menstrual weeks and is not complete until 18-20 weeks.[117, 119] Concomitantly, the septum pellucidum forms between the corpus callosum and fornices. Failure of corpus callosum development (complete or partial) results in agenesis of the corpus callosum.

The brain continues to grow and develop throughout the second and third trimester of pregnancy and during the first year of life (Fig 5-3). Development of the temporal horn during the second trimester pulls the posterior aspect of the lateral ventricles laterally and downward. Gyral and sulcal development, which are related to menstrual age, result from marked growth of the cerebral cortex (see Fig 5-3).[12] It is ob-

vious from this discussion that cranial size and normal neuroanatomic findings vary with gestational age. Correlation of head measurements with gestational age is shown in Appendix 1. Normal anatomic structure seen at term is shown in Figure 5-4.

SONOGRAPHIC APPROACH TO THE FETAL CEREBRUM

A systematic and routine sonographic approach is necessary to minimize errors in detecting cerebral malformations.[5] To this end, we suggest inclusion of three standard axial views (transthalamic, transventricular, and transcerebellar views) as part of all obstetric sonograms performed during the second and third trimesters (Fig 5-5). Two of these views (transthalamic and transventricular) are included in the basic guidelines adopted by the American Institute of Ultrasound in

Hydrocephalus

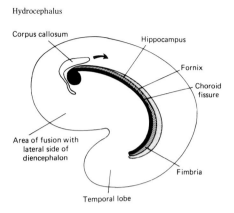

FIG 5–2.
Schematic drawing illustrating formation of the corpus callosum from anteriorly to posteriorly. (From Keeling JW (ed): *Fetal and Neonatal Pathology.* Springer-Verlag, 1987. Used by permission.)

Medicine, American College of Radiology, and the American College of Obstetricians and Gynecologists (see Chapter 1). The third view (transcerebellar) has been recommended by other authorities.[5, 13] The method for obtaining these views and their potential benefits are discussed further below. If abnormalities are demonstrated on these axial planes, then additional coronal and sagittal views may occasionally provide additional information.

The transthalamic view is the standard plane used for obtaining the biparietal diameter and head circumference (Appendix 1). At this level, one can also visual-

ize the frontal horns of the lateral ventricles, the cavum septi pellucidi between the frontal horns, and the Sylvian cisterns (Fig 5–6).[8] The cavum septi pellucidi should not be mistaken for the third ventricle, which is smaller and located more posteriorly between the thalami. Absence of the cavum septi pellucidi is a part of the malformations encompassed by holoprosencephaly and agenesis of the corpus callosum. However, the cavum septi pellucidi may also be difficult to visualize in some normal fetuses.

The transventricular view is obtained at a plane just superior to the transthalamic view (see Fig 5–5). Demonstration of the lateral cerebral ventricles in this view is essential for early detection of hydrocephalus. By 12–13 menstrual weeks, the echogenic choroid plexus should fill from side-to-side the lateral ventricle and dominate the appearance of the cerebral hemispheres (Fig 5–7). However, since the choroid plexus does not enter the frontal horn, this portion of the lateral ventricles will appear unusually prominent. The lateral and medial walls of the lateral ventricles run nearly parallel to the midline interhemispheric fissure at this time during the early second trimester. After about 18 weeks, the posterior aspect of the lateral ventricles (atria and occipital horns) are drawn laterally with the development of the temporal horns. Simultaneously, the ventricles and choroid also appear less pronounced with continued growth of the cerebral hemispheres (Fig 5–8). Although the lateral ventricles

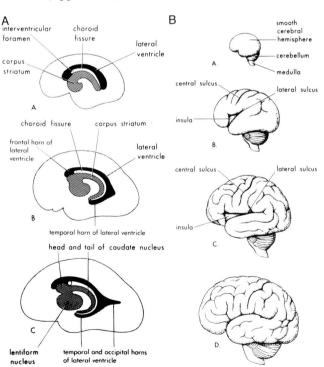

FIG 5–3.
Normal brain development. **A,** diagram showing internal development of the lateral ventricles and choroid at *A*, 15 menstrual weeks (13 fetal weeks), *B*, 23 menstrual weeks, and *C*, 34 menstrual weeks. Note development of the temporal horns. **B,** external view of brain development at *A*, 15 menstrual weeks (13 fetal weeks), *B*, 28 menstrual weeks, *C*, 37 menstrual weeks, and *D*, newborn. Note development of sulci and gyri. (From Moore KL: *The Developing Human.* Philadelphia, WB Saunders Co, 1988.)

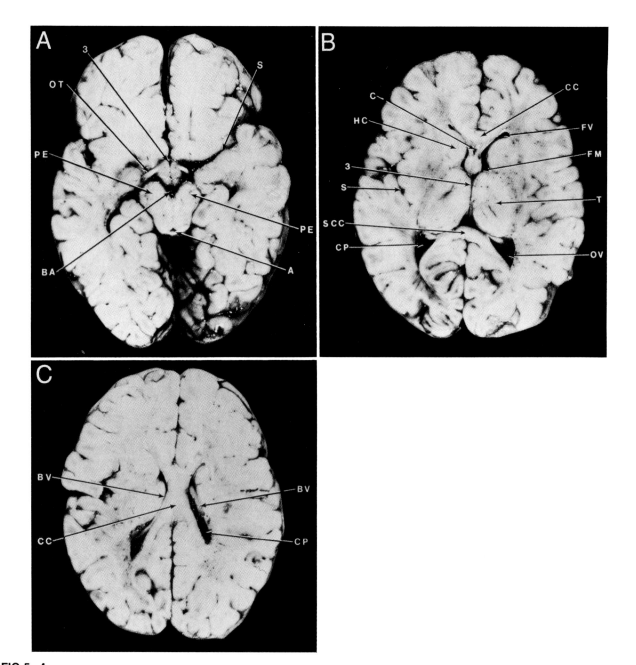

FIG 5–4.
Normal brain anatomy at term. Sections through **A,** the cerebral peduncles (midbrain), **B,** the thalami, and **C,** the lateral ventricles. *A* = aqueduct of Sylvius; *BA* = basilar artery; *BV* = body lateral ventricle; *C* = cavum septi pellucidi; *CC* = corpus callosum; *CP* = choroid plexus; *FM* = foramen of Monro; *FV* = frontal horn of lateral ventricle; *HC* = head of caudate nucleus; *OT* = optic tract; *OV* = occipital horn of lateral ventricle; *PE* = cerebral peduncle; *S* = sylvian fissure; *SCC* = splenium of the corpus callosum; *T* = thalamus; *3* = third ventricle. (From Mack LA, Alvord EC Jr: Neonatal cranial ultrasound: Normal appearances. *Seminars in Ultrasound,* vol 3. Philadelphia, Grune & Stratton, Inc, 1982, pp 216–230. Used by permission.)

NORMAL VENTRICLES

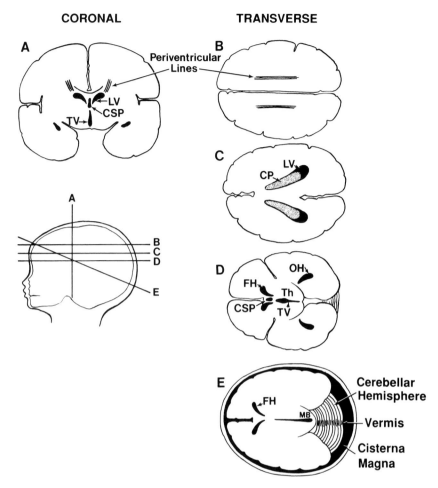

CORONAL   TRANSVERSE

FIG 5–5.
Schematic drawing of normal ventricles and intracranial anatomy. Scan planes *C, D,* and *E* are recommended as a part of all routine obstetric sonograms after the first trimester. Note that periventricular lines are seen cephalad to the later ventricles but may be mis-taken for the lateral ventricular wall. *CP* = choroid plexus; *CSP* = cavum septi pellucidi; *FH* = frontal horn; *LV* = lateral ventricle; *MB* = midbrain; *OH* = occipital horn; *Th* = thalamus; *TV* = third ventricle.

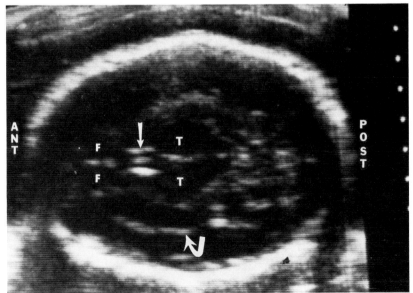

FIG 5–6.
Transthalamic view at 28 weeks' gestation. Axial scan through the thalami *(T)* also shows the septi pellucidi *(straight arrow),* frontal horns *(F),* and insula *(curved arrow). ANT* = anterior, *POST* = posterior.

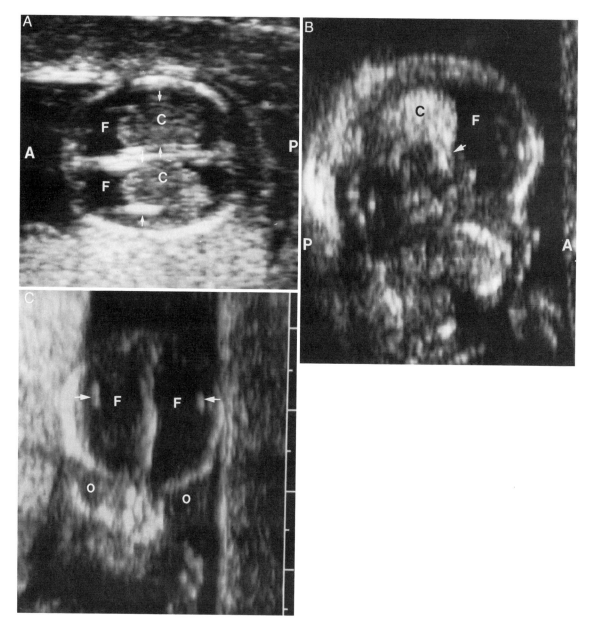

FIG 5–7.
Normal sonographic findings of the cranium at 13 weeks' gestation. **A,** axial scan shows that the echogenic choroid plexus *(C)* fills the lateral cerebral ventricles *(arrows)* and dominates the appearance of the cranium. No choroid is identified in the frontal horns *(F)*. A = anterior; P = posterior. **B,** parasagittal scan of the same fetus shows that the choroid plexus *(C)* ends abruptly at the foramen of Monro *(arrow)* and does not fill the frontal horn *(F)*. A = anterior; P = posterior. **C,** coronal scan of the same fetus through the frontal horns *(F)* confirms absence of the choroid plexus at this level. Note the relatively large size of the lateral cerebral ventricles and position of the lateral ventricular wall *(arrows)* relative to the cranial size. O = orbits.

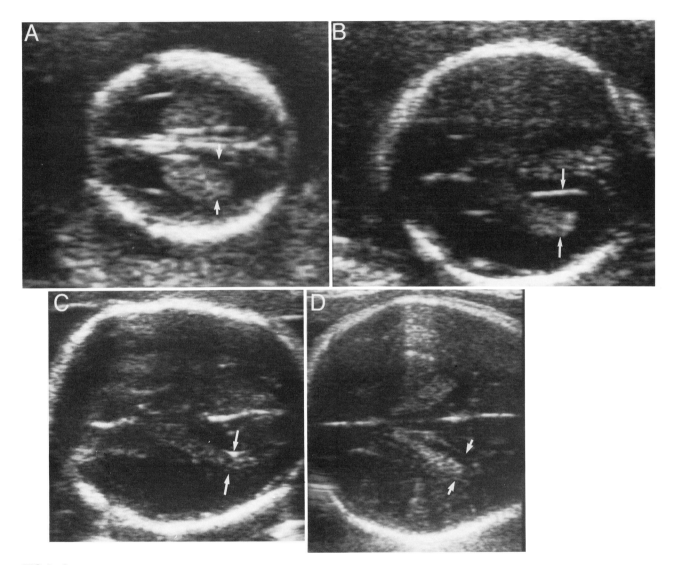

FIG 5–8.
Normal cranium ventricular development. Growth of the cranium gives the appearance that the lateral ventricles decrease in size with advancing gestational age. Actually, the transverse atrial diameter *(arrows)* remains relatively unchanged in absolute size (<10 mm) throughout gestation. Note that with development of the temporal horn, the posterior aspect of the lateral ventricles (atria and occipital horns) are progressively drawn laterally. **A,** 16 weeks; **B,** 20 weeks; **C,** 26 weeks; **D,** 37 weeks.

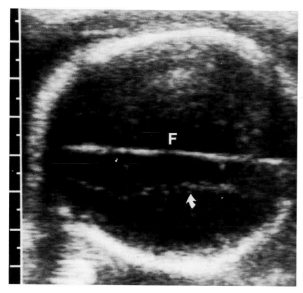

FIG 5-9.
Periventricular "lines." Axial sonogram superior to the level of the lateral cerebral ventricle shows a parallel line *(arrow)* in the far ventricle that is thought to represent intracerebral veins or fibers within the cerebral white matter. The lateral wall of the lateral ventricle is found at a slightly more caudal level. The corresponding line in the near field is obscured by noise artifact. *F* = falx.

appear relatively smaller at this time, Siedler and Filly showed that the average diameter of the lateral ventricular atrium is relatively constant (4−8 mm) between 15 to 35 weeks (see Fig 5−8).[17]

During the third trimester, parallel lines superior to the lateral ventricles once were misinterpreted to be the lateral ventricles themselves (Fig 5−9). How-

ever, these are now known to represent either deep intracerebral veins[7] or periventricular white matter tracts.[1] In either case, the periventricular line is closely adjacent to the lateral ventricular wall. Measurement from this line of the lateral ventricular wall to the midline (falx) has been used by various authors to establish the lateral ventricular ratio (Fig 5−10) (described below).

The transcerebellar view is an angled view through the posterior fossa that includes the cerebellar hemispheres and cisterna magna (Fig 5−11).[5] The cisterna magna appears as a fluid space located between the dorsum of the cerebellar hemisphere and the inner calvarium.[10, 11, 14] It should be visualized in virtually all normal fetuses during the second trimester and early third trimester. Mahony et al reported that the depth of the cisterna magna gradually increases with gestational age with an average depth of 5 + 3 mm (range, up to 10 mm).[10] The cerebellum may appear slightly more echogenic than the cerebral hemispheres and is separated from supratentorial structures by the tentorium.

The trans-cerebellar view is important for identification of small occipital encephaloceles, the Dandy-Walker malformation and cerebellar agenesis or hy-

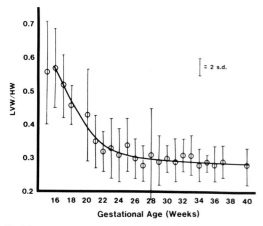

FIG 5-10.
Normal lateral ventricular/hemispheric width ratio. Graph depicting the normal lateral ventricular width/hemispheric width ratio *(LVW/HW)* relative to gestational age. Bars indicate two standard deviations about the mean. (From Johnson ML, Pretorius D, Clewell W, et al: Fetal hydrocephalus: Diagnosis and Management. Semin Perinatol 1983; 7:83−89. Used by permission.)

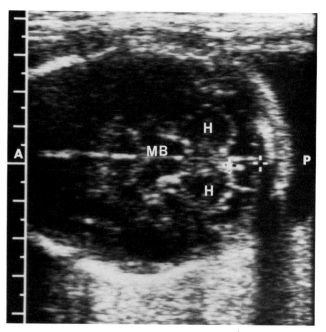

FIG 5-11.
Normal cerebellum and cisterna magna. Axial scan angled through the posterior fossa at 25 weeks shows the cisterna magna posterior to the cerebellar hemispheres *(H)* measuring 8 mm in anterior-posterior dimension *(cursors)*. The cerebellar vermis is seen as a slightly more echogenic area in the mid-cerebellum. The midline echo in the cisterna magna represents the straight sinus *(arrow)*. *MB* = midbrain; *A* = anterior; *P* = posterior.

poplasia. It also provides important indirect evidence regarding the presence or absence of spina bifida.[5, 14]

SONOGRAPHIC PITFALLS AND ARTIFACTS

1. "Pseudohydrocephalus." Developing fetal cortical mantle is normally relatively sonolucent compared to adjacent intracranial structures such as the choroid plexus, ventricular walls, and subarachnoid space. This hypoechoic cortex can be misinterpreted as hydrocephalus (Fig 5–12).[16] Further compounding the error, the more echogenic subarachnoid space is normally prominent prior to 30 weeks and can be misinterpreted as thinned brain mantle.[9] This error can be avoided easily by noting that the choroid plexus does not lie in the gravity-dependent portion of this "ventricle", but rather appears suspended in its center.[26] Careful observation will then reveal the true lateral wall of the lateral ventricle adjacent to the choroid plexus.

2. "Unilateral hydrocephalus." Acoustic noise in the near field often obscures visualization of both normal and abnormal structures in the cerebral hemisphere closest to the transducer (Fig 5–13).[15, 16] In fetuses with ventriculomegaly, this artifact can lead to the erroneous diagnosis of unilateral or asymmetric hydrocephalus. Hence, hydrocephalus should always be assumed to be symmetric unless proven otherwise. This error can be rectified by directing the transducer through the opposite cerebral hemisphere.

3. "Pseudoepidural" artifact. Reverberation artifacts may be potentially confused for abnormal fluid collections in the cerebral hemisphere farthest from the transducer.[18] Alterations in the sonographic appearance with changes in transducer position and angulation will avoid misinterpretation of this artifact.

AN OVERVIEW OF "HYDROCEPHALUS"

Etiology

Hydrocephalus ("water brain") is most commonly defined as the presence of excessive amounts of cerebrospinal fluid (CSF) within the cranial cavity. Others, however, refer to this condition as ventricular dilatation and reserve the term hydrocephalus only for conditions in which intracranial pressure is known to be elevated. While some may consider aqueductal stenosis to be the prototypical cause of hydrocephalus, the term "hydrocephalus" actually encompasses a variety of malformations with widely different pathologic and sonographic findings, pathogeneses, and prognoses (Table 5–1). Subsequent sections will discuss specific disorders that may be categorized as hydrocephalus, while this overview will discuss more general concepts related to it.

Approximately 30% of fetuses identified with hydrocephalus are associated with spina bifida as part of the Arnold-Chiari malformation or other neural tube defects.[29, 48, 57] Other central nervous system (CNS) malformations that may be associated with hydrocephalus (Table 5–2) include the Dandy-Walker malformation, agenesis of the corpus callosum, lissencephaly, intracranial neoplasm, arachnoid cyst, or vascular malformation (vein of Galen aneurysm). Many studies of hydrocephalus have also included more complex types of cranial malformations such as holoprosencephaly or disorders with no residual brain mantle (hydranencephaly). Hydrocephalus has also been associated with an increasing number of multiple anomaly syndromes, including Apert's syndrome, Robert's syndrome, Meckel-Gruber syndrome, hydrolethalus syndrome, and Walker-Warburg syndrome.[20, 31, 41, 62] Chromosome abnormalities (trisomy 18 and 13), chromosomal deletions, translocations, and chromosomal fragility (fragile X syndrome) have also been associated with hydrocephalus.[21, 36]

Whenever possible, the specific malformation re-

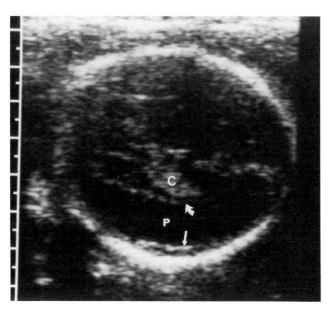

FIG 5–12.
Pseudohydrocephalus. Axial image at the level of the lateral ventricles shows choroid *(C)* in the lateral ventricle. An anechoic crescent-shaped region represents sonolucent brain parenchyma *(P)*, but could be misinterpreted as a dilated lateral ventricle. The interface with the subarachnoid space *(straight arrow)* could also be misinterpreted as thin brain mantle. The true lateral ventricular wall is shown *(curved arrow)*.

FIG 5–13.
Moderate hydrocephalus. **A,** axial image shows the choroid plexus *(C)* lying in the dependent portion of the dilated lateral ventricle, contiguous with the lateral ventricular wall *(arrow)*. Noise in the near field obscures the near ventricle. This artifact is commonly mistaken for unilateral hydrocephalus. *F* = falx. **B,** intracranial landmarks appear relatively normal at the level of the thalami *(T)*, emphasizing that specific views of the ventricles are required for detection of hydrocephalus. *A* = anterior; *P* = posterior.

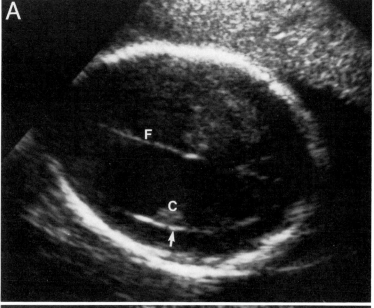

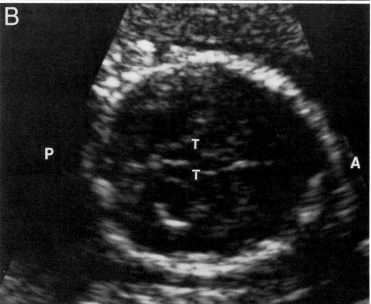

sponsible for hydrocephalus should be determined. However, most series of hydrocephalus include a large group of patients with unknown etiology. For example, in a series of 56 children with congenital hydrocephalus, Bay et al. reported the etiology as unknown (38%), aqueductal stenosis (36%), communicating hydrocephalus (18%), or Dandy-Walker malformation (9%).[20] Similarly, in a series of 23 fetuses with autopsy proven hydrocephalus, Pretorius et al. reported the cause as unknown (35%), Chiari type II (26%), aqueductal stenosis (17%), and one case each of foramen magnum stenosis, atresia of the third ventricle, Dandy-Walker malformation, holoprosencephaly, and inien-

cephaly.[50] As more specific disorders are recognized, the proportion of cases categorized as unknown will undoubtedly decrease.

The recurrence risk of hydrocephalus is widely quoted as 2% after having one child with hydrocephalus, and 8%–10% if two children were previously affected.[21, 23, 36] However, a more precise risk can be provided if the underlying etiology is known. For example, X-linked inheritance has been reported in 7%–27% of males with aqueductal stenosis.[37] If the woman is known to be a carrier for X-linked aqueductal stenosis, 50% of males will be affected and 50% of females will be carriers.

TABLE 5–1.

Causes and Associations of Hydrocephalus

Neural tube defects	Spina bifida (Arnold-Chiari malformation)
	Encephalocele
Other CNS malformations	Dandy-Walker malformation
	Agenesis of the corpus callosum
	Lissencephaly
Aqueductal stenosis	Sporadic
	Post-inflammatory
	X-linked recessive
	Autosomal recessive
Masses	Neoplasms
	Arachnoid cysts
Obstruction of CSF flow in subarachnoid space	Thanatophoric dysplasia
	Achondroplasia
	Osteogenesis imperfecta
	Post-inflammatory
	Post-hemorrhage
Vascular anomalies	Vein of Galen aneurysm
Multiple anomaly syndromes	Meckel-Gruber syndrome
	Hydrolethalus syndrome
	Walker-Warburg syndrome
	Apert syndrome
	Smith-Lemli-Opitz syndrome
	Nasal-facial-digital syndrome
	Albers Schonberg disease
	Robert's syndrome
	Fragile X syndrome
	Trisomy 18
	Trisomy 13

Pathogenesis

Most cases of hydrocephalus associated with elevated intracranial pressure are secondary to obstruction of CSF flow at the ventricular level (non–communicating obstructive hydrocephalus)[34] or in the subarachnoid space (communicating obstructive hydrocephalus). Communicating obstructive hydrocephalus may be caused by obliteration of the subarachnoid

TABLE 5–2.

CNS and Cranial Anomalies That May Be Associated With Hydrocephalus

Meningomyelocele
Holoprosencephaly
Dandy-Walker malformation
Encephalocele
Agenesis of the corpus callosum
Arachnoid cyst
Porencephalic cyst
Intraventricular hemorrhage
Microcephaly
Arteriovenous malformation
Kleeblattschadel
Lissencephaly

space (for example, from prior hemorrhage, infection, or inflammation) or a congenitally small occiput (for example, from achondroplasia or thanatophoric dwarfism). Rarely, hydrocephalus results from excessive production of CSF related to choroid plexus tumors.

Ventriculomegaly without elevated pressure (non–obstructive hydrocephalus) is less common than obstructive hydrocephalus, but is important to consider since non–obstructive hydrocephalus is not successfully treated by ventricular shunting procedures. Non–obstructive hydrocephalus may be secondary to either 1) destruction or atrophy of normal brain (for example, from porencephaly) or 2) development of subnormal amounts of brain tissue (for example, from agenesis of the corpus callosum). In either situation, the additional intracranial space may be compensated by enlarging ventricular size.[19, 39] Hydrocephalus associated with chromosomal abnormalities and certain syndromes probably also represents examples of non–obstructive hydrocephalus.

Sonographic Criteria for Hydrocephalus

Various criteria, based on either objective measurements or visual clues, have been proposed for diagnosing hydrocephalus on prenatal sonography. Two commonly used objective measurements are (1) the lateral ventricular ratio (LVR), and (2) the absolute measurement of the lateral cerebral ventricle. Before discussing these criteria, it is important for the sonographer to realize that normal or even subnormal cranial size does not exclude hydrocephalus.[24, 35, 58] Normal cranial size is commonly observed in fetuses with hydrocephalus during the second and early third trimesters, and subnormal cranial size is commonly observed in association with the Arnold-Chiari malformation before 24 weeks.[24, 58]

Normal values for the LVR have been published by various authors (see Fig 5–10).[4, 40, 51] This ratio is calculated by dividing the lateral ventricular width (measured from the middle of the midline echo to the lateral wall of the lateral ventricle in the parietal region, where the ventricular walls parallel the midline) by the hemispheric width (measured on the same scan from the middle of the midline echo to the inner table of the calvarium). The LVR is normally high during early pregnancy (71% at 15 weeks) and progressively decreases to 33% at 24 weeks and remains at this level until term. Therefore, the LVR has proved to be most helpful after 24 weeks when, as a rule, any value over 50% can be considered abnormal.[28] However, the wide normal variation during early pregnancy makes the LVR of limited usefulness for identification of ventricu-

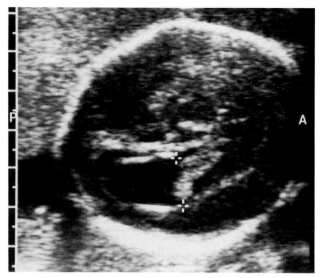

FIG 5–14.
Mild ventricular dilatation at 24 weeks. The lateral cerebral ventricles are mildly dilated, and the transverse atrial diameter measures 13 mm (normal, less than 10 mm). Early intrauterine growth retardation was also demonstrated. This fetus proved to have trisomy 21. Ventricular dilatation is an unusual manifestation of trisomy 21.

lar dilatation before 24 weeks (Fig 5–14). Further, recent evidence indicates that the ventricular measurements in normal third trimester pregnancy have been based on a periventricular echogenic line representing small vessels or white matter tracts rather than the lateral ventricular wall itself.[1, 7]

The second objective measurement of hydroceph-

alus is the transverse dimension of the lateral ventricle. Pretorius et al. suggested that hydrocephalus can be diagnosed when the lateral ventricle measures greater than 1.1 cm in transverse diameter.[50] More recently, Siedler and Filly found that the ventricular diameter, measured at the level of the ventricular atrium, normally measures 4–8 mm (range, up to 10 mm) between 15 to 35 weeks.[17] Unlike the LVR, the transverse atrial diameter remains nearly constant throughout the second and third trimesters (see Fig 5–8). Another advantage of this measurement is its sensitivity for detecting hydrocephalus, since dilatation of the atria and occipital horns is commonly considered the earliest evidence of hydrocephalus.[8, 33] For these reasons, the transverse atrial diameter is considered a more useful objective criterion for diagnosing hydrocephalus than the LVR, particularly during the second trimester.[25] However, this may be too sensitive a criterion for ventricular dilatation since we have frequently encountered normal fetuses that transiently demonstrate a transverse atrial diameter greater than 10 mm, especially between 18 to 22 weeks.[44]

Despite the usefulness of the objective criteria described above, most authorities have found that no measurements are necessary when the choroid plexus demonstrates a normal relation with the lateral ventricle. In a series of reports, Filly and co-workers found that the choroid plexus normally fills the lateral ventricle from side to side during the second trimester (see Fig 5–3) and that with development of hydrocephalus the choroid plexus in the far ventricle separates from

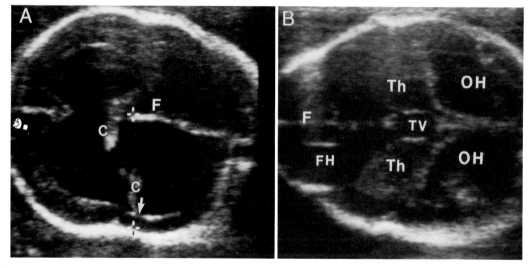

FIG 5–15.
Marked hydrocephalus secondary to the Arnold-Chiari malformation. **A,** axial sonogram at 29 weeks shows marked bilateral ventricular dilatation. Note the choroid plexus *(C)* in the far ventricle lies adjacent to the lateral ventricular wall *(arrow)*, while the choroid plexus in the near ventricle "dangles" into the contralateral ventricle. *F* = falx. **B,** axial sonogram at a level through the thalami *(Th)* shows dilatation of the third ventricle *(TV)*, occipital horns *(OH)*, frontal horns *(FH)*, and separation of the thalami. *F* = falx. (From Nyberg D, Mack L, Bronstein A, et al: Holoprosencephaly: Prenatal sonographic diagnosis. AJR 1987; 149:1050–1058. Used by permission.)

the medial wall of the lateral ventricle (see Fig 5–14).[2, 25, 26, 32, 33] More recently, this phenomenon has been shown to be related to the heavier choroid plexus sinking in the fluid-filled ventricle (Figs 5–15 and 5–16).[22, 26] Hence, the choroid plexus in the near ventricle also separates from the lateral wall of the lateral ventricle (Fig 5–17).[22, 25] This gravity-dependent property of the choroid plexus has recently been re-

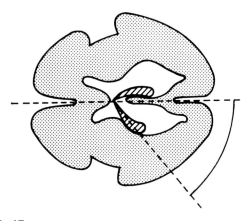

FIG 5–17.
Schematic drawing of dilated ventricles shows dangling choroid plexus and increased choroid plexus angle. (From Cardoza JD, Filly RA, Podrasky AE: The dangling choroid plexus: A sonographic observation of value in excluding ventriculomegaly. AJR 1988; 151:767–770. Used by permission.)

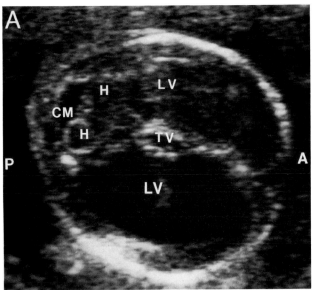

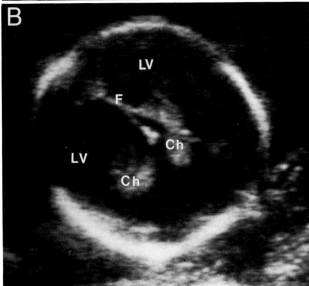

FIG 5–16.
Hydrocephalus secondary to aqueductal stenosis. **A,** axial scan angled through the posterior fossa at 20 weeks shows markedly dilated lateral ventricles *(LV)* and mildly dilated third ventricle *(TV)*. CM = cisterna magna; cerebellar hemispheres; A = anterior; P = posterior. **B,** at a slighly more cephalic level, note the "dangling" choroid plexus *(Ch)* in both the near and far ventricles. The lateral ventricles *(LV)* are markedly dilated, even though the walls are not clearly defined. *F* = falx.

ferred to as the "dangling" choroid plexus sign.[27] Since the near ventricle is often obscured, demonstration of the dangling choroid plexus is useful evidence of ventricular dilatation.

Other Sonographic Findings of Hydrocephalus

Once hydrocephalus is identified, the severity can be assessed as mild (see Fig 5–14), moderate (see Fig 5–13), or marked (see Fig 5–15). While severe hydrocephalus is not difficult to recognize, sonographers should be aware that the degree of ventricular dilatation may appear relatively subtle in the second trimester, only to appear severe by the time of delivery. Also, other clues to an underlying abnormality, such as polyhydramnios, are typically absent during the second trimester.

Obstructive hydrocephalus can be assumed to be present when marked ventricular enlargement and macrocephaly are present, when an associated abnormality is identified that is known to be associated with obstructive hydrocephalus (neural tube defect or Dandy-Walker malformation), or when progressive enlargement is shown on serial sonograms. Aqueductal stenosis occasionally can be suggested by demonstrating disproportionate dilatation of the lateral and third ventricles compared to the fourth ventricle. However, since the fourth ventricle is rarely dilated, regardless of the underlying cause, and because dilatation of the third ventricle may also accompany other causes of hydrocephalus (see Fig 5–15), this appearance should be diagnosed cautiously.

Identification of fetal hydrocephalus mandates a careful and diligent search for other malformations. As-

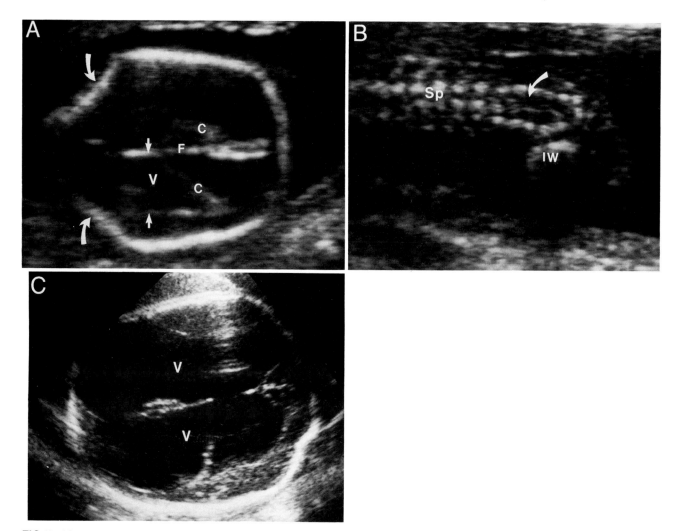

FIG 5–18.
"Lemon" sign with Arnold-Chiari malformation. **A,** axial scan at 20 weeks shows moderate dilatation *(arrows)* of the lateral ventricles *(V).* Despite the noise in the near field, the dangling choroid plexus *(C)* indicates that it is also dilated. Note the presence of a lemon-shaped frontal calvarium *(curved arrows)* which, in association with ventricular dilatation, is strong indirect evidence for spina bifida. *F* = falx. **B,** longitudinal sonogram of the spine *(Sp)* demonstrates a small dysraphic defect in the lower lumbar spine *(arrow). IW* = iliac wing. **C,** repeat sonogram at 37 weeks, after a decision was made to continue the pregnancy, shows progressive dilatation of the lateral ventricles *(V)* and resolution of the lemon sign. (From Nyberg DA, Mack LA, Hirsh JH, et al: Abnormalities of fetal contour in sonographic detection of spina bifida: Evaluation of the "lemon" sign. Radiology 1988; 167:387–392. Used by permission.)

sociated CNS malformations that should be sought include spina bifida, encephalocele, Dandy-Walker malformation, holoprosencephaly, and agenesis of the corpus callosum (see Table 5–2). Various cranial findings such as the "lemon" sign may help suggest the diagnosis of spina bifida with the Arnold-Chiari malformation, particularly before 24 weeks (Fig 5–18) (see Chapter 6). "Pointing" of the frontal horns has also been suggested as a sign of the Arnold-Chiari malformation.[40]

Identification of concurrent extra-CNS anomalies is more important for determining the survival rate, but also is more difficult. In a series of 61 fetuses with hy-

drocephalus reported by Nyberg et al., 90% of major CNS anomalies (holoprosencephaly, encephalocele, and myelomeningocele) were correctly identified, compared to only 28% of individual extra-CNS anomalies.[48] In this series, sonographic detection of any extra-CNS anomaly predicted both the presence of additional anomalies and a uniformly fatal outcome.

Associated Malformations

Associated malformations, including both CNS and extra-CNS anomalies, have been reported in 70%–85%

of fetuses with hydrocephalus.[29, 30, 48, 50, 57] Other CNS anomalies have been reported in 50%−60% of cases (see Table 5−2) including meningomyelocele in 30% of cases.[29, 43, 48, 50] Extra-CNS malformations may affect any organ system, with the heart, thorax, kidneys, abdominal wall, face, and extremities most commonly involved.

Identification of any concurrent abnormality significantly increases the likelihood of a chromosomal abnormality and should initiate chromosomal analysis.[48] Since some extra-CNS anomalies may be missed on prenatal sonography, however, karyotyping should be considered in any fetus with hydrocephalus. Identification of a single umbilical artery in association with any CNS malformation may also increase the risk of associated extra-CNS anomalies and chromosomal abnormalities.[49]

The reported frequency of chromosomal abnormalities in association with fetal hydrocephalus varies with the underlying malformation (discussed further in Chapter 17). Holoprosencephaly carries the highest risk of an abnormal karyotype, followed by the Dandy-Walker malformation or cerebellar dysgenesis, agenesis of the corpus callosum, Arnold-Chiari malformation, and aqueductal stenosis. Hydranencephaly, which superficially can mimic holoprosencephaly, has no increased risk of chromosomal abnormalities.

Prognosis

In general, the mortality rate for fetuses with hydrocephalus varies directly with the presence and severity of extra-CNS anomalies, while the neurologic outcome varies with the underlying CNS malformation.[48] In a series of 50 fetuses with hydrocephalus, Chervenak et al. reported deaths in 72% and associated anomalies (including CNS anomalies such as spina bifida) in 84%.[29] Similarly, Nyberg et al. reported that 84% of 61 fetuses with hydrocephalus had one or more major CNS anomalies (63%) and/or extra-CNS anomalies (49%).[48] The overall uncorrected mortality rate was 67% in this series with deaths occurring in all fetuses with multiple extra-CNS anomalies, 57% of fetuses with an isolated extra-CNS anomaly and 37% of fetuses with no extra-CNS anomaly.[48]

Neurologic outcome of fetal hydrocephalus is also generally poor. In a series of 40 cases, Pretorius et al. reported that only 6 infants (15%) survived (9 terminated pregnancy and 10 had ventricular decompression) and only three of these were neurologically normal (follow-up 6−18 months).[50] In reviewing 156 fetuses with hydrocephalus from the literature, Cochrane

et al. found that 75% had other CNS abnormalities, one third survived long enough to be treated postnatally, and only 7.5% were considered to have normal psychomotor development.[30] These results are considerably worse than suggested by postnatal series, which may not reflect the natural history of fetal hydrocephalus.[54]

The adverse effect of fetal hydrocephalus on the developing brain is not well understood. Histological studies have been performed that implicate acute and severe hydrocephalus in causing brain damage.[46, 60] One hypothesis proposes that increased CSF pressure leads to flattening of the ependyma and interruption of the CSF-brain barrier, followed by penetration of the periventricular white matter by CSF. Demyelination secondary to axonal degeneration results in irreversible tissue damage. However, the exact point of irreversible tissue damage is unknown.

Although some studies have suggested that neurologic outcome can be predicted by the thickness of residual cortical mantle,[54, 63] many exceptions occur. Infants with moderate to severe hydrocephalus may demonstrate normal intellectual development after shunting, whereas fetuses with mild to moderate hydrocephalus may show significant developmental delay. Also, isolated cases of ventriculomegaly have been noted to resolve later in pregnancy and result in a normal neonatal outcome without shunting.[48, 55]

Detection of apparently idiopathic mild ventricular dilatation is one of the most difficult diagnostic dilemmas to face the ultrasonographer. Some cases reflect a serious underlying disorder including chromosome abnormalities (trisomy 18,13, and even 21), whereas others may resolve spontaneously.[44] Mahony and associates reported results in 20 fetuses who demonstrated mild idiopathic lateral ventricular dilatation (MILVD), including 10 fetuses seen before 24 weeks.[44] Interestingly, no fetus proved to have obstructive hydrocephalus. Death resulted in 8 of the 20 cases (40%) and 1 fetus (5%) proved to have trisomy 21. Serial sonograms showed resolution of MILVD in 8 fetuses, and 7 of these had a normal postnatal clinical course; the remaining case developed microcephaly and bilateral posterior cerebral infarcts after demise of a co-twin.

Evidence suggests that postnatal ventricular shunting results in an improved clinical outcome in infants with obstructive hydrocephalus.[42] In a series of newborns with overt hydrocephalus, Lawrence and Coates found that less than 15% of untreated infants survived, and all of these had neurologic impairment.[42] By comparison, more than 80% of infants who underwent early shunting survived, and two thirds of these were normal at follow-up.

Management

The obstetric management of the fetus identified with hydrocephalus is influenced by a variety of factors including the age of diagnosis, the underlying malformation, presence of associated anomalies, and religious and moral beliefs. Pregnancy termination may be elected when hydrocephalus is detected before the age of fetal viability. However, because isolated hydrocephalus may occasionally be transient and associated with a normal outcome, information obtained by other tests available may also influence obstetric management.[47] Amniocentesis may be performed to measure levels of AF-AFP and acetylcholinesterase if a neural tube defect is suspected. Chromosomal analysis can be performed at the same time for identification of aneuploidy and the fragile X syndrome. Cesarean delivery may be considered when macrocephaly precludes vaginal delivery. Cephalocentesis may also be considered, although this should be considered as a destructive procedure that usually results in fetal death.[27, 68]

As noted, ventricular shunting after birth improves the survival rate and intellectual outcome for infants with obstructive hydrocephalus.[63] Prenatal shunting of hydrocephalus has generated interest, because treatment prior to brain damage could potentially improve the mental outcome of these children. However, the results to date have been somewhat disappointing. The International Fetal Surgery Registry reported clinical outcome in 41 fetuses with progressive hydrocephalus who were treated with long term ventriculo-amniotic shunt placement (n=39) or serial ventriculocentesis (n=2).[45] The best results were obtained in 32 fetuses with aqueductal stenosis (follow-up of 8.2 ± 5.8 months) who had a survival rate of 87%. However,

only 42% of survivors had normal intellectual outcome, while 7.2% had mild to moderate handicaps and 50% had severe handicaps.[45] Considering all 41 fetuses in the registry, the procedure-related mortality was 9.75%. Perhaps even more discouraging was the frequency of associated anomalies (22%) found in treated infants after birth. Based on this information, most centers have now stopped in utero treatment of hydrocephalus until more encouraging data is available.

SPECIFIC CEREBRAL MALFORMATIONS

When a cranial abnormality is suspected, recognition of typical features should lead to a correct diagnosis in nearly all cases. As a simple guide, an algorithm has been suggested for detection of major cranial malformations and cystic masses (Fig 5–19). Typical features of common intracranial malformations are also shown in Table 5–3. The following sections discuss these malformations in detail, followed by sections on unusual "acquired" mass lesions (neoplasms and intracranial hemorrhage), microcephaly, and miscellaneous abnormalities (lissencephaly, infection, and skull abnormalities).

AQUEDUCTAL STENOSIS

Pathologic and Clinical Findings

Aqueductal stenosis (Fig 5–20) comprises approximately one third of cases of hydrocephalus in postnatal series,[21, 43, 45, 61] but is relatively less common in prenatal studies. Nevertheless, aqueductal stenosis re-

FIG 5–19.
Simplified algorithm for common intracranial malformations. *ACC* = agenesis of the corpus callosum, *HP* = holoprosencephaly. Hydrocephalus includes other causes of ventricular dilatation such as the Arnold-Chiari malformation, aqueductal stenosis, agenesis of the corpus callosum, and non–obstructive hydrocephalus. While the falx is typically present with hydranencephaly, it may be absent. (Adapted from Carrasco CT, Stierman ED, Harnsberger HR, et al: J Ultrasound Med 1985; 4:163–165.)

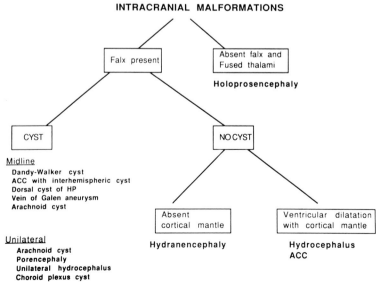

INTRACRANIAL MALFORMATIONS

Falx present — Absent falx and Fused thalami → **Holoprosencephaly**

CYST / NO CYST

Midline
Dandy-Walker cyst
ACC with interhemispheric cyst
Dorsal cyst of HP
Vein of Galen aneurysm
Arachnoid cyst

Unilateral
Arachnoid cyst
Porencephaly
Unilateral hydrocephalus
Choroid plexus cyst

Absent cortical mantle → **Hydranencephaly**

Ventricular dilatation with cortical mantle → **Hydrocephalus ACC**

TABLE 5–3.

Typical Sonographic Features of Common Cerebral Malformations

Disorder	Lateral Cerebral Ventricles	Falx	Thalami	Cerebral Cortex	Other Anomalies
Hydrocephalus (e.g., aqueductal stenosis)	Symmetrically dilated	+	Splayed	Present circumferentially (may be very thin)	Unusual
Dandy-Walker malformation	Dilated (80%)	+	Normal to splayed	Present circumferentially	Posterior fossa cyst ACC (15%)
Holoprosencephaly (alobar)	Monoventricle	−	Fused midline	Present except over dorsal sac of cup and pancake types	Common-facial, ocular anomalies: renal dysplasia, omphalocele, other extracranial anomalies, chromosome abnormalities
Hydranencepaly	Massive single fluid collection	±	Present	Absent	None
Agenesis of the corpus callosum (ACC)	Mildly dilated, particularly occipital horns	+	Normal	Normal	Common

mains one of the most common causes of hydrocephalus; Pretorius et al. reported that 17% of fetuses with hydrocephalus had aqueductal stenosis in their series.[50]

Causes of aqueductal stenosis can be categorized as acquired or congenital.[61] Acquired causes include intrauterine infection (viral and bacterial), intraventric-

AQUEDUCTAL STENOSIS

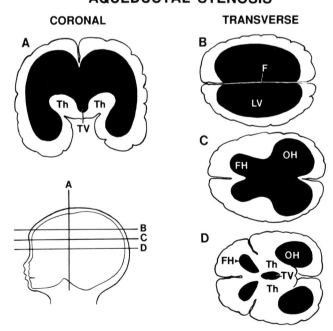

FIG 5–20.
Schematic diagram of aqueductal stenosis. *F* = falx; *FH* = frontal horn; *LV* = lateral ventricle; *OH* = occipital horn; *Th* = thalami; and *TV* = third ventricle.

ular hemorrhage, and extrinsic compression by adjacent masses; congenital causes include X-linked and autosomal recessive disorders. X-linked inheritance comprises about 2% of cases of congenital hydrocephalus and has been reported in 7%–27% of males with aqueductal stenosis.[37, 59] The majority of cases, however, are considered to be multifactorial without an identifiable cause. Aqueductal stenosis is also frequently found in association with the Arnold-Chiari malformation, but these cases should be considered separately.[53]

Russell categorized aqueductal malformations into three types: stenosis, forking ("atresia"), and membrane formation.[53] However, pathologic proof of aqueductal stenosis as the cause of obstructive hydrocephalus is frequently difficult. Although measurement of the aqueductal diameter has not been obtained by pathologic studies, the normal cross-sectional area has been determined to be 0.009 to 0.0015 cm^2 with use of magnetic resonance imaging, and a reduction in cross-sectional area to 0.0001 cm^2 or less may be necessary to restrict the flow of CSF.[52]

Sonographic Findings

The primary sonographic findings of aqueductal stenosis are dilatation of both lateral cerebral ventricles and the third ventricle (Figs 5–16 and 5–21). The degree of ventricular dilatation is usually marked and progressive. No additional CNS anomalies should be demonstrated, and extra-CNS anomalies are uncommonly seen. Congenital aqueductal stenosis is usually demonstrated during the second trimester (see Fig

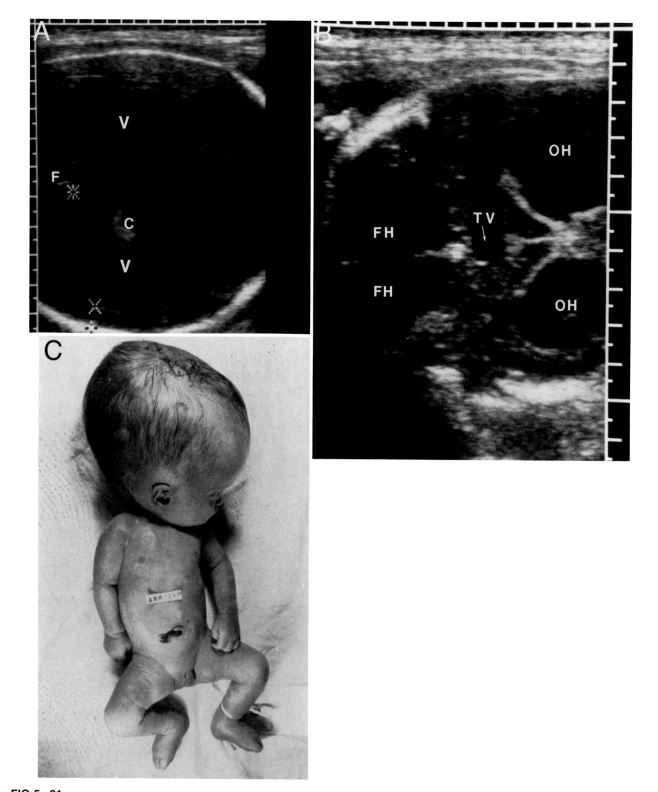

FIG 5–21.
Aqueductal stenosis. **A,** axial sonogram at 36 weeks shows massive dilatation of the lateral cerebral ventricles *(V)* and thinning of the surrounding cortical mantle. The choroid plexus *(C)* in the near ventricle is dangling into the far ventricle. *F* = falx. **B,** axial scan just superior to the thalami shows marked dilatation of the occipital horns *(OH)* and frontal horns *(FH)*. **C,** photograph after neonatal demise shows marked enlargement of the cranium.

5–16). However, because acquired aqueductal stenosis from infection or hemorrhage may occur any time during gestation, hydrocephalus may not be apparent in some cases until the third trimester.

Associated Anomalies

The precise frequency of associated anomalies is difficult to determine because most previous studies of hydrocephalus have not considered aqueductal stenosis separately. Our experience suggests that extra-CNS anomalies and chromosomal abnormalities are less common in fetuses with aqueductal stenosis than many other causes of hydrocephalus. In male fetuses with the X-linked aqueductal stenosis, flexion abnormalities of the thumbs are typically present.[59]

Prognosis

Aqueductal stenosis has a relatively favorable survival rate, but a variable neurologic outcome following ventricular shunting. In 32 fetuses with aqueductal stenosis who were treated with intrauterine shunting, the survival rate was 87%.[45] However, among the survivors, only 42% had normal intellectual outcome, while 7.2% had mild to moderate handicaps, and 50% had severe handicaps. X-linked hydrocephalus is generally associated with a worse prognosis than other causes of aqueductal stenosis. In a review of 92 infants with X-linked aqueductal stenosis, the overall mortality rate was 20.6%, and all the survivors were intellectually impaired.[56]

HOLOPROSENCEPHALY

Pathologic and Clinical Findings

Holoprosencephaly (HP) refers to a spectrum of disorders resulting from absent or incomplete diverticulation of the forebrain (prosencephalon) into cerebral hemispheres and lateral ventricles.[71, 73, 77] Since HP develops early in pregnancy (6 to 10 weeks' gestation), prenatal sonography can potentially identify all affected fetuses before the time of viability. Although many cases of HP are sporadic, a strong association between it and chromosomal abnormalities has been noted.[68, 80, 89] Maternal infections and paternal toxic exposures also have been implicated.[72]

The reported incidence of HP is between 1 in 5,200 and 1 in 16,000 live births.[81, 84, 86] Since many cases of HP spontaneously abort, the true incidence may be as high as 1 in 250 pregnancies.[78] Assuming a frequency of at least 1 in 5,200 for HP and 1 in 1,000 for other causes of fetal ventricular dilatation, HP can be expected to represent 16% or more of all cases of hydrocephalus detected prenatally.[80] A similar proportion of HP has been reported by several prenatal studies.[65, 80]

Depending on the degree of forebrain cleavage, HP has been categorized by DeMeyer into alobar (Fig 5–22), semilobar (Fig 5–23), and lobar types.[71] Alobar HP is the most severe type, in which failure of cleavage results in a monoventricular cavity and fusion of the thalami. Other pathologic findings of alobar HP include absence of the corpus callosum, falx cerebri, optic tracts, and olfactory bulbs. The semilobar

ALOBAR HOLOPROSENCEPHALY

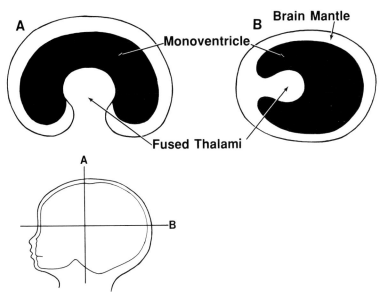

FIG 5–22.
Schematic diagram of alobar holoprosencephaly, "ball" type (see Fig 5–25). Note presence of monoventricle, fused midline thalami, and absence of falx.

SEMILOBAR HOLOPROSENCEPHALY

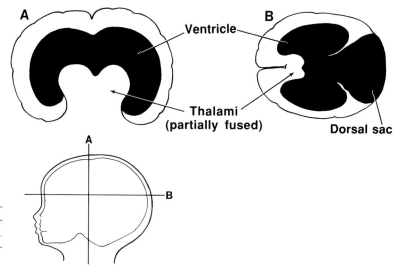

FIG 5–23.
Schematic diagram of semilobar holoprosencephaly with dorsal sac. Note absence of falx, partial fusion of thalami, and partially separated ventricles. The dorsal sac widely communicates with the ventricle.

type of HP demonstrates partial segmentation of the ventricles and cerebral hemispheres posteriorly and incomplete fusion of the thalami (Fig 5–24). Pathologists may find it difficult to distinguish alobar from semilobar HP, however, since the findings overlap to a considerable extent. Lobar HP is the least severe type, which shows normal separation of the ventricles and thalami but absence of the septi pellucidi and olfactory tracts.[76, 77]

Alobar and semilobar HP can be further categorized as "pancake," "cup," and "ball" types, terms which

THREE MORPHOLOGIC TYPES OF ALOBAR HOLOPROSENCEPHALY

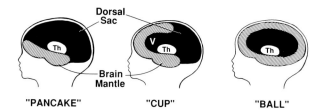

FIG 5–24.
Diagram of three morphologic types of alobar holoprosencephaly (and semilobar holoprosencephaly) in sagittal view. Pancake type: The residual brain mantle is flattened at the base of the brain. The dorsal sac *(DS)* is correspondingly large. Cup type: More brain mantle is present, but it does not cover the monoventricle. The dorsal sac communicates widely with the monoventricle. Ball type: Brain mantle completely covers the monoventricle, and a dorsal sac may or may not be present. (Modified from McGahan JP, Ellis W, Lindfors KK, et al: Congenital cerebrospinal fluid-containing intracranial abnormalities: Sonographic classification. J Clin Ultrasound 1988; 16:531–544. Used by permission.)

describe the morphologic appearance of the brain as viewed dorsally by the pathologist (see Fig 5–24).[71, 85] The specific appearance reflects the degree to which the holotelencephalon has rotated over the membranous ventricular roof. When the telencephalon incompletely covers the prosencephalic vesicle, the membranous roof expands outwardly to form a cyst ("dorsal sac") between the residual cerebral cortex and the calvarium. The pancake type has little cerebral tissue at the base of the brain and a correspondingly large dorsal sac and the cup type has more cerebral tissue and a smaller dorsal sac. The ball type is completely surrounded by brain tissue and may or may not be associated with a dorsal sac.

Facial anomalies are thought to have a common embryologic origin with the intracranial abnormalities of HP and, therefore, when present, can be considered a part of the primary malformation.[70] The well-known statement by DeMeyer that "the face predicts the brain" reflects characteristic facial anomalies of HP (in decreasing order of severity): cyclopia (fused or nearly fused orbits with supraorbital proboscis); ethmocephaly (hypotelorism with high, midline proboscis); cebocephaly (hypotelorism, single nostril in nose); median facial cleft (premaxillary agenesis); and bilateral facial cleft (see Chapter 7).[70] In general, the most severe facial anomalies occur with alobar and semilobar HP, while lobar HP is rarely associated with facial anomalies. However, sonographers should realize that facial anomalies are not universally present with HP; approximately 17% of alobar HP reported by DeMeyer had a normal or non–diagnostic face.[70]

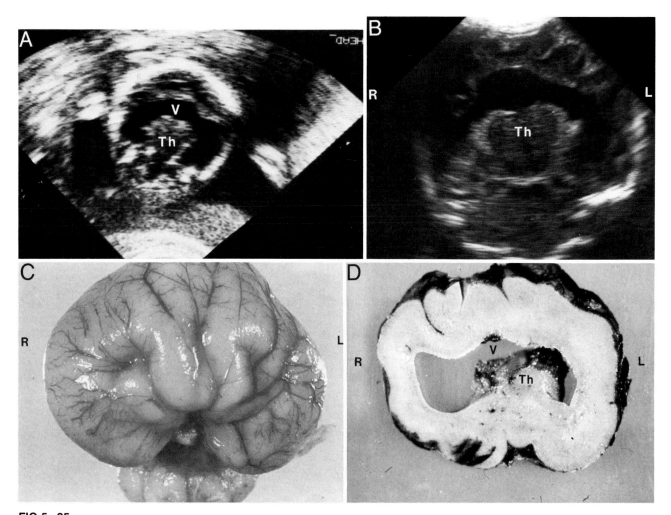

FIG 5–25.
Alobar holoprosencephaly, ball type. **A,** coronal sonogram (displayed upside down) at 19 menstrual weeks shows fused thalami *(Th)* and large monoventricular cavity *(V)*. Note absence of falx and interhemispheric cistern. **B,** coronal sonogram immediately after birth from another case demonstrates fused central thalami *(Th)* surrounded by monoventricle. *R* = right; *L* = left. **C,** corresponding pathologic specimen in frontal view shows featureless brain lacking midline structures. *R* = right; *L* = left. **D,** coronal section shows fused thalami *(Th)* and monoventricle *(V)*. *R* = right; *L* = left. (From Nyberg DA, Mack LA, Hirsch J, et al: Holoprosencephaly: Prenatal sonographic diagnosis. AJR 1987; 149:150–159. Used by permission.)

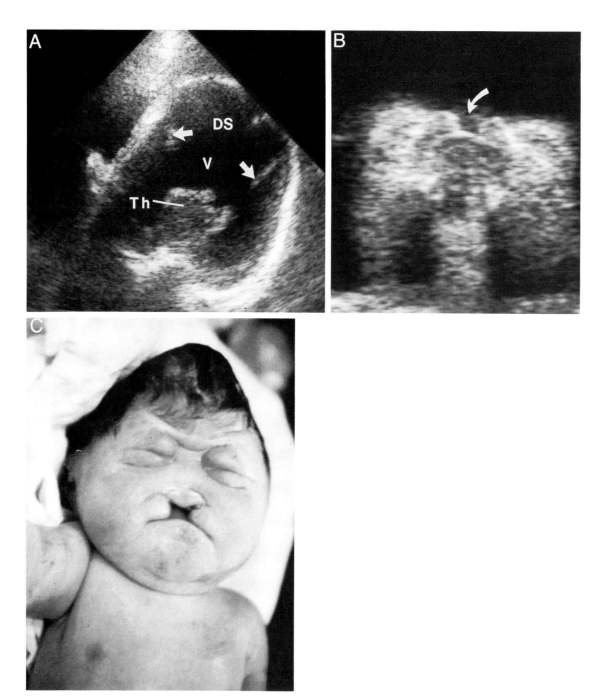

FIG 5–26.
Alobar holoprosencephaly, cup type. **A,** semicoronal scan at 34 weeks shows central fused thalami *(Th)* surrounded by a monoventricle *(V)*. Large dorsal sac *(DS)* is demarcated from the ventricle by ridge of cerebral tissue *(arrows)*. **B,** axial sonogram of the face shows midline facial cleft *(arrow)*. Flattened midface and hypotelorism were also demonstrated. **C,** photograph of face at delivery confirms midline facial cleft, hypotelorism, flattened midface, and microcephaly. A chromosome abnormality (5p+) was present. (From Nyberg DA, Mack LA, Hirsch J, et al: Holoprosencephaly: Prenatal sonographic diagnosis. AJR 1987; 149:150–159. Used by permission.)

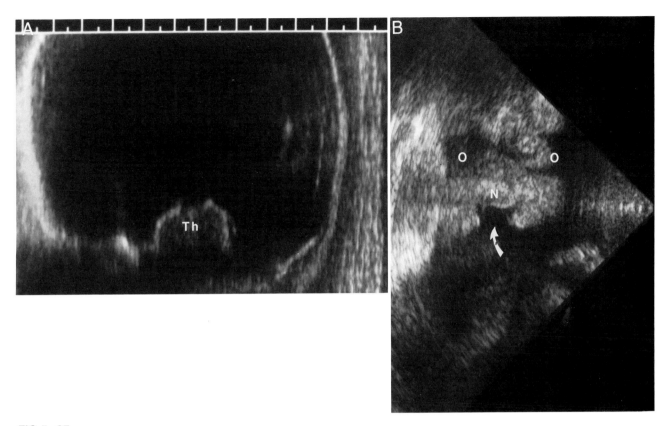

FIG 5–27.
Alobar holoprosencephaly, pancake type. **A,** coronal sonogram at 36 weeks shows fused, midline thalami *(TH)*. Little brain mantle is seen near the base of the brain. In this case, the large cystic space represents the dorsal sac. Note absence of falx and midline structures. **B,** coronal view of the face demonstrates a large midline facial cleft *(arrow)* which was confirmed following delivery. Trisomy 13 was found. *N* = nose; *O* = orbits.

Sonographic Findings

The prenatal sonographic findings of HP have been frequently reported.[66–68, 72, 75, 80, 82] Alobar HP demonstrates a featureless monoventricular cavity lacking occipital, temporal, and frontal horns (Figs 5–25 to 5–27). The midline thalami are fused, and no falx or other midline structures are demonstrated. Semilobar HP shows similar features, but the thalami are incompletely fused and some midline structures, such as the interhemispheric cistern, may be partially present (Fig 5–28)[64, 66, 80]

While some authors have emphasized demonstration of intracranial findings together with characteristic facial anomalies for diagnosing HP,[68, 75] facial malformations are not always present and so are less sensitive than the intracranial findings alone.[80, 82] Nevertheless, demonstration of facial abnormalities may add confidence to the diagnosis and help distinguish the pancake type of alobar HP (see Fig 5–27) from hydranencephaly. Knowledge of facial abnormalities may also be helpful for counseling and prognostic purposes.

In addition to variable separation of a monoventricle and variable fusion of midline thalami, the specific sonographic appearance of alobar and semilobar HP varies with the presence or absence of a "dorsal sac."[79] As noted above, a dorsal sac is present in cup and pancake morphologic types of HP, but may be absent in the ball type. When present, the dorsal sac communicates widely with the monoventricular cavity so that the distinction between them may be difficult. However, close observation will usually reveal a ridge of cerebral tissue, thought to represent the hippocampal fornix, which demarcates the boundary between the dorsal sac and ventricular cavity (see Fig 5–26).[64, 72, 80, 82, 83] A dorsal sac should be distinguished from other cystic masses such as Dandy-Walker malformation, arachnoid cyst, or porencephaly (Table 5–4).[72, 80]

Due to the variety of morphologic possibilities, HP can demonstrate a range of sonographic appearances that should be distinguished from other disorders. Hydrocephalus can be readily distinguished by demonstration of splayed thalami rather than fused thalami

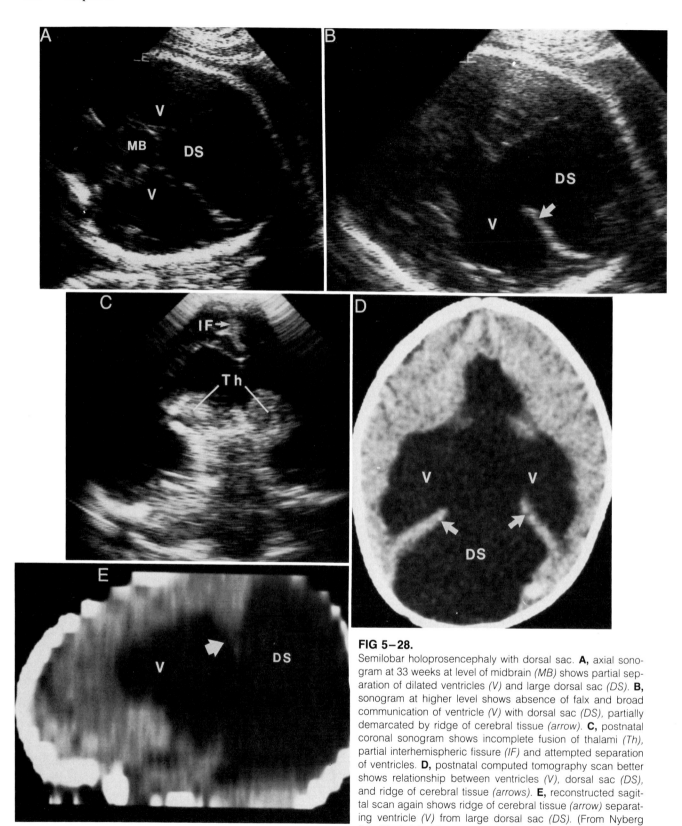

FIG 5–28.
Semilobar holoprosencephaly with dorsal sac. **A,** axial sonogram at 33 weeks at level of midbrain *(MB)* shows partial separation of dilated ventricles *(V)* and large dorsal sac *(DS)*. **B,** sonogram at higher level shows absence of falx and broad communication of ventricle *(V)* with dorsal sac *(DS),* partially demarcated by ridge of cerebral tissue *(arrow)*. **C,** postnatal coronal sonogram shows incomplete fusion of thalami *(Th),* partial interhemispheric fissure *(IF)* and attempted separation of ventricles. **D,** postnatal computed tomography scan better shows relationship between ventricles *(V),* dorsal sac *(DS),* and ridge of cerebral tissue *(arrows)*. **E,** reconstructed sagittal scan again shows ridge of cerebral tissue *(arrow)* separating ventricle *(V)* from large dorsal sac *(DS)*. (From Nyberg DA, Mack LA, Hirsch J, et al: Holoprosencephaly: Prenatal sonographic diagnosis. AJR 1987; 149:150–159. Used by permission.)

TABLE 5-4.

Differential Diagnosis of Intracranial Cystic Mass

Midline
    Agenesis of corpus callosum
        with interhemispheric cyst
    Dandy-Walker malformation
    Holoprosencephaly with dorsal
        cyst
    Prominent septi pellucidi
    Vein of Galen aneurysm
    Arachnoid cyst
Asymmetric
    Arachnoid cyst
    Porencephaly/schizencephaly
    Unilateral hydrocephalus
    Teratoma
    Choroid plexus cysts

and presence of the falx and other midline structures. Hydranencephaly may superficially appear similar to HP, especially the pancake type of alobar HP, but this disorder is characterized by complete absence of cerebral hemispheres, variable presence of the falx, and normal facial features. Also, hydranencephaly is much less commonly encountered in utero than is HP in our experience. As a practical point, the prognoses of HP and hydranencephaly are equally dismal.

Lobar HP has also been occasionally detected prenatally by demonstration of flattened frontal horns, absent septi pellucidi, and absent corpus callosum.[76] However, since a similar appearance may be seen with other cranial malformations (septo-optic dysplasia or complete agenesis of the corpus callosum), the sonographic diagnosis of lobar HP is considered less reliable than for alobar or semilobar HP.[74, 77]

Associated Abnormalities

Facial and extra-CNS anomalies should be specifically sought when HP is considered because, when present, these findings help support the diagnosis of HP (see Figs 5-26 and 5-27).[72, 80, 82, 87] Demonstration of facial anomalies and extra-CNS anomalies also provides additional prognostic information regarding the fetus. For example, cyclopia and ethmocephaly are uniformly associated with a fatal outcome, and affected infants rarely live beyond the neonatal period, while fetuses with cebocephaly or premaxillary agenesis rarely live beyond 1 year.[70] Attention is called to the fact that cyclopia does not usually demonstrate a single orbit, but rather two orbits that are very close together and share a single external opening. The characteristic proboscis should be sought superior to these orbits. Facial abnor-

malities associated with HP are discussed in greater detail in Chapter 6.

Extracranial malformations have also been identified in approximately half the fetuses with alobar or semilobar HP. Common extracranial malformations include renal cysts and dysplasia, omphalocele, cardiovascular malformations, clubfoot, myelomeningocele, and intestinal abnormalities. A relationship between the presence of facial anomalies and extracranial abnormalities has been suggested by Nyberg et al., who reported major extra-CNS anomalies in eight of nine fetuses who also had facial anomalies.[80]

Chromosome abnormalities have been identified in approximately half the fetuses with alobar or semilobar HP who underwent chromosomal analysis.[68, 75, 80] Trisomy 13 is the most common, followed by a variety of other karyotypes such as 13q-, trisomy 18, 18p-, and triploidy.[69] HP has also been associated with multiple anomaly syndromes including the Meckel-Gruber syndrome, Kallmann's syndrome, campomelic dysplasia, Hall-Pallister syndrome, and Vasadi syndrome.[69]

Prognosis

Infants with alobar and semilobar HP usually die immediately after birth or in the first year of life. Rare survivors exhibit profound mental retardation and severe developmental delay. For these reasons, prenatal diagnosis of alobar or semilobar HP may be an acceptable indication for third trimester termination or cephalocentesis.

DANDY-WALKER MALFORMATION AND CEREBELLAR DYSGENESIS

Pathologic and Clinical Findings

Approximately 5%-10% of hydrocephalus can be attributed to the Dandy-Walker malformation (DWM); conversely, 80% of fetuses with DWM demonstrate hydrocephalus.[50, 98, 102] DWM is characterized by complete or partial absence of the cerebellar vermis and cystic dilatation of the fourth ventricle (Fig 5-29). The posterior fossa is generally enlarged, with elevation of the torcula and tentorium. The Dandy-Walker "variant" is a less severe malformation with a smaller fourth ventricle cyst and less vermian hypoplasia.[95] Partial agenesis usually involves the inferior cerebellar vermis. Hydrocephalus is also less severe or absent with the DWM variant, and the posterior fossa is not as large.[95] The distinction between the DWM variant and cerebellar dysgenesis (cerebellar hypoplasia) is un-

DANDY-WALKER MALFORMATION

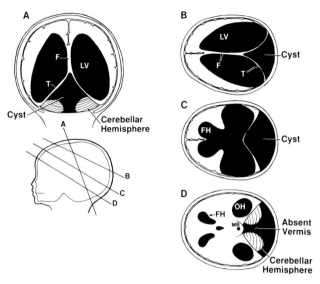

FIG 5–29.
Schematic diagram of Dandy-Walker malformation. Note the presence of a posterior fossa cyst, absence of the cerebellar vermis, and splaying of the cerebellar hemispheres. *F* = falx; *FH* = frontal horn; *LV* = lateral ventricle; *MB* = midbrain; *T* = tentorium.

clear, so cerebellar dysgenesis is included in this discussion of DWM.

In a review of 113 reported cases of DWM, Murray et al. concluded that the CNS malformation is a non–specific end-point resulting from a variety of diverse etiologies (Table 5–5).[101] These include the Meckel-Gruber syndrome (autosomal recessive), Walker-Warburg syndrome (autosomal recessive), Aicardi's syndrome (X-linked dominant), single gene disorders, chromosomal abnormalities (including trisomy 18), and multifactorial abnormalities.[101] The DWM also has been observed following exposure to rubella, CMV, toxoplasmosis, coumadin, and alcohol, as well as in association with maternal diabetes.[101]

Several hypotheses have been offered regarding the pathogenesis of DWM.[89, 92, 96, 97] Dandy and Blackfan proposed that atresia of the foramina of Magendie and Luschka was the primary etiology.[92] However, these foramina are frequently patent, and DWM is currently thought to arise from a more generalized dysembryogenesis involving the roof of the fourth ventricle.[96, 97]

Sonographic Findings

Characteristic findings of DWM have been described on prenatal sonography.[91, 94, 99, 102, 104, 105] These include (1) complete or partial agenesis of the cerebellar vermis; (2) enlargement of the fourth ventri-

TABLE 5–5.
Associations With the Dandy-Walker Malformation*†

Inherited syndromes	Mode of inheritance
Aase-Smith (arthrogryposis)	AD
Aicardi's	X-linked
Coffin-Siris	AR
Ellis-van Creveld	AR
Fraser cytophthalmos	AR
Joubert-Boltshauser	AR
Meckel-Gruber	AR
Neu-Laxova	AR
Oral-facial-digital	AR
Walker-Warburg	AR
X-linked cerebellar hypoplasia	X-linked
Teratogens and environmental factors	
Alcohol	
Coumadin	
Cytomegalovirus	
Diabetes	
Rubella	
Toxoplasmosis	
Chromosome abnormalities	
Other associations	
Facial hemangiomas	
Neural tube defects	
Midline facial cleft	
Congenital heart disease	

*Adapted from Murray et al: Clin Genet 1985; 28:272–283.
†AR = autosomal recessive, AD = autosomal dominant.

cle, which appears as a midline posterior fossa "cyst"; and (3) splaying of the cerebellar hemispheres (Figs 5–30 to 5–33). Ventricular dilatation is frequently, but not invariably, present. One study found clinically overt hydrocephalus in 20% of neonates with the DWM at birth and in 78% of infants by 1 year of life.[98] By comparison, prenatal studies have reported sonographic evidence of hydrocephalus in 50% to 70% of fetuses with DWM.[102, 105, 107] The severity of hydrocephalus appears unrelated to the size of the posterior fossa cyst, the degree of vermian hypoplasia, or the patency of the foramina.[97]

The size of the posterior fossa cyst is variable. When large, the cyst displaces the cerebellar hemispheres anteriorly against the tentorium. The primary differential diagnosis for this appearance is an arachnoid cyst, which is generally not located in the midline and is not associated with vermian agenesis. Also, posterior fossa arachnoid cysts are much rarer than DWM in utero.

When the posterior fossa cyst is small, the DWM variant or cerebellar dysgenesis should be distinguished from a large, but normal cisterna magna. The cisterna magna does not normally exceed 10 mm in depth.[10, 90] More importantly, a prominent cisterna magna is not associated with vermian agenesis. Ver-

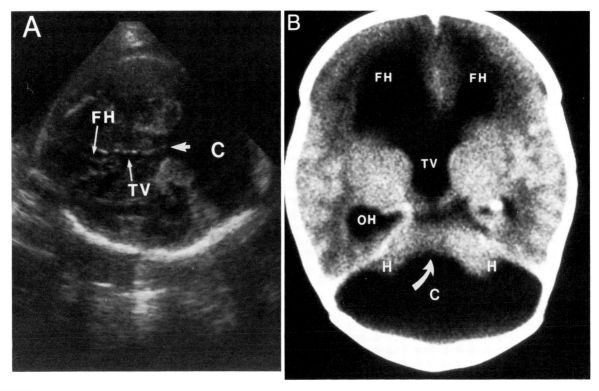

FIG 5–30.
Dandy-Walker malformation. **A,** axial scan demonstrates large posterior fossa cyst *(C)* and agenesis of the cerebellar vermis *(arrow)*. Note mild ventricular dilatation. *FH* = frontal horn; *TV* = third ventricle. **B,** cranial computed tomography of another patient with Dandy-Walker malformation shows posterior fossa cyst *(C)*, absence of the cerebellar vermis *(arrow)*, splaying of the cerebellar hemispheres *(H)*, and hydrocephalus. *FH* = frontal horns; *OH* = occipital horn; *TV* = third ventricle.

mian agenesis can be seen as the direct continuity of the posterior fossa cyst with the posterior aspect of the midbrain without an intervening vermis.

Associated Abnormalities

CNS abnormalities have been reported in 68% of DWM at autopsy, and extra-CNS anomalies have been reported in 25%–43% of cases.[97, 102] The frequency of concurrent CNS and extra-CNS anomalies supports the notion that DWM is frequently part of a generalized disorder of embryogenesis. Common associated CNS abnormalities include agenesis of the corpus callosum (see Fig 5–31), lipomas, aqueductal stenosis, microcephaly, encephalocele (see Fig 5–33) and non–specific gyral abnormalities.[97, 102, 106, 107] Myelomeningocele is uncommon. Extra-CNS anomalies commonly involve the cardiovascular and genitourinary systems. Facial anomalies and polydactyly are also frequently encountered.[97, 98, 103, 107] Chromosome abnormalities have been reported in several cases, including two of seven (29%) of fetuses with DWM or cerebellar hypoplasia reported by Nyberg et al.[90, 101, 102] Interestingly, neither fetus with chromosomal abnormalities demonstrated ventricular dilatation.

Prognosis

Neonatal studies indicate that infants with DWM have a higher mortality rate (12%–50%) and a worse intellectual outcome (IQ less than 80 in 40%–75% of survivors) than other congenital causes of hydrocephalus.[97, 100, 101, 106] Although the natural history of DWM identified in utero is largely unknown, due to the small number of cases reported,[102, 104, 105] several recent prenatal series have reported mortality rates up to 71%. Like other causes of fetal hydrocephalus, fetal mortality appears directly related to the presence of extra-CNS anomalies.[102] Ventricular shunt placement has been performed in utero for hydrocephalus associated with the DWM.[93]

AGENESIS OF THE CORPUS CALLOSUM

Pathological and Clinical Findings

The corpus callosum is a bundle of white matter tracts that decussate between the cerebral hemispheres (Fig 5–34).[12, 126] Agenesis of the corpus callosum (ACC) is an uncommon cerebral malformation that has been reported in 1 in 19,000 unselected

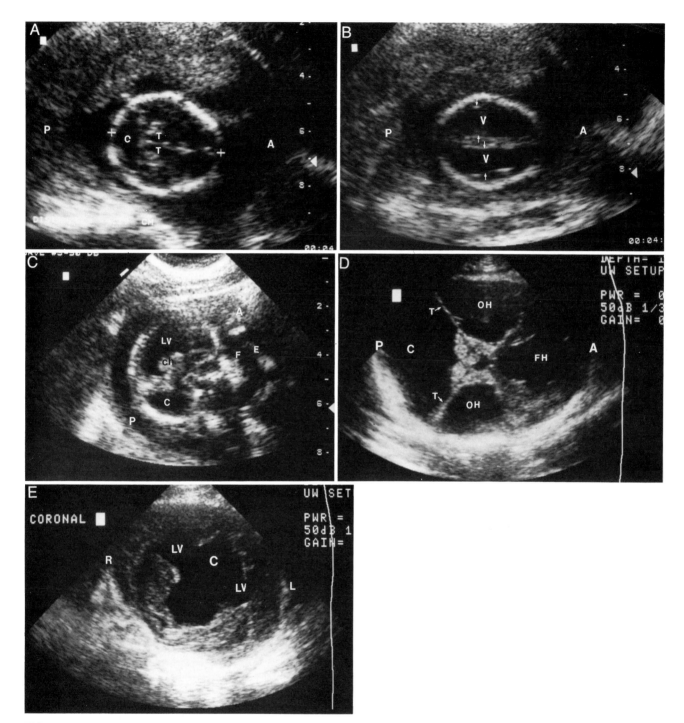

FIG 5–31.
Dandy-Walker malformation. **A,** axial scan through lower thalami *(T)* at 16 weeks shows a posterior fossa cyst *(C). A* = anterior; *P* = posterior. **B,** scan at a more cephalic level shows moderate dilatation *(arrows)* of the lateral ventricles *(V). A* = anterior; *P* = posterior. **C,** parasagittal view shows relation of the posterior fossa cyst *(C)* and dilatation of the lateral ventricle *(LV). Ch* = choroid; *F* = face; *E* = upper extremity; *A* = anterior; *P* = posterior. **D,** follow-up scan at 36 weeks shows marked enlargement of the posterior fossa cyst *(C)* and marked ventricular dilatation. Note absence of cavum septi pellucidi that normally separate the frontal horns *(FH),* suggesting agenesis of the corpus callosum. *OH* = occipital horn; *T* = tentorium; *A* = anterior; *P* = posterior. **E,** coronal scan confirms agenesis of corpus callosum with large interhemispheric cyst *(C). LV* = lateral ventricle; *R* = right; *L* = left.

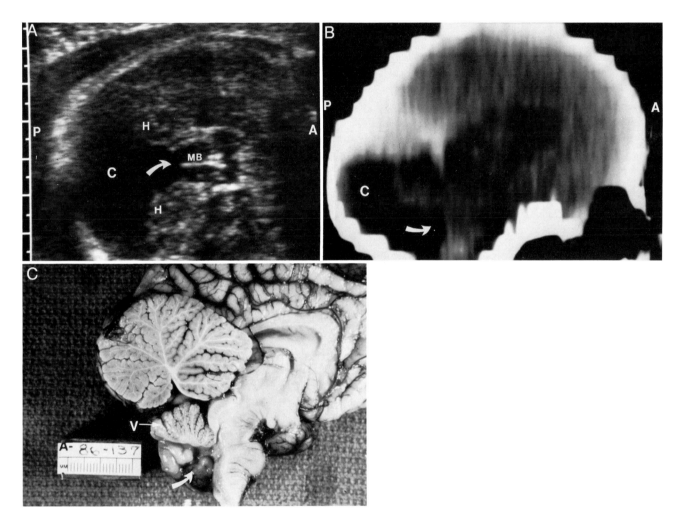

FIG 5–32.
Dandy-Walker variant. **A,** axial sonogram at 32 weeks shows posterior fossa cyst *(C),* absence of the cerebellar vermis *(curved arrow)* and splaying of the cerebellar hemispheres *(H).* Note that the posterior fossa cyst is contiguous with the midbrain *(MB).* A = anterior; P = posterior. **B,** reconstructed cranial computed tomography of the same patient after delivery shows the posterior fossa cyst *(C)* and vermian hypoplasia *(curved arrow).* A = anterior; P = posterior. **C,** sagittal view of the pathological specimen following spontaneous death at 3 days of age confirms absence of the posterior cerebellar vermis *(curved arrow).* The anterior vermis *(V)* is present. Trisomy 13, tetralogy of Fallot, and polydactyly were also present. (From Nyberg DA, Cyr D, Mack LA, et al: The Dandy-Walker malformation: Prenatal sonographic diagnosis and its clinical significance. J Ultrasound Med 1988; 7:65–71. Used by permission.)

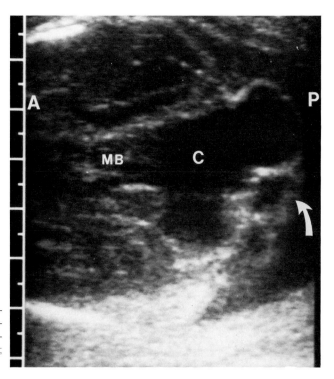

FIG 5–33.
Dandy-Walker malformation with encephalocele. Axial image of fetal head at 25 weeks showing posterior fossa cyst *(C)* that is contiguous posteriorly with the midbrain *(MB)*. A defect in the calvarium with an encephalocele is noted *(curved arrow)*. *A* = anterior; *P* = posterior.

FIG 5–34.
Normal corpus callosum. Coronal anatomic specimen shows that the corpus callosum *(CC)* forms the roof of the lateral ventricle and makes the frontal horns of the lateral ventricles *(FV)* "point" laterally. *C* = cavum septi pellucidi; *CG* = cingulate gyrus; *FL* = frontal lobe; *HC* = head of caudate nucleus; *PCA* = pericallosal artery; *S* = sylvian fissure; *T* = third ventricle; *TL* = temporal lobe. (From Mack LA, Alvord EC Jr: Neonatal cranial ultrasound: Normal appearances. *Seminars in Ultrasound,* vol 3. Philadelphia, Grune & Stratton, Inc, 1982, pp 216–230. Used by permission.)

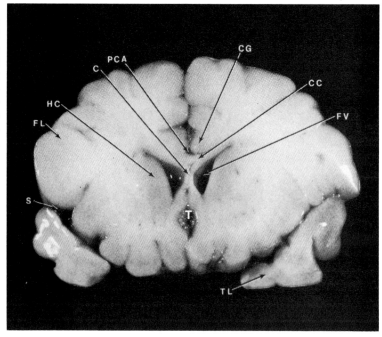

AGENESIS OF THE CORPUS CALLOSUM WITH INTERHEMISPHERIC CYST

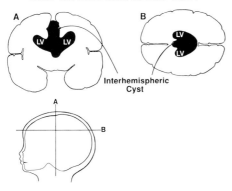

FIG 5–35.
Schematic diagram of agenesis of the corpus callosum with interhemispheric cyst. The interhemispheric cyst represents a very dilated and elevated third ventricle. *LV* = lateral ventricle.

autopsies and 2.3% of children with mental retardation.[114, 116] ACC may be complete or partial, depending on the stage at which callosal development is arrested with partial ACC involving the posterior corpus callosum (splenium).[126] Complete ACC usually occurs as a primary process before 12 menstrual weeks, but less often may be secondary to the destructive process of an already formed corpus callosum after 20 weeks.[110, 118]

Absence of the corpus callosum produces characteristic pathologic changes of the cerebral hemispheres and the ventricular system.[109, 110, 113, 124] Dilatation and superior displacement of the third ventricle (interhemispheric "cyst") is the most characteristic finding of ACC, but it also is the most variable finding (Fig 5–35).[111, 121] The lateral cerebral ventricles are displaced laterally and superiorly. Axons that normally would have formed the corpus callosum gather into two aberrant bundles of uncrossed fibers (bundles of Probst), which run longitudinally along the medial walls of the lateral ventricles.[109, 124]

Sonographic Findings

Characteristic changes of the ventricular system and cerebral hemispheres were first described by Davidoff and Dyke in 1934 from observations made on pneumoencephalography.[113] These findings include (1) lateral separation of the frontal horns and bodies of the lateral ventricles, (2) angled lateral peaks of the frontal horns and bodies of the lateral ventricles, (3) elevation and variable dilatation of the third ventricle, (4) dilatation of the occipital horns, (5) concave medial wall of the lateral ventricles related to the bundles of Probst, and (6) abnormal radial orientation of me-

dial cerebral gyri extending from the roof of the third ventricle.[113] Similar findings have been identified on sonography, most often on postnatal sonograms performed in coronal and sagittal planes.[101, 109, 112, 115, 124]

To date, relatively few cases of ACC have been diagnosed on prenatal sonography.[108, 111, 112, 120, 122, 125] The diagnosis is most evident when an interhemispheric cyst, representing a dilated and elevated third ventricle, is present (Figs 5–31 and 5–36). On the other hand, the diagnosis may be very difficult in the absence of an interhemispheric cyst (Figs 5–37 to 5–40).[111] A specific prenatal diagnosis of ACC has not been made before the third trimester, probably because the corpus callosum is not normally formed until 18 to 20 weeks.[117] Most authors have also found that detection of ACC is considerably more difficult prenatally than is possible by postnatal sonograms. This difficulty can be ascribed largely to the fact that the characteristic ventricular abnormalities, which are so obvious on coronal and sagittal views, can be quite subtle on routine transverse views of the fetal cranium.

In a series of seven fetuses with ACC, Bertino et al. reported that three demonstrated a characteristic midline cyst, including one fetus with marked hydrocephalus and the Dandy-Walker malformation, and the four remaining fetuses demonstrated more subtle abnormalities of the ventricular system.[111] Based on this experience, these authors described three findings that might lead one to suspect ACC on routine transverse views:

1. Disproportionate enlargement of the occipital horn ("colpocephaly").
2. Demonstration of both medial and lateral ventricular walls at a level where the single periventricular line is normally demonstrated.
3. A more parallel course of both ventricular walls than normally is seen (see Figs 5–37 to 5–40).[111]

These authors suggest that demonstration of these findings on axial views should stimulate additional coronal and sagittal views for evaluation of ACC.

The differential diagnosis for ACC depends on whether or not a midline cyst is demonstrated. If present, other cystic masses that should also be considered include an arachnoid cyst, porencephaly, or prominent cavum septi pellucidi/cavum septi vergae (Fig 5–41).[109, 110, 112] Distinguishing a midline cyst of ACC from an arachnoid cyst may occasionally be difficult when a suprasellar arachnoid cyst insinuates itself into the third ventricle. All types of holoprosencephaly include absence of the corpus callosum as part of the underlying malformation, although alobar and semilo-

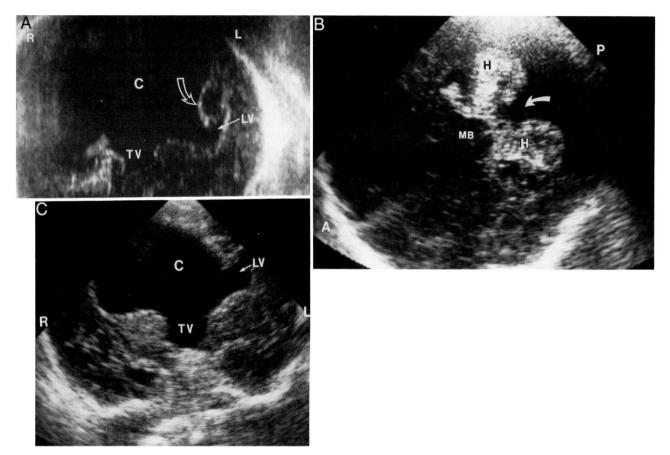

FIG 5–36.
Agenesis of the corpus callosum with interhemispheric cyst and Dandy-Walker malformation. **A,** axial sonogram at 40 weeks shows a massive interhemispheric cyst *(C)* communicating widely with the dilated third ventricle *(TV)* and laterally displaced lateral ventricles. Note the soft tissue mass in the medial wall of the lateral ventricle *(open arrow)* representing bundles of Probst. *R* = right; *L* = left. (Part **A** from Bertino RE, Nyberg DA, Cyr DR, et al: Prenatal diagnosis of agenesis of the corpus callosum. J Ultrasound Med 1988; 7:251–260. Used by permission.) **B,** angled scan through the posterior fossa in the same fetus shows splaying of the cerebellar hemispheres *(H)* and absence of the cerebellar vermis *(arrow)* indicating the presence of Dandy-Walker malformation. *MB* = midbrain; *A* = anterior; *P* = posterior. **C,** postnatal coronal sonogram shows a large interhemispheric cyst *(C)* communicating widely with the laterally displaced lateral ventricles *(LV)* and the dilated third ventricle *(TV)*. Note that the lateral ventricles point in a cephalic direction due to absence of the corpus callosum. *R* = right; *L* = left.

FIG 5–37.
Schematic diagram of agenesis of the corpus callosum without interhemispheric cyst. Note the characteristic configuration of the lateral ventricles which point superiorly on a coronal view. At scan level *B,* both walls of the lateral ventricles are identified where only periventricular lines are normally present. Also note characteristic dilatation of the occipital horns (colpocephaly). The third ventricle may or may not be dilated. *FH* = frontal horn; *LV* = lateral ventricle; *OH* = occipital horn; *TV* = third ventricle.

AGENESIS OF THE CORPUS CALLOSUM

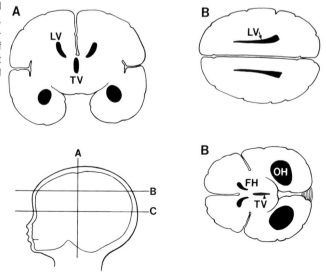

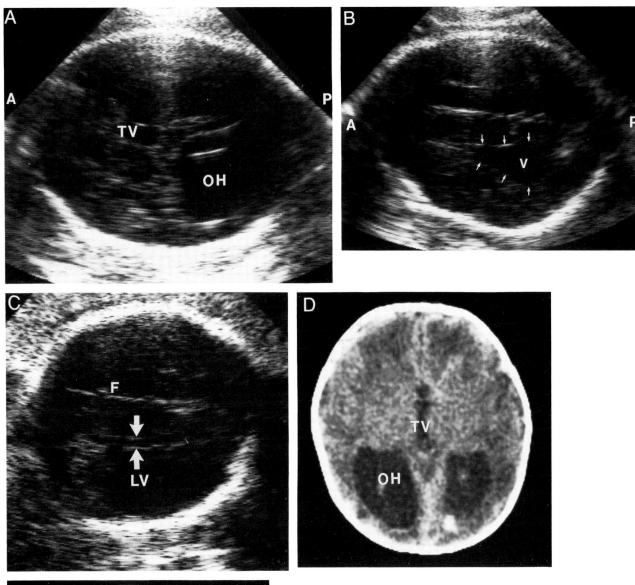

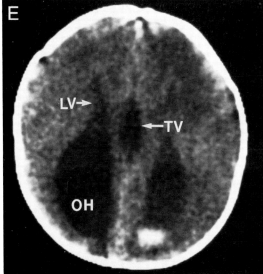

FIG 5–38.
Agenesis of the corpus callosum without interhemispheric cyst. **A,** axial sonogram at 35 weeks shows dilatation of the occipital horns *(OH)* and mild dilatation
of the third ventricle *(TV)*. A = anterior; P = posterior. **B,** scan at a slightly higher
level shows angular configuration of the lateral ventricle *(V)* due to disproportionate enlargement of the dilated occipital horn. A = anterior; P = posterior. **C,**
scan at the most cephalic level shows displacement of both the medial and lateral walls *(arrows)* of the lateral ventricles *(LV)* from the falx *(F)*. **D,** postnatal
computed tomography confirms disproportionate enlargement of the occipital
horns *(OH)* and a slightly dilated third ventricle *(TV)*. Compare with **A. E,** scan at
a slightly higher level again shows dilatation of the occipital horns *(OH)* communicating with the lateral ventricle *(LV)*. The third ventricle *(TV)* is mildly dilated.
Compare with **B.** (Parts **A, B, C,** and **D** from Bertino RE, Nyberg DA, Cyr DR, et
al: Prenatal diagnosis of agenesis of the corpus callosum. J Ultrasound Med
1988; 7:251–260. Used by permission.)

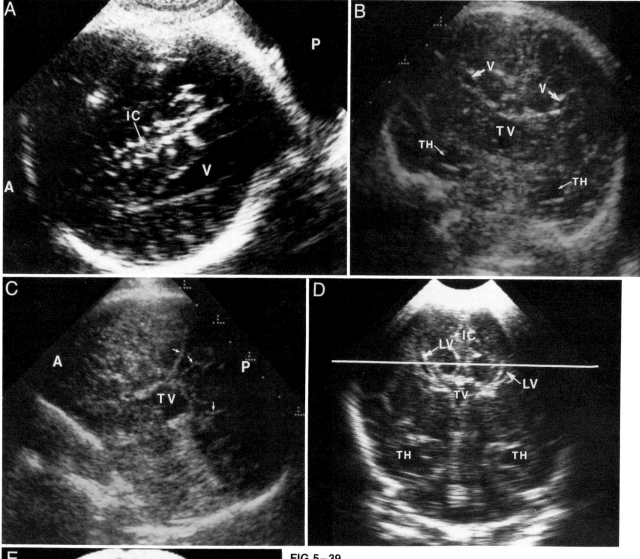

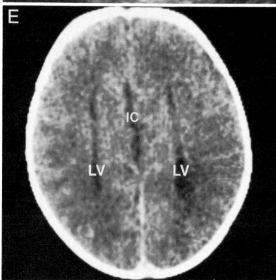

FIG 5–39.
Agenesis of the corpus callosum. **A,** transverse sonogram at 37 weeks shows angular configuration of the lateral ventricle *(V)* due to mild dilatation of the occipital horn. A prominent interhemispheric cistern *(IC)* is present. Also note abnormal sulcal and gyral pattern in the midline which is characteristic of agenesis of the corpus callosum. *A* = anterior; *P* = posterior. **B,** in utero coronal scan, performed because of abnormalities noted on transverse views, shows characteristic lateral displacement of the lateral ventricles. *TV* = third ventricle; *TH* = temporal horn. **C,** in utero sagittal scan confirms absence of the corpus callosum and shows characteristic radial array pattern of cerebral sulci *(small arrows)*. *TV* = third ventricle; *A* = anterior; *P* = posterior. **D,** postnatal coronal sonogram confirms lateral displacement of lateral ventricles *(LV)*. Note that the lateral ventricles also demonstrate an abnormal crescent shape that "points" upward, like the horns of a steer. The plane of **E** is shown by the solid line. *IC* = interhemispheric cistern; *TV* = third ventricle; *TH* = temporal horn. **E,** computed tomography shows laterally displaced lateral ventricles *(LV)* and a prominent interhemispheric cistern *(IC)*. (From Bertino RE, Nyberg DA, Cyr DR, et al: Prenatal diagnosis of agenesis of the corpus callosum. J Ultrasound Med 1988; 7:251. Used by permission.)

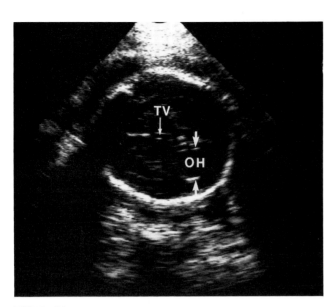

FIG 5–40.
Partial agenesis of the corpus callosum. Axial scan at 27 weeks shows only mild dilatation *(arrows)* of the occipital horns *(OH)*. The third ventricle *(TV)* is normal in size. Partial agenesis of the corpus callosum was found after delivery.

bar holoprosencephaly should not be mistaken for ACC alone, based on their distinctive sonographic features (discussed above).

If a midline cyst is not demonstrated, dilatation of the atria and occipital horns (colpocephaly) is often the initial and most prominent sonographic finding of ACC.[111] This finding is thought to result from excess space produced by the absence of the corpus callosum itself. Given this appearance, any cause of hydrocephalus should also be considered. However, ACC typically demonstrates greater enlargement of the occipital horns compared to the remaining ventricular system than is usually observed from other causes of hydrocephalus. We have found transvaginal sonography useful for distinguishing between ACC and other causes of hydrocephalus.

Associated Abnormalities

ACC is frequently associated with other malformations or syndromes.[119, 122] In an autopsy series of 47 cases of ACC, Parrish reported that 85% of patients had CNS anomalies and 62% had extra-CNS anomalies.[123] Associated CNS abnormalities may include gyral anomalies and heterotopia, midline intracerebral lipomas, encephalocele, interhemispheric arachnoid cyst, microcephaly, Dandy-Walker malformation (see Figs 5–31 and 5–36), Arnold-Chiari malformation, holoprosencephaly, septo-optic dysplasia, hydrocephalus, and aqueductal stenosis.[118, 123] Extra-CNS malformations may include abnormalities of the face, musculoskeletal system, gastrointestinal tract, genitourinary tract, cardiovascular system, and respiratory system.[123]

ACC also has been associated with multiple anomaly syndromes including the Shapiro syndrome, Rubenstein-Taybi syndrome, Aicardi's syndrome (X-linked recessive), acrocallosal syndrome, Andermann syndrome,

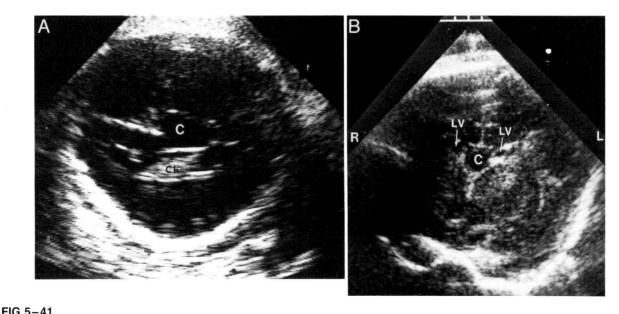

FIG 5–41.
Prominent cavum septi pellucidi. **A,** axial sonogram at 34 weeks shows a midline cyst *(C)*. *Ch* = choroid. **B,** transvaginal sonogram demonstrates that this fluid collection *(C)* represents a prominent cavum septi pellucidi normally positioned between the lateral ventricles *(LV)*. This normal structure should not be mistaken for agenesis of the corpus callosum or other midline cystic mass. *R* = right; *L* = left.

basal cell nevus syndrome (autosomal dominant), fetal alcohol syndrome, and median facial cleft syndrome.[112, 124] Like other midline cerebral malformations, ACC has been associated with chromosome abnormalities (trisomies 8, 13, and 18).[108, 111, 112, 123]

Prognosis

Isolated ACC may be asymptomatic in surviving adults. However, most children exhibit subnormal intelligence (70%) and/or seizures (60%).[121] More importantly, ACC may be associated with other CNS malformations, in which case the prognosis is determined primarily by the underlying malformation.[123]

HYDRANENCEPHALY

Pathologic and Clinical Findings

Hydranencephaly can be considered as the most severe type of destructive disorder in a continuum that also includes porencephaly and schizencephaly.[95, 130, 132] It is a rare abnormality, occurring in less than 1 in 10,000 births. Characteristic pathologic findings include total or near-total absence of the cerebral hemispheres with intact meninges and skull. The cerebellum, midbrain, thalami, basal ganglia, and choroid plexus are usually preserved.[95, 128, 132]

The most commonly accepted pathogenic mechanism for hydranencephaly is massive cerebral infarction secondary to bilateral internal carotid artery occlusion.[131] If true, this must occur in the second half of pregnancy since some portions of the brain appear normal. A possible relationship between hydranencephaly and intrauterine infection (herpes, toxoplasmosis, cytomegalovirus, and equine virus) has been occasionally reported, but in the majority of cases no etiologic factor can be identified.[127, 129]

Sonographic Findings

The sonographic diagnosis of hydranencephaly should be suspected when a large anechoic area fills the cranium with no discernible cerebral cortex (Figs 5–42 and 5–43).[65, 128, 132] The midbrain, basal ganglia, posterior fossa, and tentorium are usually normal. Occasionally, there is partial preservation of the medial occipital lobes, presumably via perfusion by the posterior communicating arteries. The falx is present, but it may be deviated or occasionally absent (see Fig 5–41). Macrocephaly is nearly always present, presumably due to continued production of CSF by the choroid

plexus.[65, 127, 128, 132] Polyhydramnios has been reported in virtually all cases. No case of hydranencephaly has been reported before the third trimester.

Intracranial contents of hydranencephaly may not appear completely anechoic, depending on the time of the sonogram relative to the vascular insult and the presence of intracranial hemorrhage. Greene et al. documented a remarkable case of hydranencephaly in evolution in which the intracranial contents initially appeared echogenic and then subsequently evolved into a hypoechoic and, finally, an anechoic appearance (see Fig 5–43).[129] This pattern is characteristic of evolving hemorrhage and is similar in appearance to hemorrhage observed in other sites, for example, periplacental hemorrhage. Aspiration of hydrancephaly may yield brown or colored fluid consistent with prior hemorrhage, even when the fluid appears anechoic.[129]

Hydranencephaly should be distinguished from massive hydrocephalus when the cerebral cortex is very thin and closely applied to the cranium. This potential confusion was more likely to occur with older ultrasound equipment when the compressed cortical rim of hydrocephalus was more difficult to appreciate. Alobar holoprosencephaly, particularly the pancake type, may also be considered in the differential diagnosis of hydranencephaly. However, alobar holoprosencephaly should be distinguished by absence of falx and midline structures, fusion of the thalami, and the presence of cerebral tissue except posteriorly overlying the dorsal sac. Also, facial anomalies and extra-CNS anomalies are usually present with alobar holoprosencephaly.

Associated Anomalies

There are no consistent anomalies associated with hydranencephaly. Also, unlike most other cerebral malformations, hydranencephaly does not carry an increased risk of chromosome abnormalities. The lack of association between concurrent anomalies and chromosomal abnormalities helps to support the vascular theory of hydranencephaly and is evidence against an embryologic basis for this malformation.

Prognosis

The prognosis for fetuses affected with hydranencephaly is uniformly dismal. In severe cases, the infant may die within a few days of birth. If the hypothalamus is preserved, however, affected infants may initially appear normal by exhibiting normal reflexes and responses. Inevitably, progressive macrocephaly develops, and few infants survive beyond 3 months. Because

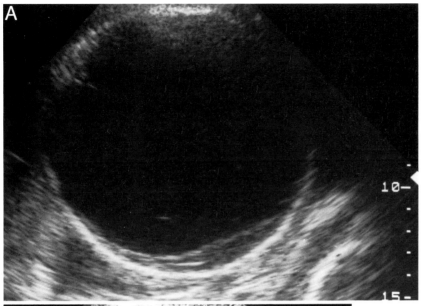

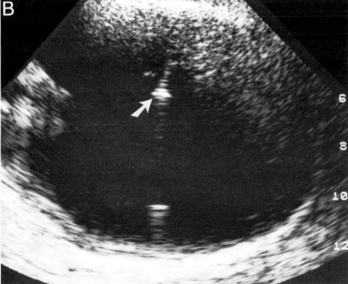

FIG 5–42.
Hydranencephaly. **A,** axial sonogram at 34 weeks demonstrates a markedly enlarged but empty cranium. Low-level echoes were seen within the fluid space consistent with hemorrhage or debris. No recognizable brain parenchyma is identified (a side-lobe artifact is noted in the far field), although thalami were identified at a more caudal level. As with this case, the falx occasionally may be absent with hydranencephaly. **B,** cephalocentesis was performed to permit vaginal delivery. The needle tip is shown *(arrow)*. Discolored fluid consistent with old blood was aspirated. A stillborn infant was delivered and hydranencephaly was confirmed. No additional anomalies were present.

of the uniformly fatal prognosis associated with hydranencephaly, cephalocentesis may be considered prior to delivery (see Fig 5–42).

PORENCEPHALY/SCHIZENCEPHALY

Clinical and Pathologic Findings

Porencephaly is a term often used for any cavitation or CSF-filled cyst in the brain. A more limited definition suggests a loss of cortical substance and communication between the cyst and the subarachnoid or ventricular spaces.[134] Porencephaly may result from vascular occlusion, birth trauma, ventricular puncture, inflammatory diseases, degeneration of the nervous system, or vascular insults from hemorrhage or embolism. In addition, there is a hereditary form of porencephaly.[134]

Congenital midline porencephaly is characterized by a triad of midline parietal scalp anomalies (alopecia or cephalocele), hydrocephalus, and a prominent midline intracranial cyst.[138] The large dorsal intracranial cyst communicates with the lateral ventricles through a mantle defect. Some authorities consider this disorder to be a form of holoprosencephaly.[138]

Like hydranencephaly and porencephaly, schizencephaly (Greek for "cleft brain") is thought by many authors to result from a destructive process.[130, 135]

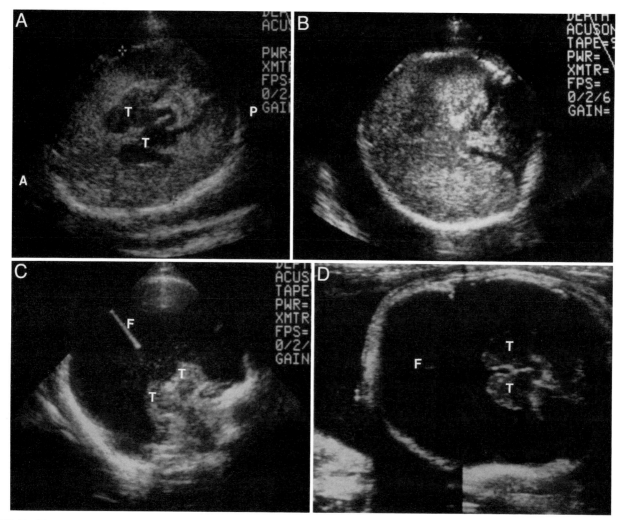

FIG 5–43.
Hydranencephaly in evolution. **A,** initial transverse sonogram made at 27 weeks at the level of the thalami *(T)* shows bright homogeneous material filling the supratentorial region. *A* = anterior; *P* = posterior. **B,** coronal sonogram confirms bright homogeneous material filling the entire supratentorial region without any recognizable brain mantle or lateral ventricles. **C,** three weeks later, coronal sonogram shows a marked change in echogenicity of supratentorial regions. The falx *(F)* is now readily identified. Low-level echoes filling the supratentorial region could be seen to swirl on real-time examination. *T* = thalami. **D,** at 40 weeks, transverse sonogram shows enlarging cranium containing only the thalami *(T)* and midbrain visible surrounded by sonolucent fluid. *F* = falx. (From Greene MF, Benacerraf BR, Crawford JM: Hydranencephaly US appearance during in utero evolution. Radiology 1985; 156:779–780. Used by permission.)

Alternatively, others believe that schizencephaly is due to abnormal neuronal migration before 6 fetal weeks.[139, 140] The term schizencephaly was originally introduced by Yakolev to describe bilateral, full-thickness clefts in the cerebral hemispheres.[139, 140] In subsequent years, however, it has become apparent that the abnormality may be unilateral and varied in degree.[133–137]

Sonographic Findings

Porencephaly appears sonographically as a fluid-filled space in the position of normal brain parenchyma. Communication with the lateral ventricles or subarachnoid space is often visible. The ipsilateral ventricle is usually enlarged to compensate for the smaller brain mass. Unlike arachoid cysts and interhemispheric cysts associated with agenesis of the corpus callosum, the porencephalic cyst produces no mass effect on the adjacent brain.

Prenatal sonographic findings of midline porencephaly include hydramnios, macrocephaly, ventriculomegaly with a common ventricle, absence of midline echo at the level of the cerebral hemispheres, and absence of facial or other associated anomalies.

Schizencephaly typically demonstrates bilateral

fluid-filled clefts extending from the cranial vault to the ventricles; however, unilateral clefts also may be demonstrated (Fig 5–44).[135] Although possibly not related in pathogenesis, the clefts are usually located in the expected distribution of the middle cerebral artery. The lateral ventricles may be dilated.

Associated Anomalies

Like hydranencephaly, associated anomalies are typically absent with porencephaly and schizencephaly.

Prognosis

Clinical symptoms of porencephaly depend on the location of the lesion. Reported symptoms include seizures, varying degrees of developmental delay, visual and sensory defects, focal motor deficits, and hydrocephalus.[134] In reviewing six cases of midline porencephaly, Vintzileos found that four had marked mental retardation, one had mild retardation, and only one had normal neurologic development.[138]

The clinical symptoms of schizencephaly also de-

pend on the amount and type of brain tissue associated with the anomaly. Typical symptoms include seizures, mental retardation, and abnormal motor function.[98]

ARACHNOID CYST

Pathologic and Clinical Findings

Arachnoid cysts represent 1% of all intracranial masses.[144, 147, 148] Two categories of arachnoid cyst are known: congenital and acquired.[141, 142, 144] Congenital arachnoid cyst probably results from abnormal leptomeningeal formation, whereas acquired arachnoid cyst is thought to develop from entrapment of CSF by arachnoid adhesions. Previous hemorrhage, trauma, or infection are contributing causes for acquired arachnoid cyst.[142] Arachnoid cysts presumably enlarge as a result of ball-valve communication with the subarachnoid space. Alternatively, heterotopic tissue similar to choroid plexus may be present within the cyst.[145]

In 30 cases of arachnoid cyst in children less than 15 years of age, 20 were supratentorial and 10 were infratentorial. Hydrocephalus was present in 20% of the supratentorial lesions and in 70% of the infratentorial lesions.[146]

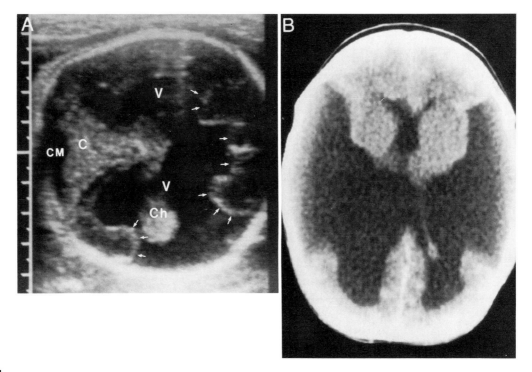

FIG 5–44.
Schizencephaly. **A,** axial sonogram angled through the posterior fossa shows large bilateral symmetric clefts of the brain mantle so that the ventricles *(V)* communicate with the subarachnoid space. Remaining brain mantle is shown *(arrows)*. The choroid plexus *(Ch)* is seen hanging within the far ventricle. *C* = cerebellum; *CM* = cisterna magna. **B,** computed tomography scan after birth confirms the prenatal findings of large, symmetric clefts of the brain mantle. (Courtesy of Laurence A Mack, MD, University of Washington, Seattle, WA.)

Sonographic Findings

An arachnoid cyst is seen as a fluid-filled, thin-walled cystic mass (see Fig 5–34) that usually displaces adjacent brain structures. It may be either asymmetric in location (Fig 5–45) or located in the midline (Fig 5–46).[143] Hydrocephalus may be demonstrated if the cyst obstructs CSF flow.

The differential diagnosis for an asymmetric arachnoid cyst includes porencephalic cyst, unilateral hydrocephalus (Fig 5–47), unilateral schizencephaly, and cystic neoplasms; the differential diagnosis for a midline arachnoid cyst includes a Dandy-Walker cyst, dorsal cyst of holoprosencephaly, agenesis of the corpus callosum with interhemispheric cyst, vein of Galen aneurysm, and prominent cavum septi pellucidi. The correct diagnosis can usually be suggested by considering the shape and precise location of the cyst as well as an evaluation of other cranial findings (see Table 5–1).

Associated Anomalies

There are no specific anomalies associated with arachnoid cysts.

Prognosis

The prognosis of arachnoid cyst is excellent if appropriate shunting and surgical therapy are performed, otherwise irreversible neurologic defects and mental retardation may occur.[141, 146]

VEIN OF GALEN ANEURYSM

Pathologic and Clinical Findings

The vein of Galen aneurysm is a rare vascular malformation that produces increased vascular flow through the vein of Galen. It is thought to arise either from a failure of maturation, with persistence of a more primitive vascular system, or from lack of development of capillaries between the arterial and venous systems.[150]

Hydrocephalus may be seen with vein of Galen aneurysm. Possible mechanisms for hydrocephalus include compression of the Sylvian aqueduct by the aneurysmal mass or defective CSF resorption resulting from intracranial venous hypertension.[149, 150] Spontaneous resolution of hydrocephalus occurred after throm-

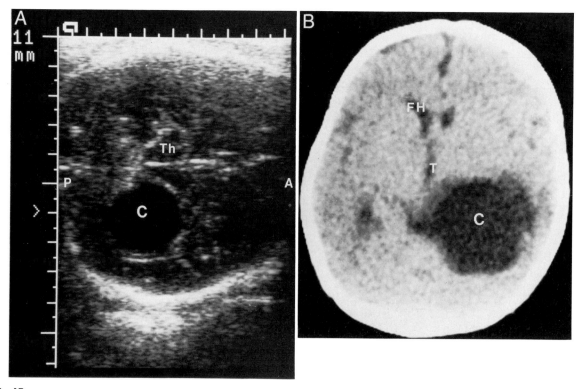

FIG 5–45.
Arachnoid cyst. **A,** axial scan at the level of the thalami *(Th)* shows an asymmetrically located arachnoid cyst *(C).* **B,** postnatal CT scan shows that the cyst *(C)* produces some mass effect on adjacent structures. *FH* = frontal horn; *T* = third ventricle. (From McGahan JP, Ellis W, Lindfors KK, et al: Congenital cerebrospinal fluid-containing intracranial abnormalities: Sonographic classification. J Clin Ultrasound 1988; 16:531–544. Used by permission.)

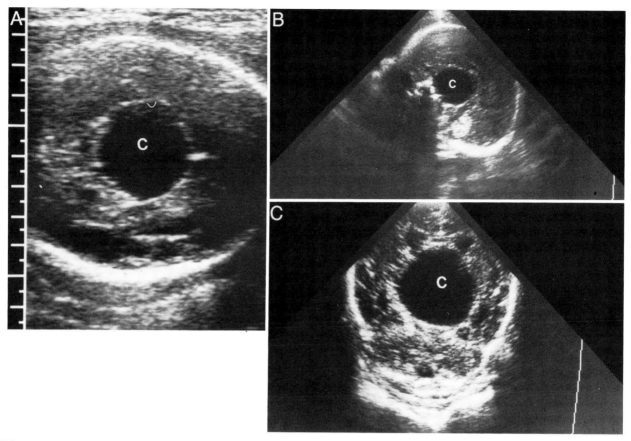

FIG 5–46.
Midline arachnoid cyst at 32 weeks' gestation. **A,** axial sonogram at the level of the cerebral peduncles shows a rounded midline cystic mass *(C)*. **B,** sagittal sonogram confirms the midline position of the cyst *(C)*. **C,** postnatal coronal sonogram confirms the midline cyst *(C)*. (From Diakoumakis EE, Weinberg B, Molin J: Prenatal sonographic diagnosis of a suprasellar arachnoid cyst. J Ultrasound Med 1986; 5:520–530. Used by permission.)

bosis of the aneurysm in three cases reported by Diebler.[149]

Patients carrying a fetus with a vein of Galen aneurysm may be referred to sonography for various clinical indications including large-for-dates secondary to polyhydramnios, fetal hydrops, elevated alpha-fetoprotein, and abnormal fetal heart rate tracing.[152, 155]

Sonographic Findings

Characteristic findings of vein of Galen aneurysm have been reported on prenatal sonography.[5, 151–156, 159] A well-defined, midline, cystic tubular structure representing the dilated vein of Galen is demonstrated in its typical location in the quadrigeminal plate cistern, superior and posterior to the thalami (Fig 5–48). A turbulent venous and/or arterial flow Doppler signal is demonstrated within the cystic structure.[151, 157, 158] Frequently, the carotid arteries and jugular veins also appear dilated and show increased flow.[153, 155, 158, 159] Areas of cerebral ischemia or in-

farction, seen as areas of increased echogenicity and smaller cysts, may occasionally be seen surrounding the vein of Galen. Extracranial sonographic findings that may be observed include polyhydramnios and signs of congestive heart failure, i.e., cardiomegaly, hydrops, and hepatomegaly.

The differential diagnosis for vein of Galen aneurysm includes other midline cystic masses such as arachnoid cyst, interhemispheric cyst associated with agenesis of the corpus callosum, and dorsal sac associated with holoprosencephaly. Distinguishing features of a vein of Galen aneurysm include its characteristic location and shape, evidence of cardiovascular disturbance, and high vascular flow observed on Doppler ultrasound.

Associated Abnormalities

CNS abnormalities related to ischemia commonly accompany the vein of Galen aneurysm. Extra-CNS abnormalities of hydrops, polyhydramnios, and cardio-

124 *Chapter 5*

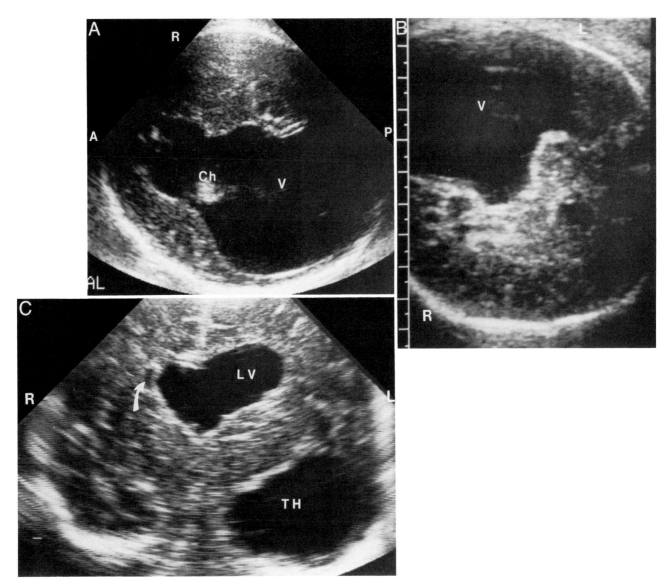

FIG 5–47.
Unilateral hydrocephalus. **A,** axial scan shows a markedly dilated left lateral ventricle *(V)* occupying much of the left hemisphere. The presence of the choroid plexus *(Ch)* confirms that the mass represents a dilated ventricle and not another cystic mass. *A* = anterior; *P* = posterior; *R* = right. **B,** scanning through the opposite hemisphere confirms that the ventricular dilatation *(V)* is unilateral and not due to a near field artifact. *R* = right; *L* = left. **C,** postnatal coronal sonogram confirms unilateral left-sided hydrocephalus with dilatation of the temporal horn *(TH)* and lateral ventricle *(LV)*. Note the compressed right lateral ventricle *(curved arrow)*. Congenital obstruction at the foramen of Monro was found in this unusual case. *R* = right; *L* = left. (Courtesy of Laurence A Mack, MD, University of Washington, Seattle, WA.)

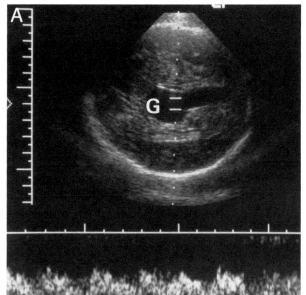

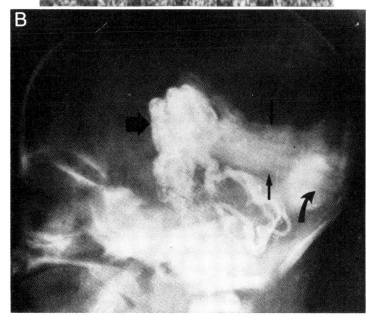

FIG 5–48.
Vein of Galen aneurysm. **A,** simultaneous real-time and duplex Doppler scan demonstrates a tubular cystic mass in the mid, posterior cranium representing a vein of Galen aneurysm *(G)*. Doppler demonstrates prominent blood flow. **B,** postnatal angiogram of another fetus diagnosed prenatally demonstrates a vein of Galen malformation with large feeding vessels *(large straight arrow)* draining into vein of Galen *(straight arrows)* and straight sinus *(curved arrow)*. (Part **A** courtesy of Roy A Filly, MD, University of California, San Francisco, CA. Part **B** from Hirsch JH, Cyr D, Eberhardt H, et al: Ultrasonographic diagnosis of an aneurysm of the vein of Galen in utero by duplex scanning. J Ultrasound Med 1983; 2:231–233. Used by permission.)

megaly can also be attributed to the underlying hemodynamic disturbance.

Prognosis

Clinical symptoms associated with a vein of Galen aneurysm fall into one of three groups, depending on the severity of the cardiovascular disturbance and the time of presentation. In group I, cyanosis, congestive heart failure, cardiomegaly, cranial bruit, and seizures develop in the first few days of life; in group II, macrocrania, hydrocephalus, subarachnoid hemorrhage, seizures, intracranial bruit, and cardiomegaly develop between 1 and 15 months of age; and in group III, headaches, seizures, subarachnoid hemorrhage and syncope develop in late childhood or adulthood.[149, 150, 154, 159] The prognosis is poor in patients in group I, variable in group II, and good in group III.

In a review of 40 cases of infants with vein of Galen aneurysm and congestive heart failure (group I), Watson et al. reported only 7 survivors, of whom 2 had hydrocephalus.[160] Death has also resulted in 5 of the 7 fetuses with vein of Galen aneurysm reported prenatally.[151, 156, 159] Embolization of the arteriovenous malformation or prompt surgical therapy may result in an improved outcome for all patient groups.

CHOROID PLEXUS CYSTS

Pathologic and Clinical Findings

Choroid cysts are thought to result from cerebrospinal fluid and cellular debris accumulating in neuroepithelial folds.[173] Histologically, small cysts are very common and have been identified in over 50% of patients at all ages in autopsy series.[167, 173] Although cysts large enough to be identified at sonography are less common, they still represent the most common intracranial "abnormality" reported prenatally.

The reported prevalence of sonographically detectable cysts has varied widely.[163, 164, 171, 174] Chan et al. detected choroid plexus cysts in 2.5% of women between 16–24 weeks who were scanned prior to genetic amniocentesis,[163] while Chitkara reported a prevalence of 0.65%, although this is undoubtedly an underestimate since all but one of the 41 choroid cysts were detected between 16–22 weeks, whereas the 6,288 sonograms used as the denominator were scanned any time between 16 to 42 weeks.[164] Other factors that undoubtedly influence the reported prevalence of choroid plexus cysts include the size criterion for "diagnosing" cysts and the thoroughness with which they are sought.

Sonographic Findings

Choroid plexus cysts have been frequently reported on prenatal sonography.[161–166, 168–172, 174] Nearly all choroid plexus cysts can be initially identified in the second trimester, between 15 to 26 weeks (Fig 5–49). Serial sonograms show that they usually resolve by 24 weeks,[161, 164, 165, 169] although occasional cysts may resolve later.[164, 171]

Choroid plexus cysts are usually small, measuring less than 1 cm in diameter (range, 0.3–2.0 cm). Since minor irregularities of the choroid plexus are commonly identified sonographically, sonolucencies smaller than 0.3 cm probably should not be considered discrete cysts. Choroid cysts are usually located in the posterior aspect of the lateral ventricles (atria). Although the cysts are often more apparent in the ventricle farthest from the transducer (see Fig 5–49), they frequently are bilateral. A multilocular appearance may be demonstrated.

The sonographic appearance of a cyst within the choroid plexus of a second trimester fetus is so characteristic that no differential diagnosis is usually required. In newborns, cysts in the germinal matrix may be related to prior hemorrhage or infection. Rarely, large choroid cysts may expand the ventricular wall and be mistaken for hydrocephalus (Fig 5–50).[162, 168] This

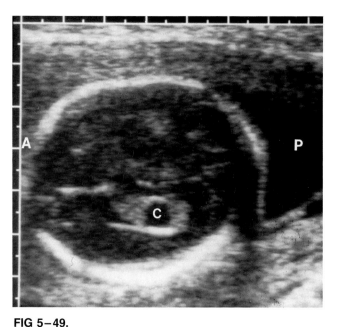

FIG 5–49.
Choroid plexus cyst. Axial scan at 20 weeks' gestation, performed prior to genetic amniocentesis, demonstrates a well-defined cyst (C) arising from the echogenic choroid plexus. The cyst resolved on a follow-up examination. No other anomalies were seen sonographically or at birth, and chromosomes were normal. A = anterior; P = posterior.

type of choroid plexus cyst appears to carry a significantly greater risk of an underlying chromosomal abnormality (trisomy 18).[162, 168]

Associated Anomalies

Choroid plexus cysts have come to clinical attention because 1) large cysts may be confused for hydrocephalus[162, 168] and 2) a possible association has been observed with chromosome abnormalities, particularly trisomy 18 (see Fig 5–50).[162, 164, 168, 170, 172] Cysts that are large or atypical in appearance or those that do not resolve on serial examinations appear to carry a greater risk of an underlying chromosome abnormality. The available data regarding a possible association between choroid plexus cysts and chromosome abnormalities is discussed further in Chapter 17.

Prognosis

Choroid cysts themselves appear to be uniformly asymptomatic and transient.[161, 164, 165] Therefore, most small cysts are ignored in clinical practice, particularly if no additional abnormalities are identified. It has been suggested that fetuses who demonstrate unusually large cysts or cysts that do not resolve by 22 menstrual weeks should be considered for chromosome analysis.

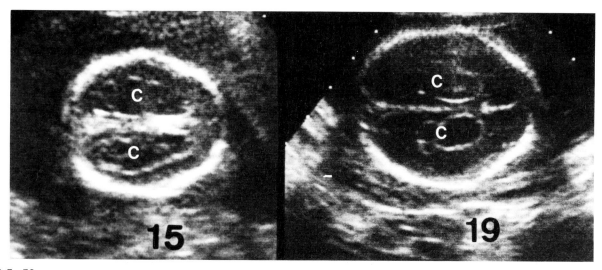

FIG 5–50.
Choroid plexus cysts associated with trisomy 18. Axial sonograms performed at 15 and 19 weeks' gestation demonstrate large, bilateral choroid plexus cysts *(C)* filling the lateral ventricles. By 36 weeks, the cysts resolved, but polyhydramnios was evident. After birth, trisomy 18, choanal atresia and small ventricular septal defects were found. (From Furness ME: Choroid plexus cysts and trisomy 18. Lancet 1987; ii:693. Used by permission.)

INTRACRANIAL NEOPLASM

Pathologic and Clinical Findings

Few cases of intracranial tumors have been reported prenatally, with the largest series reviewing ten teratomas.[177] Intracranial tumors in neonates are also considered to be rare.[173] In a review of 103 intracranial tumors in neonates less than 2 months, the types of tumors included teratoma, medulloblastoma, ependymoma, choroid plexus papilloma, astrocytoma, and other tumors.[181] The site of the tumors in the above series was supratentorial (64), subtentorial (15), supra and subtentorial (18), and unknown (6).

Sonographic Findings

Patients carrying a fetus with an intracranial neoplasm may be referred to sonography with clinical indications of large for gestational age, acute polyhydramnios, elevated MS-AFP or routine indications.[177, 182] Although most tumors have been identified in the third trimester, one case was identified as early as 20 weeks.[177]

Intracranial neoplasms are generally large tumors that demonstrate a heterogeneous, bizarre appearance (Figs 5–51 and 5–52).[175–177, 179, 180, 183] The mass is typically solid, with variable echogenicity and occasional calcification. Cystic areas may be demonstrated, although this is not typically the predominant component of the mass (see Fig 5–52).[179] Rarely, cystic neoplasms may mimic other cystic masses such as arach-

noid cysts (Fig 5–53). Hydrocephalus may be demonstrated if the mass obstructs CSF flow. Large masses may deform the cranium, and extracranial extension of the mass rarely has been demonstrated. Polyhydramnios has been reported in all cases after 20 weeks.[176, 177, 179] Serial sonograms typically show rapid enlargement of the mass and enlargement of the cranium. Rarely, extracranial extension may be demonstrated.[177, 178]

The differential diagnosis for an intracranial neoplasm includes other bizarre-appearing masses such as intracranial hemorrhage, infection, or ischemic brain necrosis. If there is a significant cystic component, other cystic masses such as arachnoid cyst and porencephaly should be considered. Meningoencephalocele and exencephaly may also be considered if the mass shows extracranial extension.

Associated Anomalies

No specific anomalies have been associated with intracranial neoplasms.

Prognosis

The prognosis for fetuses (and neonates) with intracranial tumors is dismal. In Takaku's series of 103 neonates less than 2 months of age with intracranial neoplasms, 28 were stillborn and all but 4 of the remaining infants died by 1 year of age.[181] All cases diagnosed prenatally died shortly after birth. Because of the

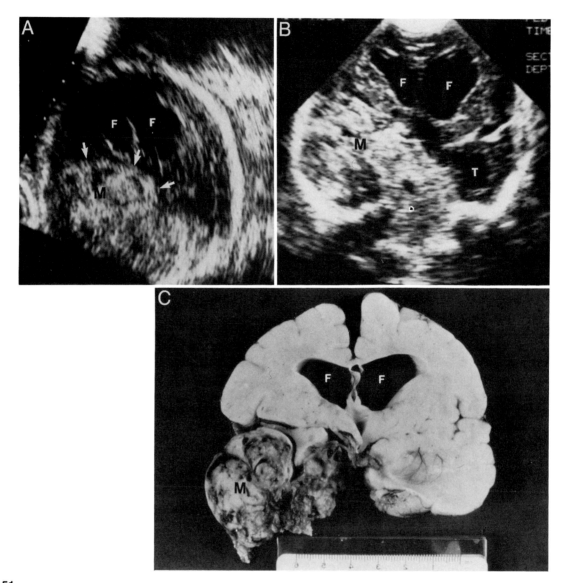

FIG 5–51.
Neoplasm (teratoma). **A,** coronal image of fetal head at 36 weeks' gestational age showing a mass *(M)* of increased echogenicity *(arrows)* in the right temporal lobe. Dilated frontal horns *(F)* are also present. **B,** coronal image of neonate showing a mass *(M)* of increased echogenicity in the right temporal lobe and dilated frontal horns *(F)* and temporal horn *(T)*. **C,** pathological specimen corresponding to sonogram. (From Lipman S, Pretorius D, Rumack C, et al: Fetal intracranial teratoma: US diagnosis of three cases and a review of the literature. Radiology 1985; 157:491–494. Used by permission.)

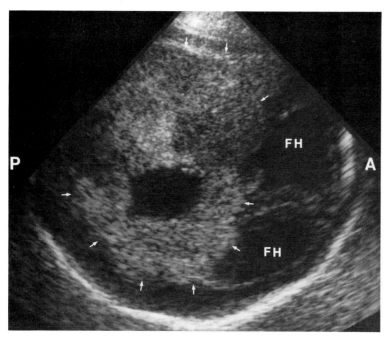

FIG 5-52.
Neoplasm (glioma). Axial sonogram demonstrates a large, bizarre appearing mass that is predominantly solid *(arrows)* but shows a central cystic component. Dilated frontal horns *(FH)* are also noted. *A* = anterior; *P* = posterior.

dismal prognosis, termination of pregnancy may be an option if the diagnosis is made prior to viability. Cesarean delivery may be necessary secondary to birth dystocia.[176] Cephalocentesis may be considered if significant hydrocephalus or a large cystic component accompanies the mass.

INTRACRANIAL HEMORRHAGE IN UTERO

Pathologic and Clinical Findings

Intracranial hemorrhage is commonly encountered in premature infants; it has been reported in 40%–60% of infants born earlier than 32 weeks' gestational age and weighing less than 1,500 gm.[189] Such hemorrhage usually originates from the germinal matrix, from which it can rupture into the ventricles. In severe cases, associated intraparenchymal hemorrhage results from extension of the germinal matrix hemorrhage or from hemorrhagic infarction. Primary hemorrhage in the posterior fossa may also occur. Alterations in blood pressure or perinatal hypoxic events are thought to be the primary stimuli for initiation of hemorrhage.

Compared to the neonatal experience, intracranial hemorrhage has rarely been observed in utero.[184–188, 190–198] Occasional case reports suggest that prenatal hemorrhage is also precipitated by anoxia or alterations in blood pressure. Risk factors that have been associated with prenatal intracranial hemorrhage

include a maternal hypertensive or hypotensive episode, maternal seizure, placental abruption, and alloimmune thrombocytopenia.[184–188, 190–198]

Alloimmune thrombocytopenia deserves a special comment as a relatively common cause of antenatal hemorrhage.[185, 188, 191, 196, 198] This disorder occurs in approximately 1 in 2,000 to 1 in 5,000 pregnancies, and intracranial hemorrhage, which may be either antenatal or postnatal, occurs in 15%–20% of cases.[185] The cause of hemorrhage is fetal and neonatal thrombocytopenia resulting from maternal antibodies to a paternally derived platelet antigen, usually PLA1. The pathophysiology is analagous to erythroblastosis fetalis (Rh disease) except that, unlike red blood cells, platelets are able to cross the placenta and isoimmunization occurs during the first pregnancy. The rate of recurrence to subsequent offspring is estimated at more than 75%.[185]

Sonographic Findings

The sonographic findings of intracranial hemorrhage vary with the location and onset of hemorrhage. Acutely, intracranial hemorrhage appears sonographically as an echogenic area within the ventricles (Fig 5–54) or within the brain parenchyma. If the fetus survives, follow-up scans or an examination remote from the onset of hemorrhage show characteristic cystic areas (Fig 5–55). Bright ependymal echoes surrounding the ventricles may be seen from associated infarction.

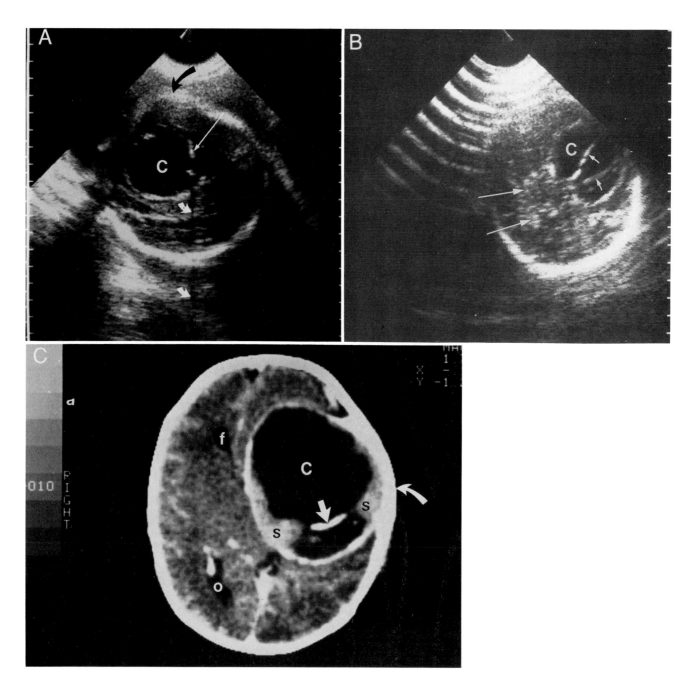

FIG 5–53.
Cystic neoplasm. **A,** axial scan at 31 weeks demonstrates a large cystic mass *(c)* in the left cerebral hemisphere, with internal septation *(long straight arrow)*. Acoustic shadow *(short arrow)* suggests calcification. Note asymmetric bulge of left cranial vault *(curved arrow)*. **B,** postnatal coronal scan shows left-sided cystic mass *(c)* with central septations *(short arrows)*. The choroid plexus *(long arrows)* lies in non–dilated occipital horn of right lateral ventricle. **C,** CT scan shows cystic mass *(c)* displacing midline structures to right. Note peripheral solid components *(s)* and calcified septation *(arrow)* of mass and asymmetric bulge of cranial vault *(curved arrow)*. *F*= frontal horn; *o* = occipital horn. (From Sauerbrei EE, Cooperberg PL: Radiology 1983; 147:689–692. Used by permission.)

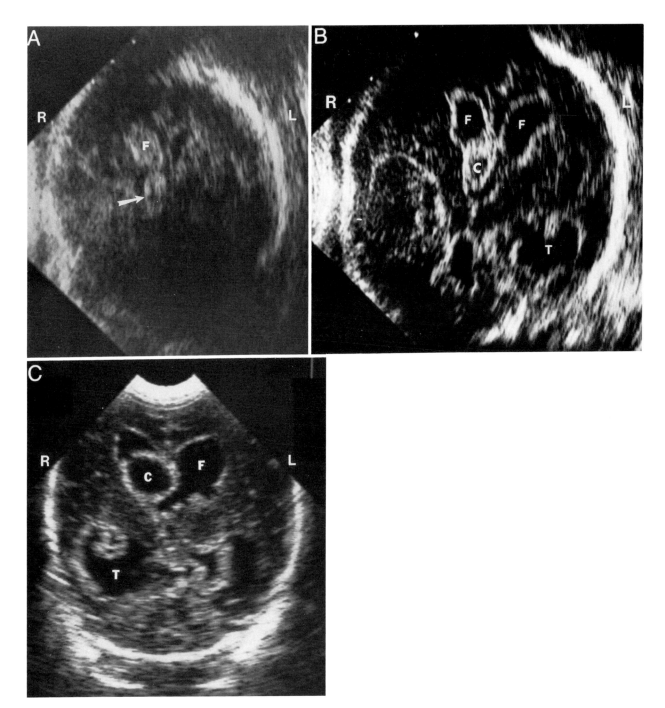

FIG 5–54.
Intracranial hemorrhage. **A,** coronal image at 33 weeks' gestational age showing increased echogenicity in the frontal horn *(F)* and caudate nucleus *(arrow)* consistent with hemorrhage. *R* = right; *L* = left. **B,** two weeks later, a subependymal cyst *(C)* has developed in the area of previous hemorrhage and dilatation of the frontal horns *(F)* and temporal horns *(T)* has occurred. *R* = right; *L* = left. **C,** postnatal coronal scan shows ventricular dilatation and a large subependymal cyst *(C)* characteristic of resolving hemorrhage. *T* = temporal horn; *F* = frontal horn; *R* = right; *L* = left. (From Pretorius D, Singh S, Manco-Johnson M: In utero diagnosis of intracranial hemorrhage resulting in fetal hydrocephalus. J Reprod Med 1986; 31:136–138. Used by permission.)

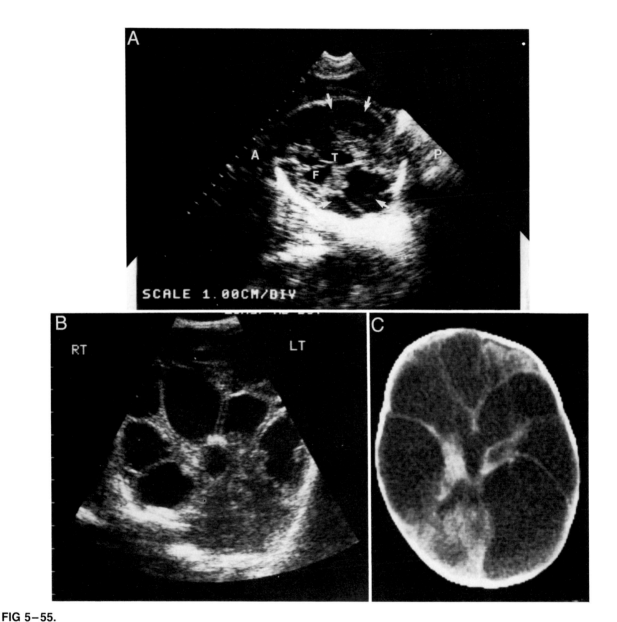

FIG 5–55.
Intracranial hemorrhage due to alloimmune thrombocytopenia. **A,** axial sonogram at 36 weeks shows multiple cysts throughout the brain parenchyma *(arrows)* and mildly dilated lateral ventricles. An earlier sonogram at 21 weeks was normal. *F* = frontal horn; *T* = third ventricle; *A* = anterior; *P* = posterior. **B,** postnatal coronal sonogram confirms multiple cysts throughout the brain mantle. **C,** computed tomography confirms sonographic findings. The cystic areas are difficult to distinguish from dilated ventricles. The etiology of hemorrhage in this case was isoimmune thrombocytopenia (maternal antibodies against fetal platelet antigens). (From Lester RB III, Sty JR: Prenatal diagnosis of cystic CNS lesions in neonatal isoimmune thrombocytopenia. J Ultrasound Med 1987; 6:479–481. Used by permission.)

Hydrocephalus may be present at the time of diagnosis or as a sequelae to intraventricular hemorrhage (see Fig 5–54).[197]

The primary differential diagnosis for intracranial hemorrhage includes intracranial neoplasm or infection. Intraventricular hemorrhage may superficially appear as an enlarged choroid plexus from an adherent clot.

Associated Anomalies

Excluding the maternal and fetal risk factors discussed above, no specific fetal anomalies are known to be associated with intracranial hemorrhage.

Prognosis

The outcome of intracranial hemorrhage in neonates is directly related to the extent of hemorrhage, with intraparenchymal hemorrhage having the worst prognosis. Due to the size of hemorrhage seen prenatally, the sonographic diagnosis of intracranial hemorrhage is often made concomitant with fetal demise[187, 190, 194] or shortly before demise.[184, 188] Two fetuses have survived with seizures and hydrocephalus,[196, 198] while 2 other fetuses have had good outcomes following ventricular shunting for hydrocephalus after birth.[193, 197]

MICROCEPHALY

Pathologic and Clinical Findings

Microcephaly signifies a decreased head size, with a reduction of the brain mass and total cell number. It has been defined variably as a head size more than 3 standard deviations (SD) below the mean by some investigators,[200] but as more than 2 SD below the mean by others.[203] One series from Sweden reported an incidence of microcephaly of 1 in 6,000 to 10,000 births.[199] The true incidence is probably higher, since these statistics do not include spontaneous abortions, stillborns, or early neonatal deaths.

The etiologies of microcephaly are diverse (Table 5–6). These may be considered either as environmental (anoxia, viral infections, radiation exposure) or congenital in origin. Congenital causes include mendelian syndromes (for example, Meckel-Gruber syndrome), chromosome abnormalities, or an underlying CNS malformation. It is important to realize that, regardless of the cause, microcephaly is usually secondary to abnor-

mal brain development; a primary calvarial disorder that restricts normal brain growth (complete craniosynostosis) is very rare.

Sonographic Findings

The sonographic findings of microcephaly include (1) small biparietal diameter and head circumference (Fig 5–56); (2) abdomen-head size discrepancy, with the head being smaller than expected; and (3) poor growth of the fetal head on serial examinations.[202–204, 206] Disorganized brain parenchyma may also be identified (see Fig 5–56).

Microcephaly may not be demonstrated until after 24 weeks, when subnormal cranial growth can be seen to fall clearly below normal values (Fig 5–57).[204, 207] Even then the diagnosis of microcephaly is often difficult, since head measurements are affected by incorrect dating and symmetric growth retardation. Chervenak et al. suggested a nomogram involving occipital frontal diameter, head circumference, and ratios involving the head circumference, abdominal circumference, and femur length to help identify fetuses with microcephaly.[201] However, an early prenatal diagnosis of microcephaly remains elusive.

The primary differential diagnosis of microcephaly is anencephaly. This distinction is occasionally difficult when the intact cranial vault of severe microcephaly is not appreciated.

Associated Abnormalities

Other anomalies that have been associated with microcephaly include encephalocele, porencephaly, lissencephaly, holoprosencephaly, macrogyria, microgyria, agyria, Kleeblattschadel, and intracranial calcification.[202] Microcephaly may be a part of various syndromes, including the Meckel-Gruber syndrome.

Prognosis

The prognosis for microcephaly varies, depending on the underlying malformation and associated anomalies. Mental retardation has been reported in 50% to 99% of fetuses with microcephaly in several series.[202, 205] In one report of 202 microcephalic children, only 7.5% to 13.5% were considered normal.[205] On the other hand, children with microcephaly resulting from intrauterine growth retardation (IUGR), congenital heart disease, or malabsorption syndromes usually have no neurologic deficits.[205] Genetic forms of

TABLE 5-6.

Causes of Microcephaly*†

CNS malformations	Holoprosencephaly
	Encephalocele
	Kleeblattschadel
	Craniosynostosis (rare)
	Lissencephaly
	Atelencephaly
Chromosome abnormalities	Trisomy 13
	Trisomy 18
	Trisomy 21
	Trisomy 22
	Triploidy
	Others
Inheritable syndromes	Bloom (AR)
	Bowen-Conradi (AR)
	Coffin-Siris (AR)
	De Barsy-cutis laxa-mr-corneal opacity (AR)
	Dubowitz (AR)
	Fanconi pancytopenia (AR)
	Johanson-Blizzard (AR)
	Joubert-cerebellar vermis aplasia (AR)
	Meckel-Gruber (AR)
	Neu-Laxova (AR)
	Rhizomelic chondrodysplasia punctata (AR)
	Robert's (AR)
	Smith-Lemli-Opitz (AR)
	Other familial (AR)
	X-linked microcephaly (X-linked)
Environmental	Chronic hypoxia
	Radiation exposure
	Infections (rubella, CMV, toxoplasmosis)
	Maternal phenylketonuria
	Drugs (alcohol, hydantoin, amninopterin)
Unknown	Brachmann-de Lange
	Rubenstein-Taybi

*Adapted from Winter RM, Knowles SAS, Bieber FR, et al: *The Malformed Fetus and Stillbirth. A Diagnostic Approach*, New York, John Wiley & Sons, Ltd, 1988.
†S = mostly sporadic, AR = autosomal recessive, AD = autosomal dominant, ASD = atrial septal defect, VSD = ventricular septal defect, TOF = tetralogy of Fallot, SVC = superior vena cava.

microcephaly, such as the Meckel-Gruber syndrome, carry a 25% risk of recurrence.

MISCELLANEOUS LESIONS

Lissencephaly

The term lissencephaly ("smooth brain") refers to total or near-total absence of gyri and sulci. Pathologically, lissencephaly has a four-layered cortex[137, 209] instead of the normal six-layered cortex found in adults. It is thought to result from an interruption of neuronal migration through the pathway from the germinal matrix to the brain surface.[208, 218] It is usually sporadic, but may also be inherited as an autosomal recessive disorder or associated with chromosomal abnormalities.

Sonographic findings of lissencephaly in the neonate include ventriculomegaly, flattening of the cortical surface without sulcal or gyral formation, and widening of the sylvian fissures and subarachnoid space.[208] Since gyri do not normally begin to form until after 4 months of gestation[220], the prenatal diagnosis of lissencephaly is not possible until the late third trimester. Lissencephaly has not yet been diagnosed prenatally.

CNS abnormalities that may be associated with lissencephaly include microcephaly, ventriculomegaly, dysgenesis of the corpus callosum, widening of the sylvian fissures, and little opercularization of the insula. A small brain stem is often associated with lissencephaly syndromes and may reflect lack of development of the corticospinal tracts. Hydrocephalus is commonly associated with lissencephaly as part of the "lissencephaly sequence".[210, 211] Various clinical syndromes

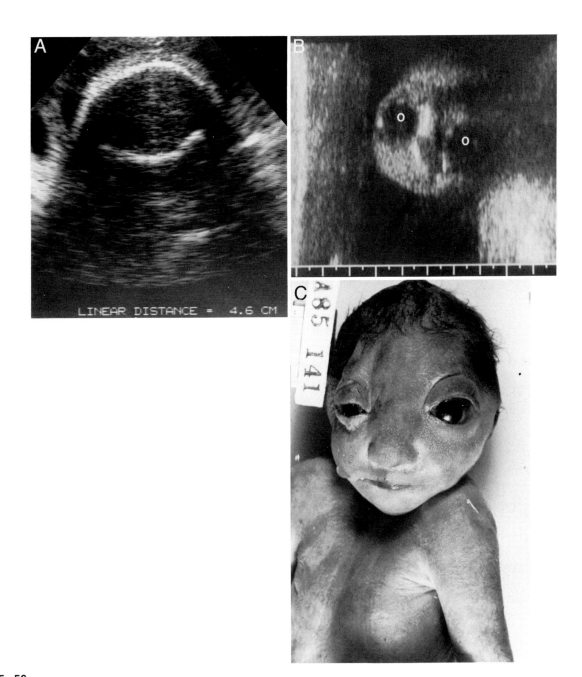

FIG 5–56.
Microcephaly **A,** axial sonogram at 29 weeks (based on menstrual history and other growth parameters) demonstrates a small cranial size, corresponding to 20 weeks. In addition, no recognizable internal landmarks are demonstrated. **B,** coronal sonogram demonstrates relative proptosis with very small cranial vault. *O* = orbits. **C,** postmortem photograph shows microcephaly, hypertelorism, and micrognathia. Other intracranial findings included lissencephaly and a Dandy-Walker cyst. The phenotype is consistent with the Neu-Laxova syndrome, an autosomal recessive disorder.

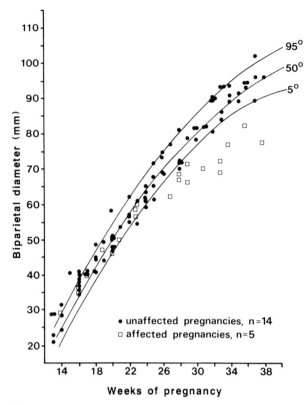

FIG 5-57.
Graph showing serial cranial measurements in 19 pregnancies (14 normal and 5 microcephalic) which were followed because of a genetic risk of recurrent microcephaly. Note that the cranial size may not fall below normal values until after 24 weeks' gestation. (From Tolmie JL, McNay M, Stephenson JBP, et al: Microcephaly: Genetic counseling and antenatal diagnosis after the birth of an affected child. Am J Med Genet 1987; 27:583-594. Used by permission.)

have been associated with lissencephaly, including the Miller-Dieker syndrome, Norman-Roberts syndrome, Walker-Warburg syndrome (autosomal recessive) and isotretinoin (Accutane) exposure.

Clinically, infants with lissencephaly typically exhibit seizures, severe mental retardation, and developmental delay. Death frequently occurs before 2 years of age.

Infection

Disseminated fetal infection may occur from cytomegalovirus, rubella, herpes, varicella, and toxoplasmosis. Microcephaly is the most commonly reported congenital abnormality resulting from such an intrauterine infection. However, the majority of fetuses exposed to maternal infections do not develop complications; Preece studied 54 children exposed prenatally to maternal cytomegolovirus and found that only nine (17%) developed congenital infection.[217]

Intracranial calcifications have been rarely identified from in utero infection, typically from cytomegalovirus or toxoplasmosis (Fig 5-58). Intracranial calcification may not necessarily demonstrate acoustic shadowing.[218]

Calvarial Abnormalities

Inadequate cranial ossification may occur with various skeletal dysplasias including achondrogenesis, osteogenesis imperfecta, and hypophosphatasia (Fig 5-59). Sonographically, the cranium may look fuzzy, poorly defined, or decreased in echogenicity, although normal echogenicity may also be observed. The falx may appear particularly prominent due to the poor mineralization of the cranium.[212]

Kleeblattschadel ("cloverleaf skull") is an unusual, but characteristic shape of the head (Fig 5-60). The precise mechanism responsible for this head shape is unknown, but premature synostosis of the coronal and lambdoidal sutures is usually present. In reviewing 27 cases of Kleeblattschadel, Partington subcategorized them into one of three types: type I coexists with thanatophoric dwarfism[213], type II is associated with less severe skeletal lesions such as ankylosis of joints, and type III has the best prognosis.[216]

Hydrocephalus is often associated with Kleeblattschadel and was found in eight of nine prenatal cases reviewed by Stamm et al.[219] All but one of the cases in this review were seen in association with thanatophoric dwarfism. Interestingly, five of nine cases were initially misinterpreted as an encephalocele.[219] Stamm et al. suggest that the bilateral temporal bulges are best demonstrated on a coronal scan through the temporal bones. Kleeblattschadel (see Fig 5-60) should not be mistaken for the lemon sign deformity (see Fig 5-19), which is seen in association with meningomyelocele (see Chapter 6).[214, 215]

SUMMARY

Optimal patient management and counseling of a suspected cranial anomaly require a specific diagnosis of the underlying malformation and identification of important associated anomalies. Prenatal sonography is remarkably sensitive for detection and classification of major intracranial malformations including hydrocephalus, holoprosencephaly, Dandy-Walker malformation, hydrancephaly, and other intracranial cystic masses (porencephaly, arachnoid cyst, neoplasms, and choroid plexus cysts). Typical sonographic findings should permit a correct diagnosis in nearly all of these cases.

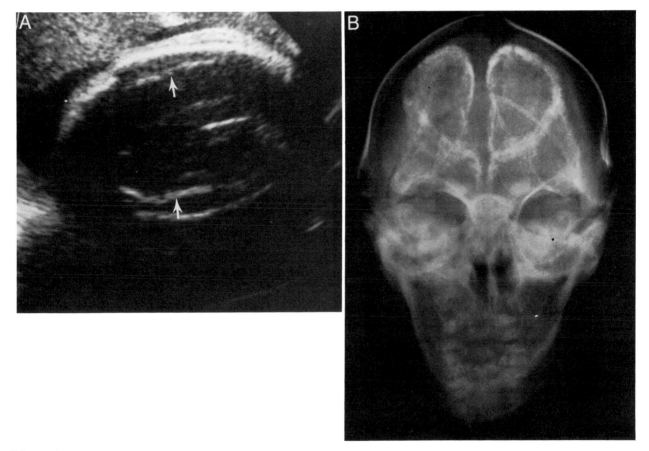

FIG 5–58.
Cytomegalovirus. **A,** axial sonogram through fetal head at 35 weeks' gestational age shows echogenic walls *(arrows)* of the dilated lateral ventricles suggesting calcification. The head was also microcephalic, consistent with 23 weeks by biparietal diameter. **B,** skull radiograph after delivery shows dense periventricular calcifications.

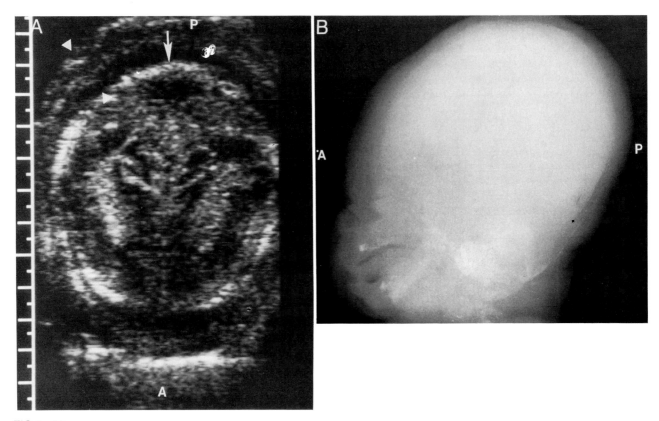

FIG 5–59.
Osteogenesis imperfecta. **A,** sonogram of fetal head shows edema *(arrowheads)* of the scalp and poor ossification of the cranium *(arrow)*. *A* = anterior; *P* = posterior. **B,** lateral radiograph after delivery shows minimal ossification of the cranium. *A* = anterior; *P* = posterior.

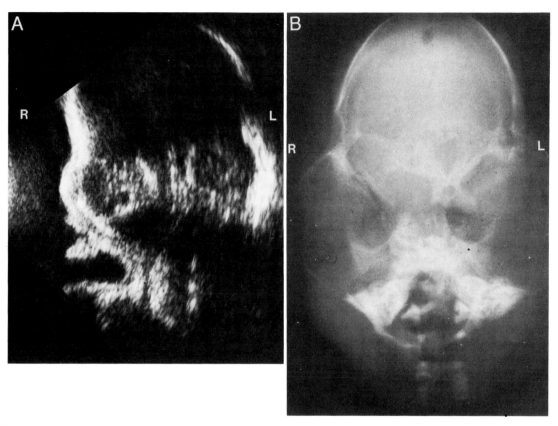

FIG 5−60.
Kleeblattschadel (cloverleaf skull). **A,** coronal prenatal scan shows cranial shape characteristic of Kleeblattschadel, with bulging temporal calvarium. The fetus also had low-set ears and multiple other anomalies. *R* = right; *L* = left. **B,** postnatal radiograph of another infant with Kleeblattschadel shows the bulging temporal calvarium. *R* = right; *L* = left.

Sonographic evaluation should also identify common causes of hydrocephalus (neural tube defects, agenesis of the corpus callosum, and aqueductal stenosis) and distinguish them from idiopathic causes.

REFERENCES

Normal Development and Sonographic Approach

1. Bowerman R, DiPietro M: Erroneous sonographic identification of fetal lateral ventricles: Relationship to the echogenic periventricular "blush". AJNR 1987; 8:661−664.
2. Chinn DC, Callen PW, Filly RA: The lateral cerebral ventricle in early second trimester. Radiology 1983; 148:529−531.
3. Cyr DR, Mack LA, Nyberg DA, et al: Fetal rhomben-cephalon: Normal ultrasound findings. Radiology 1988; 166:691−692.
4. Denkhaus H, Winsberg F: Ultrasonic measurements of the fetal ventricular system. Radiology 1979; 131:781−787.
5. Filly RA, Cardoza JD, Goldstein RB, et al: Detection of fetal CNS anomalies: A practical level of effort for a "routine" sonogram. Radiology 1989; 172; 403−408.
6. Hadlock FP, Deter RL, Park SK: Real-time sonography: Ventricular and vascular anatomy of the fetal brain in utero. AJR 1981; 136:133−137.
7. Hertzberg B, Bowie J, Burger P, et al: The three lines: Origin of sonographic landmarks in the fetal head. AJR 1987; 149:1009−1012.
8. Johnson ML, Dunne M, Mack L, et al: Evaluation of fetal intracranial anatomy by static and real-time ultrasound. J Clin Ultrasound 1980; 8:311−318.
9. Laing F, Stamler C, Jeffrey B: Ultrasonography of the fetal subarachnoid space. J Ultrasound Med 1983; 2:29−32.
10. Mahony B, Callen P, Filly R, et al: The fetal cisterna magna. Radiology 1984; 153:773−776.
11. McLeary RD, Kuhns LR, Barr M Jr: Ultrasonography of the fetal cerebellum. Radiology 1984; 151:439−442.
12. Moore KL. *The Developing Human,* ed 4. Philadelphia, WB Saunders Co, 1988, pp 364−401.
13. Nyberg DA: Recommendations for obstetric sonography in the evaluation of the fetal cranium. Radiology 1989; 172:309−311.

14. Pilu G, Romero R, DePalma L, et al: Ultrasound investigation of the posterior fossa in the fetus. Am J Perinatol 1987; 4:155–159.

15. Reuter K, D'Orsi C, Ratopoulos V, et al: Sonographic pseudyasymmetry of the prenatal cerebral hemispheres. J Ultrasound Med 1982; 1:91–95.

16. Schoenecker S, Pretorius D, Manco-Johnson M: Artifacts seen commonly on ultrasonography of the fetal cranium. J Repro Med 1985; 30:541–544.

17. Siedler DE, Filly RA: Relative growth of the higher brain structures. J Ultrasound Med 1987; 6:573–576.

18. Stanley JH, Harrell B, Horger EO III: Pseudoepidural reverberation artefact: A common ultrasound artifact in fetal cranium. J Clin Ultrasound 1986; 14:251–254.

Hydrocephalus and Aqueductal Stenosis

19. Amin NM: Normal-pressure hydrocephalus. Am Fam Pr 1983; 28:147–150.

20. Aughton DJ, Cassidy SB: Hydrolethalus syndrome: Report of an apparent mild case, literature review, and differential diagnosis. Am J Med Genet 1987; 27:935–942.

21. Bay C, Kerzin L, Hall B: Recurrence risk in hydrocephalus. Birth Defects 1979; 15:95–105.

22. Benacerraf BR, Birnholz JC: The diagnosis of fetal hydrocephalus prior to 22 weeks. J Clin Ultrasound 1987; 15:531–536.

23. Burton BK: Recurrence risk of congenital hydrocephalus. Clin Genet 1979; 16:47.

24. Callen PW, Choolijan D: The effect of ventricular dilatation upon biometry of the fetal head. J Ultrasound Med 1986; 5:17–19.

25. Cardoza JD, Goldstein RB, Filly RA: Exclusion of fetal ventriculomegaly with a single measurement: The width of the lateral ventricular atrium. Radiology 1988; 169:711–714.

26. Cardoza JD, Filly RA, Podrasky AE: The dangling choroid plexus: A sonographic observation of value in excluding ventriculomegaly. AJR 1988; 151:767–770.

27. Chayen B, Rifkin MD: Cephalocentesis: Guidance with an endovaginal probe and endovaginal needle placement. J Ultrasound Med 1987; 6:221–223.

28. Chervenak FA, Berkowitz R, Romero R, et al: The diagnosis of fetal hydrocephalus. Am J Obstet Gynecol 1983; 147:703–716.

29. Chervenak FA, Duncan C, Ment LR, et al: Outcome of fetal ventriculomegaly. Lancet 1984; ii:179–181.

30. Cochrane DD, Myles ST, Nimrod C, et al: Intrauterine hydrocephalus and ventriculomegaly: Associated abnormalities and fetal outcome. Can J Neurol Sci 1985; 12:51–59.

31. Crowe JC, Jassani M, Dickerman L: The prenatal diagnosis of the Walker-Warburg syndrome. Prenat Diagn 1986; 6:177–185.

32. Filly RA: Ultrasound evaluation of the fetal neural axis, in Callen PW (ed): *Ultrasonography in Obstetrics and Gynecology,* ed 2. Philadelphia, WB Saunders Co, 1988, pp 83–135.

33. Fiske CE, Filly RA: Ultrasound of the normal and abnormal fetal neural axis. Radiol Clin North Am 1982; 20:285–296.

34. Fitz CR, Hardwood-Nash DC: Computed tomography in hydrocephalus. J Comput Tomogr 1978; 2:91–108.

35. Gillieson MA, Hickey NM: Prenatal diagnosis of fetal hydrocephalus associated with a normal biparietal diameter. J Ultrasound Med 1984; 3:227–229.

36. Habib Z. Genetics and genetic counseling in neonatal hydrocephalus. Obstet Gynecol Surv 1981; 36:529–534.

37. Halliday J, Chow CW, Wallace D, et al: X-linked hydrocephalus: A survey of a 20-year period in Victoria, Australia. J Med Genet 1986; 23:23–31.

38. Hartung RW, Yiu-Chiu V: Demonstration of unilateral hydrocephalus in utero. J Ultrasound Med 1983; 2:369–371.

39. Hill A, Volpe JJ: Normal pressure hydrocephalus in the newborn. Pediatrics 1981; 68:623–629.

40. Johnson ML, Pretorius D, Clewell W, et al: Fetal hydrocephalus: Diagnosis and management. Sem Perinatol 1983; 7:83–89.

41. Kim H, Uppal V, Wallach R: Apert syndrome and fetal hydrocephaly. Hum Genet 1986; 73:93–95.

42. Laurence KM, Coates S: The natural history of hydrocephalus: Detailed analysis of 182 unoperated cases. Arch Dis Child 1962; 37:345–362.

43. Laurence KM: Genetic aspects of "uncomplicated" hydrocephalus and its relationship to neural tube defect. Z Kinderchir 1984; 39 (suppl 2):96–99.

44. Mahony BS, Nyberg DA, Hirsch JH, et al: Mild idiopathic lateral cerebral ventricular dilatation in utero: Sonographic evaluation. Radiology 1988; 169:715–721.

45. Manning F, Harrison M, Rodeck C, et al: Catheter shunts for fetal hydronephrosis and hydrocephalus. Report of the International Fetal Surgery Registry. N Engl J Med 1986; 315:336–340.

46. Milhorat TH, Clark RG, Hammock MK, et al: Structural, ultrastructural and permeability changes in the ependyma and surrounding brain favoring equilibrium in progressive hydrocephalus. Arch Neurol 1970; 22:397–407.

47. Murphy S, Das P, Grant DN, et al: Importance of neurosurgical consultation after ultrasonic diagnosis of fetal hydrocephalus. Br Med J 1984; 289:1212–1213.

48. Nyberg DN, Mack LA, Hirsch J, et al: Fetal hydrocephalus: Sonographic detection and clinical significance of associated anomalies. Radiology 1987; 163:187–191.

49. Nyberg DA, Shepard T, Mack L: Significance of a single umbilical artery in fetuses with central nervous system malformations. J Ultrasound Med 1988; 7:265–273.

50. Pretorius D, Davis K, Manco-Johnson M, et al: Clinical course of fetal hydrocephalus: 40 cases. AJNR 1985; 6:23–27.

51. Pretorius D, Drose J, Manco-Johnson M: Fetal lateral ventricular ratio determination during the second trimester. J Ultrasound Med 1986; 5:121–244.

52. Rorke LB: Abnormalities of brain differentiation. Birth Defects 1987; 23:215–224.

53. Russell DS: Observations on the Pathology of Hydrocephalus. London, Her Majesty's Stationery Office, 1949, pp 11–49.

54. Shurtleff DB, Foltz EL, Loeser JD: Hydrocephalus: A definition of its progression and relationship to intellectual function, diagnosis, and complications. Am J Dis Child 1973; 125:688–693.

55. Toi A: Spontaneous resolution of fetal ventriculomegaly in a diabetic patient. J Ultrasound Med 1987; 6:37–39.

56. Vintzileos AM, Ingardia CJ, Nochimson DJ: Congenital hydrocephalus: A review and protocol for perinatal management. Obstet Gynecol 1983; 62:539–549.

57. Vintzileos AM, Campbell W, Weinbaum P, et al: Perinatal management and outcome of fetal ventriculomegaly. Obstet Gynecol 1987; 69:5–11.

58. Wald N, Cuckle H, Boreham J, et al: Small biparietal diameter of fetuses with spina bifida: Implications for antenatal screening. Br J Obstet Gynecol 1980; 87:219–221.

59. Willems PJ, Brouwer OF, Dijkstra I, et al: X-linked hydrocephalus. Am J Med Genet 1987; 27:921–928.

60. Weller R, Shulman K: Infantile hydrocephalus: Clinical histological, and ultrastructural study of brain damage. J Neurosurg 1972; 36:255–265.

61. Williams B: Aqueduct stenosis, in Smith WT, Cavanaugh JB (eds): *Recent Advances in Neuropathology,* vol 2. London, Churchill Livingstone, 1982.

62. Williamson RA, Schauberger CW, Varner MW, et al: Heterogeneity of prenatal onset hydrocephalus: Management and counseling implications. Am J Med Genet 1984; 17:497–508.

63. Young HF, Nulsen FE, Weiss MH, et al: The relationship of intelligence and cerebral mantle in treated hydrocephalus (IQ potential in hydrocephalic children). Pediatrics 1973; 52:38–44.

Holoprosencephaly

64. Byrd S, Harwood-Nash D, Fitz C, et al: Computed tomography evaluation of holoprosencephaly in infants and children. J Comput Assist Tomogr 1977; 14:456–463.

65. Carrasco CR, Stierman ED, Harnsberger HR, et al: An algorithm for prenatal ultrasound diagnosis of congenital anomalies. J Ultrasound Med 1985; 4:163–165.

66. Cayea PD, Balcar I, Alberti O Jr, et al: Prenatal diagnosis of semilobar holoprosencephaly. AJR 1984; 142:401–402.

67. Chervenak FA, Isaacson G, Mahoney MJ, et al: The obstetric significance of holoprosencephaly. Obstet Gynecol 1984; 63:115–121.

68. Chervenak FA, Isaacson G, Hobbins JC, et al: Diagnosis and management of fetal holoprosencephaly. Obstet Gynecol 1985; 60:322–326.

69. Cohen MM: An update on the holoprosencephalic disorders. J Pediatr 1982; 101:865–869.

70. DeMeyer W, Zeman W, Palmer C: The face predicts the brain: Diagnostic significance of median facial anomalies for holoprosencephaly (arhinencephaly). Pediatrics 1964; 34:256–263.

71. DeMeyer W: Classification of cerebral malformations. Birth Defects 1971; VII:78–93.

72. Filly R, Chinn D, Callen P: Alobar holoprosencephaly ultrasonographic prenatal diagnosis. Radiology 1984; 151:445–459.

73. Fitz CR: Holoprosencephaly and related entities. Neuroradiology 1983; 25:225–238.

74. Fitz CR: Midline anomalies of the brain and spine. Radiol Clin North Am 1982; 20:95–104.

75. Green MF, Benacerraf BR, Frigoletto FD Jr: Reliable criteria for the prenatal diagnosis of alobar holoprosencephaly. Am J Obstet Gynecol 1987; 156:687–689.

76. Hoffman-Tietin JC, Horoupian DS, Koenigsberg M, et al: Lobar holoprosencephaly with hydrocephalus: Antenatal demonstration and differential diagnosis. J Ultrasound Med 1986; 5:691–697.

77. Manelfe C, Serely A: Neuroradiological study of holosprosencephalies. J Neuroradiology 1982; 9:15–45.

78. Matsunaga E, Shiota N: Holoprosencephaly in human embryos: Epidemiologic studies of 150 cases. Teratology 1977; 16:261–272.

79. McGahan JP, Ellis W, Lindfors KK, et al: Congenital cerebrospinal fluid-containing intracranial abnormalities: A sonographic classification. J Clin Ultrasound 1988; 16:531–544.

80. Nyberg D, Mack L, Bronstein A, et al: Holoprosencephaly: Prenatal sonographic diagnosis. AJR 1987; 149:1050–1058.

81. Osaka K, Matsumoto S: Holoprosencephaly in neurosurgical practice. J Neurosurg 1978; 48:787–803.

82. Pilu G, Romero R, Rizzo N, et al: Criteria for the prenatal diagnosis of holoprosencephaly. Am J Perinatol 1987; 4:41–49.

83. Pretorius DH, Russ PD, Rumack CM, et al: Diagnosis of brain neuropathology in utero. Neuroradiology 1986; 28:386–397.

84. Roach E, DeMeyer W, Conneally P, et al: Holoprosencephaly: Birth data, genetic and demographic analyses of 30 families. Birth Defects 1975; 11:294–313.

85. Sarwar M: *Computed Tomography of Congenital Brain Malformations.* St Louis, Warren H Green Inc, 1985.

86. Saunders E, Shortland D, Dunn P: What is the incidence of holoprosencephaly? J Med Genet 1984; 21:21–26.

87. Schnizel A, Savoldelli G, Briner J, et al: Prenatal ultrasonographic diagnosis of holoprosencephaly—two cases of cebocephaly and two of cyclopia. Arch Gynecol 1984; 236:47–53.

88. Warkany J, Passarge E, Smith CB: Congenital malformations in autosomal trisomy syndromes. Am J Dis Child 1966; 112:502–517.

Dandy-Walker Malformation

89. Benda CE: The Dandy-Walker syndrome or the so-called atresia of the foramen of Magendie. J Neuropathol Exp Neurol 1954; 13:14–29.
90. Comstock C, Boal D: Enlarged fetal cisterna magna: Appearance and significance. Obstet Gynecol 1985; 66:25S–28S.
91. Comstock CH: The posterior fossa, in Sabbagha RE (ed): *Ultrasound Applied to Obstetrics and Gynecology,* ed 2. Philadelphia, JB Lippincott Co, 1987, pp 306–314.
92. Dandy WE, Blackfan KD: Internal hydrocephalus. An experimental, clinical, and pathological study. Am J Dis Child 1914; 8:406.
93. Depp R, Sabbagha RE, Brown TJ, et al: Fetal surgery for hydrocephalus: Successful in utero ventriculoamniotic shunts for Dandy-Walker malformation. Obstet Gynecol 1983; 61:710–714.
94. Fileni A, Colosimo CC Jr, De Gaetano AM, et al: Dandy-Walker syndrome: Diagnosis in utero by means of ultrasound and CT correlations. Neuroradiol 1983; 24:233–235.
95. Fitz CR: Disorders of the ventricles and CSF spaces. Semin Ultrasound CT, MR. 1988; 9:216–230.
96. Gardner E, O'Rahilly R, Prolo D: The Dandy-Walker and Arnold-Chiari malformations. Arch Neurol 1975; 32:393–407.
97. Hart M, Malamud N, Ellis W: The Dandy-Walker syndrome: A clinicopathological study based on 28 cases. Neurology 1972; 22:771–780.
98. Hirsch J-F, Pierre-Kahn, A, Renier D, et al: The Dandy-Walker malformation. J Neurosurg 1984; 61:515–522.
99. Kirkinen P, Jouppila P, Valkeakari et al: Ultrasonic evaluation of the Dandy-Walker syndrome. Obstet Gynecol 1982; 59:18s–21s.
100. McCullough D, Balzer-Martin L: Current prognosis in overt neonatal hydrocephalus. J Neurosurg 1982; 57:378–383.
101. Murray J, Johnson J, Bird T: Dandy-Walker malformation: Etiologic heterogeneity and empiric recurrence risks. Clin Genet 1985; 28:272–283.
102. Nyberg DA, Cyr DR, Mack LA, et al: The Dandy-Walker malformation: Prenatal sonographic diagnosis and its clinical significance. J Ultrasound Med 1988; 7:65–71.
103. Olson G, Halpe D, Kaplan A, et al: Dandy-Walker malformation and associated cardiac anomalies. Child's Brain 1981; 8:173–180.
104. Pilu G, Romero R, DePalma L, et al: Antenatal diagnosis and obstetric management of Dandy-Walker syndrome. J Repro Med 1986; 31:1017–1022.
105. Russ P, Pretorius D, Johnson M: Dandy-Walker syndrome: A review of 15 cases evaluated by prenatal sonography. Am J Obstet Gynecol 1989; 161:401–406.
106. Sawaya R, McLaurin R: Dandy-Walker syndrome: Clinical analysis of 23 cases: J Neurosurg 1981; 55:89–98.
107. Tal Y, Freigang B, Dunn H, et al: Dandy-Walker syndrome: Analysis of 21 cases. Dev Med Child Neurol 1980; 22:189–201.

Agenesis of the Corpus Callosum

108. Amato M, Howald H, vonMuralt G: Fetal ventriculomegaly, agenesis of the corpus callosum and chromosomal translocation—Case report. J Perinat Med 1986; 14:271–274.
109. Atlas S, Shkolnik A, Naidich T: Sonographic recognition of agenesis of the corpus callosum. AJR 1985; 145:167–173.
110. Babcock D: The normal, absent, and abnormal corpus callosum: Sonographic findings. Radiology 1984; 151:449–453.
111. Bertino RE, Nyberg DA, Cyr DR, et al: Prenatal diagnosis of agenesis of the corpus callosum. J Ultrasound Med 1988; 7:251–260.
112. Comstock C, Culp D, Gonzalez J, et al: Agenesis of the corpus callosum in the fetus: Its evolution and significance. J Ultrasound Med 1985; 4:613–616.
113. Davidoff LM, Dyke CG: Agenesis of the corpus callosum: Its diagnosis by encephalography. AJR 1934; 32:1–10.
114. Freytag E, Lindenberg R: Neuropathic findings in patients of a hospital for the mentally deficient. A survey of 359 cases. Hopkins Med J 1967; 121:379–392.
115. Gebarski S, Gebarski K, Bowerman R, et al: Agenesis of the corpus callosum: Sonographic features. Radiology 1984; 151:443–448.
116. Grogono J: Children with agenesis of the corpus callosum. Dev Med Child Neurol 1968; 10:613–616.
117. Guibert-Tranier F, Piton J, Billerey J, et al: Agenesis of the corpus callosum. J Neuroradiology. 1982; 9:135.
118. Harwood-Nash D: Congenital malformations of the brain. Neuroradiol Infants Child 1976; 3:1019–1025.
119. Larsen P, Osborn A: Computed tomographic evaluation of corpus callosum agenesis and associated malformations. J Comput Tomogr 1982; 6:225–230.
120. Lockwood CJ, Ghidini A, Aggarwal R, et al: Antenatal diagnosis of partial agenesis of the corpus callosum: A benign cause of ventriculomegaly. Am J Obstet Gynecol 1988; 159:184–186.
121. Loeser J, Alvord E: Clinicopathological correlations in agenesis of the corpus callosum. Neurology 1968; 18:745–756.
122. Meizner J, Barhi Y, Hertzanu Y: Prenatal sonographic diagnosis of agenesis of corpus callosum. J Clin Ultrasound 1987; 15:262.
123. Parrish M, Roessmann U, Levinsohn M: Agenesis of the corpus callosum: A study of the frequency of associated malformations. Ann Neurol 1979; 6:349–354.
124. Schulman M, Dohan F, Jones T, et al: Sonographic appearance of callosal agenesis: Correlation with radiologic and pathologic findings. AJNR 1985; 6:361–368.

125. Vergani P, Ghidini A, Mariani S, et al: Antenatal sonographic findings of agenesis of the corpus callosum. Am J Perinat 1988; 5:105–108.

126. Warkany J, Lemore RJ, Cohen MM: Agenesis of the corpus callosum, in *Mental Retardation in Congenital Malformations of the Central Nervous System.* Chicago, Year Book Medical Publishers, Inc, 1981, pp 224–241.

Hydranencephaly

127. Dublin A, French B: Diagnostic image evaluation of hydranencephaly and pictorially similar entities, with emphasis on computed tomography. Radiology 1980; 137:81–91.

128. Fiske CE, Filly RA: Ultrasound of the normal and abnormal fetal neural axis. Radiol Clin North Am 1982; 20:285–296.

129. Greene MF, Benacerraf BR, Crawford JM: Hydranencephaly US appearance during in utero evolution. Radiology 1985; 156:779–780.

130. Muir CS: Hydranencephaly and allied disorders. Am J Dis Child 1959; 34:231–246.

131. Pretorius D, Russ P, Rumack C, et al: Diagnosis of brain neuropathology in utero. Neuroradiology 1986; 28:386–397.

132. Raybaud C: Destructive lesions of the brain. Neuroradiology 1983; 25:265–291.

Porencephaly/Schizencephaly

133. Barkovich AJ, Norman D: MR imaging of schizencephaly. AJR 1988; 150:1391–1396.

134. Berg R, Aleck K, Kaplan A: Familial porencephaly. Arch Neurol 1983; 40:567–569.

135. Klingensmith W, Cioffi-Ragan D: Schizencephaly: Diagnosis and progression in utero. Radiology 1986; 159:617–618.

136. Miller GR, Stears JC, Guggenheim MA, et al: Schizencephaly: A clinical and CT study. Neurol 1984; 34:997–1001.

137. Pollei SR, Boyer BR, Crawford S, et al: Disorders of migration and sulcation. Seminars US, CT and MR 1988; 9:231–246.

138. Vintzileos AM, Hovick TS, Escoto DT, et al: Congenital midline porencephaly—prenatal sonographic findings and review of the literature. Am J Perinatol 1987; 4:125–128.

139. Yakolev PI, Wadsworth RC: Schizencephalies: A study of congenital clefts in the cerebral mantle. I: Clefts with fused lips. J Neuropath Exp Neurol 1946; 5:116–130.

140. Yakolev PI, Wadsworth RC: Schizencephalies. A study of the congenital clefts in the cerebral mantel. II: Clefts with hydrocephalus and lips separated. J Neuropath Exp Neurol 1946; 5:169–206.

Arachnoid Cyst

141. Anderson F, Landing B: Cerebral arachnoid cysts in infants. J Pediatr 1966; 69:88–96.

142. Chuang S, Harwood-Nash D: Tumors and cysts. Neuroradiology 1986; 28:463–475.

143. Diakoumakis EE, Weinberg B, Molin J: Prenatal sonographic diagnosis of a suprasellar arachnoid cyst. J Ultrasound Med 1986; 5:529–530.

144. Harwood-Nash DC, Fitz CR: Intracranial cysts, in Harwood-Nash DC, Fitz CR (eds): *Neuroradiology in Infants and Children,* vol 3. St Louis, CV Mosby Co, 1976, pp 965–999.

145. Koto A, Horoupian DS, Shulman K: Choroidal epithelial cyst. J Neurosurg 1977; 47:955.

146. Locatelli D, Bonfanti N, Sfogliarini R, et al: Arachnoid cysts: Diagnosis and treatment. Childs Nerv Syst 1987; 3:121–124.

147. Menezes AH, Bell WE, Perrett GE: Arachnoid cysts in children. Arch Neurol 1980; 37:168–172.

148. Robinson RG: Congenital cysts of the brain: Arachnoid malformations. Prog Neurol Surg 1971; 4:144.

Vein of Galen Aneurysm

149. Diebler C, Dulac O, Renier D, et al: Aneurysms of the vein of Galen in infants aged 2 to 15 months. Diagnosis and natural evolution. Neuroradiology 1981; 21:185–197.

150. Gold A, Ransohoff J, Carter S: Vein of Galen malformation. Acta Neurol Scand [Suppl II] 1964; 40:5–31.

151. Hirsch JH, Cyr D, Eberhardt H, et al: Ultrasonographic diagnosis of an aneurysm of the vein of Galen in utero by duplex scanning. J Ultrasound Med 1983; 2:231–233.

152. Koh A, Grundy H: Fetal heart rate tracing with congenital aneurysm of the great vein of Galen. Am J Perinatol 1988; 5:98–100.

153. Mao K: Antenatal diagnosis of intracranial arteriovenous fistula by ultrasonography. Case report. Brit J Obstet Gynaecol 1983; 90:872–873.

154. Mendelsohn D, Hertzanu Y, Butterworth A: In utero diagnosis of a vein of Galen aneurysm by ultrasound. Neuroradiology 1984; 26:417–418.

155. Mizejewski G, Polansky S, Mondragon-Tiu F, et al: Combined use of alpha-fetoprotein and ultrasound in the prenatal diagnosis of arteriovenous fistula in the brain. Obstet Gynecol 1987; 70:452–453.

156. Reiter A, Huhta J, Carpenter R, et al: Prenatal diagnosis of arteriovenous malformation of the vein of Galen. J Clin Ultrasound 1986; 14:623–628.

157. Rodemeyer C, Smith W: Diagnosis of a vein of Galen aneurysm by ultrasound. J Clin Ultrasound 1982; 10:297–298.

158. Soto G, Daneman A, Hellman J: Doppler evaluation of cerebral arteries in a Galenic vein malformation. J Ultrasound Med 1985; 4:673–675.

159. Vintzileos A, Eisenfeld L, Campbell W, et al: Prenatal

ultrasonic diagnosis of arteriovenous malformation of the vein of Galen. Am J Perinatol 1986; 3:209–211.

160. Watson D, Smith R, Brann A: Arteriovenous malformation of the vein of Galen. Am J Dis Child 1976; 130:520–525.

Choroid Plexus Cyst

161. Benacerraf B: Asymptomatic cysts of the fetal choroid plexus in the second trimester. J Ultrasound Med 1987; 6:475–478.
162. Bundy A, Saltzman D, Prober B, et al: Antenatal sonographic findings in trisomy 18. J Ultrasound Med 1986; 5:361–364.
163. Chan L, Hixson, Laifer SA, et al: An ultrasound and karyotypic study of second trimester choroid plexus cysts. Obstet Gynecol 1989; 73:703–706.
164. Chitkara U, Cogswell C, Norton K, et al: Choroid plexus cysts in the fetus: A benign anatomic variant or pathologic entity? Report of 41 cases and review of the literature. Obstet Gynecol 1988; 72:185–189.
165. Chudleigh P, Pearce J, Campbell S: The prenatal diagnosis of transient cysts of the fetal choroid plexus. Prenat Diagn 1984; 4:135–137.
166. Fakry J, Schechter A, Tenner M, et al: Cysts of the choroid plexus in neonates: Documentation and review of the literature. J Ultrasound Med 1985; 4:561–563.
167. Findlay JW: The choroid plexuses of the lateral ventricles of the brain, their histology, normal and pathological, (in relation especially to insanity). Brain [Part II] 1899; 22:161–206.
168. Furness ME: Choroid plexus cysts and trisomy 18. Lancet 1987; ii:693.
169. Friday R, Schwartz D, Tuffli G: Spontaneous intrauterine resolution of intraventricular cystic masses. J Ultrasound Med 1985; 4:385–386.
170. Nicolaides K, Rodeck C, Gosden C: Rapid karyotyping in non–lethal fetal malformations. Lancet 1986; i:283–284.
171. Ostlere S, Irving H, Lilford R: Choroid plexus cysts in the fetus. Lancet 1987; i:1491.
172. Ricketts N, Lowe E, Patel N: Prenatal diagnosis of choroid plexus cysts. Lancet 1987; i:213–214.
173. Shuangshoti S, Roberts M, Netsky M: Neuroepithelial (colloid) cysts. Arch Path 1965; 80:214–224.
174. Toi A, Cullinan J, Blankier J, et al: Choroid plexus cysts in the fetus: Report of 62 cases. Presented to the American Institute of Ultrasound in Medicine, Washington, DC, 1988.

Intracranial Neoplasm

175. Crade M: Ultrasonic demonstration in utero of an intracranial teratoma. JAMA 1982; 247:1173.
176. Hoff N, Mackay I: Prenatal ultrasound diagnosis of intracranial teratoma. J Clin Ultrasound 1980; 8:247–249.
177. Lipman S, Pretorius D, Rumack C, et al: Fetal intracra-nial teratoma: US diagnosis of three cases and a review of the literature. Radiology 1985; 157:491–494.
178. Rostad S, Kleinschmidt-DeMasters B, Manchester D: Two massive congenital intracranial immature teratomas with neck extension. Teratology 1985; 32:163–169.
179. Sauerbrei EE, Cooperberg PL: Cystic tumors of the fetal and neonatal cerebrum: Ultrasound and computed tomographic evaluation. Radiology 1983; 147:689–692.
180. Snyder JR, Lustig-Gillman I, Milio L, et al: Antenatal ultrasound diagnosis of an intracranial neoplasm (craniopharyngioma). J Clin Ultrasound 1986; 14:304–306.
181. Takaku A, Kodama N, Ohara H, et al: Brain tumor in newborn babies. Child's Brain 1973; 4:365–375.
182. Takeuchi J, Handa H, Oda Y, et al: Alpha-fetoprotein in intracranial malignant teratoma. Surg Neurol 1979; 12:400–404.
183. Vinters HV, Murphy J, Wittman B, et al: Intracranial teratoma: Antenatal diagnosis at 31 weeks gestation by ultrasound. Acta Neuropathol 1982; 58:233–236.

Intracranial Hemorrhage

184. Bondurant S, Boehm F, Fleischer A, et al: Antepartum diagnosis of fetal intracranial hemorrhage by ultrasound. Obstet Gynecol 1984; 63:25S–27S.
185. Bussel JB, Berkowitz RL, McFarland JG, et al: Antenatal treatment of neonatal alloimmune thrombocytopenia. N Engl J Med 1988; 319:1374–1378.
186. Chinn DH, Filly RA: Extensive intracranial hemorrhage in utero. J Ultrasound Med 1983; 2:285–287.
187. Donn S, Barr M, McLeary R: Massive intracerebral hemorrhage in utero: Sonographic appearance and pathologic correlation. Obstet Gynecol 1984; 63:28S–30S.
188. Herman J, Jumbelic M, Ancona R, et al: In utero cerebral hemorrhage in alloimmune thrombocytopenia. Am J Pediatr Hematol Oncol 1986; 8:312–317.
189. Johnson M, Rumack C, Mannes E, et al: Detection of neonatal intracranial hemorrhage utilizing real-time and static ultrasound. J Clin Ultrasound 1981; 9:427–433.
190. Kim M, Elyaderani MK: Sonographic diagnosis of cerebroventricular hemorrhage in utero. Radiology 1982; 142:479–480.
191. Lester RB III, Sty JR: Prenatal diagnosis of cystic CNS lesions in neonatal isoimmune thrombocytopenia. J Ultrasound Med 1987; 6:479–481.
192. Lustig-Gillman I, Young BK, Silverman F, et al: Fetal intraventricular hemorrhage: Sonographic diagnosis and clinical implications. J Clin Ultrasound 1983; 11:277–280.
193. McGahan J, Haesslein H, Meyers M, et al: Sonographic recognition of in utero intraventricular hemorrhage. AJR 1984; 142:171–173.
194. Minkoff H, Schaeffer R, Delke I, et al: Diagnosis of intracranial hemorrhage in utero after a maternal seizure. Obstet Gynecol 1985; 65:22S–24S.
195. Mintz MC, Arger PH, Coleman BG: In utero

sonographic diagnosis of intracerebral hemorrhage. J Ultrasound Med 1985; 4:375–376.

196. Morales W, Stroup M: Intracranial hemorrhage in utero due to isoimmune neonatal thrombocytopenia. Obstet Gynecol 1985; 65:20S–21S.

197. Pretorius D, Singh S, Manco-Johnson M, et al: In utero diagnosis of intracranial hemorrhage resulting in fetal hydrocephalus. J Reprod Med 1986; 31:136–138.

198. Sadowitz D, Balcom R: Intrauterine intracranial hemorrhage in an infant with isoimmune thrombocytopenia. Clin Pediatr 1985; 24:655–657.

Microcephaly

199. Book J, Schut J, Reed S: A clinical and genetical study of microcephaly. Am J Ment Defic 1953; 57:637–660.

200. Chervenak FA, Jeanty P, Cantraine F, et al: The diagnosis of fetal microcephaly. Am J Obstet Gynecol 1984; 149:512–517.

201. Chervenak F, Rosenberg J, Brightman R, et al: A prospective study of the accuracy of ultrasound in predicting fetal microcephaly. Obstet Gynecol 1987; 69:908–910.

202. Grannum P, Pilu G: In utero neurosonography: The normal fetus and variations in cranial size. Sem Perinatol 1987; 11:85–97.

203. Kurtz A, Wapner R, Rubin C, et al: Ultrasound criteria for in utero diagnosis of microcephaly. J Clin Ultrasound 1980; 8:11–16.

204. Lenke RR, Platt LD, Koch R: Ultrasonographic failure of early detection of fetal microcephaly in maternal phenylketonuria. J Ultrasound Med 1983; 2:177–179.

205. Martin H: Microcephaly and mental retardation. Am J Dis Child 1970; 119:128–131.

206. Nguyen TH, Pescia G, Deonna T, et al: Early prenatal diagnosis of genetic microcephaly. Prenat Diagn 1985; 5:345–347.

207. Tolmie JL, McNay M, Stephenson JBP, et al: Microcephaly: Genetic counseling and antenatal diagnosis after the birth of an affected child. Am J Med Genet 1987; 27:583–594.

Miscellaneous Brain and Skull Lesions

208. Babcock D: Sonographic demonstration of lissencephaly (Agyria). J Ultrasound Med 1983; 2:465–466.

209. Dobyns WB, Stratton RF, Greenberg F: Syndromes with lissencephaly. I: Miller-Dieker and Norman-Roberts syndromes and isolated lissencephaly. Am J Med Genet 1984; 18:509–526.

210. Dobyns WB, Kirkpatrick JB, Hibbner HM, et al: Syndromes with lissencephaly. II: Walker-Warburg and cerebro-oculo-muscular syndromes and a new syndrome with type II lissencephaly. Am J Med Genet 1985; 22:157–195.

211. Dobyns WB: Developmental aspects of lissencephaly and the lissencephaly syndromes. Birth Defects 1987; 23:225–241.

212. Laughlin CL, Lee TG: The prominent falx cerebri: New ultrasonic observation in hypophosphatasia. J Clin Ultrasound 1982; 10:37–38.

213. Mahony BS, Filly RA, Callen PW, et al: Thanatophoric dwarfism with the cloverleaf skull: A specific antenatal sonographic diagnosis. J Ultrasound Med 1985; 4:151.

214. Nicolaides KH, Campbell S, Gabbe SG: Ultrasound screening for spina bifida: Cranial and cerebellar signs. Lancet 1986; ii:72–74.

215. Nyberg DA, Mack LA, Hirsch JH, et al: Abnormalities of fetal contour in sonographic detection of spina bifida: Evaluation of the "lemon" sign. Radiology 1988; 167:387–392.

216. Partington MW, Gonzales-Crussi F, Khakee SG, et al: Cloverleaf skull and thanatophoric dwarfism: Report of four cases, two in the same sibship. Arch Dis Child 1971; 46:646.

217. Preece P, Blount J, Glover J, et al: The consequences of primary cytomegalovirus infection in pregnancy. Arch Dis Child 1983; 58:970–975.

218. Rumack CM, Johnson ML: Perinatal and Infant Brain Imaging. Chicago, Year Book Medical Publishers, Inc, 1984, pp 61–90.

219. Stamm ER, Pretorius DH, Rumack CM, et al: Kleeblattschadel anomaly: In utero sonographic appearance. J Ultrasound Med 1987; 6:319–324.

220. Worthen NJ, Gilbertson V, Lan C: Cortical sulcal development seen on sonography: Relationship to gestational parameters. J Ultrasound Med 1986; 5:153–156.

6

The Spine and Neural Tube Defects

David A. Nyberg, M.D.

Laurence A. Mack, M.D.

Neural tube defects (NTDs) and spinal malformations are among the most common congenital malformations; neural tube defects alone occur in 1 per 500 to 600 births.[17] Because NTDs are also among the most devastating of malformations, enormous effort has been directed toward their prenatal detection. In the last 20 years, major technological advances have led to wide-scale screening of maternal serum alpha-fetoprotein (MS-AFP) and wide availability of high-resolution real-time ultrasound equipment. As a result, prenatal detection of nearly all NTDs is a goal that is within reach. Importantly, these fetal anomalies can be detected at a time when prospective parents have the opportunity to choose whether or not to continue the pregnancy.

For the purposes of this chapter, NTDs and spinal malformations are considered by their primary location as either primary cranial malformations (anencephaly, exencephaly, encephalocele, and iniencephaly) or primary spinal abnormalities (spina bifida, sacrococcygeal teratoma, skeletal dysplasia, and other spinal abnormalities). This is preceded by a general discussion of NTDs.

NEURAL TUBE DEFECTS

Epidemiology

The three major types of NTDs are anencephaly, encephalocele, and spina bifida.[16] Less common types of NTDs include exencephaly and iniencephaly. Anencephaly and open spina bifida occur with a nearly equal frequency of 1 in 1,000 births, with some varia-

tion, depending upon geographic location and socioeconomic factors.[17] Encephalocele occurs less often with a frequency of about 1 in 4,000 pregnancies.

The vast majority of NTDs are sporadic and are believed to be multifactorial in origin (Table 6–1).[15, 16] A marked geographic variation in the prevalence of open NTDs has been noted, with the highest rates reported in the United Kingdom and the lowest rates in Japan.[14, 16] Even within the United States, a higher prevalence of open NTDs is observed on the East Coast than on the West Coast.[16] Environmental factors include seasonal and yearly variations, low parity, and low socioeconomic status. Maternal age is probably not a factor. Specific agents that have been implicated as causing NTDs include zinc deficiency, hyperthermia, aminopterin, clomiphene citrate, and valproic acid.[15, 16]

Neural tube defects, particularly anencephaly and encephalocele, are commonly found in early pregnancy losses; approximately 3% of all spontaneous abortions show evidence of an NTD.[13] It is estimated that of all embryos with NTDs at 8 weeks' gestation, approximately one quarter will be live born, one quarter stillborn, and one half spontaneously aborted.[13]

An increased frequency of NTDs has been observed in patients with a previous fetus or child affected with an NTD, with an estimated recurrence risk of less than 5% (Table 6–2). Other patients considered to be at increased risk for carrying a fetus with an NTD include women with diabetes mellitus and parents of a fetus or child affected with other types of vertebral defects including scoliosis and sacrococcygeal teratoma.[17] Spina bifida occulta of a single vertebra

TABLE 6–1.

Recognized Causes of Neural Tube Defects*

Multifactorial inheritance
Autosomal recessive
  Meckel-Gruber syndrome (includes occipital encephalocele
    and rarely anencephaly)
  Robert's syndrome (includes anterior encephalocele)
  Jarco-Levin syndrome (includes myelomeningocele)
  Walker-Warburg syndrome (includes encephalocele)
Autosomal dominant
  Median-cleft face syndrome (includes anterior encephalocele)
  Familial anterior sacral myelomeningocele and anal stenosis
Unclear inheritance
  Syndrome of occipital encephalocele, myopia, and retinal
    dysplasia
  Anterior encephalocele among Bantus and Thais
Chromosomal abnormalities
  Trisomy 18
  Trisomy 13
  Triploidy
Environmental or maternal factors
  Maternal diabetes mellitus
  Valproic acid (spina bifida)
  Aminopterine/amethopterin
  Thalidomide (rarely)

*From Main and Mennuti: Obstet Gynecol 1986; 67:1–15. Used by permission.

TABLE 6–2.

Estimated Incidence of Neural Tube Defects Based on Specific Risk Factors in the United States*

Population	Incidence/1,000 Live Births
Mother as reference	
General incidence	1.4–1.6
Women undergoing amniocentesis for advanced maternal age	1.5–3.0
Women with diabetes mellitus	20
Women on valproic acid in first trimester	10–20
Fetus as reference	
1 sibling with NTD	15–30
2 siblings with NTD	57
Parent with NTD	11
Half sibling with NTD	8
First cousin (mother's sister's child)	10
Other first cousins	3
Sibling with severe scoliosis caused by vertebral defects	15–30
Sibling with occult spina bifida	15–30
Sibling with sacrococcygeal teratoma	15–30

*From Main and Mennuti: Obstet Gynecol 1986; 67:1–15. Used by permission.

does not appear to increase the risk of an NTD to the offspring, although it is unknown whether involvement of more than one vertebrae is a risk factor.

The pathogenesis of NTDs remains uncertain. The most commonly accepted theory involves failure of the rostral and caudal neuropores to close (Fig 6–1). This would explain the propensity of NTDs to affect the cra-

nial and caudal ends of the neural axis. The alternative theory proposes that the neural tube becomes disrupted after its formation.

AFP Screening

The association of neural tube defects and elevated levels of amniotic fluid AFP, first reported in 1972 by Brock and Sutcliffe, represented a major technological advance in prenatal detection of NTDs.[11] The United

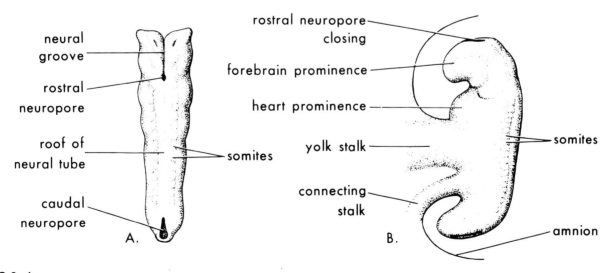

FIG 6–1.
Normal development of the spine and cranium. **A,** dorsal view of an embryo at 37 menstrual days (23 fetal days) shows fusion of the neural fold. **B,** lateral views of an embryo at 38 menstrual days (24 fetal days) shows normal prominence of the forebrain and closing of the rostral neuropore. (From Moore KL: *The Developing Human,* ed 4. Philadelphia, WB Saunders Co, 1988.)

Kingdom Collaborative Study subsequently reported that testing amniotic fluid AFP could detect 98% of anencephaly and 98% of open spina bifida.[20] This encouraging experience quickly led investigators to test for AFP in the maternal serum.[12, 18, 20, 21] Using a cutoff of 2.5 multiples of the median, screening programs have shown that elevated maternal serum AFP can detect 90% of anencephaly and approximately 80% of open spina bifida.[20]

Sonographic examination is an integral part of evaluating women with elevated MS-AFP. Conditions associated with elevated MS-AFP, such as inaccurate menstrual dating, multiple gestations, and missed abortions, can be identified readily (see Chapter 3). At the same time, a detailed sonographic examination can identify the vast majority of fetal defects that are associated with elevated AFP levels. If the sonographic examination is considered normal, patients are usually counseled regarding the benefits and risks of amniocentesis. Some centers recommend routine amniocentesis for all

such patients,[14] whereas others reserve amniocentesis for positive or inconclusive sonographic findings or for patients considered to be particularly at risk.[19] Advantages of amniocentesis include a high sensitivity and specificity of NTDs by determination of AFP and acetylcholinesterase in the amniotic fluid. Chromosome analysis can also be performed at the same time. Advantages of sonography include its lower cost, lack of risk, and the ability to provide morphologic information regarding the location and size of a neural tube defect, as well as the presence of other possible anomalies.

The Cranium

Normal Sonographic Approach to the Cranium

As recommended by the guidelines adopted by the American Institute of Ultrasound in Medicine, routine views of the cranium and spine should be incorporated into all obstetric sonograms performed during the sec-

FIG 6–2.
Schematic drawing of normal ventricles and intracranial anatomy. Scan planes C, D, and E are recommended as a part of all routine obstetric sonograms after the first trimester. *CP* = choroid plexus; *CSP* = cavum septi pellucidi; *FH* = frontal horn; *LV* = lateral ventricle; *MB* = midbrain; *OH* = occipital horn; *Th* = thalamus; *TV* = third ventricle.

NORMAL VENTRICLES

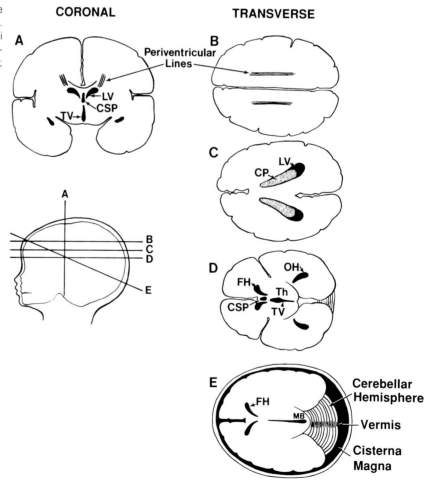

ond and third trimesters (see Chapter 1). In evaluating the cranium, the guidelines state that the examination should include, as a minimum, an axial view obtained through the thalami for cranial measurements and views of the cerebral ventricles. We suggest inclusion of one additional view, an oblique view angled through the posterior fossa, into the standard anatomic survey of the fetus (Fig 6–2). These three standard cranial views should permit a reliable prenatal diagnosis of virtually all cranial defects and the vast majority of spinal dysraphic defects before the time of viability (approximately 24 weeks).

Each of the three views described above (transthalamic, transventricular, and transcerebellar views) provides important information, both positively and negatively, regarding possible neural tube defects. A normal transthalamic view of the cranium virtually excludes anencephaly or exencephaly and also the great majority of encephaloceles (see Fig 6–2). The second view, obtained through the lateral cerebral ventricles, is essential for detecting early ventricular dilatation which frequently accompanies spina bifida as part of the Arnold-Chiari malformation. Axial views at the ventricular level also optimally demonstrate the "lemon" sign which, when present, is reliable, but indirect evidence for spina bifida. The third view, angled through the posterior fossa and cisterna magna, is necessary for visualizing small occipital encephaloceles. Also, demonstration of a normal cisterna magna virtually excludes the possibility of spina bifida, whereas obliteration of the cisterna magna (the "banana" sign) is important indirect evidence for posterior fossa compression, which usually accompanies the Arnold-Chiari II malformation (see Cranial Findings Associated With Spina Bifida below).

Cranial Disorders

Anencephaly

Pathologic, Clinical Findings.—Anencephaly is the single most common type of NTD, reported in 1 in 1,000 births.[17] Risk factors for anencephaly include a family history of an NTD and twins. Females are affected more frequently than males, with a frequency of 4 to 1.

Anencephaly is thought to result from failure of the rostral neuropore to close by 24 days of fetal life (38 menstrual days). Pathologically, anencephaly is characterized by absence of the cerebral hemispheres and accompanying cranium. However, the brain stem, portions of the mesencephalon (midbrain), and that portion of the cranium that forms from cartilage (base of the cranium) are typically present. The defect may be covered by a variable amount of angiomatous stroma (area cerebrovasculosa).[29]

Sonographic Findings.—Anencephaly (Figs 6–3 and 6–4) was the first fetal malformation detected on prenatal sonography, reported by Sunden in 1964.[33] It remained one of the most frequently reported malformations during the early experience with prenatal sonography.[22, 23, 27] Because the cranial defect occurs early in embryologic development, a diagnosis of anencephaly is potentially possible as early as 8 menstrual weeks. Typically, however, anencephaly is not reliably diagnosed until the early second trimester.[31] The sonographic diagnosis of anencephaly is highly reliable in experienced hands, with one study reporting 100% accuracy in over 100 affected fetuses.[25]

Absence of the cranial vault and brain cephalad to the orbits is a constant and diagnostic finding of anencephaly. The base of the skull is nearly always present. Coronal or sagittal views through the face optimally display the relation of the cranial defect with the the base of the skull and orbits (see Figs 6–3 and 6–4). A variable amount of soft tissue (angiomatous stroma) may be seen protruding from the cranial defect (Fig 6–5)[29].

If the cranial defect is adjacent to the uterine wall or the fetal head is low in the pelvis, the defect itself may not be immediately obvious. The correct diagnosis may be first suspected when it is realized that the standard transaxial view through the thalami is not obtainable. Inexperienced sonographers may attempt to compensate for this problem by obtaining cranial measurements from views through the base of the skull rather than through the thalami.

Polyhydramnios is reported to occur in about half the cases of anencephaly. However, the frequency of polyhydramnios appears to be related to menstrual age; Goldstein and Filly observed polyhydramnios in six of seven cases (86%) after 25 weeks, compared to 1 of 13 cases (8%) before 25 weeks.[29] These observations are consistent with the presumed mechanism of polyhydramnios caused by depressed or ineffective fetal swallowing. As with other causes of obstructed or ineffective fetal swallowing, polyhydramnios does not usually develop until the amount of amniotic fluid swallowed comprises a significant proportion of total amniotic fluid volume.

Distinguishing anencephaly from severe forms of microcephaly occasionally can be difficult. However, demonstration of an intact cranial vault, no matter how small, excludes anencephaly. Other considerations include exencephaly (absent cranium, but cerebral tissue present), encephalocele, and the amniotic band syn-

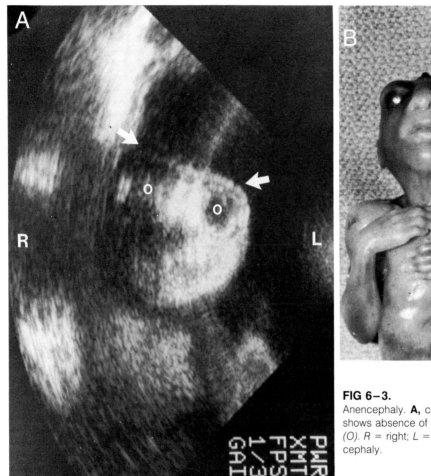

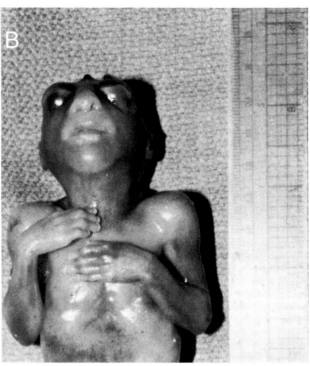

FIG 6–3.
Anencephaly. **A,** coronal view through the fetal face at 16 weeks shows absence of the cranial vault *(arrows)* cephalad to the orbits *(O). R* = right; *L* = left. **B,** postmortem photograph confirms anencephaly.

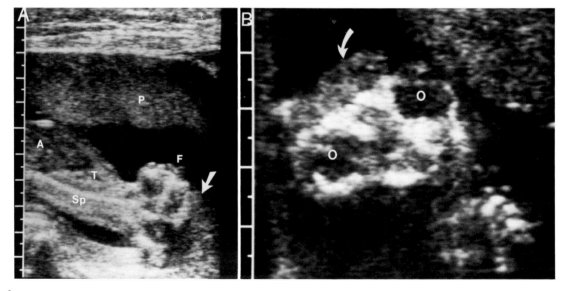

FIG 6–4.
Anencephaly. **A,** absence of calvarium *(arrow)* in sagittal scan is not optimally visualized because of fetal position with head in the maternal pelvis. *F* = face; *T* = thorax; *A* = abdomen; *Sp* = spine; *P* = placenta. **B,** coronal scan confirms absence of cranium cephalad to orbits *(O)* and shows a small amount of residual brain tissue *(arrow).*

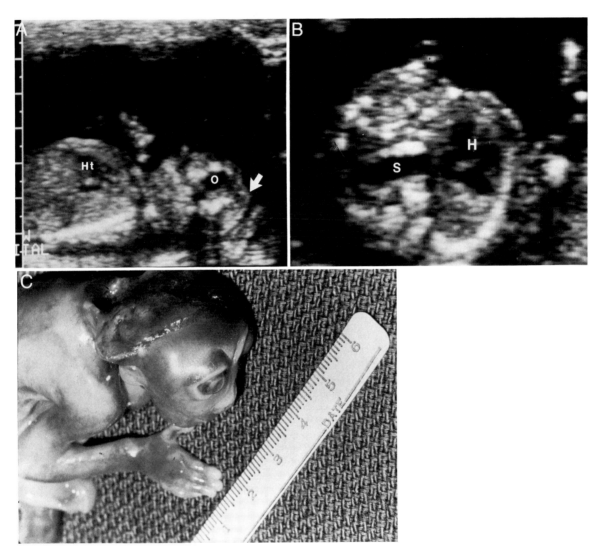

FIG 6-5.
Anencephaly with diaphragmatic hernia. **A,** sagittal view at 15 weeks shows absence of the cranial vault *(arrow)* cephalad to the orbit *(O).* *Ht* = heart. **B,** transverse view through the thorax demonstrates the stomach *(S)* and bowel in the right chest and displacement of the heart *(H)* to the right thorax. **C,** photograph of the pathologic specimen confirms anencephaly.

drome. In distinguishing anencephaly from the amniotic band syndrome, Goldstein and Filly suggest that the latter causes asymmetric cranial defects and frequent oligohydramnios and should be diagnosed only when there is evidence of other defects (abdominal wall defect or limb or digit amputations).[29]

A holoacardiac twin might be classified as anencephalic but, practically speaking, this disorder usually is not considered in the differential diagnosis, since all recognizable cranial structures are absent and diagnostic abnormalities of other organs (absent heart) are present.

Associated Anomalies.—Since anencephaly itself is uniformly fatal, further search for associated anomalies usually is not of clinical importance and, therefore, has received little attention in the literature. David and Nixon reported that 98 of 294 cases (33%) they reviewed had additional anomalies.[28] Spina bifida or rachischisis was the most common associated anomaly, found in 27% of cases.[28] Excluding the central nervous system, the urinary tract was the most commonly affected organ system (16%), with hydronephrosis being the single most common anomaly. Other anomalies in this series included diaphragmatic hernia (3%) (see Fig 6–5), cleft lip or palate (10%), cardiovascular malformations (4%), gastrointestinal anomalies (6%), and omphalocele (3%).

Prognosis.—Anencephaly is uniformly fatal. Most infants die within a few hours of birth but, rarely, survival for several months has been reported. Because anencephaly is uniformly fatal and is reliably diagnosed with sonography, it is one of the few universally accepted indications for third trimester termination.[24]

Exencephaly (Acrania)
Pathologic and Clinical Findings.—Exencephaly is characterized by complete or partial absence of the calvarium with complete, but abnormal development of brain tissue. The cartilaginous skull bones form a normal skull base. Exencephaly is much less common than anencephaly in humans.[26]

The pathogenesis of exencephaly is unclear, but recent evidence suggests that it represents an embryologic precursor to anencephaly.[26, 30] Absence of the calvarium is thought to cause brain destruction by exposing the developing brain to amniotic fluid and repeated trauma. Exposed brain may be destroyed as early as 8–10 weeks in humans.[26] This notion is supported by the observation that exencephaly is frequently observed in animals with relatively short gestational periods, and anencephaly can result if the gesta-

tion is experimentally prolonged.[26] Also, the abnormal brain tissue of exencephaly is pathologically very similar to the area cerebrovasculosa of anencephaly.

Sonographic Findings.—Several cases of exencephaly have been reported on prenatal sonography, and Hendricks et al. have recently contributed four additional cases.[26, 30, 32, 34] Sonographic findings of exencephaly include absence of the calvarial vault with exposure of cerebral tissue to the amniotic fluid (Fig 6–6). The brain parenchyma is relatively normal in amount, but heterogeneous and disorganized on pathologic examination. A "pseudo-sulcal" appearance may be demonstrated on sonography.[30]

The differential diagnosis of exencephaly includes marked undermineralization of the cranium, as seen with hypophosphatasia and osteogenesis imperfecta. However, in these conditions the cranium is present, even though diminished in echogenicity, and the underlying parenchymal pattern is normal.

Associated Anomalies.—Anomalies that have been associated with exencephaly include spinal defects, cleft lip and palate, and clubfoot.[30]

Prognosis.—Like anencephaly, exencephaly is uniformly fatal.

(En)Cephalocele
Pathologic and Clinical Findings.—The term cephalocele describes cranial defects that involve either herniation of the brain and meninges (encephalocele) or meninges and cerebrospinal fluid (meningocele).[17] In common usage, however, the term encephalocele is used to describe both conditions.[41] Meningocele probably comprises less than 10% of all cephaloceles, although a much higher frequency is observed in neonatal series, presumably because of its more favorable prognosis compared to encephalocele.[44] The reported incidence of cephalocele varies from 1 in 2,000 to 1 in 10,000 births.

Sonographic Findings.—The sonographic appearance of cephalocele varies with the location and size of the cranial defect and the presence or absence of brain involvement.[37, 43, 45, 52] Based on brain involvement, cephaloceles may have one of three sonographic appearances:

1. A purely cystic extracranial mass representing a meningocele.
2. A solid mass, usually showing a gyral pattern contiguous to the cranium (Fig 6–7).

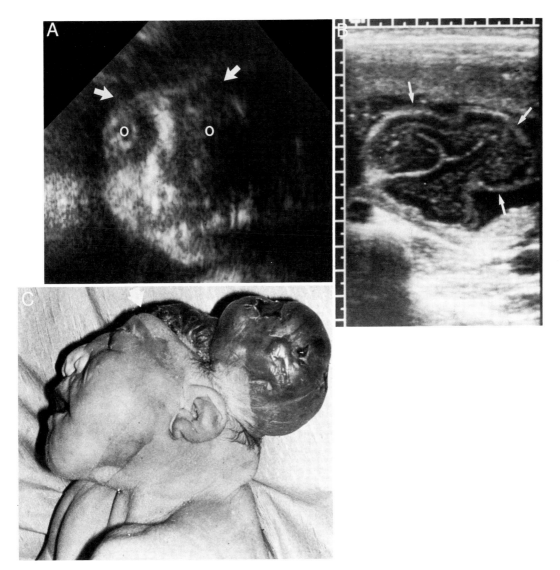

FIG 6–6.
Exencephaly. **A,** coronal sonogram through the fetal face demonstrates absence of the cranial vault *(arrows)* cephalad to the orbits *(O)*. **B,** axial sonogram cephalad to the orbits demonstrates a large amount of brain tissue *(arrows)* that protruded from the base of the brain. Note the "pseudo-sulcal" pattern. **C,** photograph of the pathologic specimen shows absence of the cranium cephalad to the orbits like anencephaly *(arrows)*, but a large amount of brain tissue is seen protruding from the defect, consistent with exencephaly.

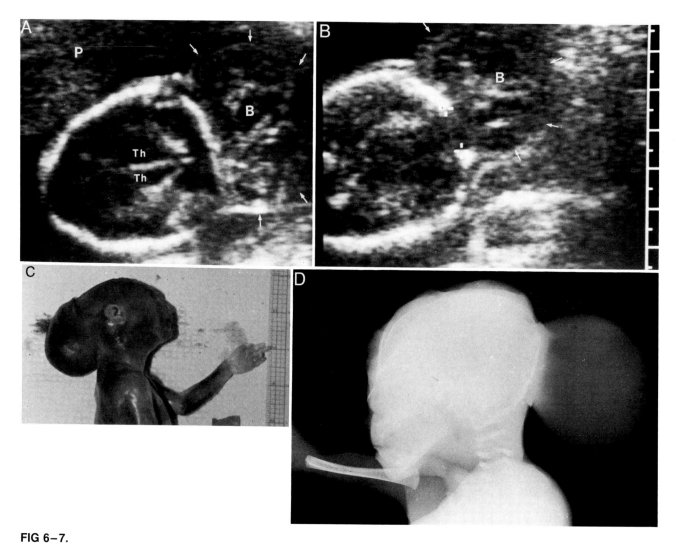

FIG 6–7.
Encephalocele. **A,** transverse scan through the mid cranium shows a large amount of brain tissue (*B,* outlined by arrows) posterior to the cranium. Note that the thalami *(Th)* appear distorted with traction towards the occiput. *P* = placenta. **B,** scan at a slightly different plane shows brain (*B,* outlined by arrows) herniated through a discrete defect of the occipital calvarium. **C,** postmortem photograph shows the large occipital encephalocele. **D,** postnatal skull radiograph shows the large calvarial defect and protruding brain tissue.

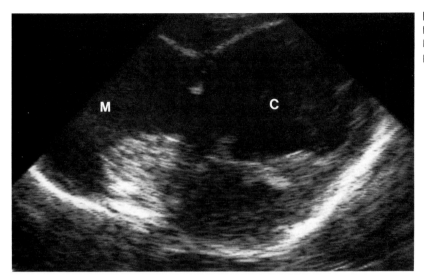

FIG 6–8.
Meningoencephalocele. Oblique scan shows a large cystic mass *(M)* with some brain tissue protruding from the occipital cranium *(C)*.

3. A combination of solid and cystic elements representing meningoencephalocele (Fig 6–8).

Most cephaloceles are large enough to be readily visible on the standard transthalamic view of the calvarium. However, small occipital cephaloceles are usually located near or just above the region of the cisterna magna and may be demonstrated only on views angled through the posterior fossa. Anterior cephaloceles are more difficult to visualize, unless they are large and produce an obvious mass. Hydrocephalus, which frequently accompanies cephalocele, may be the first clue to the underlying diagnosis. Even when ventricular dilatation is absent, intracranial anatomy usually appears distorted, with traction of normal structures toward the cranial defect (see Fig 6–7). Microcephaly may

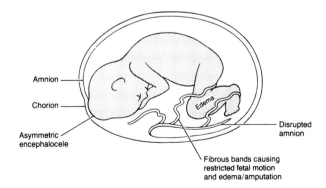

FIG 6–9.
Schematic drawing of amniotic band syndrome. Typical features include fibrous bands, asymmetric cephalocele, and amputation defects of other sites. Similar features can be seen with the limb-body wall complex, but this disorder typically demonstrates a large trunk defect and scoliosis. (From Randel SB, Filly RA, Callen PW, et al: Amniotic sheets. Radiology 1988; 166:633–636. Used by permission.)

also be an important clue to the presence of a cephalocele.

Cephaloceles in an asymmetric or atypical location should be suspected of resulting from the amniotic band syndrome (Figs 6–9 and 6–10) or limb-body wall complex (Fig 6–11). In these disorders, defects involving other anatomic sites are invariably present, and the adherant membrane may be visualized.[49] An important and common cause of cephaloceles seen prenatally is the Meckel-Gruber syndrome (Figs 6–12 and 6–13).[42, 46, 48, 53] Although prenatal studies suggest that this autosomal recessive disorder comprises less than 5% of cephaloceles, we have observed a significantly greater frequency prenatally. Hence, the Meckel-Gruber syndrome should be considered whenever a cephalocele or cystic kidneys are demonstrated.[46, 51, 55]

The differential diagnosis for a juxtacranial mass depends on the sonographic appearance (cystic or solid) and the location of the lesion. When the mass is located posteriorly, other possibilities that should be considered include cystic hygroma (Fig 6–14), exencephaly, iniencephaly (described below), and, rarely, teratoma.[30, 35, 50, 52] When the mass is located anteriorly, other considerations include teratoma and an atypical cystic hygroma. A teratoma has a predominantly solid appearance, but does not demonstrate the characteristic gyral pattern of encephalocele from eviscerated cerebrum or cerebellum. Cystic hygromata are predominantly cystic and may contain characteristic internal separations. As a diagnostic point, neither cystic hygromata nor teratomas demonstrate the calvarial defect of cephalocele. An edge refraction artifact should not be mistaken for a true calvarial defect (see Fig 6–14).

The accuracy of ultrasound for diagnosing cephalo-

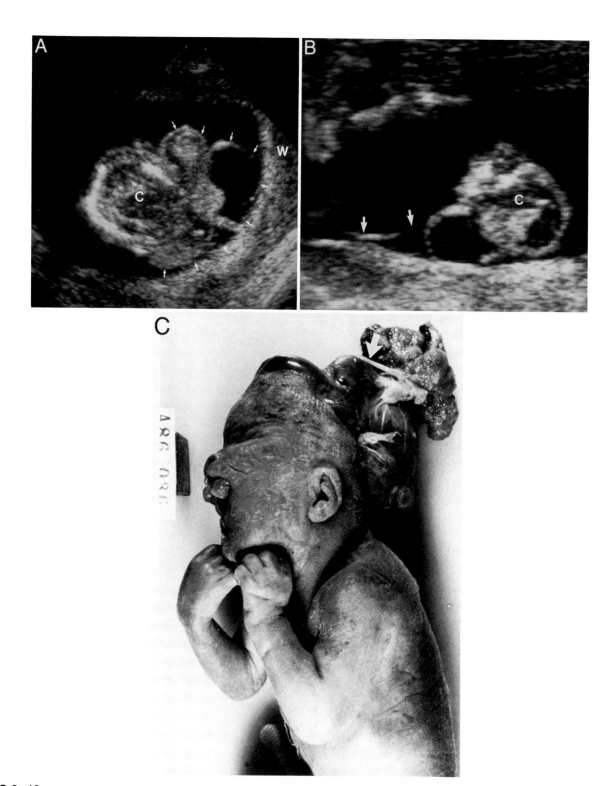

FIG 6–10.
Amniotic band syndrome. **A,** transverse scan of the cranium on transvaginal sonography at 14 weeks shows disorganized brain *(arrows)* protruding through a large calvarial defect adherent to the uterine wall *(W). C* = cranium. **B,** a portion of the ruptured amnion is contiguous with the encephalocele. *C* = cranium. **C,** postnatal photograph of another fetus with the amniotic band syndrome and exencephaly shows amniotic bands *(arrow)* attached to the protruding brain. A facial cleft is also present.

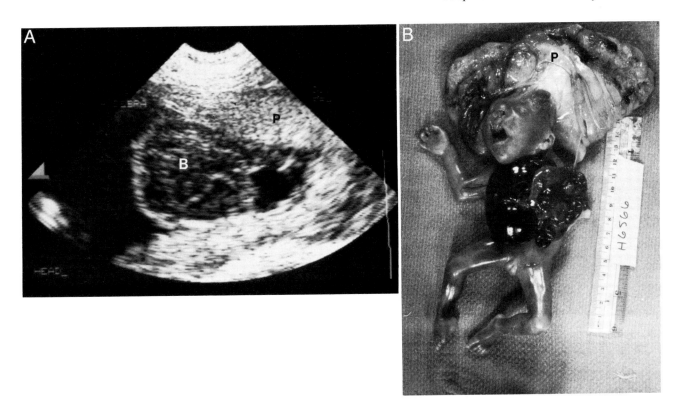

FIG 6–11.
Limb-body wall complex (body-stalk anomaly). **A,** transverse scan shows absence of much of the cranial vault with brain tissue *(B)* contiguous with the placenta *(P)*. **B,** photograph of pathologic specimen shows characteristic findings of the limb-body wall complex, with the large cranial defect intimately involved with the placenta *(P)* and placental membranes. Defects of the face, extremities, and large thoracoabdominal defect are also present. The limb-body wall complex may represent a severe and early manifestation of the amniotic band syndrome. (From Patten RM, Van Allen M, Mack LA, et al: Limb-body wall complex: In utero sonographic diagnosis of a complicated fetal malformation. AJR 1986; 146:1019–1024. Used by permission.)

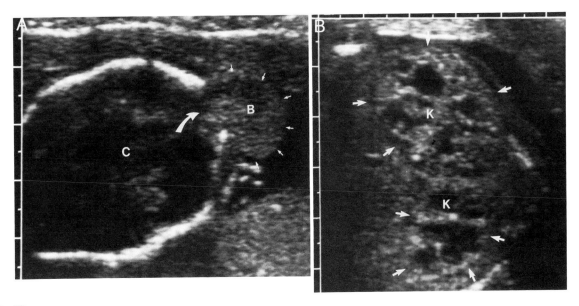

FIG 6–12.
Meckel-Gruber syndrome. **A,** axial sonogram through the cranium shows brain (*B,* demarcated by arrows) protruding through a posterior calvarial defect *(curved arrow)*. *C* = cranium. **B,** transverse scan through the abdomen shows enlarged, echogenic kidneys (*K,* demarcated by arrows) containing innumerable small cysts.

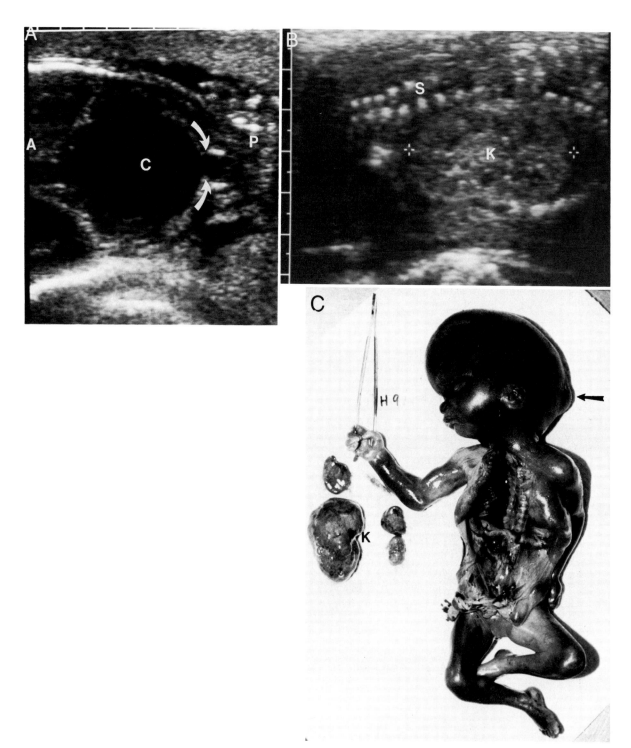

FIG 6–13.
Meckel-Gruber syndrome. **A,** axial sonogram through the posterior fossa shows a large cyst *(C)* and absence of the cerebellar vermis consistent with the Dandy-Walker malformation. A small defect is noted of the posterior calvarium *(arrows).* The cerebrospinal fluid protrudes through the defect but remains covered by skin and thickened subcutaneous tissue. *A* = anterior; *P* = posterior. **B,** longitudinal sonogram of the abdomen demonstrates a markedly enlarged and echogenic right kidney *(K).* The left kidney was similarly involved. Normal kidney length is usually less than the height of four vertebral bodies. *S* = spine. **C,** photograph of pathologic specimen shows the small occipital protrusion *(arrow),* enlarged dysplastic kidneys *(K),* and polydactyly. The Meckel-Gruber syndrome is a common cause of cephaloceles prenatally and should be considered whenever a cephalocele or cystic kidneys are demonstrated.

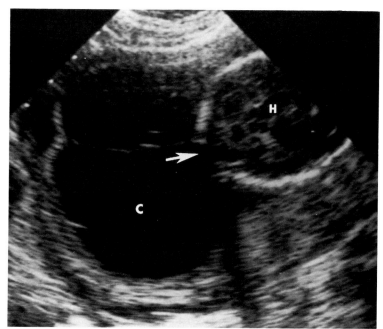

FIG 6–14.
Cystic hygroma. Transverse scan demonstrates a large cystic hygroma *(C)* posterior to the head *(H)*. The edge refraction artifact *(arrow)* should not be mistaken for a true cranial defect. The intact cranium can be shown by angling the ultrasound transducer in various planes.

celes is unknown, but is expected to be high. Small cephaloceles located in the occiput can be missed unless specific views are obtained through the posterior fossa. Cephaloceles can also be overlooked in the face of oligohydramnios, which usually accompanies the Meckel-Gruber syndrome (see Figs 6–12 and 6–13). False-positive diagnoses of cephalocele have been reported in several instances of cloverleaf skull.[36, 54] Normal fetal structures, such as hair and the external ear, also should not be confused for a cephalocele.[39]

Associated Anomalies.—Hydrocephalus has been reported in 80% of occipital meningoceles, 65% of occipital encephaloceles, and 15% of frontal cephaloceles.[44, 47] Spina bifida is present in 7% to 15% of cephaloceles,[37] and microcephaly has been reported in 20% of cases.[47] Frontal cephaloceles are often associated with facial clefts and hypertelorism.[41] Sphenoid encephaloceles are also associated with agenesis of the corpus callosum in 80% of cases.[40]

Cephalocele has been associated with a variety of multiple anomaly syndromes (Table 6–3), the most well-known of which is the Meckel-Gruber syndrome (see Figs 6–12 and 6–13).[38] This autosomal recessive disorder is characterized by renal cystic dysplasia (100%), an occipital encephalocele (80%), and polydactyly, usually involving both hands and feet.[42, 48, 53] Less common midline cranial malformations that have been associated with the Meckel-Gruber syndrome include the Dandy-Walker malformation (see Fig 6–13), agenesis of the corpus callosum, and, rarely, holoprosencephaly. The Meckel-Gruber syndrome is impor-

tant to recognize for counseling subsequent pregnancies since this condition carries a 25% chance of recurrence.

The frequency of chromosomal abnormalities associated with cephaloceles is uncertain. Of interest, Jeanty reported that three of eight fetuses with cephaloceles who underwent successful chromosomal analysis proved to have an abnormal karyotype.[45]

Prognosis.—The prognosis for cephaloceles depends primarily on whether brain tissue is present within the herniated sac.[44] In a series of 74 cases reported by Guthkelch, the mortality rate was 71% for infants with encephalocele (herniated brain) compared to a mortality rate of 11% for infants with meningocele.[44] A similar experience was reported by Jeanty et al., who described their experience with 13 cephaloceles diagnosed on prenatal sonography. In this series, all 11 fetuses with encephalocele died, whereas both fetuses with meningocele survived and are doing well following surgical correction of the defect. Intellectual outcome also is significantly worse for infants with an encephalocele compared to those with a meningocele.[44, 47] Other factors that have been associated with a worse prognosis for cephaloceles, in addition to brain involvement, are hydrocephalus and microcephaly.[44, 47]

When a cephalocele is detected before fetal viability, management options include termination of the pregnancy.[37] When detected after fetal viability, primary management decisions include determining the place, time, and mode of delivery. When a meningocele or meningoencephalocele is present, in utero aspi-

TABLE 6-3.

Syndromes Associated With Cephaloceles*

Syndrome	Mode of Inheritance	Location of Encephalocele	Frequency of Encephalocele	Other Anomalies
Amniotic band syndrome	Sporadic	Asymmetric	Uncommon	Other amputation defects
Meckel-Gruber syndrome	AR	Occipital	80%	Cystic, dysplastic kidneys, polydactyly, other midline cranial defects
Chemke syndrome	AR	Occipital	50% (3/6)	Hydrocephaly, cerebellar dysgenesis agyria
Cryptophthalmos syndrome	AR	Occipital	10%	Syndactyly, genital abnormalities
Dyssegmental dysplasia	AR	Occipital	20% (2/10)	Lethal dwarfism, metaphyseal widening, vertebral anomalies, small thorax
Knobloch syndrome	AR?	Occipital	80% (4/5)	Spina bifida, retinal detachment
von Voss syndrome	?	Occipital	100% (2/2)	Agenesis of the corpus callosum, phocomelia, urogenital anomalies, thrombocytopenia
Robert's syndrome	AR	Anterior		Micromelia
Walker-Warburg syndrome	AR	Occipital		Hydrocephalus, lissencephaly, ocular abnormalities

*Adapted from Cohen MM, Lemire RJ: Syndromes with cephaloceles. Teratology 1982; 25:161-172.

ration of the cephalocele sac has been performed. Cephalocentesis can also be performed if significant hydrocephalus is present.

Iniencephaly

Pathologic and Clinical Findings.—Iniencephaly is a rare malformation in which a defect of the occiput (inion) is usually combined with a dysraphic defect of the cervical spine. Two types of iniencephaly are recognized, those with an encephalocele (iniencephaly apertus) and those without an encephalocele (iniencephaly clausus).[56] Spina bifida may also involve the thoracic and lumbar spine, but the vertebral defect is usually closed.

Fetuses with iniencephaly demonstrate a grotesque appearance, with marked and fixed retroflexion of the head and neck as a constant feature.[56] The head is also enlarged relative to the shortened body, and the neck is absent. Abundance of hair is noted over the neck and back.[60]

Some studies suggest that iniencephaly may be a severe form of the Klippel-Feil syndrome or may belong to the spectrum of anomalies between the Dandy-Walker malformation and the Arnold-Chiari malformation.[58] Others have grouped anencephaly with retroflexion with iniencephaly.[59]

Sonographic Findings.—Iniencephaly rarely has been reported prenatally.[37, 60, 61] Foderaro et al. reported a fetus with iniencephaly at 22 menstrual weeks (18.5 weeks by femur length).[57] The head was in fixed

hyperextension, and a cystic mass was identified in the posterior fossa, suggesting the presence of the Dandy-Walker malformation (Fig 6-15). Other detectable abnormalities included a large spinal dysraphic defect of the lumbosacral spine and thoracic scoliosis. Meizner and Bar-Ziv reported another case of iniencephaly combined with anencephaly at 22 menstrual weeks.[60] Other abnormalities present included an omphalocele, facial cleft, clubfoot, and polyhydramnios.

Associated Anomalies.—Eighty four percent of infants with iniencephaly in the series of David and Nixon had associated anomalies.[28] Associated cranial anomalies include anencephaly, hydrocephalus, microcephaly, holoprosencephaly, polymicrogyria, agenesis of the cerebellar vermis, cerebellar cyst, and occipital encephalocele.[56] Extra-CNS anomalies include cyclopia, facial cleft, diaphragmatic hernia, cardiovascular and genitourinary malformations, omphalocele, anorectal atresia, arthrogryposis, clubfoot, and single umbilical artery.[28]

Prognosis.—Iniencephaly is universally fatal.

THE SPINE

Normal Embryogenesis and Sonographic Findings

Somite formation begins by the fifth menstrual week, and the neural tube is completed by the sixth menstrual week.[9] Fusion of the neural tube proceeds in

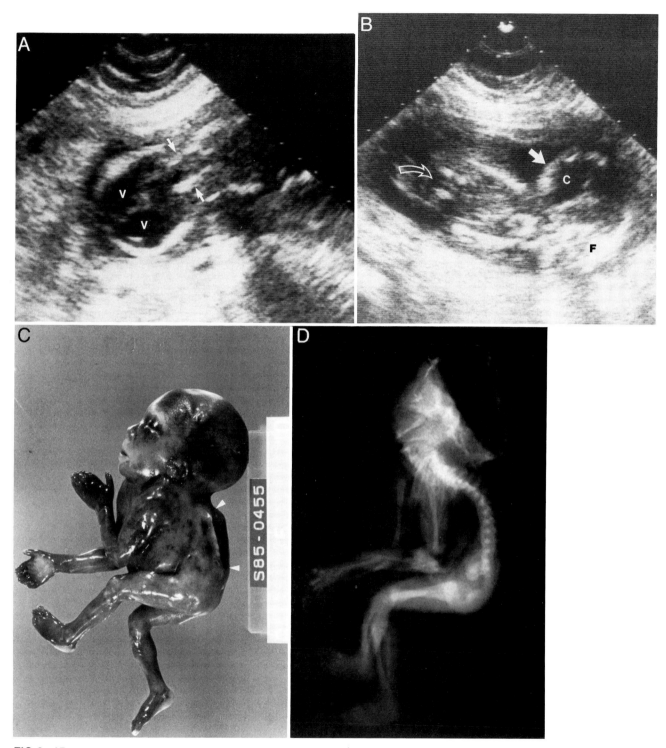

FIG 6–15.
Iniencephaly. **A,** coronal view of the cranium shows dilatation of the lateral ventricles *(V)* and suggests a dysraphic defect of the upper thoracic spine *(arrow)*. **B,** sagittal view with the face *(F)* downward shows hyperextension of the head on the cervical spine (arrow points to occiput). A cystic structure *(C)* is identified in the posterior fossa suggesting Dandy-Walker malformation. Oblique view through the abdomen and thorax (disorted due to kyposis) shows a spinal defect *(curved arrow)*. **C,** photograph of pathologic specimen shows short neck with hyperextension of the head and fusion of the occiput to the cervical and upper thoracic spine. A large dysraphic defect involves the thoracic and lumbar spine *(arrowheads)*. **D,** radiograph shows severe retroflexion of the head and cervical spine. The occiput is fused to the back of the upper thoracic spine. (From Foderaro AE, Abu-Yousef MM, Benda JA, et al: Antenatal ultrasound diagnosis of iniencephaly. J Clin Ultrasound 1987; 15:550–554. Used by permission.)

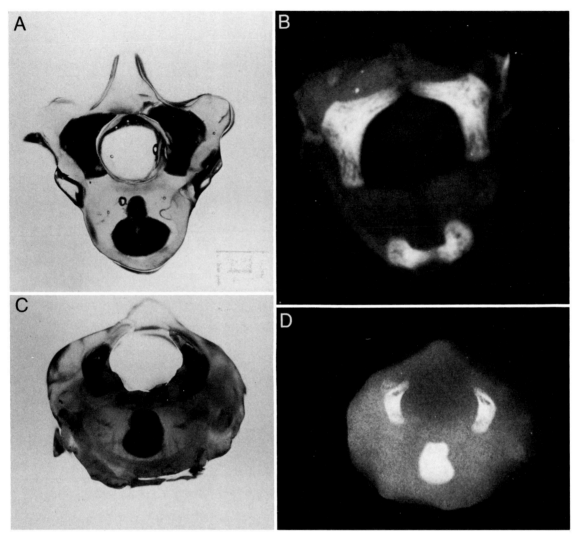

FIG 6–16.
Normal fetal spine, 18 weeks. **A,** histologic section and corresponding in vitro radiograph **(B)** of the lower thoracic spine (T–8). **C,** the lower lumbar spine (L–5) and corresponding in vitro radiograph **(D).** Note incomplete ossification of the dorsal arch of the lumbar spine. (Courtesy of Eric E Sauerbrei, MD, Department of Radiology, Kingston General Hospital, Kingston, ON.)

both a cranial and caudal direction so that temporarily the neural tube is open at both ends. The cranial opening (rostral neuropore) closes about the 25th fetal day (39th menstrual day), and the distal opening (caudal neuropore) closes about 2 days later (see Fig 6–1).[9] The neural tube caudad to the fourth pair of somites develops into the spinal cord.

Mineralization of the spine begins at 8 menstrual weeks. The three ossification centers of individual vertebrae include a single ventral center for the vertebral body (centrum) and two paired dorsal centers that will become the lateral masses and the posterior arch (Fig 6–16). Within an individual vertebra, dorsal ossification begins at the junction of the lamina and pedicles and progresses both anteriorly and posteriorly from

this point to involve the remainder of the pedicle and lamina, respectively.[3, 4] Between vertebrae, the dorsal ossification centers appear in a cephalic to caudal direction beginning in the cervical spine and progressing to the sacrum.[2] Filly et al. showed that ossification of the laminae of the lower lumbar region was not observed before 19 menstrual weeks and the arch of the upper sacral region was not consistently recognizable until after 25 weeks.[3] Sauerbrei et al. have confirmed this by correlating sonographic findings with histologic specimens (see Fig 6–16).[10]

The fetal spine and spinal cord can be rapidly and systematically examined with real-time sonography during the second and third trimesters.[1–3, 6] Transverse (axial) views have been found to be superior to longi-

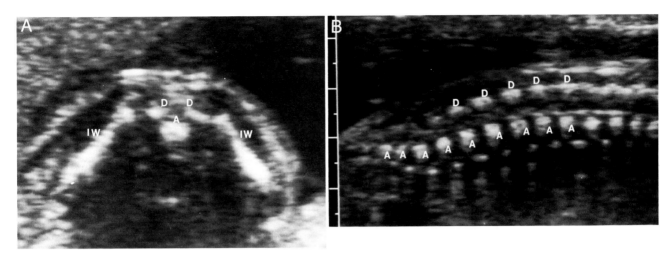

FIG 6–17.
Normal spine, 21 weeks. **A,** transverse view of the lower lumbar spine shows single anterior ossification center *(A)* and convergence of the dorsal ossification centers *(D)*. *IW* = iliac wing. **B,** parasagittal scan of the lumbosacral spine shows anterior *(A)* and dorsal *(D)* ossification centers.

tudinal (sagittal and/or coronal) views for demonstrating small spinal defects by some authors, since all three ossification centers can be imaged simultaneously (Fig 6–17).[3, 6, 72] Since it is impractical to record images of the entire spine in transverse plane, however, representative images should be recorded for documentation purposes, with attention directed to the lumbosacral spine.

Unlike axial scans, sagittal and coronal views can visualize many vertebrae on a single image (see Fig 6–17). Hence, scoliosis, hemivertebrae, and disorganized or hypomineralized vertebrae are optimally visualized on these views. Also, coronal views oriented through the dorsal ossification centers can demonstrate the extent of a dysraphic defect compared to adjacent vertebrae, and the sagittal plane can optimally demonstrate interruption of the overlying integument when a myelomeningocele is present.

High-quality sonograms can also demonstrate the spinal cord within the spinal canal. The central canal is readily detectable within the cord. The more echogenic cauda equina (nerve roots) can be seen distal to the conus medullaris (distal spinal cord). With growth of the spine, the position of the conus medullaris ascends with gestational age (Fig 6–18).[7]

Potential Pitfalls

In the evaluation of possible dysraphic defects of the lower lumbar spine, sonographers should be aware that incomplete ossification of the dorsal ossification centers can lead to false-positive diagnoses, particularly during the mid-trimester. Hence, the dorsal ossification centers may appear to be parallel to one another rather than converging to the midline on transverse views (see Fig 6–16), and no ossification center may be seen posteriorly on true sagittal views (see Fig 6–18).

The fetal position and scan angle also are important to consider when evaluating the fetal spine on axial views. Gray et al. showed that when the fetal spine is prone, the dorsal ossification centers appear to converge toward the midline as expected.[6] By contrast, when the spine is in a lateral recumbent position, the dorsal ossification centers appear nearly parallel to one another.[6] They attribute this phenomenon to the shape of the posterior elements, with the principal angle of reflection directed perpendicular to the lamina when the fetus is prone and perpendicular to the pedicle when the fetus is in a decubitus position.

Another potential difficulty is a false-positive diagnosis of a dysraphic defect ("pseudodysraphic defect") when the ultrasound beam is angled obliquely across the vertebral body of one vertebra to the dorsal ossification centers of another (Figs 6–19 and 6–20).[71] This error is particularly likely to occur when imaging the naturally curved lumbosacral spine. A normal appearance is restored when the ultrasound beam is reoriented perpendicular to the spinal axis.

Spina Bifida

Pathologic and Clinical Findings

Spina bifida is a defect that can occur anywhere along the spinal axis, but most commonly involves the lumbosacral region. Hydrocephalus eventually develops in 80%–90% of cases as part of the Arnold-Chiari

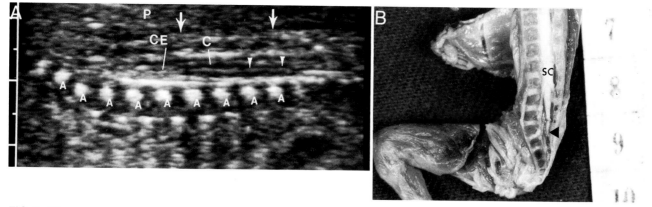

FIG 6–18.
Normal spine, 18 weeks. **A,** true sagittal scan of the lumbar spine at 18 weeks shows only the anterior ossification centers *(A)*. The dorsal ossification centers are not visualized on this midline view, since ossification of the dorsal arch is incomplete. The dermis *(arrows)* is intact, but is difficult to visualize secondary to its interface with the placenta *(P)*. Note the conus medullaris of the spinal cord *(C)* with its central canal *(arrowheads)* and the more echogenic cauda equina *(CE)* inferiorly. **B,** sagittal section of the fetal spine at 18 weeks demonstrates that the spinal cord *(SC)* extends to the upper sacrum *(arrowhead)*. With growth of the spine, the spinal cord will gradually ascend in position throughout pregnancy and infancy until its distal tip (conus medullaris) reaches its adult position at the L1–2 level. (Part **B** from Hawass ND, El-Badawi MG, Fatani JA, et al: Myelographic study of the spinal cord ascent during fetal development. AJNR 1987; 8:691–695. Used by permission.)

type II malformation.[17, 64] Although the neuromuscular outcome is variable, more children are crippled by myelomeningocele today than by poliomyelitis, muscular dystrophy, or traumatic paraplegia.[82] Survivors with spina bifida usually require enormous emotional, medical, and financial support. For these reasons, prenatal detection of spina bifida has become a major public health issue, as reflected by wide-scale screening of MS-AFP.[20]

A sacular protrusion through the spinal defect has

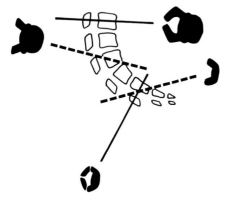

FIG 6–19.
Diagram of pseudodysraphic defect. Scanning in a true transverse plane to the lower spine *(solid lines)* demonstrates convergence of the dorsal ossification centers. By contrast, scanning obliquely across the spine *(dotted lines)* can produce a pseudodysraphic defect, with dorsal ossification centers apparently diverging from midline. (Modified from Dennis MA, Drose JA, Pretorius DH, et al: Normal fetal sacrum simulating spina bifida: "Pseudodysraphism." Radiology 1985; 155:751–754. Used by permission.)

been termed spina bifida cystica. Spina bifida cystica can be further categorized as myelomeningocele (protrusion of a sac containing cerebrospinal fluid (CSF) and neural elements) or meningocele (sac with CSF only) (Fig 6–21).[99] Over 90% of cases represent a myelomeningocele. Myelomeningocele is closely related to other spinal dysraphic abnormalities including spinal cord lipoma, diastematomyelia, neurenteric cyst, and intraspinal dermoids. All spinal dysraphic disorders share two common features: Bony spina bifida and caudal displacement of the spinal cord.[41]

Spina bifida can also be characterized as "open" (80%) or "closed" defects (20%). However, the distinction between open and closed defects is not as clear as this terminology suggests. An open defect has been defined as either uncovered or covered with a thin translucent membrane, whereas a closed defect is covered with skin or a thick, opaque membrane.[20, 21] In the following discussion, the term spina bifida refers to both open and closed spinal defects, excluding spina bifida occulta. The latter condition is a commonly encountered (2%–3% of the population) internal defect of one or more vertebrae, but is often asymptomatic and has not been identified prenatally (see Fig 6–21).[99]

The sensitivity and accuracy of sonography for detecting spina bifida have been reported from a number of studies. In evaluating these studies, important factors to consider include the method of patient selection (high risk or low risk) and the experience of the sonographer(s). Another important consideration is the time period in which the study was performed

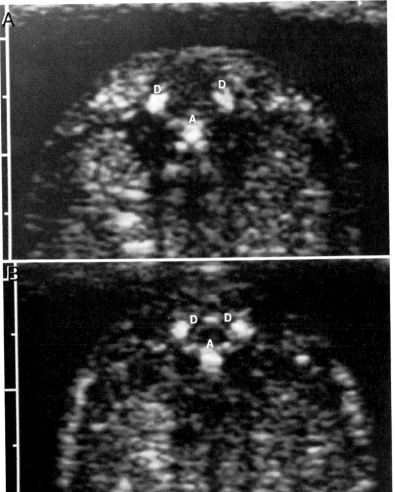

FIG 6–20.
Pseudodysraphic defect. **A,** transverse scan of the lumbar spine at 20 weeks shows absence of dorsal arch that could be mistaken for a dysraphic defect. *A* = anterior ossification center; *D* = dorsal ossification centers. **B,** scan in a true axial plane shows convergence of the dorsal ossification centers *(D)*. *A* = anterior ossification center.

since the quality of sonographic images has improved dramatically in parallel with developments in ultrasound technology. Introduction of phased-array technology and other high-resolution ultrasound equipment since 1983 represents a major advance in prenatal detection of such defects.

Initial studies detected spina bifida with a sensitivity as low as 40%, with frequent false-positive diagnoses.[67, 89, 93] This low accuracy was attributed primarily to the inexperience of the sonographers in detecting spina bifida. Roberts et al. reported that during the first three years of their experience (1977–1980), their sensitivity was only 33% and their specificity 96% for detecting spina bifida.[92] With further experience during the subsequent 3 years (1980–1983), their sensitivity rose to 80% and their specificity to 99%. Even higher sensitivity, specificity, and accuracy have been reported from referral centers that examine women in specific high-risk groups such as those with elevated MS–AFP, a family history of NTD, or sonographic demonstration of other abnormalities.

Sonographic Findings

Sonographic evaluation of spina bifida justifiably emphasizes visualization of the lower lumbar and sacral spine. In a large clinical series, spina bifida was localized to the sacral or lumbosacral spine in 63% of cases, and nearly all the remaining cases were categorized as thoracolumbar in location.[63] Therefore, excluding all but a few myelomeningoceles isolated in the thoracic or cervical spine, spina bifida nearly always involves the lower spine. Small spinal defects missed on sonography also are usually localized in the sacral or lower lumbar spine.[79] Transverse views that include the bony pelvis help ensure that this important area has been visualized.

The sonographic appearance of spina bifida varies with the location and size of the spinal defect and the

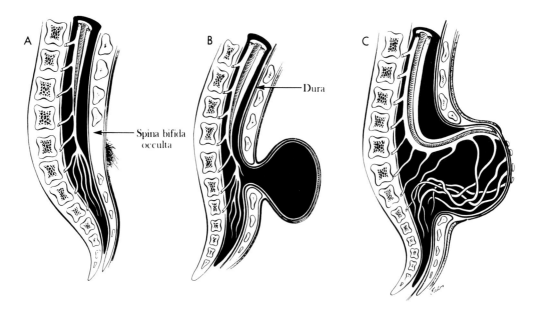

FIG 6–21.
Classification of spina bifida. **A,** spina bifida occulta is characterized by a defect in one or more vertebrae, but intact skin and no alteration in the spinal cord. Although relatively common in the adult population (2%), this is not visualized prenatally. **B,** meningocele is characterized by protrusion of meninges and cerebrospinal fluid through the spinal defect. Meningocele represents approximately 10% of spina bifida seen prenatally. **C,** myelomeningocele is characterized by protrusion of neural elements as well as meninges through the spinal defect. This type represents 90% of spina bifida seen prenatally. (From Warkany J: *Congenital Malformations: Notes and Comments.* Chicago, Year Book Medical Publishers, Inc, 1971. Used by permission.)

presence or absence of a myelomeningocele sac. The sonographic findings that are most useful for diagnosing spina bifida can be categorized as:

1. A dysraphic spinal defect.
2. Soft tissue findings (myelomeningocele sac and/ or disruption of the overlying integument).
3. Associated cranial findings (discussed below).

Demonstration of a spinal dysraphic defect is diagnostic of spina bifida (Fig 6–22). The defect usually can be seen on both transverse and longitudinal images, although small defects are demonstrated optimally on axial views with the fetus in a prone position.[6, 10, 72]

Since evaluation of only the spine can result in both false-positive and false-negative diagnoses, soft tissue findings are also important in the evaluation of suspected spina bifida. A myelomeningocele sac is present in the majority of fetuses with spina bifida, even though the sac usually appears collapsed after delivery (Fig 6–23). The myelomeningocele sac is covered by a thin translucent membrane and usually contains both CSF and neural elements. Demonstration of this finding adds considerable confidence to the sonographic diagnosis of spina bifida, particularly when the fetus is in a suboptimal position for evaluating the spine. Significant growth of the myelomeningocele sac can be observed with advancing gestational age (Fig 6–24).

Disruption of the overlying integument is another important secondary finding of spina bifida, particularly when the myelomeningocele sac is not demonstrated (Fig 6–25). Evaluation of the soft tissues is also essential in the prenatal diagnosis of an unusual lesion, lipomyelomeningocele. Seeds and co-workers described the sonographic findings in two fetuses with lipomyelomeningocele, both from the same family.[94, 95] In the second pregnancy, the only sonographic finding at 17 menstrual weeks was a 1 cm echogenic area dorsal to the fetal spine.[95] Both infants had normal neurologic outcomes following surgical excision of the fatty tumor.

It is important for the sonographer to realize that normal leg movement does not exclude spina bifida.[77] In newborns with myelomeningocele, leg movement may be secondary to neural reflexes rather than direct neuromuscular control. On the other hand, absence of leg motion or demonstration of a fixed foot or leg deformity (clubfoot) may have prognostic significance (Fig 6–26).

Once a spinal defect is identified, sonographic evaluation should include characterization of its location and size and presence or absence of a surrounding membrane. Spinal defects may occasionally be identified in the cervical or thoracic spine (Figs 6–27 and 6–28). No formal study has been undertaken to evaluate the accuracy of sonography for determining the lo-

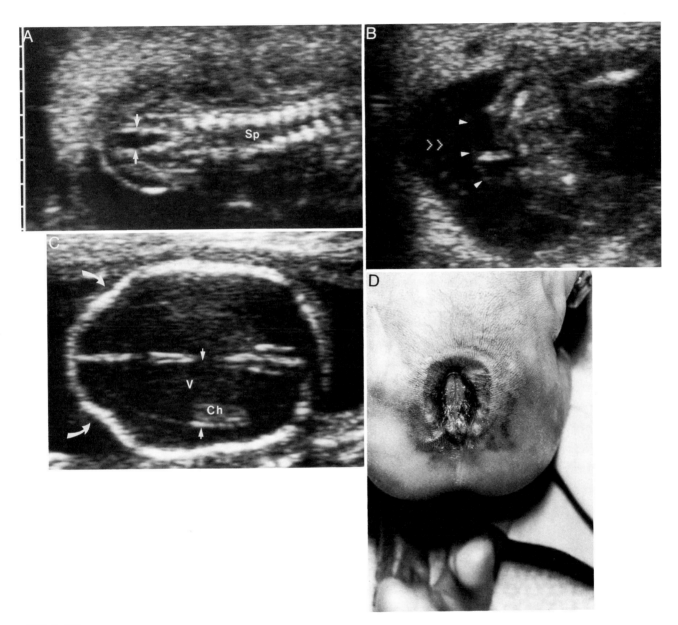

FIG 6–22.
Myelomeningocele. **A,** longitudinal sonogram of the lumbar spine *(Sp)* at 20 weeks shows dysraphic defect localized to the lower lumbar spine. **B,** transverse sonogram shows a myelomeningocele sac *(arrowhead)* containing linear neural elements. **C,** transverse sonogram of the cranium demonstrates moderate dilatation of the lateral ventricles *(V)* delineated by small arrows and a lemon-shaped frontal calvarium *(curved arrows)* (see text for Cranial findings associated with spina bifida). *Ch* = choroid. **D,** photograph at necropsy shows the low lumbar spinal defect.

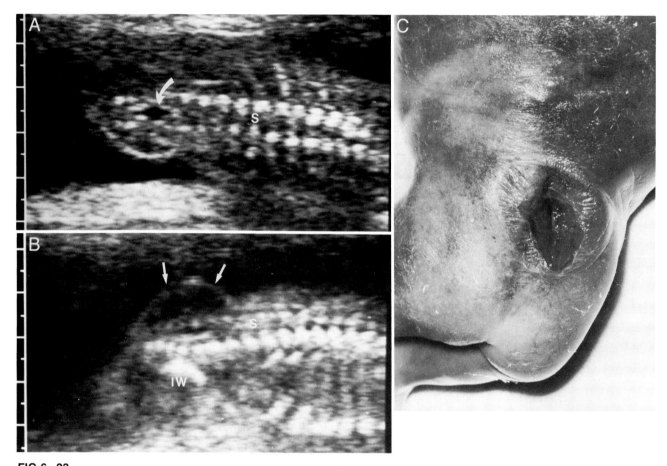

FIG 6–23.
Myelomeningocele. **A,** coronal sonogram of the lumbosacral spine at 18 weeks, performed because of elevated MS-AFP, demonstrates a dysraphic defect of the lower lumbar spine *(arrow). S* = spine. **B,** sagittal scan shows a myelomeningocele sac *(arrows). IW* = iliac wing; *S* = spine. **C,** photograph of the pathologic specimen after pregnancy termination demonstrates an open lumbosacral defect.

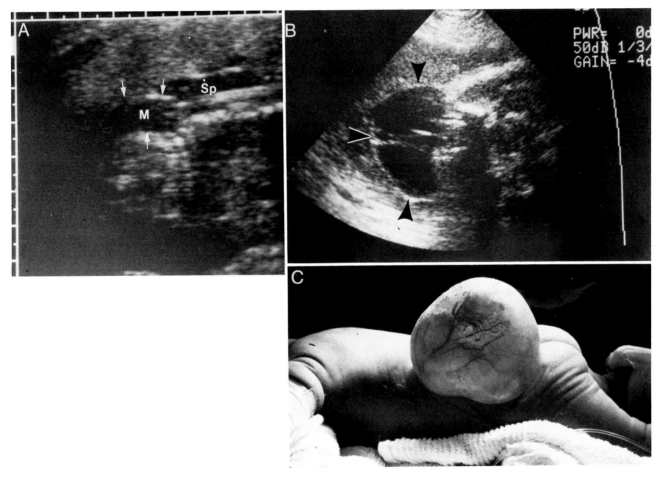

FIG 6–24.
Large myelomeningocele. **A,** longitudinal sonogram at 20 menstrual weeks demonstrates a small (1.5 cm) myelomeningocele sac (*M,* delineated by arrows) protruding from the lower lumbar spine *(Sp).* **B,** repeat sonogram at 34 weeks, after continuation of the pregnancy was elected, demonstrates a large 7 cm myelomeningocele sac *(arrowheads)* which contains neural elements. **C,** postnatal photograph of another infant diagnosed prenatally shows large myelomeningocele sac.

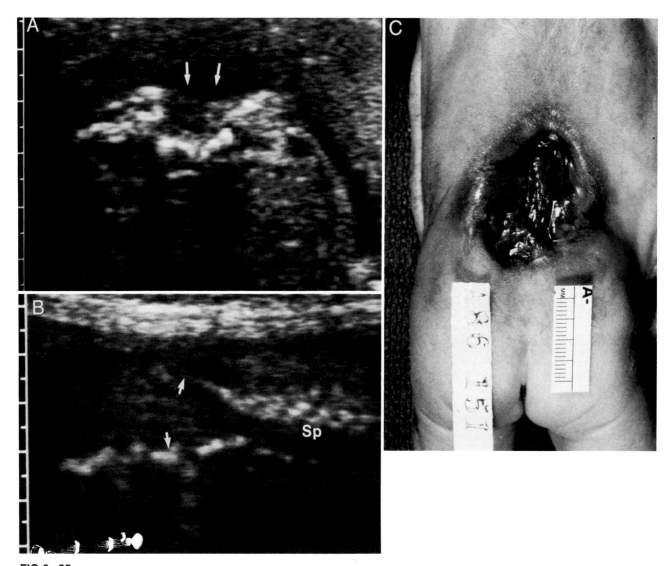

FIG 6–25.
Large lumbosacral spinal defect at 22 weeks. **A,** transverse sonogram of the mid-lumbar spine shows a large dysraphic defect *(arrows)* with divergence of the dorsal arch. A surrounding sac is not present, but disruption of the skin is noted. **B,** longitudinal sonogram demonstrates an extensive defect involving the entire lumbar spine *(arrows). Sp* = spine. **C,** photograph of the pathologic specimen confirms a large open defect involving the entire lumbar spine. Absent left kidney and single umbilical artery were also identified.

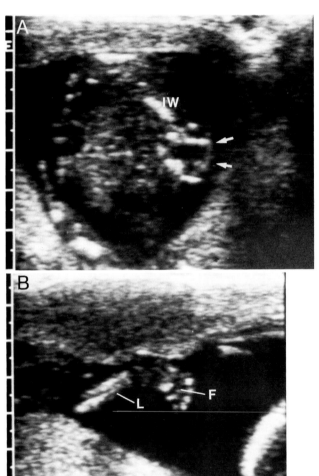

FIG 6–26.
Myelomeningocele and foot deformity. **A,** transverse scan of the lower lumbar spine demonstrates a dysraphic defect with a myelomeningocele sac *(arrows). IW* = iliac wing. **B,** examination of the lower extremities shows a clubfoot deformity. This was confirmed at the time of delivery. *F* = foot; *L* = leg.

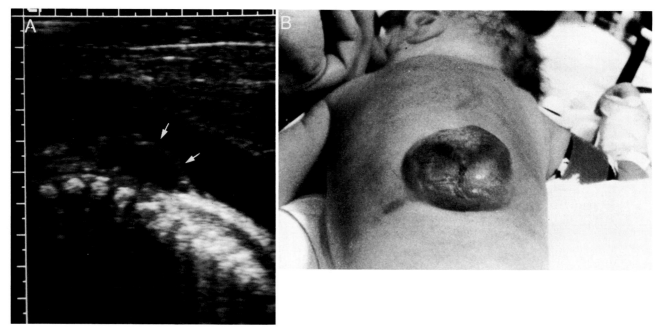

FIG 6–27.
Low thoracic myelomeningocele. **A,** longitudinal sonogram of the spine demonstrates a low thoracic myelomeningocele sac *(arrows).* **B,** postnatal photography shows the low thoracic myelomeningocele.

cation and extent of the spinal defect, although our own experience suggests sonographic estimates of the defect in utero show an excellent correlation with clinical and radiographic findings after birth.

Sonographic evaluation should also include a thorough examination for other central nervous system (CNS) anomalies and extra-CNS anomalies. Hydrocephalus has been reported in 90% of infants with the Arnold-Chiari malformation and 75% of fetuses with spina bifida seen before 24 weeks.[83, 85] If the karyotype is normal, the absence of ventricular dilatation may carry a favorable prognosis; however, this has not been specifically studied.

Identification of any extra-CNS anomaly suggests the presence of additional, undetected malformations and carries a poor prognosis.[84] In contrast, the absence of other detectable malformations is associated with a low mortality and a more favorable prognosis.

Cranial Findings Associated With Spina Bifida

False-negative diagnoses are most common before 24 weeks, when the spinal defect and myelomeningocele sac are typically small. Spinal defects can be missed even when examining women known to be at high risk for carrying a fetus with a neural tube defect. This is particularly likely when a myelomeningocele sac is absent or the spinal defect lies adjacent to the uterus or placenta. In these situations, various cranial and intracranial findings have proved to be extremely

useful for predicting the presence or absence of spina bifida. These findings can be attributed to the Arnold-Chiari malformation, which is present to some degree in nearly all cases of spina bifida. Three findings that have proved to be most useful and which are discussed in greater detail below are (Fig 6–29):

1. Ventricular dilatation.
2. The "lemon" sign.
3. Obliteration of the cisterna magna ("banana" sign).

In addition to these cranial and intracranial findings, fetuses with spina bifida examined before 24 weeks also tend to have a disproportionately small biparietal diameter compared to the menstrual age and other growth parameters (abdominal circumference and femur length), even when hydrocephalus is present.[91, 98] Because the fetal head is readily accessible to sonographic evaluation, these cranial findings may be much more apparent than the spinal defect itself, particularly during the second trimester when the spinal defect is typically small. It should be emphasized, however, that these cranial findings are indirect signs for spina bifida. If there is any question as to whether a spinal defect is present, amniocentesis should be considered for quantifying amniotic fluid AFP and acetylcholinesterase.[79]

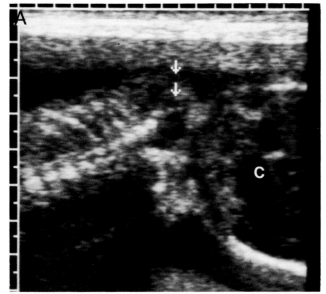

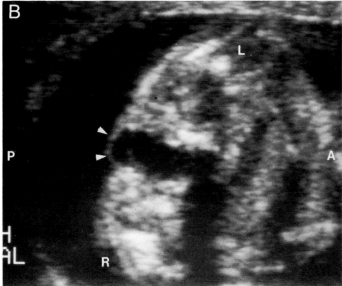

FIG 6–28.
High thoracic myelomeningocele. **A,** longitudinal sonogram of the thoracic spine demonstrates a small spinal defect *(arrows)* of the upper thoracic spine. *C* = cranium. **B,** transverse sonogram of the same patient better demonstrates the defect with protrusion of a small myelomeningocele sac *(arrowheads)*. *A* = anterior; *P* = posterior; *L* = left shoulder; *R* = right shoulder.

Ventricular Dilatation.—Identification of hydrocephalus (ventricular dilatation) is an effective means for identifying many fetuses at risk for spina bifida (Fig 6–30). Approximately one third of fetuses identified with hydrocephalus prove to have spina bifida, and 75% of fetuses with spina bifida demonstrate ventricular dilatation by 24 weeks.[83, 85] The degree of hydrocephalus is usually mild during the second trimester, seen only as incomplete filling of the ventricles by the choroid from side to side.[70] In one series of 61 fetuses identified with hydrocephalus, spina bifida was detected with an overall sensitivity of 86% with one false-positive diagnosis. During the last 3 years of this study, however, the sensitivity was 100% (13 of 13) with no false-positive diagnoses.[84]

The Lemon Sign.—The second cranial finding that has proved useful for predicting spina bifida is the "lemon" sign, so named for the cranial shape that is reminiscent of that of a lemon (Figs 6–31 and 6–33).[74, 75, 83, 85, 88] This sign was first described as such by Nicolaides et al. in 1986,[83] although its significance also was recognized a year earlier by Furness et al.[74] The lemon sign occurs at a time when the spinal defect is usually small and difficult to visualize. Resolution of the lemon sign invariably occurs by 34 weeks.[85] It is also worthwhile to note that the lemon sign is not identified in fetuses with hydrocephalus alone who lack spina bifida.[85, 87]

Presumably the lemon sign is related to the Arnold-Chiari malformation, which is present to some de-

FIG 6–29.
Cranial findings associated with spina bifida. *(1.)* Ventricular dilatation (levels A and B) is present in 75% of fetuses with spina bifida before 24 weeks. *(2.)* Frontal calvarial deformity (lemon sign) is best seen at the ventricular level *(level A)*. A mild lemon sign is also usually identified at the thalamic level *(level B)*. *(3.)* Obliteration of the cisterna magna is seen in the transcerebellar view *(level C)*. The cerebellar hemispheres may be seen wrapping around the posterior aspect of the midbrain (banana sign). *FH* = frontal horn; *Th* = thalamus; *MB* = midbrain.

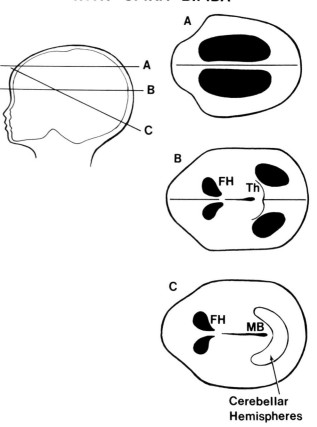

CRANIAL FINDINGS ASSOCIATED WITH SPINA BIFIDA

Cerebellar Hemispheres

gree in nearly all patients with spina bifida. It is speculated that low intraspinal pressure, which has been observed in the majority of neonates with spina bifida,[100] is somehow translated to the relatively malleable fetal cranium, and the frontal calvarium may be more susceptible to this effect than other parts of the cranium.[85, 87] With increasing maturation, a stronger calvarium may be able to resist this pressure better, explaining resolution of the lemon sign with advancing menstrual age.[85]

The lemon sign has proved to be an extremely sensitive sign for predicting spina bifida before the time of fetal viability.[83, 85, 88] In the retrospective study by Nicolaides et al., a lemon sign was demonstrated in all 54 fetuses with spina bifida examined before 24 weeks.[83] In two prospective studies of the lemon sign in high-risk patients Campbell et al. reported that the lemon sign was present in all 26 fetuses with spina bifida,[68] and Nyberg et al. reported its presence in 13 of 14 fetuses with spina bifida before 24 weeks.[68, 85] Hence, absence of a lemon sign in association with spina bifida before 24 weeks is rare (Fig 6–32).

The lemon sign is seen as a concave deformity of the cranium at approximately the level of the coronal

suture. The temporal area also tends to be the widest portion of the cranium.[85] We distinguish this appearance from a mild (intermediate) form of the lemon sign that appears as a flattened or only slightly concave shape of the cranium. By contrast, a normal cranium is convex in all portions. Our experience suggests that the lemon sign finding is optimally demonstrated on axial scans at the level of the lateral ventricles (see Fig 6–30).

While the lemon sign is sensitive for predicting the presence of spina bifida before 24 weeks, it is not specific in and of itself, since a similar finding may be found in 1% of normal patients (Fig 6–33).[68, 85] A cloverleaf skull also can potentially simulate a lemon sign, but this finding is best seen at the base of the cranium, whereas a lemon sign is best seen at the ventricular level.

If there is any question as to the significance of a lemon sign when the fetal spine appears normal, other cranial findings that are associated with spina bifida (ventricular dilatation and obliteration of the cisterna magna) also should be evaluated. A normal-appearing cisterna magna is reassuring, even when a lemon sign is

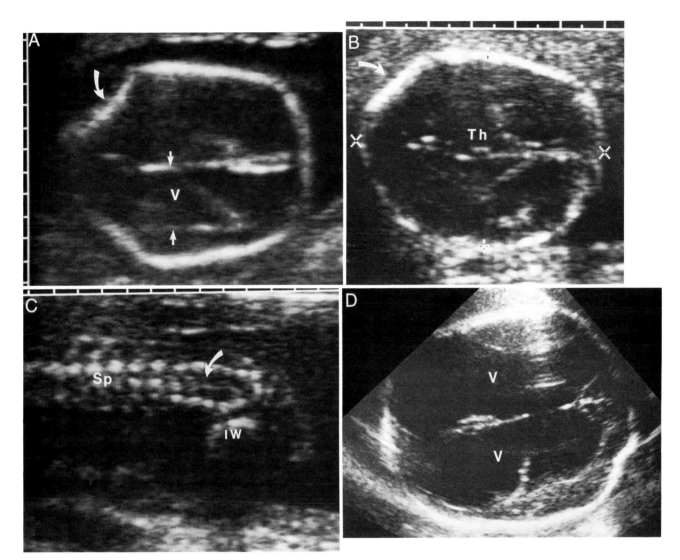

FIG 6–30.
Lemon sign. **A,** transverse cranial sonogram at 19 menstrual weeks in a woman referred to sonography because of an elevated MS-AFP level, shows a lemon-shaped frontal calvarium *(curved arrows)*. Also note moderate dilatation *(straight arrows)* of the ventricles *(V)*. **B,** scan at the level of the thalami *(Th)* shows only a mild lemon sign *(curved arrow)*, indicating that this sign is best elicited at the ventricular level. **C,** longitudinal sonogram of the spine *(Sp)* demonstrates a small dysraphic defect in the lower lumbar area *(curved arrow). IW* = iliac wing. **D,** repeat sonogram at 35 weeks, after a decision to continue the pregnancy, shows progressive dilatation of the ventricles *(V)* and resolution of the lemon sign. The infant was delivered by cesarean section at 38 weeks. (Parts **A,B,** and **C** from Nyberg DA, Mack LA, Hirsch J, et al: Abnormalities of fetal cranial contour in sonographic detection of spina bifida: Evaluation of the "lemon" sign. Radiology, 1988; 167:387–392. Used by permission.)

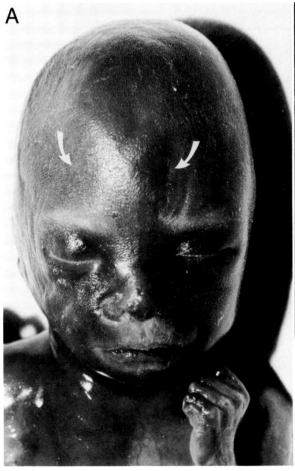

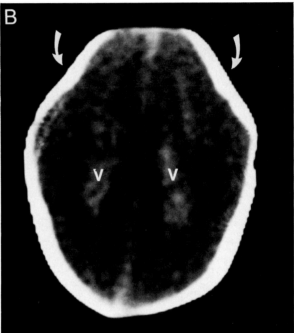

FIG 6-31.
Lemon sign. **A,** frontal photograph of 18-week fetus with a lemon sign and spina bifida identified on sonography shows mild scalloping of the frontal calvarium *(curved arrows)*, which is also readily palpable. **B,** postmortem CT shows deformity of the frontal calvarium *(curved arrows)*. *V* = ventricles.

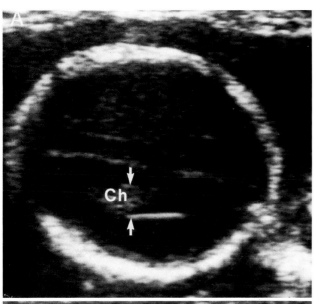

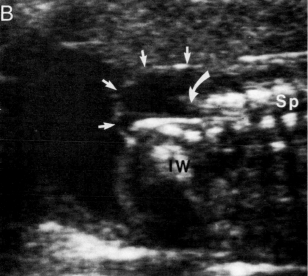

FIG 6–32.
False-negative lemon sign. **A,** transverse cranial sonogram at 20 weeks, performed because of an elevated MS-AFP level, demonstrates a normal cranial configuration. Also note normal ventricular size without ventricular dilatation, shown as choroid *(Ch)* touching the ventricular walls *(arrows).* **B,** longitudinal sonogram shows a dysraphic defect in the lower lumbar spine *(curved arrow),* covered with a membrane *(small arrows). Sp* = spine, *IW* = iliac wing. A false-negative lemon sign before 24 weeks is very unusual. (From Nyberg DA, Mack LA, Hirsch J, et al: Abnormalities of fetal cranial contour in sonographic detection of spina bifida: Evaluation of the 'lemon' sign. Radiology 1988:167; 387–392. Used by permission.)

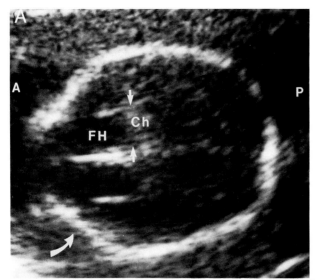

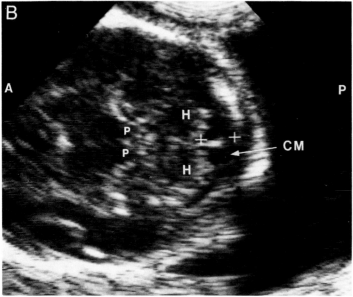

FIG 6–33.
False-positive lemon sign. **A,** transverse cranial sonogram at 18 weeks in an obese patient referred because of elevated MS-AFP, demonstrates a frontal contour deformity *(curved arrow)* but no ventricular dilatation. Note that the choroid *(Ch)* fills the ventricle from side to side *(arrows)*. FH = frontal horn; A = anterior; P = posterior. **B,** angled scan through the posterior fossa demonstrates a normal cisterna magna *(CM)* posterior to the cerebellar hemispheres *(H)*, a finding that virtually eliminates the possibility of spina bifida associated with the Arnold-Chiari malformation. P = cerebral peduncles; A = anterior; P = posterior.

thought to be present. On the other hand, a lemon sign in conjunction with ventricular dilatation and/or obliteration of the cisterna magna should be viewed as highly suspicious for spina bifida, regardless of the spinal findings (see Fig 6–30).[65, 83, 85, 90]

Obliteration of the Cisterna Magna ("Banana" Sign).—Since the cisterna magna should be readily visualized in virtually all normal fetuses during the second and early third trimester (Fig 6–34), failure to visualize it suggests compression of the posterior fossa as part of the Arnold-Chiari malformation (Fig 6–35).[65, 75a, 90] Conversely, demonstration of a normal cisterna magna is reassuring in high-risk pregnancies and nearly eliminates the possibility of the Arnold-Chiari malformation. The "banana" sign, initially de-

scribed by Nicolaides et al., is a corollary observation that describes the shape of the cerebellar hemispheres as they wrap around the posterior midbrain from posterior fossa compression (see Fig 6–35).[83] However, we and others have found that obliteration of the cisterna magna is easier to elicit than the banana-shaped cerebellum.[65, 75a, 90]

Pilu et al. observed obliteration of the cisterna magna in a prospective study of 19 fetuses with spina bifida.[90] Compared to normal measurements (Table 6–4), these authors also noted that the transverse cerebellar diameter was decreased in all 12 cases in which the cerebellar hemispheres could be visualized. Similarly, Benacerraf et al. noted obliteration of the cisterna magna in 22 of 23 fetuses with spina bifida between 16 and 27 weeks,[65] and Goldstein et al. observed efface-

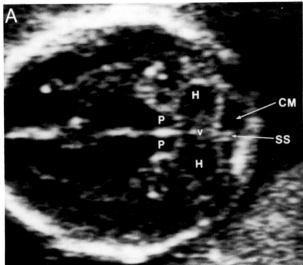

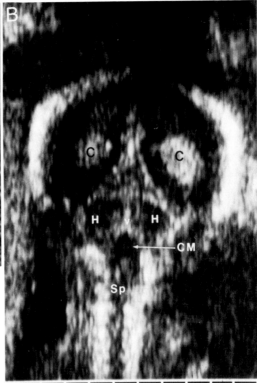

FIG 6–34.
Normal cerebellum. **A,** axial view angled through the posterior fossa (transcerebellar view) at 19 weeks shows normal cisterna magna *(CM)*, cerebellar hemispheres *(H)*, and vermis *(v)*. *P* = cerebral peduncles; *SS* = straight sinus. **B,** coronal scan shows the normal cisterna magna *(CM)*, cerebral hemispheres *(H)*, and choroid *(C)* in the atria of the lateral ventricles. *Sp* = spine.

ment of the cisterna magna in 18 of 20 fetuses with myelomeningocele before 24 weeks.[75a] These two series report a total of three fetuses with spina bifida and a normal cisterna magna, but each fetus had a skin-covered meningocele or lipomeningocele.

Associated Anomalies

Anomalies associated with spina bifida may be categorized as (1) neuromuscular deformities resulting from the spinal defect itself, (2) additional CNS anomalies, and (3) extra-CNS anomalies.

Neuromuscular anomalies caused by the spinal defect include foot deformities (see Fig 6–26), primarily clubfoot, and dislocation of the hip. These are a result of unopposed function of muscle groups because of a defect of the peripheral nerve corresponding to the involved myotomes.[96] Sonographic demonstration of absent leg movements or a fixed leg deformity may carry a worse prognosis than normal leg movement, although this is somewhat controversial and deserves further investigation.

CNS malformations that can be associated with spina bifida, other than hydrocephalus, include holoprosencephaly, agenesis of the corpus callosum, and, rarely, the Dandy-Walker syndrome. Also, tethered cord, split cord (diastematomyelia), intraspinal lipoma, and dermoid cysts are commonly associated with myelomeningocele.[41, 76]

Various non–CNS anomalies may be associated with spina bifida. In one prenatal series, 50% (10 of 20) fetuses identified with meningomyelocele had extra-CNS anomalies that involved a wide range of organs (face, kidneys, gastrointestinal tract, thorax, and extremities).[84]

Chromosome analysis should be considered, particularly if the parents are contemplating continuing the pregnancy. In a detailed analysis of 107 fetuses with CNS anomalies, Nyberg et al. reported chromosomal abnormalities in 8% (3 of 38) of fetuses with hydrocephalus and spina bifida, and 33% (3 of 9) of fetuses with spina bifida alone (see Chapter 17).[86] Considering only fetuses who underwent chromosomal analysis, these figures are 15% and 50%, respectively. The coexistence of a single umbilical artery and spina bifida was also associated with a higher frequency of both chromosomal abnormalities and extra-CNS malformations.[86]

Prognosis

In considering the prognosis for fetuses or infants diagnosed with spina bifida, the eventual outcome can be considered in four major categories (1) mortality rate, (2) physical disability, (3) intellectual disability, and (4) hindbrain dysfunction. Prognostic factors that may influence the outcome are listed in Table 6–5.

In general, the mortality rate depends on the pres-

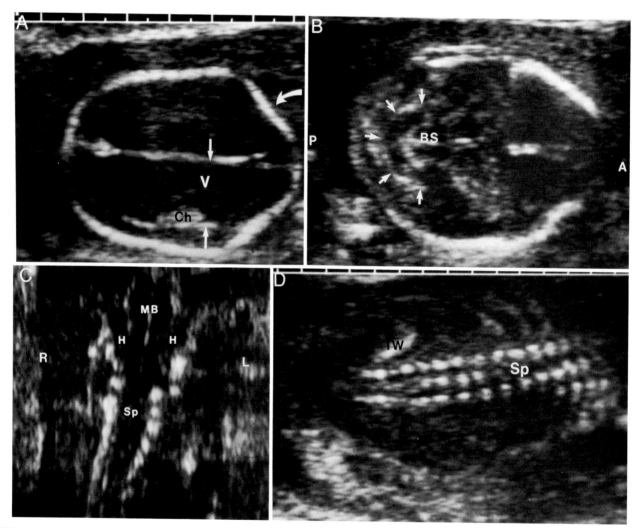

FIG 6–35.
Obliteration of cisterna magna (banana sign). **A,** transverse cranial sonogram at 20 weeks, obtained because of elevated MS-AFP level, shows a lemon sign *(curved arrow)* and marked dilatation *(straight arrows)* of the ventricles *(V)*. *Ch* = choroid. **B,** transcerebellar scan angled through the posterior fossa shows obliteration of the cisterna magna and the cerebellar hemispheres *(straight arrows)* wrapped around the brain stem (banana sign). *BS* = brain stem; *A* = anterior; *P* = posterior. **C,** coronal scan shows downward herniation of the midbrain *(MB)* and cerebellar hemispheres *(H)* into the upper cervical spine *(Sp)* which appears mildly expanded. The cisterna magna is not visualized. *R* = right; *L* = left. **D,** prolonged scanning of the fetal spine *(Sp)*, prompted by the cranial findings, failed to demonstrate a definite dysraphic defect. A small sacral defect was found on postmortem examination. *IW* = iliac wing. (Parts **A, B,** and **D** reproduced from Nyberg DA, Mack LA, Hirsch J, et al: Abnormalities of fetal cranial contour in sonographic detection of spina bifida: Evaluation of the 'lemon' sign. Radiology 1988; 167:387–392. Used by permission.)

TABLE 6–4.

Relationship Between Cerebellar and Biparietal Diameter*†

Cerebellar Diameter (mm)	Biparietal Diameter (mm)	+SE	−SE
15	34.7	38.0	31.5
16	37.2	40.6	34.0
17	39.8	43.2	36.4
18	42.2	45.7	38.8
19	44.6	48.1	41.1
20	46.9	50.5	43.4
21	49.2	52.8	45.6
22	51.4	55.0	47.8
23	53.5	57.2	49.9
24	55.6	59.3	51.9
25	57.6	61.3	53.9
26	59.6	63.3	55.8
27	61.5	65.2	57.7
28	63.3	67.1	59.5
29	65.1	68.8	61.3
30	66.8	70.6	63.0
31	68.4	72.2	64.7
32	70.0	73.8	66.3
33	71.6	75.3	67.8
34	73.0	76.8	69.3
35	74.4	78.2	70.7
36	75.8	79.5	72.1
37	77.1	80.8	73.4
38	78.3	82.0	74.7
39	79.5	83.1	75.9
40	80.6	84.2	77.0
41	81.7	85.2	78.1
42	82.6	86.2	79.1
43	83.6	87.1	80.1
44	84.4	87.9	81.0
45	85.3	88.6	81.9
46	86.0	89.3	82.7
47	86.7	89.9	83.5
48	87.3	90.5	84.2
49	87.9	91.0	84.8
50	88.4	91.4	85.4
51	88.8	91.8	85.9
52	89.2	92.1	86.4
53	89.6	92.3	86.8
54	89.8	92.5	87.2

*From Pilu G, Romero R, Reece A, et al: Subnormal cerebellum in fetuses with spina bifida. Am J Obstet Gynecol 1988; 158:1052–1056. Used by permission.
†SE = standard error.

TABLE 6–5.

Prognostic Factors Associated With Spina Bifida

Associated anomalies
Location and size of spinal defect
Open vs. closed spinal defect
Hydrocephalus
Clubfeet (possibly associated)

id.[80] Using modern surgical and shunt management in a recent series of over 800 patients with myelomeningocele, 2% of newborns died during the initial hospitalization and 15% died by age 10 years.[82] Among survivors, multiple ventricular shunt revisions often complicate recovery.

The physical and intellectual disabilities of infants with spina bifida vary considerably.[62] In an unselected series of infants treated with myelomeningocele in the 1960s, 60% had an intelligence quotient (IQ) over 80.[80] A more recent series of over 800 patients treated with myelomeningocele suggests that 73% of survivors have an IQ greater than 80 and 27% will have an IQ greater than 100.[82] However, up to 50% of patients suffer from other learning disabilities.

Three factors contributing to the eventual outcome are (1) the location and extent of the spinal defect, (2) open vs. closed defect, and (3) the presence or absence of hydrocephalus (Table 6–6).[65, 80] The most caudal and smallest defects are associated with the best prognosis and are least likely to be associated with hydrocephalus.[63, 80, 81] Mapstone et al. found that the mean IQ was 104 for infants who never required shunting (no hydrocephalus), compared to an IQ of 91 for those who were shunted without complication, and an IQ of 70 for those who were shunted with subsequent complication.[81]

Motor deficits are worse for proximal and/or open spinal defects compared to distal and closed defects. Normal ambulation can be expected for only 23% of open defects compared to 70% of closed defects.[62] Although the level of motor paralysis is relatively fixed at birth, the majority of children are able to walk with the help of crutches and braces. Bladder and bowel incontinence are common (83%) and also related to the site of the defect.[63, 80]

Hindbrain dysfunction is another serious complication of treated myelomeningocele.[88] Thirty-two percent of patients will exhibit serious symptoms of hindbrain dysfunction that include pain at the base of the skull and neck, nystagmus, weakness in the upper extremities, hypotonia, and spasticity.[82] Up to one third of patients with hindbrain dysfunction will die from this complication, usually as a result of respiratory fail-

ence of concurrent anomalies. Prior to 1950, the majority of live born patients with spina bifida died of infection. Early surgical correction of myelomeningocele decreased the mortality rate, yet the outcome remained poor because of handicaps related to hydrocephalus.[78] In 1952, patient survival was markedly improved with introduction of the one-way shunt valve that allowed controlled drainage of cerebrospinal flu-

TABLE 6–6.

Results of Aggressive Treatment of 171 Consecutive Infants With Myelomeningocele—1963 to 1968*

Level of Lesion	Percent With This Level of Lesion	Mortality (%)	IQ > 80 (%)	Hydrocephalus (%)	Ambulatory (%)	Ambulatory Without Appliances (%)
Thoracolumbar	37	35	44	91	71	0
Lumbosacral	59	11	65	62	81	16
Sacral	4	0	100	16	100	83

*From Ames MD, Schut L: Pediatrics 1972; 50:466–470.

ure, and death may be sudden.[82, 88] Symptomatic patients require surgical decompression of the brain stem. In a series of 45 symptomatic infants with hindbrain dysfunction who required laminectomy, the mortality rate was 38% after 6 years of follow-up.[88]

Management

When spina bifida is detected before fetal viability, termination of pregnancy may be elected.[69] A decision to continue the pregnancy is more likely when sonographic findings are considered favorable and no extra-CNS malformations are identified. Chromosomal analysis is considered particularly important if a decision to continue the pregnancy is made. If the pregnancy is continued, serial sonograms are performed to evaluate fetal growth and to monitor ventricular dilatation.

After the age of fetal viability, management options usually are limited to chromosomal analysis and determination of the place, time, and mode of delivery.[69] Some authorities recommend elective delivery by cesarean section to decrease the risk of contaminating or rupturing the meningomyelocele sac, although the potential benefit of this approach is controversial.[66] Elective delivery also permits the pediatricians and pediatric surgeons to prepare for subsequent management. In utero shunting of hydrocephalus is not currently performed at most centers.

Surgical closure of the meningomyelocele is performed by a pediatric neurosurgeon within hours after delivery. Ventricular shunting for infants with progressive hydrocephalus has been shown to improve the subsequent mortality significantly.[78] Severely handicapped infants require multiple surgical corrections for orthopedic deformities, extensive motor training and supervision, provisions for bladder and bowel incontinence, and, occasionally, gastroplasty for gastroesophageal reflux.

Sacrococcygeal Teratoma

Clinical and Pathologic Findings

Sacrococcygeal teratoma is a tumor arising from pleuripotential embryonic cells of the coccyx.[102, 104, 127]

Although rare, with a reported incidence of 1 in 35,000 births, sacrococcygeal teratoma is reportedly the most common tumor encountered among neonates. Females are affected four times more often than males. An association has also been noted between sacrococcygeal teratoma and twinning and other spinal defects, including NTDs. The majority of tumors occur sporadically, but a familial type has also been reported, possibly with autosomal dominant transmission.[103, 118]

Sacrococcygeal teratomas originate from an area of the primitive streak called the primitive knot or Hensen's node. The primitive streak appears as linear thickening in the ectoderm at the caudal edge of the bilaminar embryonic disc. As the mesoderm rapidly proliferates, the primitive streak comes to lie more and more caudally, until it is folded somewhat ventrally by the tail bud. The remnant of Hensen's node descends to the tip of the coccyx or its anterior surface.[107]

Pathologically, three histologic grades have been described: benign, immature, and malignant. Benign tumors are usually derived from all three germ layers. Neuroglia is the most common tissue, but respiratory, gastrointestinal, pancreatic, bronchial, and muscle tissue also can be found. Occasionally, well-formed structures such as teeth, bones, and digits may be present.[112] The presence of functioning choroid plexus, which produces cerebrospinal fluid, is thought to be responsible for cystic components of the tumor.[109] Mature and immature histologic types, which together account for 87% to 93% of sacrococcygeal teratomas, can be surgically resected with an expectation of complete cure.

Malignant tumors comprise 7% to 13% of sacrococcygeal teratoma in most postnatal series.[128] However, the specific risk is related to the age at diagnosis, with malignant elements found in 2% of patients diagnosed in the neonatal period, 10% of patients diagnosed at 2 months of age, and up to 60% of patients identified at 4 months of age. This data suggests that the prenatal diagnosis of sacrococcygeal teratoma carries a very low risk of malignancy and, in fact, the current prenatal literature supports this notion. Malignant tumors are invariably endodermal sinus or yolk sac tumors, both of which produce AFP.

TYPE I

TYPE II

TYPE III

TYPE IV

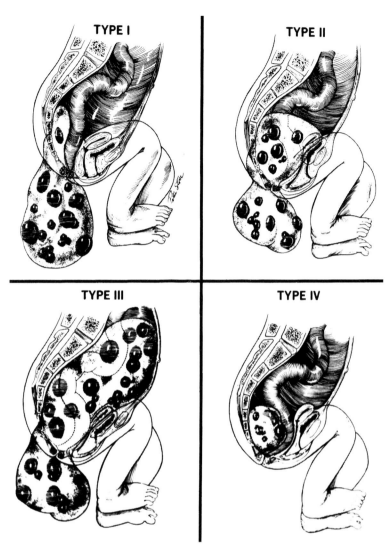

FIG 6–36.
Classification of sacrococcygeal teratoma. Type I is predominantly exterior, with only a minimal presacral component; type II is predominantly external, but with a significant intrapelvic component; type III is predominantly internal, with intra-abdominal extension; type IV is entirely internal, with no external component. (From Altman RP, Randolph JG, Lilly JR: Sacrococcygeal teratoma: American Academy of Pediatrics Surgical Section Survey—1973, vol 9. Philadelphia, Grune & Stratton, 1974, pp 389–398. Used by permission.)

The size and extension of tumor is even more important than the histology in prenatal studies. From a review of 405 cases compiled by the American Academy of Pediatrics Surgical Section, Altman classified sacrococcygeal teratomas into four types (Fig 6–36), based on their external and internal extent: type I is predominantly exterior, with only a minimal presacral component; type II is predominantly external, but with a significant intrapelvic component; type III is predominantly internal, with intra-abdominal extension; and type IV is entirely internal, with no external component.[102]

Sonographic Findings

Sacrococcygeal teratoma has been detected frequently on prenatal sonography (Table 6–7).* The majority of cases are referred to sonography because of increased uterine size, premature labor, or, in recent

*References 101, 105, 110, 111, 113, 117, 119, 121, 124–126, 129, 130

years, because of elevated MS-AFP levels. The majority of sacrococcygeal teratomas are solid or mixed cystic and solid (Figs 6–37 and 6–38); only 15% are entirely cystic (Figs 6–39 and 6–40). Radiologic evidence of calcification is present in 36% of cases.[109, 123] There is no correlation between the sonographic appearance and the histology of the tumor.

Sacrococcygeal teratoma always arises from the coccyx. In most cases, the predominant component of the mass is external to the pelvis. Demonstration of a large pelvic or intra-abdominal component makes surgical resection considerably more difficult (see Fig 6–40). Seth et al. reported sonographic visualization of a pelvic or intra-abdominal component in 6 of 15 cases.[125] An important secondary finding is anterior displacement of the urinary bladder by the mass (see Fig 6–37). The mass may also obstruct the ureters, resulting in hydronephrosis or echogenic kidneys (see Fig 6–37).

The differential diagnosis of sacrococcygeal ter-

TABLE 6–7.

Selected Literature Review of Sacrococcygeal Teratoma*

Author	No. Cases	Menstrual Age (wk)	Hydrops	Polyhydramnios	Spontaneous Mortality Rate
Holzgreve et al.[116] (1985)	6	19–33	0	6	50% (2/4)
Chervenak et al.[105] (1985)	3	28–34	0	2	33% (1/3)
Flake et al.[110] (1986)	21	16–34	9	15	28% (5/18)
Gross et al.[113] (1987)	6	19–30	0	3	0 (0/4)
Hogge et al.[115] (1987)	2	33–38	0	1†	0 (0/2)
Teal et al.[126] (1988)	3	23–32	0	1	33% (1/3)
Sheth et al.[125] (1988)	15	19–36	4	10	46% (6/13)
Total	56		13 (23%)	38 (68%)	(32%) 15/47

*Excluding 6 cases reported previously by Holzgreve et al.
†Spontaneous rupture of membranes in the second patient.

atoma depends on whether the mass is predominantly solid or cystic. A diagnosis of sacrococcygeal teratoma is assured when the mass is solid or complex in appearance and appears to arise from the coccyx. Other masses that can be found in the sacrococcygeal area include chordoma, neurogenic tumor, lipoma, rhabdomyosarcoma, hemangioma, and malignant melanoma (Fig 6–41). Bowel perforation with extension of a meconium pseudocyst to the buttock recently has been mistaken for sacrococcygeal teratoma.[120]

If the mass is predominantly or entirely cystic (see Figs 6–39 and 6–40), then a myelomeningocele must be considered and specifically excluded. Myelomeningocele is typically cystic, with internal neural elements, and always associated with a spinal dysraphic defect. By contrast, the posterior spinal elements are intact with sacrococcygeal teratoma. However, other vertebral anomalies occasionally are found with sacrococcygeal teratoma, and one of the cases reported by Seth et al. showed a widening of the lumbosacral canal from intraspinal extension.[125] If the cystic mass is entirely intra-abdominal in location (see Fig 6–39), the differential diagnosis includes an ovarian cyst, meconium pseudocyst, enteric duplication cyst, or other bowel-related abnormality.[115]

Polyhydramnios (see Fig 6–37) has been reported in 70% of prenatally diagnosed sacrococcygeal teratoma and in most cases seen after 22 weeks (Table 6–6). Polyhydramnios may develop from (1) arteriovenous shunting through the tumor, (2) high output failure from chronic anemia caused by tumor hemorrhage, or (3) transudation of fluid from the tumor mass.

Hydrops has been associated with 25% of sacrococcygeal teratoma reported prenatally (see Table 6–6), presumably on the same basis. Placentomegaly may be an early manifestation of hydrops.[106] Ten of the 15 fetuses with placentomegaly reviewed by Flake et al. also demonstrated evidence of hydrops.[110]

Development of polyhydramnios and hydrops appears to be directly related to the vascularity of the tumor; only two sacrococcygeal teratomas reported by Seth et al. demonstrated normal amniotic fluid (at 28 and 30 weeks), and both were cystic tumors with little vascularity.[125] Alter et al. propose use of Doppler ultrasound to assess vascularity of the tumor (see Fig 6–38).[101]

Oligohydramnios occasionally can occur in association with sacrococcygeal teratoma, and this also appears to be an unfavorable finding. Seth et al. observed oligohydramnios in three of 15 fetuses with hydronephrosis or renal dysplasia, presumably related to obstruction of the ureters and/or urethra by the tumor mass.[125] All three fetuses died and showed stigmata of Potter's syndrome.

Associated Anomalies

Associated anomalies, excluding hydrops, are found in approximately 18% of newborns with sacrococcygeal teratoma, most commonly involving the musculoskeletal system.[102, 109] Less frequent anomalies include renal, cardiovascular, gastrointestinal, and central nervous system anomalies. Familial sacrococcygeal teratoma is associated with anorectal stenosis and vesicoureteral reflux.[103, 118]

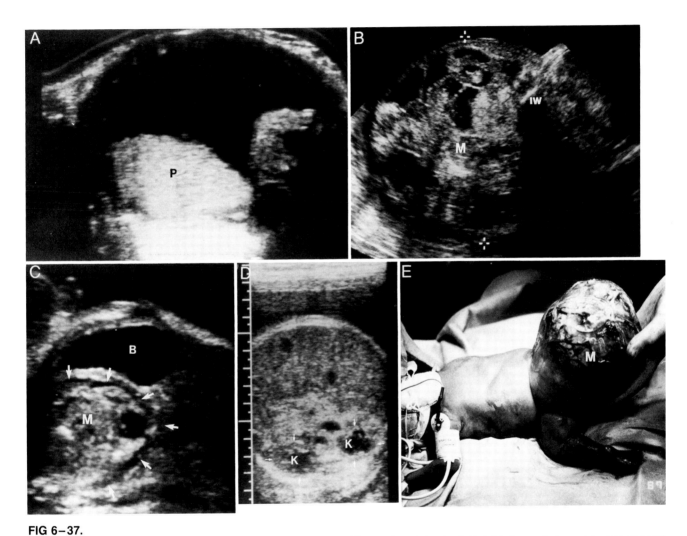

FIG 6–37.
Sacrococcygeal teratoma. **A,** scan at 34 weeks, performed because of increasing uterine fundal height, demonstrates polyhydramnios and mildly thickened placenta *(P)* (2 cm markers on left). **B,** a large 15 mass *(M)* is identified arising from the fetal buttock. The mass is predominantly solid, but contains some cystic elements. *IW* = iliac wing. **C,** longitudinal sonogram of the pelvis demonstrates intrapelvic extension *(arrows)* of the mass *(M)*. Note that the urinary bladder *(B)* is displaced anteriorly. **D,** transverse scan through the kidneys (*K,* small arrows) shows mild bilateral pelvocaliectasis. The renal cortex was also mildly echogenic relative to normal, and the retroperitoneum appears echogenic consistent with edema. **E,** photograph after cesarean delivery shows large external extent of the mass *(M)*. A large internal component was also resected at surgery. The vascular nature of the mass is shown by multiple large vessels on its surface.

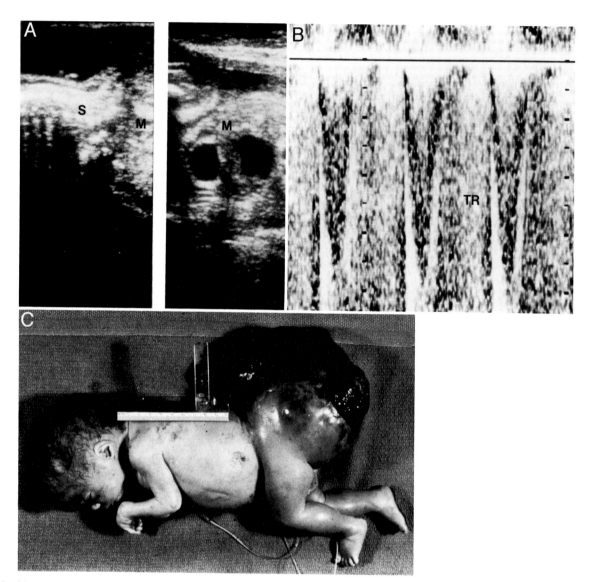

FIG 6–38.
Sacrococcygeal teratoma shown with Doppler. **A,** longitudinal view of the spine *(S)* shows a large heterogeneous mass *(M)* arising from its distal end. **B,** Doppler tracing of the tricuspid valve shows tricuspid regurgitation *(TR)* and elevated peak systolic flow (74 cm/sec) consistent with high-output cardiac failure. **C,** photograph of the pathologic specimen, following spontaneous death from fetal hydrops, shows a huge vascular tumor. (From Alter DN, Reed K, Marx GR, et al: Prenatal diagnosis of congestive heart failure in a fetus with a sacrococcygeal teratoma. Obstet Gynecol 1988; 71:978–981. Used by permission.)

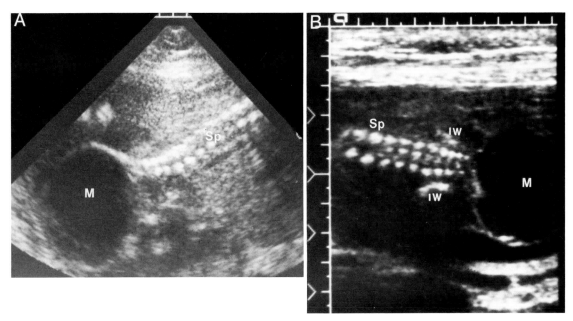

FIG 6–39.
Cystic sacrococcygeal teratoma. **A,** longitudinal sonogram of the spine *(S)* at 30 weeks shows a cystic mass *(M)* arising from the region of the coccyx. **B,** coronal view shows the distal location of the mass *(M)* and intact spine *(Sp)*. The mass was aspirated prior to delivery. *IW* = iliac wing.

Prognosis

Excluding malignant tumors, pediatric series suggest that the prognosis of sacrococcygeal teratomas is related primarily to the extension and size of the tumor. Intra-abdominal extension increases the risk of malignancy, because the diagnosis may be delayed and because surgical resection may be incomplete.[102] Since over 80% of sacrococcygeal teratomas are predominantly external (type I or II) in location, 85% to 96% of infants with sacrococcygeal teratoma come to clinical attention between birth and 1 month of age.[102] Familial sacrococcygeal teratoma has a favorable prognosis, with malignancy rarely reported.[103, 118]

Prenatal studies have reported a higher overall mortality rate (32%) than neonatal studies, with the most common causes of death related to complications of prematurity (induced by polyhydramnios), hemorrhage into the tumor, and hydrops. Hydrops and/or ascites is a particularly unfavorable finding. Only one fetus with hydrops has survived, and hydrops did not develop in this case until the third trimester, between the time of diagnosis at 32 weeks and the time of delivery at 35 weeks.[110] Flake et al. concluded that a poor prognosis was associated with symptomatic presentation prior to 30 weeks and development of hydrops and placentomegaly.[110]

There is evidence to suggest that purely cystic sacrococcygeal teratomas carry a better prognosis than solid tumors, because they are less vascular and less likely to result in hydrops. All four cystic sacrococcygeal teratomas reported by Hogge et al. (n=2) and Seth et al. (n=2) survived, and none of these demonstrated evidence of hydrops.[115, 125]

Management

Elective termination may be considered when sacrococcygeal teratoma is detected before fetal viability. Demonstration of hydrops, oligohydramnios, or renal anomalies may influence the decision to terminate the pregnancy. Serial sonograms are suggested for detection of hydrops or placentomegaly. Because of the risk of dystocia and traumatic hemorrhage to the tumor[122], cesarean delivery has been recommended for tumors larger than 5 cm.[113] When the mass is predominantly cystic, in utero aspiration of the mass has been accomplished.[121] Complete excision of the tumor is planned in the neonatal period, including resection of the coccyx; incomplete resection predisposes to malignant degeneration. Patients should be followed with clinical evaluation and AFP levels for possible recurrence.

Sacral Agenesis, Caudal Regression Syndrome

Pathologic and Clinical Findings

Sacral agenesis and the caudal regression syndrome are closely related spinal disorders. Sacral agenesis is characterized by absence of the sacrum and coccyx, whereas the vertebral abnormalities of the caudal re-

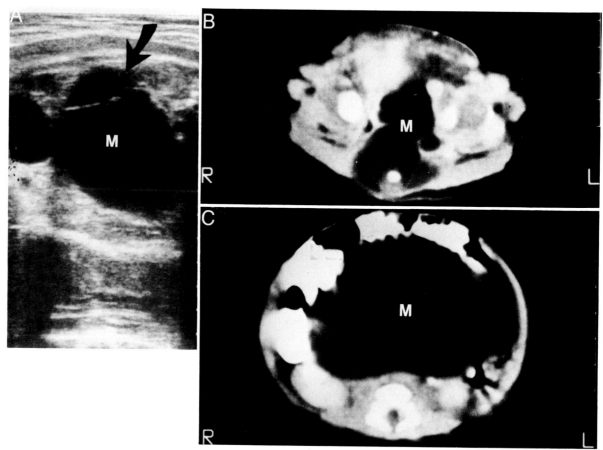

FIG 6–40.
Intra-abdominal cystic sacrococcygeal teratoma. **A,** longitudinal sonogram of the abdomen demonstrates a large 7 cm cystic mass *(M)* in the lower abdomen, superior to the urinary bladder *(B).* Internal septations are identified within the mass. **B,** postnatal computerized tomographic scan shows the cystic mass *(M)* within the pelvis with a small soft tissue area in the region of the coccyx. **C,** the mass *(M)* extends to the upper abdomen. This unusual case proved to be a cystic sacrococcygeal teratoma located entirely within the abdomen (type IV). The differential diagnosis for this appearance on prenatal sonography includes ovarian cyst or bowel-related abnormality. (From Hogge WA, Thiagarajah S, Barber VG, et al: Cystic sacrococcygeal teratoma: Ultrasound diagnosis and perinatal management. J Ultrasound Med 1987; 6:707–710.

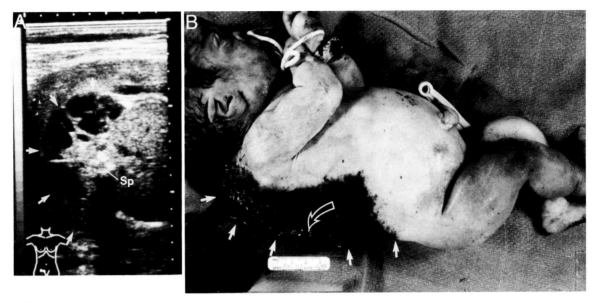

FIG 6–41.
Malignant melanoma. **A,** transverse scan of the thoracic spine *(Sp)* at 30 weeks' gestation shows a large solid mass *(arrows)* with both cystic and solid elements arising from the back. **B,** postmortem photograph shows large pigmented mass *(arrows)* arising from back. The curved arrow points to cystic hemorrhage. Metastases were also found in the spinal cord, lung, liver, and placenta. (Part **A** courtesy of Winston A Campbell, MD, Department of Obstetrics and Gynecology, University of Connecticut, Farmington, CT. Part **B** from Obstet/Gynecol 1987; 70:434–439. Used by permission).

gression syndrome vary from partial sacral agenesis to complete absence of the lumbosacral spine.[134, 140, 145] Sirenomelia (mermaid syndrome) is the most severe form of the caudal regression syndrome in which there is fusion of the lower extremities that may or may not include variable fusion of the femurs and absence of long bones. Sonography may be the only reliable method for diagnosing these disorders prenatally, since the spinal canal is closed and chromosomes are usually normal.

Wide overlap between the caudal regression syndrome and the vertebral, anal, cardiovascular, tracheoesophageal, renal, and limb (VACTERL) syndrome has been noted.[137, 151] Characteristic features of the caudal regression syndrome, in addition to the spinal deformity, include hypoplasia of the lower extremities and a wide range of associated anomalies involving the genitourinary, gastrointestinal, cardiovascular, and central nervous systems.

Maternal diabetes mellitus strongly correlates with both sacral agenesis and the caudal regression syndrome.[131, 133, 141–143] The caudal regression syndrome occurs 250 times more frequently in infants of diabetic mothers, compared with other infants,[142] and it has been estimated that 12%–16% of infants with sacral agenesis are born to mothers with diabetes mellitus.[143] Conversely, 1% of infants born to diabetic mothers have sacral agenesis. Significantly fewer anomalies are reported among diabetics in good control, suggesting

that hyperglycemia or a related metabolite is the major inciting agent.[141]

Sonographic Findings

Demonstration of markedly hypoplastic lower extremities in combination with sacral or lumbosacral agenesis is diagnostic of the caudal regression syndrome (Fig 6–42). Concurrent malformations usually dominate the sonographic appearance of the caudal regression syndrome.[136, 138] For example, Loewy reported three fetuses with the caudal regression syndrome during the second trimester: one fetus demonstrated hydrocephalus, clubfoot, and absence of the sacrum at 19 weeks; another demonstrated duodenal atresia, unilateral renal agenesis with contralateral renal dysplasia and suspected sacral agenesis at 26 weeks; and the third demonstrated unilateral renal agenesis with contralateral renal dysplasia, scoliosis, and absent sacrum.[139] The third fetus had sirenomelia with genital anomalies and severe cardiovascular anomalies.

Sonographic diagnosis of sacral agenesis is possible by showing abrupt termination of the lumbar spine without a visible sacrum (Fig 6–43). This finding, in association with bilateral renal agenesis or cystic dysplasia, may be the primary clue to the presence of sirenomelia (see Fig 6–43).[132, 135] A specific prenatal diagnosis of sirenomelia rarely has been made (see Chapter 13).[144, 145a] Sirtori et al. reported 11 cases of sirenomelia evaluated by prenatal sonography.[145a]

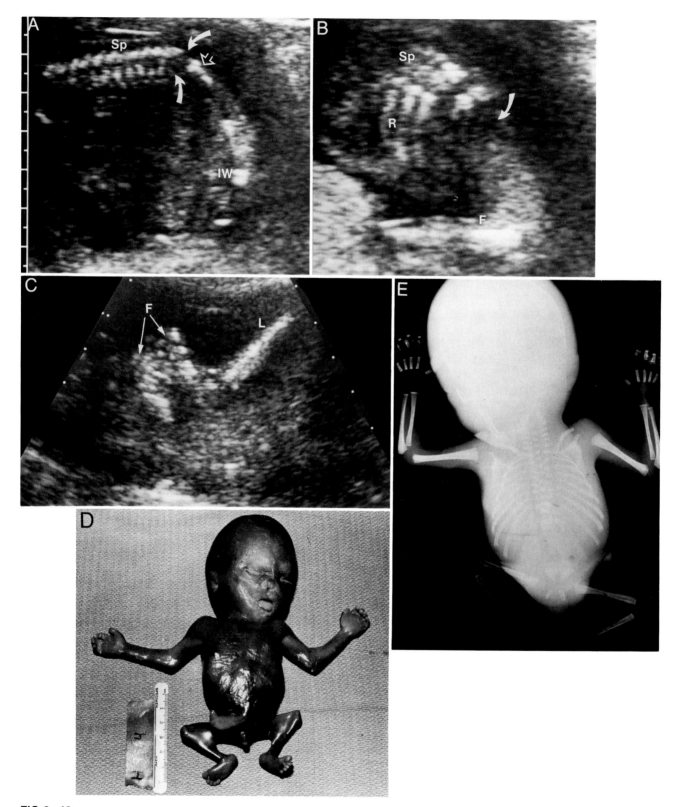

FIG 6–42.
Sacral agenesis, caudal regression syndrome. **A,** longitudinal sonogram made at 18 weeks because of a maternal history of insulin-dependent diabetes mellitus, shows abrupt termination *(arrows)* of the spine below the lower thoracic spine *(Sp)*. A small ossified focus *(open arrow)* is the only remnant of the lumbar spine. The iliac wings *(IW)* are markedly hypoplastic. **B,** coronal sonogram again demonstrates absence of the lumbar spine *(arrow)* below the thoracic spine *(Sp)* and ribs *(R)*. The femur *(F)* appears shortened and fixed in an abducted

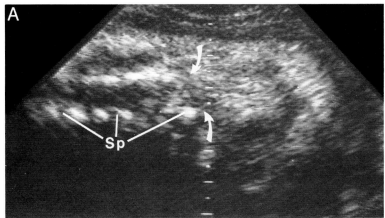

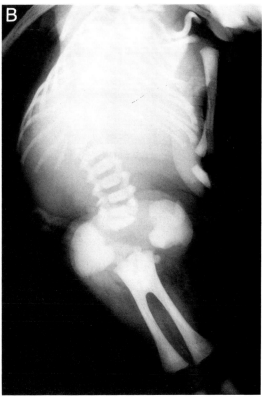

FIG 6–43.
Sacral agenesis and sirenomelia. **A,** longitudinal sonogram demonstrates abrupt termination of the lumbar spine *(Sp)*, with absence of the sacrum *(arrows)*. Absence of fetal kidneys, marked oligohydramnios, and mild dilatation of the cerebral ventricles were also noted. **B,** postnatal radiograph shows sacral agenesis, multiple vertebral and rib anomalies, and fusion of lower extremities (sirenomelia). Anorectal atresia also was present, as is true in all cases of sirenomelia. (From Harris RD, Nyberg DA, Mack LA, et al: Anorectal atresia: Prenatal sonographic diagnosis. AJR 1987; 149:395–400. Used by permission.)

Oligohydramnios was present in all cases and was severe enough to obscure a sonographic evaluation in five cases.

Associated Anomalies

Associated anomalies parallel the severity of the primary disorder. Anomalies most commonly associated with sacral agenesis include musculoskeletal deformities such as clubfoot, scoliosis, hip dislocation, and pelvic deformities; additional anomalies associated with the caudal regression syndrome include anorectal atresia, tracheoesophageal fistula, genitourinary anomalies, and spina bifida. Sirenomelia is universally associated with other major malformations, including anorectal atresia, renal agenesis or cystic dysplasia, agenesis of internal genital organs, and a single umbilical artery.[134] Cardiovascular malformations also are common. All 11 cases of sirenomelia reported by Sirtori et al. had concurrent anomalies.[145a]

Prognosis

The prognosis for sacral agenesis and the caudal regression syndrome invariably depends on the presence of associated anomalies. Among survivors, sacral agenesis usually results in bladder dysfunction and neuromuscular impairment, with motor deficits more pronounced than the sensory component.[145] Fetuses with the caudal regression syndrome have an extremely poor prognosis because of associated anomalies. Five of 12 infants died at one institution because of associated anomalies.[139] Among survivors, the degree of neurologic impairment roughly correlates with the osseous abnormality. Sirenomelia is uniformly fatal.

Other Spinal Abnormalities

Hemivertebrae, Scoliosis

Pathologic, Clinical Findings.—Congenital malformations of the vertebrae can be classified as failure of formation or failure of segmentation. The former includes unilateral formation (hemivertebrae) and anterior central defects of formation (butterfly vertebrae).[157] Failure of segmentation produces block vertebrae.

Hemivertebrae are one of the causes of congenital scoliosis,[160] and partial failure of segmentation may re-

position. **C,** scan of the lower extremities shows markedly shortened legs *(L)* and feet *(F)*. **D,** photograph of pathologic specimen shows marked shortening of lower extremities (compare with upper extremities). **E,** radiograph confirms lumbar and sacral agenesis and marked reduction of lower extremities. (Courtesy of Laurence A Mack, MD, Department of Radiology, University of Washington Hospital, Seattle, Washington.)

sult in scoliosis, kyphosis, or lordosis. Kyphoscoliosis may arise from various other conditions, including forms of arthrogryposis, some bone dysplasias, and the limb-body wall complex. The Klippel-Feil deformity consists of a short neck associated with fusion of cervical vertebrae and, often, a cervical myelomeningocele.

Vertebral anomalies are one of the hallmarks of the caudal regression syndrome and VACTERL syndrome. A diagnosis of the VACTERL syndrome is made when three or more of the cardinal anomalies are present.

Sonographic Findings.—Hemivertebrae have been diagnosed by prenatal sonography in several cases (Fig 6–44).[146, 147] The diagnosis of even an isolated defect can be made when it is unbalanced and results in scoliosis at the site of the defect. However, demonstration of vertebral defects is more difficult when the spine is normally aligned. Benacerraf re-

ported a case of hemivertebra that was subsequently associated with scoliosis (see Fig 6–44).[147] Multiple hemivertebrae and vertebral defects have been demonstrated in the Jarcho-Levin syndrome and other skeletal dysplasias (described below). Scoliosis is best recognized on longitudinal views (Fig 6–45).[1, 150]

Associated Anomalies.—Anomalies of the ribs, spinal cord, and lower limbs commonly are present as a result of the vertebral anomalies.[157] Other anomalies that are frequently associated with spinal abnormalities include malformations of the gastrointestinal, genitourinary, or central nervous systems. Scoliosis is one of the cardinal sonographic findings of the limb-body wall complex, which also includes an abdominal wall defect that most closely resembles an omphalocele.[155] Birnholz reported scoliosis in a fetus with neurofibromatosis.[1] Therefore, associated anomalies should be

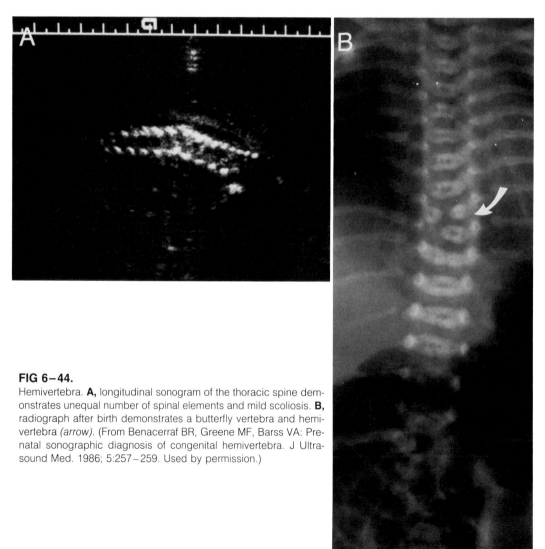

FIG 6–44.
Hemivertebra. **A,** longitudinal sonogram of the thoracic spine demonstrates unequal number of spinal elements and mild scoliosis. **B,** radiograph after birth demonstrates a butterfly vertebra and hemivertebra *(arrow).* (From Benacerraf BR, Greene MF, Barss VA: Prenatal sonographic diagnosis of congenital hemivertebra. J Ultrasound Med. 1986; 5:257–259. Used by permission.)

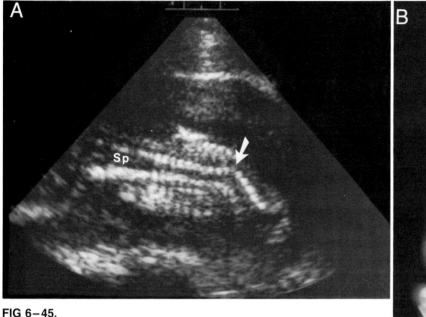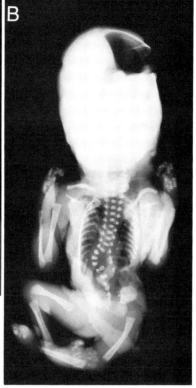

FIG 6–45.
Scoliosis from limb-body wall complex. **A,** coronal scan of the fetal spine *(Sp)* shows abrupt and marked scoliosis *(arrow).* **B,** corresponding postmortem radiograph shows marked scoliosis. Cranial and thoracoabdominal defects were also present. (From Patten RM, Van Allen M, Mack LA, et al: Limb-body wall complex: In utero sonographic diagnosis of a complicated fetal malformation. AJR 1986; 146:1019–1024. Used by permission.)

carefully sought when scoliosis or other vertebral anomalies are demonstrated.

Prognosis.—The prognosis varies with the underlying malformation. An isolated hemivertebrae carries no clinical significance when an associated spinal deformity is not present. By contrast, the limb-body wall complex is a uniformly fatal disorder.

Skeletal Dysplasia

Disorganized thoracic vertebrae and abnormal ribs are the primary manifestations of spondylothoracic dysostosis (Jarcho-Levin syndrome), also referred to as spondylocostal dysplasia, costovertebral dysplasia, and spondylothoracic dysplasia, an autosomal recessive disorder characterized by multiple fused vertebrae and hemivertebrae in the cervical, thoracic, and lumbar regions that results in a "crab-like" thorax. The rest of the skeleton is unaffected, although other associated anomalies include a single umbilical artery and genitourinary, diaphragmatic, and anorectal malformations.[166] Over 30 cases of the Jarcho-Levin syndrome have been described, and over half of these have been of Puerto-Rican descent.[165]

Several cases of the Jarcho-Levin syndrome have been described prenatally.[163, 166, 167] Tolmie et al. and Marks et al. each reported a fetus with the Jarcho-Levin syndrome in a family at risk for recurrence, and Romero et al. reported typical findings in a family not known to be at risk.[166, 167] We also have encountered a fetus with multiple hemivertebrae and marked vertebral disorganization involving the entire thoracic spine, possibly representing a form of the Jarcho-Levin syndrome (Fig 6–46).

Other considerations for multiple rib and vertebral anomalies include dyssegmental dysplasia, mesomelic dysplasia of the Robinow type, and VACTERL anomalies. Unlike Jarcho-Levin syndrome, dyssegmental dysplasia is characterized by severe micromelia (marked shortening of all extremities) and occipital encephalocele. Robinow mesomelic dysplasia is characterized by segmentation defects (hemivertebrae, butterfly vertebrae, and vertebral fusion), facial abnormalities, and mesomelia, particularly of the upper extremities.[165]

Achondrogenesis has been diagnosed prenatally by demonstration of a poorly mineralized spine (Fig 6–47).[161, 162] Mahony et al. suggested that the combination of absent vertebral body ossification, normal calvarial ossification, and severe limb reduction is diagnostic of achondrogenesis (excluding type I, which shows poor calvarial ossification) and permits reliable distinction of this disorder from other lethal short-limbed dysplasias.[162] Poor mineralization of both the spine and calvarium suggests a differential diagnosis of

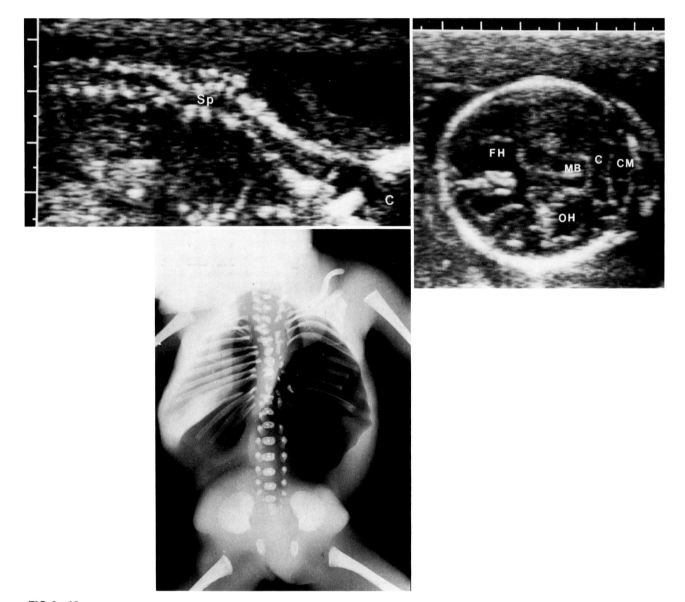

FIG 6–46.
Multiple vertebral anomalies. **A,** longitudinal sonogram of the thoracic spine *(Sp)* at 19 weeks demonstrates marked disorganization of spinal elements. *C* = cranium. **B,** transverse sonogram of the cranium shows mild bilateral ventricular dilatation. Karyotype and amniotic fluid AFP and acetylcholinesterase levels were normal. *FH* = frontal horn; *OH* = occipital horn; *C* = cerebellum; *CM* = cisterna magna, *MB* = midbrain. **C,** radiograph of pathologic specimen confirms multiple anomalies of the thoracic spine and ribs. Agenesis of the corpus callosum also was found. Although intracranial anomalies are not typically present, this may be a form of Jarcho-Levin syndrome (spondylothoracic dysostosis).

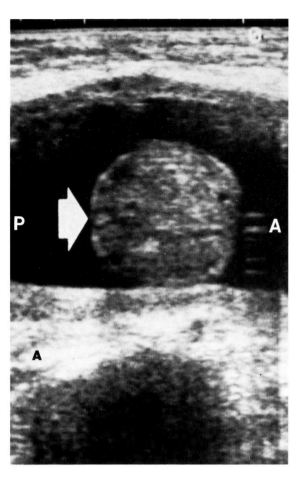

FIG 6–47.
Achondrogenesis. Transverse scan shows marked demineralization of the spine (arrow). Mineralization of the calvarium was normal, and micromelia was identified. A = anterior; P = posterior.

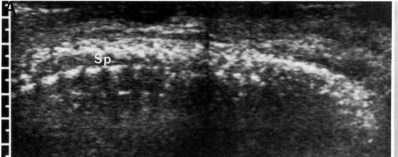

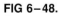

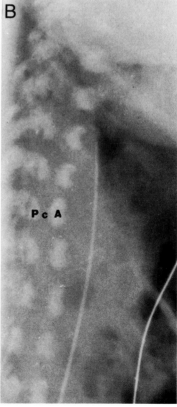

FIG 6–48.
Chondrodysplasia punctata, rhizomelic type. **A,** longitudinal scan of the spine (Sp) shows poor vertebral development with indistinct ossification centers. **B,** postnatal radiograph in lateral view shows underdeveloped vertebrae with characteristic cartilaginous bar (c) between the anterior (A) and posterior (P) ossification centers.

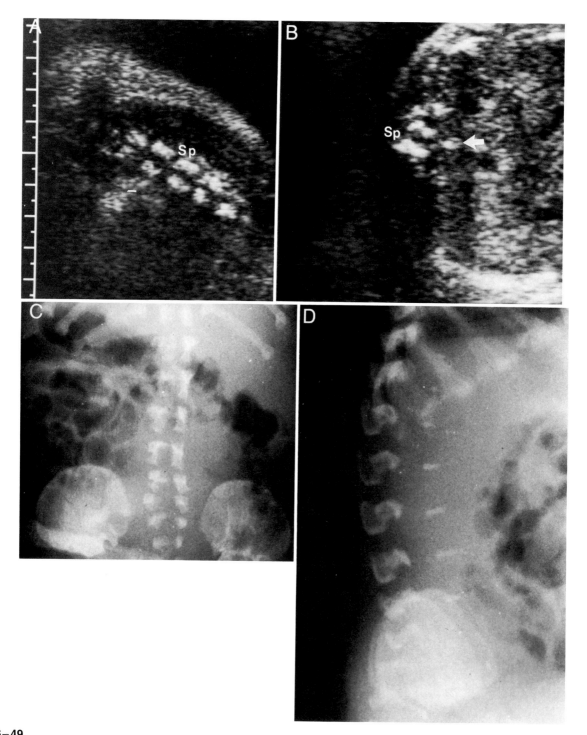

FIG 6–49.
Metatropic dysplasia. **A,** longitudinal sonogram of the lumbar spine *(Sp)* at 36 weeks demonstrates markedly narrowed spinal canal. **B,** transverse sonogram of the lumbar spine *(Sp)* confirms marked narrowing of the canal. The vertebral body is also poorly ossified *(arrow).* **C,** postnatal radiograph in anterior-posterior view shows narrowing of spinal canal in transverse dimension. **D,** lateral view shows poorly ossified vertebral bodies.

type I achondrogenesis and hypophosphatasia, and evaluation of the spine may be helpful in detecting the correct diagnosis.

Various other skeletal dysplasias may demonstrate spinal abnormalities (see Chapter 13).[167] Underdevelopment of vertebral bodies may occur with thanatophoric dwarfism, severe achondroplasia, short-rib polydactyly syndromes, and chondrodysplasia punctata (Fig 6–48). Flattened vertebrae are found in various disorders, including spondyloepiphyseal dysplasia. We have observed a narrow-appearing spinal canal, consistent with spinal stenosis, in fetuses with thanatophoric dysplasia and in one fetus with metatropic dysplasia (Fig 6–49).

SUMMARY

Neural tube defects and spinal disorders are some of the most common and clinically important congenital malformations encountered during prenatal sonography. Wide-scale screening of MS-AFP helps identify the majority of patients at risk, but will miss 20% of fetuses with open spina bifida and all closed spinal defects. Hence, AFP screening should not be considered a substitute for routine and systematic survey of the fetal cranium and spine. Recent clinical observations of cranial findings associated with spina bifida should dramatically improve the accuracy of prenatal sonography for detection of small spinal defects before the time of fetal viability. Prenatal sonography is often the primary and only method of diagnosing closed spinal deformities (sacral agenesis, scoliosis, hemivertebrae). Careful monitoring of fetuses with sacrococcygeal teratoma for potential complications, such as hydrops, may influence the obstetric managment of such cases.

REFERENCES

Normal Development

1. Birnholz JC: Fetal lumbar spine: Measuring axial growth with US. Radiology 1986; 158:805–807.
2. Cochlin DL: Ultrasound of the fetal spine. Clin Radiol 1982; 33:641–650.
3. Filly RA, Simpson GF, Linkowski G: Fetal spine morphology and maturation during the second trimester. J Ultrasound Med 1987; 6:631–636.
4. Flecker H: Time of appearance and fusion of ossification centers as observed by roentgenographic methods. AJR 1942; 47:97–159.
5. Goodwin L, Quisling RG: The neonatal cisterna magna: Ultrasonic evaluation. Radiology 1983; 149:691–695.
6. Gray DL, Crane JP, Rudloff MA: Prenatal diagnosis of neural tube defects: Origin of midtrimester vertebral ossification centers as determined by sonographic water-bath studies. J Ultrasound Med 1988; 7:421–427.
7. Hawass ND, El-Badawi MG, Fatani JA, et al: Myelographic study of the spinal cord ascent during fetal development. AJNR 1987; 8:691–695.
8. Mahony BS, Callen PW, Filly RA, et al: The fetal cisterna magna. Radiology 1984; 153:173–176.
9. Moore KL: *The Developing Human,* ed 4. Philadelphia, WB Saunders Co, pp 364–401.
10. Sauerbrei E, Nguyen K, Nolan R, et al: The fetal spine: Normal development and ossification, optimal scan planes and abnormalities. (abstract) J Ultrasound Med 1988; 7(10):598.

Overview and AFP Screening

11. Brock DJH, Sutcliffe RG: Alpha-fetoprotein in the antenatal diagnosis of anencephaly and spina bifida. Lancet 1972; ii: 197.
12. Burton BK, Sowers SG, Nelson LH: Maternal serum α-fetoprotein screening in North Carolina: Experience with more than twelve thousand pregnancies. Am J Obstet Gynecol 1983; 146:439–444.
13. Creasy MR, Albeman ED: Congenital malformations of the central nervous system in spontaneous abortions. J Med Genet 1976; 13:9.
14. Drugan A, Zador IE, Snyer FN, et al: A normal ultrasound does not obviate the need for amniocentesis in patients with elevated serum alpha-fetoprotein. Obstet Gynecol 1988; 72: 627–630.
15. Holmes LB, Driscoll SG, Atkins L: Etiologic heterogeneity of neural-tube defects. N Engl J Med 1976; 294:365–369.
16. Lemire RJ: Neural tube defects. JAMA 1988; 259:558–562.
17. Main DM, Mennuti MT: Neural tube defects: Issues in prenatal diagnosis and counseling. Obstet Gynecol 1986; 67:1–15.
18. Milunsky A, Alpert E: Results and benefits of a maternal serum alpha-fetoprotein screening program. JAMA 1984; 252:1438–1442.
19. Richards DS, Seeds JW, Katz VL, et al: Elevated maternal serum alpha-fetoprotein with normal ultrasound: Is amniocentesis always appropriate? A review of 26,069 screened patients. Obstet Gynecol 1988; 71: 203–207.
20. United Kingdom collaborative study on alpha-fetoprotein measurement in antenatal screening for anencephaly and spina bifida in early pregnancy. Lancet 1977; 1:1323–1332.
21. Wald NH, Cuckle HS: Neural tube defects: Screening and biochemical diagnosis, in Rodeck CH, Nicholaides KH (eds): *Prenatal Diagnosis.* New York, John Wiley & Sons, 1983, pp 219–241.

Anencephaly and Exencephaly (Acrania)

22. Campbell S, Johnstone FD, Holt EM, et al: Anencephaly: Early ultrasonic diagnosis and active management. Lancet 1972; ii:1226–1227.
23. Campbell S: Early prenatal diagnosis of neural tube defects by ultrasound. Clin Obstet Gynecol 1977; 20:351–359.
24. Chervenak FA, Farley MA, Walters L, et al: When is termination of pregnancy during the third trimester morally justifiable? N Engl J Med 1983; 309:822–825.
25. Chervenak FA, Isaacson G, Mahoney MJ: Advances in the diagnosis of fetal defects. N Engl J Med 1986; 315:305–307.
26. Cox GG, Rosenthall SJ, Holsapple JW: Exencephaly: Sonographic findings and radiologic-pathologic correlation. Radiology 1985; 755–756.
27. Cunningham ME, Walls WJ: Ultrasound in the evaluation of anencephaly. Radiology 1976; 118:165–167.
28. David TJ, Nixon A: Congenital malformations associated with anencephaly and iniencephaly. J Med Genet 1976; 13:263–265.
29. Goldstein RB, Filly RA: Prenatal diagnosis of anencephaly: Spectrum of sonographic appearances and distinction from the amniotic band syndrome. AJR 1988; 151:547–550.
30. Hendricks SK, Cyr DR, Nyberg DA, et al: Exencephaly—Clinical and ultrasonic correlation to anencephaly. 1988; 72:898–901.
31. Johnson A, Losure TA, Weiner S: Early diagnosis of fetal anencephaly. J Clin Ultrasound 1985; 13:503–505.
32. Mannes EJ, Crelin ES, Hobbins JC, et al: Sonographic demonstration of fetal acrania. AJR 1982; 139:181–182.
33. Sunden B: Acta Obstet Gynecol Scand 1964; 43(suppl):6.
34. Vergani P, Ghidini A, Sirtori M, et al: Antenatal diagnosis of fetal acrania. J Ultrasound Med 1987; 6:715–717.

(En)Cephalocele

35. Bieber FR, Petre RE, Beiber J, et al: Prenatal detection of a familial nuchal bleb simulating encephalocele. Birth Defects 1979; XV:51–61.
36. Chervenak FA, Blakemore KJ, Isaacson G, et al: Antenatal sonographic findings of thanatophoric dysplasia with cloverleaf skull. Am J Obstet Gynecol 1983; 146:984–985.
37. Chervenak FA, Isaacson G, Mahoney MJ, et al: Diagnosis and management of fetal cephalocele. Obstet Gynecol 1984; 64:86–90.
38. Cohen MM, Lemire RJ: Syndromes with cephaloceles. Teratology 1982; 25:161–172.
39. Fink W, Chinn DH, Callen PW: Potential pitfall in the ultrasonographic diagnosis of fetal encephalocele. Radiology 1984; 151:834–835.
40. Diebler C, Dulac O: Cephaloceles: Clinical and neuro-radiological appearance. Associated cerebral malformations. Neuroradiology 1983; 25:199–216.
41. Fitz CR: Midline anomalies of the brain and spine. Radiol Clin North Am 1982; 20:95–104.
42. Fraser FC, Lytwyn A: Spectrum of anomalies in the Meckel syndrome, or: "Maybe there is a malformation syndrome with at least one constant anomaly." Am J Med Genet 1981; 97:67–73.
43. Graham D, Johnson TRB Jr, Winn K, et al: The role of sonography in prenatal diagnosis and management of encephalocele. J Ultrasound Med 1982; 1:111–115.
44. Guthkelch AN: Occipital cranium bifidum. Arch Dis Child 1970; 45:104–109.
45. Jeanty P, Sacks G, Shah D, et al: In utero detection of fetal cephaloceles. Presented at the World Federation for Ultrasound in Medicine and Biology Meeting, Washington, DC, Oct 17–21, 1988.
46. Johnson VP, Holzwarth DR: Prenatal diagnosis of Meckel syndrome: Case reports and review of the literature. Am J Med Genet 1984; 18:699–711.
47. Lorber J: The prognosis of occipital encephalocele. Developmental Medicine Child Neurology 1967; 13(suppl):75–86.
48. Mecke S, Passarge E: Encephalocele, polycystic kidneys and polydactyly as an autosomal recessive trait simulating certain other disorders: The Meckel Syndrome. Ann Genet 1971; 14:97–103.
49. Mahony BS, Filly RA, Callen PW, et al: The amniotic band syndrome: Antenatal diagnosis and potential pitfalls. Am J Obstet Gynecol 1985; 152:63–68.
50. Nevin NC, Nevin J, Thompson W, et al: Cystic hygroma simulating an encephalocele. Prenat Diagn 1983; 3:249–252.
51. Pardes JG, Engel IA, Blomquist K: Ultrasonography of intrauterine Meckel's syndrome. J Ultrasound Med 1984; 3:33–35.
52. Sabbagha RE, Tamura RK, Cal Compo S, et al: Fetal cranial and craniocervical masses: Ultrasound characteristics and differential diagnosis. Am J Obstet Gynecol 1980; 138:511–517.
53. Salonen R: The Meckel syndrome: Clinicopathological findings in 67 patients. Am J Med Genet 1984; 18:671–689.
54. Stamm ER, Pretorius DH, Rumack CM, et al: Kleeblattschadel anomaly: In utero sonographic appearance. J Ultrasound Med 1987; 6:319–324.
55. Wapner RJ, Kurtz AB, Ross RD, et al: Ultrasonographic parameters in the prenatal diagnosis of Meckel syndrome. Obstet Gynecol 1981; 57:388–392.

Iniencephaly

56. Aleksic S, Budzilovich G, Greco MA, et al: Iniencephaly: Neuropathologic study. Clin Neuropathol 1983; 2:55–61.
57. Foderaro AE, Abu-Yousef MM, Benda JA, et al: Antenatal ultrasound diagnosis of iniencephaly. J Clin Ultrasound 1987; 15:550–554.

58. Gardner WJ: Klippel-Feil syndrome, iniencephalus, anencephalus, hindbrain hernia and mirror movements: Overdistention of the neural tube. Childs Brain 1979; 5:361–379.

59. Lemire RJ, Beckwith JB, Shepard TH: Iniencephaly and anencephaly with spinal retroflexion: A comparative study of eight human specimens. Teratology 1972; 6:27–36.

60. Meizner I, Bar-Ziv J: Prenatal ultrasonic diagnosis of a rare case of iniencephaly apertus. J Clin Ultrasound 1987; 15:200–203.

61. Shoham Z, Caspi B, Chemke B, et al: Iniencephaly: Prenatal ultrasonic diagnosis—A case report. J Perinat Med 1988; 16:139–143.

Spina Bifida

62. Althouse R, Wald N: Survival and handicap of infants with spina bifida. Arch Dis Child 1980; 55:845–850.

63. Ames MD, Schut L: Results and treatment of 171 consecutive myelomeningoceles—1963 to 1968. Pediatrics 1972; 50:466–470.

64. Bell JE, Gordon A, Maloney FJ: The association of hydrocephalus and Arnold-Chiari malformation with spina bifida in the fetus. Neuropathol Appl Neurobiol 1980; 6:29–39.

65. Benacerraf BR, Stryher J, Figoletto JD Jr, et al: Abnormal US appearance of the cerebellum (banana sign). Indirect sign of spina bifida. Radiology 1989; 171:151–153.

66. Bensen JT, Dillard RG, Burton BK: Open spina bifida: Does cesarean section delivery improve prognosis? Obstet Gynecol 1988; 71:532–534.

67. Campbell S, Pryse-Davies J, Coltart TM, et al: Ultrasound in the diagnosis of spina bifida. Lancet 1975; i:1065–1068.

68. Campbell J, Gilbert WM, Nicolaides KH, et al: Ultrasound screening for spina bifida: Cranial and cerebellar signs in a high-risk population. Obstet Gynecol 1987; 70:247–250.

69. Chervenak FA, Duncan C, Ment LR, et al: Perinatal management of meningomyelocele. Obstet Gynecol 1984; 63:376–380.

70. Chinn DH, Callen PW, Filly RA: The lateral cerebral ventricle in early second trimester. Radiology 1983; 148:529–531.

71. Dennis MA, Drose JA, Pretorius DH, et al: Normal fetal sacrum simulating spina bifida: "Pseudodysraphism." Radiology 1985; 155:751–754.

72. Elejalde MM de, Elejald BR: Visualization of the fetal spine: A proposal of a standard system to increase reliability. Am J Med Genet 1985; 21:445–446.

73. Filly RA, Golbus MS: Ultrasonography of the normal and pathologic fetal skeleton. Radiol Clin North Am 1982; 20:311–323.

74. Furness ME, Barbary JE, Verco PW: A pointer to spina bifida: Fetal head shape in the second trimester, in Gill RW, Dadd MJ (eds): WFUMB [World Federation of Ultrasound in Medicine and Biology] 1985 Proceedings. Sydney, Pergamon Press, p 296.

75. Furness ME, Barbary JE, Verco PW: Fetal head shape in spina bifida in the second trimester. JCU 1987; 15:451–453.

75a. Goldstein RB, Podrasky AE, Filly RA, et al: Effacement of the fetal cisterna magna in association with myelomeningocele. Radiology 1989; 172:409–413.

76. James HE: Intrinsically derived deformational defects secondary to spina dysraphism. Semin Perinatol 1983; 7:253–256.

77. Korenromp MJ: Early fetal leg movements in myelomeningocele. Lancet 1986; i:971–918.

78. Laurence KM: Effect of early surgery for spina bifida cystica on survival and quality of life. Lancet 1974; 1:301–304.

79. Lindfors KK, McGahan JP, Tennant FP, et al: Midtrimester screening for open neural tube defects: Correlation of sonography with amniocentesis results. AJR 1987; 149:141–145.

80. Lorber J: Results of treatment of myelomeningocele: An analysis of 524 unselected cases, with special reference to possible selection for treatment. Dev Med Child Neurol 1971; 13:279–303.

81. Mapstone TB, Rekate HL, Nulsen FE, et al: Relationship of CSF shunting and IQ in children with myelomeningocele: A retrospective analysis. Childs Brain 1984; 11:112–118.

82. Nelson MD Jr, Bracchi M, Naidich TP, et al: The natural history of repaired myelomeningocele. Radiographics 1988; 8:695–706.

83. Nicolaides KH, Campbell S, Gabbe SG: Ultrasound screening for spina bifida: Cranial and cerebellar signs. Lancet 1986; 2:72–74.

84. Nyberg DA, Mack LA, Hirsch J, et al: Fetal hydrocephalus: Sonographic detection and clinical significance of associated anomalies. Radiology 1987; 163:187–191.

85. Nyberg DA, Mack LA, Hirsch J, et al: Abnormalities of fetal cranial contour in sonographic detection of spina bifida: Evaluation of the "lemon" sign. Radiology 1988; 167:387–392.

86. Nyberg DA, Shepard T, Mack LA, et al: Significance of a single umbilical artery in fetuses with central nervous system malformations. J Ultrasound Med 1988; 9:265–273.

87. Penso C, Redline R, Benacerraf BR: A sonographic sign which predicts which fetuses with hydrocephalus have an associated neural tube defect. J Ultrasound Med 1987; 6:307–311.

88. Park TS, Hoffman HJ, Hendrick EB, et al: Experience with surgical decompression of the Arnold-Chiari malformation in young infants with myelomeningocele. Neurosurgery 1983; 13:147–152.

89. Persson PH, Kullander S, Genner G, et al: Screening for fetal malformations using ultrasound and measurements of alpha-fetoprotein in maternal serum. Br Med J 1983; 286:747–749.

90. Pilu G, Romero R, Reece A, et al: Subnormal cerebel-

lum in fetuses with spina bifida. Am J Obstet Gynecol 1988; 158:1052–1056.

91. Roberts AB, Campbell S: Fetal head measurements in spina bifida. Br J Obstet Gynaecol 1980; 87:927–928.

92. Roberts CJ, Hibbard BM, Roberts EE, et al: Diagnostic effectiveness of ultrasound in detection of neural tube defect. Lancet 1983; ii:1068–1069.

93. Robinson HP, Hood VD, Adam AH, et al: Diagnostic ultrasound: Early detection of fetal neural tube defects. Obstet Gynecol 1980; 56:705–710.

94. Seeds JW, Jones FD: Lipomyelomeningocele: Prenatal diagnosis and management. Obstet Gynecol 1986; 67(suppl):34.

95. Seeds JW, Powers SK: Early prenatal diagnosis of familial lipomyelomeningocele. Obstet Gynecol 1988; 72:469–471.

96. Sharrard WJW: The mechanism of paralytic deformity in spina bifida. Dev Med Child Neurol 1962; 4:310–313.

97. Vogt EC, Wyatt GM: Craniolacunia (luckenschadel): Report of fifty-two cases. Radiology 1941; 36:147–153.

98. Wald N, Cuckle H, Boreham J, et al: Small biparietal diameter of fetuses with spina bifida: Implications for antenatal screening. Br J Obstet Gynaecol 1980; 87:219–221.

99. Warkany J: *Congenital Malformations.* Chicago, Year Book Medical Publishers, Inc, 1971, pp 272–291.

100. Williams B: Cerebrospinal fluid pressure gradients in spina bifida cystica, with special reference to the Arnold-Chiari malformation and aqueductal stenosis. Dev Med Child Neurol 1975; 17(suppl35):138–150.

Sacrococcygeal Teratoma

101. Alter DN, Reed KL, Marx GR, et al: Prenatal diagnosis of congestive heart failure in a fetus with a sacrococcygeal teratoma. Obstet Gynecol 1988; 71:978–981.

102. Altman RP, Randolph JG, Lilly JR: Sacrococcygeal teratoma. American Academy of Pediatrics Surgical Section Survey, 1973. J Pediatr Surg 1974; 9:389–398.

103. Aschcraft KW, Holder TM: Hereditary presacral teratoma. J Pediatr Surg 1974; 9:691–697.

104. Bale PM: Sacrococcygeal developmental abnormalities and tumors in children. Perspect Pediatr Pathol 1984; 8:9–55.

105. Chervenak FA, Isaacson G, Touloukian R, et al: Diagnosis and management of fetal teratomas. Obstet Gynecol 1985; 66:666–671.

106. Cousins L, Bernirshke K, Porreco R, et al: Placentaomegaly due to fetal congestive failure in a pregnancy with a sacrococcygeal teratoma. J Reprod Med 1980; 25:142–144.

107. Donnellan WA, Swenson O: Benign and malignant sacrococcygeal teratomas. Surgery 1968; 64:834–836.

108. Edwards WR: A fetal sacrococcygeal tumour obstructing labor after attempted home confinement. Obstet Gynecol 1983; 61:19S

109. Ein SH, Adeyemi SD, Mancer K: Benign sacrococcygeal

110. Flake AW, Harrison MR, Adzick NS, et al: Fetal sacrococcygeal teratoma. J Pediatr Surg 1986; 21:563–566.

111. Gergely RZ, Eden R, Schifrin BS, et al: Antenatal diagnosis of congenital sacral teratoma. J Reprod Med 1980; 24:229–231.

112. Gonzalez-Crussi F, Winkler RF, Mirkin DL: Sacrococcygeal teratomas in infants and children: Relationship of histology and prognosis in 40 cases. Arch Pathol Lab Med 1978; 102:420–425.

113. Gross SJ, Benzie RJ, Sermer M, et al: Sacrococcygeal teratoma. Prenatal diagnosis and management. Am J Obstet Gynecol 1987; 156:393–396.

114. Hecht F, Hecht B, O'Keefe D: Sacrococcygeal teratoma: Prenatal diagnosis with elevated alpha-fetoprotein and acetylcholinesterase in amniotic fluid. Prenat Diagn 1982; 2:229–231.

115. Hogge WA, Thiagarajah S, Barber VG, et al: Cystic sacrococcygeal teratoma: Ultrasound diagnosis and perinatal management. J Ultrasound Med 1987; 6:707–710.

116. Holzgreve W, Mahony BS, Glick PS, et al: Fetal sacrococcygeal teratoma. Prenat Diagn 1985; 5:245–257.

117. Horger EO, McCarter LH: Prenatal diagnosis of sacrococcygeal teratoma. Am J Obstet Gynecol 1979; 134:228–229.

118. Hunt PT, Davidson KC, Ashcraft KW, et al: Radiography of hereditary presacral teratoma. Radiology 1977; 122:187–191.

119. Lees RF, Williamson BR, Norman A, et al: Sonography of benign sacral teratoma in utero. Radiology 1980; 134:717–718.

120. Lockwood C, Ghidini A, Romero R, et al: Fetal bowel perforation simulating sacrococcygeal teratoma. J Ultrasound Med 1988; 7:227–229.

121. Mintz MC, Mennuti M, Fishman M: Prenatal aspiration of sacrococcygeal teratoma. AJR 1983; 141:367–378.

122. Musci MN, Clark MJ, Ayres RE, et al: Management of dystocia caused by a large sacrococcygeal teratoma. Obstet Gynecol 1983; 62:10S.

123. Schey WL, Shkolnik A, White H: Clinical and radiographic considerations of sacrococcygeal teratomas: An analysis of 26 new cases and review of the literature. Radiology 1977; 125:189–195.

124. Seeds JW, Mittelstaedt CA, Cefalo RC, et al: Prenatal diagnosis of sacrococcygeal teratoma: An anechoic caudal mass. J Clin Ultrasound 1982; 10:193–195.

125. Sheth S, Nussbaum AR, Sanders RC, et al: Prenatal diagnosis of sacrococcygeal teratoma: Sonographic-pathologic correlation. Radiology 1988; 169:131–136.

126. Sherowsky RC, Williams CH, Nichols VB, et al: Prenatal ultrasonographic diagnosis of a sacrococcygeal teratoma in a twin pregnancy. J Ultrasound Med 1985; 4:159–161.

127. Teal LN, Angtuaco TL, Jiminez JF, et al: Fetal teratomas: Antenatal diagnosis and clinical management. J Clin Ultrasound 1988; 16:329–336.

128. Valdiserri RO, Yunis EJ: Sacrococcygeal teratomas: A review of 68 cases. Cancer 1981; 48:217–221.
129. Verma U, Weiss R, Almonte R, et al: Early prenatal diagnosis of soft-tissue malformations. Obstet Gynecol 1979; 53:660–663.
130. Zaleski AM, Cooperberg PL, Kliman MR: Ultrasonic diagnosis of extra fetal masses. J Can Assoc Radiol 1979; 30:55–56.

Sacral Agenesis and Caudal Regression

131. Beard RW, Lowy C: Commentary. The British survey of diabetic pregnancies. Br J Obstet Gynaecol 1982; 89:783–786.
132. Bearn JG: The association of sirenomelia with Potter's syndrome. Arch Dis Child 1960; 254–260.
133. Cousins L. Congenital anomalies among infants of diabetic mothers. Am J Obstet Gynecol 1983; 147:333–338.
134. Duhamel B. From the mermaid to anal imperforation. The syndrome of caudal regression syndrome. Arch Dis Child 1961; 36:151–155.
135. Harris RD, Nyberg DA, Mack LA, et al: Anorectal atresia: Prenatal sonographic diagnosis. AJR 1987; 149:395–400.
136. Hotston S, Carty H: Lumbosacral agenesis: A report of three new cases and a review of the literature. Br J Radiol 1982; 55:629–633.
137. Kallen B, Winberg J: Caudal mesoderm pattern of anomalies: From renal agenesis to sirenomelia. Teratology 1973; 9:99–112.
138. Kubryk N, Schmatko M, Borde M, et al: Le syndrome de regression caudale. A propos d'une observation. Ann Pediatr (Paris) 1981; 28:597–600.
139. Loewy JA, Richards DG, Toi A: In-utero diagnosis of the caudal regression syndrome: Report of three cases. J Clin Ultrasound 1987; 15:469–474.
140. Mariani AJ, Stern J, Khan AU, et al: Sacral agenesis: An analysis of 11 cases and review of the literature. J Urology 1979; 122:684–686.
141. Miller E, Hare JW, Cloherty JP, et al: Elevated maternal HB AIC in early pregnancy and major congenital anomalies in infants of diabetic mothers. N Engl J Med 1981; 304:1331–1334.
142. Mills JL: Malformations in infants of diabetic mothers. Teratology 1982; 25:385–394.
143. Passarge E, Lenz W: Syndrome of caudal regression in infants of diabetic mothers: Observation of further cases. Pediatrics 1966; 37:672–675.
144. Raabe RD, Harnsberger R, Lee TG, et al: Ultrasonographic antenatal diagnosis of "mermaid syndrome". J Ultrasound Med 1983; 2:463–464.
145. Renshaw TS: Sacral agenesis: A classification and review of twenty-three cases. J Bone Joint Surg 1978; 60A:373–383.
145a. Sirtori M, Chidini A, Romero R, et al: Prenatal diagnosis of sirenomelia. J Ultrasound Med 1989; 8:83–88.

Scoliosis, Hemivertebrae, and Other Spinal Abnormalities

146. Abrams SL, Filly RA: Congenital vertebral malformations: Prenatal diagnosis using ultrasonography. Radiology 1988; 155:762.
147. Benacerraf BR, Greene MF, Barss VA: Prenatal sonographic diagnosis of congenital hemivertebra. J Ultrasound Med 1986; 5:257–259.
148. Bond-Taylor W, Starer F, Atwell JD: Vertebral anomalies associated with esophageal atresia and tracheoesophageal fistual with reference to the initial operative mortality. J Pediatr Surg 1973; 8:9–13.
149. Claiborne AK, Blocker SH, Marin CM, et al: Prenatal and postnatal sonographic delineation of gastrointestinal abnormalities in a case of the VATER syndrome. J Ultrasound Med 1986; 5:45–47.
150. Henry RJW, Norton S: Prenatal ultrasound diagnosis of fetal scoliosis with termination of the pregnancy: Case report. Prenat Diagn 1987; 7:663–666.
151. Khoury MJ, Cordero JF, Greenberg F: A population study of the VACTERL association: Evidence for its etiologic heterogeneity. Pediatrics 1983; 71:815–820.
152. McGahan JP, Leela JM, Lindfors KK: Prenatal sonographic diagnosis of VACTERL association. J Clin Ultrasound 1988; 16:580–591.
153. Miriani AJ, Stern J, Khan AU, et al: Sacral agenesis: An analysis of 11 cases and review of the literature. J Urol 1979; 122:684–686.
154. Muraji T, Mahour GH: Surgical problems in patients with VATER-associated anomalies. J Pediatr Surg 1984; 19:550–554.
155. Patten RN, Van Allen M, Mack LA, et al: Limb-body wall complex: In utero sonographic diagnosis of a complicated fetal malformation. AJR 1986; 146:1019–1024.
156. Quan L, Smith DW: The VATER association: Vertebral defects, anal atresia, tracheoesophageal fistula with esophageal atresia, and radial dysplasia. Birth Defects 1972; VIII:75–78.
157. Roof R: *Spinal Deformities.* Philadelphia, JB Lippincott Co, 1977, pp 86–90.
158. Stevenson RE: Extravertebrae associated with esophageal atresia and tracheoesophageal fistula with reference to the intial operative mortality. J Pediatr Surg 1972; 81:1123–1129.
159. Temtamy SA, Miller JD: Extending the scope of the VATER association: Definition of the VATER syndrome. J Pediatr 1974; 85:345–349.
160. Winter RB, Moe JM, Eilers VE: Congenital scoliosis: A study of 234 patients treated and untreated. J Bone Joint Surg 1968; 50A:1–47.

Spinal Dysplasia

161. Johnson VP, Yiu-Chiu VS, Wierda DR, et al: Midtrimester prenatal diagnosis of achondrogenesis. J Ultrasound Med 1984; 3:223–226.
162. Mahony BS, Filly RA, Cooperberg PL: Antenatal sono-

graphic diagnosis of achondrogenesis. J Ultrasound Med 1984; 3:333–335.

163. Marks F, Hernanz-Schulman M, Horii S, et al: Spondylothoracic dysplasia. J Ultrasound Med 1989; 8:1–5.

164. Robinow M, Silverman FN, Smith HD: A newly recognized dwarfing syndrome. Am J Dis Child 1969; 117:645–651.

165. Romero R, Ghidini A, Eswara MS, et al: Prenatal findings in a case of spondylocostal dysplasia type I (Jarcho-Levin syndrome). Obstet Gynecol 1988; 71:988–991.

166. Rouse G, Zager J, Toumey F, et al: Sonographic and idiopathic evaluation of the fetal spine in short-limb dysplasia. Presented at the World Federation for Ultrasound in Medicine and Biology Meeting, Washington, DC, Oct 17–21, 1988.

167. Tolmie JL, Whittle MJ, McNay MB, et al: Second trimester prenatal diagnosis of the Jarcho-Levin syndrome. Prenat Diagn 1987; 7:129–134.

The Face and Neck

Barry S. Mahony, M.D.

Frederick N. Hegge, M.D.

Many sonologists regard the fetal face as a complex and unrewarding region of the fetus to examine in their anatomic survey. Although the official guidelines of the American Institute of Ultrasound in Medicine do not specifically recommend an examination of the fetal face and neck, they do state that suspected abnormalities may require a specialized evaluation to permit diagnosis of numerous anomalies which otherwise would remain unrecognized until after birth.[7]

Prenatal sonographic examination of the fetal face and neck need not be an excessively time-consuming task, but in the appropriate setting it may provide diagnostic information which significantly alters perinatal management.[5] Furthermore, a brief survey of the face and neck on all obstetric sonograms facilitates the expertise and familiarity necessary for accurate diagnosis in anomalous pregnancies.[5]

The first portion of this chapter discusses the basic embryogenesis of the face and neck followed by a discussion of the prevalence of facial abnormalities and the accuracy of their sonographic detection. Then it explores the facial abnormalities detected with prenatal ultrasound. The second portion of this chapter concerns the fetal neck, including a discussion of the sonographic approach to the neck and the numerous masses affecting the neck.

EMBRYOLOGY OF THE FACE AND NECK

By the time the face and neck have attained adequate size to permit sonographic examination, the embryo has acquired all of its basic morphologic charac-

teristics. Therefore, the sonologist need not possess a detailed knowledge of the complex embryogenesis of this region in order to diagnose most facial abnormalities. However, an understanding of the basic embryology of this region assists in predicting patterns of malformation.

Most malformations of the face and neck involve anomalous development of the facial processes, pharyngeal pouches, branchial apparatus, or the optic vesicles (Fig 7–1).[18, 19, 20] By 14 days after fertilization, the embryo has developed a Hensen node, which eventually gives rise to many of the primordia of the face.[20] At 21 to 31 days the cranial portion of the embryo develops several mesenchymal elevations which form the facial processes and pharyngeal arches. The differential growth of these processes soon obliterates the grooves between them, but it is along these grooves that facial clefts typically develop. By approximately 24–26 days post-fertilization, the optic vesicles appear as evaginations from the forebrain. These are the precursors of the eyes. At about the same time the branchial apparatus and pharyngeal pouches begin to form, which give rise to many of the individual structures of the face and neck.[19]

Changes in proportion and relative position of individual structures characterize later stages of embryogenesis of the face and neck.[19] Initially directed laterally, the eyes gradually become directed anteriorly. The nasal fossae, initially widely separated, gradually come closer together as the nasal septum thins and the medial nasal folds fuse. The external ears, which initially develop caudal to the face, gradually assume a more cephalic orientation. Throughout the fetal period

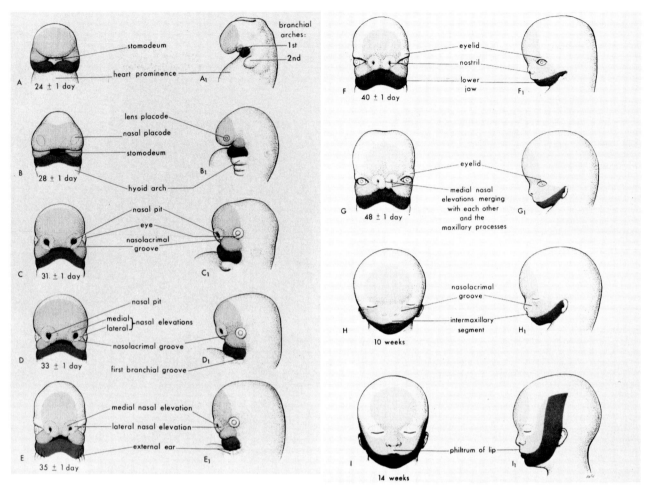

FIG 7–1.
Embryologic development of the face. Frontal **(A)** and lateral **(B)** drawings of the face illustrate the progressive developmental stages of the face. *Hatched area* = frontonasal prominence; *light shaded area* = maxillary prominence; *dark shaded area* = mandibular prominence. (From Moore KL: *The Developing Human: Clinically Oriented Embryolgy,* ed 4. Philadelphia, WB Saunders Co, 1988. Used by permission.)

the face and neck continue their process of growth and maturation, with changes in proportion and relative position of their individual structures.

During early to mid embryogenesis genetic factors play the predominant role in development of the face and neck, but during the latter stages of the embryonic period environmental influences increase in importance. Therefore, malformations of the face and neck frequently result from chromosomal aberrations or environmental insults. Throughout the fetal period, development continues to be influenced by environmental factors.

PREVALENCE OF ANOMALIES AND ACCURACY OF ULTRASOUND

Although several major dysmorphology textbooks document the large number of malformations and syn-

dromes involving the face, the prevalence figures for many specific anomalies are either unknown or quite low.[3, 4, 12, 13] Two series discuss the accuracy of prenatal ultrasound in detection of facial abnormalities and the frequency of detection of these anomalies.[5, 9] Numerous other publications concerning the fetal face and neck involve case reports or smaller series.[1, 2, 8, 10, 11]

Among approximately 7,100 low-risk and high-risk obstetric examinations, Hegge et al. detected 11 fetuses (0.15%) with facial abnormalities at 20–39 weeks' gestation.[5] All of the affected fetuses had concomitant structural anomalies, polyhydramnios, or a history of maternal teratogen exposure. Eight of the fetuses with detected facial abnormalities had coexistent anomalies, and seven had polyhydramnios. The coexistent anomalies frequently dominated the sonographic impression and indicated a high likelihood for facial abnormalities. For example, four of the fetuses had holoprosencephaly, and one had the amniotic band syndrome. During the course of the survey, the following facial anomalies were detected: Absent eyes, hypertelorism, proptosis, proboscis, absent nose, single nostril, flattened or sunken nose, micrognathia, and a large facial cleft. Two cases with cleft lip, four with cleft palate, and one with a flattened nose were known to have been missed.

Pilu et al. examined the accuracy of prenatal ultrasound for the detection of facial anomalies among 223 fetuses at risk for craniofacial abnormalities, based upon detection of extrafacial anomalies, chromosomal aberrations, or a family history of craniofacial malformation or maternal teratogen exposure.[9] In 11% of these targeted high-risk pregnancies, the face could not be visualized at 18–40 weeks' gestation on two separate occasions because of inopportune fetal positioning, severe oligohydramnios, or maternal obesity. Eighteen fetuses had facial anomalies, yielding a prevalence of 8% in this high-risk population, and prenatal ultrasound detected facial anomalies in 14 of 18 (78%) fetuses. Among the 18 anomalous fetuses, 12 (67%) had holoprosencephaly and three others had readily detected cranial abnormalities (anencephaly, microcephaly, or hydrocephalus). Only two cases had a positive family history (the Robin anomalad or maternal diabetes). Polyhydramnios was present in 61% of cases. The sonographic findings included the predictable median cleft lip and palate, hypotelorism, proboscis, and absent nasal bridge in cases with holoprosencephaly, as well as other cases with micrognathia. In this series, prenatal sonography did not detect four cases with cleft palate, three with cleft lip, and one with cyclops. No fetuses with a normal face were diagnosed as abnormal prenatally.

These two series indicate that prenatal ultrasound is quite accurate in detection of many facial abnormalities, but that most facial anomalies detected prenatally occur in the setting of polyhydramnios, obvious extrafacial anomalies, or a history of maternal teratogen exposure. Only occasionally does a family history of craniofacial malformation signal the presence of a recurrent facial anomaly. Even in fetuses at high risk for facial anomaly, ultrasound is not highly sensitive for detection of cleft lip or palate.

SONOGRAPHIC APPROACH TO THE FACE

Ultrasound evaluates the face and neck quite well as early as 16 weeks of gestation.[15, 16] Extensive and time-consuming sonographic investigation may demonstrate remarkable and beautiful detail of the fetal face and neck anatomy, including, but certainly not limited

to various muscles, nerves, and arteries.[14, 17] A meticulous examination of the face is neither warranted nor useful in the vast majority of cases, however, and is unlikely to be productive in low-risk obstetrical sonography. On the other hand, targeted examination of the face is a productive and accurate means of detecting facial anomalies in fetuses with concomitant structural abnormalities or in pregnancies complicated by polyhydramnios or a maternal history of teratogen exposure.[5, 9]

The external anatomy of the fetus provides the foundation for organizing and interpreting the ultrasound of the face, and the sonographic technique does not differ from that utilized for evaluation of other fetal parts. In fetuses for whom concomitant anomalies or maternal history of teratogen exposure indicate a high likelihood of facial abnormalities, evaluation of the following facial structures and associated questions may prove useful in the detection of the majority of facial anomalies.

A. The orbits and nose (Fig 7–2).
1. *Is hypotelorism, hypertelorism, microphthalmia, or anophthalmia present?*
2. *Is a proboscis or cebocephaly present?*
3. *Are any periorbital masses or intraocular abnormalities present?*

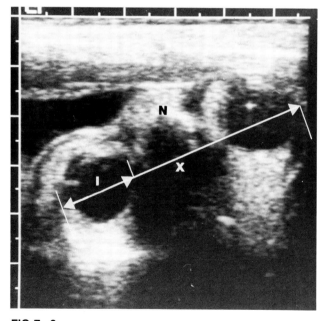

FIG 7–2.
Orbits. Axial scan through the level of the normal orbits at 31 weeks shows the nasal bridge *(N)*, binocular distance *(X)*, and intraocular diameter *(I)*. In this case the binocular distance = 51 mm and the intraocular distance = 17 mm.

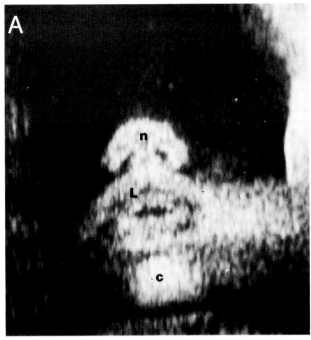

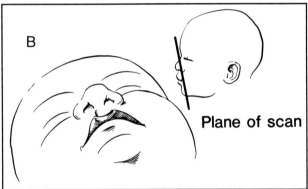

FIG 7–3.
Upper lip, mouth, chin, and nose. **A,** frontal view of the upper lip and mouth demonstrates the intact upper lip, normal nose and chin, and absence of protuberance of the tongue. **B,** this drawing illustrates the approximate frontal plane of section through the upper lip. L = upper lip; n = nose; c = chin. (Part **B** from Meininger MG, Christ JE: Real-time ultrasonography for the prenatal diagnosis of facial clefts. Birth Defects 1982; 18:161–167. In Salinas C (ed): Craniofacial anomalies: New perspectives. New York, Alan R Liss, Inc, for the March of Dimes Birth Defects Foundation. Used by permission.)

B. The upper lip and mouth (Fig 7–3).
   1. *Is the upper lip cleft?*
   2. *Is the tongue protuberant or the mouth widely open?*
C. The facial profile (Fig 7–4).
   1. *Is the nose flattened, the chin abnormally small, or the nasal bridge absent?*
   2. *Is an abnormal mass present?*

D. The ears (Fig 7–5).
   1. *Are the ears low set or of abnormal size?*
   2. *Are the ears obviously deformed?*

The vast majority of facial anomalies detected prenatally involve the orbital and periorbital region or the mouth. The facial profile views and images of the ears occasionally may be useful in fetuses with a large craniofacial mass or with multiple malformations.

THE ORBITS/PERIORBITAL REGION

Visualization of the orbital region requires very little scanning time in most cases, but documentation of the presence and size of two eyes and of the distance between them may provide useful diagnostic information (Table 7–1).[21, 22, 23] The binocular distance, determined by measurement between the lateral orbital rims, provides information regarding hypotelorism or hypertelorism and, in rare cases, may assist in pregnancy dating if severe distortion of other biometric parameters has occurred (i.e., cloverleaf skull and micromelia in thanatophoric dysplasia) (Fig 7–6).[22]

Attention to detail of the periorbital and intraorbital anatomy occasionally will detect rare anomalies and may provide useful data regarding ocular dynamics. At least in the third trimester of pregnancy, it also may be possible to detect intraocular abnormalities which suggest a specific diagnosis in a fetus with other detected anomalies, even in the absence of familial risk.

Diprosopus

Clinical and Pathologic Findings

An extremely rare form of conjoined twinning, diprosopus results in a single body but duplication of craniofacial structures ranging from isolated duplication of the nose to complete facial duplication.[25] The two midline globes may be fused or separate within a central orbit or may occupy completely separate orbits. As with other forms of conjoined twinning, diprosopus arises from a single fertilized ovum with subsequent incomplete fission of the embryo before the third week of gestation. Diprosopus has a poor prognosis.

Sonographic Findings

Prenatal sonographic findings in three reported cases of diprosopus at 20–28 weeks' gestation include polyhydramnios and hydrocephaly with partial duplication of the intracranial structures.[24, 25, 26] Following

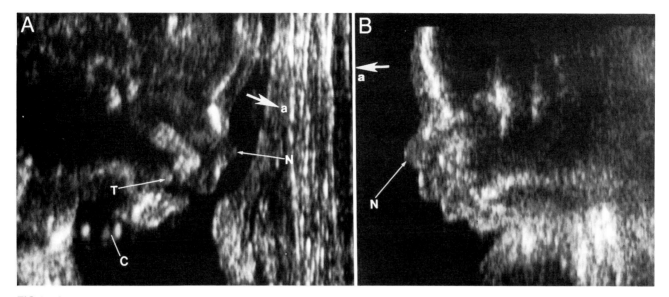

FIG 7–4.
The normal facial profile. **A** and **B,** midsagittal normal facial profile scans demonstrate the variability of the normal facial profile. Abnormal facial profile view may assist in the accurate diagnosis of syndromes with multiple malformations. However, distinction between the normal and abnormal facial profile may be quite subtle. *A* = anterior; *N* = nose; *T* = tongue; *C* = segment of umbilical cord adjacent to the neck.

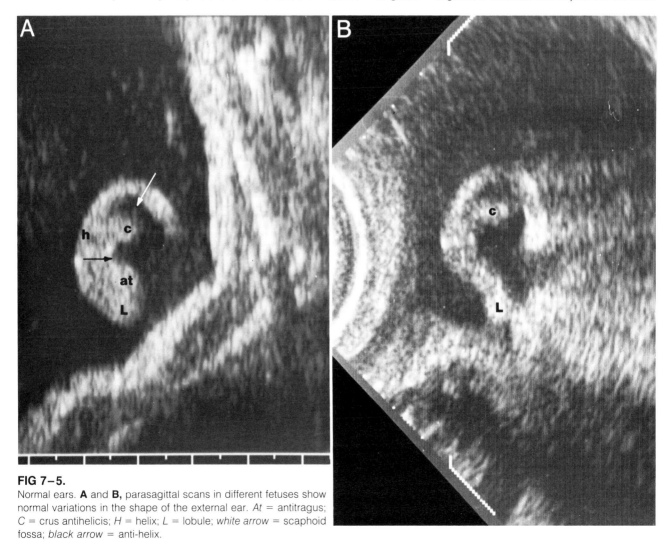

FIG 7–5.
Normal ears. **A** and **B,** parasagittal scans in different fetuses show normal variations in the shape of the external ear. *At* = antitragus; *C* = crus antihelicis; *H* = helix; *L* = lobule; *white arrow* = scaphoid fossa; *black arrow* = anti-helix.

TABLE 7–1.

Estimated Gestational Age (in Weeks Plus Days)
From the Binocular Distance (BD)*

BD (mm)	Gestational Age Percentile		
	5th	50th	95th
15	7 + 1	10 + 3	13 + 6
16	7 + 5	11 + 0	14 + 3
17	8 + 2	11 + 4	15 + 0
18	8 + 6	12 + 1	15 + 4
19	9 + 4	12 + 6	16 + 1
20	10 + 1	13 + 3	16 + 5
21	10 + 5	14 + 0	17 + 2
22	11 + 2	14 + 4	17 + 6
23	11 + 6	15 + 1	18 + 4
24	12 + 4	15 + 6	19 + 1
25	13 + 1	16 + 3	19 + 5
26	13 + 5	17 + 0	20 + 2
27	14 + 2	17 + 4	20 + 6
28	14 + 6	18 + 1	21 + 4
29	15 + 4	18 + 6	22 + 1
30	16 + 1	19 + 3	22 + 5
31	16 + 4	20 + 0	23 + 2
32	17 + 1	20 + 4	23 + 6
33	17 + 6	21 + 1	24 + 4
34	18 + 3	21 + 5	25 + 1
35	19 + 0	22 + 2	25 + 5
36	19 + 4	22 + 6	26 + 2
37	20 + 1	23 + 4	26 + 6
38	20 . 6	24 + 1	27 + 3
39	21 + 3	24 + 5	28 + 0
40	22 + 0	25 + 2	28 + 4
41	22 + 4	25 + 6	29 + 1
42	23 + 1	26 + 4	29 + 6
43	23 + 6	27 + 1	30 + 3
44	24 + 3	27 + 5	31 + 0
45	25 + 0	28 + 2	31 + 4
46	25 + 4	28 + 6	32 + 1
47	26 + 1	29 + 4	32 + 6
48	26 + 6	30 + 1	33 + 3
49	27 + 2	30 + 5	34 + 0
50	27 + 6	31 + 2	34 + 4
51	28 + 4	31 + 6	35 + 1
52	29 + 1	32 + 4	35 + 6
53	29 + 5	33 + 0	36 + 3
54	30 + 2	33 + 4	37 + 0
55	30 + 6	34 + 1	37 + 4
56	31 + 4	34 + 6	38 + 1
57	32 + 1	35 + 3	38 + 5
58	32 + 5	36 + 0	39 + 2
59	33 + 2	36 + 4	39 + 6
60	33 + 6	37 + 1	40 + 4
61	34 + 4	37 + 6	41 + 1
62	35 + 1	38 + 3	41 + 5
63	35 + 5	39 + 0	42 + 2
64	36 + 2	39 + 4	42 + 6
65	36 + 6	40 + 1	43 + 4

*From Jeanty P, Cantraine F, Cousaert E, et al: The binocular distance: A new way to estimate gestational age. J Ultrasound Med 1984; 3:241–243. Used with permission.

therapeutic amniocentesis in one case, the fetal facial structures were examined and showed two mouths, two noses, two ears, and four eyes (Fig 7–7).[25] Each of the cases detected prenatally died.

In the absence of anencephaly, visualization of duplication of intracranial contents distinguishes this entity from others. Even in anencephalic fetuses, however, the characteristic duplication of facial structures is specific for diprosopus. Sagittal and parasagittal scans of the facial profile, as well as coronal scans through the level of the orbits and of the nose show three or four orbits and two noses. Detection of the two noses separating the central orbits from the two lateral orbits distinguishes diprosopus from other periorbital structures, such as lacrymal duct cysts.

Associated Findings

The incidence of neural tube defects, especially anencephaly, is high in diprosopus. Each of the reported cases with diprosopus had concomitant spinal dysraphism, and one also had a diaphragmatic hernia in addition to the polyhydramnios, hydrocephaly, and partial duplication of intracranial structures.

Otocephaly

Clinical and Pathologic Findings

Otocephaly is a rare spectrum of malformations always associated with agnathia or micrognathia.[27] It represents a failure of ascent of the auricles during embryogenesis, but in the more severe cases complete failure of neural crest development and migration occurs resulting in absence of the eyes and forebrain. Absence of the mouth also may occur. Otocephaly is reported to be incompatible with life.[27]

Sonographic Findings

Cayea et al. reported a case of otocephaly at 26 weeks in which no normal facial anatomy was evident (Fig 7–8).[27] An anterior encephalocele protruded in the midline at the level of the forehead. Two obliquely angled structures resembling ears were noted near the midline in the midfacial region. No orbits or mouth were present.

Associated Findings

Other reported anomalies in association with otocephaly include adrenal hypoplasia, single umbilical artery, alobar holoprosencephaly, hypoplastic tongue, tracheoesophageal fistula, and cardiac defects.[27] The case detected prenatally also had polyhydramnios.

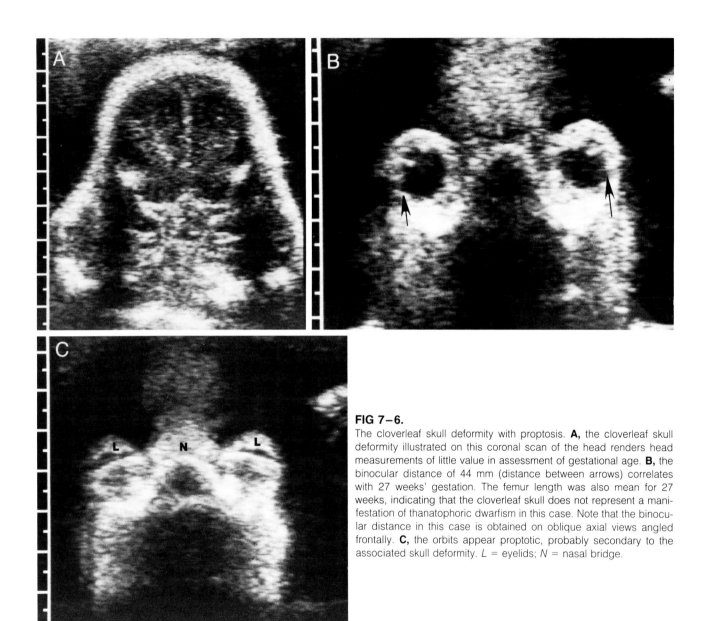

FIG 7–6.
The cloverleaf skull deformity with proptosis. **A,** the cloverleaf skull deformity illustrated on this coronal scan of the head renders head measurements of little value in assessment of gestational age. **B,** the binocular distance of 44 mm (distance between arrows) correlates with 27 weeks' gestation. The femur length was also mean for 27 weeks, indicating that the cloverleaf skull does not represent a manifestation of thanatophoric dwarfism in this case. Note that the binocular distance in this case is obtained on oblique axial views angled frontally. **C,** the orbits appear proptotic, probably secondary to the associated skull deformity. *L* = eyelids; *N* = nasal bridge.

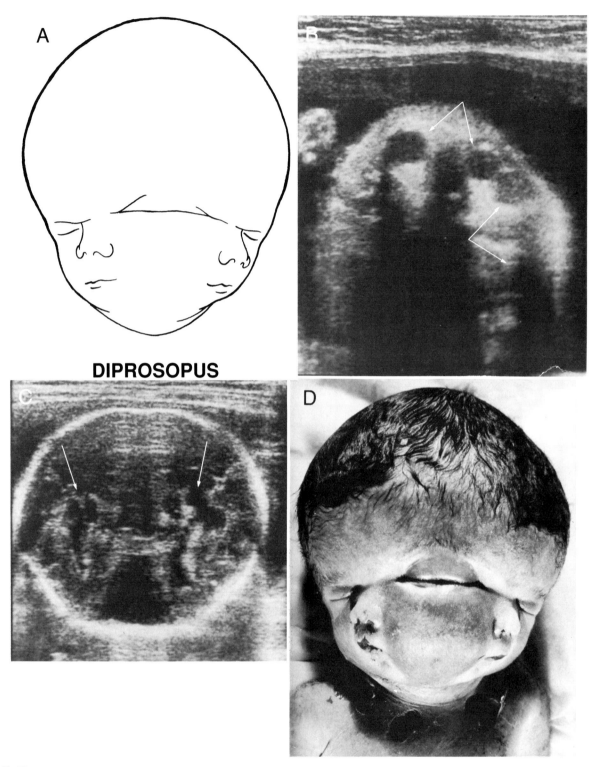

DIPROSOPUS

FIG 7–7.
Diprosopus. **A,** this drawing illustrates partial or complete craniofacial duplication indicative of diprosopus. The degree of facial duplication varies. **B,** scan of the face at 28 weeks shows four globes *(arrows)*. The two median globes share a single orbit. **C,** angled axial scan of the head displays duplication of the lateral ventricles *(arrows)*. **D,** postmortem photograph illustrates the duplication of facial structures with a single sarge midline orbit. (From Okazaki JR, Wilson JL, Holmes SM, et al: Diprosopus: Diagnosis in utero. AJR 1987; 149:147–148. Used by permission.)

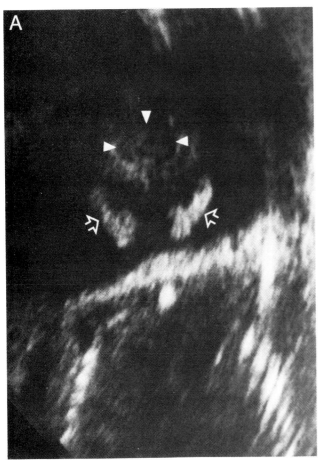

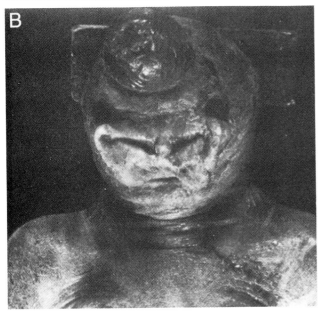

FIG 7–8.
Otocephaly. **A,** coronal scan of the face at 26 weeks shows absence of the eyes with an anterior encephalocele *(arrowheads)* and two soft tissue structures resembling ears obliquely positioned near the midline *(open arrows).* **B,** postmortem photograph illustrates the absence of orbits and nose with midline ears and anterior encephalocele. (From Cayea PD, Bieber FR, Ross MJ, et al: Sonographic findings in otocephaly (synotia). J Ultrasound Med 1985; 4:377–379. Used by permission.)

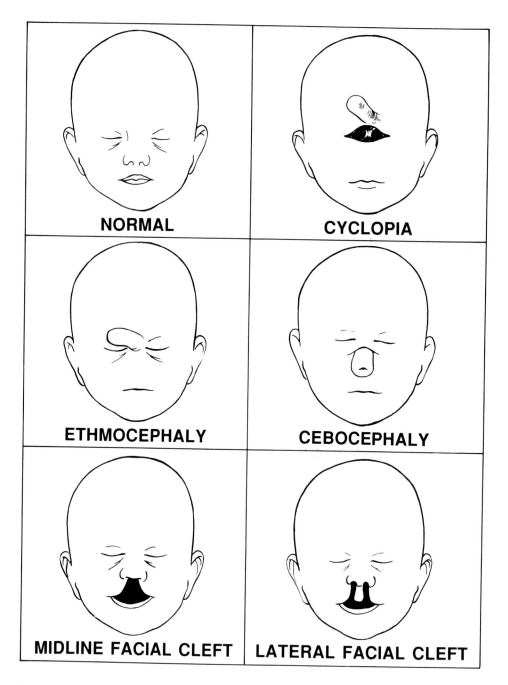

NORMAL   **CYCLOPIA**

ETHMOCEPHALY   **CEBOCEPHALY**

MIDLINE FACIAL CLEFT   **LATERAL FACIAL CLEFT**

FIG 7–9.
Facial features of holoprosencephaly. These drawings illustrate the normal facial features in contrast with the variable facial features of holoprosencephaly. In cyclopia, the proboscis projects from the lower forehead superior to one median orbit and the nose is absent. Ethmocephaly is very similar to cyclopia, but has two narrowly-placed orbits with a proboscis and absent nose. In cebocephaly, a rudimentary nose with a single nostril and hypotelorism are present. Hypotelorism may occur with a median cleft lip or bilateral cleft lip.

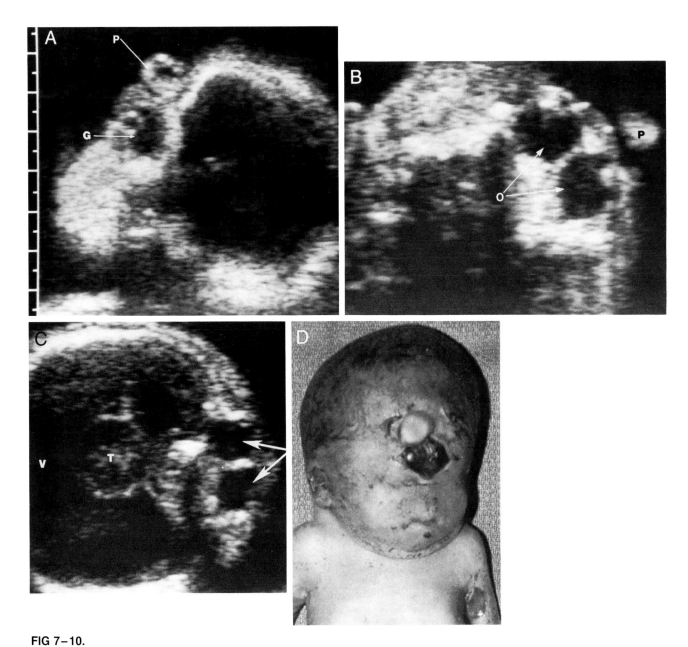

FIG 7–10.
Cyclopia with alobar holoprosencephaly. **A,** sagittal scan of the face displays the proboscis (*P*) projecting from the forehead above a single median globe (*G*) with absence of the nose. **B,** oblique axial scan again shows the proboscis and the two orbits (*O*) within one median globe. **C,** axial scan of the head demonstrates the two paramedian orbits within one globe (*arrows*) fused thalami (*T*), and single ventricle (*V*) indicative of alobar holoprosencephaly with cyclopia. **D,** postmortem photograph confirms the prenatal facial findings. (Courtesy of Laurence A Mack, MD, University of Washington Hospital, Seattle, WA.)

Hypotelorism/Holoprosencephaly

Clinical and Pathologic Findings

In the vast majority of cases in which hypotelorism has been detected prenatally, the decreased interorbital distance has been part of the holoprosencephaly sequence.[29–31, 35, 37, 38, 40–43] Other causes for hypotelorism include chromosomal aberrations, microcephaly, maternal phenylketonuria, Meckel-Gruber syndrome, myotonic dystrophy, the Williams syndrome, oculodental dysplasia and trigonocephaly.[3, 4, 12, 13]

Holoprosencephaly results from variable but incomplete median cleavage of the prosencephalon during organogenesis. Facial malformations secondary to aplasia or hypoplasia of the median facial bones are extremely common in the holoprosencephaly sequence.[33, 34, 36, 39] The most severe facial deformities occur with alobar holoprosencephaly in which there has been complete absence of cleavage of the prosencephalon into cerebral hemispheres. This produces characteristic intracranial and facial findings including (Fig 7–9):

1. Cyclopia with one median orbit, proboscis from the lower forehead, and absent nose (Fig 7–10).
2. Ethmocephaly, with proboscis between two narrowly placed orbits, and absent nose.
3. Cebocephaly with hypotelorism and rudimentary nose (Figs 7–11 and 7–12).
4. Hypotelorism, median cleft lip, and flat nose (Fig 7–13).
5. Bilateral cleft lip.

Following the dictum that "the face predicts the brain," all cases with cyclopia, ethmocephaly, cebocephaly, or hypotelorism with median cleft lip have holoprosencephaly, and most are of the alobar type.[33] However, not all patients with holoprosencephaly, even the severe alobar type, have facial deformity. Semilobar holoprosencephaly, a less severe form than the alobar type, is often associated with hypotelorism and median cleft lip or bilateral cleft lip. Facial deformities are usually absent in lobar holoprosencephaly, the least severe form.

Sonographic Findings

Three series concerning prenatal sonographic diagnosis of holoprosencephaly that concentrate on facial findings describe a total of 32 cases, 28 with the alobar type, and 4 with the semilobar form of holoprosencephaly (Table 7–2).[37, 40, 41] Although the menstrual

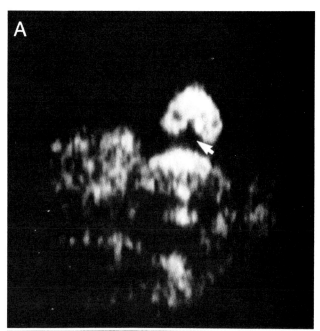

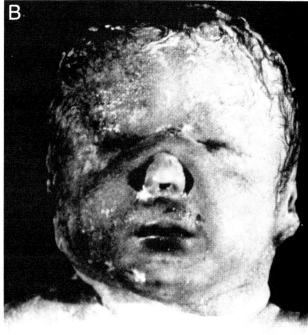

FIG 7–11.
Cebocephaly. **A,** coronal scan of the nose and lips at 29 weeks demonstrates a single nostril *(arrow)*. Additional scans showed hypotelorism, alobar holoprosencephaly, and polyhydramnios. **B,** postmortem photograph confirms the prenatal findings. (From Bundy AL, Lidov H, Soliman M, et al: Antenatal sonographic diagnosis of cebocephaly. J Ultrasound Med 1988; 7:395–398. Used by permission.)

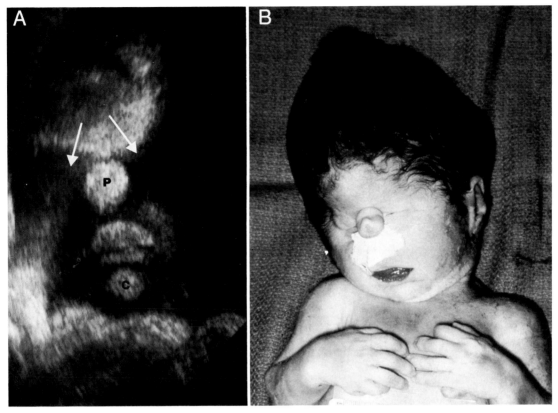

FIG 7–12.
Cebocephaly. **A,** coronal scan of the face demonstrates an unusually protuberant nose and hypotelorism. Other scans showed intracranial features typical of holoprosencephaly. **B,** postmortem photograph confirms the cebocephaly and hypotelorism. *P* = proboscis; *C* = chin; *arrows* = orbits. (From Nyberg DA, Mack LA, Hirsch J, et al: Fetal hydrocephalus: Sonographic detection and clinical significance of associated anomalies. Radiology 1987; 163:187–191. Used by permission.)

age at diagnosis ranged from 14 to 38 weeks, 27 of 32 cases were diagnosed after 20 weeks. Chromosomal analysis among 26 fetuses showed abnormal karyotype in 12 cases, 9 of which had trisomy 13. The predominant facial features detected sonographically included hypotelorism (13 cases) and facial cleft (12 cases). Postnatally, 15 cases had hypotelorism with a facial cleft. Six cases also had cyclopia, five of which had been detected prenatally. Four fetuses had normal facial anatomy by ultrasound and confirmed at birth. In only one fetus was the face inaccessible to sonographic examination because of fetal positioning.

Associated Anomalies

Extrafacial anomalies dominate the sonographic findings in holoprosencephaly.[40] Chapter 5 discusses the specific intracranial and extracraniofacial findings of holoprosencephaly in detail. However, detection of facial anomalies in holoprosencephaly warrants a detailed search for concomitant extracraniofacial abnormalities, reported to occur in 8 of 9 cases in one series.[40]

Although specific intracranial findings permit accurate diagnosis of holoprosencephaly and are typically more obvious than are facial anomalies, detection of facial abnormalities in holoprosencephaly helps predict the outcome as well as the likelihood of concomitant extracraniofacial malformations.[40] Cyclopia, ethmocephaly, cebocephaly, and median facial cleft all signify a poor prognosis, with survival rarely extending beyond 1 year of age, probably because most fetuses with these findings have alobar or semilobar holoprosencephaly rather than the less severe lobar type.

Hypertelorism/Anterior Cephalocele

Clinical and Pathologic Findings

Increased interorbital distance (hypertelorism) may occur sporadically as a primary defect or may be secondary to other malformations of the cranium and face. Secondary hypertelorism occurs as part of many syndromes or malformations, such as anterior cephalocele. Smith lists 47 associated syndromes, many of which are chromosomal or inherited entities or occur

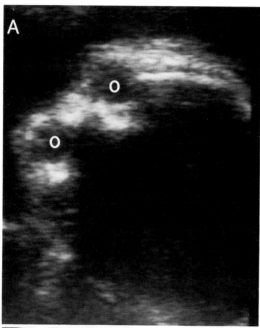

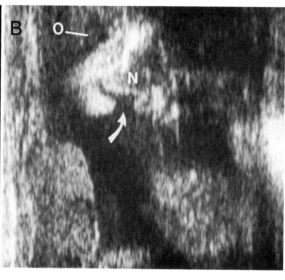

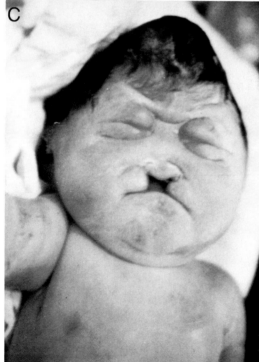

FIG 7–13.
Midline facial cleft with holoprosencephaly. **A,** axial scan through the orbits of this 34-week fetus with alobar holoprosencephaly and midline facial cleft shows the hypotelorism and flattened midface. Other scans showed the intracranial findings characteristic of alobar holoprosencephaly. **B,** frontal scan of the face from a similar case demonstrates midline facial cleft. **C,** postnatal photograph illustrates the prenatal findings. *N* = flattened nose; *O* = orbit; curved arrow = midline facial cleft. (Parts **A** and **C** from Nyberg DA, Mack LA, Bronstein A, et al: Holoprosencephaly: Prenatal sonographic diagnosis. AJR 1987; 149:1051–1058. Used by permission.)

TABLE 7–2.

Summary of Facial and Karyotype Features in 32 Fetuses
With the Holoprosencephaly Sequence*

	Alobar	Semilobar
N	28	4
Prenatal facial features		
No abnormalities seen	6	3
Cyclopia	5	-
Ethmocephaly	-	-
Cebocephaly	-	-
Proboscis	2	1
Hypotelorism	12	1
Microphthalmia/anophthalmia	4	-
Facial cleft	12	-
Absent nasal bridge	6	-
Postnatal diagnosis		
Normal	2	2
Cyclopia	6	-
Ethmocephaly	1	2
Cebocephaly	3	-
Hypotelorism/facial cleft	15	-
Macerated fetus	1	-
Karyotype		
Normal	13	1
Trisomy 13	8	1
Other abnormal	2	1
Not performed	5	1

* Data from references 37, 40, and 41.

as a result of maternal teratogen exposure.[12] Detection of unequivocal hypertelorism in a fetus at risk for a specific syndrome provides convincing evidence of recurrence.

With rare exceptions, the few cases of hypertelorism detected prenatally have occurred in the setting of an anterior cephalocele.[44, 45, 46] Most cephaloceles occur in the occipital region and only rarely in the frontonasal region, where they project through a defect in the ethmoid, sphenoid, or frontal bone. Frontal cephaloceles often displace the globe downward and outward and produce hypertelorism. They are generally smaller than cephaloceles in other locations and tend to have a much better prognosis, unless they are a part of a multiple malformation syndrome such as atelosteogenesis.[44]

Sonographic Findings

A fronto-ethmoidal cephalocele protruding through a calvarial defect frontally may produce hypertelorism and a mass visible on the sagittal profile view or on axial views through the periorbital region (Fig 7–14).[44, 46] Visualization of the calvarial defect assures the diagnosis and distinguishes cephaloceles from other frontonasal masses or structures such as lacrymal duct cysts, or-

bital duplication (diprosopus), facial hemangioma, or dermoid cysts.

Associated Anomalies

Whereas occipital cephaloceles typically result from incomplete closure of the rostral portion of the neural tube, frontal cephaloceles often appear to arise from intrinsic calvarial defects. For example, failure of endochondral bone development at the base of the skull in atelosteogenesis may result in a frontal calvarial defect.[44] In such cases or in other cases with microcephaly or multiple malformations, the underlying malformation syndrome characteristically determines the prognosis and recurrence risk, as well as the predominant sonographic findings.[44]

Microphthalmia/Anophthalmia

Clinical and Pathologic Findings

Measurement of the intraocular diameter may detect recurrence of one of approximately 25 syndromes associated with microphthalmos.[3, 4, 12, 13] Routine measurement of ocular diameters, however, would not be expected to provide more than a low diagnostic yield. Nevertheless, since the eyes derive embryologically from neural folds of the forebrain, assessment for the presence or absence of microphthalmia when intracranial abnormalities are present or in a fetus at familial risk may provide useful data, especially since a clinical association exists between microphthalmia and mental retardation.[21, 47]

Anophthalmia results from failure of the optic vesicle to form. It occurs more rarely than microphthalmia, but its manifestations are more obvious than microphthalmia, assuming the orbital region is accessible to scanning. Taybi lists the causes for anophthalmia as trisomy 13, Lenz's syndrome (X-linked microphthalmia), Goldenhar-Gorlin syndrome, and microphthalmia with digital anomalies.[13] Among the several etiologies that may result in anophthalmia, only the Goldenhar-Gorlin syndrome has associated ipsilateral ear and facial abnormalities. This syndrome probably results from diminished unilateral embryonic vascular supply to the first and second branchial arches and occurs in approximately 1 in 5,000 births.

The prognosis for microphthalmia and anophthalmia varies with the underlying etiology and severity of associated malformations. In general, however, it is frequently associated with mental retardation.[21, 48]

Sonographic Findings

During the second and third trimesters, the ocular diameter increases progressively but not linearly in

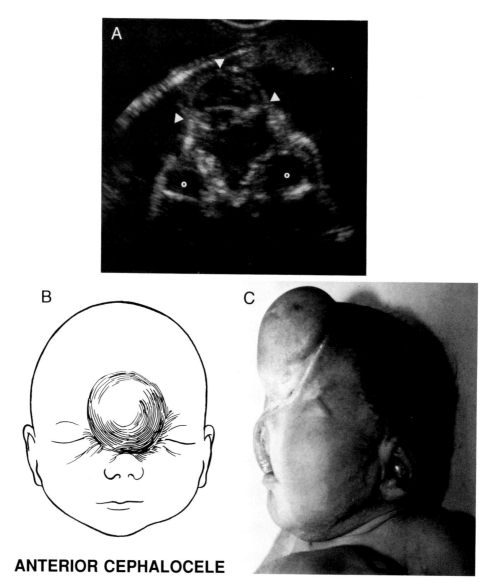

ANTERIOR CEPHALOCELE

FIG 7–14.
Hypertelorism with frontal encephalocele. **A,** axial sonogram through the level of the orbits shows hypertelorism with the orbits displaced laterally by a large frontal encephalocele. **B,** frontal drawing illustrates the hypertelorism secondary to an anterior cephalocele. **C,** postnatal photograph confirms the prenatal findings. *O* = orbits; *arrow heads* = encephalocele. (Courtesy of Philippe Jeanty, M.D., Vanderbilt University, Nashville, TN.)

size.[21] Data regarding ocular diameters published by Jeanty et al. for outer dimensions of the orbit compare with those for the diameter of the spherical globe itself published by Birnholz.[21, 22] Although normal eye size becomes progressively more variable in the third trimester, Birnholz states that a transverse globe diameter of 15 mm or more excludes microphthalmia.[21]

Unless the orbits are unequivocally small, diagnosis of microphthalmia during the second trimester may be considerably more difficult than in the third trimester. In such cases ocular measurements provide evidence to confirm the sonologist's impression of abnormality.

Feldman et al. reported unmistakable microphthalmia as a manifestation of recurrent Fraser syndrome (autosomal recessive cryptophthalmus, usually with microphthalmus or anophthalmus, hypoplastic nares, and ambiguous genitalia) in a fetus with concomitant hydrocephalus at 18 weeks' gestation.[47] In this case, the severe microphthalmia in the setting of familial risk for recurrence enabled accurate diagnosis.

Anophthalmia demonstrates striking absence of the globe and often the orbit on the axial view through the expected level of the orbits (Fig 7–15). It has been detected prenatally in a case with the Goldenhar-Gorlin

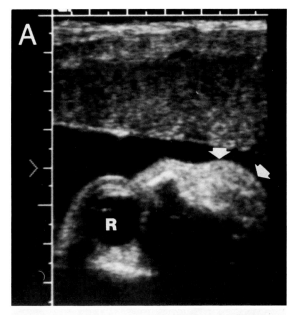

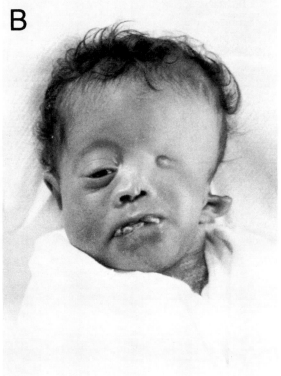

FIG 7–15.
Hemifacial microsomia (Goldenhar-Gorlin syndrome) at 30 weeks. **A,** axial scan through the level of the orbit demonstrates absence of the left orbit. Additional scans showed low-set and malformed ipsilateral ear (see Fig 7–36). **B,** postnatal photograph confirms the prenatal findings. *Arrows* = absent left orbit; *R* = right orbit. (From Tamas DE, Mahony BS, Bowie JD, et al: Prenatal sonographic diagnosis of hemifacial microsomia (Goldenhar-Gorlin syndrome). J Ultrasound Med 1986; 5:461–463. Used by permission.)

syndrome (hemifacial microsomia).[48] Cayea et al. described absence of the orbits in a case of otocephaly.[27]

Associated Findings

Because of the potential association between anophthalmia or severe microphthalmia and chromosomal, extremity, or other craniofacial abnormalities, detection of the absence of the globe or severe micophthalmia should prompt a chromosomal analysis as well as careful search of the fetus, especially for other potentially subtle facial or extremity malformations.

Periorbital Masses

Clinical and Pathologic Findings

Lacrimal duct cysts (dacryocystoceles) result from impatency of the distal portion of the nasolacrimal duct.[49] The nasolacrimal duct usually becomes patent by the eighth intrauterine month, but approximately 30% of all newborns have an impatent nasolacrimal duct. Only 2% of newborns have a symptomatic cyst. Even when symptomatic, dacryocystoceles are typically isolated findings.

Dacryocystoceles occur inferomedial to the orbit. This typical location suggests the diagnosis over other much less common periorbital masses, including anterior encephalocele, dermoid, or hemangioma. An anterior encephalocele typically displaces the globe downward and outward and has an underlying calvarial defect with hydrocephaly. A periorbital dermoid cyst typically occurs superolateral to the globe and only rarely occurs inferomedially.

A periorbital hemangioma may resemble a dacryocystocele in size and location, but typically exhibits the characteristic Doppler signal. Cutaneous hemangiomata are common at birth, and most remain small and clinically insignificant. Although they remain histologically benign, occasionally an hemangioma may enlarge rapidly, progressively distort normal structures, and obstruct the airway, esophagus, or auditory canal.[50–52]

Sonographic Findings

Antenatal sonographic reports of dacryocystoceles have documented their typical location inferomedial to the globe (Fig 7–16).[49] They exhibit hypoechoic texture without concomitant displacement of the globe but with synchronous eye movements. In reported cases, the cysts measured approximately one cm in diameter and had not been evident at 20–23 weeks, but became apparent at 30–33 weeks.[49] Their hypoechoic echotexture differentiates dacryocystoceles from periorbital hemangiomata, which are typically highly echogenic. In addition, hemangiomata detected prena-

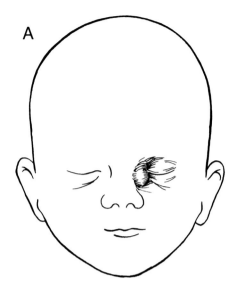

DACROCYSTOCELE

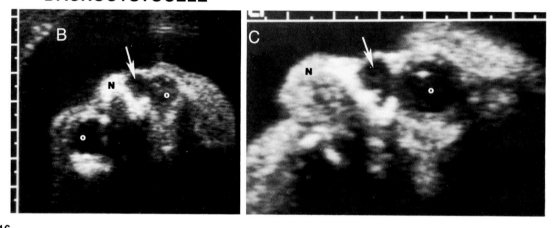

FIG 7–16.
Dacryocystoceles. **A,** this drawing illustrates the characteristic location of a lacrimal duct cyst (dacryocystocele). **B** and **C,** these two fetuses each have a small lacrimal duct cyst (dacryocystocele) that resolved spontaneously postnatally. Both scans are slightly oblique from the axial plane to show the dacryocystocele along the inferomedial margin of the orbit adjacent to the nose. In both cases, the globe is not displaced and synchronous eye movements were noted. Mild idiopathic polyhydramnios, but no other detectable abnormalities are present. *Arrow* = dacryocystocele; *O* = orbit; *N* = nose. (From Davis WK, Mahony BS, Carroll BA, et al: Antenatal sonographic detection of benign dacryocystoceles (Lacrimal duct cysts). J Ultrasound Med 1987; 6:461–465. Used by permission.)

tally tend to be larger and exhibit characteristic Doppler signal.[51]

The facial hemangioma reported by Meizner et al. at 32 weeks described a 6 cm homogeneously echogenic cheek mass with concomitant severe polyhydramnios and subsequent intrauterine demise (Fig 7–17).[50] In this unusual case, the etiology for the polyhydramnios and demise remained idiopathic. Lasser et al. reported a giant cystic cavernous hemangioma of the frontotemporal region detected at 25 weeks.[51] At 35 weeks the mass measured 12 × 24 cm and Doppler velocimetry of the mass showed evidence for blood flow through low-resistance channels. Despite extensive therapy, the newborn died at 10 days of age.

Conversely, Pennell et al. reported a case at 30 weeks without associated polyhydramnios and with a normal outcome.[52] The well-defined 3.5 cm exophytic mass anterior to the ear had similar echotexture to the placenta and contained numerous pulsating vascular spaces. Although it grew to 4 cm in diameter 3 weeks later and to 6 cm at term, it regressed to 2.5 cm at 6.5 months of age. This example demonstrates the more typical benign course of regression of hemangiomata.

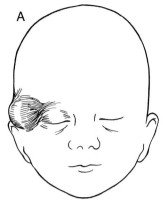

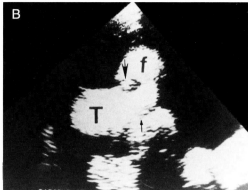

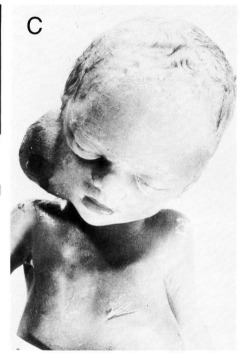

DERMOID/HEMANGIOMA

FIG 7–17.
Cavernous hemangioma of the cheek. **A,** A hemangioma may resemble a dacryocystocele in location (inferomedial to the orbit) but has characteristic Doppler signal. It may also occur in a variety of other locations, including the cheek or superolateral to the orbit. A periorbital dermoid typically occurs superolateral to the orbit. **B,** frontal sonogram of the face at 32 weeks in a fetus with polyhydramnios and a facial cavernous hemangioma shows the 6 cm echogenic tumor mass of the right cheek. **C,** postnatal photograph confirms the prenatal findings. X-ray demonstrated multiple small calcifications within the cavernous hemangioma. T = hemangioma; *large arrow* = eye; f = forehead; *smaller arrow* = mouth region. (From Meizner I, Bar-Ziv J, Holcberg G, et al: In utero prenatal diagnosis of fetal facial tumor—hemangioma. J Clin Ultrasound 1985; 13:435–437. Used by permission.)

Intraocular Findings

Clinical and Pathologic Findings

The Walker-Warburg syndrome, a rare autosomal recessive condition, includes severe abnormalities of cortical gyrations (type 2 lissencephaly), hydrocephaly, and abnormalities of the eyes.[56] Approximately 50% of cases have an occipital encephalocele, and some fetuses with the syndrome also have microphthalmia. However, retinal dysplasia and detachment are considered essential for the diagnosis.

Since the eye derives embryologically from the forebrain, several investigators have suggested that observation of fetal eye movement patterns and regression of the hyaloid artery of the eye may provide useful information regarding concomitant brain growth and functional development of the central nervous system.

Sonographic Findings

Farrell et al. diagnosed the Walker-Warburg syndrome in utero on the basis of detection of retinal detachment in the setting of a small occipital encephalo-cele and hydrocephalus but an unremarkable family history (Fig 7–18).[56] The retinal detachment was not apparent at 30 weeks, but at 32 weeks the orbit contained an abnormal echogenic ring initially felt to represent an unusually small globe. At 35 weeks a conical echogenic structure within the globe was clearly present, indicative of retinal detachment. Crowe et al. diagnosed recurrent Walker-Warburg syndrome at 15 weeks on the basis of visualization of an encephalocele, but did not detect orbital or intraorbital abnormalities.[55]

Birnholz reported that slow eye movements normally occur by 16 weeks' gestation and that rapid eye movements begin at 23 weeks.[53] The rapid eye movements become more frequent between 24 and 35 weeks, after which eye inactivity becomes more common.[53] Birnholz also detected abnormal fetal eye movement patterns in eight fetuses between 16 and 39 weeks, all of whom had obvious abnormalities of brain structure.[53]

The hyaloid artery originates from the main ophthalmic artery and terminates at the posterior surface

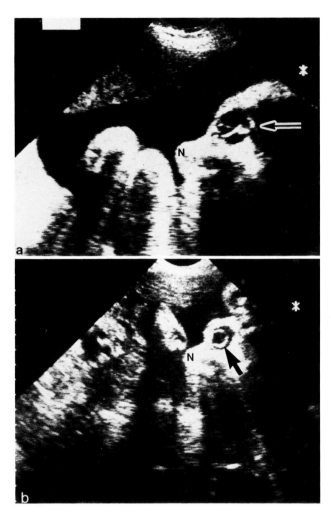

FIG 7–18.
The Walker-Warburg syndrome at 35 weeks. Coronal **(A)** and axial **(B)** views of the right orbit display the echogenic detached retina as a conical structure within the globe. The detached retina has its base toward the lens and its apex pointing posteriorly toward the optic nerve. Other scans showed hydrocephalus, absence of the cerebellar vermis, and occipital encephalocele. *Arrow* = detached retina; *N* = nose. (From Farrell SA, Toi A, Leadman ML, et al: Prenatal diagnosis of retinal detachment in Walker-Warburg syndrome. Am J Med Genet 1987; 28:619–624. Used by permission.)

of the lens. It appears as an echogenic line coursing centrally through the eye and becomes beaded in appearance as it begins to regress.[54] Birnholz and Farrell reported that the hyaloid artery normally regresses by 30 weeks' gestation but remained visible beyond 30 weeks in 9 of 25 abnormal pregnancies (trisomy 21, 3 cases; isolated microcephaly, 2 cases; trisomy 13, trisomy 18, fetal alcohol syndrome, fetal hydantoin syndrome, 1 case each).[54] Therefore, delayed regression of the hyaloid artery may indicate retarded brain development.[54]

THE UPPER LIP, MOUTH, AND TONGUE

Evaluation of the mouth, upper lip, and tongue provides useful information regarding cleft lip or macroglossia, especially in the setting of a positive family history, polyhydramnios, or concomitant anomalies. Detection of facial clefts, macroglossia, or an unusually shaped mouth may suggest the presence of a syndrome. For example, Witt et al. described a fetus with a small mouth fixed in the open position as one manifestation of recurrent restrictive dermopathy at 32 weeks.[67] Occasionally, a mass protruding into the mouth may be visible or produce an unusual facial expression, with

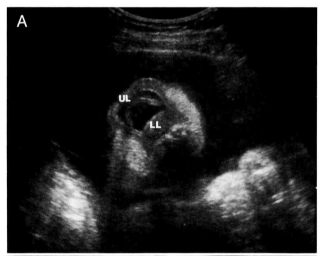

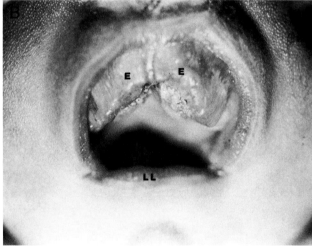

FIG 7–19.
Anterior encephalocele extending into the mouth. **A,** frontal sonogram of the mouth demonstrates the mouth to be widely open secondary to a large anterior encephalocele which extended partially into the mouth. **B,** postnatal photograph confirms the prenatal findings. *UL* = upper lip; *LL* = lower lip; *E* = encephalocele. (Courtesy of Philippe Jeanty, MD, Vanderbilt University, Nashville, TN.)

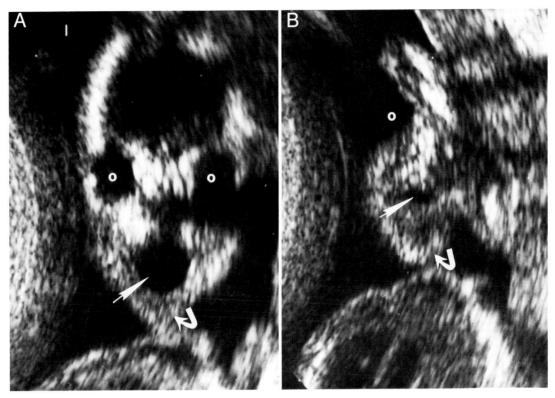

FIG 7–20.
Normal mouth opening and closing. Unlike the fetus illustrated in Figure 7–20, the normal fetus may intermittently open its mouth widely **(A)** but then closes the mouth spontaneously **(B),** as these frontal scans obtained within several seconds of each other illustrate. *Straight arrow = mouth; curved arrow = chin; O = orbit.*

persistent opening of the mouth (Figs 7–19 and 7–20). Furthermore, detection of fetal regurgitation in the setting of otherwise unexplained polyhydramnios provides corroborative information to suggest esophageal atresia.[60]

CLEFT LIP/CLEFT PALATE

Clinical and Pathologic Findings

Cleft lip (and/or palate), the most common congenital facial deformity at birth, results from failure of fusion of the frontal prominence with the maxillary process during embryogenesis.[19, 20] Cleft lip and/or palate may be complete or incomplete, unilateral or bilateral, symmetric or asymmetric. Approximately two thirds of those with cleft lip also have cleft palate.[3]

Over 100 syndromes are associated with cleft lip/palate.[12] The etiology remains idiopathic in most cases, however, and syndromes probably account for less than 10% of all cases.[3, 12] In cases not associated with a syndrome, the etiology probably represents a multifactorial combination of environmental and genetic factors with a threshold effect.[3] Recurrence risk ranges

from 4% with one affected sibling to 17% with both an affected sibling and parent.[3] In cases associated with multiple malformations or a syndrome, the likelihood of having cleft lip and/or cleft palate depends upon the associated malformations or syndrome (Table 7–3).

Although the incidence of cleft lip/palate apparently varies widely among various races and geographic locations, the incidence for non–syndromic cases is frequently cited in the range of 1 in 800 for cleft lip with or without cleft palate, 1 in 1,300 for cleft lip and palate, and 1 in 2,000 for isolated cleft lip or palate.[66] Japanese and certain native American tribes may have a higher incidence, whereas Afro-American blacks apparently have a lower incidence.[3] Males are affected more commonly than females, especially in more severe cases.[3]

Antenatal detection of a facial cleft may help prepare the parents for the visually disturbing, but frequently repairable deformity so that the birth becomes a process of confirmation of diagnosis with a treatment plan in place rather than one of surprise. Christ has even proposed in utero repair of facial clefts, a procedure which has been accomplished in mice without any recognizable deformity at birth.[63]

TABLE 7–3.

Some Common Associations With Cleft Lip and/or Palate.
(Partial List Concentrating on the Entities That the Sonologist
May Encounter With Relative Frequency)*

	% With CL/CP
Familial	
1 affected sib	4
1 affected parent	4
2 affected sibs	9
1 affected sib and 1 affected parent	17
Chromosomal abnormalities	
Trisomy 13	60
Trisomy 18	15
Trisomy 21	0.5
Triploidy	30
Many translocation syndromes	20–40
Selected malformations and syndromes	
Acrocephalopolysyndactyly	32
Amniotic band syndrome	common
Anencephaly	10
Congenital heart disease	2
Diastrophic dysplasia	20–50
Holoprosencephaly	50
Kniest dysplasia	40
Meckel-Gruber syndrome	90–100
Multiple pterygium syndrome	90–100
Roberts' syndrome	100
Spondyloepiphyseal dysplasia congenita	35

*Modified from Bergsma D: *Birth Defects Compendium,* ed 2. For The
National Foundation—March of Dimes. New York, Alan R Liss, Inc,
1979.
CL/CP = cleft lip and/or cleft palate.

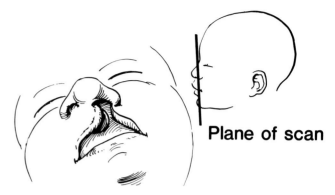

FIG 7–21.
Facial cleft. This drawing illustrates a plane of section which visualizes clefts of the upper lip well. (From Meininger MG, Crist JE: Real-time ultrasonography for the prenatal diagnosis of facial clefts. Birth Defects 1982; 18:161–167. In Salinas C (ed): Craniofacial anomalies: New perspectives. New York, Alan R Liss, Inc for the March of Dimes Birth Defects Foundation. Used by permission.)

Sonographic Findings

Facial clefts constitute a special category of congenital abnormality with significant connotations regarding psychologic and social adaptation. These connotations and the relatively high incidence of non-syndromic clefting, even in the absence of familial risk, may render useful a routine survey of the lip for clefting. A positive family history of facial clefts increases the chance of recurrent facial cleft approximately 40 to 170-fold and warrants a careful search for facial cleft.

Despite the prevalence of cleft lip/palate, very few sonographic reports of isolated cleft lip and/or palate exist. Meizner detected one case at 27 weeks and Salzman reported another case at 36 weeks, and in neither case was the familial risk stated (Fig 7–21).[8, 64] Seeds reported a case detected at 17 weeks with a positive family history, and Christ reported two other cases detected at 28 and 33 weeks.[62, 65] We have seen two cases with isolated cleft lip at 17–18 weeks without familial risk (Fig 7–22). Increased surveillance will undoubtedly detect additional cases.

Statistics regarding sensitivity, specificity, and accuracy of prenatal ultrasound for detection of cleft lip and/or palate are not yet available. Although some facial structures become visible by the end of the first trimester, development of soft tissue features of the face probably limit detection of clefts to approximately 16 weeks, and the rate of detection can reasonably be expected to increase thereafter until fetal position limits visualization.

When detected, cleft lip tends not to be subtle, although one must guard against a false-positive diagnosis based upon visualization of the normal philtrum (the midline groove of the upper lip) or frenulum labii superioris (Figs 7–23 and 7–24).[59] Frontal scans provide the optimal views of the face for visualization of clefts (see Fig 7–21). Placement of the transducer beneath the chin, above the forehead, or lateral to the cheek, followed by subtle changes in transducer angulation, permits sequential scans through the soft tissues of the lips, chin, alveolar ridge, and nose. Parasagittal and sagittal profile views only occasionally lend corroborative information. Frequently, the fetus holds its hands near the face, and the sonologist must wait for the hands to move.

Because of shadowing from facial bones, the findings of cleft palate may be much more subtle than cleft lip. Following detection of cleft lip, frontal scans obtained more posteriorly may demonstrate incomplete formation of the maxillary ridge indicating cleft palate. Again, one should exercise caution to avoid false-positive diagnosis of the basis of shadowing from maxillary ossification.

To our knowledge, isolated cleft palate has not been diagnosed prenatally, although Meizner reported one case with Pierre Robin syndrome, whose only finding detected prenatally was cleft palate.[8] However, Bundy described polyhydramnios with a small non-vi-

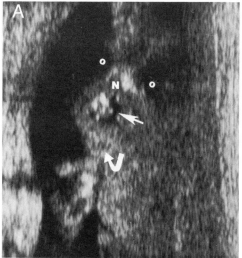

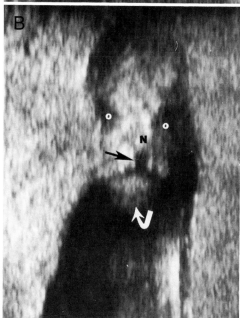

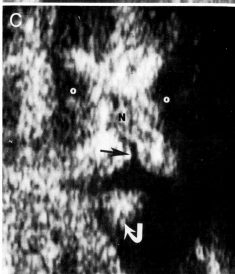

sualized fetal stomach as ancillary signs of cleft palate, presumably secondary to an abnormal swallowing mechanism.[61] Obviously, these ancillary signs may alternatively result from any cause for proximal gastrointestinal tract obstruction.

Associated Findings

Most cases of cleft lip/cleft palate diagnosed in utero have been detected as a manifestation of a syndrome, usually the holoprosencephaly sequence in conjunction with trisomy 13.[45, 57, 58, 64] Occasional cases with trisomy 18 have shown a cleft lip/cleft palate on prenatal ultrasound. Both of these syndromes have a dismal prognosis. The concomitant manifestations of the trisomy typically dominate the sonographic picture, and detection of the facial clefts only corroborates the impression. Nevertheless, detection of a facial cleft in the setting of holoprosencephaly correlates with a poor prognosis and may help prepare the parents to view their child at birth.

In trisomy 13, which occurs with an incidence of approximately 1 in 6,000 births, 60% of cases have cleft lip and cleft palate or cleft palate without cleft lip (Fig 7–25). In a series of 9 cases of trisomy 13 detected prenatally 5 of 9 (56%) had a facial cleft identified sonographically, and 4 of these also had holoprosencephaly.[58] Other common features of trisomy 13 include cystic kidneys, omphalocele, cardiac structural defects, and polydactyly. In trisomy 18, which occurs with an incidence of approximately 1 in 3,000 births, approximately 15% of cases have cleft lip and/or cleft palate. Among a series of 15 cases detected prenatally, the only facial abnormality seen was micrognathia, and none had a facial cleft.[58]

Cleft lip and/or palate also occurs in approximately 0.5% of cases with trisomy 21 and 30% of triploidy cases.[3] They occur in more than 90% of cases with the Meckel syndrome (encephalocele with enlarged and multicystic kidneys) and the multiple pterygium syndrome and are essential to the diagnosis of numerous other syndromes but uncommon in many others (see Table 7–3).[3] Prenatal detection of cleft lip and/or palate, therefore, should initiate careful search for other anomalies and may warrant chromosomal analysis.

FIG 7–22.
Isolated cleft lip/palate at 17–18 weeks. **A** and **B,** routine scanning of the face at 17 weeks' gestation demonstrates an isolated cleft lip and palate on these frontal scans. **C,** similar frontal scans at 18 weeks in another fetus show an isolated cleft lip. Most facial clefts detected prenatally occur as a manifestation of a syndrome in which more obvious findings indicate a high probability for facial cleft. *Straight arrow* = cleft lip/palate; *O* = orbits; *N* = nose; *curved arrow* = chin.

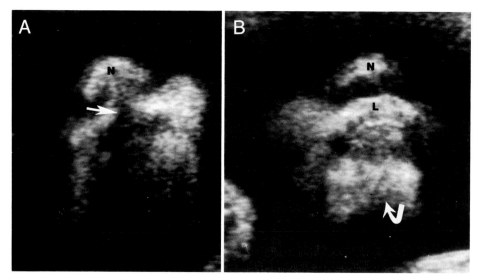

FIG 7–23.
The normal philtrum or frenulum of the upper lip simulating a cleft lip. **A,** frontal scan of the upper lip and nose suggests the possibility of a cleft lip. **B,** in such cases, scanning slightly anteriorly or posteriorly or at slightly different angles demonstrates the intact upper lip, This fetus was confirmed to be normal at birth. *Straight arrow* = philtrum; *L* = intact upper lip; *N* = nose; *curved arrow* = chin.

AMNIOTIC BAND SYNDROME

Clinical and Pathologic Findings

The amniotic band syndrome is a common non-recurrent cause of various fetal malformations involving the craniofacial region, limbs, and trunk. It occurs in approximately 1 in 1,200 live births and as many as 1 in 56 spontaneous abortions.[76, 79] Extremely protean clinical manifestations of the syndrome may produce bizarre facial clefts, fissures, or slash defects in non–embryologic distributions. Rupture of the amnion, with subsequent entanglement of the fetus by fibrous mesodermic bands that emanate from the chorionic side of the amnion, probably causes the clinical features of the syndrome, although some authors propose a teratogen effect.[70, 71, 77, 81]

The facial defects in the amniotic band syndrome probably result from fetal swallowing of the fibrous bands. The swallowed portion of the band presumably tethers the unswallowed portion, which then cuts across the face in random fashion and causes the bizarre slash defects. The prognosis for the amniotic band syndrome varies widely, ranging from death secondary to disruption of the umbilical cord or discordant anencephaly to minor facial clefts, extremity amputations, or lymphedema.[76, 82]

Sonographic Findings

Detection of facial clefts in locations other than the common embryologic paramedian or median sites suggests the amniotic band syndrome and warrants a careful search for other manifestations of the syndrome including lymphedema, amputation, asymmetric encephalocele, and gastropleural schisis (Fig 7–26).[72, 78] Visualization of the fibrous bands attached to the fetus with characteristic deformities and restriction of motion is diagnostic of the amniotic band syndrome and precludes the need for chromosomal analysis. Even visualization of the characteristic fetal deformities when the bands cannot be seen provides strong evidence of the syndrome.[75, 78, 79, 80, 82, 83, 96]

MACROGLOSSIA

Clinical and Pathologic Findings

The Beckwith-Wiedemann syndrome is probably the most common cause for an enlarged tongue prenatally. This syndrome usually occurs sporadically, but may recur as a dominant trait with incomplete penetrance and variable expressivity.[12] The most common congenital findings include macroglossia, gigantism, and omphalocele but hepatomegaly, renal hyperplasia and dysplasia, distinctive ear creases, and prolonged neonatal hypoglycemia are also commonly present.[84] Macroglossia occurs in 97.5% of cases, whereas 60% have other anomalies.[87]

Sonographic Findings

Detection of an unmistakably enlarged and protuberant tongue has permitted the prenatal diagnosis of the Beckwith-Wiedemann syndrome, especially when

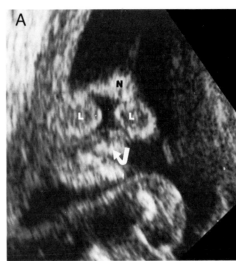

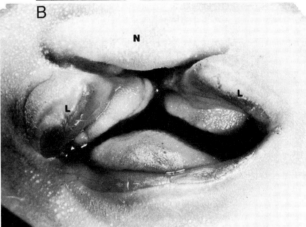

FIG 7–25.
Trisomy 13 with a midline cleft lip and palate. **A,** frontal sonogram
of the mouth at 21 weeks demonstrates the midline cleft upper lip
separating the two sides of the lip. Additional scans showed an
omphalocele. **B,** postnatal photograph confirms the prenatal facial
features. *L* = portions of upper lip separated by cleft; *N* = nose;
curved arrow = tongue.

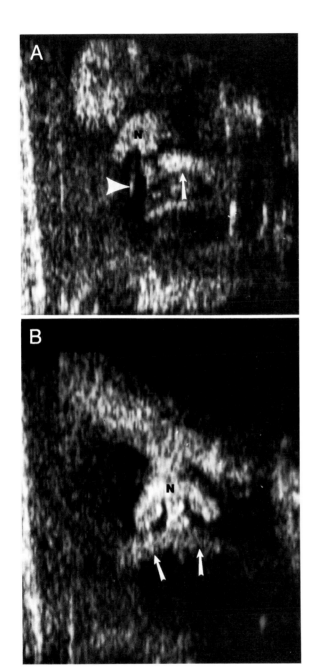

FIG 7–24.
Umbilical vein mimicking cleft lip. **A,** partial volume artifact of the
umbilical vein immediately adjacent to the upper lip may mimic a
cleft lip. **B,** scanning at slight obliquity or documentation of venous
Doppler signal avoids this pitfall. *Arrow head* = umbilical vein; *arrows* = intact upper lip; *N* = nose.

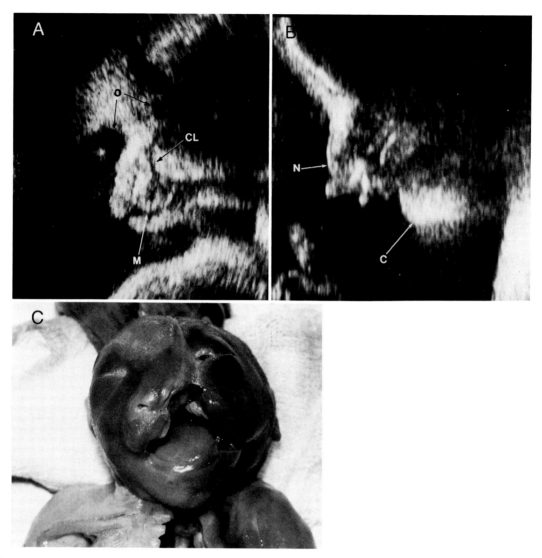

FIG 7–26.
Facial clefts with the amniotic band syndrome. **A,** frontal scan of the face at 35 weeks shows a large cleft extending from the mouth to the orbit. **B,** parasagittal scan of the face demonstrates anomalous tissue adjacent to the mouth and nose. **C,** postmortem photograph of a similar case illustrates bizarre facial clefts indicative of the amniotic band syndrome. The amniotic band syndrome has extremely variable manifestations, but may create bizarre facial clefts or slash defects in non–embryologic distributions. *M* = mouth; *CL* = cleft; *O* = orbits; *N* = nose; *C* = chin.

seen in a fetus with a positive family history or in conjunction with large for gestational age measurements, polyhydramnios, omphalocele, or visceromegaly.[84] Prenatal detection of the Beckwith-Weidemann syndrome permits planned glossectomy after birth and delivery in a setting capable of managing prolonged and often severe hypoglycemia.

Among five cases of the Beckwith-Weidemann syndrome detected at 18–35 weeks, macroglossia was detected prenatally in only one case in which a large for gestational age fetus and a family history of the disorder alerted the sonologist to search for macroglossia (Fig 7–27).[84, 85, 86, 89] Among the three cases detected

beyond 20 weeks' gestation, all had polyhydramnios, large for gestational age measurements, and enlarged kidneys; one had an omphalocele. The case detected at 18 weeks occurred in a fetus with a familial risk for the syndrome; ultrasound detected an omphalocele and large for dates measurements.[90] Another recurrent case of the Beckwith-Wiedemann syndrome had no abnormalities detected prenatally, but the newborn had macroglossia.[88]

The anomalies associated with the Beckwith-Wiedemann syndrome (omphalocele, visceromegaly, etc.) most commonly occur in entities other than the Beckwith-Wiedemann syndrome. However, to to our

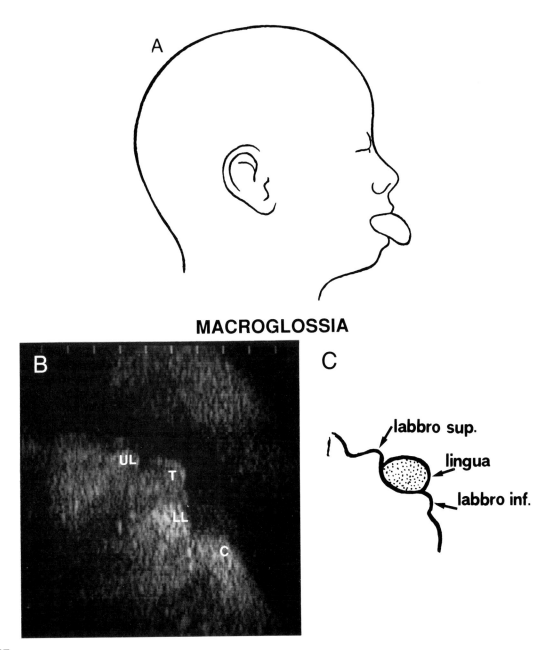

MACROGLOSSIA

FIG 7–27.
Macroglossia. **A,** large tongue protruding through the open mouth may suggest the Beckwith-Wiedemann syndrome, especially in the setting of a positive family history or other features of the syndrome (visceromegaly, omphalocele, large for gestational age, and polyhydramnios). Rare tumors also may produce tongue enlargement. **B** and **C,** sagittal sonogram **(B)** and corresponding drawing **(C)** of the mouth shows a protuberant tongue extending through the open mouth in this 30-week fetus with the Beckwith-Wiedemann syndrome. *UL* = upper lip (labbro sup); *T* = enlarged tongue (lingua); *LL* = lower lip (labbro inf); *C* = chin. (From Cobellis G, Iannoto P, Stabile M, et al: Prenatal ultrasound diagnosis of macroglossia in the Wiedemann-Beckwith syndrome. Prenat Diagn 1988; 8:79–81. Used by permission.)

knowledge, macroglossia has not been described prenatally in entities other than the Beckwith-Wiedemann syndrome. Nevertheless, it might occur in several of the mucopolysaccharide syndromes, athyrotic hypothyroidism, chromosomal abnormalities, or tumors of the tongue.[91] Occasionally, an anterior encephalocele may extend through the ethmoid sinuses into the mouth and resemble an enlarged tongue (see Fig 7–19).

THE FACIAL PROFILE VIEW

The midsagittal view of the face demonstrates the fetal profile optimally. This scan plane may visualize large facial or neck masses as well as more subtle abnormalities, including abnormal or absent nose, micrognathia, enlarged tongue, or absent nasal bridge. The profile view demonstrates most large masses, including epignathus, anterior cephaloceles, cervical teratoma, and hemangiomata. Occasionally, detection of smaller tumors not extending to the midline, such as hemangioma or sarcoma, requires parasagittal scans.

The profile images of the face may be especially helpful in fetuses with a positive family history for facial abnormalities or maternal ingestion of teratogens. For example, Hegge et al. diagnosed the fetal coumadin syndrome at 20 weeks based on visualization of a sunken nose in a fetus whose mother had a history of coumadin use.[5] They also detected flattened nose in a fetus with recurrent Conradi type of chondrodysplasia punctata (Fig 7–28). Pilu et al. diagnosed the Robin anomalad at 35 weeks, based on visualization of micrognathia of a fetus with polyhydramnios and a previously affected sibling.[9] Distinction between the normal and abnormal profile of the nose and chin has not been well defined, however, and undoubtedly changes at different stages of pregnancy. Indeed, a midsagittal facial scan at 23 weeks of the fetus with the Robin anomalad was interpreted as normal, whereas the similar scan at 35 weeks showed marked micrognathia.[97]

Therefore, unequivocal facial deformity of a fetus at risk for a specific syndrome permits accurate diagnosis, but absence of detectable abnormality does not exclude recurrence. Crane and Beaver reported sonographic diagnosis of recurrent autosomal dominant mandibulofacial dysostosis (Treacher Collins syndrome) based upon visualization of micrognathia and

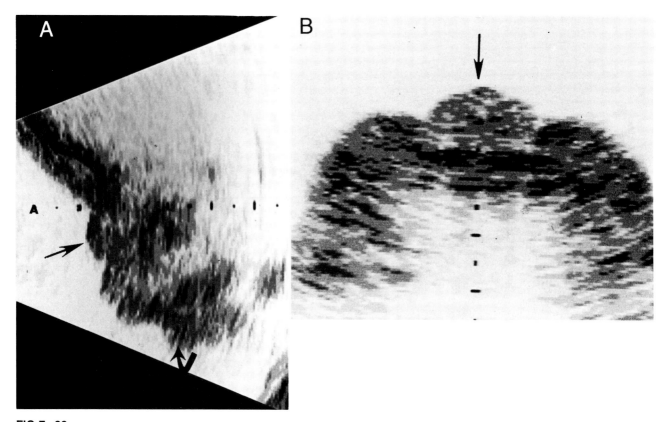

FIG 7–28.
Flattened nose at 24 weeks in recurrent chondrodysplasia punctata, dominant type (Conradi). **A** and **B,** facial profile scan **(A)** and axial view at the level of the nose **(B)** show an unmistakably flattened nose. *Straight arrow* = flattened nose; *curved arrow* = chin; *A* = anterior.

microtia at 17 weeks and confirmed later in gestation and at birth.[94] The same report documents a fetus at risk for the same syndrome but with normal facial and auricular structure on the prenatal sonogram and confirmed to be normal at birth. Two other reports document micrognathia as one manifestation of recurrent Pena-Shokeir phenotype in utero.[93, 98] In another report, detection of severe micrognathia, in conjunction with severe growth retardation at 18 weeks, enabled accurate prenatal diagnosis of recurrent Seckel-like syndrome.[95]

Even in the absence of genetic or teratogen risk, abnormalities seen on a facial profile view may assist in accurate diagnosis in multiple malformation syndromes (Fig 7–29). For example, Benson et al. reported a case of Nager acrofacial dysostosis syndrome at 30 weeks, with severe micrognathia, polyhydramnios, malformed ear, and severely shortened and deformed upper extremities (Figs 7–30 and 7–35).[92] Malinger et al. documented micrognathia and a facial amniotic band in a fetus with polyhydramnios at 31 weeks who had the Pierre Robin sequence.[96]

In cases with multiple malformations, the profile view may also detect absence of the nasal bridge and/or frontal bossing (Fig 7–31). Unfortunately, neither of these findings is a specific sign; each occurs in over 25 different syndromes.[12, 13] Nevertheless, each of these cases underscores the utility of scanning the facial profile in pregnancies complicated by a positive familial history, polyhydramnios, or other detected fetal anomalies.

EPIGNATHUS

Clinical and Pathologic Findings

Epignathus represents a rare pharyngeal teratoma arising from the palate in the region of Rathke's pouch. Although it may vary greatly in size and texture, epignathus generally extends through the mouth and creates a mass anteriorly. There is no known genetic or recurrence risk or predisposing factors. Perinatal management usually involves planned cesarean section to avoid dystocia and fetal trauma with immediate establishment of an airway followed by surgical excision. Even with optimal management, survival rates are only approximately 30%–40%.[103]

Sonographic Findings

Among the six reported cases of epignathus detected prenatally, the earliest diagnosis was made at 21 weeks' gestation.[101–106] In each case, the complex cystic and solid mass measured approximately 6–12 cm

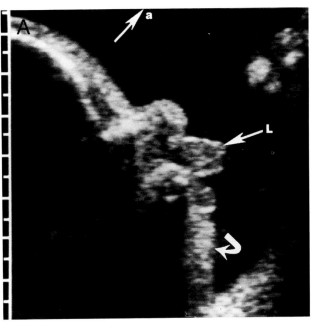

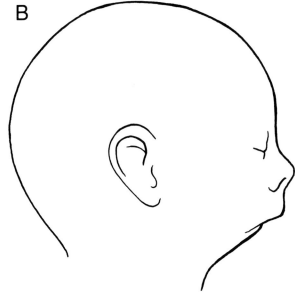

MICROGNATHIA

FIG 7–29.
Micrognathia at 29 weeks with the femoral hypoplasia syndrome. **A,** midsagittal facial profile view shows prominence of the upper lip and micrognathia. Other scans showed clubfoot, short femora, and polyhydramnios. *a* = anterior. **B,** drawing showing the degree of micrognathia often present when detected prenatally. *L* = upper lip; *curved arrow* = micrognathia.

in diameter adjacent to the anterior portion of the face, although the large size of the mass made it difficult to establish the exact site of origin (Fig 7–32). One case showed calcification within the mass, and another caused noticeable hyperextension of the head.[101, 106]

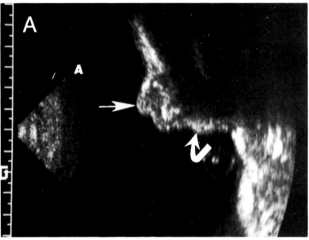
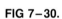
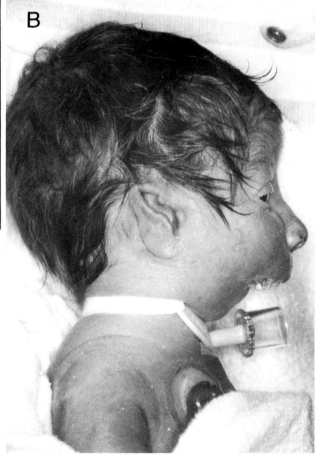

FIG 7–30.
Micrognathia with Nager acrofacial dysostosis syndrome. **A,** sagittal scan of the face documents marked micrognathia. Other scans showed polyhydramnios, marked extremity shortening, four digits on the hand, and deformed external ear (see Fig. 7–35). **B,** postnatal photograph confirms the prenatal findings of micrognathia. *A* = anterior; *straight arrow* = nose; *curved arrow* = micrognathic chin. (From Benson CB, Pober BR, Hirch MP, et al: Sonography of Nager acrofacial dysostosis syndrome in utero. J Ultrasound Med 1988; 7:163–167. Used by permission.)

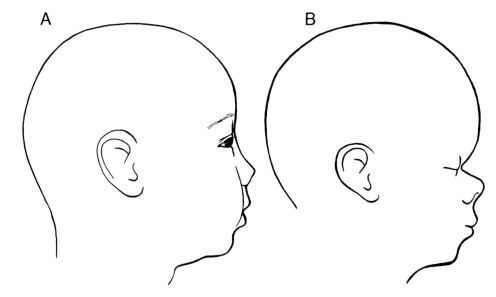

NORMAL   **ABSENT NASAL BRIDGE**

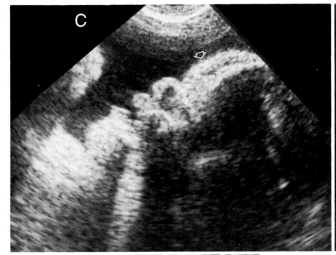

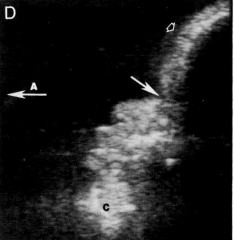

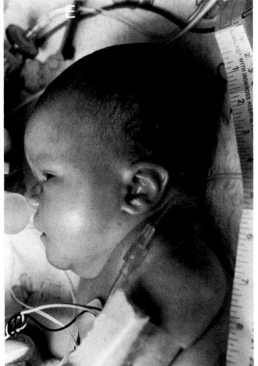

FIG 7–31.
Absent nasal bridge and frontal bossing. Drawings show the normal facial profile **(A)** and absence of the nasal bridge **(B)**. **C,** corresponding sagittal facial profile view (facing left) shows absence of the nasal bridge and frontal bossing. Other scans of this fetus showed extremity shortening in this fetus with meta-tropic dysplasia. Absence of the nasal bridge also can occur in heterozygous achondroplasia, asphyxiating thoracic dysplasia, and chondrodysplasia punctata, as well as in over 20 other syndromes. **D** and **E,** similar sagittal facial sonogram of a different fetus and its postnatal photograph show frontal bossing. Although the sonogram accurately depicts the fetal external morphology, these findings are not specific. *Solid arrow* = absent nasal bridge; *C* = chin; *open arrow* = frontal bossing; *A* = anterior.

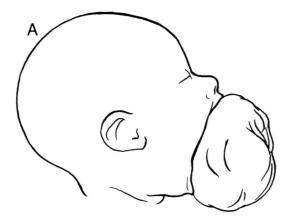

EPIGNATHUS

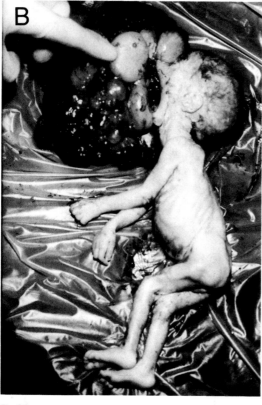

FIG 7–32.
Epignathus. **A,** epignathus often creates a large complex mass that extends through the open mouth anteriorly. **B,** the complex cystic and solid epignathus arises from the ethmoid sinus in this 29-week fetus. It produced polyhydramnios and neonatal death. (From Holmgren G, Rydnert J: Male fetus with epignathus originating from the ethmoidal sinus. Eur J Obstet Gynecol 1987; 24:69–72. Used by permission.)

None of the cases detected prenatally survived the neonatal period. Conversely, two cases with polyhydramnios, but relatively small tumors not detected prenatally, survived following postnatal surgical resection.[99, 100]

Associated Findings

All six reported cases of epignathus detected prenatally had concomitant polyhydramnios, presumably because of obstruction of the oropharynx. Occasionally, a large and vascular epignathus may lead to high-output cardiac failure and hydrops fetalis. Otherwise, it is typically an isolated anomaly with benign histology.

THE EARS

Sonographic examination of the fetal external ears rarely provides useful information in the absence of more obvious concomitant abnormalities. The striking clarity of detail when amniotic fluid outlines the ear structures, however, is often readily recognizable to the parents.[17, 109] As with a survey of other features of the fetal facial region, routine identification of the ears renders evaluation in anomalous cases less difficult. At most one can usually examine only one ear because of fetal positioning.

Clinical and Pathologic Findings

Smith lists 61 causes for malformation of the external ear and 21 for low-set ears.[12] Many of these occur as a manifestation of a variety of syndromes.

Sonographic Findings

Despite the large number of potential causes for malformation or malposition of the ears, few sonographic reports document abnormalities of the fetal external ear.[48, 92, 98, 109, 113] The paucity of reports regarding the external fetal ear probably results primarily from lack of routine survey of the ears. Usually the deformities must be gross to be recognized prenatally or occur as a part of a syndrome with much more obvious sonographic findings (Figs 7–33 to 7–35). Nevertheless, targeted examination of the ears may provide useful corroborative information to enable a specific antenatal diagnosis when other structural anomalies have been detected.

Based upon detection of unmistakably low-set ears, polyhydramnios, acrocephaly, syndactyly, and dextrocardia at 32 weeks, Hill et al. correctly diagnosed the rare (1 in 160,000 live births) Apert syndrome in a fetus with a normal karyotype and an unremarkable family history.[113] Detection of an ipsilateral low-set and malformed external ear in the setting of unilateral anophthalmia and polyhydramnios at 30 weeks permitted accurate diagnosis of the Goldenhar-Gorlin syndrome in a fetus with a normal karyotype and an unremarkable family history (Fig 7–36).[48] Birnholz has described edema of the eternal ear in

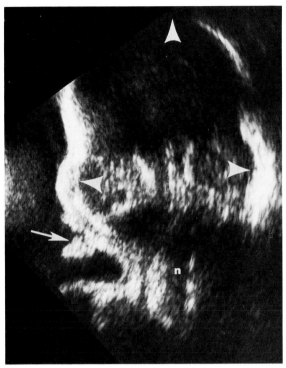

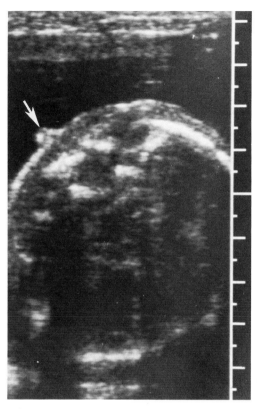

FIG 7–33.
Low-set ears with the cloverleaf skull deformity. Coronal scan of the head and neck of a fetus with the cloverleaf skull deformity demonstrates very low-set ear, probably at least in part secondary to the gross distortion of the skull. *Arrowheads* = cloverleaf skull deformity; *arrow* = low-set ear; *n* = neck.

FIG 7–34.
Small ear at 20 weeks in the Roberts syndrome. Scan of the ear region shows only a nubbin of tissue *(arrow)*. This fetus had the Roberts syndrome and multiple obvious congenital anomalies (see also Fig. 13–33).

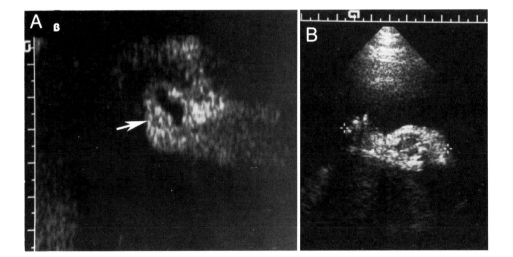

FIG 7–35.
Poor development of the external ear in Nager acrofacial dysostosis syndrome. **A,** scan of the external ear at 30 weeks displays poor development of the pinna. **B,** this fetus also had numerous other more obvious abnormalities, including severe polyhydramnios and marked shortening of the upper extremities with only four digits. Additional scans showed severe micrognathia (see Fig. 7–30). *Arrow* = poorly formed pinna of the ear; *graticules* = foreshortened right arm with only four digits on the hand. (From Benson CB, Pober BR, Hirsh MP, et al: Sonography of Nager acrofacial dysostosis syndrome in utero. J Ultrasound Med 1988; 7:163–167. Used by permission.)

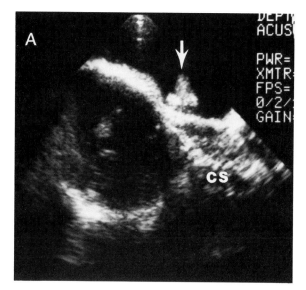

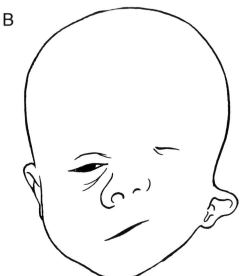

ANOPHTHALMIA
HEMIFACIAL MICROSOMIA

FIG 7–36.
Low-set, deformed ear with Goldenhar-Gorlin syndrome at 30 weeks. **A,** parasagittal scan of the head and neck displays an unmistakably low-set and malformed left external ear. Other scans showed absence of the ipsilateral orbit (see Fig. 7–15). **B,** drawing illustrating the features of hemifacial microsomia (Goldenhar-Gorlin syndrome). This syndrome probably occurs as a result of a unilateral vascular accident to the first and second branchial arches during embryogenesis. *Arrow* = low-set, malformed left external ear. CS = cervical spine. (From Tamas DE, Mahony BS, Bowie JD, et al: Prenatal sonographic diagnosis of hemifacial microsomia (Goldenhar-Gorlin syndrome). J Ultrasound Med 1986; 5:461–463. Used by permission.)

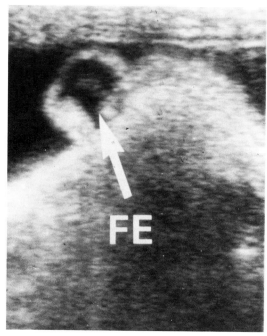

FIG 7–37.
Prominent external ear that might simulate an encephalocele. Scan of the side of the head demonstrates amniotic fluid outlining the external ear. Documentation of the characteristic ear morphology and absence of calvarial defect precludes the diagnosis of a rare parietal cephalocele. *FE* = fetal external ear. (From Fink IJ, Chinn DH, Callen PW: A potential pitfall in the ultrasonographic diagnosis of fetal encephalocele. J Ultrasound Med 1983; 2:313–314. Used by permission.)

hydrops fetalis, thickened ear in diabetic-induced macrosomia, rounded pinnae in achondrogenesis, and prominent mid-helix in thanatophoric dysplasia and osteogenesis imperfecta.[109] In each of these cases, however, the ear findings did not lead the sonologist to the correct antenatal diagnosis. Fink et al. warn against mistaking the external ear for a rare parietal encephalocele (Fig 7–37).[112] Documentation of the characteristic external ear anatomy in the absence of calvarial defect avoids this error.

Diagnosing low-set ears may be very difficult in all but the very obvious cases, primarily because it may be difficult to obtain the exact horizontal section which shows the corner of the orbit and the point where the helix of the ear meets the cranium.[113] Normally the helix meets the cranium above this point. A coronal scan showing the position of the ear relative to the neck and mandible may demonstrate a low-set position of the ear more clearly (see Figs 7–33 and 7–36).

Birnholz and Farrell found a linear correlation between the maximal normal fetal ear length and gestational age as follows:[110] ear length (mm) = 1.1011 X gestational age (wk) − 9.5089. They also describe abnormally short ears (defined as more than 1.5 SD less than the age-corrected mean) in three fetuses with trisomy 13 and two with trisomy 18.[110] They therefore suggest that ear length be determined in any pregnancy with a risk or suspicion of a chromosomal disorder or when a fetal anomaly has been detected.[107, 110] At least pending additional corroborative studies and further delineation of when retarded ear length manifests, blanket recommendation for ear length measurement in all pregnancies at risk for a chromosomal abnormality seems quite premature.

Based upon the assumption that the auditory system is functional by the beginning of the third trimester, many authors have utilized a wide variety of modifications of the auditory evoked response to assess fetal condition, usually as an adjunct to the biophysical profile and non-stress tests. A fetal blink-startle response to vibro-acoustic stimulation applied to the maternal abdomen occurs as early as 24 weeks' gestation in some fetuses, with a consistent response in virtually all normal fetuses by 29–31 weeks.[108, 111, 114] Lack of standardization of the technique for the auditory evoked response among various studies limits the value of its interpretation.[115]

SONOGRAPHIC APPROACH TO THE NECK

The official guidelines of the American Institute of Ultrasound in Medicine recommend documented examination of the fetal cervical spine during the second and third trimesters of pregnancy.[7] However, numerous structures of the neck can be visualized in approximately 95% of cases (Figs 7–38 and 7–39).[14] Most neck abnormalities detected antenatally create a mass effect which distorts normal internal anatomy as well as the external contour of the neck. In such cases, detailed or targeted examination is not necessary to detect the mass. Following detection of a neck abnormality, however, narrowing the differential diagnosis may be a more difficult task. Information regarding location and echocharacteristics of the mass, associated findings, maternal and family history, and amniocentesis data assists in narrowing the list and often renders a definitive diagnosis (Table 7–4).[10, 11]

Cystic hygroma colli probably represent the most common cause for a neck mass detected prenatally. Case reports document that antenatal ultrasound occasionally can detect other neck masses, including cervical meningomyelocele, hemangioma, teratoma,

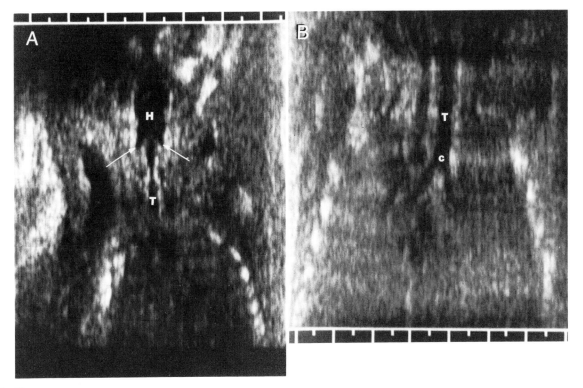

FIG 7–38.
Normal airway. Coronal scans of the neck **(A)** and upper thorax **(B)** show the hypopharynx, piriform sinuses, larynx, trachea, and carina. The esophagus is usually collapsed and not well seen, although with fetal deglutition the hypopharynx collapses, the larynx elevates, and a bolus of fluid can sometimes be seen transiently within the esophagus. *H* = hypopharynx; *arrows* = piriform sinuses; *T* = trachea; *C* = carina.

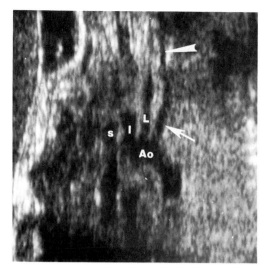

FIG 7–39.
Normal aortic arch vessels. Oblique coronal sonogram of the lower neck at 34 weeks demonstrates the aortic arch, innominate artery, left common carotid, left subclavian artery, left vertebral artery, and superior vena cava. *Ao* = aortic arch; *I* = innominate artery; *L* = left common carotid artery; *arrow* = left subclavian artery; *arrow head* = left vertebral artery; = superior vena cava.

goiter, sarcoma, and metastatic adenopathy. Occasionally, a large encephalocele may mimic a neck mass. In most of these rare cases, polyhydramnios, hydrops fetalis, or other clinical features signals a careful search of the fetal neck. In several reported cases of neck hemangioma, however, the routine amniotic survey revealed the abnormality. To our knowledge, other neck masses (branchial cleft cyst, thyroglossal duct cyst, laryngocele, fibroma, lipoma, etc.) have not yet been detected antenatally.

Even when the sonologist cannot predict the exact histology of a neck mass, detection of a tumor permits optimal perinatal management since large but histologically benign tumors may cause dystocia or obstruct the upper respiratory tract and necessitate emergency intubation at birth. In other cases, detection of a neck abnormality (i.e., cystic hygroma colli) may indicate a high likelihood of chromosomal abnormality or biochemical disturbance (i.e., goiter). Attempts at definitive antenatal diagnosis of fetal neck abnormalities, therefore, is by no means merely a mental exercise but provides useful clinical information.

Since most fetal neck abnormalities tend to be quite large rather than subtle, routine examination of the cervical spine region will frequently detect many neck anomalies, especially during the second trimester when the fetus often holds the head in a neutral position. Different angles of insonation and adjacent amniotic fluid during the second trimester usually enable visualization of the neck anteriorly as well as posteriorly.

Polyhydramnios with excessive fetal motion, extreme maternal obesity, or flexion of the neck with fetal crowding during the third trimester may limit visualization of the neck in approximately 5% of cases.[14]

The most useful parameters to assess following detection of a neck abnormality include (see Table 7–4):

A. *Is an abnormal neck mass present?* If so:
   1. *Is the mass unilateral or bilateral, posterior, or anterior?*
   2. *Is the mass centered in the midline or not?*
   3. *What are its echotexture and Doppler characteristics?*
      a. Most bilateral posterior masses are cystic hygroma colli, especially multicystic masses with a midline septation.
      b. Most unilateral anterior masses are teratomas.
      c. Most bilateral anterior masses are goiter.
      d. Hemangiomas can occur anywhere with variable echotexture, but have typical arterial and venous Doppler signal.
B. *Is polyhydramnios or a concomitant anomaly present?* These signs often indicate a poor prognosis.
C. *Is the neck abnormally positioned?* Hyperextension occurs with face presentation but can occasionally signify the presence of an anterior mass of the face or neck or fusion of the back of the head to the spine.

CYSTIC HYGROMA COLLI

Clinical and Pathologic Findings

Cystic hygroma probably results either from abnormal embryonic sequestration of lymphatic tissue or from abnormal budding of lymphatic endothelium between the sixth and ninth weeks of gestation.[144] Failure of the jugular lymphatic sacs to drain into the internal jugular vein probably results in the dilatation of the lymphatic sacs into cystic spaces and may lead to the jugular lymphatic obstruction sequence and hydrops fetalis (Fig 7–40).[12, 133]

Cystic hygroma occurs in the neck in approximately 80% of cases in which it is termed cystic hygroma colli (CHC). It typically involves the posterior and lateral portions of the neck and often occurs bilaterally in an asymmetric fashion, although the left posterior triangle is the most frequent single location postnatally. The incidence of CHC is not well defined. Reports range from 1 in 6,000 pregnancies to 1 in 120 pregnancies at risk for having a structural anomaly.[123, 139, 142, 147]

TABLE 7–4.

Helpful Sonographic Features in the Differential Diagnosis of Fetal Neck Masses

Neck Mass	Relative Frequency	Typical Location	Echotexture	Size	Associated Findings	Concomitant Anomalies
Cystic hygroma colli	Common	Posterolateral bilateral but asymmetric	Multicystic with midline septation	Large (85% larger than head)	Hydrops (75%), oligohydramnios (60%)	Common chromosome abnormality
Occipital cephalocele	Less Common	Posterior, midline	Complex (brain tissue) Cystic (meningocele)	Variable	Calvarial defect; ± microcephaly; polyhydramnios (33%)	Meckel-Gruber (5%–14%) Spinal defect (4%–15%)
Meningomyelocele	Uncommon	Posterior, midline	Complex or cystic if sac intact	Variable	Spinal dysraphism	Clubfoot, arthrogryposis; other neural tube defects
Hemangioma	Uncommon	Variable	Variable, low-level echoes	Variable	Arterial and venous Doppler signals; ± hydrops	Rare
Teratoma	Uncommon	Anterolateral; unilateral	Complex	5–10 cm; broad-based	Polyhydramnios (30%)	Rare
Goiter	Uncommon	Anterior; bilateral	Solid or complex	Bi-lobed 2–6 cm	Polyhydramnios; maternal goiter or thyrotoxicosis	Rare
Metastases (neuroblastoma)	Rare	Asymmetric	Solid	6 cm	Maternal tachycardia, nausea, adrenal enlargement, placental metastases	Rare
Sarcoma	Rare	Variable	Solid	8–12 cm		Rare
Melanoma	Rare	Variable	Mixed	4–8 cm	Hydrocephalus if spinal cord involved	Rare
Branchial cleft cyst	Rare	Anterior; unilateral	Cystic	?	?	Rare
Thyroglossal duct cyst	Rare	Anterior; submandibular	Cystic	?	?	Rare
Laryngocele	Rare	Anterior; laryngeal	Cystic	?	?	Rare
Fibroma, lipoma, etc.	Rare	Variable	Solid	?	?	Rare
Pseudo-mass: a. nuchal umbilical cord b. trapped amniotic fluid c. subchorionic cyst d. fetal hair	Common	Adjacent to neck	Dependent upon artefact	Variable	a. Umbilical cord Doppler signal; b. Changes with maternal position; c. Within placenta; d. Attached to scalp	Rare

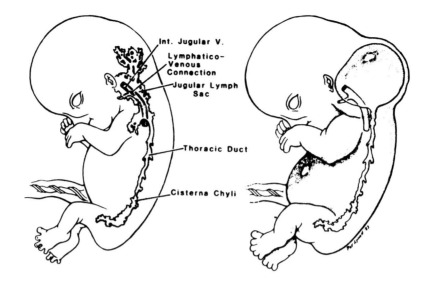

FIG 7–40.
Cystic hygroma colli. This drawing illustrates that the jugular lymphatic sacs normally drain into the internal jugular vein (left portion of drawing). Cystic hygroma colli (right portion of drawing) probably result from failure of the jugular lymphatic sacs to drain. (From Chervenak FA, Isaacson G, Blakemore KJ, et al: Fetal cystic hygroma: Cause and natural history. N Engl J Med 1983; 308:822–825. Used by permission.)

Sonographic Findings

CHC usually manifests as an unexpected finding on the antenatal ultrasound upon survey of the neck during the second trimester.[155] Although is has been detected as early as 12 weeks' gestation, the mean age of diagnosis is approximately 19 weeks.[132, 133, 135, 138, 149] The findings may regress and disappear later in gestation.[126, 150]

The ultrasound of CHC typically shows asymmetric, thin-walled, multiseptate, cystic masses of the posterolateral aspects of the neck, but cystic hygroma may localize anteriorly or extend into the axilla or mediastinum (Fig 7–41).* The loculations range in size but in 85% of cases are as large or larger than the head (Fig 7–42).[124] Occasionally the CHC may have a more complex echotexture with solid components interspersed with the multicystic areas, if the obstructed lymphatics occur among muscle and fibrous tissue or if portions of the abnormal lymphatics remain clumped together and non-dilated.[152]

Identification of the midline septation extending from the posterior neck and representing the nuchal ligament outlined by bilateral cysts constitutes the most specific sign for the diagnosis of CHC (see Fig 7–41).[125] Grundy et al., however, reported a case of fetal neck hemangioma outlining the nuchal ligament in the absence of CHC.[134] In this case the cysts were thick-walled, contained low level echos, and extended

*References 119, 124, 125, 131, 136, 144, 147, and 151.

into the thorax and upper abdomen, but their distinction from CHC was quite subtle.

Occasionally a CHC may mimic a cervical meningocele or low occipital cephalocele, but identification of the characteristic nuchal ligament in the absence of spinal dysraphism or calvarial defect discriminates CHC from a neural tube defect.[120, 140, 143] Furthermore, a mass created by a meningocele or cephalocele tends to occur in the midline in association with distortion of intracranial anatomy and cerebral ventricular dilatation or microcephaly, whereas CHC typically occurs asymmetrically and does not produce intracranial distortion or ventriculomegaly.

Other processes which may potentially mimic a CHC upon initial inspection, but become recognizable with changes in fetal position or transducer angulation, include a segment of umbilical cord behind the neck, prominent fetal hair, a pocket of amniotic fluid temporarily trapped against the neck, or adjacent subchorionic cyst.[146, 157] With these pitfalls in mind, the sonologist should diagnose CHC reliably and accurately in virtually all cases during the second trimester of pregnancy.[143]

Associated Findings

CHC often progresses to hydrops fetalis (Fig 7–43). In four of the largest series reported, 59 of 79 (76%) fetuses with CHC had hydrops.[124, 133, 143, 145] Oligohydramnios complicates 60% of pregnancies with CHC, whereas polyhydramnios is unusual.[124, 143] Al-

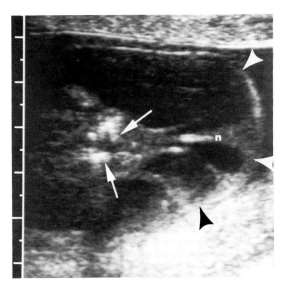

FIG 7–41.
Cystic hygroma colli in monosomy X. This axial scan through the posterior neck at 16 weeks illustrates the characteristic appearance of cystic hygroma colli in this fetus with monosomy X (Turner syndrome). The multiseptate, cystic, thin-walled, asymmetric masses outline the midline nuchal ligament. Note that the posterior elements of the cervical spine converge, which excludes a rare cervical meningomyelocele as the cause for the posterior neck mass. *Arrowheads* = multiseptated cystic hygroma colli; *n* = nuchal ligament; *arrows* = converging posterior elements of cervical spine.

though polyhydramnios has been reported to occur in up to 20% of cases, the sonologist must beware not to mistake the large fluid-filled loculations of CHC for polyhydramnios (see Fig 7–42).[124, 157] The etiology for oligohydramnios remains conjectural but possibly results from fetal hypoperfusion leading to decreased renal output; the polyhydramnios probably represents a manifestation of hydrops rather that esophageal compression. Given the common association between CHC and hydrops, the discordantly low incidence of polyhydramnios and high incidence of oligohydramnios suggests that factors leading to oligohydramnios predominate in the vast majority of cases.

Excluding hydrops fetalis and aberrations of amniotic fluid volume, other detectable anomalies associated with CHC are rare. For example, CHC has been described in rare cases with cardiac defects, diaphragmatic hernia, or hydronephrosis, and as a manifestation of the Noonan and Roberts syndromes.[128, 130, 139, 156]

Approximately 45%–50% of fetuses with CHC have monosomy X (Table 7–5).[122, 124, 133, 145] Only one of every 150 fetuses with the Turner syndrome do not undergo a spontaneous abortion.[132] CHC may also occur as a manifestation of other chromosomal abnormalities, especially trisomy 21, 18, or 13,

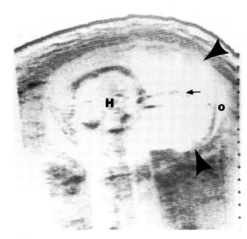

FIG 7–42.
Cystic hygroma colli with oligohydramnios. Axial scan through the head and neck shows a cystic hygroma colli that is larger than the head. In 85% of cases, the cystic loculations in cystic hygroma colli are as large or larger than the head and should not be confused with polyhydramnios. This pregnancy has oligohydramnios, which complicates approximately 60% of cases with cystic hygroma colli. Note the midline nuchal ligament. *Arrowheads* = cystic hygroma colli; *H* = head; *O* = oligohydramnios; *arrow* = nuchal ligament.

which account for 10%–15% of cases with CHC (Fig 7–44).[127, 130, 142, 145, 148] One cannot assume, therefore, that a fetus with CHC has monosomy X. Furthermore, 10%–15% of fetuses with CHC have a normal 46,XX karyotype, and an additional 5%–10% have a normal 46,XX karyotype.[127, 129, 133, 139, 145] Those with a male karyotype often have female external genitalia.[133] Although some authors state that CHC with a normal karyotype implies an excellent prognosis, the series reported by Chervenak et al. described two of three such cases that also had multiple congenital anomalies.[124]

The risk of recurrence for aneuploidy is low, but CHC with a normal karyotype may be inherited as an autosomal recessive trait with 25% recurrence (Figs 7–43 and 7–45).[129, 130, 133, 145] Although most aneuploid fetuses with CHC have hydrops, most non-hydropic fetuses with CHC also are aneuploid.[124, 133] The absence of hydrops with CHC, therefore, is of little value in predicting the karyotype, and accurate counseling following detection of CHC requires chromosomal analysis.

Elevated levels of amniotic fluid alpha-fetoprotein (AFP) occur in 40%–50% of cases with CHC, probably on the basis of a) sampling the hygroma fluid rather than amniotic fluid, b) transudation of the α-fetoprotein through the thin membrane covering the CHC, or c) imminent fetal death.[121, 122, 137, 141] Concomitant CHC and neural tube defect or anterior abdominal wall

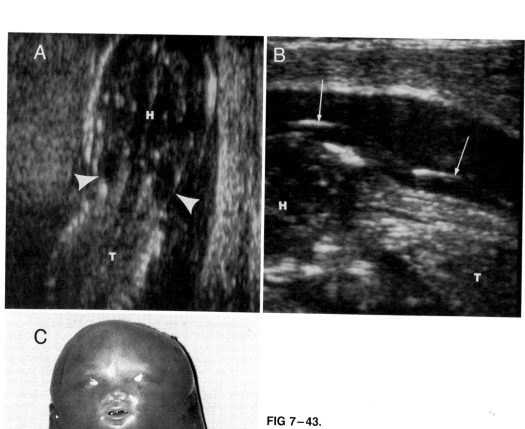

H·7653

FIG 7–43.
Recurrent cystic hygroma colli with a normal karyotype. **A,** coronal scan of the head, neck, and thorax
at 13 weeks demonstrates the bilateral cystic neck
masses. **B,** parasagittal scan of the similar region
shows the subcutaneous edema extending onto the
scalp and body wall, indicative of hydrops. The
presence of hydrops is of little value in predicting
karyotype. This fetus had a normal karyotype and a
family history of cystic hygroma colli with a normal
karyotype. Most fetuses with cystic hygroma colli
are aneuploid with a low recurrence risk, but those
with a normal karyotype may have autosomal recessive recurrence. **C,** postnatal photograph of another
case shows cystic hygroma colli. *Arrowheads* =
cystic hygroma colli; *arrows* = subcutaneous
edema; *H* = head; *T* = thorax.

TABLE 7–5.

Karyotypes of 84 Fetuses With Cystic Hygroma Colli Diagnosed Prenatally*

Karyotype	N	%
45, X	39	46
46, XX	11	13
46, XY	6	7
Trisomy 18	5	6
Trisomy 21	4	5
Trisomy 13	1	1
47, XXY	1	1
Unknown	17	20

*Modified from Pijpers L, Reuss A, Stewart PA, et al: Fetal cystic hygroma: Prenatal diagnosis and management. Obstet Gynecol 1988; 72:223–224.

defect is rare. Acetylcholinesterase activity can be absent in amniotic fluid but present in fluid aspirated from the hygroma itself.[121, 124, 137] Measurement of alkaline phosphatase isoenzymes may distinguish cystic hygroma fluid (which has virtually no intestinal isoenzymes) from amniotic fluid (which contains approximately 80% intestinal isoenzymes) during the second trimester.[121]

Occasionally, hydrops fetalis may manifest as a predominant edema of the back of the neck, mimicking CHC in a fetus with a normal karyotype.[133] Such cases require additional evaluation for other causes of hydrops.[130] On the other hand, predominant nuchal thickening may also manifest in the second trimes-

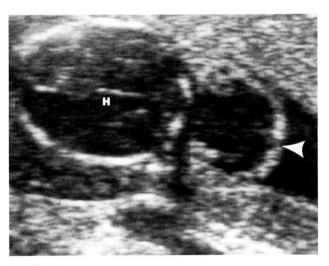

FIG 7–44.
Cystic hygroma colli with trisomy 21. Axial scan of the nuchal region at 14–15 weeks displays a cystic hygroma colli in a fetus with trisomy 21. Approximately 10%–15% of cases with cystic hygroma colli occur in trisomy 21, 18, or 13. The absence of calvarial defect distinguishes the hygroma from an occipital encephalocele. *H* = head; *arrowhead* = hygroma.

ter of pregnancy and has been described in trisomy 21.[116, 117, 118, 150] The loose skin folds or webbing which occasionally manifest at birth in monosomy X, trisomy 21, and trisomy 18 probably represent residual of intrauterine CHC. Nuchal thickening ($\geq$ 5 mm) in the absence of true CHC has been described during the second trimester in association with trisomy 21 (see Chapter 17).[116–118, 154] This finding was not described in any of the abortuses with trisomy 21 studied by Stevens and Shepard.[153] Furthermore, this sign requires meticulous technique to avoid spuriously increasing the nuchal thickness measurement by angling the transducer caudally.[154]

Prognosis
Because the majority of reported cases have undergone elective termination of pregnancy, the mortality rate of CHC detected with prenatal ultrasound cannot be stated with certainty. However, a compilation of small series and case reports of fetuses not electively terminated suggests a spontaneous mortality rate of approximately 80%–90%.* The presence of hydrops fetalis or lymphangiectasia in CHC portends a grave prognosis, with death usually occuring within several weeks of the time of diagnosis.[124] Two reports suggest that isolated cystic hygromas in atypical locations in the neck or axilla may have a better prognosis (Figs 7–46 and 7–47).[119, 136]

OCCIPITAL CEPHALOCELE/CERVICAL MENINGOMYELOCELE

Clinical and Pathologic Findings
A large occipital encephalocele may extend into the nuchal region and resemble a neck mass. Occipital encephalocele occurs with a frequency of approximately 1 in 2,700 pregnancies, and most encephaloceles occur in the occiput.[159] It results from lack of midline fusion of the neural tube during embryogenesis.

A cervical meningomyelocele represents a cause for a posterior neck mass often written about but rarely demonstrated in published prenatal sonographic reports unless it is large and extensive.[10, 11, 164] A midline sac may cover the defect or the sac may have ruptured (Fig 7–48).

Sonographic Findings
Although upon initial inspection an occipital encephalocele may mimic other posterior neck masses,

*References 122, 124, 129, 133, 138, 139, 142–145, 147, 148, and 151.

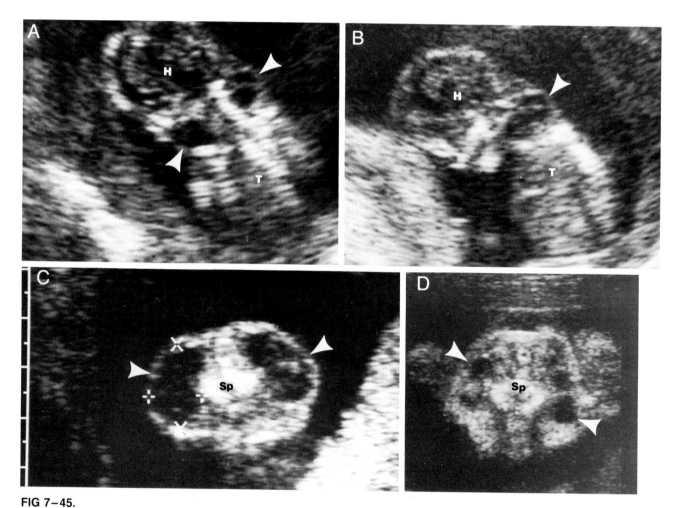

FIG 7–45.
Cystic hygroma colli with normal karyotype with subsequent resolution then fetal demise. Coronal **(A),** parasagittal **(B),** and axial **(C),** scans of the neck demonstrate bilateral cystic hygroma colli at 14 weeks. **D,** axial scan of the neck at 20 weeks shows the hygroma almost completely resolved. No hydrops was present at that time, and the fetus has a normal karyotype. However, the fetus was delivered at 27 weeks with massive hydrops and died shortly after birth. The spontaneous mortality rate for cystic hygroma colli is approximately 80%–90%. *H* = head; *T* = thorax; *arrowheads* = cystic hygroma; *Sp* = spine.

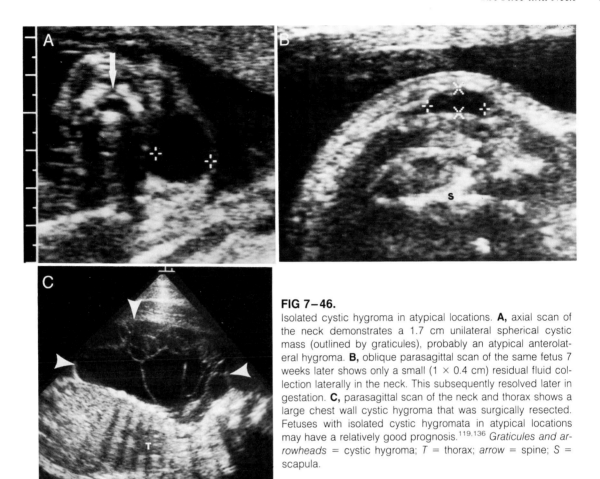

FIG 7–46.
Isolated cystic hygroma in atypical locations. **A,** axial scan of the neck demonstrates a 1.7 cm unilateral spherical cystic mass (outlined by graticules), probably an atypical anterolateral hygroma. **B,** oblique parasagittal scan of the same fetus 7 weeks later shows only a small (1 × 0.4 cm) residual fluid collection laterally in the neck. This subsequently resolved later in gestation. **C,** parasagittal scan of the neck and thorax shows a large chest wall cystic hygroma that was surgically resected. Fetuses with isolated cystic hygromata in atypical locations may have a relatively good prognosis.[119, 136] *Graticules and arrowheads* = cystic hygroma; *T* = thorax; *arrow* = spine; *S* = scapula.

careful analysis with demonstration of the midline calvarial opening reliably distinguishes an encephalocele from other neck masses. An ultrasound performed during the second trimester detects approximately 95% of occipital encephaloceles. Often such cases have an elevated maternal serum alpha-fetoprotein (MS-AFP) level, unless the defect is covered by skin.[143]

A midline septation, if present, extends through the calvarial defect into the brain, and this distinguishes the midline septation of CHC from that of an encephalocele (Fig 7–49). The calvarial opening also distinguishes an occipital encephalocele from bizarre calvarial distortion of a cloverleaf skull deformity as well as from other neck masses or normal structures (branchial cleft cyst, teratoma, hemangioma, nuchal umbilical cord, trapped pocket of amniotic fluid, etc.). The echotexture of cephaloceles ranges from cystic (meningocele) to solid with visualization of the herniated brain into the mass (encephalocele).

As with other dysraphic neural tube defects,

the pathognomonic sign of splaying of the posterior elements of the spine differentiates a cervical myelomeningocele from other neck masses and artifacts.[146, 157]

Associated Findings

Other frequent associated findings in cases with an occipital encephalocele include polyhydramnios in 33%, spinal dysraphism in 4%–15%, and polycystic kidneys with polydactyly in 5%–14% (autosomal recessive Meckel-Gruber syndrome).[143, 158–162] Occipital encephalocele may also occur in association with other rare syndromes.[160] An encephalocele occurring in association with the amniotic band syndrome may localize anywhere, but typically occurs off-midline, and detection of any off-axis calvarial opening mandates a careful search for other manifestations of the amniotic band syndrome.[78] In a recent series, three of nine cases with an encephalocele occurred as a part of the amniotic band syndrome.[159] Herniated brain through an en-

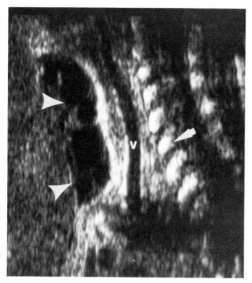

FIG 7–47.
Nuchal umbilical cord mimicking cystic hygroma. Coronal scan of the neck shows the umbilical cord adjacent to the neck resembling a multiloculated cystic neck mass. Documentation of the characteristic Doppler wave form avoids confusion between the nuchal umbilical cord and a potential neck mass. The internal jugular vein is quite prominent in this normal 34-week fetus. *Arrowheads = nuchal umbilical cord; V = internal jugular vein; arrow = cervical spine.*

cephalocele often results in microcephaly or hydrocephaly.

Neural elements extending through the dysraphism of a cervical neural tube defect indicate a myelomeningocele and a poorer prognosis than for a meningocele. The presence of hydrocephaly and a compressed posterior fossa imply the Arnold-Chiari III malformation. Detection of a cervical meningomyelocele warrants a careful anatomic search with an expected increased incidence of club feet, arthrogryposis, and other neural tube defects. As with other neural tube defects, detection of concomitant anomalies increases the likelihood of an underlying chromosomal aberration.

Prognosis

Herniated brain though an encephalocele, with concomitant microcephaly, carries a dismal prognosis.[159] In the series reported by Pearce et al., 84% of 21 fetuses with encephalocele had microcephaly.[143] On the other hand, approximately 50% of cases with an isolated occipital meningocele without herniated brain or microcephaly have a normal outcome following surgical correction.[159, 163] Similarly, a cervical myelomeningocele has a worse prognosis than does a meningocele without herniation of neural elements.

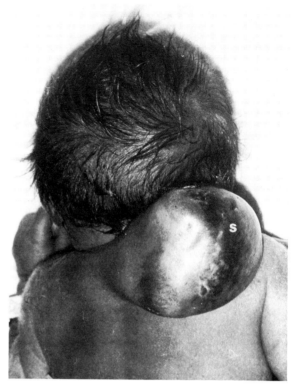

FIG 7–48.
Cervical myelomeningocele. A cervical myelomeningocele represents a rare cause for a midline posterior neck mass. A sac may cover the spinal defect, as this posterior photograph of a newborn illustrates, or the sac may have ruptured. However, the pathognomonic sign of dysraphism is splaying of the posterior elements of the spine. *S = sac covering cervical myelomeningocele.*

HEMANGIOMA

Clinical and Pathologic Findings

Hemangiomas comprise one of the most common tumors of childhood, but hemangiomatous malformation presenting as a neck mass on prenatal ultrasound is rare.[165, 166, 169]

Sonographic Findings

Among four case reports at 16–24 weeks and one near term, the sonographic features of a hemangiomatous neck mass ranged from a homogeneously echogenic to a mixed cystic and solid appearance.[165, 166, 169, 170] Doppler evaluation of one case demonstrated arterial and venous pulsations, and another case showed a central pulsating vessel within confluent cystic areas (Fig 7–50).[169, 170] Two cases occurred in the nuchal region and spread to the chest and upper extremities in association with hydrops, whereas one spread to the chest from the anterior portion of the neck in association with the Klippel-Trenaunay-Weber syn-

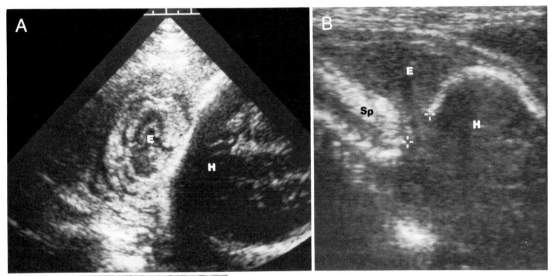

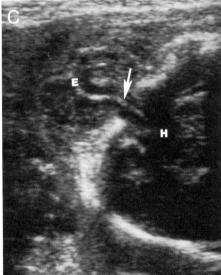

FIG 7–49.
Occipital encephalocele. **A,** oblique scan of the back of the head and neck shows a complex mass extending over the posterior portion of the neck but does not demonstrate the calvarial defect. **B,** Documentation of the calvarial defect confirms the diagnosis of encephalocele, as this coronal scan of the neck and occiput displays. **C,** visualization of the midline structure extending through the calvarial defect into the brain on this axial scan through the occiput provides convincing evidence for an encephalocele and distinguishes an encephalocele from other neck masses. *E* = encephalocele; *H* = head; *Sp* = cervical spine; *graticules* = calvarial defect; *arrow* = midline brain structure extending through calvarial defect into encephalocele.

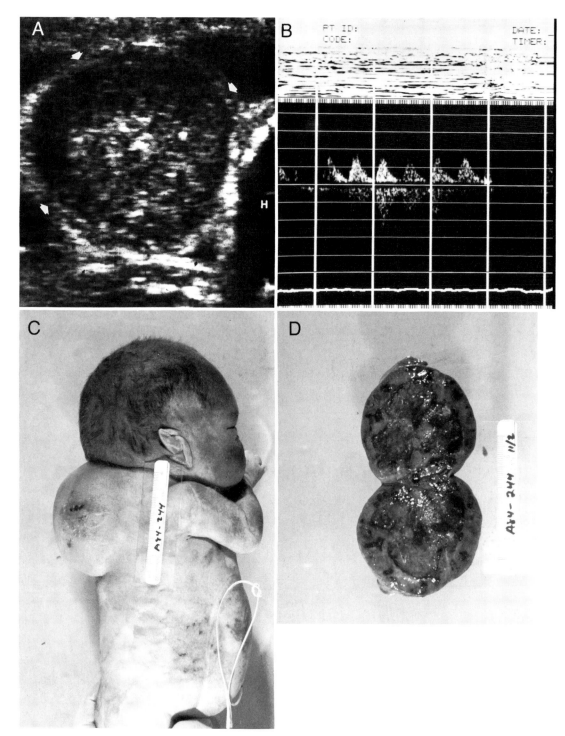

FIG 7–50.
Hemangioma. **A,** sagittal scan through the back of the neck shows a large mass with mid-range echoes projecting from the nuchal region. **B,** doppler wave form demonstrates arterial pulsations within the mass. **C,** postmortem photograph illustrates the mass extending from the nuchal region onto the upper back. **D,** cut cross-section of the mass shows its solid texture. *Arrows* = mass; *H* = head. (From McGahan JP, Schneider JM; Fetal neck hemangioendothelioma with secondary hydrops fetalis: Sonographic diagnosis. J Clin Ultrasound 1986; 14:384–388. Used by permission.)

drome (vascular abnormalities with associated limb hypertrophy).[166, 169, 170] A paratracheal hemangioma in another case caused hydrops near term.[167] The hemangioma arose from the back of the neck, measured two thirds the size of the head, and had echotexture similar to the placenta.

Among the three cases of neck hemangiomas detected with prenatal ultrasound that did not undergo elective termination, two died in utero with hydrops during the third trimester, and the third died shortly following birth from hemorrhage secondary to attempted surgical removal of the mass.[165, 166, 169]

Because of its location, a nuchal hemangioma may mimic a cystic hygroma or asymmetric edema from hydrops fetalis. However, the internal echos, thicker septa, or extent of the tumor and especially the Doppler signals within a hemangiomatous malformation help to exclude other entities. Furthermore, three of four cases with a neck hemangioma detected prenatally had a normal amount of amniotic fluid. On the other hand, cystic hygroma colli is often associated with oligohydramnios, whereas hydrops is frequently associated with polyhydramnios. Chromosomal analysis in a fetus with a neck hemangioma would be expected to be normal.

Associated Findings

Given the overall prevalence of hemangiomas postnatally, most neck hemangiomas are probably isolated abnormalities. On the other hand, hemangiomas detected prenatally tend to be large and associated with concomitant signs of hydrops fetalis.

CERVICAL TERATOMA

Clinical and Pathological Findings

Teratoma of the neck is a rare neoplasm, with only approximately 140 cases having been reported since 1854.[171, 173, 175] The vast majority of cervical teratomas have benign histology, and they usually occur as an isolated anomaly.[173, 180, 182] Fortunately, no recurrence has been reported.[183]

Sonographic Findings

The ultrasound features of a cervical teratoma detected at 16–32 menstrual weeks in six case reports include a large unilateral well-defined, broad-based mass of the anterolateral portion of the neck causing hyperextension of the neck (Figs 7–51 to 7–53).[174, 177, 179, 183, 184] Although 40%–50% of neck teratomas of infants have pathognomonic calcifications identified radiographically, none of the antenatal sono-

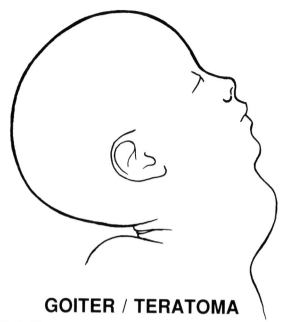

GOITER / TERATOMA

FIG 7–51.
Anterior neck mass. A large anterior neck mass typically causes distortion of the external contour of the neck anteriorly and produces hyperextension of the neck. Most anterior neck masses detected in utero are either cervical teratomas or goiter.

grams have shown this finding.[172, 173] Nevertheless, a large, complex, unilateral, cystic, and solid tumor of the anterolateral portion of the fetal neck strongly suggests the diagnosis of cervical teratoma. Other less likely possibilities include a) an atypically located cystic hygroma or a branchial cleft cyst, both of which would be cystic or multicystic; b) a goitrous thyroid, which typically is symmetrically enlarged bilaterally; or c) a rare sarcoma. Many authors believe that cervical teratomas arise from the thyroid, which explains their anterolateral locations.[173, 175] Gundry et al. reported elevated levels of thyroid-stimulating hormone (TSH) in two of three patients with cervical teratoma.[173]

In one case of a cervical teratoma detected on routine ultrasound, a hypoechoic teratoma measured 1.7 cm at 16–17 weeks but progressively enlarged to 5 cm at 25 weeks and 8 cm at 34 weeks and developed definite solid components.[184] The amniotic fluid volume remained normal, but fetal demise occurred at 34 weeks. Other cases detected at 25–29 weeks have shown a well-defined, large (8–10 cm), unilateral, anterolateral cystic and solid mass in conjunction with marked polyhydramnios, presumably from esophageal compression (see Figs 7–52 and 7–53). Each of these cases died at birth. A fifth case at 32 weeks only described the mass as huge and involving the entire neck in a fetus who died at birth.[182] Following prenatal diagnosis in one case, however, planned cesarean section

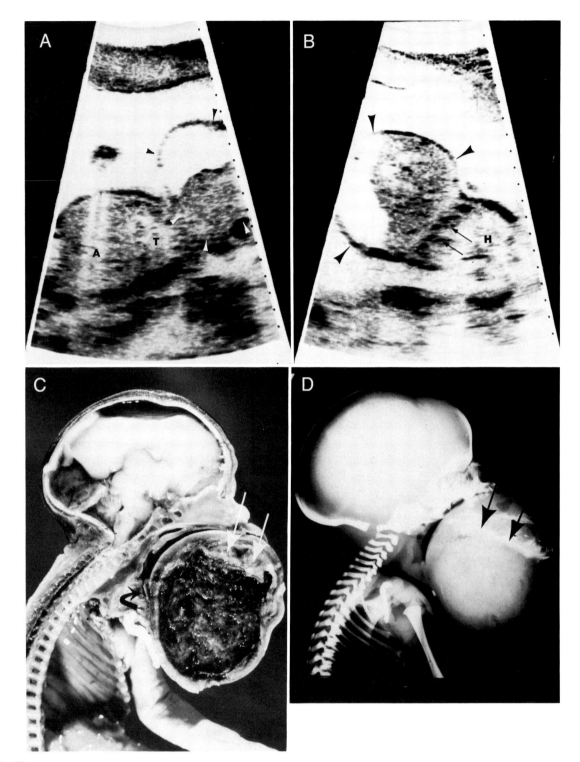

FIG 7–52.
Cervical teratoma. **A,** sagittal scan of the neck and trunk at 29 weeks shows polyhydramnios, absence of fluid in the stomach, and an 8 cm anterolateral complex cystic and solid neck mass. **B,** oblique scan through the neck mass and head demonstrates hyperextension of the neck and deformity of the mandible by the mass. The mass prevented resuscitation, and death occured shortly after birth. **C** and **D,** sagittal hemisection and postmortem radiograph confirm the prenatal findings. *Arrowheads* = complex cystic and solid teratoma; *T* = thorax; *A* = abdomen; *H* = head; *arrows* = mandible invaded by the teratoma; *curved arrow* = obstructed proximal esophagus and upper airway. (From Patel RB, Gibson JY, D'Cruz CA, et al: Sonographic diagnosis of cervical teratoma in utero. AJR 1982; 139:1220–1222. Used by permission.)

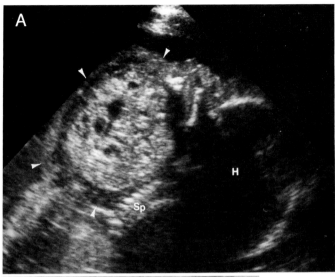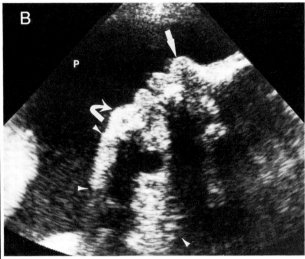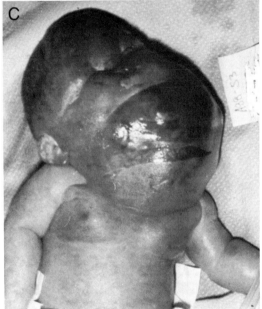

FIG 7–53.
Cervical teratoma. **A,** coronal scan of the neck at 33 weeks shows a large, complex anterolateral neck mass. **B.** sagittal profile view of the face demonstrates that the mass causes hyperextension of the neck and polyhydramnios. **C,** postnatal photograph confirms the prenatal findings. *Arrowheads* = teratoma; *curved arrow* = chin; *arrow* = nose; *Sp* = cervical spine; *H* = head; *P* = polyhydramnios.

with immediate establishment of a patent airway permitted survival with no central or peripheral neurologic defects.[174]

Associated Findings

Cervical teratoma typically occurs as an isolated anomaly. Approximately 30% of cases have associated polyhydramnios.[173] Isolated reports have documented one case each of concomitant cystic fibrosis, imperforate anus, chondrodystrophia fetalis, and hypoplastic left ventricle.[173, 176, 181]

Prognosis

Without prompt postnatal surgical resection, approximately 80% of newborns with cervical teratoma die, usually from respiratory obstruction.[173] However, with immediate resuscitation and surgical removal, the mortality is 9%–17%.[171, 173, 179] The favorable prognosis if surgical excision and satisfactory respiratory exchange can be maintained warrants consideration of early delivery following documentation of fetal lung maturity.

The prognosis may correlate inversely with the size of the tumor.[178] For example, one case with a relatively small tumor (5 × 4 cm) not detected with prenatal ultrasound survived following postnatal surgical resection of the well-encapsulated cervical teratoma.[178] It is interesting to note that, although only approximately 4% of cervical teratomas are histologically malignant, two of the four cases detected prenatally were malignant.[180, 183]

GOITER

Clinical and Pathologic Findings

Congenital hypothyroidism occurs in approximately 1 in 3,700 births.[188] In most cases of fetal goiter, the pregnancy has been complicated by maternal thyroid-blocking therapy.[188, 189, 192] Since the fetal thyroid and hypothalamo-pituitary-thyroid axis begin to function by 12–14 weeks of gestation and are crucial to normal development, placental transfer of iodine or antithyroid agents can disturb the thyroid homeostasis throughout the second and third trimesters of pregnancy.[188] With appropriate prenatal or prompt postnatal medical therapy, the prognosis for fetal goiter is good.[188]

Sonographic Findings

Fetal goiter produces a bi-lobed anterior neck mass displacing the common carotid arteries posterolaterally (Figs 7–54 and 7–55). In five case reports initially scanned at 26–33 weeks, three cases had a solid goiter, one had a goiter with cystic and solid components, and one goiter was described as being cyst-like.[185–187, 191, 193] Cases were examined because of maternal thyrotoxicosis and fetal tachycardia (two cases), polyhydramnios (two cases), and a family history of goiter (one case).

The following case summaries of fetal goiter are presented in some detail to highlight the utility of (1) examining the thyroid in pregnancies complicated by treatment of the mother with iodine-containing compounds, a strong family history of goiter, or unexplained polyhydramnios, and (2) evaluating the amniotic fluid TSH level in a pregnancy with a bi-lobed anterior neck mass.

One case occurred in a fetus exposed to large dosages of propylthiouracil via the mother since 16 weeks of gestation.[193] Following intra-amniotic instillation of thyroxine, the 4 × 6 cm mixed cystic/solid goiter decreased in size, and the fetus was born with a small goiter (2 × 3 cm.) but normal thyroid functions studies.

The second and third cases also involved a hyperthyroid woman being treated with thyrostatic medication.[191] Three weeks following subtotal thyroidectomy and cessation of medical therapy, this woman's fetus developed tachycardia, and ultrasound at 33 weeks showed a 2 × 2 cm cyst-like thyroid. Following documentation of a low amniotic fluid thyroxine level but elevated reverse triiodothyronine level, thyrostatic medication was reinstated with resultant normal fetal heart rate. At birth, redundant neck folds suggested the presence of a prior neck mass, but none was palpable. The subsequent pregnancy also resulted in fetal tachy-

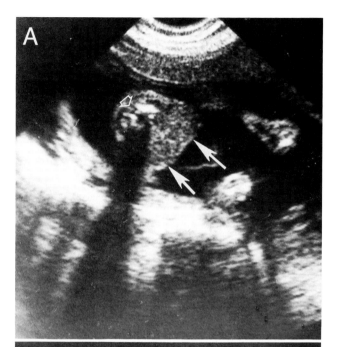

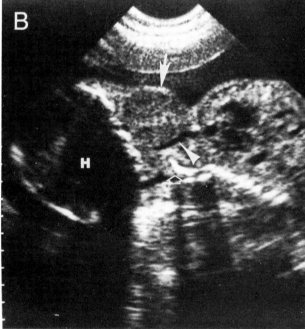

FIG 7–54.
Goiter. **A,** axial sonogram of the neck shows bi-lobed solid anterior neck masses indicating goiter. The masses distort the external contour of the fetal neck. **B,** sagittal scan of the left thyroid lobe demonstrates posterior displacement of the carotid artery and distortion of the anterior contour of the neck by the goiter. Other scans showed polyhydramnios. *Arrows* = goiter; *arrowhead* = carotid artery; *open arrow* = cervical spine; *H* = head. (From Barone CM, Van Natta FC, Kourides IA, et al: Sonographic detection of fetal goiter, an unusual cause of hydramnios. J Ultrasound Med 1985; 4:625–627. Used by permission.)

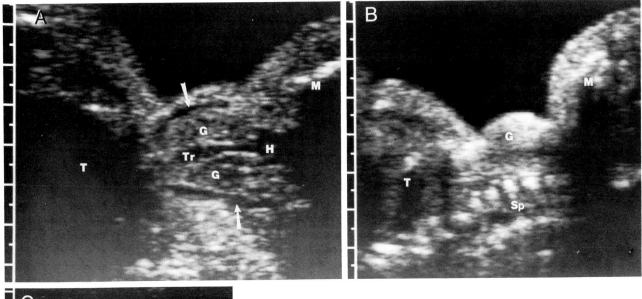

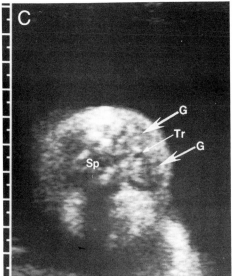

FIG 7–55.
Goiter. **A,** coronal scan of the neck at 32 weeks shows a bi-lobed solid goiter adjacent to the midline trachea and larynx. The mass distorts the contour of the neck and displaces the neck vasculature laterally. **B,** parasagittal scan demonstrates that the mass distorts the anterior contour of the neck. **C,** axial scan of the neck displays the bi-lobed goiter adjacent to the trachea. Polyhydramnios is present. Fetal umbilical blood sampling documented normal TSH and T4 levels, and the above findings gradually resolved over the next month. The newborn was euthyroid. G = goiter; M = mandible; T = thorax; arrows = neck vasculature; H = hypopharynx; Tr = trachea; Sp = cervical spine.

cardia and thyroid enlargement (1.9 × 3.1 cm) treated with maternal thyrostatic medication. Although the fetal heart rate returned to normal for approximately 6 weeks, tachycardia recurred at 33 weeks, and the fetus was stillborn with an "extremely large" goiter.

The fourth case occurred in a fetus without maternal goiterogens but with polyhydramnios and elevated amniotic fluid levels of TSH (see Fig 7–54).[185, 186] This case had primary hypothyroidism at birth with a 5 × 1.3 cm goiter immediately treated with thyroid hormone resulting in subsequent normal development. The fifth case occurred in a fetus with a family history of goiter.[187] This fetus had a small goiter (2.1 × 1.8 × 1.3 cm) and did not have polyhydramnios, but was born with macroglossia, an elevated TSH level, and a disorder of organification.

We have also seen a case at 32 weeks' gestation without maternal thyroid disease or goiterogens but with marked polyhydramnios and mild, but unmistakable thyroid enlargement (see Fig 7–55). This fetus had normal TSH and T4 levels. The goiter and polyhydramnios gradually resolved, and the newborn was euthyroid.

Associated Anomalies
Most cases of fetal goiter are isolated anomalies, but occur in the setting of polyhydramnios, family history of goiter, or maternal therapy with iodine-containing compounds. Cases with fetal thyrotoxicosis typically have tachycardia and may become hydropic.[190]

METASTATIC TUMOR OR ADENOPATHY

Adenopathy from metastatic tumor represents another rare cause for a neck mass on the prenatal sonogram. For example, adenopathy from metastatic neuroblastoma is the most common tumor to present in this manner at birth.[197] Neuroblastoma accounts for approximately 25% of congenital malignancies, and 60%–70% of neonates with congenital neuroblastoma have metastases at initial presentation, usually to the adrenals but occasionally to the sympathetic chain in the neck.[194, 199, 200]

Sonographic Findings

Metastatic neuroblastoma to the neck has been reported following in utero detection at 32 weeks of a 6–7 cm solid neck mass extending asymmetrically across the anterior portion of the neck in a fetus with hydrops and tachycardia.[197] The reported case of metastatic neuroblastoma died in utero with hydrops shortly following the diagnosis.[197] However, disseminated neuroblastoma (type IV–S) without bone metastasis at birth has a relatively favorable prognosis.[200]

Associated Findings

Since disseminated neuroblastoma may cause hydrops and tachycardia, detection of a solid neck mass in the fetus of a woman with symptoms of catecholamine excess suggests the possibility of metastatic neuroblastoma.[197, 198, 201, 202] The mother of the fetus with metastatic neuroblastoma detected prenatally had tachycardia and complained of third trimester nausea and vomiting.[197] The maternal symptoms probably resulted from catecholamine excess produced by the fetal neuroblastoma, which crossed the placenta into the maternal circulation. Toxemia or thyrotoxicosis may cause similar symptoms.

Additional findings might include an enlarged and nodular fetal adrenal and placental metastases. Fetal umbilical blood sampling would yield elevated levels of vanillylmandelic acid (VMA).

OTHER ANTERIOR NECK MASSES

Bulic et al. reported a congenital sarcoma discovered by ultrasound at 30 weeks' gestation as a 12 × 12 × 8 cm mass projecting from the neck anteriorly and associated with polyhydramnios.[195] Campbell et al. reported a case of malignant melanoma of the fetal neck and back at 30 weeks' gestation.[196] The melanoma measured 8.4 × 5.4 × 3.5 cm and had cystic and solid components. It arose from tissue beneath the skin surface of the neck, but extended into the spinal cord and meninges and created hydrocephaly.

Although not uncommon postnatally, to our knowledge other anterior neck masses have not yet been described prenatally and might be difficult to diagnose definitively. For example, a branchial cleft cyst occurs anterolaterally in the neck where it might mimic a teratoma in location but would probably be more cystic. A thyroglossal duct cyst localizes within the midline of the submandibular region where it could resemble a hemangioma or other mass. In such cases, correlation with Doppler, clinical, biochemical, and historical data may assist in diagnosis.

ABNORMAL POSITIONING OF THE NECK

Normally, the fetus holds the neck in a relatively neutral or "military" position. Hyperextension of the neck can occur with face presentation but warrants a search for a mass anteriorly. Rarely, the back of the head may be fused to the thoracic spine with iniencephaly.

TUBULAR STRUCTURES IN THE NECK

Visualization of the trachea and vasculature may be helpful in evaluation of many mass lesions of the fetal neck. Displacement of the trachea or carotid by a mass, for example, may indicate the source of the mass and may imply the presence of compression upon these structures resulting in obstructive symptoms at birth.

The fetal esophagus remains collapsed and not visible in its resting state and only distends during deglutition.[14] A dilated and fluid-filled esophagus has been documented prenatally in two cases with polyhydramnios and absence of fluid in the stomach that were documented to have esophageal atresia.[204] It is probably not a frequent finding, however, and was not described among 22 cases with esophageal atresia evaluated retrospectively.[205] Nevertheless, detection of polyhydramnios, especially in the absence of gastric fluid, warrants a search for a dilated esophagus.

Doppler evaluations suggest that growth retardation from placental insufficiency may result in an increase in the end-diastolic flow through the intracranial internal carotid arteries at the bifurcation of the middle and anterior cerebral arteries.[203, 206] This implies the "brain-sparing" effect of growth retardation.[206] The sensitivity of this test is quite low, perhaps in part because of technical difficulties related to the Doppler signal at the intracranial internal carotid artery bifurcation. The sensitivity might increase with Doppler evaluation of the straight portion of the extracranial internal carotid artery.

SUMMARY

Survey of the fetal face and neck need not be an elaborate or time-consuming task and may provide corroborative or essential information for prenatal diagnosis. Since most abnormalities of this region affect external anatomy, they are grossly obvious to the parent and clinician at birth. Prenatal detection of a face and/or neck anomaly helps prepare the parents to deal with the deformity involving this highly emotionally charged anatomic location and enables the clinician to plan the delivery and perinatal care optimally. Furthermore, survey of the face and neck in the absence of abnormality provides reassurance to the parents and frequently may serve as the focal point in parental bonding and enjoyment during their prenatal sonogram.

REFERENCES

Introduction and Prevalence of Anomalies

1. Benacerraf BR, Frigoletto FD, Bieber FR: The fetal face: Ultrasound examination. Radiology 1984; 153:495–497.
2. Benacerraf BR, Frigoletto FD, Greene MF: Abnormal facial features and extremities in human trisomy syndromes: Prenatal US appearance. Radiology 1986; 159:243–246.
3. Bergsma D (ed): *Birth Defects Compendium,* ed 2. New York, Alan R Liss, Inc, 1979.
4. Gorlin RJ, Pindborg JJ: *Syndromes of the Head and Neck.* New York, McGraw-Hill Book Co, 1964.
5. Hegge FN, Prescott GH, Watson PT: Fetal facial abnormalities identified during obstetric sonography. J Ultrasound Med 1986; 5:679–684.
6. Koontz WL: The detection of facial anomalies with ultrasound (letter). Am J Obstet Gynecol 1987; 157:1316.
7. Leopold GR: Antepartum obstetrical ultrasound examination guidelines. J Ultrasound Med 1986; 5:241–242.
8. Meizner I, Katz M, Bar-Ziv J, et al: Prenatal sonographic detection of fetal facial malformations. Isr J Med Sci 1987; 23:881–885.
9. Pilu G, Reece A, Romero R, et al: Prenatal diagnosis of craniofacial malformations with ultrasonography. Am J Obstet Gynecol 1986; 155:45–50.
10. Rempen A, Feige A: Differential diagnosis of sonographically detected tumors of the fetal cervical region. Eur J Obstet Gynecol Reprod Biol 1985; 20; 89–105.
11. Sabbagha RE, Tamura RK, Dal Compo S, et al: Fetal cranial and craniocervical masses: Ultrasound characteristics and differential diagnosis. Am J Obstet Gynecol 1980; 138:511–517.
12. Smith DW: *Recognizable Patterns of Human Malformations,* ed 3. Philadelphia, WB Saunders Co, 1982.
13. Taybi H: *Radiology of Syndromes and Metabolic Disorders,* ed 2. Chicago, Year Book Medical Publishers, Inc, 1983.

Embryology and Normal Development

14. Cooper C, Mahony BS, Bowie JD, et al: Ultrasound evaluation of the normal fetal upper airway and esophagus. J Ultrasound Med 1985; 4:343–346.
15. Escobar LF, Bixler D, Padilla LM, et al: Fetal craniofacial morphometrics: In utero evaluation at 16 weeks' gestation. Obstet Gynecol 1988; 72:674–679.
16. Hata K, Hata T, Takamiya O, et al: Ultrasonographic measurement of the fetal neck correlated with gestational age. J Ultrasound Med 1988; 7:333–337.
17. Jeanty P, Romero R, Staudach A, et al: Facial anatomy of the fetus. J Ultrasound Med 1986; 5:607–616.
18. Johnston MC, Sulik KK: Some abnormal patterns of development in the craniofacial region. Birth Defects 1979; 15:23–42.
19. Moore KL: *The Developing Human,* ed 4. Philadelphia, WB Saunders Co, 1988.
20. Stewart RE: Craniofacial malformations: Clinical and genetic considerations. Pediatr Clin N Am 1978; 25:485–515.

Normal Orbital Dimensions

21. Birnholz JC: Ultrasonic fetal ophthalmology. Early Hum Dev 1985; 12:199–209.
22. Jeanty P, Cantraine F, Cousaert E, et al: The binocular distance: A new way to estimate fetal age. J Ultrasound Med 1984; 3:241–243.
23. Mayden KL, Tortora M, Berkowitz RL, et al: Orbital diameters: A new parameter for prenatal diagnosis and dating. Am J Obstet Gynecol 1982; 144:289–297.

Diprosopus

24. Chervenak FA, Pinto MM, Heller CI, et al: Obstetric significance of fetal craniofacial duplication: A case report. J Reprod Med 1985; 30:74–76.
25. Okazaki JR, Wilson JL, Holmes SM, et al: Diprosopus: Diagnosis in utero. AJR 1987; 149:147–148.
26. Strauss S, Tamarkin M, Engelberg S, et al: Prenatal sonographic appearance of diprosopus. J Ultrasound Med 1987; 6:93–95.

Otocephaly

27. Cayea PD, Bieber FR, Ross MJ, et al: Sonographic findings in otocephaly (synotia). J Ultrasound Med 1985; 4:377–379.

Hypotelorism/Holoprosencephaly

28. Blackwell DE, Spinnato JA, Hirsch G, et al: Antenatal ultrasound diagnosis of holoprosencephaly: A case report. Am J Obstet Gynecol 1982; 143:848–849.
29. Bundy AL, Lidov H, Soliman M, et al: Antenatal sonographic diagnosis of cebocephaly. J Ultrasound Med 1988; 7:395–398.
30. Byrne PJ, Silver MM, Gilbert JM, et al: Cyclopia and congenital cytomegalovirus infection. Am J Med Genet 1987; 28:61–65.
31. Cayea PD, Balcar I, Alberti O, et al: Prenatal diagnosis of semilobar holoprosencephaly. AJR 1984; 142:401–402.
32. Chervenak FA, Isaacson G, Mahoney MJ, et al: The obstetric significance of holoprosencephaly. Obstet Gynecol 1984; 63:115–121.
33. De Meyer W, Zeman W, Palmer CG: The face predicts the brain: Diagnostic significance of median facial anomalies for holoprosencephaly (arhinencephaly). Pediatrics 1964; 34:256–263.
34. De Meyer W. Classification of cerebral malformations. Birth Defects 1971; 7:78–93.
35. Filly RA, Chinn DH, Callen PW: Alobar holoprosencephaly: Ultrasonographic prenatal diagnosis. Radiology 1984; 151:455–459.
36. Fitz CR: Holoprosencephaly and related entities. Neuroradiology 1983; 25:225–238.
37. Greene MF, Benacerraf BR, Frigoletto FD: Reliable criteria for the prenatal sonographic diagnosis of alobar holoprosencephaly. Am J Obstet Gynecol 1987; 156:687–689.
38. Lev-Gur M, Maklad NF, Patel S: Ultrasonic findings in fetal cyclopia. J Reprod Med 1983; 28:554–557.
39. Manelfe C, Sevely A: Neuroradiological study of holoprosencephalies. J Neuroradiol 1982; 9:15–45.
40. Nyberg DA, Mack LA, Bronstein A, et al: Holoprosencephaly: Prenatal sonographic diagnosis. AJR 1987; 149:1051–1058.
41. Pilu G, Romero R, Rizzo N, et al: Criteria for the prenatal diagnosis of holoprosencephaly. Am J Perinatol 1987; 4:41–49.
42. Schinzel A, Savoldelli G, Briner J, et al: Prenatal ultrasonographic diagnosis of holoprosencephaly: Two cases of cebocephaly and two of cyclopia. Arch Gynecol 1984; 236:47–53.
43. Toth Z, Csecsei K, Szeifert G, et al: Early prenatal diagnosis of cyclopia associated with holoprosencephaly. J Clin Ultrasound 1986; 14:550–553.

Hypertelorism/Anterior Cephalocele

44. Chervenak FA, Isaacson G, Rosenberg JC, et al: Antenatal diagnosis of frontal cephalocele in a fetus with atelosteogenesis. J Ultrasound Med 1986; 5:111–113.
45. Chervenak FA, Tortora M, Mayden K, et al: Antenatal diagnosis of median cleft face syndrome: Sonographic demonstration of cleft lip and hypotelorism. Am J Obstet Gynecol 1984; 149:94–97.

46. Donnenfield AE, Hughes H, Weiner S: Prenatal diagnosis and perinatal management of frontoethmoidal meningoencephalocele. Am J Perinatol 1988; 5:51–53.

Micropthalmia/Anophthalmia

47. Feldman E, Shalev E, Weiner E, et al: Micropthalmia: Prenatal ultrasonic diagnosis: A case report. Prenat Diagn 1985; 5:205–207.
48. Tamas DE, Mahony BS, Bowie JD, et al: Prenatal sonographic diagnosis of hemifacial microsomia (Goldenhar-Gorlin syndrome). J Ultrasound Med 1986; 5:461–463.

Periorbital Masses

49. Davis WK, Mahony BS, Carroll BA, et al: Antenatal sonographic detection of benign dacrocystoceles (lacrimal duct cysts). J Ultrasound Med 1987; 6:461–465.
50. Meizner I, Bar-Ziv J, Holcberg G, et al: In utero prenatal diagnosis of fetal facial tumor-hemangioma. J Clin Ultrasound 1985; 13:435–437.
51. Lasser D, Preis O, Dor N, et al: Antenatal diagnosis of giant cystic cavernous hemangioma by Doppler velocimetry. Obstet Gynecol 1988; 72:476–477.
52. Pennell RG, Baltarowich OH: Prenatal sonographic diagnosis of fetal facial hemangioma. J Ultrasound Med 1986; 5:525–528.

Intraocular Findings

53. Birnholz JC: Fetal eye movement patterns. Science 1981; 213:679–681.
54. Birnholz JC, Farrell EE: Fetal hyaloid artery: Timing of regression with US. Radiology 1988; 166:781–783.
55. Crowe C, Jassani M, Dickerman L: The prenatal diagnosis of the Walker-Warburg syndrome. Prenatal Diagn 1986; 6:177–185.
56. Farrell SA, Toi A, Leadman ML, et al: Prenatal diagnosis of retinal detachment in Walker-Warburg syndrome. Am J Med Genet 1987; 28:619–624.

The Mouth and Upper Lip

57. Benacerraf BR, Frigoletto FD, Greene MF: Abnormal facial features and extremities in human trisomy syndromes: Prenatal US appearance. Radiology 1986; 159:243–246.
58. Benacerraf BR, Miller WA, Frigoletto FD: Sonographic detection of fetuses with trisomies 13 and 18: Accuracy and limitations. Am J Obstet Gynecol 1988; 158:404–409.
59. Birnholz JC: AIUM Newsletter. February 1988, pp 3–4.
60. Bowie JD, Claire MR: Fetal swallowing and regurgitation: Observation of normal and abnormal activity. Radiology 1982; 144:877.
61. Bundy AL, Salzman DH, Emerson D, et al: Sonographic features associated with cleft palate. J Clin Ultrasound 1986 14:486–489.

62. Christ JE, Meininger MG: Ultrasound diagnosis of cleft lip and cleft palate before birth. Plast Reconst Surg 1981; 68:854–859.

63. Christ JE: Fetal surgery: A frontier for plastic surgery. Plast Reconstr Surg 1986; 77:645–647.

64. Saltzman DH, Benacerraf BR, Frigoletto FD: Diagnosis and management of fetal facial clefts. Am J Obstet Gynecol 1986; 155:377–379.

65. Seeds JW, Cefalo RC: Technique of early sonographic diagnosis of bilateral cleft lip and palate. Obstet Gynecol 1983; 62:2S–7S.

66. Tolarova M: Orofacial clefts in Czechoslovakia. Incidence, genetics and prevention of cleft lip and palate over a 19-year period. Scand J Plast Reconstr Surg 1987; 21:19–25.

67. Witt DR, Hayden MR, Holbrook KA, et al: Restrictive dermopathy: A newly recognized autosomal recessive skin dysplasia. Am J Med Genet 1986; 24:631–648.

Amniotic Band Syndrome

68. Borlum K-G: Amniotic band syndrome in second trimester associated with fetal malformations. Prenat Diagn 1984; 4:311–314.

69. Chen H, Gonzalez E: Amniotic band sequence and its neurocutaneous manifestations. Am J Med Genet 1987; 28:661–673.

70. Donnenfeld AE, Dunn LK, Rose NC: Discordant amniotic band sequence in monozygotic twins. Am J Med Genet 1985; 20:685–694.

71. Fiedler JM, Phelan JP: The amniotic band syndrome in monozygotic twins. Am J Obstet Gynecol 1983; 146:863–864.

72. Fiske CE, Filly RA, Golbus MS: Prenatal ultrasound diagnosis of amniotic band syndrome. J Ultrasound Med 1982; 1:45–47.

73. Fried AW, Woodring JH, Shier RW, et al: Omphalocele in limb-body wall deficiency syndrome: Atypical sonographic appearance. J Clin Ultrasound 1982; 10:400–402.

74. Herbert WNP, Seeds JW, Cefalo RD, et al: Prenatal detection of intra-amniotic bands: Implications and management. Obstet Gynecol 1985; 65:36S–38S.

75. Hill LM, Kislak S, Jones N: Prenatal ultrasound diagnosis of a forearm constriction band. J Ultrasound Med 1988; 7:293–295.

76. Kalousek DK, Bamforth S: Amnion rupture sequence in previable fetuses. Am J Med Genet 1988; 31:63–73.

77. Lockwood C, Ghidini A, Romero R: Amniotic band syndrome in monozygotic twins: Prenatal diagnosis and pathogenesis. Obstet Gynecol 1988; 71:1012–1016.

78. Mahony BS, Filly RA, Callen PW, et al: The amniotic band syndrome: Antenatal diagnosis and potential pitfalls. Am J Obstet Gynecol 1985; 152:63–68.

79. Rushton DI: Amniotic band syndrome. Br Med J 1983; 286:919–920.

80. Seeds JW, Cefalo RC, Herbert WNP: Amniotic band syndrome. Am J Obstet Gynecol 1982; 144:243–248.

81. Torpin R: *Fetal Malformations Caused by Amnion Rupture During Gestation.* Springfield, IL, Charles C Thomas, 1968, pp 1–76.

82. Worthen NJ, Lawrence D, Bustillo M: Amniotic band syndrome: Antenatal ultrasonic diagnosis of discordant anencephaly. J Clin Ultrasound 1980; 8:453–455.

83. Yamaguchi M, Yasuda H, Kuroki T, et al: Early prenatal diagnosis of amniotic band syndrome. Am J Perinatol 1988; 5:5–8.

Macroglossia

84. Cobellis G, Iannoto P, Stabile M, et al: Prenatal ultrasound diagnosis of macroglossia in the Wiedemann-Beckwith syndrome. Prenat Diagn 1988; 8:79–81

85. Grundy H, Walton S, Burlbaw J, et al: Beckwith-Wiedemann syndrome: Prenatal ultrasound diagnosis using standard kidney to abdominal circumference ratio. Am J Perinatol 1985; 2:236–239.

86. Koontz WL, Shaw LA, Lavery JP: Antenatal sonographic appearance of Beckwith-Wiedemann syndrome. J Clin Ultrasound 1986; 14:57–59.

87. Pettenati MJ, Haines JL, Higgins RR, et al: Wiedemann-Beckwith syndrome: Presentation of clinical and cytogenetic data on 22 cases and review of the literature. Hum Genet 1986; 74:143–154.

88. Shapiro LR, Duncan PA, Davidian MM, et al: The placenta in familial Beckwith-Wiedemann syndrome. Birth Defects 1982; 18:203–206.

89. Weinstein L, Anderson C: In utero diagnosis of Beckwith-Wiedemann syndrome by ultrasound. Radiology 1980; 134:474.

90. Winter SC, Curry CJR, Smith JC, et al: Prenatal diagnosis of the Beckwith-Wiedemann syndrome. Am J Med Genet 1986; 24:137–141.

91. Zanetti B, Signori E, Consolaro, et al: Congenital fibrosarcoma of the tongue. Z Kinderchir 1982; 35:7–8.

The Facial Profile

92. Benson CB, Pober BR, Hirsch MP, et al: Sonography of acrofacial dysostosis syndrome in utero. J Ultrasound Med 1988; 7:163–167.

93. Chen H, Blumberg B, Immken L, et al: The Pena-Shokeir phenotype: Report of five cases and further delineation of the syndrome. Am J Med Genet 1983; 16:213–224.

94. Crane JP, Beaver HA: Midtrimester sonographic diagnosis of mandibulofacial dysostosis. Am J Med Genet 1986; 25:251–255.

95. Majoor-Krakauer DF, Wladimiroff JW, Stewart PA, et al: Microcephaly, micrognathia, and bird-headed dwarfism: Prenatal diagnosis of a Seckel-like syndrome. Am J Med Genet 1987; 27:183–188.

96. Malinger G, Rosen N, Achiron R, et al: Pierre Robin sequence associated with amniotic band syndrome: Ultrasonographic diagnosis and pathogenesis. Prenat Diagn 1987; 7:455–459.

97. Pilu G, Romero R, Reece EA, et al: The prenatal diagnosis of Robin anomalad. Am J Obstet Gynecol 1986; 154:630–632.

98. Shenker L, Reed K, Anderson C, et al: Syndrome of camptodactyly, ankyloses, facial anomalies, and pulmonary hypoplasia (Pena-Skokeir syndrome): Obstetric and ultrasound aspects. Am J Obstet Gynecol 1985; 152:303–307.

Epignathus

99. Alter AD, Cove JK: Congenital nasopharyngeal teratoma: Report of a case and review of the literature. J Pediatr Surg 1987; 22:179–181.

100. Anderson RL, Simpson GF, Sherman S, et al: Fetal pharyngeal teratoma—another cause of elevated amniotic fluid alpha-fetoprotein. Am J Obstet Gynecol 1984; 150:432–433.

101. Chervenak FA, Tortora M, Moya FR, et al: Antenatal sonographic diagnosis of epignathus. J Ultrasound Med 1984; 3:235–237.

102. Chervenak FA, Isaacson G, Touloukian R, et al: Diagnosis and management of fetal teratomas. Obstet Gynecol 1985; 66:666–671.

103. Holmgren G, Rydnert J: Male fetus with epignathus originating from the ethmoidal sinus. Eur J Obstet Gynecol Reprod Biol 1987; 24:69–72.

104. Kang KW, Hissong SL, Langer A: Prenatal ultrasound diagnosis of epignathus J Clin Ultrasound 1978; 6:330–331.

105. Kaplan C, Perlmutter S, Molinoff S: Epignathus with placental hydrops. Arch Pathol Lab Med 1980; 104:374–375.

106. Teal LN, Angtuaco TL, Jimenez JF, et al: Fetal teratomas: Antenatal diagnosis and clinical management. J Clin Ultrasound 1988; 16:329–336.

The Ear

107. Aase JM, Wilson AC, Smith DW: Small ears in Down's syndrome: A helpful diagnostic aid. J Pediatr 1973; 82:845–847.

108. Birnholz JC, Benacerraf BR: The development of human fetal hearing. Science 1983; 222:516–518.

109. Birnholz JC: The fetal external ear. Radiology 1983; 147:819–821.

110. Birnholz JC, Farrell EE: Fetal ear length. Pediatr 1988; 81:555–558.

111. Crade M, Lovett S: Fetal response to sound stimulation: Preliminary report exploring use of sound stimulation in routine obstetrical ultrasound examinations. J Ultrasound Med 1988; 7:499–503.

112. Fink IJ, Chinn DH, Callen PW: A potential pitfall in the ultrasonographic diagnosis of fetal encephalocele. J Ultrasound Med 1983; 2:313–314.

113. Hill LM, Thomas ML, Peterson CS: The ultrasonic detection of Apert syndrome. J Ultrasound Med 1987; 6:601–604.

114. Kuhlman KA, Burns KA, Depp R, et al: Ultrasonic imaging of normal fetal response to external vibratory acoustic stimulation. Am J Obstet Gynecol 1988; 158:47–51.

115. Romero R, Mazor M, Hobbins JC: A critical appraisal of fetal acoustic stimulation as an antenatal test for fetal well-being. Obstet Gynecol 1988; 71:781–786.

Cystic Hygroma Colli

116. Benacerraf BR, Frigoletto FD, Cramer DW: Down syndrome: Sonographic sign for diagnosis in the second-trimester fetus. Radiology 1987; 163:811–813.

117. Benacerraf BR, Frigoletto FD, Laboda LA: Sonographic diagnosis of Down syndrome in the second trimester. Am J Obstet Gynecol 1985; 153:49–52.

118. Benacerraf BR, Frigoletto FD: Soft tissue nuchal fold in the second-trimester fetus: Standards for normal measurements compared with those in Down syndrome. Am J Obstet Gynecol 1987; 157:1146–1149.

119. Benacerraf BR, Frigoletto FD: Prenatal sonographic diagnosis of isolated congenital cystic hygroma, unassociated with lymphedema or other morphologic abnormality. J Ultrasound Med 1987; 6:63–66.

120. Bieber FR, Petres RE, Biebar JM, et al: Prenatal detection of a familial nuchal bleb simulating encephalocele. Birth Defects 1979; 15:51–61.

121. Brock DJ, Barron L, Bedgood D, et al: Distinguishing hygroma and amniotic fluid. Prenatal Diagn 1985; 5:363–366.

122. Brown BSJ, Thompson DL: Ultrasonographic features of the fetal Turner syndrome. J Can Assoc Radiol 1984; 35:40–46.

123. Byrne J, Blanc WA, Warburton D, et al: The significance of cystic hygroma in fetuses. Hum Pathol 1984; 15:61–67.

124. Chervenak FA, Isaacson G, Blakemore KJ, et al: Fetal cystic hygroma: Cause and natural history. N Engl J Med 1983; 308:822–825.

125. Chervenak FA, Isaacson G, Tortora M: A sonographic study of fetal cystic hygromas. J Clin Ultrasound 1985; 13:311–315.

126. Chodirker BN, Harman CR, Greenberg CR: Spontaneous resolution of a cystic hygroma in a fetus with Turner syndrome. Prenat Diagn 1988; 8:291–296.

127. Cowchock FS, Wapner RJ, Kurtz A, et al: Not all cystic hygromas occur in the Ullrich-Turner syndrome. Am J Med Genet 1982; 12:327–331.

128. Cumming WA, Ohlsson A, Ali A: Campomelia, cervical lymphocele, polycystic dysplasia, short gut, polysplenia. Am J Med Genet 1986; 25:783–790.

129. Dallapiccola B, Zelente L, Perla G, et al: Prenatal diagnosis of recurrence of cystic hygroma with normal chromosomes. Prenat Diagn 1984; 4:383–386.

130. Elejalde BR, de Elejalde MM, Leno J: Nuchal cysts syndromes: Etiology, pathogenesis, and prenatal diagnosis. Am J Med Genet 1985; 21:417–432.

131. Frigoletto FD, Birnholz JC, Driscoll SG, et al:

Ultrasound diagnosis of cystic hygroma. Am J Obstet Gynecol 1980; 136:962–964.

132. Exalto N, Van Zalen RM, Van Brandenburg WJA: Early prenatal diagnosis of cystic hygroma by real-time ultrasound. J Clin Ultrasound 1985; 13:655–658.

133. Garden AS, Benzie RJ, Miskin M, et al: Fetal cystic hygroma colli: Antenatal diagnosis, significance, and management. Am J Obstet Gynecol 1986; 154:221–225.

134. Grundy H, Glasmann A, Burlbaw J, et al: Hemangioma presenting as a cystic mass in the fetal neck. J Ultrasound Med 1985; 4:147–150.

135. Gustavii B, Edvall H: First-trimester diagnosis of cystic nuchal hygroma. Acta Obstet Gynecol Scand 1984; 63:377–378.

136. Hoffman-Tretin J, Koenigsberg M, Ziprkowski M: Antenatal demonstration of axillary cystic hygroma. J Ultrasound Med 1988; 7:233–235.

137. Holzgreve W, Rempen A, Beller FK: Fetal lymphangiectasia—Another cause for a positive amniotic fluid acetylcholinesterase test. Arch Gynecol 1986; 239:123–125.

138. Lyngbye T, Huagaard L, Klebe JC: Antenatal sonographic diagnoses of giant cystic hygroma of the neck: A problem for the clinician. Acta Obstet Gynecol Scand 1986; 65:873–875.

139. Marchese C, Savin E, Dragoue E, et al: Cystic hygroma: Prenatal diagnosis and genetic counselling. Prenatal Diagn 1985; 5:221–227.

140. Nevin NC, Nevin J, Thompson W, et al: Cystic hygroma simulating an encephalocele. Prenat Diagn 1983; 3:249–252.

141. Pawlowitzki IH, Wormänn B: Elevated amniotic alpha-fetoprotein in a fetus with Turner's syndrome due to puncture of a cystic hygroma. Am J Obstet Gynecol 1979; 133:584–585.

142. Pearce JM, Griffin D, Campbell S: Cystic hygroma in trisomy 18 and 21. Prenat Diagn 1984; 4:371–375.

143. Pearce JM, Griffin D, Campbell S: The differential prenatal diagnosis of cystic hygroma and encephalocele by ultrasound examination. J Clin Ultrasound 1985; 13:317–320.

144. Phillips HE, Mc Gahan JP: Intrauterine fetal cystic hygromas: Sonographic detection. AJR 1981; 136:799–802.

145. Pijpers L, Reuss A, Stewart PA, et al: Fetal cystic hygroma: Prenatal diagnosis and management. Obstet Gynecol 1988; 72:223–224.

146. Quinlan RW: A sonographic artifact, fetal hair, mimicking a craniocervical meningocele in pregnancy complicated by hydramnios. J Reprod Med 1984; 29:354–356.

147. Rahmani MR, Fong KW, Connor TP: The varied sonographic appearance of cystic hygroma in utero. J Ultrasound Med 1986; 5:165–168.

148. Redford DHA, Mc Nay MB, Ferguson-Smith ME, et al: Aneuploidy and cystic hygroma detectable by ultrasound. Prenat Diagn 1984; 4:377–382.

149. Reuss A, Pijpers L, Schampers PTFM, et al: The impor-

tance of chorionic villus sampling after first trimester diagnosis of cystic hygroma. Prenat Diagn 1987; 7:299–301.

150. Rodis JF, Vintzileos AM, Campbell WA, et al: Spontaneous resolution of fetal cystic hygroma in Down's syndrome. Obstet Gynecol 1988; 71:976–977.

151. Shaub M, Wilson R, Collea J: Fetal cystic lymphangioma (cystic hygroma): Prepartum ultrasonic findings. Radiology 1976; 121:449–450.

152. Sheth S, Nussbaum AR, Hutchins GM, et al: Cystic hygromas in children: Sonographic-pathologic correlation. Radiology 1987; 162:821–824.

153. Stevens TD, Shepard TH: The Down syndrome in the fetus. Teratology 1980; 22:37–41.

154. Toi A, Simpson GF, Filly RA: Ultrasonically evident fetal nuchal skin thickening: Is it specific for Down syndrome? Am J Obstet Gynecol 1987; 156:150–153.

155. Zagoria RJ, Machen BC, King GT, et al: Unsuspected fetal abnormality. Invest Radiol 1986; 21:282–284.

156. Zarabi M, Mieckowski GC, Mazer J: Cystic hygroma associated with Noonan's syndrome. J Clin Ultrasound 1983; 11:398–400.

Occipital Encephalocele/Cervical Myelomeningocele

157. Callen PW, Mahony BS: Obstetrics, in Vogler JB, Helms CA, Callen PW (eds): *Normal Variants and Pitfalls in Imaging.* Philadelphia, WB Saunders Co, 1986, pp 335–363.

158. Chatterjee MS, Bondoc B, Adhate A: Prenatal diagnosis of occipital encephalocele. Am J Obstet Gynecol 1985; 153:646–647.

159. Chervenak FA, Isaacson G, Mahoney MJ, et al: Diagnosis and management of fetal cephalocele. Obstet Gynecol 1984; 64:86–90.

160. Cohen MM, Lemire RJ: Syndromes with cephaloceles. Teratology 1982; 25:161–172.

161. Holmes LB, Driscoll SG, Atkins L: Etiologic heterogeneity of neural-tube defects. N Engl J Med 1976; 294:365–369.

162. Karjalainen O, Aula P, Seppala M, et al: Prenatal diagnosis of the Meckel syndrome. Obstet Gynecol 1981; 57:13S–15S.

163. Lorber J, Schofield JK: The prognosis of occipital encephalocele. Z Kinderchir 1979; 28:347–351.

164. Sabbagha RE, Depp R, Grasse D, et al: Ultrasound diagnosis of occipitothoracic meningocele at 22 weeks gestation. Am J Obstet Gynecol 1978; 131:113–114.

Hemangioma

165. Bell RL: Ultrasound of hemangioma of the neck in a newborn. J Tenn Med Assoc 1978; 70:289.

166. Grundy H, Glasman A, Burlbaw J, et al: Hemangioma presenting as a cystic mass in the fetal neck. J Ultrasound Med 1985; 4:147–150.

167. Lenke RR, Cyr DR, Mack LA, et al: Fetal hydrops sec-

ondary to a paratracheal hemangiomatous malformation. J Ultrasound Med 1986; 5:223–225.
168. Lewis BD, Doubilet PM, Heller VL, et al: Cutaneous and
visceral hemangiomata in the Klippel-Trenaunay-Weber
syndrome: Antenatal sonographic detection. AJR 1986;
147:598–600.
169. Mc Gahan JP, Schneider JM: Fetal neck hemangioendothelioma with secondary hydrops fetalis: Sonographic
diagnosis. J Clin Ultrasound 1986; 14:384–388.
170. Seoud M, Santos-Ramos R, Friedman JM: Early prenatal
ultrasonic findings in Klippel-Trenaunay-Weber syndrome. Prenat Diagn 1984; 4:227–230.

Cervical Teratoma

171. Batsakis JG, Littler ER, Oberman HA: Teratomas of the
neck. Arch Otolaryngol 1964; 79:619–624.
172. Goodwin BD, Gay BB: The roentgen diagnosis of teratoma of the thyroid region. AJR 1965; 95:25–31.
173. Gundry SR, Wesley JR, Klein MD, et al: Cervical
teratomas in the newborn. J Pediatr Surg 1983;
18:382–386.
174. Holinger LD, Birnholz JC: Management of infants with
prenatal diagnosis of airway obstruction by teratoma.
Ann Otol Rhinol Laryngol 1987; 96:61–64.
175. Hajdu SI, Faruque AA, Hajdu ED, et al: Teratoma
of the neck in infants. Am J Dis Child 1966;
111:412–416.
176. Jordan RB, Gauderer WL: Cervical teratomas: An analysis, literature review and proposed classification. J Pediatr Surg 1988; 23:583–591.
177. Patel RB, Gibson JY, D-Cruz CA, et al: Sonographic diagnosis of cervical teratoma in utero. AJR 1982;
139:1220–1222.
178. Rosenfeld CR, Coln CD, Duenhoelter JH: Fetal cervical
teratoma as a cause of polyhydramnios. Pediatrics
1979; 64:176–178.
179. Schoenfeld A, Edelstein T, Joel-Cohen SJ: Prenatal ultrasonic diagnosis of fetal teratoma of the neck. Br J Radiol 1977; 51:742–744.
180. Schoenfeld A, Ovadia J, Edelstein T, et al: Malignant
cervical teratoma of the fetus. Acta Obstet Gynecol
Scand 1982; 61:7–12.
181. Silberman R, Mendelson IR: Teratoma of the neck. Report of two cases and review of the literature. Arch Dis
Child 1960; 35:159–170.
182. Suita S, Ikeda K, Nakano H, et al: Teratoma of the neck
in a newborn infant—a case report. Z Kindershir
1982; 35:9–11.
183. Thurkow AL, Visser GHA, Oosterhuis JW, et al: Ultrasound observations of a malignant cervical teratoma of
the fetus in a case of polyhydramnios: Case history and
review. Eur J Obstet Gynecol Reprod Biol 1983;
14:375–384.
184. Trecet JC, Claramunt V, Larraz J, et al: Prenatal ultrasound diagnosis of fetal teratoma of the neck. J Clin
Ultrasound 1984; 12:509–511.

Goiter

185. Barone CM, Van Natta FC, Kourides IA, et al:
Sonographic detection of fetal goiter, an unusual cause
of hydramnios. J Ultrasound Med 1985; 4:625–627.
186. Kourides IA, Berkowitz RL, Pang S, et al: Antepartum
diagnosis of goitrous hypothyroidism by fetal ultrasonography and amniotic fluid thyrotropin concentration. J Clin Endocrinol Metab 1984; 59:1016–1018.
187. Leger J, Le Guern H, Plouhinec C, et al: Antenatal diagnosis of fetal goiter by ultrasonography. Presse Med
1987; 16:1521–1524.
188. Mehta PS, Mehta SJ, Vorherr H: Congenital iodide goiter and hypothyroidism: A review. Obstet Gynecol
Surv 1983; 38:237–247.
189. Packard GB, Williams ET, Wheelock SE: Congenital obstructing goiter. Surgery 1960; 48:422–430.
190. Page DV, Brady K, Mitchell J, et al: The pathology of
intrauterine thyrotoxicosis: Two case reports. Obstet
Gynecol 1988; 72:479–481.
191. Pekonen F, Teramo K, Makinen T, et al: Prenatal diagnosis and treatment of fetal thyrotoxicosis. Am J Obstet Gynecol 1984; 150:893–894.
192. Theodoropoulos T, Braverman LE, Vagenakis AG: Iodine induced hypothyroidism: A potential hazard during perinatal life. Science 1979; 205:502–503.
193. Weiner S, Scharf JI, Bolognese RJ, et al: Antenatal diagnosis and treatment of a fetal goiter. J Reprod Med
1980; 24:39–42.

Metastases/Other Neck Masses

194. Birner WF: Neuroblastoma as a cause of antenatal
death. Am J Obstet Gynecol 1961; 82:1388–1391.
195. Bulic VM, Urbanke A, Ciglar S, et al: Bösartiger tumor
(Sarkom) am hals eines fetus, durch ultraschall
während der gravidität festgestellt. Zbl Gynäk 1975;
97:747–753.
196. Campbell WA, Storlazzi E, Vintzileos AM, et al: Fetal
malignant melanoma: Ultrasound presentation and review of the literature. Obstet Gynecol 1987; 70:434–
439.
197. Gadwood KA, Reynes CJ: Prenatal sonography of metastatic neuroblastoma. J Clin Ultrasound 1983; 11:512–
515.
198. Moss TJ, Kaplan L: Association of hydrops fetalis with
congenital neuroblastoma. Am J Obstet Gynecol 1978;
132:905–906.
199. Schneider KM, Becker JM, Krasna IH: Neonatal neuroblastoma. Pediatrics 1965; 36:359–366.
200. Schwischuk LE: *Radiology of the Newborn and Young
Infant,* ed 2. Baltimore, Williams & Wilkins Co, 1980,
pp 602–609.
201. Van der Slikke JW, Balk AG: Hydramnios with hydrops
fetalis and disseminated fetal neuroblastoma. Obstet
Gynecol 1980; 55:250–251.
202. Voute PA, Wadman SK, Van Putten WJ: Congenital neu-

roblastoma. Symptoms in the mother during pregnancy. Clin Pediatr 1970; 9:206–207.

Tubular Neck Structures

203. Clapp JF, Mc Laughlin MK, Gellis J, et al: Regional distribution of cerebral blood flow in experimental intrauterine growth retardation. Am J Obstet Gynecol 1984; 150:843–846.
204. Eyheremendy E, Pfister M: Antenatal real-time diagnosis of esophageal atresia. J Clin Ultrasound 1983; 11:395–397.
205. Pretorius DH, Drose JA, Dennis MA, et al: Tracheoesophageal fistula in utero: Twenty-two cases. J Ultrasound Med 1987; 6:509–513.
206. Wladimiroff JW, Wijngaard JAGW, Degani S, et al: Cerebral and umbilical arterial blood flow velocity waveforms in normal and growth retarded pregnancies. Obstet Gynecol 1987; 69:705–709.

8

The Thorax

Pamela L. Hilpert, M.D., Ph.D.

Dolores H. Pretorius, M.D.

Arrested, disordered, or delayed maturation of the fetal lung frequently results in postnatal respiratory distress or death. Derangements of the intrauterine environment, thorax, or extrathoracic fetal organ systems are common and profoundly affect the prenatal development of the lungs.

This chapter discusses the embryogenesis of normal lung development followed by a discussion of the sonographic approach to thoracic abnormalities. This precedes a more detailed discussion of the individual pathologic entities affecting the thorax, excluding intrinsic cardiac abnormalities. Please see Chapter 9 for a detailed discussion of the heart.

NORMAL LUNG DEVELOPMENT

Four sequential stages of fetal lung development occur, with a gradual transition between each subsequent stage (Figs 8–1 and 8–2).[1, 6–9] An understanding of these normal stages of prenatal lung development provides insight regarding the sequelae of various abnormalities which affect the thorax at different stages of gestation and with varying degrees of severity.

First, the embryonic period lasts from conception until the fifth week of gestation. During this phase, the lung bud develops as an outgrowth from the ventral aspect of the primitive foregut. Alteration in development during the embryonic period leads to pulmonary agenesis (bilateral or unilateral).

Second, the pseudoglandular period lasts from 5 to 17 weeks of gestation. Surrounding mesenchyme induces growth and development of the bronchial tree during this phase of lung development.[10] A series of dichotomous branchings of the initial lung bud occur to form the trachea and the bronchial branches to the level of the terminal bronchioles by about 16 weeks' gestation. At this time the airways consist of narrow tubules with thick columnar or cuboidal lining surrounded by loose mesenchymal stroma. Although the pre-acinar airways continue to increase in size as gestation progresses, further branching cannot occur. An insult to the developing lung during the pseudoglandular period leads to a decrease in the number of bronchial divisions, with or without an overgrowth of the columnar or cuboidal lining characteristic of this period.

Third, the canalicular phase lasts from 17 to 24 weeks' gestation. An insult that persists into these later stages of lung development typically results in abnormally small size of the conducting airways as well as a decreased number and size of acini and accompanying blood vessels. Differentiation of the airways begins with enlargement of the lumina and thinning of the cuboidal epithelial lining during the canalicular phase of lung development. The capillary network, which serves for future gas exchange, becomes intimately associated with the epithelium of the primitive respiratory bronchioles. Cartilage, connective tissue, muscle, and lymphatics form at this time.

And fourth, the terminal sac or alveolar phase lasts from 24 weeks until term. Great variability in lung maturity exists during this stage of lung development. During this stage, the epithelial lining further differentiates into type I and II pneumocytes, surfactant appears, the blood-gas barrier thins, and progressive branching of the respiratory airways occurs until term.

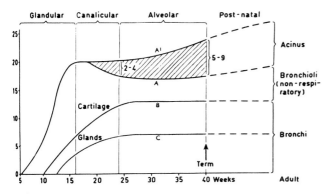

FIG 8–1.
Developmental stages of the intrasegmental bronchial tree. *Line A* represents the increase in the number of bronchial generations; *shaded area* between *A* and *A¹* represents the respiratory part of the bronchial tree (i.e., respiratory bronchioles and alveolar ducts). *Line B* shows the extension of cartilage along the bronchial tree, and *Line C,* the extension of mucous glands. The diagram includes adult values, showing the increase in total generations in the postnatal period. The verticle axis indicates number of generations. (From Bucher U, Reid L: Development of the intrasegmental bronchial tree: The pattern of branching and development of cartilage at various stages of intrauterine life. Thorax 1961; 16:207–218. Used by permission.)

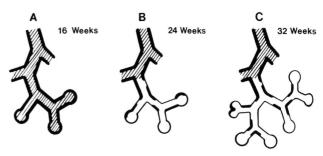

FIG 8–2.
Development of the bronchial tree. **A,** 16 weeks: at the end of the pseudoglandular period, all the nonrespiratory airways exist to the level of the terminal bronchioles. They are lined by thick columnar or cuboidal cells. **B,** 24 weeks: branching and differentiation of the respiratory airways begins during the canalicular phase. The epithelium is interrupted by ingrowth of capillaries. **C,** 32 weeks: progressive branching and differentiation of the respiratory airways occurs during the alveolar phase. (From Bucher U, Reid L: Development of the intrasegmental bronchial tree: The pattern of branching and development of cartilage at various stages of intrauterine life. Thorax 1961; 16:207-218. Used by permission.)

Lung growth continues postnatally, with continued formation of alveoli until about 8 years of age.

Normal fetal lung growth depends on several factors (1) adequate intrathoracic space to allow pulmonary parenchymal growth and development; (2) adequate intrauterine space (sufficient amniotic fluid) to allow thoracic growth and motion; (3) normal balance of fluid volume and pressure within the trachea and airspaces; and (4) normal fetal breathing movements.[8] Deficiency of any of these factors may result in abnormal lung development.[8, 29]

THE SONOGRAPHIC APPROACH

Sonography routinely visualizes the fetal lungs by the mid second trimester. They create homogeneous mid-range echoes, although their echogenicity varies and subtle differences in echogenicity have not been proven to be useful in prenatal diagnosis (Fig 8–3).[2, 5] The lungs grow at a rate commensurate to that of the heart and thorax, such that the ratio between the diameter of the heart and the thoracic circumference normally remains constant throughout the second and third trimesters.[4]

Normally, the cardiac position and axis both remain constant throughout the second and third trimesters.[3] Since intrathoracic space-occupying lesions often displace the heart or mediastinum and potentially pro-

duce pulmonary hypoplasia by compression or replacement of normal lung parenchyma, determination of the cardiac position and axis provides useful information in the evaluation of the normal and abnormal fetal thorax.[3] The four-chamber view of the heart best evaluates the cardiac position and axis (Fig 8–4). Furthermore, the thoracic circumference is derived on the plane of section for the four-chamber view of the heart (Fig 8–5). For these reasons, the four-chamber view is useful in detection and initial evaluation of both the normal and abnormal fetal thorax.

On the four-chamber view, the heart normally lies anterior to a line dividing the chest into equal anterior and posterior portions and to the left of a line drawn from the spine to the anterior chest wall (see Fig 8–4). Only a small portion of the right and left atria lies outside the left anterior quadrant. The apex of the normal fetal heart touches the inner aspect of the left chest wall. The cardiac axis is the angle that the interventricular septum makes with the line drawn from the spine to the anterior chest wall. The range of normal cardiac axes is 22 to 75 degrees, with a mean of 45 degrees.[3]

Deviation of the fetal heart from the expected normal position warrants a search for either an intrathoracic mass or fluid collection (Table 8–1). Deviation of the normal fetal cardiac axis also should initiate a search for intracardiac anomalies. In such cases, location of the inferior and superior vena cavae, stomach, and liver (fetal situs) must be determined. Abnormal fetal cardiac axis without an abnormal cardiac position also may indicate a primary lung abnormality or be a normal variant. For example, in four fetuses with only abnormal cardiac axis, two died with severe congenital

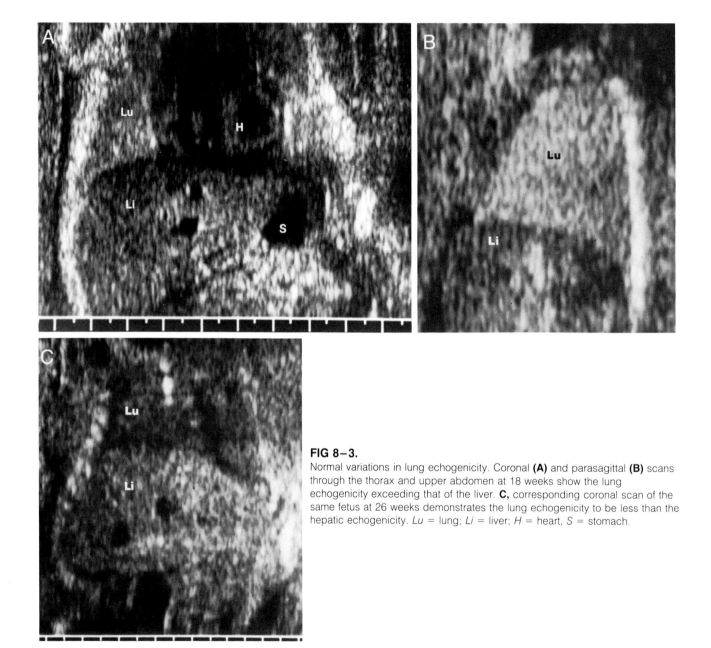

FIG 8–3.
Normal variations in lung echogenicity. Coronal **(A)** and parasagittal **(B)** scans through the thorax and upper abdomen at 18 weeks show the lung echogenicity exceeding that of the liver. **C,** corresponding coronal scan of the same fetus at 26 weeks demonstrates the lung echogenicity to be less than the hepatic echogenicity. *Lu* = lung; *Li* = liver; *H* = heart, *S* = stomach.

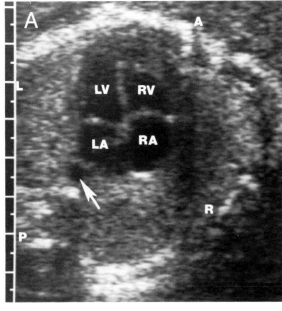

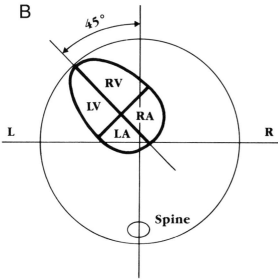

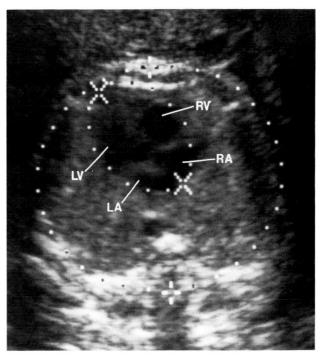

FIG 8–5.
Normal thoracic circumference. Scan of the thorax at the level of the four-chamber view of the heart shows the thoracic circumference. + *graticules* = thoracic circumference; × *graticules* = cardiac circumference; *LA* = left atrium; *LV* = left ventricle; *RA* = right atrium; *RV* = right ventricle.

FIG 8–4.
Normal four-chamber view of the heart. Sonogram **(A)** and corresponding schematic drawing **(B)** through the normal fetal thorax shows the four cardiac chambers with appropriate cardiac axis, position, and size. Documentation of normal relationships on this single view helps to exclude many thoracic abnormalities. *A* = anterior; *P* = posterior; *R* = right; *L* = left; *RA* = right atrium; *RV* = right ventricle; *LA* = left atrium; *LV* = left ventricle; *arrow* = descending aorta. (Part **B** from Comstock CH: Normal fetal heart axis and position. Obstet Gynecol 1987; 70:255–259. Used by permission.)

anomalies (congenital alveolar hypoplasia and bilateral bronchomalacia), and two are alive and well.[3]

Subsequent to the detection or suspicion of a thoracic abnormality or mass on the prenatal ultrasound, the following series of questions may assist in differential diagnosis and prediction of outcome:

1. *Is there evidence for pulmonary hypoplasia?*
2. *Is an abnormal thoracic fluid collection or mass present? If so, what is the size and echogenicity of the abnormality? Does it appear to arise from the pleural space, chest wall, lung, pericardium, or abdomen?*
3. *Are concomitant anomalies or hydrops present?*

Pulmonary hypoplasia detected prenatally usually occurs in prolonged and severe oligohydramnios secondary to oliguria or intrauterine growth retardation. Many other cases, however, result from primary thoracic abnormalities (Table 8–2). In the case of an abnormal thoracic mass or pleural fluid collection, evaluation of the size and associated mass effect of the abnormality may assist in prediction of its etiology and associated pulmonary hypoplasia. Unfortunately, how-

TABLE 8–1.

Causes for Mediastinal Shift

Unilateral or asymmetric pleural fluid collection
Thoracic mass (see Tables 8–3 to 8–5)
Unilateral bronchial atresia, stenosis, or compression
Unilateral agenesis of the lung

TABLE 8–2.

Primary Thoracic Abnormalities Affecting Prenatal Lung Development

A. Pleural fluid collections
 1. Chylothorax
 2. Hydrops fetalis
B. Developmental abnormality of the lung and foregut
 1. Cystic adenomatoid malformation of the lung
 2. Bronchopulmonary sequestration
 3. Bronchial atresia
 4. Pulmonary agenesis
 5. Bronchogenic cyst
 6. Neurenteric cyst
 7. Gastroenteric or duplication cyst
C. Developmental abnormality of the diaphragm
 1. Diaphragmatic hernia
 2. Diaphragmatic eventration
D. Neoplasms
 1. Mediastinal teratoma; neuroblastoma; chest wall hamartoma, etc.
E. Cardiac and pericardiac abnormalities
 1. Cardiomyopathy
 2. Cardiomegaly
 3. Teratoma, rhabdomyoma, fibroma, etc.
 4. Pulmonary vein atresia
 5. Pulmonic stenosis or atresia
F. Developmental abnormality of the thoracic cage or vertebrae
 1. Skeletal dysplasia involving the ribs
  a. Asphyxiating thoracic dysplasia
  b. Thanatophoric dysplasia
  c. Osteogenesis imperfecta, etc.
 2. Vertebral or paravertebral deformity
  a. Skeletal dysplasia (Jarcho-Levin dysplasia, etc.)
  b. Chromosomal abnormality (trisomy 13, 18)
  c. Kyphoscoliosis (limb-body wall complex, etc.)

ever, the sonographic characteristics of many thoracic masses are often not adequately distinctive to permit a specific diagnosis antenatally (Tables 8–3 to 8–5). For example, numerous etiologies create an abnormal intrathoracic mass effect characterized by increased echogenicity. In such cases, attempts to determine the location and source of the mass (i.e., chest wall, pericardium, lung, or abdomen) may limit the diagnostic possibilities or provide a specific diagnosis (Table

TABLE 8–3.

Major Etiologies for an Echogenic Thoracic Mass

Diaphragmatic hernia or eventration
Cystic adenomatoid malformation type III
Bronchopulmonary sequestration
Bronchogenic cyst with bronchial compression
Bronchial atresia
Pericardial teratoma
Chest wall hamartoma
Neuroblastoma

TABLE 8–4.

Major Etiologies for a Cystic Thoracic Mass

Diaphragmatic hernia or eventration
Cystic adenomatoid malformation types I and II
Large or loculated pleural or pericardial fluid collection
Foregut duplication cyst
 Neurenteric, bronchogenic, or gastroenteric cyst
Cystic teratoma
Pericardial cyst
Enlarged cardiac chamber (Ebstein's anomaly, etc.)

8–6). In cases with hydrops fetalis, skeletal dysplasia, or other associated anomalies indicative of a syndrome, detection of thoracic abnormalities often provides useful prognostic and diagnostic information.

PULMONARY HYPOPLASIA

Clinical and Pathologic Findings

Pulmonary hypoplasia has been defined as an absolute decrease in lung volume and weight for gestational age or as a decreased ratio of lung weight to body weight.[30, 32] It is relatively common, occurring with an incidence of 1.4% of all live births.[23] The incidence increases to 6.7% of all stillborn infants and constitutes approximately 10% to 15% of all neonatal autopsies.[23, 29, 34]

As reflected in the clinical presentation and outcome, pathologic changes in pulmonary hypoplasia vary in degree from a mild reduction in acinar number to complete absence of acini.[11, 21] Analysis of lung DNA content correlates well with morphometric measurements of pulmonary hypoplasia.[34] Since the time of onset and type of causative event determine the histologic findings, histologic analysis may provide information regarding the timing of the insult that resulted in severe lung hypoplasia. The severity of pulmonary hypoplasia depends upon the gestational age at onset, duration of the inciting conditions, and severity of the insult.

For example, renal agenesis may produce histologically very immature lung tissue with severe pulmonary

TABLE 8–5.

Major Etiologies for a Complex Thoracic Mass

Diaphragmatic hernia or eventration
Cystic adenomatoid malformation type I, II, or III
Bronchopulmonary sequestration
Bronchogenic, neurenteric, or gastroenteric cyst
Mediastinal cystic hygroma, lymphangiectasia
Pericardial teratoma

TABLE 8–6.

Helpful Sonographic Features in the Differential Diagnosis of Thoracic Masses and Mass Effect*

Mass	Mediastinal Shift	Location	Echogenicity	Other Features	Associated Abnormalities and Hydrops
Hydrothorax	Often, if asymmetric or unilateral	Pleural space	Anechoic		Common
Cystic adenomatoid malformation	Common	Intrapulmonary	Variable: Multicystic—type I,II Echogenic—type III	May resolve spontaneously	Common
Bronchopulmonary sequestration	Uncommon	Usually inferior portion of thorax or upper abdomen	Echogenic	Spherical or triangular shape	Common in extra-lobar type
Diaphragmatic hernia	Common	Often left-sided	Variable	Peristalsing bowel in thorax. Absence of normally positioned stomach. Scaphoid abdomen	Common
Pericardial teratoma	Common	Directly adjacent to the heart	Echogenic, occasional cystic components	Displacement of the heart	Common
Bronchial atresia, stenosis, or compression	Common		Echogenic	May change or resolve	Uncommon
Bronchogenic cyst	Uncommon	Often mediastinal or centrally in lower lobe	Often simple cyst	Mediastinal shift, if associated bronchial compression	Rare
Neurenteric cyst	Occasional	Extrapulmonary, posterior mediastinum	Often simple cyst		Vertebral anomalies
Gastroenteric or duplication cyst	Occasional	Extrapulmonary	Often simple cyst		Rare
Chest wall hamartoma	Occasional	Chest wall	Echogenic	Rib destruction, shift of mediastinum, if large intrathoracic component	Uncommon

*Adapted from Albright EB, Crane JP, Shackelford GD: Prenatal diagnosis of a bronchogenic cyst. J Ultrasound Med 1988; 7:91–95.

hypoplasia, since the causative event occurs early in gestation and produces severe chronic oligohydramnios. On the other hand, diaphragmatic hernia or large pleural effusions that arise later in gestation in association with a normal amniotic fluid volume may produce histologically normal and mature acini but small lungs.[18, 34] Cystic adenomatoid malformation of the lung leads to maturational arrest and morphologic disorganization of the lung, with a decrease in the number of airway generations and accompanying pulmonary artery branches.[18]

Most commonly, pulmonary hypoplasia results from prolonged oligohydramnios or a structural or chromosomal abnormality leading to a small thorax (Fig 8–6).[24] In such cases, the prenatal clinical presentation relates to the underlying condition. However, approximately 10%–15% of all cases with pulmonary hypoplasia occur with no associated abnormality of the fetus or intrauterine environment.[23, 29]

Several factors may contribute to the development of pulmonary hypoplasia. In the case of pulmonary hypoplasia related to renal agenesis or severe bilateral dysplasia, for example, the morphologic changes in the lungs indicate that the initial insult occurred between 12 and 16 weeks' gestation at a time when amniotic fluid is often markedly decreased but may be normal.

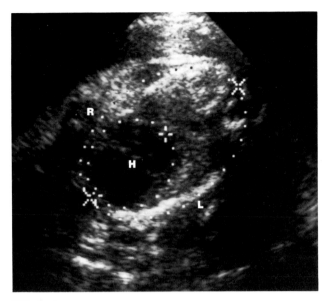

FIG 8–6.
Pulmonary hypoplasia secondary to severe oligohydramnios associated with intrauterine growth retardation. Transverse scan through the thorax at 32 weeks shows compression of the chest into an oblong shape with severe oligohydramnios. Although the heart circumference of 11.5 cm is near the mean for 32 weeks, the chest circumference of 19.8 cm is only mean for 26 weeks and more than 2 SD below the mean for 32 weeks. *H* = heart; *L* = left; *R* = right; × *graticules* = thoracic circumference; + *graticules* = heart circumference.

This finding suggests that factors other than oligohydramnios, such as pulmonary fluid dynamics, fetal breathing movements, and hormonal influences, may contribute to the resultant pulmonary hypoplasia.[21] In prolonged premature rupture of membranes, the histologic changes in the lungs and the degree of pulmonary hypoplasia correlate with the time of onset, duration, and severity of oligohydramnios.[26, 33]

Sonographic Findings

Ultrasound offers the hope of prenatal detection of pulmonary hypoplasia and associated conditions. Therefore, in the appropriate clinical setting (i.e., prolonged rupture of membranes, growth retardation, or associated fetal abnormalities suggesting the possibility of compromised lung development) sonographic diagnosis or confirmation of abnormally small lungs indicative of pulmonary hypoplasia may be useful (Table 8–7).

Since the fetal thorax normally grows at a regular rate from 16 to 40 weeks, a linear correlation exists between thoracic size and gestational age (Tables 8–8 and 8–9).[14, 15, 19, 27] For this reason, ratios between the thoracic size and other biometric parameters

TABLE 8–7.
Major Etiologies of Pulmonary Hypoplasia

A. Oligohydramnios
  1. Renal
    a. Bilateral renal agenesis
    b. Bilateral multicystic dysplastic kidney disease
    c. Severe obstructive uropathy
    d. Unilateral renal agenesis with contralateral multicystic dysplastic kidney
    e. Unilateral renal agenesis or multicystic dysplasia with contralateral severe obstruction
    f. Autosomal recessive (infantile) polycystic kidney disease
  2. Non–renal
    a. Severe intrauterine growth retardation
    b. Premature rupture of membranes
    c. Idiopathic
B. Intrathoracic mass effect
  1. Pleural fluid collections
  2. Diaphragmatic hernia or eventration
  3. Cystic adenomatoid malformation of the lung
  4. Bronchopulmonary sequestration
  5. Large foregut cyst
  6. Thoracic neuroblastoma
C. Cardiovascular
  1. Cardiomyopathy
  2. Hypoplastic right heart
  3. Pulmonary stenosis
  4. Ebstein's anomaly
D. Musculoskeletal
  1. Skeletal dysplasia
  2. Chest wall hamartoma
E. Nervous system
  1. Anencephaly
  2. Intrauterine anoxic or ischemic damage
  3. Congenital myopathy
  4. Pena-Shokeir syndrome
  5. Phrenic nerve abnormalities
F. Chromosomal aberration
  1. Trisomy 13, 18, 21
G. Idiopathic

(abdominal circumference, head circumference, biparietal diameter, and femur length) remain constant, with a high correlation coefficient in normal pregnancies.[4, 14, 15, 19, 27] Comparison of the measured thoracic size with the predicted size, therefore, permits assessment of appropriateness of thoracic size at different gestational ages and may assist in the prediction of small lungs indicative of pulmonary hypoplasia.

The reported measurements for thoracic circumference (TC) vary among different series, probably because of differences in the plane of section and in the amount of tissue included in the measurement. For example, some series apparently include the skin and subcutaneous tissues of the thorax in measurements of TC, while others measure the TC at the outer, mid or inner perimeter of the rib cage. We choose to measure

TABLE 8–8.

Fetal Thoracic Circumference Measurements*†

Gestational Age (wk)	No.	Predictive Percentiles								
		2.5	5	10	25	50	75	90	95	97.5
16	6	5.9	6.4	7.0	8.0	9.1	10.3	11.3	11.9	12.4
17	22	6.8	7.3	7.9	8.9	10.0	11.2	12.2	12.8	13.3
18	31	7.7	8.2	8.8	9.8	11.0	12.1	13.1	13.7	14.2
19	21	8.6	9.1	9.7	10.7	11.9	13.0	14.0	14.6	15.1
20	20	9.5	10.0	10.6	11.7	12.9	13.9	15.0	15.5	16.0
21	30	10.4	11.0	11.6	12.6	13.7	14.8	15.8	16.4	16.9
22	18	11.3	11.9	12.5	13.5	14.6	15.7	16.7	17.3	17.8
23	21	12.2	12.8	13.4	14.4	15.5	16.6	17.6	18.2	18.8
24	27	13.2	13.7	14.3	15.3	16.4	17.5	18.5	19.1	19.7
25	20	14.1	14.6	15.2	16.2	17.3	18.4	19.4	20.0	20.6
26	25	15.0	15.5	16.1	17.1	18.2	19.3	20.3	21.0	21.5
27	24	15.9	16.4	17.0	18.0	19.1	20.2	21.3	21.9	22.4
28	24	16.8	17.3	17.9	18.9	20.0	21.2	22.2	22.8	23.3
29	24	17.7	18.2	18.8	19.8	21.0	22.1	23.1	23.7	24.2
30	27	18.6	19.1	19.7	20.7	21.9	23.0	24.0	24.6	25.1
31	24	19.5	20.0	20.6	21.6	22.8	23.9	24.9	25.5	26.0
32	28	20.4	20.9	21.5	22.6	23.7	24.8	25.8	26.4	26.9
33	27	21.3	21.8	22.5	23.5	24.6	25.7	26.7	27.3	27.8
34	25	22.2	22.8	23.4	24.4	25.5	26.6	27.6	28.2	28.7
35	20	23.1	23.7	24.3	25.3	26.4	27.5	28.5	29.1	29.6
36	23	24.0	24.6	25.2	26.2	27.3	28.4	29.4	30.0	30.6
37	22	24.9	25.5	26.1	27.1	28.2	29.3	30.3	30.9	31.5
38	21	25.9	26.4	27.0	28.0	29.1	30.2	31.2	31.9	32.4
39	7	26.8	27.3	27.9	28.9	30.0	31.1	32.2	32.8	33.3
40	6	27.7	28.2	28.8	29.8	30.9	32.1	33.1	33.7	34.2

*From Chitkara U, Rosenberg J, Chervenak FA, et al: Prenatal sonographic assessment of the fetal thorax: Normal values. Am J Obstet Gynecol 1987; 156:1069–1074. Used by permission.
†Measurements in centimeters.

the TC in axial view at the level of the four-chamber view of the heart (Figs 8–5 and 8–6). We exclude the skin and subcutaneous tissues in TC measurements for two reasons (1) the size of the thoracic cage, rather than the thickness of the subcutaneous tissues, probably affects underlying lung development, and (2) abnormalities which adversely affect the thorax (for example, thanatophoric dysplasia, achondrogenesis, etc.) also may produce thickening of the subcutaneous tissues.

An absolute thoracic circumference measurement less than the 5th percentile for expected values or a declining TC/AC ratio has been suggested as evidence for pulmonary hypoplasia.[4, 15, 22, 31] Both methods have potential limitations for diagnosing pulmonary hypoplasia in certain malformations. For example, malformations that produce an intrathoracic mass (herniated intra-abdominal contents, pleural effusions, cystic adenomatoid malformation of the lung, etc.) may compromise lung growth by direct compression but still result in a normal or near normal chest circumference.[27, 28]

However, the TC/AC ratio may be altered by malformations that produce either an abnormally small abdominal circumference (severe growth retardation, diaphragmatic hernia, gastroschisis, etc.) or abnormally large abdominal circumference (ascites or abdominal mass, most commonly of renal origin).

Measurements of normal fetal cardiac size are also available (see Chapter 9).[4] The biventricular outer dimension (the transverse diameter of the heart at the level of the atrioventricular valves measured at end-diastole) increases linearly with advancing gestational age. The ratio between the biventricular outer dimension and the thoracic diameter or circumference remains constant throughout the second and third trimester in the normal fetus. Therefore, comparison of thoracic circumference and heart size measurements at a known gestational age may permit determination of normalcy or abnormalcy of cardiac or lung size. Since an increased cardiothoracic ratio may result from cardiomegaly without pulmonary hypoplasia or small lungs with a normally sized heart, a combination of ab-

TABLE 8–9.

Fetal Thoracic Length Measurements*†

Gestational Age (wk)	No.	Predictive Percentiles								
		2.5	5	10	25	50	75	90	95	97.5
16	6	0.9	1.1	1.3	1.6	2.0	2.4	2.8	3.0	3.2
17	22	1.1	1.3	1.5	1.8	2.2	2.6	3.0	3.2	3.4
18	31	1.3	1.4	1.7	2.0	2.4	2.8	3.2	3.4	3.6
19	21	1.4	1.6	1.8	2.2	2.7	3.0	3.4	3.6	3.8
20	20	1.6	1.8	2.0	2.4	2.8	3.2	3.6	3.8	4.0
21	30	1.8	2.0	2.2	2.6	3.0	3.4	3.7	4.0	4.1
22	18	2.0	2.2	2.4	2.8	3.2	3.6	3.9	4.1	4.3
23	21	2.2	2.4	2.6	3.0	3.4	3.8	4.1	4.3	4.5
24	27	2.4	2.6	2.8	3.1	3.5	3.9	4.3	4.5	4.7
25	20	2.6	2.8	3.0	3.3	3.7	4.1	4.5	4.7	4.9
26	25	2.8	2.9	3.2	3.5	3.9	4.3	4.7	4.9	5.1
27	24	2.9	3.1	3.3	3.7	4.1	4.5	4.9	5.1	5.3
28	24	3.1	3.3	3.5	3.9	4.3	4.7	5.0	5.4	5.4
29	24	3.3	3.5	3.7	4.1	4.5	4.9	5.2	5.5	5.6
30	27	3.5	3.7	3.9	4.3	4.7	5.1	5.4	5.6	5.8
31	24	3.7	3.9	4.1	4.5	4.9	5.3	5.6	5.8	6.0
32	28	3.9	4.1	4.3	4.6	5.0	5.4	5.8	6.0	6.2
33	27	4.1	4.3	4.5	4.8	5.2	5.6	6.0	6.2	6.4
34	25	4.2	4.4	4.7	5.0	5.4	5.8	6.2	6.4	6.6
35	20	4.4	4.6	4.8	5.2	5.6	6.0	6.4	6.6	6.8
36	23	4.6	4.8	5.0	5.4	5.8	6.2	6.5	6.8	7.0
37	22	4.8	5.0	5.2	5.6	6.0	6.4	6.7	7.0	7.1
38	21	5.0	5.2	5.4	5.8	6.2	6.6	6.9	7.1	7.3
39	7	5.2	5.4	5.6	6.0	6.4	6.8	7.1	7.3	7.5
40	6	5.4	5.6	5.8	6.1	6.5	6.9	7.3	7.5	7.7

*From Chitkara U, Rosenberg J, Chervenak FA, et al: Prenatal sonographic assessment of the fetal thorax: Normal values. Am J Obstet Gynecol 1987; 156:1069–1074. Used by permission.
†Measurements in centimeters.

solute measurements and ratios determines which organ system is abnormal in size.

Deviation of cardiac position or axis may result either from an intrathoracic mass or an abnormality of the thoracic cage. Both of these conditions have a high incidence of resultant pulmonary hypoplasia.[3] For example, among 11 fetuses with abnormal cardiac position, 9 had congenital diaphragmatic abnormalities on the left side pushing the heart to the right, 1 had right-sided pulmonary hypoplasia with the heart in the right hemithorax, and 1 was normal on follow-up sonogram near term and upon postnatal examination.[3] Only two of these 11 infants survived the neonatal period (mortality = 81%). Enlargement of the heart secondary to cardiomyopathy or Ebstein's anomaly may also cause pulmonary hypoplasia secondary to mass effect of the large heart.

The implications of fetal breathing activity during the sonographic examination remain controversial with regard to the prenatal diagnosis of pulmonary hypoplasia and the prediction of fetal outcome. Many factors affect fetal respiratory activity, including time of day, maternal smoking, drugs, and glucose load. Blott et al. followed 11 pregnancies complicated by prolonged oligohydramnios resulting from second trimester rupture of membranes; all five fetuses without breathing movements underwent intrauterine or early postnatal demise from pulmonary hypoplasia.[13] However, Fox reported three cases of lethal pulmonary hypoplasia which demonstrated fetal breathing activity in utero.[20] Absence of fetal breathing movements may help to differentiate true from false preterm labor; if breathing movements are absent, true labor and subsequent delivery are more likely to occur than if breathing movements are present.[12, 17]

Associated Abnormalities

The majority of cases with pulmonary hypoplasia result from associated major structural or chromosomal abnormalities, and half of all cases of pulmonary hypoplasia are attributed to a space-occupying lesion in the thorax that compresses or replaces normal lung parenchyma (Table 8–7).[23, 28, 35] Diaphragmatic hernia is the most common of these processes. Large pleural effusions or rare intrathoracic tumors (neuroblastoma, foregut abnormalities, teratomas) may act in a similar fashion. Primary parenchymal abnormalities of the lungs, such as cystic adenomatoid malformation of the lung, sequestration, and bronchial atresia, may also lead to pulmonary hypoplasia by replacing normal pulmonary parenchyma.[120] With any intrathoracic mass lesion, the mass effect may result in a normal thoracic circumference but significant pulmonary hypoplasia.

Excluding intrathoracic masses, bilateral renal disease with resultant severe oligohydramnios is a common cause of pulmonary hypoplasia and accounts for 20%–25% of cases in some series (Fig 8–7).[23, 28, 35] Less common etiologies include (1) cardiovascular abnormalities which restrict pulmonary blood flow (right-sided cardiac obstructing lesions); (2) skeletal abnormalities producing a small or deformed thoracic cage; (3) neural abnormalities leading to reduced or absent fetal breathing activity at either a central nervous system or diaphragmatic level; and (4) other causes of oligohydramnios, such as extramembranous pregnancy (Fig 8–8). Chromosomal anomalies resulting in pulmonary hypoplasia are usually associated with one of the aforementioned structural defects. In approximately 10%–15% of cases, no structural or chromosomal abnormality to account for pulmonary hypoplasia can be identified.[23, 28, 35] The majority of these cases are probably fetuses with prolonged oligohydramnios secondary to ruptured membranes or growth retardation.

Prognosis and Management

Although pulmonary hypoplasia varies in severity, the overall mortality rate is high; approximately 80% of newborns with the clinical diagnosis of pulmonary hypoplasia die.[13, 16, 22, 27, 32] Such infants present with severe respiratory distress immediately following delivery and frequently succumb shortly thereafter, either as a result of respiratory difficulties or associated anomalies. In cases with an intrathoracic mass, therefore, surgical correction usually must be performed immediately after birth. Drainage or surgical repair of an intrathoracic mass in utero may permit re-expansion of the lung and prevent the development of pulmonary hypoplasia.[48, 56]

HYDROTHORAX

Clinical and Pathologic Findings

Abnormal fetal pleural fluid collections develop from various etiologies (Table 8–10). Excluding hydrops, the most common cause is undoubtedly chylothorax. Chylothorax is particularly likely when the pleural effusion is unilateral, with the right side affected more often than the left. It affects males twice as often as females.[47] Fetal age at presentation ranges from 19 weeks to term. Most cases with large pleural effusions present because of large-for-dates measurements with polyhydramnios, probably from compression by the effusion upon the fetal esophagus, superior vena cava, or heart.[46, 47]

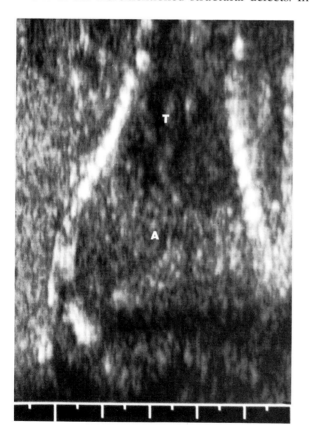

FIG 8–7.
Pulmonary hypoplasia from bilateral renal agenesis. Compression of the thorax by severe prolonged oligohydramnios produces pulmonary hypoplasia and a bell-shaped thorax, as this coronal scan of the trunk demonstrates at 28 weeks. *T* = thorax; *A* = abdomen.

TABLE 8–10.
Major Etiologies for Pleural Fluid Collections

Hydrops fetalis
Chylothorax
Chromosome (trisomy 21, monosomy X)
Pulmonary lymphangiectasia
Cystic adenomatoid malformation of the lungs
Bronchopulmonary sequestration
Diaphragmatic hernia
Chest wall hamartoma (uncommon)
Pulmonary vein atresia
Idiopathic

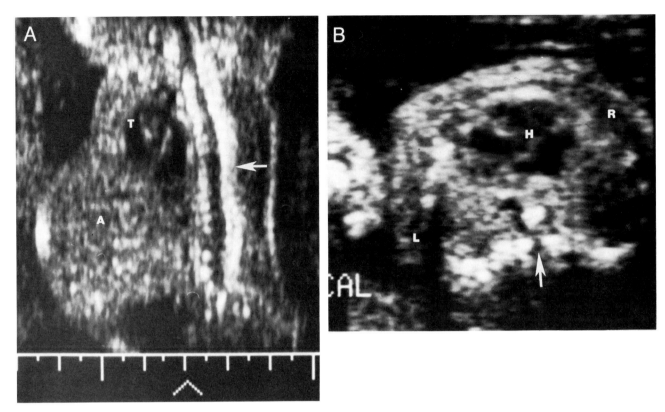

FIG 8–8.
Pulmonary hypoplasia associated with osteochondrodysplasia. Sagittal **(A)** and axial **(B)** scans at 23 weeks show the chest to be small relative to the abdomen, but the heart has a normal size, position, and axis. Abnormalities of thoracic size and shape occur with numerous osteochondrodysplasias. When unmistakably present, they correlate with the presence of pulmonary hypoplasia and poor prognosis. *T* = thorax; *A* = abdomen; *H* = heart; *arrow* = spine; *L* = left; *R* = right.

Congenital chylothorax probably results from a malformation of or rent in the fetal thoracic duct.[47] The thoracic duct normally drains into the left internal jugular vein. However, during embryonic development, bilateral thoracic channels exist. The upper third of the right duct and the lower two thirds of the left duct subsequently obliterate, producing multiple cross-communicating channels draining into the permanent thoracic duct. Because of this anatomic arrangement, leakage from the lower portion of the duct more often results in a right pleural effusion, but leakage from the upper portion of the duct produces a left pleural effusion.

The diagnosis of chylothorax is readily made postnatally by the characteristic chylous appearance of the pleural fluid. However, the prenatal diagnosis is more difficult because, prior to oral milk feeding, the fluid appears clear and colorless because of the absence of chylomicrons. Lipoprotein electrophoresis of pleural fluid obtained by fetal thoracentesis may show typical predominance of high-density lipoprotein and allow a confident prenatal diagnosis of chylothorax.[45]

Sonographic Findings

Hydrothorax produces an anechoic space located peripherally within the thoracic cavity (Figs 8–9 to 8–12). Large pleural fluid collections may occupy the entire thoracic cavity, producing mediastinal shift, cardiac compression, or inversion of the diaphragm. The presence of significant septations or solid components within an intrathoracic fluid collection indicates a diagnosis other than pleural fluid, such as diaphragmatic hernia, cystic adenomatoid malformation, or sequestration. The partially collapsed lungs generally retain their normal shape, whereas hypoplastic lungs may appear as tiny, dense rounded masses on each side of the heart.[38, 48, 51]

Pleural fluid frequently represents one of several features of hydrops fetalis. Other sonographic signs of hydrops fetalis include generalized ascites, pericardial effusion, subcutaneous edema, polyhydramnios, and placental enlargement.[44] Hydrops fetalis can result from fetal-maternal blood group incompatibility (immune hydrops) or many other fetal and maternal non–immune factors (see Chapter 13). Approximately 25% of cases of non-immune hydrops fetalis are idiopathic, while the remainder have associated abnormali-

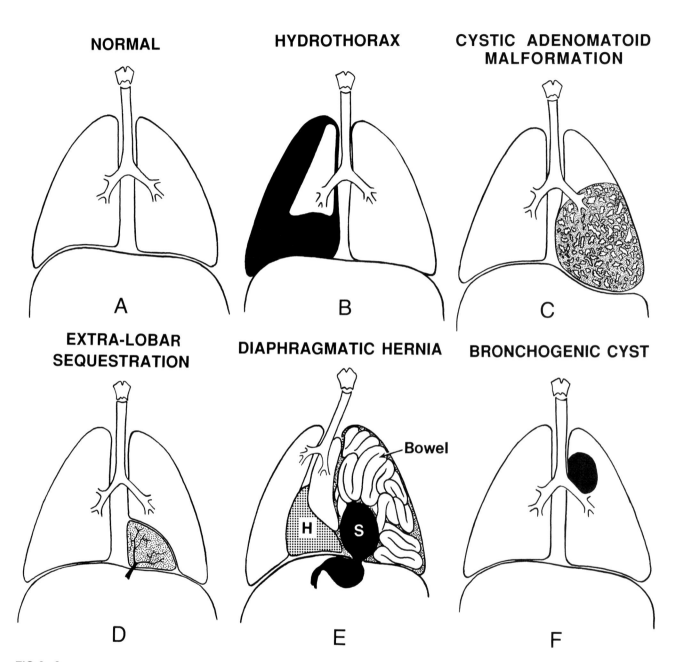

NORMAL

HYDROTHORAX

CYSTIC ADENOMATOID MALFORMATION

A

B

C

EXTRA-LOBAR SEQUESTRATION

DIAPHRAGMATIC HERNIA

BRONCHOGENIC CYST

Bowel

H   S

D

E

F

FIG 8–9.
Schematic drawings of thoracic masses and mass effect. **A,** normal thorax. The lungs have convex margins anterolaterally. **B,** hydrothorax. Anechoic pleural fluid displaces the lungs away from the chest wall and compresses the lungs. **C,** cystic adenomatoid malformation. An intrapulmonary mass of variable echogenicity may shift the mediastinum and create hydrops. **D,** bronchopulmonary extra-lobar sequestration. A spherical or triangular echogenic mass is evident in the inferior portion of the thorax or upper abdomen. **E,** diaphragmatic hernia. A complex mass (usually left-sided) creates mediastinal shift. Peristalsing bowel in the thorax provides convincing evidence of the diagnosis. Displaced stomach or scaphoid abdomen is an ancillary finding. **F,** bronchogenic cyst. A simple cyst near the mediastinum or centrally in the lung may produce mediastinal shift, if it causes bronchial compression.

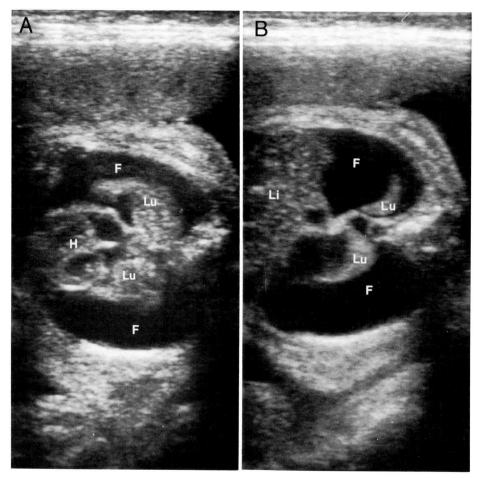

FIG 8–10.
Hydrothorax. Axial **(A)** and coronal **(B)** scans of the thorax show large bilateral pleural fluid collections in a fetus with hydrops from tachycardia. *F* = pleural fluid; *H* = heart; *Lu* = lungs.

ties, most often cardiovascular, chromosomal, hematologic, or infectious.[41, 44] Therefore, identification of a pleural effusion warrants a directed examination of the fetus and placenta, fetal chromosomal analysis, and maternal physical and laboratory examination.

Associated Abnormalities

Chylothorax may occur as an isolated finding, but it also can be seen in a variety of syndromes including trisomy 21, monosomy X, and syndromes involving lymphatic or vascular abnormalities (Figs 8–11 and 8–12).[16, 49, 52] Rare causes of congenital chylothorax include congenital pulmonary lymphangiectasia, hypoplastic lungs, and lung tumors.[42]

Prognosis and Management

Hydrothorax has an overall perinatal mortality of more than 50%, with a higher mortality rate in fetuses who have hydrops than in fetuses for whom the effusion is an isolated finding.[48] The outcome of a fetus with an abnormal pleural fluid collection depends upon the underlying cause of the effusion and the degree of associated pulmonary hypoplasia (see Pulmonary Hypoplasia section above). The prognosis is good for a fetus with an effusion not associated with hydrops fetalis or presenting in the latter portion of the third trimester, unlike the dismal prognosis for the fetus with severe hydropic changes, associated structural or chromosomal abnormalities, or significant pulmonary hypoplasia.[16, 38, 40, 43, 45, 50] Fluid accumulation in the thoracic cavity functions as any space-occupying lesion; if large or chronic it may restrict fetal lung development. Accumulation of a large fluid collection during the second trimester signifies a high likelihood of significant pulmonary hypoplasia.[16] Conversely, the pediatric literature indicates that chylothorax identified in the neonatal period carries only a 20% mortality rate.[39]

Prenatal thoracentesis of a large pleural fluid collection is a relatively simple and benign procedure that may be useful for a variety of reasons.[36, 37, 46, 48, 50]

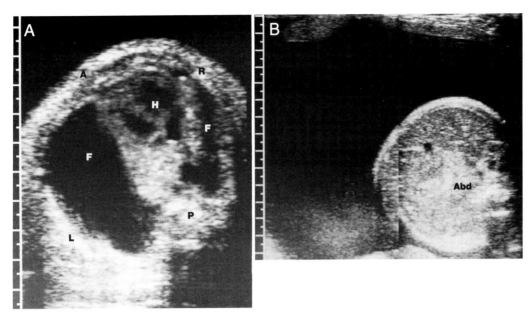

FIG 8-11.
Hydrothorax associated with trisomy 21. **A,** axial scan of the thorax at 32 weeks shows a large left pleural fluid collection which shifts the mediastinum to the right. A smaller right pleural fluid collection also is present. The left pleural fluid collection was drained in utero but reaccumulated within 48-72 hours. **B,** transverse scan of the abdomen (A) shows moderate to severe polyhydramnios. Other scans showed fluid within the stomach. No other signs of hydrops were present. *F* = pleural fluid; *H* = heart; *A* = anterior; *P* = posterior; *R* = right; *L* = left; *Abd* = abdomen.

First, thoracentesis immediately before delivery with re-expansion of the lung to fill the hemithorax may facilitate resuscitation postnatally. The re-expansion of the lung indicates that marked pulmonary hypoplasia has not occurred.[50] Second, fetuses with a large pleural effusion detected early in gestation also may benefit from removal of the mass effect created by the hydrothorax, especially during the critical period of lung

development during the second trimester. Because the fluid reaccumulates within 6-48 hours following thoracentesis, two to five thoracenteses or indwelling thoracoamniotic shunt placements may be necessary to maintain lung re-expansion.[48, 51] Third, relief of the mass effect created by a large pleural effusion may lead to resolution of polyhydramnios and uterine distension. It may also permit improved visualization of car-

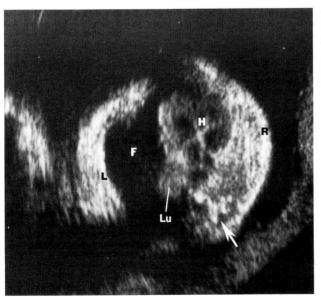

FIG 8-12.
Hydrothorax associated with pulmonary sequestration. Axial scan at 35 weeks shows a large left pleural fluid collection with shift of the mediastinum to the right. Polyhydramnios is also present. The fetus had pulmonary sequestration. *F* = pleural fluid; *H* = heart; *Lu* = lungs; *arrow* = spine; *L* = left; *R* = right.

diac anatomy. And fourth, culture of fetal lymphocytes may reveal a chromosomal abnormality (see Fig 8–10).

Rodeck et al. recently reported their experience with placement of pleuroamniotic shunts in utero.[48] Expansion of the lung immediately after aspiration implies that lung compression was relatively brief and that severe pulmonary hypoplasia had not occurred.[48] Among eight fetuses with hydrothorax in whom pleuroamniotic shunts were inserted prenatally, all six survivors had nearly complete re-expansion of the lung, whereas both non–survivors failed to re-expand the lung.[48] Blott et al. successfully utilized thoracoamniotic shunting at 24 weeks to drain a cystic adenomatoid malformation type 1.[37] The lung rapidly re-expanded, and this infant had normal postnatal respiratory function.

CYSTIC ADENOMATOID MALFORMATION

Clinical and Pathologic Findings

Cystic adenomatoid malformation of the lung (CAML) is a hamartomatous lesion resulting from cessation of bronchiolar maturation with overgrowth of mesenchymal elements. It typically presents with respiratory distress in the neonatal period or with chronic infection in the older infant.[69, 74] Since CAML frequently communicates with the tracheobronchial tree, air may be present within the lesion in the early postnatal pe-

riod.[74] However, numerous cases have been identified prenatally as early as 20 weeks' gestation either as an incidental finding or because of size-dates discrepancy related to acute maternal hydramnios.[53] It shows no preference for location or sex. Two or more lobes are affected in 20% of cases.[69]

CAML is thought to result from arrested cellular development at an early stage.[69, 74] Proliferation of polypoid glandular tissue without normal alveolar differentiation produces the "adenomatoid" histology. Arterial and venous connections are typically normal, but CAML lacks a well-defined bronchial system. Absence of bronchial cartilage differentiates CAML from a bronchogenic cyst and indicates that the insult occurred before the tenth week of gestation.

CAML has been classified into three subtypes based upon clinical, gross, and histologic features (Fig 8–13).[69, 74] Histologic features common to all types of CAML include (1) adenomatoid increase in structures resembling terminal bronchioles; (2) polypoid configuration of columnar (type I), mixed (type II), or cuboidal (type III) epithelial lining of cystic structures; (3) proliferation of smooth muscle and elastic tissue in cyst walls; (4) absence of cartilage; and (5) absence of inflammation.

Type I lesions contain relatively well-differentiated bronchial components but no bronchial cartilage. The absence of bronchial cartilage, which normally develops during embryogenesis, indicates that the insult occurred before the tenth week of gestation. Type II le-

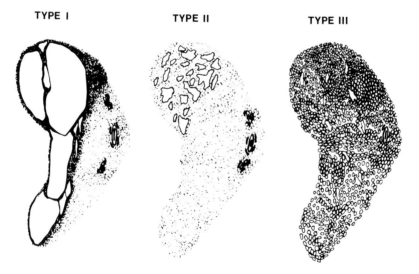

TYPE I   TYPE II   TYPE III

FIG 8–13.

Classification of congenital cystic adenomatoid malformation. Type I is composed of a small number of large cysts. Relatively normal alveoli are seen between and adjacent to these cysts. Type II contains numerous smaller cysts (<1 cm in diameter). The area between the cysts is occupied by large alveolus-like structures. Type III occupies the entire lobe or lobes and is composed of regularly spaced bronchiole-like structures separated by masses of cuboidal epithelium-lined, alveolus-like structures. (From Stocker JT, Madewell JE, Drake RM: Congenital cystic adenomatoid malformation of the lung. Classification and morphologic spectrum. Hum Pathol 1977; 8:155–171. Used by permission.)

sions probably occur prior to 31 days of gestation, based upon the high frequency of associated structural anomalies involving other organ systems developing at this time. Type III lesions have minimal differentiation of epithelial and mesenchymal structures, suggesting that the embryologic insult occurred after the appearance of the two lung buds, between 26 and 28 days.

Type I CAML contains one or several large cysts ranging from 2 to 10 cm in diameter with smaller cysts along the periphery. Type I lesions are large and frequently present with symptoms of respiratory distress in the early postnatal period, but the infant typically does well following surgical resection. Because the smaller cysts blend imperceptibly with normal lung tissue, the distinction between normal and abnormal tissue may be difficult when only a portion of the lung is involved.

Type II CAML, on the other hand, has multiple small macroscopic cysts, each measuring less than 1 cm in diameter and scattered evenly throughout the mass. Each of these small cysts histologically resembles a dilated terminal bronchiole. Concurrent severe structural or chromosomal anomalies frequently dominate the clinical picture and overshadow the degree of respiratory difficulty postnatally.[69, 74]

Type III CAML typically creates a large solid mass affecting an entire lobe with a mixture of structures resembling bronchioles and alveoli of the early canilicular stage of fetal development. Infants with Type III lesions present in the immediate postnatal period because of the bulk of the mass. The prognosis is poor, and death frequently ensues from pulmonary hypoplasia.

Sonographic Findings

Thirty-five reported cases of CAML are available for review (see Table 8–11). The earliest case reported to date was at 20 weeks.[53] Fitzgerald reported a type I CAM at 23 weeks' menstrual age in a fetus who had a normal sonogram at 15 weeks.[61] Most reported cases (57%) have type I CAML, and most of these (65%) are alive and well; the remainder died in utero during the third trimester. Only two cases of type II CAML have been reported to date, and both are alive and well. Type III CAML represents 37% of reported cases detected prenatally. Among these fetuses, seven died in utero, five underwent elective termination, and only one is alive and well.

Type I CAML may produce either a single cyst or, more commonly, multiple large cysts (>2 cm) within the hemithorax (Fig 8–14). These cysts often involve an entire pulmonary lobe. The multiple large cysts distinguish this entity from a bronchogenic cyst, which

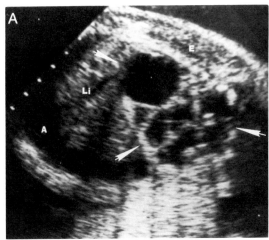

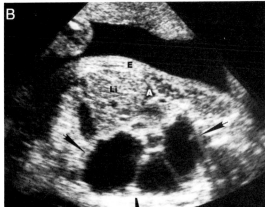

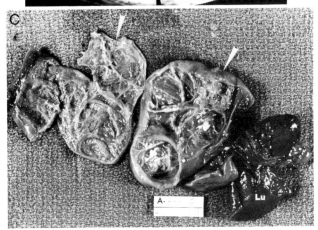

FIG 8–14.
Cystic adenomatoid malformation, Type I. **A,** parasagittal scan of the trunk at 28 weeks shows multiple thoracic cysts creating a mass effect which displaces the diaphragm inferiorly. Ascites, subcutaneous edema, and polyhydramnios also are present. **B,** similar scan in a different fetus shows multiple thoracic cystic masses. This fetus has only a trace amount of ascites, mild subcutaneous edema, and polyhydramnios. **C,** corresponding pathologic specimen demonstrates the numerous deflated cystic masses arising from the lung. *Arrowheads* = cystic adenomatoid malformation; *Lu* = lungs; *Li* = liver; *A* = ascites; *E* = subcutaneous edema. (Part **B** courtesy of Lawrence A Mack, MD, University of Washington Hospital; Washington, DC.)

typically is small, solitary, and near the midline. Furthermore, the delicate internal septations distinguish a type I CAML from a duplication cyst. Macrocystic type II CAML creates a mass with numerous small cysts. Confident distinction from other types of hemithoracic masses may be difficult. The concomitant structural anomalies, however, frequently dominate the sonographic picture.

Microcystic type III CAML produces a homogeneously echogenic mass without discernible individual cysts (Fig 8–15). The echogenic mass may closely resemble pulmonary sequestration or intrathoracic

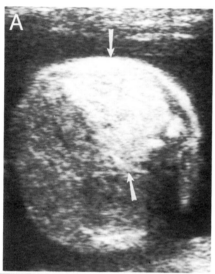

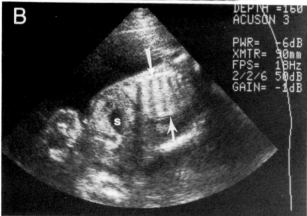

FIG 8–15.
Cystic adenomatoid malformation, Type III. Transverse **(A)** and coronal **(B)** scans of the thorax at 26 weeks shows a homogeneously echogenic left lung mass displacing the mediastinum to the right and the hemidiaphragm inferiorly. Polyhydramnios is present. Follow-up scans at 27 and 30 weeks were unchanged. *Arrows* = cystic adenomatoid malformation; *S* = stomach. (From Adzick NS, Harrison MR, Glick PL, et al: Fetal cystic adnomatoid malformation: Prenatal diagnosis and natural history. J Pediatr Surg 1985; 20:483–488. Used by permission.)

bowel from a diaphragmatic hernia. Unlike type III CAML, however, pulmonary sequestration rarely causes polyhydramnios or hydrops, and diaphragmatic hernia often produces a scaphoid abdomen with peristalsing bowel in the hemithorax. Occasionally, both CAML and diaphragmatic hernia may coexist in the same fetus.

Associated Abnormalities

Among 35 reported cases with CAML detected prenatally, 68% had polyhydramnios, 6% had oligohydramnios, and 26% had normal amniotic fluid volume (Table 8–11). CAML caused mediastinal shift in 16 of 18 (89%) cases and ascites in 15 of 24 (62%) cases for whom this information was reported. Unequivocal hydropic changes were present in 15 of 24 (62%) cases detected prenatally, unlike the 6% incidence of hydrops among cases diagnosed postnatally.[69, 74] Polyhydramnios, ascites, and particularly hydrops correlate with a poor fetal outcome. Most cases with a normal amniotic fluid volume had type I CAML.

Approximately 25% of cases with CAML detected postnatally have associated anomalies.[69, 74] Associated anomalies occur most commonly with type II CAML and include (1) other malformations of the pulmonary system, (2) renal anomalies (usually renal agenesis), and (3) gastrointestinal abnormalities (congenital diaphragmatic hernia and bowel atresia).

Prognosis and Management

As with all intrathoracic space-occupying lesions, survival of the fetus with CAML correlates with the presence or absence of pulmonary hypoplasia and associated anomalies. In the absence of lethal pulmonary hypoplasia, the prognosis for a type I CAML is excellent following resection. For a type II lesion, associated structural or chromosomal abnormalities produce an overall poor survival rate. Type III lesions present in the early postnatal period, because of the bulk of the mass, and have a poor prognosis based upon fetal hydrops or pulmonary hypoplasia. The presence of fetal hydrops, more common in type III CAML, generally is associated with fetal or neonatal death. All fetuses with CAML and hydrops detected prenatally died or were electively terminated. Blott et al. reported successful thoracoamniotic shunting of type I CAML at 24 weeks' gestation with re-expansion of the lung and normal postnatal respiratory function.[56] However, CAML may occasionally improve or resolve spontaneously in utero and yield a good outcome (Figs 8–16 to 8–18).[60, 75]

TABLE 8–11.

Review of 35 Reported Prenatal Cases of Cystic Adenomatoid Malformation of the Lung*

	Menstrual Age (wk)	Mediastinal Shift	Amniotic Fluid Volume	Ascites	Hydrops	Type	Outcome	Reference
1	23	+	Oligo	+	−	III	TOP	72
2	23		Oligo	+	+	III	TOP	72
3	30	+	Poly	+	+	III	Died 30 wk	66
4	25		Poly	+	−	I	Died 33 wk	53
5	33	+	Poly	−	−	I	A&W	53
6	26	+	NL	−	−	III	A&W	53
7	24		NL	−	−	I	A&W	53
8	20		NL		−	I	A&W	53
9	26		NL		−	I	A&W	53
10	27		NL		−	I	A&W	53
11	33		Poly		−	I	Died 36 wk	53
12	32		Poly		+	III	Died 34 wk	53
13	30		Poly		+	III	Died 36 wk	53
14	22		Poly		+	III	TOP	53
15	24		Poly		+	III	TOP	53
16	35	+	Poly	+	−	I	Died 35 wk	64
17	24	+	Poly	+	+	III	Died 24 wk	64
18	25		Poly	+	−	I	A&W	64
19	29	+	Poly	+	−	I	Died 31 wk	59
20	36	+	Poly	−	−	I	A&W	71
21	23	+	NL	+	+	I	Died 27 wk	61
22	32		Poly		+	III	Died 32 wk	58
23	32		Poly	+	+	III	Died 34 wk	62
24	26		Poly	+	+	I	Died 29 wk	55
25			Poly		+	I	Died 31 wk	70
26	27		NL		−	I	A&W	73
27	28	+	Poly	+	+	III	Died 29 wk	68
28	23	+	NL	−	−	I	A&W	54
29	25	+	Poly	+	+	I	A&W	67
30	32	+	Poly	+	−	I	A&W	63
31	30	−	NL	−	−	I	A&W	57
32	34	−	Poly	+	+	III	TOP	65
33	24	+	Poly	−	−	II	A&W	60
34	32	+	Poly	−	−	I	A&W	75
35	33	+	Poly	−	−	II	A&W	75

*Oligo = oligohydramnios; NL = normal amniotic fluid volume; Poly = polyhydramnios; TOP = termination of pregnancy; A&W = alive and well; all blanks = unreported in original source.

BRONCHOPULMONARY SEQUESTRATION

Clinical and Pathologic Findings

Bronchopulmonary sequestration, a congenital pulmonary malformation in which a portion of the bronchopulmonary mass is separated from the normal bronchial system, probably results from development of anomalous vascular connections during embryogenesis.[7] As the developing lung bud arises from the ventral surface of the foregut, it normally shares its vascular supply from the splanchnic plexus with the foregut. As the pulmonary artery develops from the sixth embryonic arch, the branches of the splanchnic plexus persist as bronchial arteries. In bronchopulmonary seques-

tration, an anomalous vessel from a systemic artery supplies a bronchopulmonary mass separate from the normal bronchial system.[7, 78, 84] This anomalous vessel usually arises from the descending aorta and drains into the pulmonary vein. Although typically fleshy on gross examination and histologically homogeneous, the sequestered bronchopulmonary tissue may exhibit cystic changes postnatally.

Bronchopulmonary sequestrations are uncommon, with an overall incidence of 0.15%–6.4% of congenital pulmonary malformations.[86] Two types of bronchopulmonary sequestration occur, with classification based upon the extent of pleural covering. An extra-lobar sequestration has its own separate pleural covering and

FIG 8–16.
Resolving cystic adenomatoid malformation, type I. **A,** parasagittal scan of the trunk at 32 weeks shows a large chest mass expanding the right hemithorax with flattening of the right hemidiaphragm. A macroscopic cyst is present within the otherwise homogeneously echogenic mass. Polyhydramnios is present. **B,** corresponding sonogram at 39 weeks demonstrates that the mass has decreased markedly in size. The cystic component is still evident, but the polyhydramnios and thoracic expansion have resolved. Elective postnatal surgery at 6 weeks of age showed a right upper lobe cystic adenomatoid malformation, type I. *Arrows* = right chest mass with single cystic component. (From Saltzman DH, Adzick NS, Benacerraf BR: Fetal cystic adenomatoid malformation of the lung: Apparent improvement in utero. Obstet Gynecol 1988; 71:1000–1002. Used by permission.)

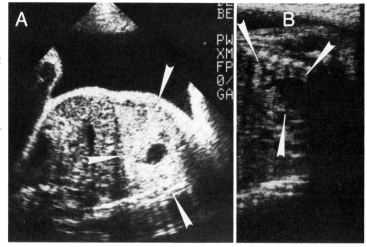

frequently presents in infancy because of associated congenital abnormalities or pulmonary hypoplasia. An intralobar sequestration, on the other hand, shares a visceral pleural surface with normal lung tissue and typically presents in adulthood with an acute or recurrent infection. Intralobar sequestration occurs three times more commonly than does extra-lobar sequestration.

Bronchopulmonary sequestration most often occurs in the lower lobes, particularly the posterior basal segments. Both intralobar and extra-lobar sequestrations may appear simultaneously and bilaterally. Whereas intralobar sequestration occurs with equal frequency on the right and left sides, approximately 80% of extra-lobar sequestrations occur in the left hemithorax (see Fig 8–18).[86] Approximately 5% of sequestrations occur below the diaphragm (Fig 8–19).[76, 82] Males and females are affected with equal frequency.[86]

Sonographic Findings

Bronchopulmonary sequestration may be noted incidentally on prenatal sonographic examination or may be identified during the survey of a fetus with hydrops fetalis. A single case of intralobar sequestration and several reports of extra-lobar sequestration document their prenatal appearance.[76, 80, 81, 82, 83, 85, 87] A seques-

FIG 8–17.
Resolving cystic adenomatoid malformation, type II. Transverse scan of the thorax at 33 weeks shows a large heterogeneous left lung mass with numerous small cystic areas. The mass displaces the heart to the right. The mass was stable in size 3 weeks later. However, 6 to 7 weeks later it became significantly smaller. Left lower lobectomy at 1 day of age showed type II cystic adenomatoid malformation. The infant recovered normally. *Arrowheads* = left chest mass; *H* = heart. (From Adzick NS, Harrison MR, Glick PL, et al: Fetal cystic adenomatoid malformation: Prenatal diagnosis and natural history. J Pediatr Surg 1985; 20:483–488. Used by permission.)

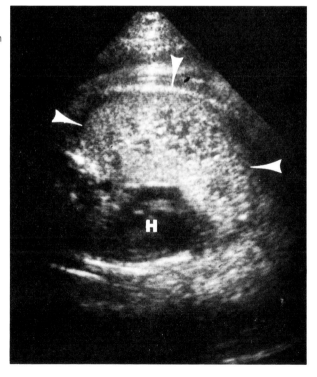

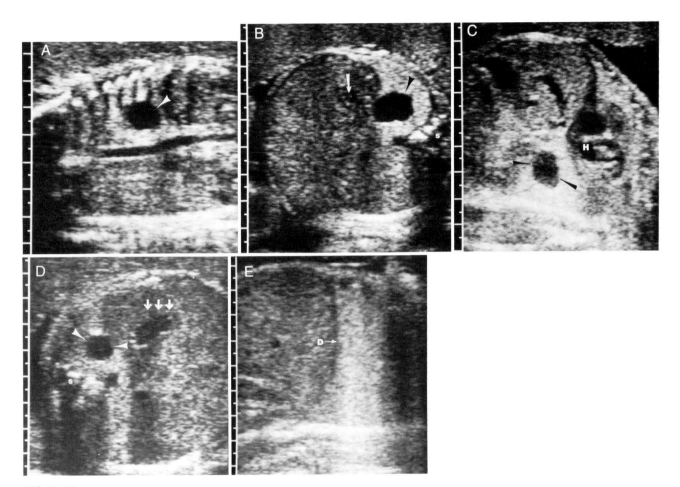

FIG 8–18.
Resolved cystic adenomatoid malformation (presumed). Transverse **(A)**, coronal **(B)**, and oblique parasagittal **(C)** scans at 27 weeks show a 13 mm cystic mass of the left lung base. The inferior left lung also appears echogenic relative to the remainder of the lung. **D,** transverse scan of the inferior thorax 3 weeks later demonstrates the cystic component to have decreased in size to 10 mm. The adjacent lung is no longer intensely echogenic. **E,** parasagittal scan of the left lung base at 33 weeks shows interval resolution of the cyst. Postnatal radiographs and clinical course were normal. *Arrowhead* = cystic mass of left lung base; *Arrow* = stomach; *S* = Spine; *H* = heart; *D* = diaphragm.

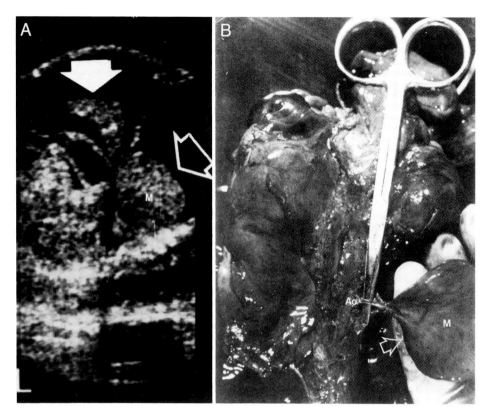

FIG 8–19.
Extra-lobar pulmonary sequestration. **A,** left parasagittal scan of the lower thorax and upper abdomen shows a triangular left hemithorax mass *(open arrow)* surrounded by pleural fluid. The mass is in the posteromedial aspect of the left hemithorax. Ascites outlines the liver *(solid arrow).* Polyhydramnios is present. **B,** autopsy specimen shows the 4 × 2.5 × 2 cm extra-lobar pulmonary sequestration attached by a narrow pedicle to the descending aorta. The scissors demarcate the vascular pedicle. *Open arrow* = extralobar pulmonary suquestration; *closed arrow* = liver; *Ao* = aorta; *M* = mass. (From Thomas CS, Leopold GR, Hilton S, et al: Fetal hydrops associated with extralobar pulmonary sequestration. J Ultrasound Med 1986; 5:668–671. Used by permission.)

tration typically produces a well-defined, homogenous, highly echogenic mass in the inferior aspect of the hemithorax or upper abdomen (Figs 8–19 and 8–20). The reported intralobar sequestration was spherical in shape, whereas the fetuses with extra-lobar sequestration had a conical or triangular shaped mass. This conical or triangular shape of extra-lobar sequestration probably results from its complete pleural investment and narrow vascular pedicle and may be a helpful differentiating feature. The solid mass of bronchopulmonary sequestration, however, may closely resemble other echogenic masses, especially CAML type III. Occasional cystic components of the mass may produce further diagnostic confusion with CAML type II or, possibly, diaphragmatic hernia.[86]

Associated Abnormalities

As with any intrathoracic mass, bronchopulmonary sequestration may cause pulmonary hypoplasia. Other extrathoracic anomalies are more common and severe in extra-lobar sequestration than in intralobar seques-

tration. Approximately 60% of fetuses with extra-lobar sequestration have associated anomalies, including diaphragmatic anomalies (28%), other pulmonary abnormalities (10%), cardiac and pericardiac malformations (8%), epiphrenic diverticula (2%), tracheoesophageal fistula (1.5%), and miscellaneous anomalies (10%).[86] Non-immune hydrops fetalis frequently complicates extra-lobar sequestration and leads to preterm labor or fetal demise.[85, 87] Approximately 14% of patients with intralobar sequestration have other associated congenital abnormalities, including skeletal (4%), foregut (4%), diaphragmatic (3%), cardiac, renal, or cerebral anomalies.[86]

Prognosis

The postnatal outcome of bronchopulmonary sequestration correlates with the presence or absence and severity of associated anomalies, pulmonary hypoplasia, and hemodynamic disturbances. Overall, intralobar sequestration holds an excellent prognosis. Extra-lobar sequestration has a poor prognosis, based

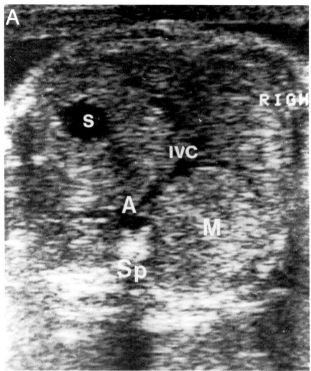

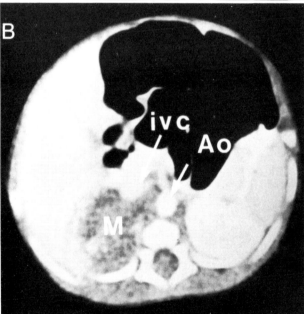

FIG 8–20.
Extra-lobar pulmonary sequestration. **A,** transverse sonogram of the upper abdomen at 34 weeks shows a large right retroperitoneal mass displacing the inferior vena cava anteriorly. **B,** computed tomography of the neonatal upper abdomen confirms the prenatal findings. The mass has peripheral and focal contrast enhancement. An en bloc resection showd a 4 cm periadrenal extralobar sequestered lung. *M* = extra-lobar pulmonary sequestration; *IVC* = inferior vena cava; *Ao* = descending aorta; *S* = stomach; *Sp* = spine. (From Mariona F, McAlpin G, Zador I, et al: Sonographic detection of fetal extrathoracic pulmonary sequestration. J Ultrasound Med 1986; 5:283–285. Used by permission.)

upon a higher incidence of serious concomitant anomalies and development of hydrops fetalis.

CONGENITAL DIAPHRAGMATIC ABNORMALITIES

Clinical and Pathologic Findings

Congenital diaphragmatic defects occur in approximately 1 in 2,000 to 3,000 births.[98, 99, 106] They typically occur as a sporadic malformation with little or no increased risk of recurrence, but rare families with recurrent cases exist.[94] Congenital diaphragmatic defects include:

1. Bochdalek hernias.
2. Foramen of Morgagni hernias.
3. Diaphragmatic eventrations.
4. Diaphragmatic agenesis.
5. Esophageal hiatal hernias.

This section discusses the first three entities. It does not discuss diaphragmatic agenesis and esophageal hiatal hernias, because of the lack of prenatal clinical information and sonographic correlation regarding these two entities.

Although the clinical outcome and frequency of associated abnormalities are similar for all diaphragmatic defects, features related to embryologic development may aid in antenatal differential diagnosis. Cullen describes the embryological development of the diaphragm as follows (Figs 8–21 and 8–22).[197]

"The diaphragm has four developmental components. The ventral component is formed in the third to fifth week of gestation by the septum transversum, arising from a mesodermal plate of the cephalic fold that grows dorsally from the developing anterior body wall. It envelops the esophagus, inferior vena cava, and aorta and fuses with the foregut mesentery by the eighth week of development to form the posterior and medial portions of the diaphragm. The lateral margins of the diaphragm are then developed from muscular components of the body wall. The pleuroperitoneal canals are the last areas to close from fusion of the membranous portions of the components already discussed. Muscular fibers from the third, fourth, and fifth cervical myotomes reinforce these membranous folds, completing diaphragmatic closure by the ninth week of gestation."

Bochdalek hernias comprise more than 90% of all diaphragmatic abnormalities affecting the fetus. This abnormality occurs during the eighth to tenth week of gestation, the time at which bowel normally returns to the abdominal cavity. It represents failure or incom-

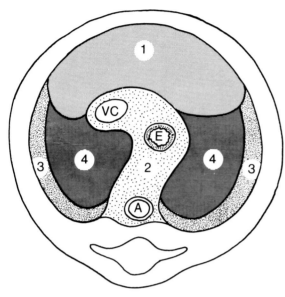

FIG 8-21.
Developmental components of the diaphragm: *1,* Anterior component from the septum transversum; *2,* Posterior component from the foregut mesentery; *3,* Lateral components from the body wall muscles; *4,* Pleuroperitoneal canals. *A* = aortic hiatus; *E* = esophageal hiatus; *VC* = vena cava hiatus. (From Cullen MC, Klein MD, Philippart AI: Congenital diaphragmatic hernia. Surg Clin N Am 1985; 65:1115-1138. Used by permission.)

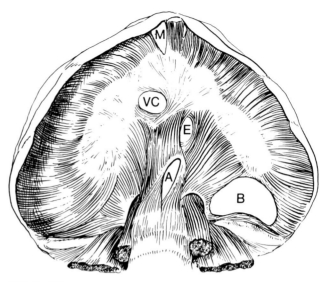

FIG 8-22.
The diaphragm as seen from below. *B* = potential site of Bochdalek's hernia; *M* = potential site for Morgagni's hernia; *A* = aortic hiatus; *E* = esophageal hiatus; *VC* = vena cava hiatus. (From Cullen MC, Klein MD, Philippart AI: Congenital diaphragmatic hernia. Surg Clin N Am 1985; 65:1115-1138. Used by permission.)

plete closure of the pleuroperitoneal reflections which normally form the diaphragm. The Bochdalek defect characteristically occurs posterolaterally and on the left side (75%), but infrequently involves the right hemidiaphragm or both hemidiaphragms (Figs 8-22 to 8-25).[88, 97, 98] Bowel typically herniates into the hemithorax, especially with a left-sided defect. Herniation of the liver, gallbladder, or spleen occurs less commonly.[88, 95, 98]

Foramen of Morgagni hernias occur in the anteromedial retrosternal portion of the diaphragm as a result of maldevelopment of the septum transversum (see Figs 8-21 and 8-22).[97] These hernias often lack a hernia sac composed of abdominal peritoneal layers. Depending on the integrity of the pericardium, abdominal contents may herniate into the pericardial space.

Eventration of the diaphragm, although not a true hernia, is characterized by an elevated diaphragm that can lead to compression of the developing lung, pulmonary hypoplasia, and postnatal respiratory compromise. The herniated viscera are covered by a sac composed of abdominal peritoneal layers as well as thinned fibrous or muscular components of the diaphragm.

Sonographic Findings

The sonographic diagnosis of congenital diaphragmatic hernias has been made as early as 18 weeks'

menstrual age.[91] When recognized prenatally, it is usually on the basis of routine screening or in the work-up for size-dates discrepancy because of polyhydramnios related either to generalized hydrops or to upper gastrointestinal obstruction by the herniated viscera.[88] The early recognition of this condition and its associated abnormalities has important implications for obstetrical management.

The typical sonographic finding of Bochdalek diaphragmatic hernia is mediastinal shift produced by herniated bowel or liver (Figs 8-23 to 8-25).[95, 96] Diaphragmatic hernia occurs on the left side much more commonly than on the right. The heart usually retains its normal axis, despite its abnormal position in the right hemithorax.[3] With the less common right-sided diaphragmatic abnormalities, the mediastinum may shift to the left or remain midline (Fig 8-25). Peristalsis of bowel within the fetal chest confirms the diagnosis, although this finding is not always apparent.[3]

Identification of an apparently intact diaphragmatic outline does not exclude this diagnosis (see Fig 8-25). Indirect signs of diaphragmatic hernia include (1) absence of visualization of the stomach or gallbladder within the abdomen; (2) abnormal position of the stomach, gallbladder, or hepatic and umbilical veins within the abdomen; (3) scaphoid shape of the abdomen secondary to displacement of viscera into the chest; (4) paradoxical motion of the abdominal contents into the ipsilateral hemithorax during fetal respiratory motion, with concomitant descent of

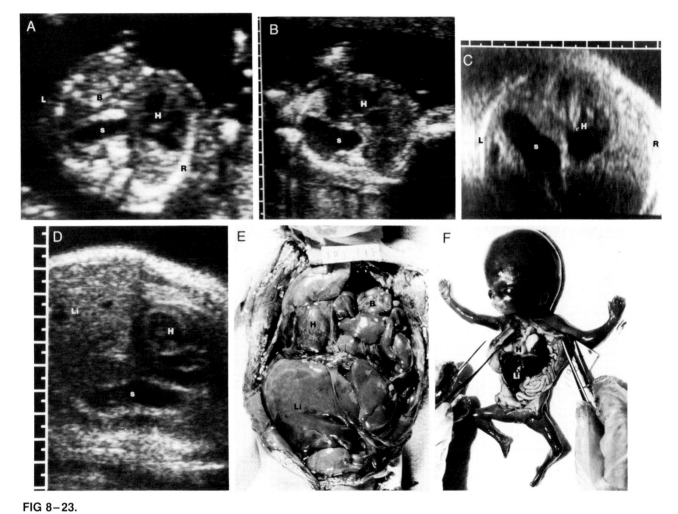

FIG 8–23.
Diaphragmatic hernia. left Bochdalek. **A,** transverse scan of the thorax shows the heart displaced to the right by the stomach and echogenic small bowel. Polyhydramnios is present. **B,** similar scan in another fetus demonstrates the heart displaced anteriorly and to the right by herniated bowel. **C** and **D,** transverse and left parasagittal scans of the lower thorax and upper abdomen show the heart displaced anteriorly and to the right by the stomach, a portion of which remains within the abdomen. **E** and **F,** postnatal photographs of two different fetuses illustrate herniated bowel displacing the heart to the right. The amount of herniated bowel varies. *H* = heart; *S* = stomach; *B* = herniated bowel; *Li* = liver; *R* = right; *L* = left.

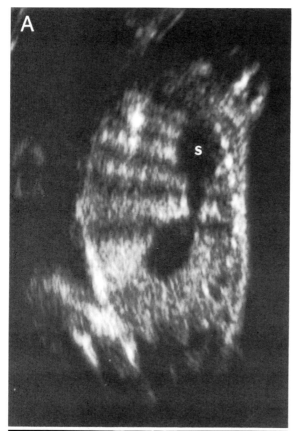

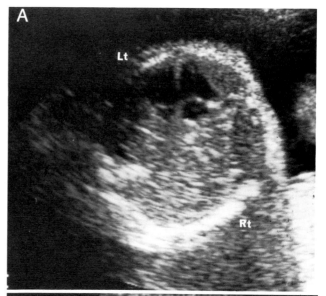

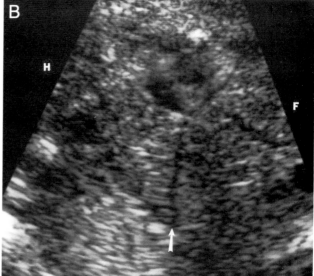

FIG 8–25.
Diaphragmatic hernia, right Bochdalek. **A,** transverse scan of the thorax at 25 weeks shows mild deviation of the heart to the left, with subtle increased echogenicity of the right hemithorax but no focal mass effect. **B,** coronal scan of the right upper abdomen and lower thorax shows an apparently intact diaphragmatic outline. However, upon delivery at 33 weeks, a right diaphragmatic hernia was found, with liver and bowel in the right hemithorax. The neonate died at 24 hours of age from bilateral pulmonary hypoplasia. Visualization of an apparently intact diaphragmatic outline does not exclude diaphragmatic hernia. *Lt* = left; *Rt* = right; *H* = toward fetal head; *F* = toward fetal feet; *arrow* = right diaphragmatic outline.

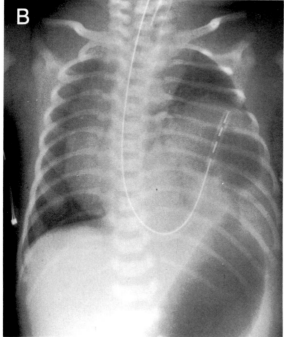

FIG 8–24.
Diaphragmatic hernia, left Bochadalek. **A,** parasagittal scan of the trunk shows the stomach extending from the abdomen into the left hemithorax. **B,** postnatal chest radiograph with nasogastric tube in place confirms the location of the stomach extending into the left hemithorax. *S* = stomach.

non–herniated contralateral abdominal contents; and (5) polyhydramnios, which often develops during the third trimester (Figs 8–23 and 8–24).[95, 96] A disproportionately small abdominal circumference may result from abdominal contents herniated into the thorax or from intrauterine growth retardation. Diaphragmatic hernia in association with intrauterine growth retardation strongly indicates the presence of other associated anomalies.[96, 98]

A Morgagni hernia typically causes herniation of the liver through the anteromedial diaphragmatic defect. The stomach may remain below the diaphragm. Ascites, pleural effusion, or pericardial effusion may outline the herniated viscera, because these hernias often lack a peritoneal covering.[104a]

The differential diagnosis for diaphragmatic hernia includes cystic adenomatoid malformation, bronchogenic and enteric cysts, mediastinal cystic teratoma, pulmonary sequestration, bronchial atresia, large chest wall or pleural-based masses, and unilateral agenesis of the lung (Fig 8–26).[88] In cases where the diagnosis is uncertain or confirmation is required, plain film or CT-assisted amniography may be performed.[91, 95, 96]

Associated Abnormalities

Congenital diaphragmatic abnormalities may create an intrathoracic mass effect which compresses the developing lungs and leads to pulmonary hypoplasia. Abdominal viscera initially herniate into the chest during the formation of the conducting airways, leading to a reduction in the number of bronchial divisions.[100] Persistence of significant intrathoracic mass effect for extended periods of fetal development results in reduction in number of pulmonary vascularity and alveoli. Although it predominantly affects the ipsilateral lung, bilateral pulmonary hypoplasia often occurs. The decreased area of the pulmonary vascular bed also results in pulmonary hypertension.

Associated anomalies commonly occur in all types of congenital diaphragmatic abnormalities.[88, 98, 106] More than half of all affected infants have associated structural or chromosomal abnormalities (Table 8–12). Puri and Gorman found that 56% of infants with diaphragmatic hernia had concomitant lethal nonpulmonary anomalies at autopsy.[106] When a diaphragmatic hernia occurs in association with growth retardation, the incidence of a concurrent major abnormality increases to 80% to 90%.[96, 98] The overwhelming association with major congenital anomalies warrants a thorough examination for associated structural defects and fetal chromosomal analysis. No clear hereditary features of diaphragmatic hernias have been identified, although several familial cases have been reported.

The major abnormalities associated with Bochdalek hernias include those of the cardiovascular system, genitourinary tract, central nervous system, musculoskeletal system, and gastrointestinal tract (Table

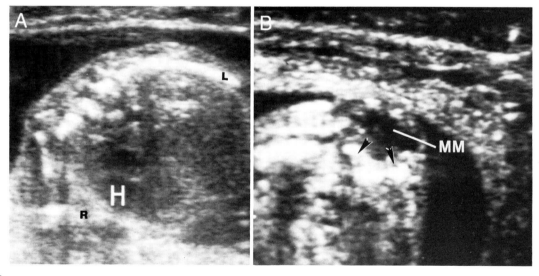

FIG 8–26.
Unilateral agenesis of the lung. **A,** transverse scan of the thorax at 19 weeks shows the heart displaced into the right hemithorax. No left hemithorax masses were evident. **B,** transverse scan of the lumbar spine demonstrates splaying of the posterior elements with a small cystic meningomyelocele. Postmortem examination revealed unilateral agenesis of the right lung, lumbar meningomyelocele, anal atresia, abnormal thumb buds, and atresia of the external ears. H = heart; *arrowheads* = splayed lumbar posterior elements; *MM* = meningomyelocele; *L* = left; *R* = right. (From Nyberg DA, Mack LA, Hirsch JH, et al: Fetal hydrocephalus: Sonographic detection and clinical significance of associated anomalies. Radiology 1987; 163:187–191. Used by permission.)

TABLE 8–12.

Recognizable Conditions Associated With Congenital Diaphragmatic Hernia*

Chromosomal abnormalities
  Trisomy 21
  Trisomy 13
  Trisomy 18
  45,X
  46,XX, 13 q−
  46,XX,−p+der(1)
Asplenia/polysplenia
Beckwith-Wiedemann syndrome
Caudal regression
DeLange syndrome
Fryns syndrome
Goldenhar anomaly
Klippel-Feil anomaly
Myelodysplasia complex
Pierre Robin sequence
Rubenstein-Taybi syndrome
Stickler syndrome
Tuberous sclerosis

*Modified from Benjamin DR, Juul S, Siebert JR: Congenital posterolateral diaphragmatic hernia: Associated malformations. J Pediatr Surg 1988; 23:899–903.

a higher incidence of affected males and bilateral defects but a lower incidence of concomitant life-threatening malformations compared with sporadic cases.[94] In the series of familial congenital diaphragmatic hernias reported by Crane, only 3.6% of cases had associated severe malformations, compared with 47% of cases that occurred without familial risk for recurrence.[94]

Unilateral eventration of the diaphragm also has an increased incidence of the Beckwith-Wiedemann syndrome and associated chromosomal abnormalities, particularly trisomies 13, 15, and 18.[88, 90] Bilateral eventration has been associated with congenital infection (rubella, toxoplasmosis, cytomegalovirus), arthrogryposis multiplex congenita, and Werdnig-Hoffman disease.[104]

Prognosis and Management

Variations in associated structural or chromosomal abnormalities and in the size, location, and chronicity of the mass effect created by a diaphragmatic hernia in utero all lead to protean clinical manifestations of this entity. However, almost all newborns with diaphragmatic hernia experience at least some respiratory insufficiency from pulmonary hypoplasia, although rare cases do not manifest until later in the first year of life. The 75% mortality rate for infants with a diaphragmatic hernia has not changed significantly despite advances in perinatal and postnatal care, although variations in reporting bias may affect this figure.[88, 98, 105]

Associated lethal anomalies and degree of pulmonary hypoplasia correlate directly with outcome of the infant with diaphragmatic hernia. The infant with an

8–13). Malrotation is the most commonly associated gastrointestinal tract abnormality. More than 50% of infants with a Morgagni hernia have an associated anomaly, including chromosomal defects, mental retardation, and cardiovascular defects. In one survey involving 94 cases of prenatally diagnosed diaphragmatic hernia, 4% had trisomy (see Chapter 17).[88] Reported familial cases of congenital diaphragmatic hernia show

TABLE 8–13.

Frequency of Associated Anomalies Among 108 Cases of Congenital Diaphragmatic Hernia*†

No. of Occurrences (%)	Organ System	Selected Examples
23	Cardiovascular	Coarctation, tetralogy of Fallot, transposition, pulmonic stenosis
15	Urinary	Renal agenesis, cystic renal dysplasia, ureteropelvic junction obstruction with hydronephrosis
10	Central Nervous	Arrhinencephaly, holoprosencephaly, hydrocephalus, myelodysplasia
9	Musculoskeletal	Talipes equinovarus, hemivertebrae, absent ribs
8	Genital	Ambiguous genitalia, bicornuate uterus, microphallus, cryptorchidism, uterovaginal atresia
7	Gastrointestinal	Annular pancreas, imperforate anus, absent gallbladder

*Some had more than one anomaly.
†From Benjamin DR, Juul S, Siebert JR: Congenital posterolateral diaphragmatic hernia: Associated malformations. J Pediatr Surg 1988; 23:899–903. Used by permission.

isolated diaphragmatic defect has a 34% survival rate following prompt postnatal surgical correction, but the infant with associated anomalies has only a 7% survival rate.[88, 90, 98] Approximately 50% of those with diaphragmatic hernia and associated anomalies are stillborn.

Sonographic detection of diaphragmatic hernia and presence or absence of associated abnormalities may assist in predicting those fetuses who have a relatively favorable prognosis, thereby optimizing perinatal management.[95, 96] Sonographic indicators of a poor prognosis for a fetus with a diaphragmatic hernia include (1) a large intrathoracic mass with marked mediastinal shift; (2) intrauterine growth retardation; (3) polyhydramnios; (4) hydrops fetalis; (5) detection prior to 24 weeks; and (6) detection of concurrent anomalies.[88, 98] Adzick et al. found that fetuses with a diaphragmatic hernia and polyhydramnios had a mortality rate of 89%.[88]

Since the current postnatal surgical approach involves immediate reduction of the herniated viscera, detection of a diaphragmatic hernia warrants delivery at a perinatal center staffed by pediatric surgeons and neonatologists.[102, 105] Extracorporeal membrane oxygenation may provide adequate oxygenation to permit non–emergency surgical repair later in the neonatal period. Prenatal correction of diaphragmatic hernia has also generated interest. An animal model indicates that pulmonary hypoplasia associated with diaphragmatic hernia may be partially reversible following removal of the compressive mass effect upon the developing lung in utero.[100, 101] At least in theory, sonography may assist in selection of fetuses with an isolated diaphragmatic hernia who may benefit from this procedure.

PERICARDIAL TERATOMA

Clinical and Pathologic Findings

Teratoma arising from the pericardium represents a rare cause for an intrathoracic mass but can cause severe cardiorespiratory compromise, including hydrops fetalis and pulmonary hypoplasia.[109–112, 114, 115] It usually attaches to the aortic root or pulmonary vessels via a pedicle.[111] Calcifications and cystic areas frequently occur within the teratoma.[114] Pericardial teratoma is further discussed in Chapter 9.

Sonographic Findings

Pericardial teratoma typically produces a predominantly solid intrathoracic mass in intimate association with the heart (Fig 8–27).[111] The mass displaces the heart and usually produces mediastinal shift and hy-

drops fetalis. Differentiation between a large pericardial teratoma and other solid intrathoracic masses may be difficult. Attempts to determine if the mass appears to arise from the lungs (CAML, pulmonary sequestration, etc.), abdomen (diaphragmatic hernia), or myocardium (rhabdomyoma, fibroma, etc.) rather than from the pericardium may assist in the differential diagnosis (see Chapter 9).[111, 113]

FOREGUT ABNORMALITIES

Clinical and Pathologic Findings

The primitive bronchial tree arises as a ventral diverticulum of the foregut early in embryogenesis.[9] This close association between the tracheobronchial tree and the esophagus during early embryologic development results in a wide spectrum of uncommon malformations involving both organ systems. Most of these foregut malformations are incidental findings detected postnatally, but rare reports document their prenatal appearance.

Bronchogenic cysts result from abnormal budding of the ventral foregut diverticulum between 26 and 40 days of embryogenesis, the period of most active tracheal and bronchial development.[7, 86] They occur at or near the carina within the mediastinum, centrally within the lung or, rarely, below the diaphragm; such cysts are more common on the right and in males. Respiratory epithelium lines the cyst, and the wall usually contains mucous glands, cartilage, elastic tissue, and smooth muscle. Typically, the cyst does not communicate with the tracheobronchial tree and is an incidental radiographic finding during childhood, although infants may occasionally present with stridor, dysphagia, or pneumonia.

Bronchial atresia probably results from a vascular insult to the developing bronchus.[120] Although it does not communicate with the gastrointestinal tract, and therefore is not a true foregut malformation, bronchial atresia is discussed here for the sake of comparison. This rare abnormality usually occurs in segmental or lobar bronchi and, as such, rarely is fatal unless concomitant stenosis or atresia of the main-stem bronchi or trachea occurs. The bronchi distal to the atresia become dilated and mucus-filled.

Neurenteric cysts result from incomplete separation of the endodermal elements of the notochordal plate. The cyst wall contains both gastrointestinal and neural elements and connects to the meninges, with a high association of concomitant vertebral body anomalies which determine the prognosis. Although the cyst commonly attaches to a portion of the gastrointestinal

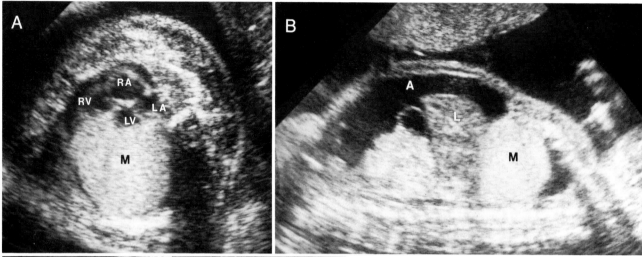

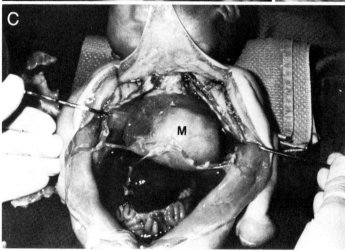

FIG 8-27.
Pericardial teratoma. **A,** transverse scan of the thorax shows a large homogeneously echogenic mass immediately adjacent to the left ventricle, left atrium, and right ventricle, with displacement of the heart to the right. Subcutaneous edema is present. **B,** sagittal scan of the trunk demonstrates the thoracic mass, as well as ascites, body-wall edema, and mild polyhydramnios. **C,** postmortem photograph shows the large pericardial teratoma. *M* = pericardial teratoma; *LV* = left ventricle; *LA* = left atrium; *RV* = right ventricle; *RA* = right atrium; *L* = liver; *A* = ascites. (Courtesy of Frederick N Hegge, MD, Emanuel Hospital, Portland, OR.)

tract, it rarely communicates with the gut lumen within the thorax.

Gastroenteric or duplication cysts result from failure of the esophagus to undergo complete vacuolation from its solid anlage into a hollow tube. Gastrointestinal mucosa lines these lesions which occur in the middle or posterior mediastinum, usually on the right side and in males. They generally produce no symptoms and are incidental findings noted during infancy or early childhood.

Sonographic Findings

Several prenatal sonographic reports of bronchogenic cysts as early as 22 weeks' gestation describe a small (1.5–2.5 cm), well-defined, unilocular intrathoracic cystic lesion adjacent to the mediastinum without associated mediastinal shift, hydramnios, or hydropic changes.[55, 116, 123] Two of these cases were identified as incidental findings, one was associated with an elevated maternal serum alpha-fetoprotein (MS-AFP) level, and

two were associated with other anomalies. Young et al. reported an echocenic left hemithoracic mass caused by a 1.5 cm mediastinal bronchogenic cyst that compressed the left mainstem bronchus (Fig 8–28).[124] The bronchogenic cyst was not apparent on the prenatal sonogram, and the overall appearance resembled another case of main-stem bronchial atresia (Fig 8–29).[120]

The prenatal appearance of a neurenteric cyst has not yet been described. One case report of a gastroenteric cyst described a 3×6 cm posterior thoracic mass with large cystic loculi separated by thick septations in a 34-week fetus who had a normal amount of amniotic fluid, appropriate fetal growth, and no associated abnormalities.[121]

Associated Abnormalities

Bronchogenic and gastroenteric cysts typically occur as isolated findings without associated anomalies. However, Reece et al. reported two cases of bron-

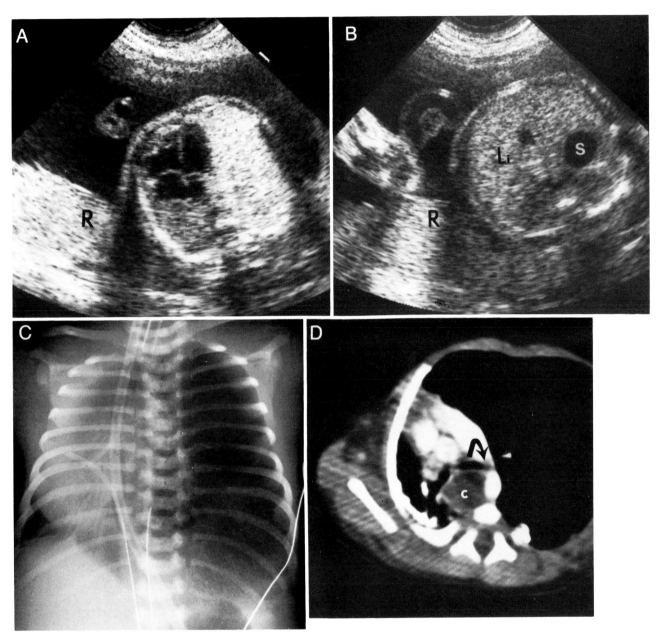

FIG 8–28.
Bronchogenic cyst with bronchial compression. **A,** transverse scan of the thorax at 23 weeks shows an enlarged and echogenic left lung displacing the heart to the right. This remained stable at 30 weeks. **B,** transverse scan of the upper abdomen shows normal relationships. **C,** postnatal chest radiograph demonstrates unilateral hyperexpansion and decreased pulmonary vascularity of the left lung with mediastinal shift to the right. **D,** contrast-enhanced postnatal computed tomography of the chest demonstrates a water-density mass posterior to the carina and compression of the left mainstem bronchus. *R* = right; *S* = stomach; *Li* = liver; *C* = mediastinal bronchogenic cyst; *curved arrow* = compressed left mainstem bronchus. (From Young G, L'Heureux PR, Kruekeberg ST, et al: Mediastinal bronchogenic cyst: Prenatal sonographic diagnosis. AJR 1989; 152:125–129. Used by permission.)

chogenic cysts with severe concomitant anomalies.[123] One 34-week fetus had truncus arteriosis, esophageal atresia, meningomyelocele, and multicystic kidneys, and another 22 week-fetus had a congenital diaphragmatic hernia. These probably represent exceptions to the rule, and the bronchogenic cysts may have been incidental findings. On the other hand, neurenteric cysts frequently associate with spinal anomalies (scoliosis, spina bifida, or hemivertebra) located at the same level or cranial to the cyst.

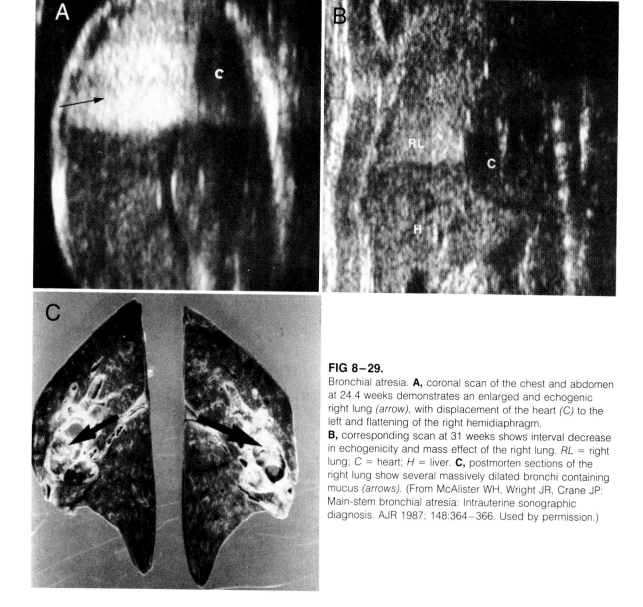

FIG 8–29.
Bronchial atresia. **A,** coronal scan of the chest and abdomen at 24.4 weeks demonstrates an enlarged and echogenic right lung *(arrow),* with displacement of the heart *(C)* to the left and flattening of the right hemidiaphragm.
B, corresponding scan at 31 weeks shows interval decrease in echogenicity and mass effect of the right lung. *RL* = right lung; *C* = heart; *H* = liver. **C,** postmorten sections of the right lung show several massively dilated bronchi containing mucus *(arrows).* (From McAlister WH, Wright JR, Crane JP: Main-stem bronchial atresia: Intrauterine sonographic diagnosis. AJR 1987; 148:364–366. Used by permission.)

CHEST WALL ABNORMALITIES

Clinical and Pathologic Findings

Normal fetal lung growth requires appropriate growth of the thoracic cage.[7, 8] A small but otherwise morphologically normal thoracic cage, therefore, frequently results in pulmonary hypoplasia. Although a variety of causes may produce a small thorax, it most commonly occurs in the setting of prolonged oligohydramnios related to bilateral renal disease or rupture of membranes. Morphologic abnormalities of the thoracic cage, usually secondary to skeletal dysplasia or chromosomal anomaly, may also result in a small thorax and pulmonary hypoplasia. In such cases, deformity or collapse of the thoracic cage or connective tissue abnormalities result in the small thorax and pulmonary hypoplasia.[7]

Focal enlargement of the chest wall rarely occurs. A hamartoma may arise within the rib and extend into the fetal thorax. This is a benign tumor which generally occurs as an isolated malformation and can be cured by surgical resection postnatally. Occasionally a cystic hygroma may extend onto the chest wall or a large cutaneous hemangioma may occur with the Klippel-Trenaunay-Weber syndrome. Other tumors, such as melanoma or neuroblastoma, are rare causes of a focal mass. On the other hand, diffuse subcutaneous thickening of the chest wall frequently occurs in hydrops fetalis and in a variety of skeletal dysplasias.

Sonographic Findings

Most cases with an abnormally small or deformed thoracic cage detected prenatally occur in the setting of obvious oligohydramnios or in cases with either obvious extremity shortening or a documented familial risk for skeletal dysplasia.[30, 125, 128, 132] The 25%–50% recurrence risk for an autosomal recessive or dominant skeletal dysplasia, the discordant extremity measurements, or the lack of amniotic fluid alert the sonologist to examine the thoracic cage carefully. In apparent de novo cases with skeletal dysplasia, on the other hand, the configuration and size of the thoracic cage usually are not as distinctive as other features in defining the specific type of dwarfism antenatally (see Chapter 12). Nevertheless, documentation of an unequivocally small thorax in the setting of skeletal dysplasia or extreme oligohydramnios correlates with the presence of pulmonary dysplasia and a poor prognosis.

The normal configuration of the fetal thoracic cage is that of convex borders laterally, anteriorly, and superiorly. Coronal scans at the level of the anterior mediastinum demonstrate the thoracic contour best (Fig 8–30). Coronal scans through the posterior thorax may be misleading in the assessment of thoracic configuration, since the posterior thorax frequently maintains a relatively normal configuration, even in the face of gross distortion anterolaterally. An abnormally small fetal thorax typically creates a concave border of the thoracic cage anterolaterally, frequently described as "bell-shaped" and often associated with pulmonary hypoplasia from restriction of lung growth (see Fig 8–30). Many skeletal dysplasias create more distinctive shapes on postnatal radiographs, but these distinctions have not yet proven useful in prenatal diagnosis. Flaring of the lower ribs or abnormal spacing of the ribs may be seen.[30] Sharp concave deformity of the thoracic cage may imply rib fractures, usually indicative of osteogenesis imperfecta type IIA (see Fig 8–31).[131]

Other chest wall abnormalities sometimes occur as an unexpected finding on a routine sonographic exam or on an examination performed for maternal hydramnios or fetal hydrops.[126, 127] A chest wall hamartoma may present sonographically as a highly echogenic

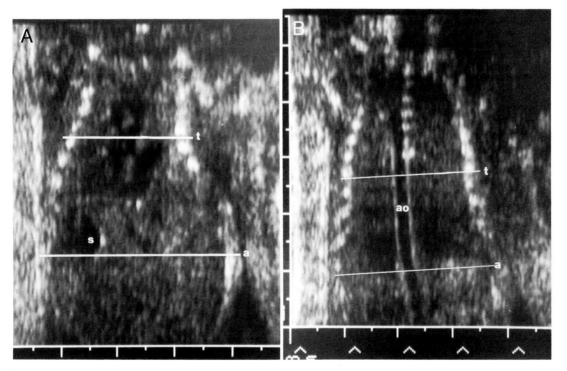

FIG 8–30.
Bell-shaped thorax, **A,** coronal scan through the anterior chest shows the concave configuration of the thoracic cage anterolaterally in association with severe oligohydramnios. This thoracic configuration often indicates the presence of pulmonary hypoplasia. **B,** coronal scan through the posterior thorax of the same fetus shows the thoracic diameter almost equal to the abdominal diameter. *T* = thoracic diameter; *a* = abdominal diameter; *s* = stomach; *ao* = aorta.

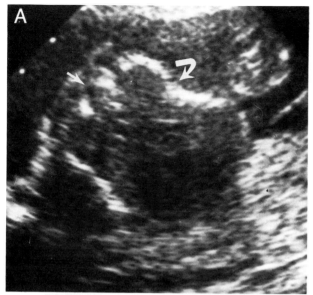

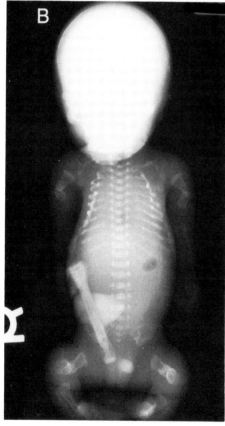

FIG 8–31.
Osteogenesis imperfecta: type II. **A,** transverse scan of the thorax
at 22 weeks shows rib fractures *(curved arrow)*, with concavity of
the chest. *Straight arrow* = spine. **B,** postnatal radiograph demonstrates multiple fractures. (From Pretorius DH, Rumack CM,
Manco-Johnson ML, et al: Specific skeletal dysplasias in utero:
Sonographic diagnosis. Radiology 1986; 159:237–242. Used by
permission.)

mass with posterior shadowing suggesting calcification.
The mass may extend into the thoracic cavity, in which
case it may be difficult to differentiate it from a calcified thoracic neuroblastoma (see Fig 8–32). The multiseptated fluid-filled mass of a cystic hygroma that extends onto the chest wall resembles hygroma in other
locations. Lymphangiectasia involves the chest wall in a
similar fashion, but its marked involvement of the subcutaneous tissues diffusely distinguishes this entity
from cystic hygroma and subcutaneous edema from hydrops fetalis. The rare hemangiomata of Klippel-
Trenaunay-Weber syndrome may have thick septations
and usually extend onto an extremity, whereas other
rare masses such as melanoma would presumably be
homogeneously solid.

Associated Abnormalities

In cases with severe oligohydramnios, skeletal dysplasias, or other rare chest wall abnormalities, the thoracic findings help to define the prognosis, but the associated findings dominate the sonographic impression
far more than do the thoracic abnormalities. For example, in bilateral renal agenesis or multicystic dysplastic
kidneys, the severe oligohydramnios and absence of
bladder-filling is usually more striking than is the small
thorax. In short-limbed dysplasias, on the other hand,
striking micromelia connote a dismal prognosis, especially in the setting of an unmistakably small thorax.
Enlargement of the chest wall often occurs in association with gross hydrops fetalis or with other concomitant masses of the neck or extremities.

Prognosis

An unmistakably small or deformed thoracic cage
generally connotes pulmonary hypoplasia and a lethal
or grave prognosis. The prognosis for enlargement of
the chest wall depends upon the underlying etiology.
For example, cystic hygroma frequently results in
death, and lymphangiectasia has a uniformly lethal outcome. On the other hand, postnatal surgical resection
often cures a chest wall hamartoma.

SUMMARY

The four-chamber view of the heart enables detection of many thoracic abnormalities that frequently occur in the setting of severe oligohydramnios, skeletal
dysplasia, or hydrops fetalis. In such cases, delineation
of thoracic size and shape may assist in predicting the
presence of pulmonary hypoplasia. The four-chamber
view of the heart also permits detection of most other

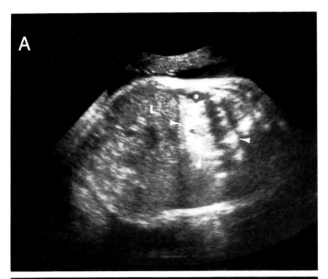

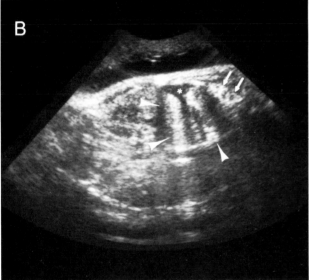

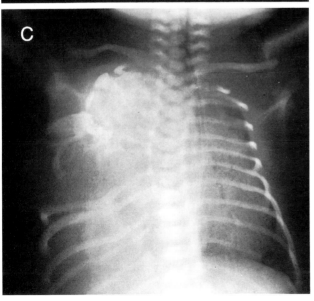

thoracic abnormalities, including hydrothorax and masses.

Following detection of an abnormal thoracic mass or fluid collection, assessment of the size, echocharacteristics, and location of the abnormality assists in determining its etiology. Occasionally, the prenatal sonogram can render a specific diagnosis of a thoracic mass. For example, intrathoracic peristalsis indicates a diaphragmatic abnormality, usually a diaphragmatic hernia. On the other hand, intrathoracic masses from a variety of etiologies may create variable but quite similar ultrasound findings, and definitive diagnosis often requires postnatal evaluation.

REFERENCES

Normal Lung Development and the Sonographic Approach

1. Bucher U, Reid L: Development of the intrasegmental bronchial tree: The pattern of branching and development of cartilage at various stages of intrauterine life. Thorax 1961; 16:207–218.
2. Carson PL, Meyer CR, Bowerman RA: Prediction of fetal lung maturity with ultrasound. Radiology 1985; 155:533.
3. Comstock CH: Normal fetal heart axis and position. Obstet Gynecol 1987; 70:255–259.
4. DeVore GR, Horenstein J, Platt LD: Fetal echocardiography: Assessment of cardiothoracic disproportion—A new technique for the diagnosis of thoracic hypoplasia. Am J Obstet Gynecol 1986; 155:1066–1071.
5. Fried AM, Loh FK, Umer MA, et al: Echogenicity of fetal lungs: Relation to fetal age and maturity. AJR 1985; 145:591–594.
6. Hislop A, Reid L: Development of the acinus in the human lung. Thorax 1974; 29:90–96.
7. Inselman LS, Mellins RB: Growth and development of the lung. J Pediatr 1981; 98:1–15.
8. Kitterman JA: Fetal lung development. J Devel Physiol 1984; 6:67–82.

FIG 8–32.
Chest wall hamartoma. **A,** coronal scan from the right side at 34.5 weeks shows an echogenic mass *(arrow heads)* of the right hemithorax. Acoustic shadowing from ribs obscures portions of the mass. A small portion of compressed lung is seen between the mass, a small pleural effusion *(asterisk)*, and the liver *(L)*. **B,** coronal scan through the posterior chest wall demonstrates that a portion of the mass involves the chest wall *(arrows)*. Arrowheads = mass; Asterisk = small pleural effusion. **C,** postnatal chest radiograph illustrates characteristic destruction of the second through fifth right ribs and deformity of the right sixth through ninth ribs by the hamartoma which deviates the mediastinum to the left. (From Brar MK, Cubberley DA, Baty BJ, et al: Chest wall hamartoma in a fetus. J Ultrasound Med 1988; 7:217–220. Used by permission.)

9. Moore KL: *The Developing Human: Clinically Oriented Embryology,* ed 4. Philadelphia, WB Saunders Co, 1988.

10. Wessels NK: Mammalian lung development: Interactions in formation and morphogenesis of tracheal buds. J Exp Zool 1970; 175:455–466.

Pulmonary Hypoplasia

11. Askenazi SS, Perlman M: Pulmonary hypoplasia: Lung weight and radial alveolar count as criteria of diagnosis. Arch Dis Child 1979; 54:614–618.

12. Besinger RE, Compton AA, Hayashi RH: The presence or absence of fetal breathing movements as a predictor of outcome in preterm labor. Am J Obstet Gynecol 1987; 157:753–757.

13. Blott N, Greenough A, Nicolaides KH, et al: Fetal breathing movements as a predictor of favorable pregnancy outcome after oligohydramnios due to membrane rupture in second trimester. Lancet 1987; ii:129–131.

14. Callan NA, Otis C, Colmorgen G, et al: The ultrasonic measurements of normal fetal thoracic parameters: Implication in fetal compression, in proceedings of the thirty-first annual meeting of the Society for Gynecologic Investigation, San Francisco, CA, March 21–24, 1984.

15. Fong K, Ohlsson A, Zalev A: Fetal thoracic circumference: A prospective cross-sectional study with real-time ultrasound. Am J Obstet Gynecol 1988; 158:1154–1160.

16. Castillo RA, Devoe LD, Falls G, et al: Pleural effusions and pulmonary hypoplasia. Am J Obstet Gynecol 1987; 157:1252–1255.

17. Castle BM, Turnbull AC: The presence or absence of fetal breathing movements as a predictor of outcome in preterm labor. Lancet 1983; ii:471–472.

18. Chamberlain D, Hislop A, Hey E, et al: Pulmonary hypoplasia in babies with severe rhesus isoimmunization: A quantitative study. J Pathol 1977; 122:43–52.

19. Chitkara U, Rosenberg J, Chervenak FA, et al: Prenatal sonographic assessment of the fetal thorax: Normal values. Am J Obstet Gynecol 1987; 156:1069–1074.

20. Fox HE, Moessinger AC: Fetal breathing movements and lung hypoplasia: Preliminary human observations. Am J Obstet Gynecol 1985; 151:531–533.

21. Hislop A, Hey E, Reid L: The lungs in congenital bilateral renal agenesis and aplasia. Arch Dis Child 1979; 54:32–38.

22. Johnson A, Callan NA, Bhutani VK, et al: Ultrasonic ratio of fetal thoracic to abdominal circumference: An association with fetal pulmonary hypoplasia. Am J Obstet Gynecol 1987; 157:764–769.

23. Knox WF, Barson AJ: Pulmonary hypoplasia in a regional perinatal unit. Early Hum Dev 1986; 14:33–42.

24. Lawrence S, Rosenfeld CR: Fetal pulmonary development and abnormalities of amniotic fluid volume. Semin Perinatol 1986; 10:142–153.

25. Nimrod C, Varela-Gittings F, Machin G, et al: The effect of very prolonged membrane rupture on fetal development. Am J Obstet Gynecol 1984; 148:540–543.

26. Nimrod C, Davies D, Iwanicki S, et al: Ultrasound prediction of pulmonary hypoplasia. Obstet Gynecol 1986; 68:495–497.

27. Nimrod C, Nicholson S, Davies D, et al: Pulmonary hypoplasia testing in clinical obstetrics. Am J Obstet Gynecol 1988; 158:277–280.

28. Page DV, Stocker JT: Anomalies associated with pulmonary hypoplasia. Am Rev Respir Dis 1982; 125:216–221.

29. Reale FR, Esterly JR: Pulmonary hypoplasia: A morphometric study of the lungs of infants with diaphragmatic hernia, anencephaly, and renal malformations. Pediatrics 1973; 51:91–96.

30. Schinzel A, Savodelli G, Briner J, et al: Prenatal sonographic diagnosis of Jeune syndrome. Radiology 1985; 154:777–778.

31. Songster GS, Gray DL, Crane JP: Prenatal prediction of lethal pulmonary hypoplasia using ultrasonic fetal chest circumference. Obstet Gynecol 1989; 73:261–266.

32. Swischuk LE, Richardson CJ, Nichols MM, et al: Primary pulmonary hypoplasia in the neonate. J Pediatr 1979; 95:573–577.

33. Vintzileos AM, Campbell WA, Nochimson DJ, et al: Degree of oligohydramnios and pregnancy outcome in patients with premature rupture of the membranes. Obstet Gynecol 1985; 66:162–167.

34. Wigglesworth JS, Desia R: Use of DNA estimation for growth assessment in normal and hypoplastic fetal lungs. Arch Dis Child 1981; 56:601–605.

35. Wigglesworth JS, Desia R: Is fetal respiratory function a major determinant of perinatal survival? Lancet 1982; i:264–267.

Hydrothorax

36. Benacerraf BR, Frigoletto FD, Wilson M: Successful midtrimester thoracentesis with analysis of the lymphocyte population in the pleural effusion. Am J Obstet Gynecol 1986; 155:398–399.

37. Blott M, Nicolaides KH, Greenough A: Pleuroamniotic shunting of fetal pleural effusions. Obstet Gynecol 1988; 71:798–799.

38. Bovicelli L, Rizzo N, Orsini LF, et al: Ultrasonic real-time diagnosis of fetal hydrothorax and lung hypoplasia. J Clin Ultrasound 1981; 9:253–254.

39. Chernick V, Reed MH: Pneumothorax and chylothorax in the neonatal period. J Pediatr 1970; 76:624–632.

40. Defoort P, Thiery M: Antenatal diagnosis of congenital chylothorax by gray scale sonography. J Clin Ultrasound 1978; 6:47–48.

41. Hutchinson AA, Drew JH, Yu VYH, et al: Nonimmunologic hydrops fetalis: A review of 61 cases. Obstet Gynecol 1982; 59:347–352.

42. Jaffe R, DiSegni E, Altaras M, et al: Ultrasonic real-time

diagnosis of transitory fetal pleural and pericardial effusion. Diagn Imag Clin Med 1986; 55:373–375.

43. Lange IR, Manning FA: Antenatal diagnosis of congenital pleural effusions. Am J Obstet Gynecol 1981; 140:839–840.

44. Mahony BS, Filly RA, Callen PW, et al: Severe nonimmune hydrops fetalis: Sonographic evaluation. Radiology 1984; 151:757–761.

45. Meizner I, Carmi R, Bar-Ziv J: Congenital chylothorax—Prenatal ultrasonic diagnosis and successful post partum management. Prenat Diagn 1986; 6:217–221.

46. Petres RE, Redwine FO, Cruikshank DP: Congenital bilateral chylothorax: Antepartum diagnosis and successful intrauterine surgical management. JAMA 1982; 248:1360–1361.

47. Randolph JG, Gross RE: Congenital chylothorax. AMA Arch Surg 1957; 74:405–419.

48. Rodeck CH, Fisk NM, Fraser DI, et al: Long-term in utero drainage of fetal hydrothorax. N Engl J Med 1988 319:1135–1138.

49. Samuel N, Sirotta L, Bar-Ziv J, et al: The ultrasonic appearance of common pulmonary vein atresia in utero. J Ultrasound Med 1988; 7:25–28.

50. Schmidt W, Harms E, Wolf D: Successful prenatal treatment of nonimmune hydrops fetalis due to congenital chylothorax. Brit J Obstet Gynecol 1985; 92:685–687.

51. Seeds JW, Bowes WA: Results of treatment of severe hydrothorax with bilateral pleuroamniotic catheters. Obstet Gynecol 1986; 68:577–579.

52. Wilson RHJ, Duncan A, Hume R, et al: Prenatal pleural effusion associated with congenital pulmonary lymphangectasia. Prenat Diagn 1985; 5:73–76.

Cystic Adenomatoid Malformation

53. Adzick NS, Harrison MR, Glick PL, et al: Fetal cystic adenomatoid malformation: Prenatal diagnosis and natural history. J Pediatr Surg 1985; 20:483–488.

54. Asher JB, Sabbagha RE, Tamura RK, et al: Fetal pulmonary cyst: Intrauterine diagnosis and management. Am J Obstet Gynecol 1985; 15:97.

55. Avni EF, Vandereslt A, Van Gansbeke D, et al: Antenatal diagnosis of pulmonary tumors: Report of two cases. Pediatr Radiol 1986; 16:190–192.

56. Blott M, Nicolaides KH, Greenough A: Postnatal respiratory function after chronic drainage of fetal pulmonary cyst. Am J Obstet Gynecol 1988; 159:858–859.

57. Cohen RA, Moskowitz PS, McCallum WD: Sonographic diagnosis of cystic adenomatoid malformation in utero. Prenat Diagn 1983; 3:139.

58. Diwan RV, Brennan JN, Philipson EH, et al: Ultrasonic prenatal diagnosis of Type III congenital cystic adenomatoid malformation of the lung. J Clin Ultrasound 1983; 11:218–221.

59. Donn SM, Martin JN, White SJ: Antenatal ultrasound findings in cystic adenomatoid malformation. Pediatr Radiol 1981; 10:180–182.

60. Fine C, Adzick NA, Doubilet PM: Decreasing size of a congenital adenomatoid malformation in utero. J Ultrasound Med 1988; 7:405–408.

61. Fitzgerald EJ, Toi A: Antenatal ultrasound diagnosis of cystic adenomatoid malformation of the lung. J Can Assoc Raiol 1986; 37:48–49.

62. Garrett WJ, Kossoff G: Gray scale echocardiography in the diagnosis of hydrops due to fetal lung tumor. J Clin Ultrasound 1975; 3:45–50.

63. Glaves J, Baker JL: Spontaneous resolution of maternal hydramnios in congenital cystic adenomatoid malformation of the lung. Br J Obstet Gynecol 1983; 90:1065.

64. Graham D, Winn K, Dex W, et al: Prenatal diagnosis of cystic adenomatoid malformation of the lung. J Ultrasound Med 1982; 1:9–12.

65. Hansmann M, Redel DA: Prenatal symptoms and clinical management of heart diseases, in Premier Symposium International d'Echocardiologie Foetale, Berger-Levrault, 1982, pp 137–149.

66. Johnson JA, Rumack CM, Johnson ML, et al: Cystic adenomatoid malformation: Antenatal diagnosis. AJR 1984; 142:483–484.

67. Kronpab L, Heilmann KL: Prenatale ultraschallbefunde bei einem fall von zystisch-adenomatoider malformation der lunge mit generalisiertem hydrops des feten. Geburtsh Frauenheilkd 1984; 44:689.

68. Mayden KL, Tortora M, Chervenak FE, et al: The antenatal sonographic detection of lung masses. Am J Obstet Gynecol 1984; 148:349.

69. Miller RK, Sieber WK, Yunis EJ: Congenital cystic adenomatoid malformation of the lung: A report of 17 cases and review of the literature. Pathol Annu, I 1980; 387–407.

70. Oster AG, Fortune DW: Congenital cystic adenomatoid malformation of the lung. Am J Clin Pathol 1978; 70:595–604.

71. Pezzuti RT, Isler RJ: Antenatal ultrasound detection of cystic adenomatoid malformation of the lung. Report of a case and review of the recent literature. J Clin Ultrasound 1983; 11:342–346.

72. Rempen A, Feige A, Wunsch P: Prenatal diagnosis of bilateral cystic adenomatoid malformation of the lung. J Clin Ultrasound 1987; 15:3–8.

73. Stauffer UG, Savoldelli G, Mieth D: Antenatal ultrasound diagnosis in cystic adenomatoid malformation—Case report. J Pediatr Surg 1984; 19:141–142.

74. Stocker JT, Madewell JE, Drake RM: Congenital cystic adenomatoid malformation of the lung. Hum Pathol 1977; 8:155–171.

75. Saltzman DH, Adzick NS, Benacerraf BR: Fetal cystic adenomatoid malformation of the lung: Apparent improvement in utero. Obstet Gynecol 1988; 71:1000–1002.

Bronchopulmonary Sequestration

76. Baumann H, Kirkinen P, Huch A: Prenatal ultrasonographic findings in extralobar subdiaphragmatic lung sequestration—A case report. J Perinat Med 1988; 16:67–68.
77. Carter R: Pulmonary sequestration. Ann Thorac Surg 1969; 7:68.
78. Clements BS, Warner JO, Shinebourne EA: Congenital bronchopulmonary vascular malformations: Clinical application of a simple anatomic approach in 25 cases. Thorax 1987; 42:409–416.
79. Collin PP, Desjardins JG, Khan AH: Pulmonary sequestration. J Pediatr Surg 1987; 22:750–753.
80. Davies RP, Ford WDA, Lequesne GW, et al: Ultrasonic detection of subdiaphragmatic pulmonary sequestration in utero and postnatal diagnosis by fine-needle aspiration biopsy. J Ultrasound Med 1989; 8:47–49.
81. Kristofferson SE, Ipsen L: Ultrasonic real time diagnosis of hydrothorax before delivery in an infant with extralobar lung sequestration. Acta Obstet Gynecol Scand 1984; 63:723.
82. Mariona R, McAlpin G, Zador I, et al: Sonographic detection of fetal extrathoracic pulmonary sequestration. J Ultrasound Med 1986; 5:283–285.
83. Maulik D, Robinson L, Daily DK, et al: Prenatal sonographic depiction of intralobar pulmonary sequestration. J Ultrasound Med 1987; 6:703–706.
84. Pare JAP, Fraser RG: *Synopsis of Disease of the Chest.* Philadelphia, WB Saunders Co, 1983.
85. Romero R, Chervenak FA, Kotzen J, et al: Antenatal sonographic findings of extralobar pulmonary sequestration. J Ultrasound Med 1982; 1:131–132.
86. Savic B, Birtel FJ, Tholen W: Lung sequestration: Report of seven cases and review of 540 published cases. Thorax 1979; 34:96–101.
87. Thomas CS, Leopold GR, Hilton S, et al: Fetal hydrops associated with extralobar pulmonary sequestration. J Ultrasound Med 1986; 5:668–671.

Congenital Diaphragmatic Abnormalities

88. Adzick NS, Harrison MR, Glick PL, et al: Diaphragmatic hernia in the fetus: Prenatal diagnosis and outcome in 94 cases. J Pediatr Surg 1985; 20:357–361.
89. Bell MJ, Ternberg JL: Antenatal diagnosis of diaphragmatic hernia. Pediatrics 1977; 60:738–740.
90. Benacerraf BR, Greene MF: Congenital diaphragmatic hernia: US diagnosis prior to 22 weeks gestation. Radiology 1986; 158:809–810.
91. Benacerraf BR, Adzick NS: Fetal diaphragmatic hernia: Ultrasound diagnosis and clinical outcome in 19 cases. Am J Obstet Gynecol 1987; 156:573–576.
92. Benjamin DR, Juul S, Siebert JR: Congenital posterolateral diaphragmatic hernia: Associated malformations. J Pediatr Surg 1988; 23:899–903.
93. Berman L, Stringer D, Ein SH, et al: The late-presenting pediatric Bochdalek hernia: A 20 year review. J Pediatr Surg 1988; 23:735–739.
94. Crane JP: Familial congenital diaphragmatic hernia: Prenatal diagnostic approach and analysis of twelve families. Clin Genet 1979; 16:244–252.
95. Chinn DH, Filly RA, Callen PW, et al: Congenital diaphragmatic hernia diagnosed prenatally by ultrasound. Radiology 1983; 148:119–123.
96. Comstock CH: The antenatal diagnosis of diaphragmatic anomalies. J Ultrasound Med 1986; 5:391–396.
97. Cullen ML, Klein MD, Philippart AI: Congenital diaphragmatic hernia. Surg Clin N Am 1985; 65:1115–1138.
98. David TJ, Illinsworth CA: Diaphragmatic hernia in the southwest of England. J Med Genet 1976; 13:253–262.
99. Harrison MR, deLorimier AA: Congenital diaphragmatic hernia. Surg Clin N Amer 1981; 61:1023–1035.
100. Harrison MR, Jester JA, Ross NA: Correction of congenital diaphragmatic hernia in utero. I: The model: Intrathoracic balloon produces fatal pulmonary hypoplasia. Surgery 1980; 88:174–182.
101. Harrison MR, Bressack MA, Churg AM, et al: Correction of congenital diaphragmatic hernia in utero. II: Simulated correction permits fetal lung growth with survival at birth. Surgery 1980; 88:260–268.
102. Harrison MR, Adzick NS, Nakayama DK, et al: Fetal diaphragmatic hernia: Pathophysiology, natural history and outcome. Clin Obstet Gynecol 1986; 29:490–500.
103. Langer JC, Filler RM, Bohn DJ, et al: Timing of surgery for congenital diaphragmatic hernia: Is emergency operation necessary. J Pediatr Surg 1988; 23:731–734.
104. Liggins GC, Kitterman JA: Development of the fetal lung, in Elliot K, Whelan J (eds): *The Fetus and Independent Life.* London, Pittman Ciba Foundation Symposium. 86;1981:308–322.
104a. Whittle MJ, Gilmore DH, McNay MB, et al: Diaphragmatic hernia presenting in utero as a unilateral hydrothorax. Prenat Diag 1989, 9:115–118.
105. Nakayama DK, Harrison MR, Chinn DH, et al: Prenatal diagnosis and natural history of the fetus with a congenital diaphragmatic hernia: Initial clinical experience. J Pediatr Surg 1985; 20:118–124.
106. Puri P, Gorman F: Lethal nonpulmonary anomalies associated with congenital diaphragmatic hernia: Implications for early intrauterine surgery. J Pediatr Surg 1984; 19:29–32.
107. Redmond C, Heaton J, Calix J, et al: A correlation of pulmonary hypoplasia, mean airway pressure, and survival in congenital diaphragmatic hernia treated with extracorporeal membrane oxygenation. J Pediatr Surg 1987; 22:1143–1149.
108. Stiller RJ, Robert NS, Weiner S, et al: Congenital diaphragmatic hernia: Antenatal diagnosis and obstetrical management. J Clin Ultrasound 1985; 13:212–215.

Pericardial or Intracardial Teratoma

109. Arciniegas E, Hakami M, Farooki ZQ, et al: Intrapericardial teratoma in infancy. J Thoracic Cardiovasc Surg 1980; 79:306.

110. Bower RJ, Kiesewetter WB: Mediastinal masses in infants and children. Arch Surg 1977; 112:1003.

111. Cyr DR, Guntheroth WG, Nyberg DA, et al: Prenatal diagnosis of an intrapericardial teratoma. A cause for nonimmune hydrops. J Ultrasound Med 1988; 7:87.

112. DeGeeter B, Kretz JG, Nisand I, et al: Intrapericardial teratoma in a newborn infant: Use of fetal echocardiography. Ann Thorac Surg 1983; 35:664.

113. Edwards JE: Cardiac tumors, in Adams FH, Emmanouilides GC (eds): *Heart Disease in Infants and Children,* ed 3. Baltimore, Williams & Wilkens Co, 1983, p 742.

114. Farooki ZQ, Arciniegas E, Hakimi M, et al: Real-time echocardiographic features of intrapericardial teratoma. J Clin Ultrasound 1985; 10:125.

115. Zerella JT, Kalpe CE: Intrapericardial teratoma— Neonatal cardiorespiratory distress amenable to surgery. J Pediatr Surg 1980; 15:961.

Foregut Abnormalities and Bronchial Atresia

116. Albright EB, Crane JP, Shackelford GD: Prenatal diagnosis of a bronchogenic cyst. J Ultrasound Med 1988; 7:91–95.

117. Doi O, Hutson JM, Myers NA, et al: Bronchial remnants: A review of 58 cases. J Pediatr Surg 1988; 23:789–792.

118. Fowler CL, Pokorny WJ, Wagner ML, et al: Review of bronchopulmonary foregut malformations. J Pediatr Surg 1988; 23:793–797.

119. Hobbins JC, Grannum PT, Berkowitz RL, et al: Ultrasound in the diagnosis of congenital anomalies. Am J Obstet Gynecol 1979; 134:331–345.

120. McAlister WH, Wright JR, Crane JP: Main-stem bronchial atresia: Intrauterine sonographic diagnosis. AJR 1987; 148:364–366.

121. Newnhan JP, Crues JV, Vinstein AL, et al: Sonographic diagnosis of thoracic gastroenteric cyst in utero. Prenat Diagn 1984; 4:467–471.

122. Ramenofsky ML, Leape LL, McCauley RGK: Bronchogenic cyst. J Pediatr Surg 1979; 14:219–224.

123. Reece EA, Lockwood CJ, Rizzo N, et al: Intrinsic intrathoracic malformations of the fetus: Sonographic and clinical presentation. Obstet Gynecol 1987; 70:627–632.

124. Young G, L'Heureaux P, Kruekeberg JT, et al: Mediastinal bronchogenic cyst: Prenatal sonographic diagnosis. AJR 1989; 152:125–127.

Chest Wall Abnormalities

125. Apuzzio JJ, Diamond N, Ganesh V, et al: Difficulties in the prenatal diagnosis of Jarcho-Levin syndrome. Am J Obstet Gynecol 1987; 156:916–918.

126. Brar MK, Cubberley DA, Baty BJ, et al: Chest wall hamartoma in a fetus. J Ultrasound Med 1988; 7:217–220.

127. de Filippi G, Canestri G, Bosio U, et al: Thoracic neuroblastoma: Antenatal demonstration in a case with unusual postnatal radiologic findings. Br J Radiol 1986; 59:704–706.

128. Graham D, Tracey J, Will D, et al: Early second trimester sonographic diagnosis of achondrogenesis. J Clin Ultrasound 1983; 11:336–338.

129. Hobbins JC, Mahoney MJ: The diagnosis of skeletal dysplasias with ultrasound, in Sanders RD, James AE (eds): *The Principles and Practice of Ultrasonography in Obstetrics and Gynecology.* New York, Appleton-Century-Crofts, 1980, p 198.

130. Kurtz AB, Wapner RJ: Ultrasonographic diagnosis of second trimester skeletal dysplasias: A prospective analysis in a high-risk population. J Ultrasound Med 1983; 2:99–106.

131. Pretorius DH, Rumack CM, Manco-Johnson ML, et al: Specific skeletal dysplasias in utero: Sonographic diagnosis. Radiology 1986; 159:237–242.

132. Skiptunas SM, Weiner S: Early pregnancy diagnosis of ashpyxiating thoracic dysplasia (Jeune's syndrome): Value of fetal thoracic measurement. J Ultrasound Med 1987; 6:41–43.

9

Cardiac Malformations

David A. Nyberg, M.D.

Donald S. Emerson, M.D.

Congenital heart disease (CHD) is the most common severe congenital abnormality found among live births, with a prevalence of 8 per 1,000.[7,8] It is an important cause of perinatal mortality with a rate of 27 per 1,000 stillbirths.[7] CHD is also responsible for more than half the deaths due to congenital anomalies in childhood. For these reasons, prenatal detection of major CHD is an important goal of prenatal sonography. This chapter presents an overview of CHD, including structural and valvular disorders, cardiomyopathies, arrhythmias, and cardiac tumors. The sonographic approach to the normal and abnormal heart is then presented.

RISK FACTORS

The etiologies of CHD are heterogeneous and include chromosomal, Mendelian, teratogenic, and multifactorial causes.[8,9,11] Certain groups of patients are at increased risk for carrying a fetus with CHD (Table 9–1). Risk factors can be considered either as a maternal or familial risk factor (family history, maternal diabetes, teratogen exposure) or a fetal risk factor (known chromosome abnormality, hydrops and extracardiac malformations).

Family History

CHD is usually a sporadic occurrence, but 5% of cases can be attributed to familial inheritance or an inheritable disorder. A positive family history for CHD is one of the most common clinical indications for fetal echocardiography.[15] The empiric recurrence risk is 1 in 50 if one previous child had CHD, and this risk increases to 1 in 10 if two children have been affected.[15] When a parent is affected, the risk to the next generation is also on the order of 1 in 10.[12] The recurrence risk may be as high as 25%–50% if an inheritable syndrome with an autosomal recessive or autosomal dominant inheritance is known to be present.[9]

The specific type of CHD also may influence the empiric recurrence risk. Nora and Nora suggest that the recurrence risk is 2.5% for tetralogy of Fallot, 2% for transposition of the great vessels, and 1% for truncus arteriosus.[11] Boughman et al. noted the highest recurrence rate (13.5%) in cases of hypoplastic left heart, suggesting an autosomal recessive inheritance for this anomaly.[2] Allan and associates found the risks of recurrence for the following types of CHD: aortic valve atresia, 1 in 28; coarctation of the aorta, 1 in 15; "complex" CHD, 1 in 11; and truncus arteriosus, 1 in 13.[1] However, only the rates for aortic coarctation and complex anomalies were significantly different (p<.05) than expected when compared to previously reported risk rates in children.

Maternal Diabetes

The incidence of CHD among infants of diabetic mothers is five times greater than the baseline rate.[14] The overall frequency of congenital anomalies among women with diabetes has been related to poor glucose control, reflected by hemoglobin A_{1c} levels in the first trimester.[10] Specific malformations that have been associated with maternal diabetes include ventricular septal defects and transposition of the great arteries.[14] Hy-

TABLE 9–1.

Risk Factors for Congenital Heart Disease

Maternal risk factor
  Family history of CHD
    Inheritable syndrome
    Parent
    Siblings
  Maternal diabetes
  Other maternal conditions
    Collagen vascular disease (arrhythmias)
    Phenylketonuria
  Teratogen exposure during pregnancy
    Alcohol
    Amphetamines
    Infections (rubella)
    Isoretinoin
    Lithium
    Trimethadione
Fetal risk factor
  Known chromosome abnormality
  Fetal arrhythmia
  Known sonographic abnormality (see
    Table 9–4)

pertrophic cardiomyopathy is also associated with maternal diabetes, although this disorder normally regresses in the neonatal period.

Teratogens

Exposure to certain teratogens in early pregnancy is reported to be associated with a 1 in 50 risk of heart malformation. Known cardiac teratogens include alcohol, lithium, vitamin A, anticonvulsants, thalidomide, steroids, amphetamines, narcotics, and oral contraceptives.[6, 23]

Chromosome Abnormality

Fetuses with a known chromosome abnormality are at significantly increased risk for CHD (Table 9–2). Conversely, a known cardiac anomaly significantly increases the likelihood of an underlying chromosome abnormality. In a population-based study of 1,484 live born infants with CHD, Ferencz et al. found chromosome abnormalities in 12.5% of cases, a frequency 100 times greater than a control group.[5] An even higher frequency of chromosome abnormalities (30%) has been reported in prenatal series. Trisomy 21 comprises 78% of chromosome abnormalities in infants with CHD, followed by trisomy 13 (8%), trisomy 18 (5%), 45 X (4%), and various other karyotypes (5%).[4, 5, 13] A further discussion of the risk of a chromosome abnormality associated with a cardiac defect can be found in Chapter 17.

Non-immune Hydrops

Fetal hydrops is secondary to an underlying cardiac disorder in up to 25% of cases.[43, 72] The presence of hydrops is also a very poor prognostic finding in association with CHD. For example, 14 of 74 cardiac

TABLE 9–2.

Congenital Heart Disease and Chromosome Syndromes Among Live Births*†

Chromosomal Abnormality	Prevalence in Live Births	Frequency of Congenital Heart Disease (%)	Typical Defect
Trisomy 21	1:800	50	VSD, ECD
Trisomy 18	1:5000	99	VSD, ECD, DORV
Trisomy 13	1:20,000	90	VSD
45X	1:5000	35	Coarct, Bic AOV
Triploidy	rare	?	VSD
Trisomy 8	rare	50	VSD
Trisomy 22	rare	67	ASD
Trisomy 9	rare	50	VSD
5p−	1:20,000	20	VSD
4p−	rare	40	ASD
13q−	rare	25	VSD
18q−	rare	<50	VSD

*Adapted from Copel JA, Pilu G, Kleinman CS: Congenital heart disease and extracardiac anomalies: Associations and indications for fetal echocardiography. Am J Obstet Gynecol 1986; 154:1121–1132. Used by permission.
†VSD = ventricular septal defect; ASD = atrial septal defect; ECD = endocardial cushion defect (atrioventricular communis); DORV = double-outlet right ventricle; Coarct = coarctation of the aorta; Bic AOV = bicuspid aortic valve.

TABLE 9–3.

Cardiac Anomalies That May Cause Fetal Hydrops

Hypoplastic left ventricle
Atrioventricular septal defect
Truncus arteriosus
Double-outlet right ventricle
Tetralogy of Fallot with absent pulmonary valve
Tricuspid valvular dysplasia
Ebstein's anomaly
Coarctation of the aorta
Total anomalous pulmonary venous return
Supraventricular arrhythmias
Bradyarrhythmias
Cardiac tumors

anomalies identified by Crawford et al. presented with hydrops, and only one of these (7%) was still alive at the time of their report.[57] On the other hand, hydrops resulting from cardiac arrhythmias has a more favorable prognosis with medical management. The types of cardiac abnormalities that may be associated with fetal hydrops are shown in Table 9–3.

Extracardiac Malformations

Concurrent extracardiac anomalies are present in 25%–30% of live born infants with CHD,[6, 7] and in nearly 50% of fetuses with CHD detected prenatally.[5, 49, 57] The gastrointestinal, genitourinary, and central nervous systems are most frequently involved

(Table 9–4).[5, 49, 57] Coexisting anomalies may be either randomly related or may be part of an underlying chromosome abnormality or multiple anomaly syndrome (Table 9–5).[5]

Prenatal detection of an extracardiac anomaly should initiate a search for possible cardiac defects. However, the specific risk of CHD varies with the type of malformation detected. For example, CHD is frequently associated with omphalocele, but is infrequently associated with gastroschisis. Abnormalities in more than one organ system should suggest the possibility of an underlying chromosome defect.

Fetal Arrhythmias

An underlying structural defect or cardiac tumor may be associated with a fetal arrhythmia, particularly complete heart block. Approximately 50% of fetuses with complete heart block are found to have a cardiac defect,[109] and the remaining cases are usually associated with a maternal connective tissue disorder.

Suspected Abnormalities on Routine Sonograms

The increasing use of "routine" obstetric sonography provides the opportunity for prenatal detection of cardiac anomalies that might otherwise remain unsuspected. Since the majority of cardiac defects occur in the absence of known risk factors, such a screening evaluation could have a significant impact on prenatal

TABLE 9–4.

Sonographic Abnormalities That Are Associated With Cardiac Defects*

Abnormalities of cardiac position	Cardiosplenic syndromes
Central nervous system	Holoprosencephaly
	Dandy-Walker malformation
	Agenesis of the corpus callosum
	Encephalocele (Meckel-Gruber syndrome)
	Microcephaly
Gastrointestinal	Situs abnormality
	Esophageal atresia
	Duodenal atresia
	Anorectal atresia
Ventral wall	Omphalocele
	Ectopia cordis
Diaphragmatic hernia	
Renal	Renal agenesis
	Dysplastic kidneys
Twins	Conjoined
	Monoamniotic
Amniotic fluid	Unexplained marked polyhydramnios
Growth	Early symmetric growth retardation

*Adapted from Copel JA, Pilu G, Kleinman CS: Congenital heart disease and extracardiac anomalies: Associations and indications for fetal echocardiography. Am J Obstet Gynecol 1986; 154:1121–1132.

TABLE 9-5.

Syndromes Associated With Cardiac Anomalies*†

Beckwith-Wiedemann	AD	ASD, VSD
		Omphalocele, macroglossia, hypoglycemia
CHARGE	S	Colobomas
		Heart defects
		Atresia of choanae
		Retarded growth or mental development
		Genital anomalies
		Ear anomalies
Cornelia de Lange	S	VSD, TOF, complex heart defects
di George	S	Aortic arch abnormalities, VSD, PDA, cellular immunodeficiency, hypoparathyroidism
Ellis-Van Creveld syndrome	AR	ASD, polydactyly, limb shortening
Goldenhar	S	Unspecified cardiac defects, facial abnormalities, micrognathia, renal abnormalities
Holt-Oram	AD	ASD or VSD, upper limb abnormalities
Noonan	AD	Pulmonary stenosis, ASD, septal hypertrophy, mental retardation, short stature, short webbed neck, low-set ears
Pierre Robin	X-linked	ASD, persistence of left SVC, cleft palate, micrognathia
Rubenstein-Taybi	S	Complex heart defects, microcephaly, mental retardation, beaked nose, glaucoma
Radial aplasia-thrombocytopenia (TAR)	AR	Unspecified cardiac defects, radial aplasia, lower limb defects
VACTERL association	S	Unspecified cardiac defects
Williams	S	Supravalvular aortic stenosis, hypercalcemia, elfin facies

*Modified from Copel JA, et al.[3] ; Ferencz C, et al.[5] ; and Winter RM, et al.[16]
†S = mostly sporadic; AR = autosomal recessive; AD = autosomal dominant; ASD = atrial septal defect; VSD = ventricular septal defect; TOF = tetralogy of Fallot; SVC = superior vena cava.

detection of CHD. Indeed, suspicion of a cardiac abnormality during routine scanning is rapidly becoming one of the most common indications leading to prenatal detection of CHD.[42]

SONOGRAPHIC TECHNIQUE AND EQUIPMENT

The technique and thoroughness with which the fetal heart is evaluated will inevitably vary with the clinical indications for the examination. A thorough, "targeted" fetal echocardiogram is appropriate for patients considered to be at significant risk for carrying a fetus with a cardiac anomaly (described above). A targeted echocardiogram is a specialized study, often done by or in conjunction with a pediatric cardiologist.

In many centers, it is performed independent of the remainder of the obstetric sonogram and is scheduled at a separate time. The examination requires patience on the part of the examiner, since often it may take as long as 60–90 minutes to perform a complete study on an abnormal fetal heart. In addition to cross-sectional imaging, a targeted fetal echocardiogram usually includes M-mode echocardiography and may also include other sophisticated tests, such as duplex Doppler or color-flow Doppler.[17, 26, 33, 35, 90]

In contrast to a targeted echocardiogram, a screening examination of the fetal heart may be performed in conjunction with an obstetric sonogram for routine clinical indications. Such a screening examination usually includes a four-chamber view of the heart (see Cross-Sectional Imaging below), although many authorities also urge inclusion of views of the great vessels.[34, 43, 49] A

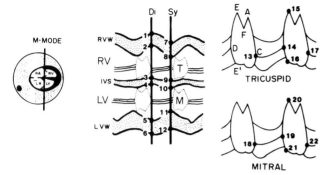

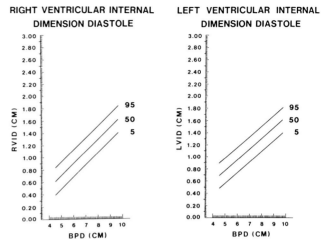

FIG 9–1.

Normal M-mode. *RVW* = right ventricular wall; *RRV* = right ventricle; *IVS* = interventricular septum; *LV* = left ventricle; *LVW* = left ventricular wall; *T* = tricuspid valve; *M* = mitral valve; *Di* = diastole; *Sy* = systole; *D* = opening point of atrioventricular valve; *E* = opening excursion of atrioventricular leaflets; *F* = beginning of rapid filling phase of ventricle; *A* = end of rapid filling phase of ventricle; *C* = closure of atrioventricular valve. Numbers refers to points of normal computer measurements. (From DeVore GR, Siassi B, Platt LD IV: M-mode assessment of ventricular size and contractility during the second and third trimesters of pregnancy in the normal fetus. Am J Obstet Gynecol 1984; 150:981–998. Used by permission.)

FIG 9–2.

Normal values and confidence limits for ventricular chamber dimensions during diastole. (From DeVore GR: Cardiac imaging, in Sabbagha RE (ed): *Diagnostic Ultrasound Applied to Obstetrics and Gynecology,* ed 2. Philadelphia, JB Lippincott Co, 1987, pp 324–363. Used by permission.)

Previous studies have reported percentiles of ventricular size and arterial diameters relative to gestational age, femur length, and BPD (Figs 9–2 to 9–4).[2, 23, 24, 27, 28] Small pericardial effusions also may be better demonstrated with M-mode than cross-sectional imaging.

M-mode echocardiography is very useful for evaluating fetal arrhythmias by simultaneously displaying movements from an atrial and ventricular wall or from an atrioventricular and semilunar valve. The start of an atrial contraction is defined by either (1) contraction of the atrial wall, or (2) start of the a-component of atrioventricular valve motion. The start of ventricular

screening evaluation of the fetal heart does not include M-mode ultrasound, duplex Doppler, or other sophisticated techniques.

M-mode

Real-time directed M-mode echocardiography is a useful supplement to cross-sectional imaging for evaluating myocardial wall thickness, cavity dimension, and valve and wall motion (Fig 9–1, and Table 9–6).[18, 25]

TABLE 9–6.

Mean, 5%, and 95% Confidence Limits for M-mode Computations of Cardiac Ventricular Contractility (n=82)*

	3%	Mean	95%	SD
Right ventricle				
Fractional shortening (%)	24.73	32.14	39.54	3.78
Left ventricle				
Fractional shortening (%)	25.69	33.12	40.54	3.79
Biventricular				
Inner fractional change (%)	19.69	26.57	33.45	3.51
Outer fractional change (%)	5.48	11.27	17.05	2.95
Heart rate	122	142	162	10
Right/left ratios				
Internal dimension—diastole	0.80	0.98	1.15	0.08
Fractional shortening	0.74	0.98	1.21	0.12
Mean circumferential shortening	0.70	0.98	1.26	0.14
Tricuspid/mitral excursion	0.83	0.99	1.15	0.08
Wall thickness—diastole	0.58	1.12	1.65	0.27

*Modified from DeVore GR, Siassi B, Pratt LD: Fetal echocardiography. IV. M-mode assessment of ventricular contractility during the second and third trimesters of pregnancy in the normal fetus. Am J Obstet Gynecol 1984; 150:981–988. Used by permission.

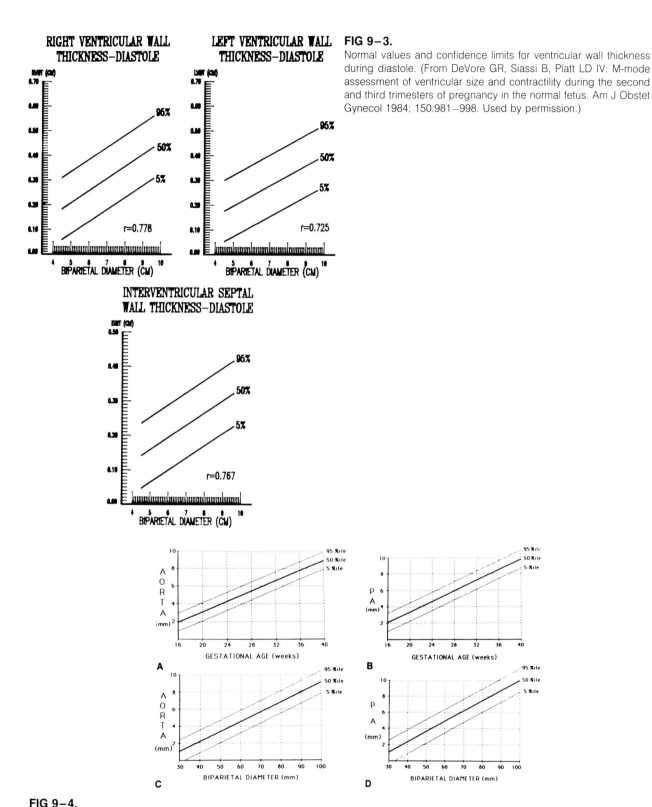

FIG 9-3.
Normal values and confidence limits for ventricular wall thickness during diastole. (From DeVore GR, Siassi B, Platt LD IV: M-mode assessment of ventricular size and contractility during the second and third trimesters of pregnancy in the normal fetus. Am J Obstet Gynecol 1984; 150:981–998. Used by permission.)

FIG 9-4.
Normal values and confidence limits for **A,** aortic root diameter vs. menstrual age. **B,** pulmonary artery *(PA)* diameter vs. menstrual age. **C,** aortic root diameter vs. biparietal diameter. **D,** pulmonary artery diameter vs. biparietal diameter. (From Cartier MS, Davidoff A, Warneke LA, et al: The normal diameter of the fetal aorta and pulmonary artery: Echocardiographic evaluation in utero. AJR 1987; 149:1003–1006.

TABLE 9–7.

Flow Measurement in the Normal Fetal Heart*

	Peak Velocity (cm/sec) ±SE	Mean Temporal Velocity (cm/sec) ±SE
Tricuspid valve	51± 1.2 (range, 34.1–78.2)	11.8 ± .4 (range, 7.2–16.9)
Mitral valve	47 ± 1.1 (range, 20.8–67.6)	11.2 ± .3 (range, 6.6–16.5)
Pulmonary valve	60 ± 1.9 (range, 24.1–81.6)	16 ± .6 (range, 9.2–25.7)
Aortic valve	70 ± 2.6 (range, 56.0–94.0)	18 ± .7 (range, 13.7–22.5)
Right ventricular output	307 ± 127 ml/kg/min	
Left ventricular output	232 ± 106 ml/kg/min	

*Adapted from Reed KL, Meijboom EJ, Sahn DJ, et al: Cardiac Doppler flow velocities in human fetuses. Circulation 1986; 73:41–46.

contraction is defined by (1) the onset of ventricular wall motion, (2) opening of a semilunar valve, or (3) closure of an atrioventricular valve.

Doppler

If the fetal echocardiographic study is abnormal, duplex Doppler or, more recently, by color-flow Doppler is sometimes performed.[17, 26, 33, 35, 90] Normal flow velocity profiles across both atrioventricular and semilunar valves have been described.[33, 35] The atrioventricular valves in the fetus typically demonstrate a small v-component (due to venous filling) and a higher a-component (due to atrial contraction). This pattern is opposite that observed in the adult, possibly due to diminished ventricular compliance.

Normal values for both peak and mean flow velocities across the valves have also been reported by Reed and others (Table 9–7).[33, 35] When the ultrasound beam is oriented along the plane of blood flow at the valves, an estimation of the pressure difference across the valve can be obtained. This estimation uses the modified Bernoulli equation which states that: $P = 4V^2$, where P is the pressure drop (in mm of mercury) and V is the velocity in the stenotic area.

Cross-sectional Imaging

Cross-sectional imaging is the mainstay of fetal echocardiography.[19, 22, 23, 30, 32, 36] Both linear and sector transducers may be used. In performing targeted fetal echocardiograms, image magnification, cineloop capability, and videotape recording have also proved to be useful.

Determining the location and axis of the heart should be the initial step in any fetal echocardiogram. Identification of left and right sides can be quickly performed by determining the fetal lie (vertex, breech, or transverse) and localization of the spine. The stomach should be identified on the left side, and the heart

should lie mainly in the left chest, with the apex pointing toward the left anterior chest wall.[21]

Specific views of the heart that are sought on cross-sectional imaging will vary from institution to institution and the clinical indications for the examination (Figs 9–5 and 9–6). The four-chamber view is recommended by many authorities from 18 weeks' gestation onward as part of a screening evaluation. This view can be obtained with generally available real-time equipment in the vast majority of cases. As part of a more thorough screening examination or a targeted fetal

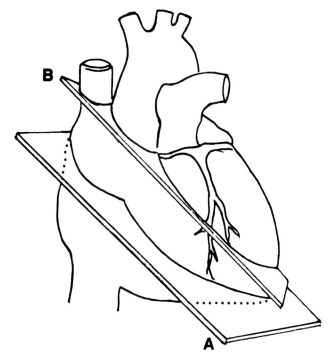

FIG 9–5.

Normal cross-sectional planes. Four-chamber view *(plane A)* is obtained by directing the ultrasound beam parallel to the long axis of the heart. The left ventricular long-axis view *(plane B)* is obtained by directing the ultrasound beam toward the fetal right shoulder. (From Perone N: A practical guide to fetal echocardiography. Contemporary Ob/Gyn 1988; Jan: 55–81. Used by permission.)

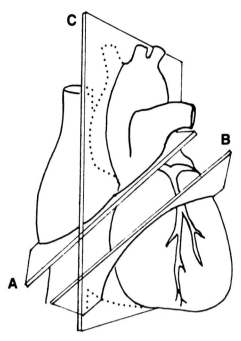

FIG 9–6.
Normal cross-sectional planes. Short-axis view of the great vessels *(plane A)* is obtained by directing the ultrasound beam toward the fetal left shoulder with cephalic angulation. The short-axis view of the ventricles *(plane B)* is obtained by moving toward the apex of the heart. The aortic arch view *(plane C)* is obtained by aligning the aortic root with the descending aorta. (From Perone N: A practical guide to fetal echocardiography. Contemporary Ob/Gyn 1988; Jan: 55–81. Used by permission.)

TABLE 9–8.

Fetal Cardiac Abnormalities That May Be Detected on a Four-Chamber View*

Hypoplastic left heart
Hypoplastic right heart
Single ventricle
Atrioventricular septal defect
Ventricular septal defect (large)
Double-inlet ventricle (single ventricle)
Ebstein's anomaly
Tetralogy of Fallot
Valve atresia or stenosis—tricuspic, mitral, pulmonic, aortic
Coarctation of the aorta
Ventricular wall hypertropy
Atrial isomerism
Situs inversus
Ectopia cordis
Cardiomyopathy
Cardiac tumors
Pericardial effusion
Arryhythmias

*Modified from Reed KL[33]; Reed, et al.[35]

echocardiogram, additional views that may be sought include an axial view of the great vessels (short-axis view), left ventricular outflow tract, long-axis right ventricle, right atrial inflow, and longitudinal view of the aortic arch (see Figs 9–5 and 9–6). The method for obtaining these views and their potential value is described in detail below.

The Four-Chamber View

The four-chamber view can evaluate the size, location and axis of the heart, the relative size of the ventricular and atrial chambers, the thickness and continuity of the ventricular and atrial septa, and the atrioventricular valves. Familiarity with the normal appearance of this plane of section can lead to the possibility of screening for major forms of congenital heart disease (Table 9–8).[43, 45] For example, Copel and associates reported that 96% (71 of 74) of sonographically detectable heart anomalies showed one or more abnormalities on the four-chamber view.[55]

The four-chamber view (Figs 9–7 and 9–8) is obtained in a horizontal section just above the level of the diaphragm. Regardless of fetal position (see Fig 9–7) the apex normally points at approximately a 45-degree angle toward the left anterior chest wall.[21] The two atria are of approximately equal size, and the two ventricles are of approximately equal size until 32 weeks, when the right ventricle may look slightly larger than the left. The atrioventricular valves are oriented nearly perpendicular to the ventricular and atrial septa, forming a "cross" with them. The septal leaflet of the tricuspid valve is inserted slightly lower in the ventricular septum than is the mitral valve.

The interatrial septum is a thin structure that separates the atria. The flap of the foramen ovale can be visualized opening toward the left atrium. The pulmonary veins may be visualized as they empty into the left atrium.

Short-Axis View of the Great Vessels

Moving cranially from the four-chamber view, the aortic root can be identified in the center of the chest as it arises from the left ventricle. This scan plane has been referred to as the "five-chamber" view. Slight cranial angulation can demonstrate the aorta as it sweeps to the right, and the pulmonary artery as it arises anteriorly from the right ventricle and is directed straight back toward the spine. Slightly further cranially, the aortic arch can be seen.

The short-axis view of the great vessels can be obtained by turning the transducer slightly from the transverse section so that the ultrasound plane is directed toward the fetal left shoulder (Fig 9–9).[32] This view, sometimes referred to as a "sausage and egg" appearance, demonstrates the right ventricular outflow tract, pulmonic valve, main pulmonary artery, and the

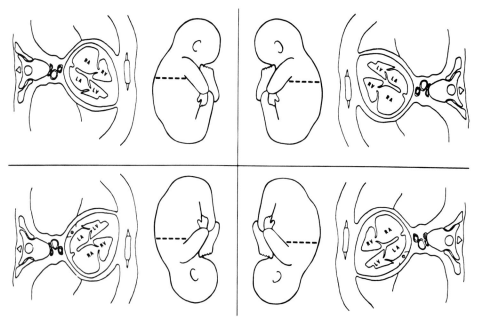

FIG 9–7.
Four-chamber view depicted in different fetal positions. The dotted line indicates the plane of section through which the accompanying image is obtained. *LA* = left atrium; *LV* = left ventricle; *RA* = right atrium; *RV* = right ventricle. (From Perone N: A practical guide to fetal echocardiography. Contemporary Ob/Gyn 1988; Jan: 56–81. Used by permission.)

pulmonary bifurcation encircling the aortic root (Figs 9–9 and 9–10). The ductal junction with the descending aorta may also be seen in this view (see Fig 9–10). Sliding the transducer from this position toward the fetal apex will demonstrate the right and left ventricles

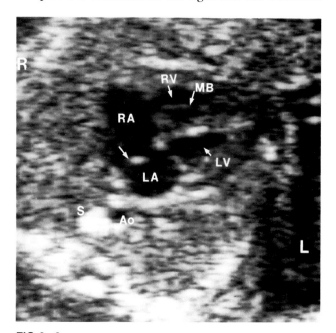

FiG 9–8.
Normal four-chamber view (22 weeks). *RV* = right ventricle; *LV* = left ventricle; *RA* = right atrium; *LA* = left atrium; *MB* = moderator band; *Ao* = aorta; *S* = spine; *L* = left; *R* = right.

in a short axis-view (transventricular view) (Fig 9–11).

Normal features to recognize during imaging of the great vessels include (1) the great vessels course nearly perpendicular to one another near their origin; (2) the pulmonary artery is anterior and to the left of the aortic root; (3) the pulmonary artery diameter is slightly larger than the aortic root (ratio of 1.2 to 1),[34, 36] and (4) the root of the aorta arises only from the left ventricle.

Long-Axis Left Ventricle

The long-axis view of the left ventricle is obtained by turning the transducer slightly from the four-chamber view so that the ultrasound plane is directed toward the right shoulder of the fetus (Fig 9–12).[32] This view demonstrates the aortic valves, left atrium, left ventricle, mitral valve, interventricular septum, and proximal aortic root (Figs 9–13 and 9–14). Since the aortic wall should be continuous with the interventricular septum, this view is useful for evaluating membranous ventricular septal defects.

Long-Axis Right Ventricle

The long-axis view of the right ventricle can be obtained by continuing to turn the transducer from the long-axis view of the left ventricle to nearly a straight sagittal view of the fetus. This shows the right ventricular outflow tract, pulmonary valve, main pulmonary artery, and ductus arteriosus (Fig 9–15). The pulmo-

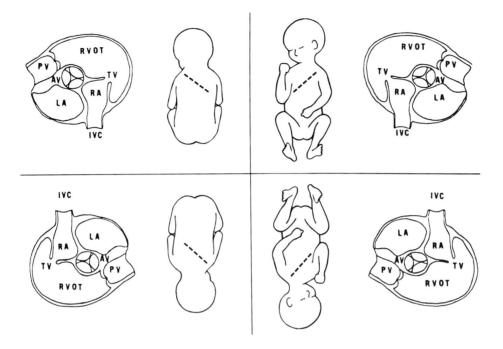

FIG 9–9.
Short-axis view of the great vessels in different fetal positions. The dotted line indicates the plane of section through which the accompanying image is obtained. *AV* = aortic valve; *LA* = left atrium; *IVC* = inferior vena cava; *PV* = pulmonic valve; *RA* = right atrium; *RVOT* = right ventricular outflow tract; *TV* = tricuspid valve. (From Perone N: A practical guide to fetal echocardiography. Contemp Ob/Gyn 1988; Jan: 55–81. Used by permission.)

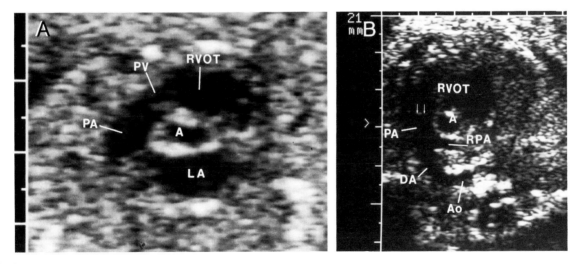

FIG 9–10.
Short-axis view of the great vessels (22 weeks). **A,** this view demonstrates the typical "sausage and egg" view as the pulmonary artery *(PA)* and right ventricular outflow tract *(RVOT)* drape around the aortic root *(A)* seen in cross section. *PV* = pulmonic valve; *LA* = left atrium. **B,** slight cephalic angle in another fetus demonstrates the bifurcation of the pulmonary artery *(PA)* into the right pulmonary artery *(RPA)* and the ductus arteriosus *(DA)*, which courses to the descending aorta *(Ao)*. *A* = aortic root; *RVOT* = right ventricle outflow tract; *small arrows* = pulmonic valve.

FIG 9–11.

Transventricular short axis view (22 weeks). The right ventricle *(RV)* is separated from the left ventricle *(LV)* by the interventricular septum *(IVS)*. The papillary muscles of the mitral valve *(mv)* are seen within the body of the left ventricle.

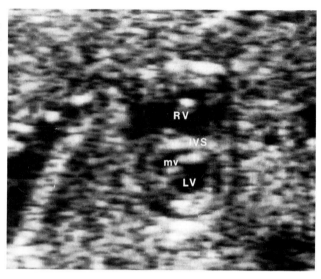

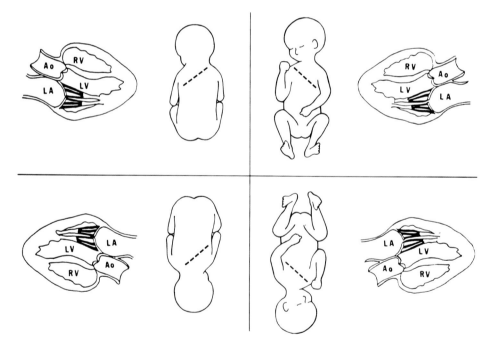

FIG 9–12.

Long-axis view of left ventricle in different fetal positions. The dotted line indicates the plane of section through which the accompanying image is obtained. *Ao* = aortic root; *LA* = left atrium; *LV* = left ventricle; *RV* = right ventricle. (From Perone N: A practical guide to fetal echocardiography. Contemp Ob/Gyn 1988; Jan: 55–81. Used by permission.)

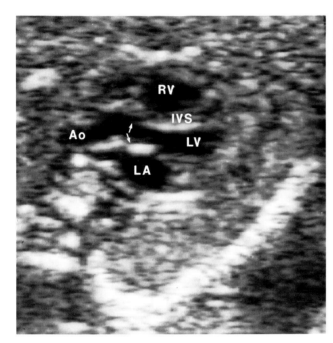

FIG 9–13.
Long-axis view of left ventricle. This view demonstrates the aortic root *(Ao)* arising from the left ventricle *(LV)*. Note continuity of the interventricular septum *(IVS)* and aortic wall. *LA* = left atrium; *RV* = right ventricle; arrows indicate region of aortic valve.

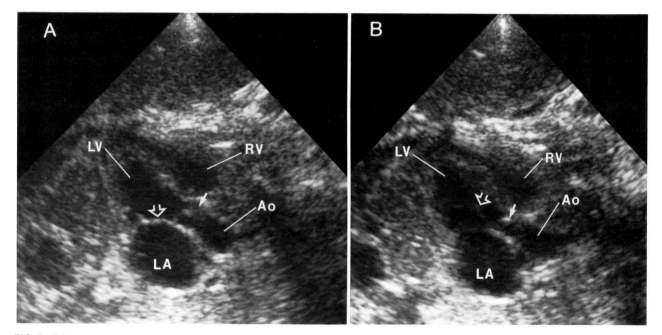

FIG 9–14.
Long-axis view of left ventricle. In systole (A), the aortic valve *(straight arrow)* is open and the mitral valve *(open arrow)* is closed, and in diastole (B), the mitral valve is open and the aortic valve is closed. *Ao* = aortic root; *LA* = left atrium; *LV* = left ventricle; *RV* = right ventricle.

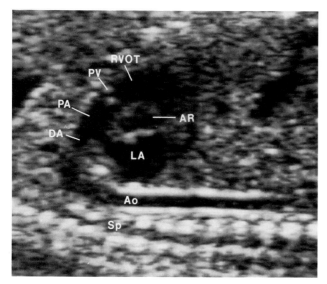

FIG 9–15.
Longitudinal view of the pulmonary artery, ductal arch (22 weeks). This view demonstrates the right ventricular outflow tract *(RVOT)*, pulmonic valve *(PV)*, pulmonary artery *(PA)*, and ductus arteriosus *(DA)* coursing straight back toward the spine *(Sp)* and joining the descending aorta *(Ao)*. *LA* = left atrium; *AR* = aortic root.

nary artery can be seen to course straight back toward the fetal spine. After bifurcating into left and right pulmonary branches, the pulmonary artery continues as the ductus arteriosus. Hence, this view best demonstrates the ductus arteriosus and "ductal arch".

Right Atrial Inflow

The right atrial inflow view is obtained in a section sagittal to the fetus over the right heart. This view

demonstrates the inferior and superior vena cava, the right atrium, and tricuspid valve. The eustachian valve may be seen as a linear echogenic contour from the junction of the inferior vena cava and right atrium to the foramen ovale.

Longitudinal View of the Aortic Arch

The aortic arch view can be obtained either from a right-anterior approach or a left-posterior approach and aligning the ascending and descending aorta (see Fig 9–6). When properly aligned, this view includes the ascending and descending aorta, aortic arch, and the major vessels arising from the aortic arch (Fig 9–16). The "candy cane" shape of the aortic arch should be distinguished from the less rounded "hockey stick" appearance of the ductus as it enters the descending aorta. Also, no neck vessels arise from the superior border of the ductus.

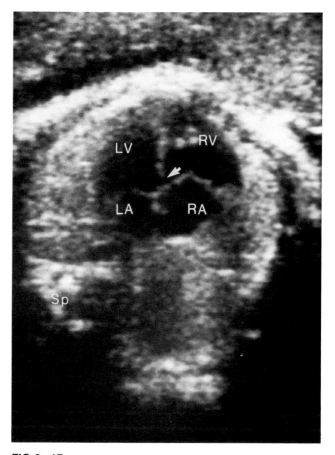

FIG 9–17.
Pseudoventricular septal defect. Four-chamber view with interventricular septum aligned parallel to the ultrasound beam demonstrates an area of echo dropout *(arrow)* that could be mistaken for a ventricular septal defect. *LA* = left atrium; *LV* = left ventricle; *RA* = right atrium; *RV* = right ventricle; *Sp* = spine.

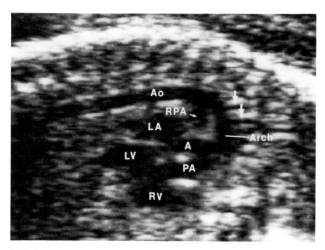

FIG 9–16.
Aortic arch. Longitudinal scan demonstrates the aortic root *(A)*, aortic arch *(Arch)*, and descending aorta *(Ao)*. Note the presence of neck vessels *(arrows)* arising from the aortic arch. *LV* = left ventricle; *RV* = right ventricle; *PA* = pulmonary artery; *RPA* = right pulmonary artery; *LA* = left atrium.

Potential Pitfalls

The interventricular septum is thickest at the apex of the heart and tapers as it approaches the atrioventricular valves. The thinner region of the interventricular septum may appear artifactually absent on the four-chamber view, especially when the interventricular system lies parallel to the direction of the ultrasound beam (Fig 9–17).[45] This potential pitfall probably results from a refractive shadow arising from the muscular region of the interventricular septum. In such cases, a more perpendicular orientation should reveal the intact septum.

The moderator band can be identified in the right ventricle, coursing from the interventricular septum to the lower free wall. The moderator band may appear prominent in size; it should not be mistaken for an intracardiac tumor or other mass. Bright reflections from the papillary muscle are occasionally seen within the left ventricle (Fig 9–18).[31, 37] This finding should not be confused with other abnormalities such as intraventricular tumors, aberrant fibromuscular bands, or endocardial fibroelastosis.

The normal hypoechoic myocardium can be mis-

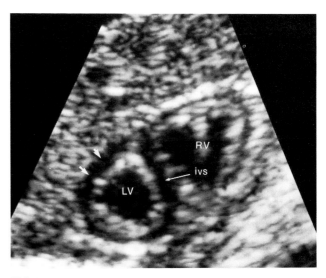

FIG 9–19.
Pseudopericardial effusion. Short-axis transventricular view demonstrates hypoechoic myocardium *(arrows)* that could be mistaken for pericardial effusion. Note that this hypoechoic rim extends into the interventricular septum *(ivs)*, thereby confirming that it represents myocardium and not pericardial fluid. *LV* = left ventricle; *RV* = right ventricle. (Courtesy of Douglas L Brown, MD, Department of Radiology, University of Tennessee, Memphis, TN.)

taken for small amounts of pericardial effusion (Fig 9–19). Therefore, the diagnosis of definite pericardial effusion requires a clear separation between the pericardium and epicardium. This appearance can be confirmed on M-mode ultrasound. When larger pericardial effusion develops, the heart may demonstrate a rocking motion within the cavity. Pericardial effusion should be distinguished from pleural effusion.

OVERVIEW OF CARDIAC MALFORMATIONS

Sonographic Accuracy and Limitations

The sonographic accuracy for detecting cardiac malformations prenatally has now been reported by several centers.[49, 57, 75, 87] Factors that influence the reported accuracy include the clinical indication for the sonogram (high-risk vs. low-risk), gestational age, the experience of the sonographer, and the type of equipment used. Other important technical factors include fetal position, the amount of amniotic fluid present, and maternal size.

Malformations of the cardiovascular system are clearly some of the most difficult anomalies to diagnose on prenatal sonography. This is due, in part, to the rapidity of the fetal heart rate, which hinders visualization of cardiac structures. A rapid heart rate superimposed on fetal motion and suboptimal position further restrict evaluation of cardiac defects. Gestational age at

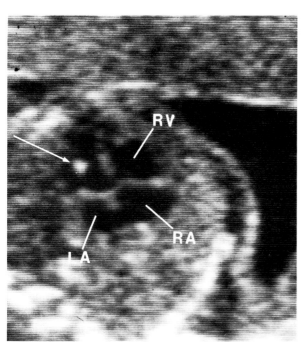

FIG 9–18.
Echogenic cordae tendinae. Four-chamber view demonstrates an echogenic focus *(arrow)* arising from a thickened posterior chordae tendinae in the left ventricle. This should not be mistaken for an intraventricular tumor or other mass. *LA* = left atrium; *RA* = right atrium; *RV* = right ventricle. (From Schechter AG, Fakhry J, Shapir LR, et al: In utero thickening of the chordae tendinae. A cause of intracardiac echogenic foci. J Ultrasound Med 1987; 6:691–695. Used by permission.)

the time of the sonogram also limits early prenatal diagnosis of CHD. Due to the small size of cardiac structures, a reliable diagnosis of cardiac anomalies before 18 weeks is extremely difficult.

The difficulties in diagnosing cardiac malformations, even in high-risk patients on targeted echocardiograms, have been emphasized.[75, 87] Some centers have attempted to minimize errors by routinely repeating the echocardiogram a few weeks later.[90] Sandor et al. suggest that each center must determine its own statistics with regard to the sensitivity, specificity, and predictive value of echocardiography.[87]

The accuracy of fetal echocardiography improves with the severity of the cardiac defect. Defects that can be readily detected include atrioventricular septal defect, single ventricle, hypoplastic left heart, hypoplastic right heart, and Ebstein's anomaly. On the other hand, defects that are consistently missed in most series include isolated atrial septal defects, small to moderate ventricular septal defects, aortic stenosis, pulmonic stenosis, total anomalous pulmonary venous return, and aortic coarctation.[49, 57, 75, 87]

The sonographic accuracy for detecting cardiac defects in low-risk patients during routine obstetric sonography is largely unknown. Among 49 fetuses who had proven CHD and who were scanned after 18 weeks' gestation by Benacerraf and associates, 29 patients were referred for low-risk indications and 20 patients for high-risk indications.[49] Of the 29 low-risk patients, 16 (55%) were correctly identified as having CHD, and 14 of the 29 cases were diagnosed before 24 weeks.[49] Further studies are needed to determine whether these favorable results are representative of other centers.

Overall Prognosis

CHD detected prenatally encompasses more severe anomalies and carries a higher spontaneous mortality rate (>80%) than cardiac defects that are first detected at birth.[40, 41, 49, 57] (Table 9–9) These differences can be explained primarily by two factors (1) prenatal series include more severely anomalous fetuses who die in utero or shortly after birth and who are excluded from neonatal series and (2) fetuses with more severe cardiac and associated anomalies are more likely to be detected prenatally. For example, Crawford et al. reported that the survival rate was only 17% for sonographically detected cardiac anomalies compared to a survival rate of 81% for cardiac lesions that were

TABLE 9–9.

Comparison of Type and Frequency of Heart Defects in a Neonatal, Prenatal, and Autopsy Series*

	Live Born Series† (n=3104) (%)	Stillbirth Series† (n=265) (%)	Prenatal Series‡ (n=72) (%)
VSD	30.3	34.7	9.7
Complete transposition	4.7	9.1	5.5
Tetralogy of Fallot	5.1	3.4	8.3
Hypoplastic left heart	1.3	3	5.5
Double-outlet right ventricle	.2	.4	1.3
Atrioventricular septal defect	3.2	6.8	13.8
Ebstein's anomaly	-	-	5.6
Interrupted aortic arch	-	-	4.1
Coarctation	5.7	9.4	6.8
Aortic stenosis or aortic atresia	5.2	0	2.7
Pulmonic stenosis	7.4	1.1	-
Truncus arteriosus	1	6	1.3
Single ventricle	.3	6.4	10.9³
TAPVR§	1.1	-	-
Myocardial disease	-	-	11.1
Tumor	-	-	4.1
Patent ductus	8.6	-	-
Miscellaneous	17.1	8.3	1.3

*Includes absent left connection (5.5%), double-inlet (2.7%), and tricuspid atresia (2.7%).
†Hoffman JIE, Christianson R: Congenital heart disease in a report of 19,502 births with long-term follow-up. Am J Cardiol 1978; 42:641–664.
‡Allan LD, Crawford DC, Handerson R, et al: Spectrum of congenital heart disease detected echocardiographically in prenatal life. Br Heart J 1985; 54:523–526.
§TAPVR = total anomalous pulmonary venous return.

missed on prenatal sonography.[57] Differences between the types and frequency of cardiac anomalies observed in prenatal, neonatal, and autopsy series are shown in Table 9–8.

Classification of CHD

The traditional method of classifying cardiac anomalies has been in the form of malformation patterns such as hypoplastic left heart, tetralogy of Fallot, Ebstein's anomaly, etc. Since many authors continue to classify cardiac anomalies in this way, similar terms are used to describe specific types of anomalies further in this chapter. However, a large proportion of cardiac defects examined at autopsy are complex and may not necessarily fit into one of these diagnoses.

The limitations of an anatomic classification have led to a classification of CHD based on sequential analysis of the cardiac chambers and great arteries and their connections to one another. This classification was developed by Shinebourne and others after the segmental approach of cardiac anatomy introduced by Van Praagh.[48, 91, 92, 95] CHD can be described by this sequential approach by evaluating:

1. Atrial situs.
2. Atrioventricular connections.
3. Ventriculoarterial connections.
4. Associated anomalies.

Atrial situs can be described as situs solitus, situs inversus, or situs ambiguous.[95] Atrial situs solitus is described when the morphologic right atrium is on the fetal right side, and atrial situs inversus is described when the morphologic right atrium is on the fetal left side. With the exception of situs ambiguous, the atrial situs corresponds to the visceral situs; therefore, the right atrium is located opposite the side of the fetal stomach. The flap of the foramen ovale opens into the left atrial cavity, which helps further to identify the right from the left atria. This can be confirmed by following the inferior vena cava to the right atrium, but this is rarely necessary.

Determination of the atrioventricular connections requires recognition of the morphologic features of the left and right ventricles. The right ventricle may be identified by the more trabeculated appearance of the ventricular cavity and the presence of the moderator band near the apex of the right ventricular cavity. Normally, the right atrium connects with the morphologic right ventricle, and the left atrium connects with the morphologic left ventricle. If the reverse is true, atrioventricular discordance is said to be present.

The ventriculoarterial connections can be considered as one of four possibilities:[95]

1. Arterial concordance. The aorta arises from the morphologic left atrium, and the pulmonary trunk arises from the morphologic right ventricle.
2. Arterial discordance (transposition). The aorta arises from the morphological right ventricle and the pulmonary trunk from the left ventricle. In d-transposition the aortic valve is to the right of the pulmonary valve and in l-transposition the aortic valve is to the left of the pulmonary artery.
3. Double-outlet connection. More than half of both great arteries arise from the same ventricle.
4. Single-outlet connection. Only one great vessel arises from the ventricles.

Associated anomalies refer to various other cardiac defects not described by the segmental analysis. These include[95]:

1. Anomalies of venous return.
2. Anomalies of atrial anatomy.
3. Anomalies of the atrioventricular junction.
4. Anomalies of ventricular anatomy.
5. Anomalies of infundibular anatomy.
6. Anomalies of the aortic arch and its derivatives.

SPECIFIC CARDIAC DEFECTS

Situs Ambiguous (Cardiosplenic Syndromes)

Clinical and Pathologic Findings

In situs ambiguous, both atria are morphologically right atria (dextroisomerism) or morphologically left atria (levoisomerism); these patterns are associated with asplenia and polysplenia syndromes, respectively. Both asplenia syndrome (bilateral right-sidedness) and polysplenia syndrome (bilateral left-sidedness) are also characterized by complex CHD and various intraabdominal and intrathoracic abnormalities.[79, 83]

Other features of the polysplenia syndrome usually include (1) bilateral left bronchi and pulmonary arteries, (2) interruption of the inferior vena cava with drainage via the azygous or hemiazygous vein, (3) two or more spleens, and (4) abnormalities of the superior vena cava.[79, 83] Additional features of the asplenia syndrome usually include (1) bilateral right bronchi and pulmonary arteries, (2) ipsilateral location of both the aorta and the inferior vena cava (either left side or right side),

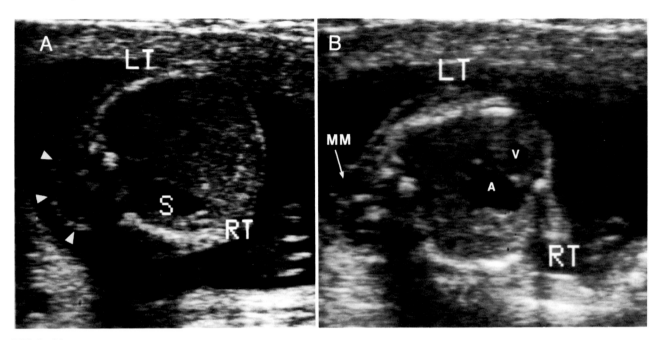

FIG 9–20.
Situs ambiguous and polysplenia syndrome **A,** transverse view of the abdomen in a fetus referred with bradycardia (complete heart block) at 19 weeks demonstrates the stomach *(S)* on the fetal right. A large myelomeningocele *(arrowheads)* is also demonstrated. *RT* = right; *LT* = left. **B,** transverse view of the thorax shows a common atrium *(A)* and ventricle *(V).* Other abnormalities found at autopsy included polysplenia, absent gallbladder, absent inferior vena cava, single umbilical artery, facial cleft, and absent right kidney. Complete heart block in association with structural abnormalities of the atrioventricular valve have been strongly associated with left atrial isomerism and the polysplenia syndrome. *MM* = myelomeningocele.

(3) absence of the spleen with a midline, horizontal liver, and (4) bilateral superior venae cavae.[79, 83]

Sonographic Findings

The asplenia and polysplenia syndromes can be detected prenatally by recognizing discordancy between the location of the fetal stomach and heart, which normally are both located on the left (Fig 9–20).[53, 60, 61] Some form of CHD is found in 40% of patients with abdominal situs inversus (stomach on the right). Fetuses with the asplenia and polysplenia syndromes can also be detected by demonstration and CHD and an arrhythmia. Patients with the asplenia syndrome often have an ambiguous atrioventricular connection, usually a common atrioventricular valve.[60] The combination of atrioventricular septal defect with complete heart block has been found to be highly suggestive of left atrial isomerism (polysplenia syndrome).[60, 83, 109]

Absence of the inferior vena cava with continuation of the azygous vein (a right-sided structure) is associated with the asplenia syndrome. De Araujo and associates recognized interruption of the inferior vena cava with azygous continuation prenatally in a fetus with the polysplenia syndrome.[60] Demonstration of both the aorta and the inferior vena cava on the same side may also suggest the asplenia syndrome.

Associated Anomalies

Complex cardiac defects are commonly associated with both the asplenia and polysplenia syndromes, although they are typically more common and are usually more complex with the asplenia syndrome.[79, 83] Types of defects include atrioventricular septal defect, transposition of the great vessels, pulmonary stenosis or atresia, persistent truncus arteriosus, and abnormalities of the pulmonary veins. As noted, congenital heart block has been strongly associated with the asplenia syndrome and may be the initial clue to its presence.[60, 67] Genitourinary anomalies and spina bifida are also associated with these syndromes.

Prognosis

Due to the severity of complex cardiovascular malformations, infants with asplenia syndrome have a 90% to 95% mortality rate during the first year of life, and infants with polysplenia syndrome have an 80% mortality rate.[79, 83]

Ventricular Septal Defect

Clinical and Pathologic Findings

Ventricular septal defects (VSDs) represent the most common cardiac defect in most postnatal series, accounting for 25% to 30% of all structural defects.[5, 7] They can be present in various sizes and positions or be part of more complex anomalies. VSDs may involve any of the four parts of the ventricular septum: the inlet, trabecular, infundibular, or membranous portions. The membranous type is most common, accounting for 75% of VSDs.

Malformations of the central nervous system, the genitourinary tract, and gastrointestinal tract (including tracheoesophageal fistula) are the most common extracardiac anomalies associated with VSDs.[49] Extracardiac or chromosome abnormalities were found in 11 of 19 fetuses with a VSD detected prenatally by Crawford and associates.[57]

Sonographic Findings

A VSD appears sonographically as an interruption of the interventricular septum. VSDs that are large (Figs 9–21 and 9–22) or associated with more complex cardiac anomalies are more easily demonstrated than isolated or small defects. A VSD located in the outlet or membranous portion of the septum can be missed on routine scanning, since this area is not included on the standard four-chamber view (Fig 9–23). Subaortic axial views or longitudinal views of the left ventricular outflow tract may be helpful in demonstrating such defects.

The sonographic accuracy for detecting ventricular

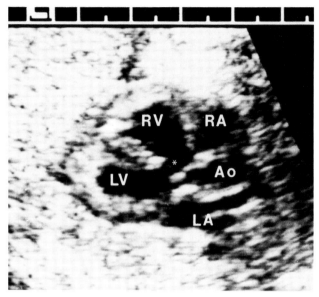

FIG 9–22.
Ventricular septal defect. Left parasternal view at 30 weeks demonstrates a subaortic ventricular septal defect (*) which creates partial obstruction of the left ventricular outflow tract. Examination of the kidneys also demonstrated unilateral hydronephrosis. Amniocentesis identified a chromosomal translocation. *Ao* = aorta; *LA* = left atrium; *LV* = left ventricle; *RA* = right atrium; *RV* = right ventricle.

septal defects has been reported by several authors. Crawford et al. reported detection of ventricular septal defects in 19 fetuses; all were moderate or large in size, and only 2 were isolated.[57] At the same time, 10 additional ventricular septal defects were missed, four of which closed spontaneously. Similarly, Benacerraf et al. reported missing nine of 13 isolated atrioseptal or ventricular septal defects.[49] Two cases diagnosed at 28 and 26 weeks' gestation were not seen on earlier examinations.

Associated Anomalies

Approximately 60% of all VSDs are isolated, and most small VSDs discovered after birth are isolated defects.[64] By contrast, all 19 VSDs detected prenatally by Crawford et al. were moderate to large, and 17 of these were part of a complex cardiac anomaly (n=15) and/or had associated extracardiac anomalies.[57] Other cardiac anomalies in this series included tetralogy of Fallot (n=6), double-outlet right ventricle and mitral atresia (n=3), coarctation of the aorta (n=2), tricuspid insufficiency (n=2), and one case each of transposition of the great arteries and left atrial isomerism. Other cardiac anomalies that may be associated with VSD include pulmonic atresia and atrioventricular septal defect.[64]

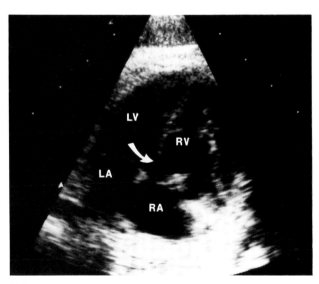

FIG 9–21.
Ventricular septal defect. Four-chamber view at 30 weeks demonstrates a defect *(arrow)* in the ventricular septum near the crux of the heart. *LA* = left atrium; *LV* = left ventricle; *RA* = right atrium; *RV* = right ventricle. (From Brown DL, Emerson DS, Cartier MS, et al: Congenital cardiac anomalies: Prenatal sonographic diagnosis. AJR 1989; 153:109–114. Used by permission.)

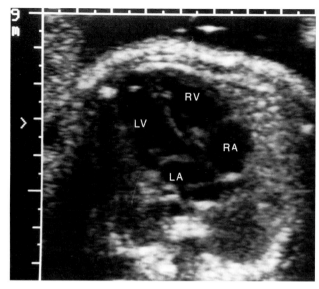

FIG 9–23.
False-negative ventricular septal defect. Four-chamber view in a fetus with cloacal exstrophy shows an apparently intact interventricular septum. However, a moderate-sized ventricular septal defect was found after delivery. Since only a portion of the interventricular septum is shown on the four-chamber view, sweeping the heart from the apex to the base in short-axis projection may help in evaluating the entire interventricular septum. *LA* = left atrium; *LV* = left ventricle; *RA* = right atrium; *RV* = right ventricle.

Prognosis

Since the ventricular pressures are nearly equal, an isolated VSD does not result in shunting in utero. Infants are usually asymptomatic immediately after birth but develop left-to-right shunting as the systemic arterial pressure increases and the pulmonary vascular pressure decreases. Large VSDs may lead to pulmonary hypertension and eventually result in reversal of the shunt.

The prognosis for VSDs depends on associated cardiac and extracardiac anomalies. The prognosis for isolated small to moderate-sized VSDs is good. Postnatal series suggest that 40% of such defects close spontaneously within 2 years, and 60% close within 5 years. However, since many small or isolated VSDs remain undetected, prenatal detection of a VSD is less favorable. In one prenatal series, only 3 of 19 (16%) of fetuses with a sonographically detected VSD survived.[57]

Atrioventricular Defect (Endocardial Cushion Defect)

Clinical and Pathologic Findings

Atrioventricular septal defect (ASD), also known as endocardial cushion defect or canal defect, results from persistence of the primitive atrioventricular canal that is present during embryologic development. Ana-

tomically, this malformation is characterized by a defect in the atrial and ventricular septa at the crux of the heart. The atrioventricular valves have abnormal anterior and posterior leaflets which bridge the septal defect.

Several types of atrioventricular septal defect are recognized according to the mode of attachment of the bridging leaflets. A complete atrioventricular canal (type III) is the most common.[82] In a series of 357 cases of CHD studied by Fontana and Edwards, 48 (13.4%) were an atrioventricular septal defect and 33 of these were of the complete type.[64]

Sonographic Findings

The sonographic appearance of atrioventricular septal defect is characteristic. A large defect is noted at the crux of the heart (Figs 9–24 and 9–25). A single atrioventricular valve typically is present, which also demonstrates exaggerated excursion upon real-time examination.

Atrioventricular septal defect is one of the most common serious cardiac defects detected prenatally. Among 29 cases identified in one prenatal series,[76] clinical indications for referral included non-immune hydrops (n=11), family history of CHD (n=7), fetal bradycardia (n=5), and identification of extracardiac fetal anomalies (n=6).

Bradycardia, in combination with complete heart block, appears to be highly associated with left atrial isomerism (polysplenic syndrome).[57, 60, 74] Machado et al. reported complete heart block in 11 of 29 fetuses (38%) with atrioventricular septal defect, and all had left atrial isomerism.[74] Similarly, Crawford et al. reported congenital heart block in 5 of 18 fetuses (28%) with atrioventricular septal defect, and all 5 had left atrial isomerism.[57]

Associated Anomalies

Atrioventricular septal defect is frequently associated with other cardiac defects and has been strongly linked to trisomy 21 (see Fig 9–25). A prenatal study found that 14 of 29 fetuses with atrioventricular septal defect had a chromosome abnormality, and 9(64%) of these had trisomy 21.[74] In a larger study of 128 live born infants with atrioventricular septal defect, 70% had trisomy 21.[5] Conversely, nearly half of the 187 infants with CHD and a chromosome abnormality had atrioventricular septal defect as the primary diagnosis.[5]

Additional cardiac anomalies that may be associated with atrioventricular septal defect include tetralogy of Fallot, double-outlet right ventricle, coarctation of the aorta, and pulmonary stenosis or atresia, among

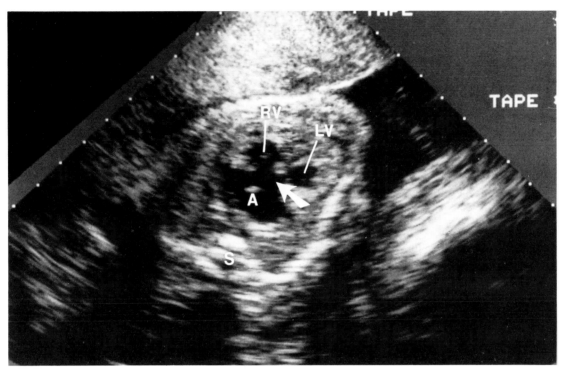

FIG 9–24.
Atrioventricular septal defect (endocardial cushion defect). Four-chamber view at 28 weeks demonstrates a large defect *(arrow)* at the crux of the heart. *RV* = right ventricle; *LV* = left ventricle; *A* = atria; *S* = spine. (From Brown DL, Emerson DS, Cartier MS, et al: Congenital cardiac anomalies: Prenatal sonographic diagnosis. AJR 1989; 153:109–114. Used by permission.)

others. Machado et al. found additional cardiac malformations in 21 of 29 fetuses (72%) with atrioventricular septal defect identified prenatally.[74] Only 1 fetus (3.4%) had no additional defects or chromosome abnormality. Similarly, all 18 fetuses with atrioventricular septal defect reported by Crawford et al. had additional anomalies.[57]

Prognosis

The prognosis for fetuses with atrioventricular septal defect is poor because of the high rate of additional anomalies and/or chromosome abnormalities. Only 4 survivors were reported among 29 fetuses (14%) with atrioventricular septal defect in the series of Machado et al., and this included two infants with trisomy 21

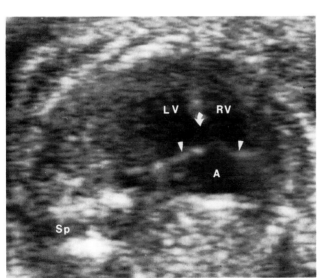

FIG 9–25.
Atrioventricular septal defect and trisomy 21. Transverse image at 18 weeks shows large ventricular septal defect *(curved arrow)* at the crux of the heart and absence of interatrial septum. A large, single atrioventricular valve *(arrowhead)* is present. Chromosome analysis yielded trisomy 21. *RV* = right ventricle; *LV* = left ventricle; *A* = atria; *Sp* = spine.

and a third with inoperable defects.[74] Similarly, only 4 survivors (22%) were reported by Crawford et al., and all of these had additional anomalies.[57] By contrast, postnatal series report that survival rates up to 83% can be expected following surgical correction.[52]

Double-Inlet (Single Ventricle, Cor Biloculare)

Clinical and Pathologic Findings

Double-inlet connection is an unusual defect where both atrioventricular valves drain into one ventricle. This defect apparently results from failure of development of the interventricular septum.

Sonographic Findings

The sonographic appearance of double-inlet shows an absence of the interventricular septum. Both atrioventricular valves are present, however. The differential diagnosis includes a large ventricular septal defect, hypoplastic right heart, and hypoplastic left heart.

Associated Anomalies

Aortic and pulmonic stenosis, transposition of the great vessels, and absence of the spleen are frequently associated with double-inlet.[64] Conduction defects may also be present.

Prognosis

The prognosis for double-inlet depends primarily on the presence of associated anomalies. Left-to-right shunting develops after birth, but this is influenced by the presence of pulmonic stenosis. Postnatal studies suggest that with palliative procedures the survival rate is 50% to 70%.[77, 80] The outcome for fetuses identified prenatally would be expected to be significantly worse.

Ebstein's Anomaly

Clinical and Pathologic Findings

Ebstein's anomaly is a malformation of the tricuspid valve, where the septal leaflet of this valve is displaced into the cavity of the right ventricle and the valve is frequently dysplastic.

Sonographic Findings

Ebstein's anomaly alters the normal appearance of the crux of the heart, with inferior displacement of the tricuspid valve (Fig 9–26). The valve is usually incompetent, producing gross right atrial dilatation. Marked right atrial enlargement may also result from tricuspid dysplasia and regurgitation without displacement of the atrioventricular valve inferiorly (Fig 9–27).

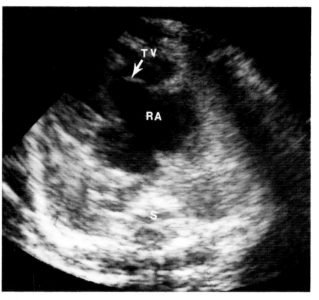

FIG 9–26.
Ebstein's anomaly. Transverse image at 34 weeks demonstrates marked dilatation of the right atrium *(RA)* and inferior displacement of the tricuspid valve leaflet *(TV). S =* spine. (From Brown DL, Emerson DS, Cartier MS, et al: Congenital cardiac anomalies: Prenatal sonographic diagnosis. AJR 1989; 153:109–114. Used by permission.)

Associated Anomalies

Ebstein's anomaly may be associated with other severe anomalies, including pulmonary atresia or pulmonary stenosis, atrioventricular canal, and transposition of the great vessels. Arrhythmias are a common problem.[101] The frequency of chromosome abnormalities in prenatal series is unknown, although no chromosome abnormalities were reported among 16 infants with Ebstein's anomaly in one postnatal series.[5]

Prognosis

Surgical procedures, with replacement of the atrioventricular valve, have resulted in significantly improved outcome for Ebstein's anomaly.[101] However, congestive heart failure frequently develops in utero or during the neonatal period from tricuspid regurgitation, which portends a poor prognosis. Arrhythmias may remain a persistent problem following surgical correction.[101]

Hypoplastic Left Heart

Clinical and Pathologic Findings

Hypoplastic left heart syndrome results from aortic atresia in association with mitral atresia or mitral hypoplasia. In its severest form, the aortic root ends

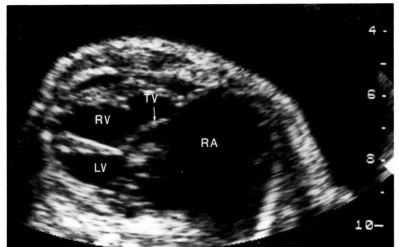

FIG 9–27.
Tricuspid dysplasia. Transverse view demonstrates a markedly enlarged right atrium *(RA)* that obscured visualization of the left atrium. The tricuspid valve *(TV)* appeared thickened but not displaced inferiorly. Duplex Doppler demonstrated marked tricuspid regurgitation. *RV* = right ventricle; *LV* = left ventricle.

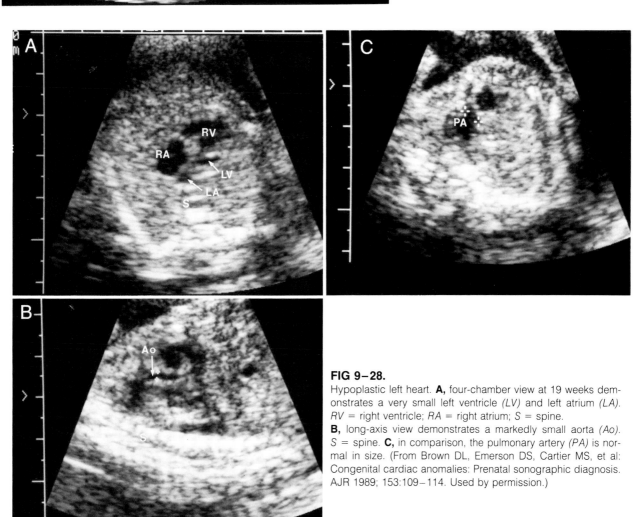

FIG 9–28.
Hypoplastic left heart. **A,** four-chamber view at 19 weeks demonstrates a very small left ventricle *(LV)* and left atrium *(LA)*. *RV* = right ventricle; *RA* = right atrium; *S* = spine.
B, long-axis view demonstrates a markedly small aorta *(Ao)*. *S* = spine. **C,** in comparison, the pulmonary artery *(PA)* is normal in size. (From Brown DL, Emerson DS, Cartier MS, et al: Congenital cardiac anomalies: Prenatal sonographic diagnosis. AJR 1989; 153:109–114. Used by permission.)

blindly within the cardiac muscle just below the coronary arteries without formation of the valve. When the mitral valve is atretic, the left ventricular chamber is only a slit-like pouch within the myocardium. This type constitutes one form of univentricular heart with absent atrioventricular connections.

Sonographic Findings

The primary sonographic feature of hypoplastic left heart is the diminutive left ventricle (Fig 9–28).[92] The left atrium is small to normal in size, and the aorta is tiny and may be difficult to visualize. The mitral valve is absent or hypoplastic. A mild form of hypoplastic left heart may result from mitral and aortic stenosis (Fig 9–29).

Associated Anomalies

Hypoplastic left heart is associated with coarctation of the aorta in 80% of cases with aortic atresia.

Only 2 chromosome abnormalities were found among 85 cases of hypoplastic left heart reported by Ferencz et al.[5] However, one case reported prenatally had trisomy 13.[85]

Prognosis

Hypoplastic left heart in its severest is uniformly fatal if untreated. It carries an extremely poor prognosis, even with palliative procedures. Ischemia and myocardial dysfunction result from hypoperfusion of the aorta and coronary arteries; congestive heart failure usually develops from myocardial ischemia or from right ven-

tricular overload. Cyanosis may also develop if the left-to-right shunt at the atrial level is not adequate.

Hypoplastic Right Heart

Clinical and Pathologic Findings

Hypoplastic right heart is usually due to pulmonary atresia with intact ventricular septum. Tricuspid atresia may or may not be present.

Sonographic Findings

The primary sonographic finding of hypoplastic right heart is a small right ventricle. The pulmonary root either will not be seen in its usual position or it will be tiny in relation to the aorta. The differential diagnosis of a hypoplastic right heart includes a single ventricle.

Associated Anomalies

Atrial septal defects, ventricular septal defects and transposition of the great vessels are the most common defects associated with tricuspid atresia. Extracardiac anomalies appear to be uncommonly associated with hypoplastic right heart; no chromosome abnormalities were found among 20 cases of tricuspid atresia or among 28 cases of pulmonary atresia reported by Ferencz et al.[5]

Prognosis

Fetal hydrops frequently develops in utero or after birth from tricuspid regurgitation. Following birth, tri-

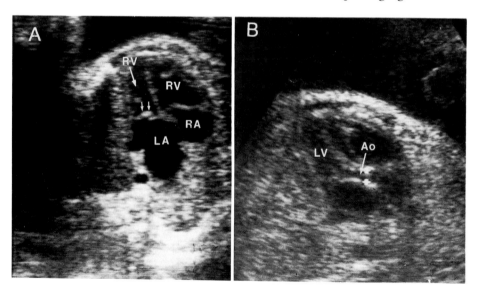

FIG 9–29.
Mitral and aortic valvular stenosis. **A,** transverse scan at 31 weeks shows enlarged left atrium *(LA)* and small right ventricle *(RV)*. Also note that the mitral valve *(small arrows)* appears small and thickened. **B,** longitudinal view demonstrates a small left ventricle *(LV)* and aortic root *(Ao)*. The pulmonary artery was normal in size. Findings after delivery included stenosis of the mitral valve and aortic valve and mildly hypoplastic left ventricle. (Courtesy of Fred N Hegge, MD, Emanuel Hospital, Portland, OR.)

cuspid atresia carries a poor prognosis, with few patients surviving infancy.

Tetralogy of Fallot

Clinical and Pathologic Findings

Tetralogy of Fallot is a common malformation, representing 5%–10% of congenital heart defects among live borns.[5] This anomaly is characterized by (1) a VSD, (2) overriding aorta, (3) stenosis of the right ventricular outflow tract, and (4) hypertrophy of the right ventricle. Some cases are also associated with absence of the pulmonary valve.

Sonographic Findings

Tetralogy of Fallot is characterized by an enlarged aorta that overrides a ventricular septal defect (Fig 9–30). A similar appearance may be seen in pulmonary atresia with a ventricular septal defect and in truncus arteriosus. In tetralogy of Fallot, the pulmonary outflow is usually small, but it can be massively dilated from absence of the pulmonic valve. By comparison, the pulmonary outflow tract is absent with pulmonary atresia. In truncus arteriosus, the pulmonary artery arises from the common arterial trunk, and the right ventricular conus is absent.

DeVore and associates have stressed that the ventricular septal defect in tetralogy of Fallot is usually not visible on the four-chamber view and that recognition of aortic dilatation is the key to the correct diagnosis.[62] All seven fetuses with tetralogy of Fallot studied by these authors demonstrated dilatation of the aorta when compared with other cardiac (biventricular dimension) or extracardiac (biparietal diameter, head circumference, and femur length) parameters.[62]

Associated Anomalies

As noted, absence of the pulmonary valve may accompany tetralogy of Fallot. Other cardiac and extracardiac abnormalities often are present (see Fig 9–30). A chromosome abnormality was found in 17 of 138 (12%) live born infants with tetralogy of Fallot[5] and in 3 of 6 fetuses (50%) reported in a prenatal series.[57]

Prognosis

The prognosis for tetralogy of Fallot with intact pulmonary valves has significantly improved with advances in cardiac surgery. Congestive heart failure may develop in utero or after birth secondary to pulmonic regurgitation when the pulmonary valve is absent.

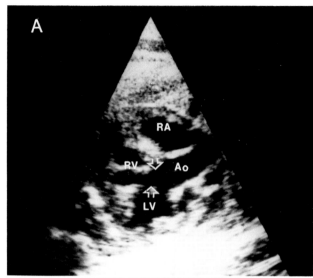

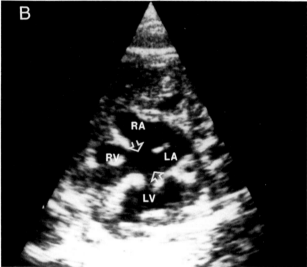

FIG 9–30.
Tetralogy of Fallot with atrioventricular septal defect. **A,** dilated aorta *(Ao)* is demonstrated overriding an atrioventricular septal defect *(arrows).* The pulmonary outflow tract was small. *RV* = right ventricle; *LV* = left ventricle; *RA* = right atrium. **B,** four-chamber view demonstrates the large atrioventricular septal defect *(arrows).* RV, right ventricle; LV, left ventricle; RA, right atrium; *LA;* left atrium.

Transposition of the Great Vessels

Clinical and Pathologic Findings

Complete transposition of the great vessels (d-transposition) is defined as discordance of the ventriculoarterial connection with the aorta connected to the right ventricle and the pulmonary artery connected to the left ventricle.

Sonographic Findings

In most cases of complete transposition, the aorta arises anterior and to the right of the pulmonary artery

FIG 9–31.
Transposition of the great vessels. Longitudinal view at 34 weeks demonstrates the aorta *(Ao)* ascending anterior and parallel to the pulmonary artery *(PA)*, rather than crossing perpendicular to it. The aorta connected to the right ventricle. *LV* = left ventricle; *arrow* = innominate artery. (From Brown DL, Emerson DS, Cartier MS, et al: Congenital cardiac anomalies: Prenatal sonographic diagnosis. AJR 1989; 153:109–114. Used by permission.)

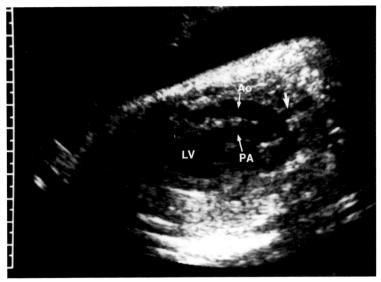

(Figs 9–31 and 9–32). Both great vessels may appear parallel to one another rather than being perpendicular at their origin. A ventricular septal defect may or may not be present.

Associated Anomalies

Other cardiac anomalies that may be associated with complete transposition include ventricular septal defect (see Fig 9–32), pulmonic stenosis, hypoplastic left or right heart, and coarctation of the aorta.[100]

Prognosis

Palliative procedures and early surgical correction have significantly improved the prognosis for infants with complete transposition. Most recently, 5-year survival rates up to 89% have been reported.[100] However, as with most cardiac defects, the prognosis varies with the presence of other cardiac anomalies (ventricular septal defect, pulmonic stenosis, and coarctation of the aorta).

Double-Outlet Right Ventricle

Clinical and Pathologic Findings

Double-outlet right ventricle is a rare condition forming less than 1% of CHD. It is characterized by origination of both great vessels from the right ventricle. However, since a ventricular septal defect is usually present, it may be difficult to clearly determine the origin of both vessels. A commonly accepted definition of double-outlet right ventricle is when more than one and one-half semilunar valves arise from a single ventricle.[71] Several types of double-outlet right ventricle are recognized. The ventricular septal defect may be subaortic or subpulmonic in location, and the aorta may

be either normally positioned or inversely positioned relative to the pulmonary artery.

Sonographic Findings

In double-outlet right ventricle, both great arteries arise from the right ventricle (Figs 9–33 and 9–34). The position of the great arteries relative to each varies, but their normal perpendicular course usually is lost. The differential diagnosis includes tetralogy of Fallot or transposition of the great vessels with a VSD. The distinction between these disorders is often difficult.

Associated Anomalies

Other cardiac malformations are always present with double-outlet right ventricle and multiple abnormalities frequently coexist. These may include ventricular septal defect, pulmonary or left ventricular outflow obstruction, and major atrioventricular valve abnormalities. Extracardiac anomalies that have been reported include tracheoesophageal fistula, facial cleft, and chromosome abnormalities.[84]

Prognosis

The prognosis for double-outlet right ventricle varies with the presence of associated abnormalities.[65] In a surgical series of 46 patients with double-outlet right ventricle, 12 had subpulmonic ventricular septal defect, and 5 had additional abnormalities (4 of these died).[65] The prognosis would be expected to be significantly worse in prenatal series.

Truncus Arteriosus

Clinical and Pathologic Findings

Truncus arteriosus is characterized by a single arterial vessel (truncus) arising from the heart, which sup-

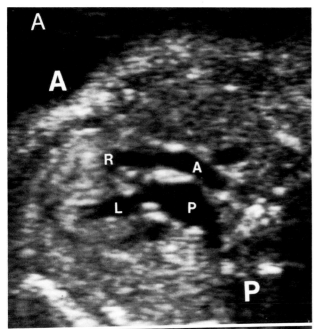

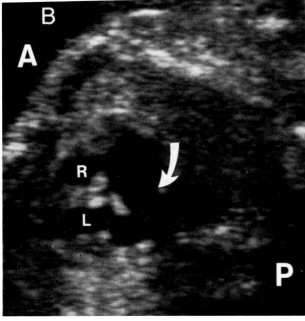

FIG 9–32.
Transposition of the great vessels and atrioventricular septal defect. **A,** coronal view shows parallel course of aorta *(A)* and pulmonary artery *(P)*, rather than the normal perpendicular course. *R* = right ventricle; *L* = left ventricle; *A* = anterior; *P* = posterior. **B,** four-chamber view shows atrial septal defect *(curved arrow)*. Alobar holoprosencephaly was also identified and chromosome analysis yielded trisomy 13. *R* = right ventricle; *L* = left ventricle; *A* = anterior; *P* = posterior. (Courtesy of John McGahan, MD, Radiology Department, University of California, Sacramento, CA.)

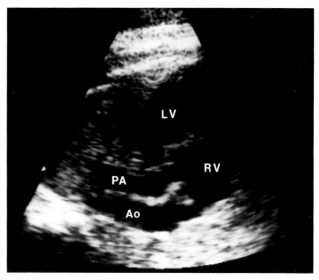

FIG 9–33.
Double-outlet right ventricle. Scan at 27 weeks shows both the aorta *(Ao)* and the pulmonary artery *(PA)* arising in parallel from the right ventricle *(RV)*. *LV* = left ventricle. (From Brown DL, Emerson DS, Cartier MS, et al: Congenital cardiac anomalies: Prenatal sonographic diagnosis. AJR 1989; 153:109–116. Used by permission.)

plies the coronary, pulmonary, and systemic arterial circulations.[96] Four types of truncus arteriosus are recognized with types I and II being the most common:[54]

1. Type I, a pulmonary trunk arises from the truncus.
2. Type II, two pulmonary arteries arise from the posterior aspect of the truncus.
3. Type III, two pulmonary arteries arise from the lateral aspects of the truncus.
4. Type IV, the pulmonary arteries are absent, and the pulmonary circulation is supplied by systemic collateral arteries arising from the descending aorta.

Sonographic Findings

Truncus arteriosus can be identified as a single trunk arising from the heart (Figs 9–35 and 9–36).[40, 59] The right ventricular outflow tract is absent. The pulmonary branches may be difficult to visualize, but demonstration of their origin from the arterial trunk is diagnostic and helps distinguish truncus arteriosus from pulmonary atresia and tetralogy of Fallot.

Associated Anomalies

Truncus arteriosus is frequently associated with other cardiac lesions including ventricular septal defect, atrioventricular septal defect, abnormalities of the semilunar valves, and abnormal number of pulmonary

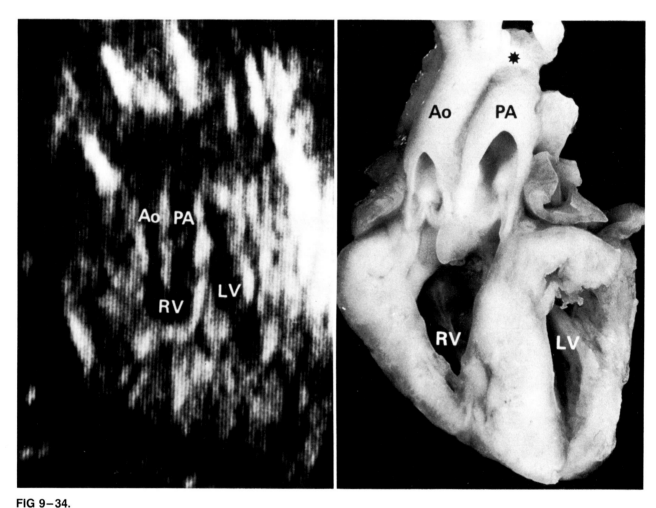

FIG 9–34.
Double-outlet right ventricle. **A,** longitudinal view shows both the aorta *(Ao)* and pulmonary artery *(PA)* arising from the right ventricle *(RV)*. *LV* = left ventricle. **B,** photograph of pathologic specimen confirms origin of both great vessels from the right ventricle *(RV)*. The outflow into the aorta *(Ao)* is narrow, and the ascending aorta slightly underdeveloped. Aortic hypoplasia *(asterisk)* is also noted at the aortic arch. *LV* = left ventricle; *PA* = pulmonary artery. (From Stewart PA, Wladimiroff JW, Becker AE: Early prenatal detection of double-outlet right ventricle by echocardiography. Br Heart J 1985; 54:340–342. Used by permission.)

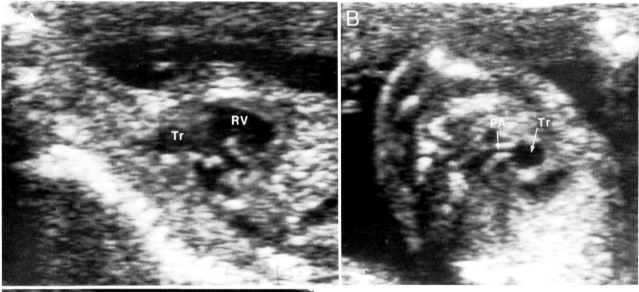

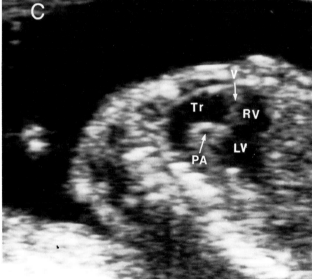

FIG 9–35.
Truncus arteriosus. **A,** longitudinal view demonstrates a single large arterial trunk *(Tr)* arising from the right ventricle *(RV)*. **B,** slightly different view demonstrates a large ventricular septal defect with communication of the right ventricle *(RV)* and left ventricle *(LV)*. The large trunk *(Tr)* arises from the ventricles without an intervening right ventricular outflow tract. Note tiny pulmonary artery *(PA)* and absence of outflow tract. *RV* = right ventricle; *V* = truncus valve. **C,** short axis demonstrates that the small pulmonary artery *(PA)* arises from the main arterial trunk *(Tr)*. Truncus arteriosus can be differentiated from tetralogy of Fallot by absence of right ventricular outflow tract and by origin of the pulmonary artery from the truncus. (Courtesy of Dale R Cyr, RDMS, and Laurence A Mack, MD, Department of Radiology, University of Washington Hospital, Seattle, WA.)

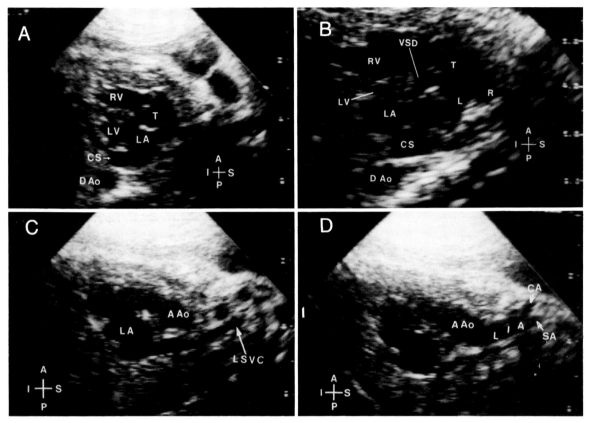

FIG 9–36.
Truncus arteriosus. **A,** longitudinal view shows large arterial trunk *(T)* arising from both the right ventricle *(RV)* and left ventricle *(LV)* and overriding a ventricular septal defect *(VSD)*. Also noted is an enlarged coronary sinus just behind the left atrium *(LA)*. *DAo* = descending aorta; *A* = anterior; *P* = posterior; *I* = inferior; *S* = superior. **B,** left *(L)* and right *(R)* branches of pulmonary artery are identified arising from the larger arterial trunk *(T)*. A VSD is noted between the right ventricle *(RV)* and left ventricle *(LV)*. *LA* = left atrium; *CS* = coronary sinus; *DAo* = descending aorta. **C,** sagittal view left superior vena cava *(LSVC)* is identified draining into the left atrium *(LA)* via the coronary sinus. *AAo* = ascending aorta arising from trunk. **D,** view just to right of Figure **C** shows the length of ascending aorta *(Ao)*, left innominate artery *(LIA)* and their division into left carotid artery *(CA)*, and left subclavian artery *(SA)*. This configuration on the fetal left indicates the presence of right-sided aortic arch. (From De Araujo J, Schmidt KG, Silverman NH, et al: Prenatal detection of truncus arteriosus by ultrasound. Pediatr Cardiol 1987; 8:261–263. Used by permission.)

veins.[54, 96] The truncal valve is often dysplastic, which may result in fetal hydrops.

Extracardiac anomalies that may be associated with truncus ateriosus include genitourinary anomalies, situs inversus, and asplenia syndromes.[54] Only 1 of 22 infants with truncus arteriosus had a chromosome abnormality[5] although trisomy 13 was found in a case detected prenatally.[59]

Prognosis

The prognosis for fetuses or infants with truncus arteriosus is generally poor. However, early surgical correction (< 6 months) helps avoid problems related to pulmonary hypertension and has resulted in a significantly improved outcome compared to infants corrected after 18 months. Ebert et al. reported a 19% overall mortality rate (including six infants who died prior to

surgery) for 106 infants who underwent physiologic correction of the defect before 6 months of age.[63] Eight of 11 infants who died following surgery had truncal valve insufficiency, indicating that this problem is associated with a significantly worse prognosis than infants without truncal valve insufficiency.

Pulmonic Stenosis

Clinical and Pathologic Findings

Pulmonic stenosis results from either stenosis of the pulmonic valves or narrowing of the infundibular outflow tract.

Sonographic Findings

Sonographic detection of pulmonic stenosis is difficult on cross-sectional sonography alone. The pulmonary artery may be enlarged from poststenotic dilatation, and the right ventricle may show hypertrophied walls. Right atrial enlargement may occur from tricuspid regurgitation. Careful evaluation may demonstrate thickening of the pulmonic valve, with incomplete opening during systole.

Duplex Doppler offers the hope of improved prenatal diagnosis of valvular stenoses and regurgitation. Color-flow Doppler may also be useful by demonstrating poststenotic turbulent flow.

Associated Anomalies

Other cardiac lesions that may be associated with pulmonic stenosis include atrial septal defect, ventricular septal defect, total anomalous pulmonary venous return, and aortic stenosis.

The risk of an associated chromosome abnormality appears to be low; only one abnormal karyotype was reported among 105 cases of pulmonic stenosis.[5]

Prognosis

The prognosis of pulmonic stenosis depends on the severity of stenosis and the presence of additional anomalies. In general, a good outcome can be expected following surgical repair of the defect.

Aortic Stenosis

Clinical and Pathologic Findings

Congenital obstruction of the aorta or aortic outflow tract may be divided into three types: valvular, subvalvular, or supravalvular. Valvular aortic stenosis may be due to dysplasia, thickened valves, or fused aortic cusps and may be associated with a bifid aortic valve. A male predominance has been observed for valvular aortic stenosis. Subvalvular aortic stenosis includes inherited disorders (autosomal dominant) of asymmetric septal hypertrophy and idiopathic hypertrophic subaortic stenosis. Supravalvular stenosis includes (1) isolated types, (2) an association with peripheral pulmonary arterial stenosis and a familial tendency, and (3) an association with Williams syndrome.

Sonographic Findings

Like pulmonic stenosis, aortic stenosis is difficult to recognize prenatally with cross-sectional sonography alone. The aortic valve may appear thickened, but this is difficult to demonstrate. The aorta may be small in supravalvular aortic stenosis or large in valvular stenosis, with poststenotic dilatation. Severe stenosis may lead to myocardial dysfunction and ventricular enlargement. Endocardial fibroelastosis secondary to aortic valvular stenosis has been demonstrated prenatally.[38]

Duplex Doppler may prove to be helpful in diagnosing aortic stenosis by demonstrating accelerated flow and turbulence at or distal to the obstruction.

Associated Anomalies

Valvular aortic stenosis and valvular dysplasia are known to be associated with chromosome abnormalities; three of 49 infants with aortic stenosis had an abnormal karyotype.[5]

Subvalvular aortic stenosis may be associated with various inheritable disorders, including asymmetric septal hypertrophy and idiopathic hypertrophic subaortic stenosis; these are usually transmitted in an autosomal dominant pattern. Subvalvular aortic stenosis may also result from hypertrophic cardiomyopathy associated with maternal diabetes.

Supravalvular aortic stenosis is known to be associated with Williams syndrome whose other features include hypercalcemia, peripheral pulmonary stenosis, elfin facies, psychomotor and growth retardation, dental anomalies, and inguinal hernia.[68]

Prognosis

Aortic stenosis has a good prognosis in the absence of other significant anomalies. Newborns who present with congestive heart failure have experienced a high operative mortality rate, but rates as low as 9% recently have been reported.[78]

Interruption of the Aortic Arch/Coarctation

Clinical and Pathologic Findings

Coarctation of the aorta can be a simple shelf region at the distal end of the arch or severe hypoplasia of the arch. Complete interruption of the aortic arch may also occur.

Sonographic Findings

Direct visualization of the aortic arch appears to be relatively insensitive for detection of aortic coarctation. In a prenatal series of aortic arch abnormalities, Machado et al. failed to demonstrate a discrete coarctation "shelf" in any case, although hypoplasia was seen in eight cases and interruption was seen in two cases.

Recently, enlargement of the right ventricle and pulmonary artery relative to the left ventricle and aorta has been recognized as a possible clue to the diagnosis of aortic arch anomalies (Fig 9–37).[39, 44, 49] Among 24 fetuses with dilatation of the right ventricle and pulmonary artery reported by Allan et al., 18 proved to have coarctation or interruption of the aorta (see Fig 9–23), with the earliest age of diagnosis at 18 weeks.[39]

Doppler evaluation may be a useful adjunct in the

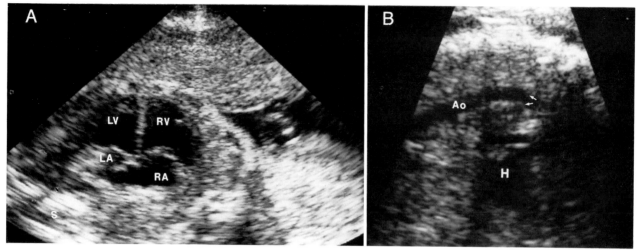

FIG 9–37.
Coarctation of the aorta. **A,** transverse scan at 25 weeks demonstrates slight decrease in the size of the left ventricle *(LV)* compared to the right ventricle *(RV)*. This is a non–specific finding, but is suggestive of aortic coarctation. *RA* = right atrium, *LA* = left atrium; *S* = spine. **B,** longitudinal view of the aortic arch suggests narrowing in the isthmic region *(arrows)*. The actual narrowing from coarctation is usually difficult to image. *Ao* = descending aorta; *H* = heart. (From Brown DL, Emerson DS, Cartier MS, et al: Congenital cardiac anomalies: Prenatal sonographic diagnosis. AJR 1989; 153:109–116. Used by permission.)

detection of aortic coarctation/interruption by demonstrating greater than 2 to 1 flow across the tricuspid valve relative to the mitral valve (upper normal, 1.8 to 1).[17]

Associated Anomalies

Additional cardiac anomalies are present in the vast majority of fetuses with aortic coarctation or interruption. These include aortic stenosis, bicuspid aortic valve (25%–50%) ventricular septal defect, atrioventricular septal defects, transposition of the great arteries, double-outlet right ventricle, and truncus arteriosus. Extracardiac anomalies that may be associated with aortic coarctation include diaphragmatic hernia, Di George syndrome, and chromosome abnormalities, especially Turner's syndrome (45,X).[5, 44] A chromosome abnormality was found in 10 of 101 infants (10%) with aortic coarctation.[5]

Prognosis

The outlook for successful surgery in aortic coarctation depends on its severity and the presence of associated anomalies.

Total Anomalous Pulmonary Venous Return

Clinical and Pathologic Findings

Total anomalous pulmonary venous return (TAPVR) is characterized by an abnormal venous-atrial connection resulting from failure of the intrapulmonary veins to connect with the left side of the primitive atrium during embryologic development. As a result,

the pulmonary veins may unite with one of a number of other venous channels. TAPVR may be subcategorized by the site of anomalous drainage as:

1. Above the diaphragm into the coronary sinus, superior vena cava, persistent left superior vena cava, or directly into the right atrium.
2. Below the diphragm into the inferior vena cava or the portal veins.

The anomalous veins may be obstructed, especially when they drain below the diaphragm.

Sonographic Findings

Sonographic identification of TAPVR is difficult. Only one case has been correctly identified prenatally.[57, 60] The prenatal features of TAPVR include right ventricular dilatation and failure to identify the normal insertion of the pulmonary veins into the left atrium. The left atrium also is usually smaller than normal.

Associated Anomalies

TAPVR is associated with a variety of other cardiac and extracardiac anomalies, including atrioventricular septal defect, situs ambiguous, asplenia, and polysplenia.

Prognosis

The prognosis for TAPVR varies with the presence of additional anomalies. In general, other cardiac lesions usually are absent, and an excellent prognosis can be expected following early surgical correction. Hammon reported that the immediate postoperative survival rate was 80% in 25 infants.[69] The single most important risk factor associated with a higher perioperative mortality was the presence of pulmonary venous obstruction.[69]

Cardiomyopathy and Endocardial Fibroelastosis

Clinical and Pathologic Findings

Cardiomyopathies represent a heterogeneous group of disorders expressed as severe myocardial dysfunction. Causes of cardiomyopathy include congenital heart defects, myocardial ischemia, myocarditis, infectious agents, glycogen storage diseases, and familial causes.

Endocardial fibroelastosis is characterized by grossly thickened endocardium and subendocardium, with an increase in collagen and elastin fibers. Two types are recognized: primary and secondary. Primary endocardial fibroelastosis is a type of cardiomyopathy resulting in gross cardiac hypertrophy. Most cases are sporadic, but some are familial. Secondary endocardial fibroelastosis may result from certain types of CHD which cause increased turbulence, such as aortic stenosis with aortic insufficiency or aortic atresia with mitral stenosis and intact ventricular septum.[38, 85]

Sonographic Findings

Cardiomyopathy demonstrates an enlarged heart with poor contractility of the myocardium. Endocardial fibroelastosis typically demonstrates an abnormally echogenic endocardium. This appearance should be distinguished from an echogenic pericardium, which could result from pericarditis (Fig 9–38).

Associated Anomalies

Associated anomalies of cardiomyopathy or endocardial fibroelastosis depend on the underlying cause.

Prognosis

The prognosis varies with the underlying primary disorder. Prenatal detection would be expected to carry a poor prognosis. All five cases of cardiomyopathy or endocardial fibroelastosis reported by Crawford et al. resulted in fetal death.[57]

FETAL ARRHYTHMIAS

Fetal arrhythmias frequently are observed with increasing use of fetal monitoring and prenatal ultrasonography. Characterization of fetal rhythm distur-

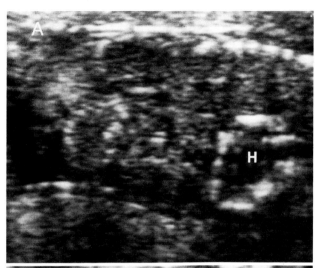

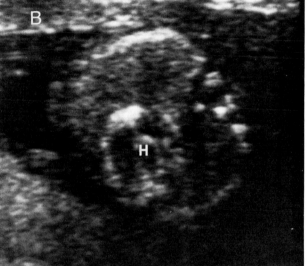

FIG 9–38.
Pericarditis? Longitudinal **(A)** and transaxial **(B)** views of the heart at 16 weeks demonstrates markedly echogenic outline of heart *(H)*. This was initially thought to represent endocardial fibroelastosis, but follow-up scan suggested it arose from the pericardium. This finding completely reverted to normal on serial examinations. A healthy infant was delivered without apparent cardiac abnormalities. This unusual, transient sonographic finding was thought perhaps to reflect pericarditis in utero.

bances requires use of M-mode echocardiography and/ or pulsed Doppler ultrasound. It is also important to exclude an underlying structural defect that may be associated with some arrhythmias. For these reasons, evaluation of fetal arrhythmias is one of the more common reasons for referral for a targeted fetal echocardiogram.

In simple terms, arrhythmias can be categorized as an abnormally fast (tachycardia), slow (bradycardia), or irregular rhythm. The normal heart rate at 20 weeks' gestation is 140 ($\pm$ 20) beats per minute (bpm), falling to 130 ($\pm$ 20) bpm near term.[117] A rate greater than

180 is generally considered tachycardia, and a rate less than 100 is considered bradycardia.[105, 116]

Tachycardia

Clinical and Pathologic Findings

Tachycardia may originate from a site within the ventricle or above the ventricle (sinoatrial node, atrium, or atrioventricular node). Supraventricular tachycardias are much more common and include paroxysmal supraventricular tachycardia (commonly referred to as supraventricular tachycardia), atrial flutter, and atrial fibrillation.

Sonographic Findings

Using M-mode or duplex Doppler, supraventricular tachycardia is characterized by an atrial rate of 180–300 beats per minute (bpm); atrial flutter by an atrial rate of 300–400 bpm; and atrial fibrillation by a rate of 400 to 700 bpm (Fig 9–39). Variable degrees of atrioventricular block result in a ventricular rate ranging from 60–200 bpm.

Fetal hydrops may be the initial manifestation of supraventricular tachyarrhythmia in utero. This may be due to ineffective atrial contraction, which appears to

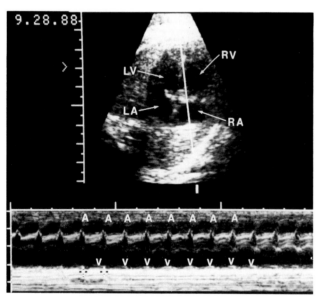

FIG 9–39.
Supraventricular tachycardia. Simultaneous real-time four-chamber view and M-mode tracing (solid line indicates direction of M-mode) through the right ventricle *(RV)*, tricuspid valve, and right atrium *(RA)* in a 36-week fetus with supraventricular tachycardia (heart rate, 300 bpm). There is one-to-one concordance of atria contractions *(A)* and ventricular contractions *(V)*. Rhythm converted to normal with maternal digoxin therapy. *LV* = left ventricle; *LA* = left atrium.

be more important for ventricular filling in utero than after birth, and the rapid ventricular rate.

Associated Abnormalities

Cardiac anomalies are not typically associated with supraventricular tachycardias. However, a possible association has been noted between supraventricular arrhythmias, including supraventricular tachycardia or atrial flutter, and redundancy or aneurysm of the foramen ovale.[107, 120, 121] Stewart and Wladimiroff showed evidence of an atrial septal aneurysm bulging into the left atrium in eight of 148 fetuses investigated for fetal arrhythmia.[121] All eight showed some form of atrial arrhythmia, including three with atrial flutter and two with supraventricular tachycardia. Some of the atrial aneurysms are restrictive and may result in fetal hydrops. Supraventricular tachycardia has also been associated with Ebstein's anomaly.[101]

Some types of supraventricular tachycardia are associated with Wolff-Parkinson-White syndrome. In this disorder, a reentry rhythm is established by an anomalous atrioventricular connection through the bundle of Kent. Tachyarrhythmias have also been associated with cardiac tumors.[72, 108]

Prognosis

The prognosis varies with the presence or absence of fetal hydrops. Development of fetal hydrops carries a poor prognosis and is more difficult to treat in utero. In a series of 21 fetuses treated in utero (16 with supraventricular tachycardia, three with atrial flutter, and two with atrial fibrillation), deaths occurred in two cases (10%), both with atrial flutter.[111]

Treatment

A number of publications have described pharmacologic treatment of supraventricular tachycardia using maternally administered antiarrhythmic drugs. Treatment of tachyarrhythmia is recommended to avoid complications of fetal hydrops. Also, successful conversion of the arrhythmia is easier if treated before the development of hydrops.

Digoxin is the initial drug of choice for treatment of supraventricular tachycardia.[111] Other agents that have been tried with varying degrees of success include propranolol,[110] procainamide,[72] verapamil,[105] quinidine,[110, 117] and flecainide (Table 9–10).[114] Kleinman and associates reported that 15 of 16 fetuses with supraventricular tachycardia were successfully converted to sinus rhythm using pharmacologic therapy.[111] Six patients responded to digoxin alone, one to combined digoxin and propranolol, and eight to a combination of digoxin and verapamil.[111]

TABLE 9–10.
Antiarrhythmic Therapy*

	Digoxin	Verapamil	Propranolol	Procainamide
Loading				
PO	1.0–2.5 mg			
IV	0.5–2.0 mg	5.0–10.0 mg	0.5 mg q 5 min	12 mg/kg
Maintenance				
PO	0.25–0.75 mg/day	80–120 mg q 6–8 hrs	20–160 mg q 6–8 hrs	6 mg/kg q 4 hrs
IV	0.25 mg			
Protein bound	20%	90%	90%–95%	15%
Eliminating organ	Kidney	Liver	Liver	Kidney
Transplacental passage (cord/maternal serum level)	0.8–1.0	0.3–0.4	0.1–0.3	0.8–1.3
Therapeutic plasma concentration	0.5–2.0 ng/ml	50–100 ng/ml	50–1000 ng/ml	4–14 mcg/ml
Comments	Level may increase when verapamil is added; fetus may tolerate (need?) higher level than adult	Extensive first pass metabolism: may cause heart block; negative inotropic agent: DO NOT give with propranolol	Extensive first pass metabolism; DO NOT give with verapamil; fetal bradycardia, hypoglycemia, growth retardation; maternal bronchospasm can occur	Active metabolite, Nacetyl procainamide (NAPA); may accumulate in fetus or neonate; in atrial fib/flutter should treat first with digoxin or verapamil

*From Kleinman CS, Lopel JA, Weinstein EM, et al: Semin Perinatol 1985; 9:113–129. Used by permission.

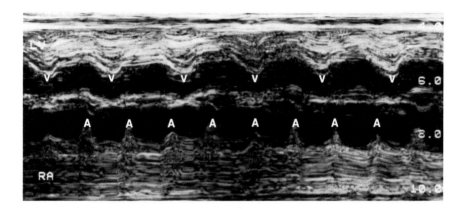

FIG 9–40.
Complete heart block. M-mode tracing through the right ventricle and right atrium in a woman with systemic lupus erythematosus demonstrates complete dissociation of atrial rate (150 bpm) and ventricular rate (70 bpm). *A* = atrial contractions; *V* = ventricular contractions.

Bradycardia

Clinical and Pathologic Findings

Transient bradycardia is commonly observed during the course of routine obstetric scanning. This may be induced by the act of scanning itself from manual compression of the fetus [131] This response presumably represents a vasovagal reaction. Therefore, fetal bradycardia is important only if it is sustained.[105]

Complete heart block is the most important cause of sustained fetal bradycardia. In one prenatal series, ten of 12 fetuses with persistent bradycardia had complete heart block.[109]

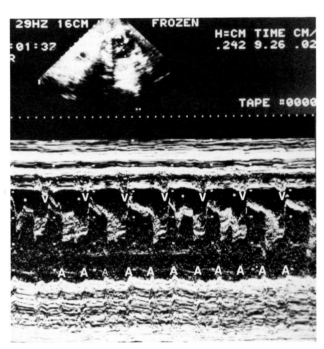

FIG 9–41.
Complete heart block and atrioventricular septal defect. Simultaneous real time and M-mode tracing through the right ventricle, atrioventricular valve, and right atrium in a fetus referred for bradycardia shows dissociation between atrial contractions (A), occurring at 100 bpm, and the ventricular contractions (V), occurring at 55 bpm. A large atrioventricular septal defect was also identified and polysplenia syndrome was found at autopsy. The combination of atrioventricular septal defect and complete heart block is strongly associated with left atrial isomerism and the polysplenia syndrome.

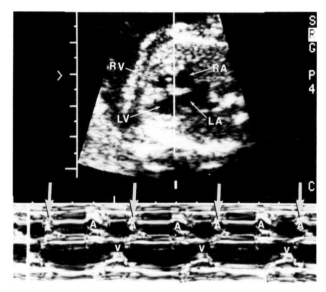

FIG 9–42.
Group beating (atrial bigeminal rhythm) causing bradycardia. Simultaneous real-time and M-mode tracing through the tricuspid valve, interventricular septum, and left ventricle *(solid line)* indicates direction of M-mode) in a fetus at 19 weeks with bradycardia. Atrial contractions *(A)* are indicated by opening of tricuspid valve, with alternative atrial contractions *(arrows)* not conducted to the ventricles (*V* = ventricular contractions), resulting in an atrial rate of 150 bpm and ventricular rate of 75 bpm. This rhythm may be secondary to premature atrial contractions with non–conduction to the ventricles or to atrioventricular block of the Wenckebach type. *RV* = right ventricle; *LV* = left ventricle; *RA* = right atrium; *LA* = left atrium.

Sonographic Findings

Complete heart block is diagnosed as independent atrial and ventricular rates on M-mode echocardiography (Figs 9–40 and 9–41). The atrial rate is typically 120–140 bpm, while the ventricular rate is 40–60 bpm. Complete heart block should be distinguished from sinus bradycardia, which can occur as a sign of fetal distress.

Other causes of bradycardia include frequent non–conducted premature atrial or junctional contractions or incomplete heart block of the Wenckebach type (Fig 9–42).

Associated Anomalies

In approximately 50% of cases, complete heart block is accompanied by one or more structural abnormalities such as atrioventricular septal defect, corrected transposition, cardiac tumors, and cardiomyopathies. Complete heart block in combination with atrioventricular septal defect is strongly suggestive of atrial levoisomerism and the polysplenia syndromes (see Fig 9–41).[56, 60, 74] The remaining fetuses are frequently associated with maternal collagen vascular disease, most commonly systemic lupus erythematosus (see Fig 9–41).[115] In these patients, circulating antinuclear antibodies of the SSA or SSB types appear to damage the developing conduction tissue.[115] Anti-SSA antibodies are found in the great majority of mothers who have delivered infants with congenital heart block, even though the maternal disorder may not be clinically evident. Occasionally, fetal bradycardia and heart block may also be associated with cardiac tumors.

Prognosis

The prognosis for bradycardia depends on the presence of associated anomalies and fetal hydrops. The prognosis is very poor when a cardiac defect is present, whereas the prognosis in isolated complete heart block is good if antenatal management and delivery are carefully monitored. In one series of eight fetuses with bradycardia, two presented with hydrops and both died.[119]

Irregular Rhythms

Clinical and Pathologic Findings

Irregular arrhythmias are usually due to escape (ectopic) beats of atrial or ventricular origin (Fig 9–43). These are commonly observed to some degree in most fetuses during the third trimester. While most fetuses have only occasional ectopic beats that are not detected, some fetuses have frequent beats that pro-

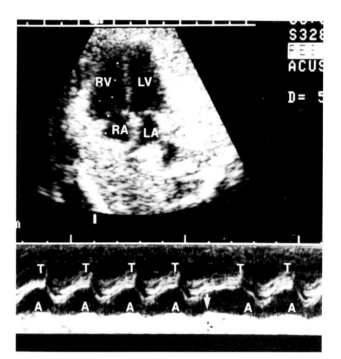

FIG 9–43.
Premature atrial contraction. Simultaneous real-time four-chamber view and M-mode tracing through right ventricle *(RV)*, tricuspid valve, and right atrium (dotted line indicates direction of M-mode) demonstrates a premature atrial contraction *(arrow)* that is not conducted to the tricuspid valve or ventricle. The compensatory pause between openings of the tricuspid valve *(V)* is incomplete; a complete pause would last twice as long as the atrial interval. *LV* = left ventricle; *RA* = right atrium; *LA* = left atrium.

duce an obvious arrhythmia (see Fig 9–39). The great majority of irregular beats originate from the atria.

Sonographic Findings

By directing M-mode ultrasound simultaneously through an atrial and ventricular chamber, it can be determined whether the premature beat is atrial or ventricular in origin and, if atrial, whether the beat is conducted to the ventricle.

Associated Anomalies

No significant anomalies have been associated with premature atrial or ventricular contractions. An increased number of premature contractions may be induced by maternal use of caffeine, cigarettes, or alcohol.

Prognosis

Isolated premature atrial or ventricular contractions are rarely associated with morbidity or mortality, and no treatment is necessary. Rarely, isolated premature atrial contractions will develop sustained paroxysmal tachycardia.[116]

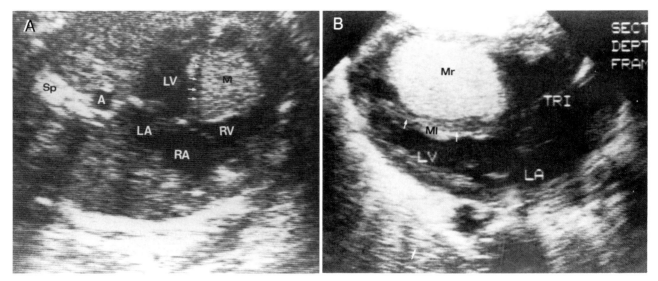

FIG 9–44.
Rhabdomyoma. **A,** transverse scan at 37 weeks shows echogenic mass (*M*) in right ventricle (*RV*). A smaller mass is suggested in the left ventricle (*LV*). *Arrows* = interventricular septum; *LA* = left atrium; *RA* = right atrium; *A* = aorta; *Sp* = spine. **B,** postnatal scan confirms large mass in right ventricle (*Mr*) and smaller mass in left ventricle (*MI*). *LV* = left ventricle; *LA* = left atrium; *TRI* = tricuspid valve. (From Schaffer RM, Cabbad M, Minkoff H, et al: Sonographic diagnosis of fetal cardiac rhabdomyoma. J Ultrasound Med 1986; 5:531–533. Used by permission.)

TUMORS

Clinical and Pathologic Findings

Congenital cardiac tumors are rare. The most common cardiac tumor in infancy is the cardiac rhabdomyoma which typically arises from the interventricular septum.[132] The vast majority of cases are associated with tuberous sclerosis.[124] Other types of cardiac tumors include fibroma, mesothelioma, hemangioma, and teratoma. Intrapericardial teratomas are usually benign, pedunculated tumors with attachment to the aortic root or pulmonary vessels.

Sonographic Findings

A variety of cardiac tumors have been described on prenatal sonography including rhabdomyomas, angiomas, and teratomas.[72, 123–128, 131, 133–137] A rhabdomyoma appears as a solid, echogenic mass located within the heart (Fig 9–44). Multiple tumors may be identified.[127] The earliest prenatal diagnosis of a rhabdomyoma was reported by Crawford et al. at 22 menstrual weeks in a family with known tuberous sclerosis and a 50% risk for recurrence.[124] An earlier examination at 18 weeks reportedly was normal in this case.

Intrapericardial teratoma is the second most common cardiac tumor reported prenatally; at least 3 cases of intrapericardial teratoma have been reported to date.[125, 126, 135] Cyr et al. reported one case at 26 weeks in association with a large pericardial effusion (Fig 9–45).[125] The mass appeared to be separate from

both the lung and myocardium, permitting the correct diagnosis. Marked growth of the mass led to fetal hydrops 3 weeks later, and death occurred following induced vaginal delivery.

The differential diagnosis for an intrathoracic mass includes cystic adenomatoid malformation of the lung (CAML), bronchopulmonary sequestration, and bronchogenic cyst. However, these masses are extracardiac in location.

Associated Anomalies

As noted, a strong association has been observed between rhabdomyomas and tuberous sclerosis. Tuberous sclerosis is inherited as an autosomal dominant condition with variable penetrance. Typical clinical features include subependymal hamartomas with characteristic intracranial calcification, retinal hamartomas, characteristic skin lesions (adenoma sebaceum), renal tumors (primarily angiomyolipomas), seizures, and mental retardation. Two of 36 infants (6%) with rhabdomyomas reported by Fenoglio et al. had additional symptomatic congenital heart defects.[129]

Prognosis

Intracavitary cardiac tumors may produce obstruction of blood flow, congestive heart failure, and intrauterine death, whereas intramural tumors are unlikely to result in congestive heart failure.[129] Other complications include arrhythmia, pericardial effusion, and embolic phenomena.[72] In one of the largest reported au-

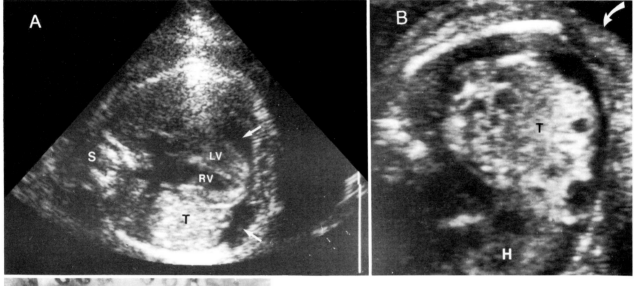

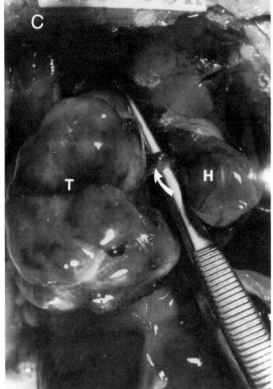

FIG 9–45.
Intrapericardial teratoma. **A,** transverse scan through the thorax at 26 weeks demonstrates a tumor *(T)* that appears to be outside the heart but within the pericardium. Pericardial effusion is identified *(arrows)*. *RV* = right ventricle; *LV* = left ventricle; S = spine. **B,** follow-up scan at 29 weeks shows increasing size of the mass *(T)* and onset of hydrops *(curved arrow)*. Ascites was also demonstrated. *H* = heart. **C,** postmortem photograph shows the teratoma *(T)* arising from the heart *(H)* by a pedicle *(arrow)*. (From Cyr DR, Guntheroth WG, Nyberg DA, et al: Prenatal diagnosis of an intrapericardial teratoma. A cause for non–immune hydrops. J Ultrasound Med 1988; 7:87–90. Used by permission.)

topsy series of cardiac rhabdomyomas (n=36), Fenoglio and associates observed that 78% infants died by 1 year of age, with the majority dying within the first few hours of life.[129]

SUMMARY

Cardiac defects detected prenatally are more severe and are more frequently associated with extracardiac anomalies than are cardiac defects that are first detected at birth. Fetal echocardiography is useful for detection of cardiac defects and for monitoring complications such as fetal hydrops. In addition to detection of structural defects, prenatal sonography can detect cardiomyopathies and cardiac tumors and characterize fetal arrhythmias. Routine evaluation of the fetal heart during "routine" obstetric sonography should significantly improve our ability to detect cardiac abnormalities in utero.

REFERENCES

Risk Factors and General Reference

1. Allan LD, Crawford DC, Chita SK, et al: Familial recurrence of congenital heart disease in a prospective series of mothers referred for fetal echocardiography. Am J Cardiol 1986; 58:334–337.
2. Boughman JA, Berg KA, Astemborski JA, et al: Familial risks of congenital heart defect assessed in a population-based epidemiologic study. Am J Med Genet 1987; 26:839–849.
3. Copel JA, Pilu G, Kleinman CS: Congenital heart disease and extracardiac anomalies: Associations and indications for fetal echocardiography. Am J Obstet Gynecol 1986; 154:1121–1132.
4. Evans PR: Cardiac anomalies in mongolism. Br Heart J 1950; 12:258–262.
5. Ferencz C, Rubin JD, McCarte RJ, et al: Cardiac and non–cardiac malformations: Observations in a population-based study. Teratology 1987; 35:367–378.
6. Greenwood RD, Rosenthall A, Parisi L, et al: Extracardiac abnormalities in infants with congenital heart disease. Pediatrics 1975; 55:485–492.
7. Hoffman JIE, Christianson R: Congenital heart disease in a cohort of 19,502 births with long-term followup. Am J Cardiol 1978; 42:641–647.
8. Mitchell SC, Korones SB, Berendes HW: Congenital heart disease in 56,109 births: Incidence and natural history. Circulation 1971; 43:323–332.
9. McKusick VA: Mendelian inheritance in man, in *Catalogs of Autosomal Dominant, Autosomal Recessive, and X-Linked Phenotypes,* ed 7. Baltimore, The Johns Hopkins Press, 1986.
10. Miller E, Hare JW, Cloherty JP, et al: Elevated maternal hemoglobin A1c in early pregnancy and major congenital anomalies in infants of diabetic mothers. N Engl J Med 1981; 304:1331–1334.
11. Nora JJ, Nora AH: The genetic contribution to congenital heart diseases, in Nora JJ, Takao A (eds): *Congenital Heart Disease: Causes and Processes.* Mt Kisco, New York, Futura, 1984, pp 3–13.
12. Rose V, Gold RJM, Lindsey G, et al: A possible increase in the incidence of congenital heart defects among the offspring of affected parents. JACC 1985; 6:376–382.
13. Rowe RD, Uchida IA: Cardiac malformations in mongolism. Am J Med 1961; 31:726–735.
14. Rowland TW, Hubbell JP Jr, Nadas AS: Congenital heart disease in infants of diabetic mothers. J Pediatr 1973; 83:815–820.
15. Sanchez-Cascos A. The recurrence risk in congenital heart disease. Eur J Cardiol 1978; 7:197–210.
16. Winter RM, Knowles SAS, Bieber FR, et al: *The Malformed Fetus and Stillbirth: A Diagnostic Approach.* John Wiley & Sons, New York, 1988.

Normal Anatomy and Sonographic Studies

17. Allan LD, Chita SK, Al-Ghazali W, et al: Doppler echocardiographic evaluation of the normal human fetal heart. Br Heart J 1987; 57:528–533.
18. Allan LD, Joseph MC, Boyd EGCA: M-mode echocardiography in the developing human fetus. Br Heart J 1982; 47:573–583.
19. Axel L. Real-time sonography of fetal cardiac anatomy. AJR 1983; 141:283–288.
20. Cartier MS, Davidoff A, Warneke LA, et al: The normal diameter of the fetal aorta and pulmonary artery: Echocardiographic evaluation in utero. AJR 1987; 149:1003–1007.
21. Comstock CH: Normal fetal heart axis and position. Obstet Gynecol 1987; 70:255–259.
22. Cyr DR, Guntheroth WG, Mack LA, et al: A systematic approach to fetal echocardiography using real-time/two-dimensional sonography. J Ultrasound Med 1986; 5:343–350.
23. DeVore GR: The prenatal diagnosis of congenital heart disease—A practical approach for the fetal sonographer. J Clin Ultrasound 1985; 13:229–245.
24. DeVore GR, Siassi B, Platt LD: Fetal echocardiography. IV: M-mode assessment of ventricular size and contractility during the second and third trimesters of pregnancy in the normal fetus. Am J Obstet Gynecol 1984; 150:981–988.
25. DeVore GR, Siassi B, Platt LD: M-mode echocardiography of the aortic root and aortic valve in second and third trimester normal human fetuses. Am J Obstet Gynecol 1985; 152:543–550.
26. Huhta JC, Strasburger JF, Carpenter RJ, et al: Pulsed Doppler fetal echocardiography. J Clin Ultrasound 1985; 13:247–254.
27. Jeanty P, Romero R, Cantraine F, et al: Fetal cardiac dimensions: A potential tool for the diagnosis of congenital heart defects. J Ultrasound Med 1984; 3:359–364.
28. Jordaan HVF: Cardiac size during prenatal development. Obstet Gynecol 1987; 69:854–858.
29. Kleinman CS, Santulli TV Jr: Ultrasonic evaluation of the fetal human heart. Semin Perinatol 1983; 7:90–101.
30. Lange LW, Sahn DJ, Allen HD, et al: Qualitative real-time cross-sectional echocardiographic imaging of the human fetus during the second half of pregnancy. Circulation 1980; 62:799–806.
31. Levy DW, Mintz MC: The left ventricular echogenic focus: A normal finding. AJR 1988; 150:85–86.
32. Perone N: A practical guide to fetal echocardiography. Contemp Ob Gyn 1988; 1:55–81.
33. Reed KL. Fetal and neonatal cardiac assessment with Doppler: Semin Perinatol 1987; 11:347–356.
34. Reed KL, Anderson CF, Shenker L: Fetal pulmonary artery and aorta: Two-dimensional Doppler echocardiography. Obstet Gynecol 1987; 69:175–178.
35. Reed KL, Meijboom EJ, Sahn DJ, et al: Cardiac Doppler

flow velocities in human fetuses. Circulation 1986; 73:41–46.

36. Sahn DJ, Lange LW, Allen HD, et al: Quantitative real-time cross-sectional echocardiography in the developing normal fetus and newborn. Circulation 1980; 62:588–597.

37. Schecter AG, Fakhry J, Shapiro LR, et al: In utero thickening of the chordae tendinae. J Ultrasound Med 1987; 6:691–695.

Structural Abnormalities/Cardiomyopathies

38. Achiron R, Malinger G, Zaidel L, et al: Prenatal sonographic diagnosis of endocardial fibroelastosis secondary to aortic stenosis. Prenat Diagn 1988; 8:73–77.

39. Allan LD, Chita SK, Anderson RH, et al. Coarctation of the aorta in prenatal life: An echocardiographic, anatomical, and functional study. Br Heart J 1988; 59:356–360.

40. Allan LD, Crawford DC, Anderson RH, et al: Echocardiographic and anatomic correlates in fetal congenital heart disease. Br Heart J 1984; 52:542–548.

41. Allan LD, Crawford DC, Anderson RH, et al: Spectrum of congenital heart disease detected echocardiographically in prenatal life. Br Heart J 1985; 54:523–526.

42. Allan LD, Crawford DC, Chita SK, et al: Prenatal screening for congenital heart disease. Br Med J 1986; 292:1717–1719.

43. Allan LD, Crawford DC, Sheridan, et al: Aetiology of non–immune hydrops: The value of echocardiography. Br J Obstet Gynecol 1986; 93:223–225.

44. Allan LD, Crawford DC, Tynan M: Evolution of coarctation of the aorta in intrauterine life. Br Heart J 1984; 52:471–473.

45. Allan LD, Tynan M, Campbell S, et al: Identification of congenital cardiac malformations by echocardiography in the midtrimester fetus. Br Heart J 1981; 46:358–362.

46. Allan LD, Tynan MJ, Campbell S, et al: Echocardiographic and anatomical correlates in the fetus. Br Heart J 1980; 44:444–451.

47. Allan LD: *Manual of Fetal Echocardiography.* Lancaster, England, MTP Press, 1986.

48. Becker AE, Anderson RH: *Pathology of Congenital Heart Disease.* London, Butterworth, 1981.

49. Benacerraf BR, Pober BR, Sanders SP: Accuracy of fetal echocardiography. Radiology 1987; 165:847–849.

50. Berger TJ, Blackstone EH, Kirklin JW, et al: Survival and probability of cure without and with operation in complete atrioventricular canal. Ann Thorac Surg 1979; 27:104–111.

51. Bovicelli L, Picchio FM, Pilu G, et al: Prenatal diagnosis of endocardial fibroelastosis. Prenat Diagn 1984; 4:67–72.

52. Chin AJ, Keane JF, Norwood WI, et al: Repair of complete common atrioventricular canal in infancy. J Thorac Cardiovasc Surg 1982; 84:437–445.

53. Chitayat D, Lao A, Wilson D, et al: Prenatal diagnosis of asplenia/polysplenia syndrome. Am J Obstet Gynecol 1988; 158:1085–1087.

54. Collett RW, Edwards JE: Persistent truncus arteriosus: A classification according to anatomic types. Surg Clin N Am 1949; 29:1245.

55. Copel JA, Pilu G, Green J, et al: Fetal echocardiographic screening for congenital heart disease: The importance of the four-chamber view. Am J Obstet Gynecol 1987; 157:648–655.

56. Crawford DC, Chapman MG, Allan LD: The evaluation of persistent bradycardia in prenatal life. Br J Obstet Gynecol 1985; 92:941–944.

57. Crawford DC, Chita SK, Allan LD: Prenatal detection of congenital heart disease: Factors affecting obstetric management and survival. Am J Obstet Gynecol 1988; 159:352–356.

58. Crawford DC, Drake DP, Kwaitkowski D, et al: Prenatal diagnosis of reversible cardiac hypoplasia associated with congenital diaphragmatic hernia: Implications for postnatal management. J Clin Ultrasound 1986; 14:718–721.

59. deArujo LML, Schmidt KG, Silverman NH: Prenatal detection of truncus arteriosus by ultrasound. Pediatr Cardiol 1987; 8:261–263.

60. deArujo LML, Silverman NH, Filly RA: Prenatal detection of left atrial isomerism by ultrasound. J Ultrasound Med 1987; 6:667–670.

61. DeVore GR, Sarti DA, Siassi B, et al: Prenatal diagnosis of cardiovascular malformations in the fetus with situs inversus invescerum during the second trimester of pregnancy. J Clin Ultrasound 1986; 14:454–457.

62. DeVore GR, Siassi B, Platt LD. Fetal echocardiography. VIII: Aortic root dilatation-A marker for tetralogy of Fallot. Am J Obstet Gynecol 1988; 159:129–136.

63. Ebert PA, Turley K, Stanger P, et al: Surgical treatment of truncus arteriosis in the first 6 months of life. Ann Surg 1984; 200:451–456.

64. Fontana RS, Edwards JE: *Congenital Cardiac Disease. A Review of 357 Cases Studied Pathologically.* Philadelphia, WB Saunders Co, 1962.

65. Franks R, Lincoln C: Surgical management of the double outlet right ventricle, in Anderson RH, MacCartney FL, Shinebourne EA, et al (eds): *Paediatric Cardiology,* vol 5. London, Churchill Livingstone, 1983, pp 441–450.

66. Fyler DC, Buckley LP, Hellenbrand WE, et al: Report of the New England Regional Infant Cardiac Program. Pediatrics 1980; 65:375–461.

67. Garcia OL, Mehta AV, Pickoff AS, et al: Left isoinversion and complete atrioventricular block: A report of 6 cases. Am J Cardiol 1981; 48:1103.

68. Gray SW, Skandalakis JE: *Embryology for Surgeons.* Philadelphia, WB Saunders Co, 1972, pp 741–793.

69. Hammon JW, Bender HW, Graham TP, et al: Total anomalous pulmonary venous connection in infancy. Ten years' experience including studies of postoperative ventricular function. J Thorac Cardiovasc Surg 1980; 80:544–551.

70. Hoffman JIE, Rudolph AM: The natural history of ventricular septal defects in infancy. Am J Cardiol 1965; 16:634–653.

71. Kirklin JW, Pacifico AD, Bargeron LM, Soto B: Cardiac repair in anatomically corrected malposition of the great arteries. Circulation 1973; 48:153–159.

72. Kleinman CS, Donnerstein RL, DeVore GR, et al: Fetal echocardiography for evaluation of in utero congestive heart failure. N Engl J Med 1982; 306:568–575.

73. Laks H, Milliken JC, Perloff JK, et al: Experience with the Fontan procedure: J Thorac Cardiovasc Surg 1984; 88:939–951.

74. Machado MVL, Crawford DC, Anderson RH, et al: Atrioventricular septal defect in prenatal life. Br Heart J 1988; 59:352–355.

75. Marasini M, Cordone M, Pongiglione G, et al. In utero ultrasound diagnosis of congenital heart disease. J Clin Ultrasound 1988; 16:103–107.

76. Matsuoka R, Misugi K, Goto A, et al: Congenital heart anomalies in the trisomy 18 syndrome, with reference to congenital polyvalvular disease. Am J Med Genet 1983; 14:657–668.

77. McKay R, Pacifico AD, Blackstone EH, et al: Septation of the univentricular heart with left anterior subaortic outlet chamber. J Thorac Cardiovasc Surg 1982; 84:77–87.

78. Messina LM, Turley K, Etanger P, et al: Successful aortic valvotomy for severe congenital valvular aortic stenosis in the newborn infant. J Thorac Cardiovasc Surg 1984; 88:92–96.

79. Miller JH, Nakib A, Anderson RC, et al: Congenital cardiac disease associated with polysplenia syndrome. A developmental complex of bilateral "left-sidedness." Circulation 1967; 36:789–799.

80. Moodie DS, Ritter DG, Tajik AH, et al: Long-term followup after palliative operation for univentricular heart. Am J Cardiol 1984; 53:1648–1651.

81. Norwood WI, Lang P, Hansen DD: Physiologic repair of aortic atresia-hypoplastic left heart syndrome. N Engl J Med 1983; 308:23–26.

82. Omeri MA, Bishop M, Aokley C, et al: The mitral valve in endocardial cushion defects. Br Heart J 1965; 27:161–176.

83. Rose V, Izukawa T, Moes CAF: Syndromes of asplenia and polysplenia. A review of cardiac and noncardiac malformations in 60 cases with special reference to diagnosis and prognosis. Br Heart J 1975; 37:840–852.

84. Rowe RD, Freedom RM, Mehrizi A, et al: *The Neonate With Congenital Heart Disease,* ed 2. Philadelphia, WB Saunders Co, 1981.

85. Sahn DJ, Shenker L, Reed KL, et al: Prenatal ultrasound diagnosis of hypoplastic heart syndrome in utero associated with hydrops fetalis. Am Heart J 1982; 104:1368–1372.

86. Samuel N, Sirotta L, Bar-Ziv J, et al: The ultrasonic appearance of common pulmonary vein atresia in utero. J Ultrasound Med 1988; 7:25–28.

87. Sandor GGS, Farquarson D, Wittman B, et al: Fetal echocardiography: Results in high-risk patients. Obstet Gynecol 1986; 67:358–364.

88. Scott DJ, Rigby ML, Miller GAH, et al: The presentation of symptomatic heart disease in infancy based on 10 years experience (1973–82). Implications for the provision of services. Br Heart J 1984; 52:248–257.

89. Shart M, Abinader EG, Shapiro I, et al: Prenatal echocardiographic diagnosis of Ebstein's anomaly with pulmonary atresia. Am J Obstet Gynecol 1983; 147:300–303.

90. Shenker L, Reed KL, Marx GR, et al: Fetal cardiac Doppler flow studies in prenatal diagnosis of heart disease. Am J Obstet Gynecol 1988; 158:1267–1273.

91. Shinebourne EA, MacCartney FJ, Anderson RH: Sequential chamber localization—logical approach to diagnosis in congenital heart disease. Br Heart J 1976; 38:327–340.

92. Silverman NH, Enderlein MA, Golbus MS: Ultrasonic recognition of aortic valve atresia in utero. Am J Cardiol 1984; 53:391–392.

93. Stewart PA, Wladimiroff JW, Becker AE: Early prenatal detection of double outlet right ventricle by echocardiography. Br Heart J 1985; 54:340–342.

94. Stewart PA, Buis-Liem T, Verney RA, et al: Prenatal ultrasonic diagnosis of familial asymmetric septal hypertrophy. Prenat Diagn 1986; 6:249–256.

95. Tynan MJ, Becker AE, MacCartney FJ, et al: Nomenclature and classification of congenital heart disease. Br Heart J 1979; 41:544–553.

96. VanPraagh R, VanPraagh S: The anatomy of common aorticopulmonary trunk (truncus arteriosus communis) and its embryologic implications: A study of 97 necropsy cases. Am J Cardiol 1965; 16:406–426.

97. VanPraagh R: The segmental approach to diagnosis in congenital heart disease. Birth Defects 1972; 8:4–23.

98. VanPraagh S, Antoniadis E, Otero-Coto RD, et al. Common atrioventricular canal with and without conotruncal malformations: An anatomical study of 251 postmortem cases, in Nora JJ, Takao A (eds): *Congenital Heart Disease: Causes and Processes,* New York, Futura, 1984, pp 636–637.

99. Veille JC, Sivakoff M: Fetal echocardiographic signs of congenital endocardial fibroelastosis. Obstet Gynecol 1988; 72:219–222.

100. Vogel M, Freedom RM, Smallhorn JF, et al: Complete transposition of the great arteries and coarctation of the aorta. Am J Cardiol 1984;53:1627–1632.

101. Westaby S, Karp RB, Kirklin JW, et al: Surgical treatment in Ebstein's malformation. Ann Thorac Surg 1982; 34:338–395.

102. Yagel S, Hochner-Celnikier D, Hurwitz A, et al: The significance and importance of prenatal diagnosis of fetal cardiac malformations by Doppler echocardiography. Am J Obstet Gynecol 1988; 158:272–277.

103. Yagel S, Mandelberg A, Hurwitz A, et al: Prenatal diagnosis of hypoplastic left ventricle. Am J Perinatol 1986; 3:6–8.

104. Yagel S, Sherer D, Hurwitz A: Significance of ultrasonic

prenatal diagnosis of ventricular septal defect. J Clin Ultrasound 1985; 13:588–590.

Arrhythmias

105. Allan LD, Anderson RH, Sullivan ID, et al: Evaluation of fetal arrhythmias by echocardiography. Br Heart J 1983; 50:240–245.
106. Allan LD, Crawford DC, Anderson RH: Evaluation and treatment of fetal arrhythmias. Clin Cardiol 1984; 7:467–473.
107. Buis-Liem TN, Ottenkamp J, Meerman RH, et al: The concurrence of fetal supraventricular tachycardia and obstruction of the foramen ovale. Prenat Diagn 1987; 7:425–431.
108. Cameron A, Nicholson S, Nimrod C, et al: Evaluation of fetal cardiac disrhythmias with two-dimensional, m-mode, and pulsed Doppler ultrasonography. Am J Obstet Gynecol 1988; 158:286–290.
109. Crawford D, Chapman M, Allan LD: The assessment of persistent bradycardia in prenatal life. Br J Obstet Gynecol 1985; 92:941–944.
110. Dumesic DA, Silverman NH, Tobias S, et al: Transplacental cardioversion of fetal supraventricular tachycardia with procainamide. N Engl J Med 1982; 307:1128.
111. Kleinman CS, Copel JA, Weinstein EM, et al: In utero diagnosis and treatment of supraventricular tachycardia. Semin Perinatol 1985; 9:113–129.
112. Kleinman CS, Hobbins JC, Jaffe CC, et al: Echocardiographic studies of the human fetus: Prenatal diagnosis of congenital heart disease and cardiac dysrhythmias. Pediatrics 1980; 65:1059.
113. Lingman G, Marsall K: Circulatory effects of fetal cardiac arrhythmias. Pediatr Cardiol 1986; 7:67–74.
114. Maxwell DJ, Crawford DC, Curry PVM, et al: Obstetric significance, diagnosis and management of fetal tachycardias. Br Med J 1988; 197:110–113.
115. McCue CM, Mantakas ME, Tinglestad JB, et al: Congenital heart block in newborns of mothers with connective tissue disease. Circulation 1977; 56:82–89.
116. Silverman NH, Enderlein MA, Stanger P, et al: Recognition of fetal arrhythmias by echocardiography. J Clin Ultrasound 1985; 13:255–263.
117. Southall DP, Richards J, Hardwick RA, et al: Prospective study of fetal heart rate and rhythm patterns. Arch Dis Child 1980; 55:506.
118. Spinnato JA, Shaver DC, Flinn GS, et al: Fetal supraventricular tachycardia: In utero therapy with digoxin and quinidine. J Am Coll Cardiol 1984; 64:730–735.
119. Steinfeld L, Rappaport HL, Rossbach HC, et al: Diagnosis of fetal arrhythmias using echocardiography and Doppler techniques. J Am Coll Cardiol 1986; 8:1425–1433.
120. Stewart PA, Tonge HM, Wladimiroff JW: Arrhythmia and structural abnormalities of the fetal heart. Br Heart J 1983; 50:550–554.
121. Stewart PA, Wladimiroff JW: Fetal atrial arrhythmias

associated with redundancy/aneurysm of the foramen ovale. J Clin Ultrasound 1988; 16:643–650.

Tumors

122. Banfield F, Dick M, Behrendt DM, et al: Intrapericardial teratoma: A new and treatable cause of hydrops fetalis. Am J Dis Child 1980; 134:1174–1175.
123. Boxer BA, Seidman S, Singh S, et al: Congenital intracardiac rhabdomyoma: Prenatal detection by echocardiography, perinatal management, and surgical treatment. Am J Perinatol 1986; 3:303–305.
124. Crawford DC, Garrett C, Tynan M, et al: Cardiac rhabdomyoma as a marker for the antenatal detection of tuberous sclerosis. J Med Genet 1983; 20:303–312.
125. Cyr DR, Guntheroth WG, Nyberg DA, et al: Prenatal diagnosis of an intrapericardial teratoma. A cause for nonimmune hydrops. J Ultrasound Med 1988; 7:87–90.
126. DeGeeter B, Kretz JG, Nisand I, et al: Intrapericardial teratoma in a newborn infant: Use of fetal echocardiography. Ann Thorac Surg 1983; 35:664–666.
127. Dennis MA, Apparetti K, Manco-Johnson ML, et al: The echocardiographic diagnosis of multiple fetal cardiac tumors. J Ultrasound Med 1985; 4:327–329.
128. DeVore GR, Hakim S, Kleinman CS, et al: The in utero diagnosis of an interventricular septal cardiac rhabdomyoma by means of real-time directed, m-mode echocardiography. Am J Obstet Gynecol 1982; 143:967–969.
129. Fenoglio JJ, McAllister HA, Ferrans VJ: Cardiac rhabdomyoma: A clinicopathologic and electron microscopic study. Am J Cardiol 1976; 38:241–251.
130. Journel H, Roussey M, Plais MH, et al: Prenatal diagnosis of familial tuberous sclerosis following detection of cardiac rhabdomyoma by ultrasound. Prenat Diagn 1986; 6:283–289.
131. Leithiser RE Jr, Fyfe D, Weatherby E III, et al: Prenatal sonographic diagnosis of atrial hemangioma. AJR 1986; 147:1207–1208.
132. Nadas AS, Ellison RC: Cardiac tumors in infancy. Am J Cardiol 1968; 21:363–366.
133. Platt LD, DeVore GR, Horenstein J, et al: Prenatal diagnosis of tuberous sclerosis: The use of fetal echocardiography. Prenat Diagn 1987; 7:407–411.
134. Platt LD, Geierman C, Turkel SB, et al: Atrial hemangioma and hydrops fetalis. Am J Obstet Gynecol 1987; 141:107–109.
135. Rasmussen SL, Hwang WS, Harder J, et al: Intrapericardial teratoma. J Ultrasound Med 1987; 6:159–162.
136. Riggs T, Sholl JS, Ilbawi M, et al: In utero diagnosis of pericardial tumor with successful surgical repair. Pediatr Cardiol 1984; 5:23–26.
137. Schaffer RM, Cabbad M, Minkoff H, et al: Sonographic diagnosis of fetal cardiac rhabdomyoma. J Ultrasound Med 1986; 5:531–533.

Intra-abdominal Abnormalities

David A. Nyberg, M.D.

Intra-abdominal anomalies present a particular challenge to the obstetric sonographer since they can arise from a variety of different organs and anatomic sites. Potential sites of intra-abdominal abnormalities include the urinary tract (kidneys, ureter, and bladder), adrenal glands, gastrointestinal tract (stomach, duodenum, jejunoileum, and colon), liver, spleen, gallbladder, pancreas, female reproductive tract (uterus and ovaries), and mesentery or peritoneal cavity.[10] Despite the diversity of causes of intra-abdominal abnormalities, a likely diagnosis or a limited differential diagnosis can usually be suggested after carefully considering the location and sonographic appearance of the abnormality. The length of this chapter and related chapters attests to the variety of intra-abdominal disorders that can now be identified sonographically.[2, 4, 6] Abnormalities of the urinary tract can usually be distinguished from other sites and are discussed separately in Chapter 12. Also discussed separately are related topics of fetal ascites (see Chapter 14), anterior abdominal wall defects (see Chapter 11), and diaphragmatic hernia (see Chapter 7).

As with other congenital malformations, correct interpretation of intra-abdominal anomalies depends on a thorough understanding of normal embryologic development and normal sonographic appearances. Following this discussion, major groups of abnormalities that will be discussed in the present chapter include:

1. Bowel abnormalities.
2. Non-bowel related cystic masses.
3. Intra-abdominal calcifications and meconium peritonitis.
4. Disorders of the liver, spleen, and biliary tract.

NORMAL EMBRYOLOGIC DEVELOPMENT AND FUNCTION

The primitive gut forms at the end of the fifth menstrual week (20 days post-fertilization), when the dorsal part of the yolk sac invaginates into the growing embryonic disc.[5] It can be considered as three parts (1) foregut, (2) midgut, and (3) hindgut, which are supplied by the celiac artery, superior mesenteric artery, and inferior mesenteric artery, respectively.[5] Derivatives of the foregut include the pharynx, respiratory tract, esophagus, stomach, proximal duodenum, liver, and pancreas; derivatives of the midgut include the small bowel and proximal large bowel; and derivatives of the hindgut include the distal colon, rectum, and portions of the vagina and urinary bladder.

Intestinal peristalsis begins by 11 menstrual weeks, and fetal swallowing begins shortly thereafter.[3] Radioisotope dilution techniques have estimated that the fetus swallows 2–7 ml per day at 16 weeks, 16 ml/day by 20 weeks, and 450 ml/day by term.[1, 9] Small bowel peristalsis propels the swallowed fluid to the large bowel where it is resorbed, leaving a residual of material called meconium. Meconium begins to accumulate in the bowel by 4–5 months and completely fills the colon by term. In this regard, the large bowel may be considered a natural reservoir for accumulating meconium. Shortly after birth, meconium normally is evacuated from the colon.

Simply stated, meconium may be considered a refuse of sloughed cells, lanugo hairs, mucoproteins, vernix caseosa, steroids, urea, and a sufficient amount of biliverdin to give it a green coloration.[3] However, it also contains a large portion of mucopolysaccharide

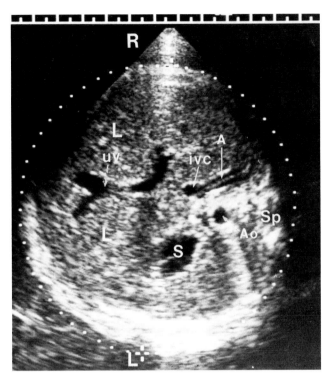

FIG 10–1.
Normal abdomen at 38 weeks. Transverse scan in a plane where abdominal circumference is measured demonstrates the liver *(L),* spleen *(Sp),* stomach *(S),* umbilical portion of the left portal vein *(uv),* and right adrenal *(A)* gland. Note that the liver comprises most of the upper abdomen. *Ao* = aorta; *ivc* = inferior vena cava; *Sp* = spine; *L* = left; *R* = right.

that probably originates from the gastrointestinal tract by active secretion. The function of meconium is a mystery that remains largely unsolved. Our current understanding is not much clearer than that of Aristotle, who thought that meconium (mekonium=poppy) had a role in keeping the fetus asleep until delivery.

NORMAL SONOGRAPHIC APPEARANCE

The sonographic appearance of the abdomen varies with menstrual age (Figs 10–1 and 10–2). At any age, however, the liver comprises most of the upper abdomen in the fetus (see Fig 10–1). Due to its greater supply of oxygenated blood in utero, the left lobe of the liver is larger than the right, a relationship that is reversed in the adult. The spleen is visualized on a transverse plane just posterior and to the left of the fetal stomach.

The gallbladder is normally visualized as an ovoid fluid-filled structure to the right and inferior to the intrahepatic portion of the umbilical vein. It can be mistaken for the umbilical vein unless the characteristic

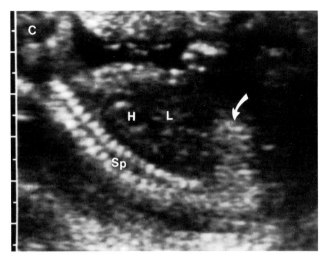

FIG 10–2.
Normal abdomen at 16 weeks. Longitudinal sonogram demonstrates ill-defined area of increased echogenicity representing normal bowel *(arrow)* in the abdominal cavity. Individual segments of bowel are not identified at this time. *L* = liver; *H* = heart; *Sp* = spine; *C* = cranium.

course of the umbilical vein or its intrahepatic branches are visualized.

By 11 menstrual weeks, the fetus is capable of swallowing sufficient amounts of amniotic fluid to permit sonographic visualization of the stomach.[9] By 16 weeks, the stomach should be demonstrated in nearly all normal fetuses. In a frequently quoted study of over 5,000 obstetrical ultrasound examinations, the stomach was identified in all but one case of esophageal atre-

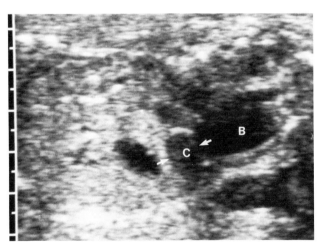

FIG 10–3.
Normal bowel. Longitudinal scan of fetal pelvis at 22 weeks demonstrates a loop of sigmoid colon *(C)* adjacent to the urinary bladder *(B).* The colon measures 7 mm in diameter *(arrows).* (From Nyberg DA, Mack LA, Patten RM, et al: Fetal bowel: Normal sonographic findings. J Ultrasound Med 1987; 6:3–6. Used by permission.)

NORMAL

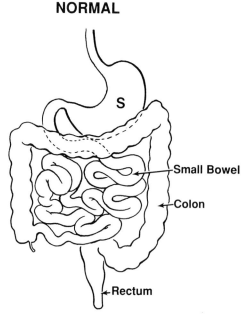

FIG 10–4.
Line drawing of normal bowel. The colon courses around the abdominal cavity and is significantly larger than the more central small bowel.

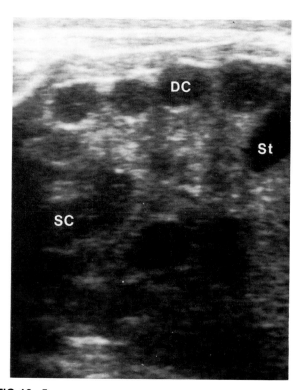

FIG 10–5.
Normal bowel. Longitudinal scan at 34 weeks demonstrates the descending colon *(DC)* parallel to the flank and the sigmoid colon *(SC)* in the pelvis. *ST* = stomach. (From Nyberg DA, Mack LA, Patten RM, et al: Fetal bowel: Normal sonographic findings. J Ultrasound Med 1987; 6:3–6. Used by permission.)

sia.[18] In a more recent prospective study, Pretorius et al. failed to identify the stomach sonographically in 20 of 1,065 fetuses (2%) examined after 12 weeks, and nearly half these fetuses proved to be normal.[8] Because stomach size varies significantly between patients and even within the same fetus over time, non–visualization of the stomach may require repeat scanning a few hours or even days later.[8]

During the first and second trimester, the bowel is normally visualized as an ill-defined area of increased echogenicity in the mid to lower abdomen (see Fig 10–2). Distinguishing large bowel from small bowel is possible after 20 menstrual weeks (Fig 10–3), and this distinction becomes more obvious with advancing gestational age.[7] Characteristically, the large bowel appears as a continuous tubular structure located in the periphery of the abdomen that is filled with hypoechoic meconium (Figs 10–4 and 10–5).[7,11] By comparison, the small bowel is located centrally and remains more echogenic in appearance until the late third trimester. Unlike the colon, the small bowel also undergoes continuous, active peristalsis that can be observed sonographically during the third trimester (Fig 10–6).

The large bowel progressively enlarges with meconium throughout pregnancy, measuring 3 to 5 mm at 20 weeks and reaching 20 mm or occasionally even larger near term (Fig 10–7).[7] Although the small

bowel also becomes more prominent with gestational age, individual segments do not normally exceed 5 mm in diameter or 15 mm in length even near term. The discrepancy between large and small bowel is lost soon after birth, when swallowed air distends the poorly muscularized small bowel at the same time the colon is evacuated.

Unless correctly recognized, normal colon can be mistaken for abnormally dilated bowel or other pathological processes including renal cysts and pelvic masses. This potential pitfall is especially likely when the meconium, which is usually hypoechoic compared to the bowel wall, has a more sonolucent appearance (Fig 10–8). Sonolucent meconium presumably reflects a greater content of water but, in our experience, has no clinical significance as long as the colon diameter remains normal in size. We rarely have observed unusually echogenic meconium in the colon in some post-dates fetuses, probably due to increased water resorption of fluid over time, and in some fetuses with a proximal bowel obstruction, presumably due to diminished transit of amniotic fluid (Fig 10–9).

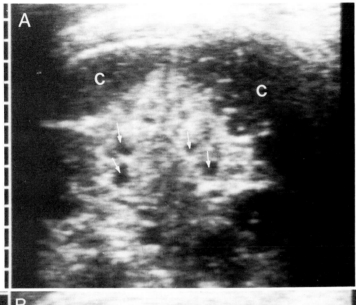

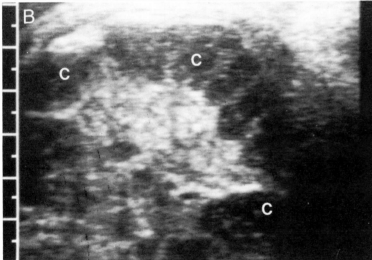

FIG 10–6.
Normal small bowel. **A,** longitudinal scan shows multiple small bowel loops *(arrows)* which demonstrated active peristalsis on real-time examination. *C* = colon. **B,** seconds later, small bowel loops have changed in appearance while the colon *(C)* is unchanged. (From Nyberg DA, Mack LA, Patten RM, et al: Fetal bowel: Normal sonographic findings. J Ultrasound Med 1987; 6:3–6. Used by permission.)

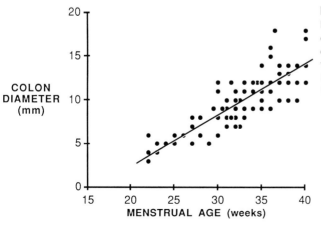

FIG 10–7.
Maximum colon diameter compared with menstrual age *(MA).* The colon diameter is usually less than 20 mm in preterm fetuses, but occasionally can be greater than 20 mm in term or postterm fetuses. (From Nyberg DA, Mack La, Patten RM, et al: Fetal bowel: Normal sonographic findings. J Ultrasound Med 1987; 6:3–6. Used by permission.)

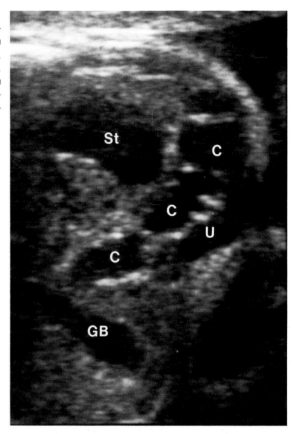

FIG 10–8.
Normal colon. Oblique scan of the abdomen at 32 weeks demonstrates the transverse colon *(C)* coursing across the abdomen. In some fetuses, the colon demonstrates a sonolucent appearance, presumably due to increased water content of meconium. *St* = stomach; *U* = umbilical vein; *GB* = gallbladder fossa. (From Nyberg DA, Mack LA, Patten RM, et al: Fetal bowel: Normal sonographic findings. J Ultrasound Med 1987; 6:3–6. Used by permission.)

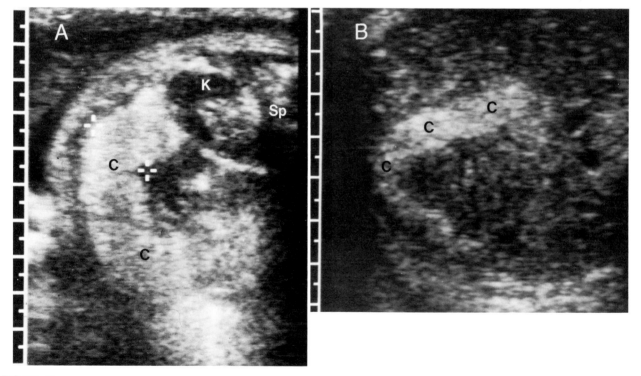

FIG 10–9.
Causes of echogenic meconium within colon. **A,** post-term. Transverse scan at 42 weeks shows prominent colon *(C)* filled with echogenic meconium. The colon diameter measures 22 mm in diameter, which may be normal for a term or post-term fetus. However, the echogenic appearance of meconium is unusual and is presumably related to decreased fluid content secondary to fluid resorption by the colonic mucosa *(K* = kidney; *Sp* = spine). **B,** proximal bowel obstruction. Transverse sonogram demonstrates an unusually echogenic colon *(C)* in a fetus with duodenal atresia (same fetus as in Fig 10–15).

TABLE 10–1.

Typical Features of Common Gastrointestinal Abnormalities

Abnormality	Typical US Findings	Associated Anomalies	Chromosomes, Genetics
Esophageal atresia	Polyhydramnios, absent stomach	Cardiovascular, intestinal, genitourinary	Tri 21, Tri 18
Duodenal atresia	"Double bubble", polyhydramnios	Cardiovascular, genitourinary	Tri 21 (30%)
Jejunoileal atresia	Dilated bowel, polyhydramnios	Bowel abnormalities	
Meconium ileus	Echogenic bowel, dilated bowel, polyhydramnios	Cystic fibrosis	Autosomal recessive
Meconium peritonitis	Peritoneal calcification, ascites, polyhydramnios, dilated bowel	Bowel atresia, cystic fibrosis <10%	Usually sporadic, autosomal recessive
Anorectal atresia	Dilated colon (sometimes), normal amniotic fluid	Vertebral, cardiovascular, tracheoesophageal fistula, genitourinary, limb abnormalities, central nervous system, caudal regression syndrome	None

APPROACH TO BOWEL DISORDERS

The normal appearance of fetal bowel can be altered by a number of pathological processes (Table 10–1). Most commonly, a mechanical or functional bowel obstruction results in proximal bowel dilatation that is characteristically recognized as one or more tubular structures within the fetal abdomen (Table

TABLE 10–2.

Causes of Dilated Bowel

Small bowel
  Jejunoileal atresia
  Volvulus
  Meconium ileus
  Meconium peritonitis
  Hirschsprung's disease
  Enteric duplications
  Congenital choridorrhea
Large bowel (Also consider causes of small bowel dilatation)
  Anorectal atresia
  Meconium plug syndrome
  Hirschsprung's disease
Pitfall
  Normal bowel
  Hydroureter

10–2). Dilated bowel segments are usually sonolucent in appearance, but may be normal or even increased in echogenicity. Before a bowel segment is diagnosed as abnormal, however, normal bowel should be specifically considered and excluded. In this regard, it is important to recognize that a sonolucent appearance of bowel is not necessarily abnormal and that bowel diameter is a more reliable criterion for diagnosing bowel dilatation.

Other intra-abdominal cystic masses should also be considered when dilated bowel is thought to be present (Table 10–3). Cystic masses arising from the kidney should be excluded by their characteristic paraspinal location. Demonstration of a cystic mass that has a round or spherical shape should suggest the possibility of a non–bowel related mass. Duodenal atresia is a notable exception to this generalization because the dilated duodenum may appear as a cystic mass, but in this situation continuity between the dilated duodenum and stomach is readily demonstrated. Distinguishing hydroureter from dilated bowel may occasionally be a difficult problem, particularly when cystic tubular structures are localized to the pelvis.

Ideally, sonographic evaluation would be able to distinguish dilated small bowel from dilated large

TABLE 10–3.

Causes of Intra-abdominal Cystic Masses

Renal cyst, hydronephrosis, urinoma
Urinary bladder
Hydroureter
Dilated bowel
Persistent cloaca
Ovarian cyst
Meconium pseudocyst
Hydrometrocolpos
Mesenteric cyst (lymphangioma)
Enteric duplication cyst
Choledochal cyst
Liver, splenic cysts
Hemangioma

bowel and estimate the level of obstruction. In actual practice, distinguishing *abnormal,* dilated small bowel from large bowel may be very difficult, probably because obstructed small bowel may assume a peripheral location and become aperistaltic, thereby mimicking large bowel.[83] Therefore, small bowel dilatation often cannot be confidently diagnosed until the bowel diameter exceeds normal colon measurements for age.

Despite these limitations, sonographic findings frequently can suggest whether dilated bowel represents small or large bowel. The presence of multiple bowel loops and/or localization to the mid to upper abdomen suggests small bowel dilatation. A dilated bowel segment located in the pelvis or periphery of the abdomen might suggest possible large bowel dilatation. However, it should also be realized that causes of small bowel dilatation are much more common than causes of large bowel dilatation.

Polyhydramnios is a common and important associated finding of bowel dilatation, particularly when due to small bowel obstruction.[13] Polyhydramnios may develop from obstruction at any level along the small bowel but does not, as a rule, accompany large bowel dilatation alone. These observations are consistent with the hypothesis that the large bowel is the major site of amniotic fluid resorption in the fetus.

It is important to note that many causes of bowel dilatation do not usually become apparent until after 24 weeks. An earlier age of diagnosis is occasionally possible for some proximal sites of obstruction, such as duodenal atresia, although polyhydramnios rarely develops before 24 weeks from any gastrointestinal cause. These observations reflect the increasing contribution of fetal swallowing and bowel function to normal fluid dynamics during the third trimester.[1, 9]

In the following section, major bowel disorders that can be identified sonographically will be discussed

as they arise along the course of the gastrointestinal tract, from proximal to distal. These can be considered as three major groups:

A. Proximal gastrointestinal abnormalities.
   1. Esophageal atresia.
   2. Abnormalities of the stomach (including situs inversus).
   3. Duodenal atresia.
B. Small bowel dilatation.
   1. Jejunoileal atresia.
   2. Volvulus.
   3. Meconium ileus.
   4. Non-obstructive causes of small bowel dilatation.
C. Large bowel abnormalities.
   1. Colon atresia.
   2. Anorectal atresia.
   3. Hirschsprung's disease.

PROXIMAL GASTROINTESTINAL DISORDERS

Esophageal Atresia

Clinical and Pathologic Findings

Esophageal atresia occurs in 1 in 2,500 to 4,000 live births as a sporadic disorder with no known pattern of inheritance. It is associated with tracheoesophageal fistula in over 90% of cases.[19] Esophageal malformations (esophageal atresia and/or tracheoesophageal fistula) result from incomplete division of the foregut into the ventral respiratory portion and the dorsal digestive portion by the tracheoesophageal septum, a process that normally is complete by 8 weeks.[19]

The pathologic classification of esophageal malformations as described by Gross is as follows (Fig 10–10):[21]

   A. Atresia without tracheoesophageal fistula.
   B. Atresia with fistula of the upper esophageal segment.
   C. Atresia with fistula of the lower esophageal segment.
   D. Atresia with fistula of both proximal and distal segments.
   E. Fistula without esophageal atresia.

Type C is by far the most common, comprising 88% of cases. Esophageal atresia alone (type A) accounts for 8% of cases and the remaining types (B,D, and E) are found in only 1%–2% of cases each.[27]

Sonographic Findings

Esophageal atresia alone (type A) would be expected to cause polyhydramnios and failure to visualize

ESOPHAGEAL ATRESIA
TRACHEOESOPHAGEAL FISTULA

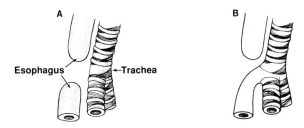

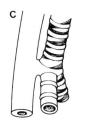 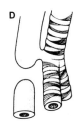 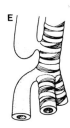

FIG 10–10.
Types of esophageal malformations. Type C (esophageal atresia with fistula of lower esophageal segment) accounts for 88% of cases.

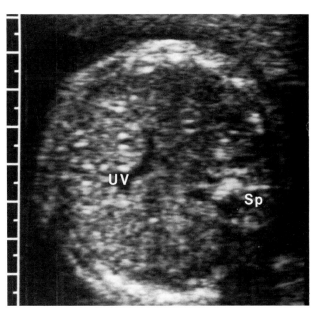

FIG 10–11.
Esophageal atresia. Transverse scan of the abdomen at 28 weeks shows no evidence of a stomach, and delayed scans failed to show a stomach. Polyhydramnios was also noted. Esophageal atresia with trachesoesphageal fistula was found at autopsy. *SP* = spine; *UV* = umbilical vein.

a fluid-filled stomach (Fig 10–11). This constellation of findings was first suggested by Hobbins et al. in 1979[24] and was confirmed by Farrant in 1980.[18] Other authors have reported similar findings.[29, 30, 35] However, demonstration of fluid in the stomach does not necessarily exclude esophageal atresia, since enough fluid may be excreted by the gastric mucosa to make it visible. Conversely, absence of a visible stomach and polyhydramnios can be demonstrated, even when a tracheoesophageal fistula is present.[29, 30] This apparently is because the narrowed fistula and distal esophageal segment obstructs flow of amniotic fluid in utero, even though it may not obstruct passage of air following birth.[34]

In a series of 22 fetuses with tracheoesophageal fistula, polyhydramnios was present in 62% of cases, and both polyhydramnios and failure to visualize the stomach were observed in 32% of cases.[30] No case of esophageal atresia has been diagnosed before 24 weeks, probably because fetal swallowing contributes relatively little to amniotic fluid dynamics at this time.

The differential diagnosis for polyhydramnios and non–visualization of the fetal stomach in its usual location includes diaphragmatic hernia, situs inversus, facial cleft, and central nervous system anomalies (Table 10–4). Facial clefts probably cause ineffective fetal swallowing, and central nervous system disorders presumably result in depression of swallowing on a neurologic basis. Oligohydramnios from any cause also may result in failure to visualize the stomach because little

amniotic fluid is available to swallow.[8] Finally, the stomach may not be visible in some normal fetuses on initial scans only to appear on a repeat examination. The likelihood that non–visualization of the stomach represents a true malformation increases with the degree of polyhydramnios.

Other sonographic findings also may occasionally suggest the diagnosis of esophageal atresia. Rarely, a dilated esophageal segment proximal to the point of atresia can be identified.[17] A dilated distal esophageal segment has also been reported both prenatally and postnatally, and in these cases a proximal bowel obstruction (duodenal or gastric atresia) was also present.[16, 22] Visualization of regurgitation after swallowing has been observed and is presumptive evidence for esophageal atresia;[15, 34] however, hyperactive swallowing alone has been observed in association with

---

TABLE 10–4.

Causes of Nonvisualization of the Stomach

Esophageal atresia/tracheoesophageal fistula
Diaphragmatic hernia
Facial cleft
Central nervous system disorders
Other swallowing disorders
Oligohydramnios from other causes

Pitfall: Transient non-visualization of stomach in normal fetuses.

---

other causes of polyhydramnios.[15] Finally, intrauterine growth retardation is often found in association with esophageal atresia.[26]

Associated Malformations

Concurrent malformations are associated with esophageal atresia in 50%–70% of cases.[20] In a series of over 1,000 cases reviewed by Holder et al.,[25] half had associated anomalies in the following sites:

Gastrointestinal: 28%.
Cardiac: 24%.
Genitourinary: 13%.
Musculoskeletal: 11%.
Central nervous system: 7%.
Facial anomalies: 6%.
Other: 12%.

Common gastrointestinal anomalies associated with esophageal malformations include malrotation, anorectal atresia, duodenal atresia, Meckel diverticulum, and annular pancreas. Anorectal atresia comprised 9% of concurrent gastrointestinal anomalies in the series of 500 infants reported by Louhimo and Lindahl.[27] The association between esophageal atresia and anorectal atresia has been included as a group of malformations recognized by the acronym VACTERL (vertebral anomalies, anorectal atresia, cardiovascular malformations, tracheo-esophageal fistula, renal anomalies, and limb abnormalities).

Both trisomy 21 and trisomy 18 have been associated with esophageal atresia,[19, 30, 31] and affected fetuses may demonstrate anomalies of other organs (see Chapter 18). Although the precise frequency of chromosomal abnormalities is uncertain, Pretorius et al. reported abnormal karyotypes in four of 22 (19%) fetuses with tracheoesophageal fistulas evaluated prenatally (2 cases each of trisomy 21 and trisomy 18). Two neonatal series reported chromosomal abnormalities in 3%–4% of infants with esophageal atresia, although this is undoubtedly an underestimate for the fetal population.[20, 27]

Prognosis

Waterston devised a clinical classification (groups A, B, and C) for esophageal malformations based on the presence of other anomalies, the birth weight, and development of respiratory complications.[33] However, other authors have omitted pulmonary complications from this classification, because they develop after birth and are not an intrinsic part of the disorder.[27]

With the availability of modern surgical techniques, neonatal care, and ventilatory support, the mortality rate for live borns with esophageal atresia has been reduced from 100% to 7%–15% when significant other anomalies are absent.[14, 23, 27] The mortality rate for infants with low birth weights and prematurity, who are commonly encountered because of polyhydramnios, has particularly improved.[32] By comparison, infants with concurrent anomalies have a survival rate of 0% to 58%, depending on the type and severity of anomalies.[27] For surviving infants, gastroesophageal reflux may produce repeated pneumonitis and recurrent stricture.[12]

Stomach and Duodenum

As previously noted, the stomach can be visualized as early as 11 menstrual weeks. Normal stomach measurements have been described;[36] however, marked variation in stomach size can be seen, even within the same fetus. An enlarged stomach alone has been reported in association with an antral web[38] or congenital pyloric stenosis. However, how one reliably distinguishes an abnormally dilated stomach from a normal, but prominent stomach has not been established.

Echogenic debris can sometimes be seen lying in the dependent portion of the stomach. This has been termed a gastric "pseudomass".[37] This finding has been observed in association with intra-amniotic hemorrhage, in which case it is thought to represent accumulation of swallowed blood. Identical findings have also been observed in normal fetuses, in which case it is thought to represent swallowed vernix.

Situs Inversus

Clinical and Pathologic Findings

The prevalence of situs inversus is estimated at 1 in 10,000 adults.[39, 42] Situs inversus may be classified into two major categories:

1. Complete (situs inversus totalis).
2. Partial.

Situs inversus totalis involves reversal of both the abdominal and thoracic viscera so they form a mirror image of normal. In partial situs inversus, the thoracic viscera may be reversed, while the abdominal viscera are normally positioned; or the abdominal viscera may be reversed, while the thoracic viscera are normal. Rarely, isolated situs inversus of the stomach and duodenum may occur. Partial situs inversus is commonly categorized as bilateral right-sidedness (asplenia syndrome) or bilateral left-sidedness (polysplenia syndrome).

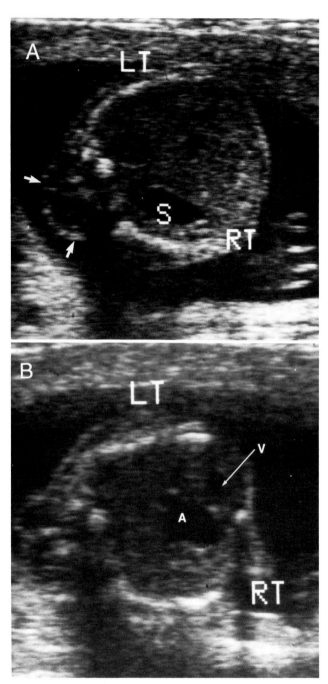

FIG 10–12.
Abdominal situs inversus and polysplenia syndrome. **A,** transverse view of the abdomen at 19 weeks demonstrates the stomach *(S)* on the fetal right. A large myelomeningocele *(arrows)* extending from the thoracic spine to the sacrum is also demonstrated. *RT* = right; *LT* = left. **B,** transverse view of the thorax in the same fetus demonstrates a single ventricle *(V)* and atrium *(A)*. Other abnormalities at autopsy included a single umbilical artery, facial cleft, absent right kidney, polysplenia, absent gallbladder, and inferior vena cava. *LT* = left; *RT* = right.

The pathogenesis of situs inversus is uncertain, although it is clear that it must occur before development of the spleen, an asymmetrical organ that normally appears at 6 menstrual weeks. During the same time period, the cardiovascular system is in a critical process of development and is susceptible to the same potential teratogenic effects that presumably cause situs inversus.

Sonographic Findings

In total situs inversus, the heart axis and the aortic arch also are on the right, the liver and spleen are transposed, and the gallbladder is on the left. In partial situs inversus, the stomach also is usually identified on the right side (Figs 10–12 and 10–13).[40, 46] In asplenia syndrome, the spleen is absent, the liver is horizontal and midline, the gallbladder is midline, the heart has a normal axis or is midline, and the inferior vena cava and aorta are on the same side (either left- or right-sided). In polysplenia syndrome, the liver and spleen are usually transposed, the gallbladder is absent, and the inferior vena cava is interrupted at the liver with continuation of the azygous or hemizygous vein. Cardiac and other anomalies usually dominate the appearance of both the asplenic and polysplenic syndrome (see Fig 10–12).

Associated Anomalies

About 20% of patients with situs inversus totalis prove to have Kartagener's syndrome (total situs inversus, bronchiectasis, nasal polyposis).[42, 43] In the remaining cases, however, situs inversus totalis is often an incidental finding in otherwise normal patients. There is less than a 3% risk of cardiac malformation with situs inversus totalis (mirror image dextrocardia).

In contrast to the low risk of concurrent anomalies from total situs inversus, partial situs inversus is associated with severe concurrent anomalies in 40% of cases. Of these, cardiovascular malformations are among the most common and severe (see Fig 10–12).[44, 45] Complex cardiac defects, including common atrioventricular septal defect (endocardial cushion defect), transposition of the great vessels, pulmonary stenosis or atresia, and persistent truncus arteriosus, are associated with both the polysplenia syndrome and the asplenia syndrome, although they are usually more complex and more common in the asplenia syndrome. Congenital heart block has been associated with the polysplenic syndrome and may be the initial clue to its presence.[40, 41] Genitourinary anomalies and spina bifida (see Fig 10–12) are also associated with partial situs inversus.[42]

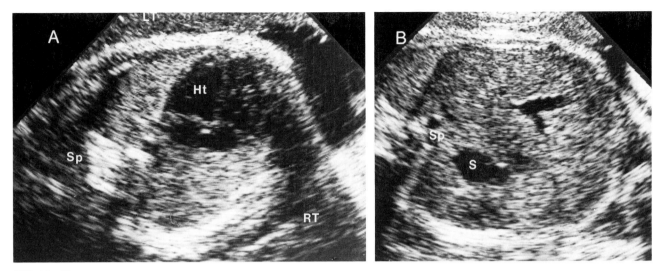

FIG 10–13.
Abdominal situs inversus, isolated. **A,** transverse view of the thorax at 35 weeks demonstrates normal orientation of the heart *(HT)* to the left thorax. *LT* = left; *RT* = right; *Sp* = spine. **B,** transverse scan slightly caudal to figure A demonstrates the stomach *(S)* on the fetal right side. No additional abnormalities were identified on sonography or at birth. *Sp* = spine.

Prognosis

Due to the severity of complex cardiovascular malformations, infants with asplenia syndrome have a 90% to 95% mortality rate during the first year of life, and infants with polysplenia syndrome have an 80% mortality.

In contrast to partial situs inversus, patients with isolated situs inversus totalis are usually asymptomatic and have a normal outcome. About 20% of patients with situs inversus totalis prove to have Kartagener's syndrome (total situs inversus, bronchiectasis, nasal polyposis).[42, 43] Kartagener's syndrome may be familial in some cases.

Duodenal Atresia

Clinical and Pathologic Findings

Duodenal atresia (Fig 10–14) is estimated to affect 1 in 5,000 pregnancies, and approximately 30% of these are associated with trisomy 21.[50] The etiology is usually a diaphragm or membrane that interrupts the duodenal lumen.[62] Less often the proximal and distal bowel segment end in a blind loop connected by a fibrous band. The site of obstruction typically is near the ampulla of Vater with 80% distal to the ampulla and 20% proximal to it.[62] Atresia of the common bile duct may be an associated abnormality. Annular pancreas is found in conjunction with duodenal atresia in 21% of cases, although this is not considered the primary cause of obstruction by most authorities.[62]

The most frequently cited explanation for develop-

ment of duodenal atresia is failure to recanalize the duodenal lumen after a temporary solid state during early embryologic development. However, other authors suggest that, similar to other small bowel atresias, duodenal atresia results from vascular impairment during gut development.[62] Thalidomide exposure be-

DUODENAL ATRESIA

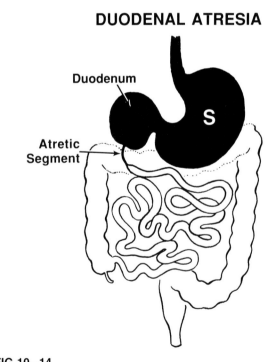

FIG 10–14.
Schematic drawing of duodenal atresia. The fluid-filled stomach *(S)* and duodenum proximal to the site of atresia cause the characteristic double bubble appearance.

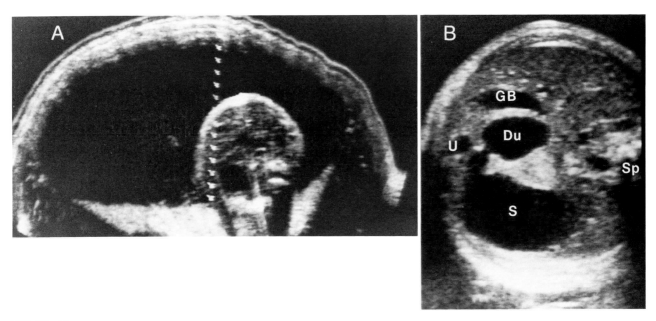

FIG 10–15.
Duodenal atresia. **A,** articulated scan at 34 weeks demonstrates marked polyhydramnios. **B,** transverse scan of the abdomen in the same patient demonstrates the double bubble appearance with fluid-filled stomach *(S)* communicating with the duodenum *(Du)*. *GB* = gallbladder; *U* = umbilical vein; *Sp* = spine.

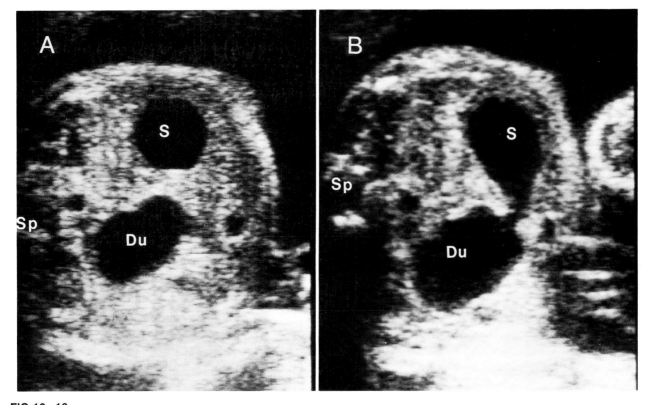

FIG 10–16.
Duodenal atresia. **A,** transverse sonogram at 30 weeks demonstrates a characteristic double bubble appearance representing the fluid filled-stomach *(S)* and duodenum *(Du)*. Mild polyhydramnios was also present. *Sp* = spine. **B,** scan at a slightly more caudal level demonstrates communication between the stomach *(S)* and dilated duodenum *(Du)*. Such continuity should be demonstrated to ensure that the abnormal fluid collection represents the duodenum. *Sp* = spine.

tween the 30th and 40th day of gestation may also result in duodenal atresia.

Because of its association with trisomy 21, detection of duodenal atresia is a well-accepted indication for prenatal chromosomal analysis. Unfortunately, since sonographic detection of duodenal atresia usually is not possible until after 24 weeks, termination of pregnancy is infrequently considered a therapeutic option by the time of diagnosis. Nevertheless, knowledge of a fetus with a chromosomal malformation is important information that may influence the place, mode, or time of delivery.[56]

Sonographic Findings

Duodenal atresia frequently has been detected on prenatal sonography[48, 49, 52, 53] since its initial report by Loveday.[55] Polyhydramnios develops in most cases, presumably at a point in gestation when the amount of swallowed amniotic fluid exceeds the absorptive capacity of the stomach and proximal duodenum (Fig 10–15).[54] Because the obstruction is complete, the characteristic "double bubble" sign representing the fluid-filled stomach and duodenum should always be seen with duodenal atresia (Figs 10–15 and 10–16). Nearly all prenatally diagnosed cases of duodenal

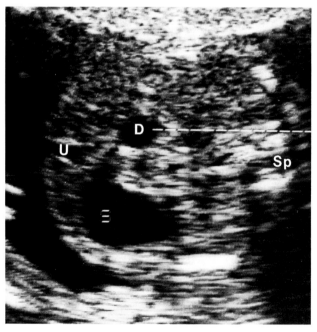

FIG 10–17.
Duodenal atresia at 18 weeks. Transverse sonogram at 18 menstrual weeks prior to genetic amniocentesis demonstrates a fluid-filled duodenum *(D)* communicating with the stomach *(S)*. Chromosome analysis yielded trisomy 21. A fluid-filled duodenum should not normally be visualized. *Sp* = spine; *U* = umbilical vein.

atresia have been reported after 24 weeks. Recently, however, Romero et al. reported a double bubble finding in a fetus with duodenal atresia and a normal karyotype at 22 weeks.[56] We have also observed two fetuses with duodenal atresia between 18 to 20 weeks, and each demonstrated a fluid-filled proximal duodenum without polyhydramnios (Fig 10–17). This suggests that, with careful observation, duodenal atresia can occasionally be diagnosed before 24 weeks, even though polyhydramnios does not develop until later.[54] Duodenal stenosis may demonstrate a similar appearance (Fig 10–18).

Continuity with the stomach should be demonstrated to distinguish a distended duodenum from other cystic masses in the right upper quadrant, such as choledochal cyst and hepatic cysts (see Fig 10–16). Other causes of duodenal or proximal bowel obstruction that could potentially produce a double bubble appearance include duodenal stenosis (see Fig 10–18), annular pancreas, obstructing bands (Ladd's bands), volvulus, or intestinal duplications (Table 10–5). However, our experience suggests that virtually all fetuses who demonstrate a typical double bubble finding prove to have duodenal atresia; other causes of duodenal obstruction are usually incomplete and would be expected to result in less prominent dilatation of the duodenum.

A prominent, but normal stomach should not be mistaken for duodenal atresia.[51] This potential pitfall is possible when a prominent incisura angularis is confused for the dilated duodenum and can be avoided by scanning in a transverse plane. Also, an enlarged stomach alone is located to the left of midline, while a dilated duodenum is located to the right of midline. It should be noted that an enlarged stomach alone has been reported from congenital pyloric stenosis.[38] The gallbladder potentially could be confused for the duodenum.

Associated Anomalies

About half the fetuses with duodenal atresia have concurrent malformations[50] including:

Skeletal: 36%.
Gastrointestinal: 26%.
Cardiovascular: 20%.
Genitourinary: 8%.
Chromosomal: 30%.

Associated skeletal abnormalities include vertebral and rib anomalies, sacral agenesis, radial abnormalities, and talipes equinovarus.[47, 50] Concurrent gastrointestinal abnormalities include esophageal atresia/

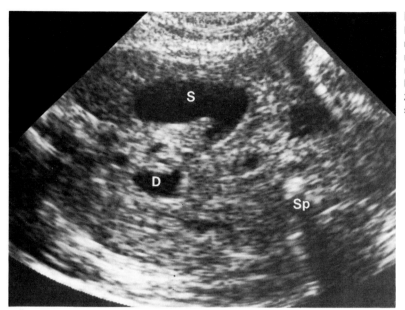

FIG 10–18.
Duodenal stenosis. Transverse sonogram at 31 menstrual weeks demonstrates a fluid-filled duodenum communicating with the stomach *(S)*. Mild cerebral ventricular dilatation was also noted. At birth, bladder exstrophy also was identified, and trisomy 21 was found on chromosome analysis. *Sp* = spine; *D* = duodenum.

tracheoesophageal fistula (7%), intestinal malrotation (20%), malrotation, jejunoileal atresia, Meckel diverticulum, and anorectal atresia (3%).[62]

Cardiovascular malformations, often present in conjunction with trisomy 21, are found in 20% of cases and are a leading cause of infant mortality. Endocardial cushion defects are so characteristic of trisomy 21 that the presence of both duodenal atresia and an endocardial cushion defect is virtually pathognomonic of this disorder.[50]

Prognosis

The overall mortality rate of duodenal atresia has been reported as 36%, with associated malformations as the leading cause of death.[50] Those fetuses who do not have trisomy 21 or major concurrent anomalies have a favorable prognosis. Because significant fluid and electrolyte imbalances develop soon after birth, the atretic site should be surgically bypassed with a gastrojejunostomy as soon as possible. For this reason, awareness of duodenal atresia before birth may result in an improved clinical outcome.[56]

TABLE 10–5.

Possible Causes of the "Double Bubble"

Duodenal atresia
Duodenal stenosis
Annular pancreas
Ladd's bands
Proximal jejunal atresia

Pitfall: Prominent incisura angularis.

SMALL BOWEL ABNORMALITIES

Jejunoileal Atresia, Stenosis

Clinical and Pathologic Findings

Small bowel (jejunoileal) atresia (Fig 10–19) is slightly more common than duodenal atresia, with an estimated prevalence of approximately 1 in 3,000 to 1 in 5,000 births.[62, 69] The sites of small bowel atresia are proximal jejunum (31%), distal jejunum (20%), proximal ileum (13%), and distal ileum (36%).[59] More than one site is involved in 6% of cases.[59]

Jejunoileal atresia (Fig 10–20) is commonly categorized as follows: type I, a mucosal diaphragm with in-

JEJUNOILEAL ATRESIA

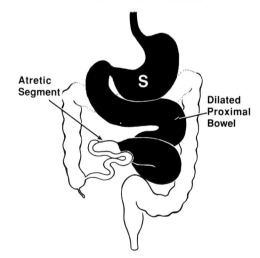

Atretic Segment

S

Dilated Proximal Bowel

FIG 10–19.
Schematic drawing of jejunoileal atresia. Dilated loops of bowel are demonstrated proximal to the site of atresia. *S* = stomach.

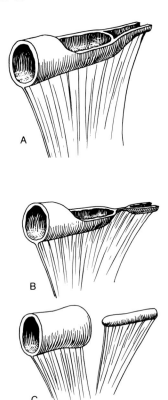

FIG 10–20.
Types of intestinal atresia. **A,** type I, is characterized by a mucosal diaphragm and intact bowel; **B,** type II, is characterized by blind ends of bowel connected by a fibrous band; and **C,** type III, is characterized by a mesenteric defect. Some authors have included diffuse bowel atresia (apple peel atresia) as type IV. (From Gray SW, Skandalakis JE: *Embryology for Surgeons.* Philadelphia, Saunders Co, 1972. Used by permission.)

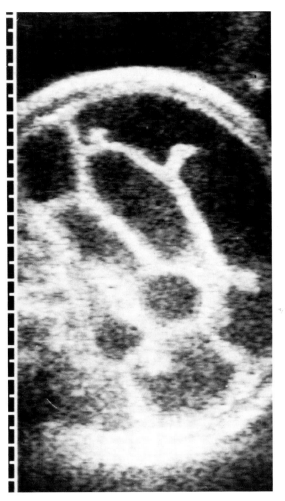

FIG 10–21.
Ileal atresia. Transverse sonogram of the abdomen at 36 weeks demonstrates multiple loops of dilated bowel. An isolated ileal atresia was found at the time of surgery.

tact bowel wall (20%); type II, blind ends of intestine connected by a fibrous band (32%); or type III, blind ends of intestine separated by a mesenteric gap (48%).[62, 67] A modified classification proposed by Grossfeld and associates includes: type IIIb, "apple peel" atresia, a rare type of atresia that affects the entire jejunum, proximal ileum, and distal duodenum; and type IV, multiple atresias.[63]

Overwhelming clinical and experimental evidence indicates that jejunoileal atresia and stenoses usually result from vascular impairment during embryologic development.[72] These vascular "accidents" may be sporadic or secondary to a predisposing disorder such as volvulus or gastroschisis. Apple peel atresia, which may be familial, probably results from occlusion of a branch of the superior mesenteric artery.[60]

Volvulus may occur when the mesentery is incompletely affixed to the retroperitoneum. Normally, the rapidly growing midgut herniates into the body stalk after 7 weeks and completes a 270-degree counterclockwise rotation before returning to the abdominal cavity by 12 weeks. From the 12th week until after birth, the bowel and mesentery undergo a process of fixation to the retroperitoneum, with the duodenum, ascending colon, and descending colon becoming retroperitoneal structures.

Sonographic Findings

Both jejunal and ileal atresia have been detected prenatally as dilated small bowel segments proximal to the site of atresia, usually in association with polyhydramnios (Figs 10–21 and 10–22).[61, 64–66, 68, 71, 85] These findings are indistinguishable when midgut volvulus is also present.[57, 70] The sensitivity of ultrasound for demonstrating these findings from jejunoileal atresia is unknown, but is probably low. Polyhydramnios is more likely from a proximal atresia. Rarely, dilated bowel material can be identified before 24 weeks (Fig 10–23).

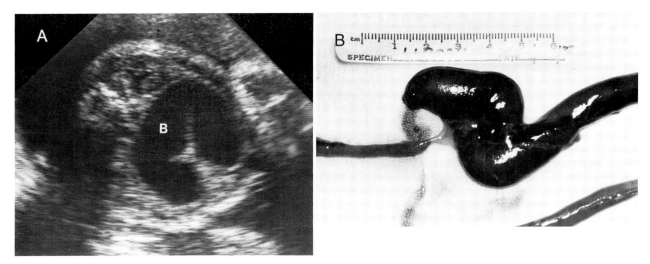

FIG 10–22.
Jejunal atresia. **A,** transverse sonogram at 32 weeks shows an abnormally dilated bowel *(B)* segment. **B,** pathologic specimen in another case shows bowel atresia connected by a fibrous band (type II).

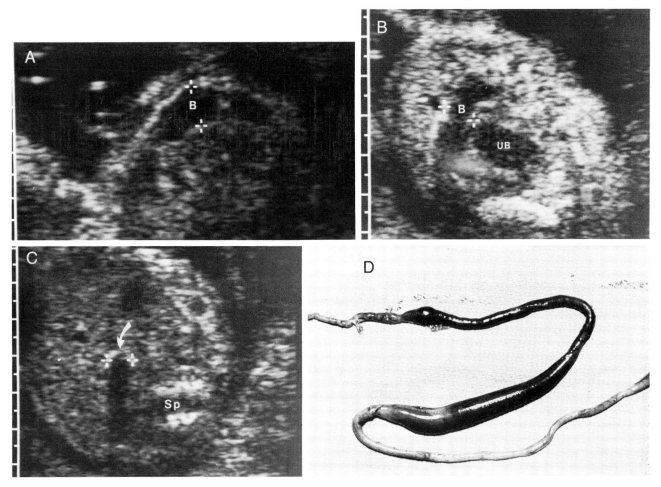

FIG 10–23.
Jejunal stenosis. **A,** transverse sonogram at 22 menstrual weeks demonstrates a mildly dilated bowel *(B)* segment in the periphery of the abdomen measuring 7 mm in diameter. **B,** semi-coronal scan demonstrates the bowel *(B)* segment coursing across the abdomen. The course of the bowel loop initially suggested that it represented colon. *UB* = urinary bladder. **C,** focal area of increased echogenicity and acoustic shadowing *(arrow)* is demonstrated at the presumed site of obstruction within the bowel lumen. Termination of pregnancy was elected by the parents, due to the potential risk of meconium ileus. *Sp* = spine. **D,** pathologic specimen shows dilatation of the proximal jejunum with abrupt narrowing. Despite the sonographic finding, no calcified focus was found pathologically, and the echogenic area presumably represented inspissated meconium. This case is unusual, since bowel dilatation is usually not detected prior to 24 weeks.

When dilated small bowel is demonstrated, meconium ileus should be considered in addition to jejunoileal atresia and volvulus. Rare causes of small bowel dilatation and polyhydramnios include Hirschsprung's disease and congenital chloridorrhea. The sonographic distinction between these possibilities is difficult, if not impossible. Unfortunately, measurement of amniotic fluid microvillar enzyme levels is also unlikely to be helpful in identification of meconium ileus, since low levels would be expected from any cause of bowel obstruction.

Care should be taken to distinguish dilated bowel from hydroureter, in which case oligohydramnios and/or hydronephrosis are often present. Dilated bowel also should be distinguished from other intra-abdominal cystic masses including ovarian cysts, enteric duplication cysts, and mesenteric cysts.

Associated Anomalies

Unlike esophageal atresia or anorectal atresia, extra-intestinal anomalies are found in less than 7% of small bowel atresias.[59] This is consistent with the hypothesis that small bowel atresia is an acquired defect due to vascular impairment, whereas esophageal and anorectal atresia result from fundamental disorders of embryogenesis.

Other bowel abnormalities, however, are frequently associated with jejunoileal atresia.[59, 66] Associated bowel abnormalities that have been reported include the probable cause of atresia (malrotation, volvulus, intestinal duplications, meconium ileus, or gastroschisis) in 27%, complications of atresia (meconium peritonitis) in 6%,[58] and concurrent bowel abnormalities (colon atresia, esophageal atresia, anorectal atresia, enteric duplications) in 5%.[72]

Prognosis

All patients with small bowel atresia present with symptoms of bowel obstruction, typically within a few days of life. The prognosis depends primarily on the site and extent of bowel involvement and other anomalies or complications. The primary complication of bowel obstruction from small bowel atresia is ischemia and infarction. This leads to in utero bowel perforation and menonium peritonitis in about 6% of cases of jejunoileal atresia. Conversely, approximately 40% of cases of meconium peritonitis are associated with small bowel atresia.[202]

Without surgery, the mean survival time for infants with intestinal atresia is less than 6 days, but with surgical correction the overall mortality rate has been reduced to 12%.[58] Distal ileal atresia carries an excellent

prognosis, with a survival rate approaching 100%. Jejunal atresia has a less favorable prognosis, possibly due to the greater rate of premature delivery.[58] The mortality rate is also increased with concurrent malformations (43%),[58] meconium peritonitis (62%), and congenital volvulus (80%). Multiple sites of atresia and apple-peel atresia have a poor prognosis.

Meconium Ileus

Clinical and Pathologic Findings

Meconium ileus (Fig 10–24) is characterized by impaction of abnormally thick and sticky meconium in the distal ileum.[92, 94] Virtually all newborns who develop meconium ileus prove to have cystic fibrosis, an autosomal recessive disorder that affects 1 in 2,000 caucasian births.[94] Conversely, meconium ileus affects 10%–15% of patients with cystic fibrosis and is the earliest clinical manifestation of this disorder.[94] Cystic fibrosis is rare among black and Asian populations.

Characteristic pathologic findings of meconium ileus include a dilated ileum, relatively normal jejunum, and a collapsed empty colon.[62] Up to 50% of infants with meconium ileus develop other gastrointestinal complications including volvulus, atresia, bowel perforation, or meconium peritonitis.[94] Analysis of meconium from fetuses with meconium ileus shows an abnormally high protein and mucous content, increased mucous, and decreased water content compared with normal meconium.[78] Abnormal meconium composition probably results from increased mucous secretion by the gas-

MECONIUM ILEUS

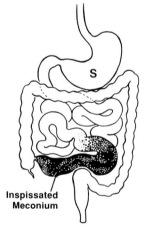

FIG 10–24.
Schematic drawing of meconium ileus. Thick, inspissated meconium obstructs the distal ileum. Findings that may be demonstrated on sonography are (1) echogenic areas representing inspissated meconium, or (2) proximal bowel dilatation.

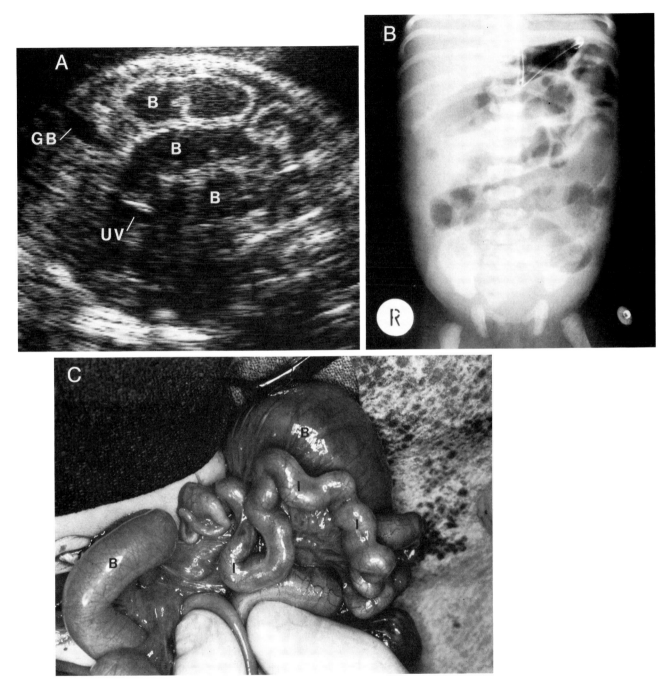

FIG 10-25.
Dilated bowel and meconium ileus. **A,** transverse scan of the abdomen at 35 weeks' gestation demonstrates several loops of dilated small bowel *(B)* in the central abdomen, which measured 13 mm in diameter. No mass, ascites, or calcification was observed. *GB* = gallbladder; *UV* = umbilical vein. **B,** abdominal radiograph after birth demonstrates multiple air-filled loops of small bowel, and a barium enema showed a microcolon. Meconium ileus was found at the time of surgery. A sweat-chloride test at 7 weeks was positive for cystic fibrosis. **C,** intra-operative photograph of a similar case shows abnormal concretions of meconium obstructing the distal ileum *(I)* with dilatation of more proximal small bowel *(B).* (Parts **A** and **B** from Nyberg DA, Hastrup W, Watts H, et al: Dilated fetal bowel: A sonographic sign of cystic fibrosis. J Ultrasound Med 1987; 6:257-260. Used by permission. Part **C** courtesy of Robert T Schaller, Jr, MD, Department of Pediatric Surgery, Childrens Hospital Medical Center, Seattle, WA.)

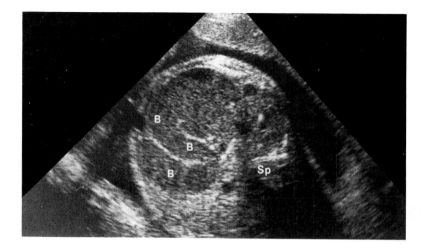

FIG 10–26.
Dilated bowel and meconium ileus. Transverse sonogram at 34 weeks demonstrates abnormally dilated loops of bowel *(B)* filled with meconium. The location and course of the bowel loops suggested they represented small bowel. At surgery, meconium ileus and bowel perforation with meconium peritionitis were identified. *Sp* = spine. (From Kurtz AB: AIUM film reading session. J Ultrasound Med 1986; 5:537. Used by permission.)

trointestinal tract and abnormalities of electrolytes that are characteristic of cystic fibrosis.

Inspissated meconium may also obstruct the colon, resulting in the mucous plug syndrome. In this disorder, transient colonic obstruction and failure to pass meconium in the first few days of life results from distal meconium impaction. While not as strongly linked to cystic fibrosis as is meconium ileus, as many as 25% of infants with the mucous plug syndrome have been reported to have cystic fibrosis.[94]

Sonographic Findings

Meconium ileus has been demonstrated in utero as 1) dilated bowel (Figs 10–25 to 10–27) [79, 83, 85, 91]

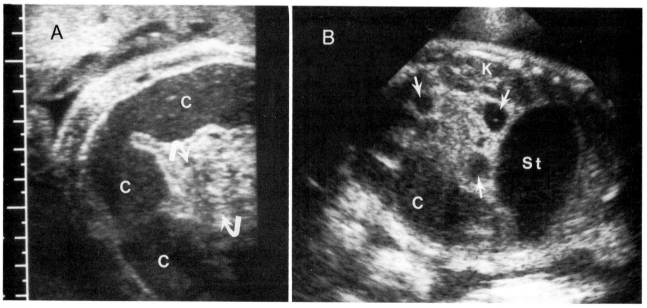

FIG 10–27.
Meconium plug syndrome and cystic fibrosis. **A,** transverse scan at 34 weeks demonstrates dilated colon *(C)* coursing around the more echogenic and non–dilated small bowel *(arrows)*. The colon measures 23 mm in diameter, which is abnormally dilated at this age. **B,** repeated sonogram 2 weeks later demonstrates dilated colon *(C)*, stomach *(St)*, and small bowel loops *(arrows)*. Spontaneous perforation of the distal ileum occurred on day 3 of life, requiring small bowel resection and an ileostomy. Cystic fibrosis was confirmed at one month of age. *K* = kidney. (From Nyberg DA, Hastrup W, Watts H, et al: Dilated fetal bowel: A sonographic sign of cystic fibrosis. J Ultrasound Med 1987; 6:257–260. Used by permission.)

and/or 2) echogenic meconium (Fig 10–28).[73, 81, 87–89] Small bowel dilatation develops secondary to the impacted meconium which is characteristic of meconium ileus. Most cases have been diagnosed after 26 weeks (see Figs 10–24 and 10–25),[91] although bowel dilatation in the second trimester has also been observed.[79] Colon dilatation from the mucous plug syndrome has also been noted in association with cystic fibrosis (see Fig 10–27).[91] Polyhydramnios usually accompanies the bowel dilatation.

The association between echogenic intra-abdominal "masses" and meconium ileus has been reported in both the second and third trimesters among fetuses with cystic fibrosis (Fig 10–28).[73, 81, 88, 89] Although initially observed in families with a 25% recurrence risk for cystic fibrosis,[88, 89] similar observations have been made in non–selected patients.[73, 81, 87] In these cases, the echogenic "masses" probably represent the impacted meconium itself. However, it is important for the sonographer to realize that echogenic intra-abdominal areas are not specific for meconium ileus and also can be observed in some normal fetuses as well as in association with other fetal abnormalities (see Fig 10–28).[80, 84, 86]

The significance of echogenic bowel probably varies with its location (small bowel vs. colon), menstrual age, and degree of echogenicity. Decreased water content and/or inspissation of meconium is the probable explanation for this echogenic appearance in most fetuses with echogenic bowel, regardless of the underlying etiology. In normal fetuses before 20 weeks, meconium inspissation within the small bowel can be tran-

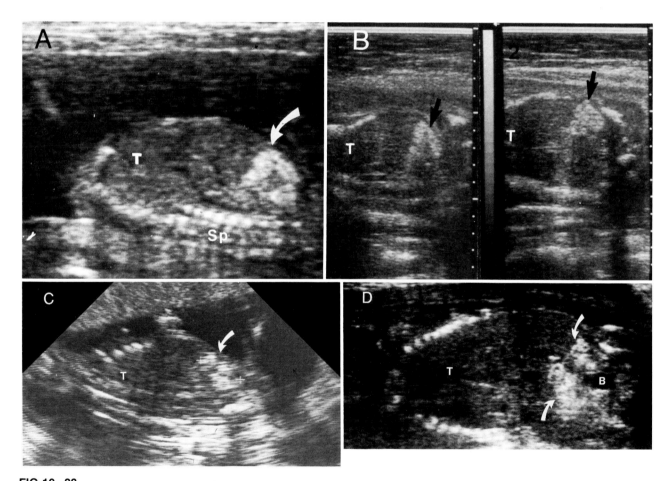

FIG 10–28.
Causes of echogenic small bowel (intraluminal echogenic meconium). **A,** normal. Longitudinal scan demonstrates echogenic bowel *(arrow)* in the lower abdomen at 18 weeks. *Sp* = spine; *T* = thorax. **B,** cystic fibrosis. Longitudinal scans show echogenic bowel *(arrows)* in the lower abdomen. *T* = thorax. **C,** trisomy 21. Longitudinal scan shows echogenic bowel *(arrow)* within the lower abdomen. Trisomy 21 has not yet been associated with echogenic bowel, although we have noted several similar cases. *T* = thorax. **D,** cytomegalovirus. Longitudinal sonogram demonstrates echogenic bowel *(arrow)* within the lower abdomen. *B* = urinary bladder; *T* = thorax. (Part **A** from Fakhry J, Reiser M, Shapiro LR, et al: Increased echogenicity in the lower fetal abdomen: A common normal variant in the second trimester. J Ultrasound Med 1986; 5:489–492. Part **B** from Meizner I: J Clinic Ultrasound 1987; 5:94. Used by permission.)

sient, whereas in fetuses with meconium ileus it may be persistent and obstructive. Our preliminary experience suggests that echogenic small bowel may also occasionally be observed in association with chromosome disorders, presumably due to delayed bowel transit.[82] This observation is of interest, because amniotic fluid microvillar enzymes are known to be decreased in fetuses with trisomy syndromes as well as in fetuses with cystic fibrosis.[75]

Associated Anomalies

Meconium ileus is virtually always associated with cystic fibrosis.[94] The specific genetic defect of cystic fibrosis remains obscure, although elevated concentrations of sweat sodium and chloride are integral and diagnostic features of the disorder in children and adults. In recent years, antenatal evaluation of cystic fibrosis became possible by noting that the majority of affected fetuses demonstrate decreased levels of various intestinal microvillar enzymes (alkaline phosphotase, gamma-glutamyltranspeptidase amnionpeptidase M, maltase, and sucrase) in the amniotic fluid.[75–77] This data suggests that bowel transit in fetuses with cystic fibrosis becomes impaired from inspissated meconium. Since intestinal microvillar analysis carries an 8% false-negative rate and a 2% false-positive rate, this method has been used almost exclusively for evaluating patients with a family history of cystic fibrosis.[81]

Intestinal microvillar enzyme analysis is probably of limited usefulness for determining the cause of echogenic meconium in patients lacking a family history of cystic fibrosis since inspissated meconium from any cause may result in decreased microvillar enzymes.[82] In this situation, DNA probes hold some promise for identifying affected fetuses with cystic fibrosis in the future.[74, 81, 90, 95, 96] Recent data provide realistic hope that the specific mutation of cystic fibrosis may be identified in the near future and permit screening of the general population to detect heterozygous carriers.[81]

Prognosis

The prognosis for patients with cystic fibrosis has improved considerably in recent decades with improved antibiotic and medical therapy. Nevertheless, patient morbidity is significant, as 80% of patients develop pancreatic insufficiency and 95% develop recurrent respiratory infections and chronic lung disease. Affected males are invariably infertile. Since cystic fibrosis is an autosomal recessive disorder, the recurrence risks for those patients with a previously affected pregnancy is 25%.

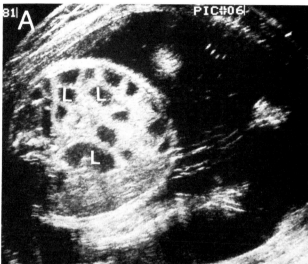
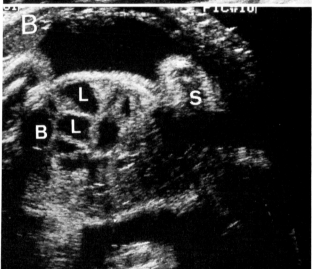

FIG 10–29.
Congenital chloridorrhea. **A,** transverse scan at 33 weeks demonstrates multiple loops of dilated small bowel *(L)* and polyhydramnios. **B,** longitudinal sonogram from the same case again demonstrates multiple loops of dilated small bowel loops *(L)*. Severe watery diarrhea began during the first day of life, and congenital chloridorrhea was found requiring continued electrolyte replacement. *B* = urinary bladder; *S* = shoulder. (Part **A** from Kirkinen P, Jouppila P: Prenat Diagnosis 1984; 4:457–461. Used by permission. Part **B** courtesy of Dr Kirkenen, University of Oulu, Finland.)

Non–obstructive Small Bowel Dilatation

Rarely, bowel dilatation may be seen in the absence of obstruction from congenital chloridorrhea (Fig 10–29). This is an autosomal recessive disorder characterized by absent or impaired cellular transport of chloride from the distal ileum and colon.[98, 99] It is thought to be secondary to deficiency of the chloride-bicarbonate ion-exchange pump. Postnatal clinical features of congenital chloridorrhea include profuse watery diarrhea, dehydration, and metabolic alkalosis. Congenital chloridorrhea has been observed as multiple loops of dilated bowel and polyhydramnios in several cases prenatally.[98, 99] This disorder can be fatal after birth if not correctly diagnosed and treated with volume replacement.

Megacystis-microcolon intestinal hypoperistalsis syndrome (MMIHS) is another rare case of functional bowel obstruction.[97] However, in all cases reported prenatally, an enlarged non-obstructed urinary bladder has dominated the sonographic picture (see Chapter 13).[100, 101, 103, 104] Failure to empty the urinary bladder also results in hydronephrosis and a thickened urinary bladder wall. Over 90% of reported cases are females, unlike urethrovesical obstruction, which occurs predominantly in males.[104] Also, unlike urethrovesical obstruction, amniotic fluid is normal to increased in amount with MMIHS. Although the pathogenesis remains uncertain, some authors believe that MMIHS is secondary to a degenerative disease of smooth muscle resulting in absent peristalsis.[102] The prognosis is poor, with long-term survivors reported in only 11% of cases.[104]

LARGE BOWEL ABNORMALITIES

Colon Atresia

Clinical and Pathologic Findings

Colon atresia accounts for 5% to 10% of all gut atresias.[105, 106] Like small bowel atresia, the presumed pathogenesis for colonic atresia is vascular insufficiency.[107] Colon atresia should be distinguished from anorectal atresia which has a very different pathogenesis and prognosis (see below).

Sonographic Findings

Colonic atresia has not yet been reported prenatally. Findings would be expected to include dilated colon during the third trimester and normal amniotic fluid.

Associated Anomalies

As with jejunoileal atresia, extra-intestinal anomalies are rare, but other intestinal anomalies are not uncommon. Small bowel atresia and colon atresia may coexist.

Prognosis

The prognosis for isolated colonic atresia is excellent following surgical resection of the involved bowel segment.

Anorectal Atresia

Clinical and Pathologic Findings

Anorectal malformations (Fig 10–30) occur in about 1 in 5,000 live births. A number of complex pathologic classifications have been derived for describing anal or rectal atresia. For simplification these are referred to here as anorectal atresia. Anorectal atresia can be categorized into two groups: high (supralevator) lesions that terminate above the levator sling and low (infralevator) lesions that terminate below the levator sling.[111, 114] High lesions are more common and are more frequently associated with fistulas and genitourinary malformations. Membranous atresia (imperforate anus), in its simplest form, is a rare condition that results from failure of the anal membrane to perforate. An especially complex type of atresia is a persistent cloaca (discussed below), in which the rectum, vagina, and urinary tract communicate with the perineum through a single opening.

Anorectal malformations result from abnormal partitioning of the cloaca by the urorectal septum (Fig 10–31).[111] The cloaca represents the distal confluence of (1) the distal hindgut, (2) the allantois, and (3) the mesonephric ducts. During the ninth menstrual week, downgrowth of the urorectal septum separates the cloaca into the dorsal rectum and the ventral urogenital

ANORECTAL ATRESIA

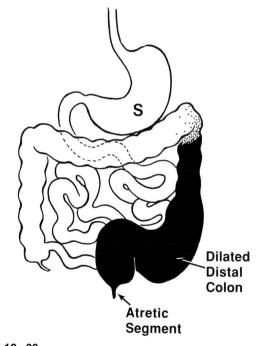

FIG 10–30.
Schematic drawing of anorectal atresia. Distal obstruction may result in dilatation of the colon. S = stomach.

FIG 10–31.
Embryogenesis of the rectum. **A,** the cloaca *(CL)* receives the allantois *(AL)* ventrally and the hindgut *(HG)* dorsally. The arrow indicates the developing urorectal septum, which will extend caudally to meet the cloaca membrane *(CM)*. **B,** downward growth of the urorectal septum completely separates the urogenital sinus *(U-G)* from the rectum *(R)*. The urogenital sinus will form the urinary bladder. Anorectal malformations result from abnormal formation of the urorectal septum and abnormal development of the cloacal membrane *(CM)*. (From Boles ETB Jr: *Clinics in Perinatology,* vol 5. Philadelphia, WB Saunders Co, 1978, pp 149–161. Used by permission.)

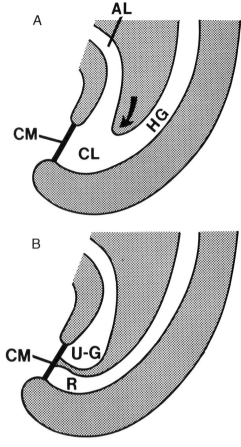

sinus (see Fig 10–31).[111] The urogenital sinus subsequently forms the urinary bladder and urethra, and the rectum remains a blind pouch until the anal membrane perforates by the tenth week. As the urorectal septum develops, the mesonephric ducts fuse into the cloaca laterally. These form the seminal vesicles in males, but atrophy in females. Induced by the mesonephric ducts, the paired paramesonephric ducts (mullerian ducts) fuse in the midline to form the uterovaginal cord.

Sonographic Findings

Anorectal atresia occasionally has been recognized on prenatal sonography as dilated colon in the lower abdomen or pelvis (Figs 10–32 and 10–33).[108, 109, 114]

FIG 10–32.
Anorectal atresia. Coronal sonogram at 35 weeks shows a segment of dilated colon *(C)* in the fetal pelvis measuring 22 mm in diameter. Note V configuration of dilated bowel segment. Absence of amniotic fluid was also noted. Other abnormalities at postmortem examination (following spontaneous death at 1 week of age) included esophageal atresia with tracheoesophageal fistula, right renal cystic dysplasia, left renal agenesis, tetralogy of Fallot, short extremities, and rocker-bottom feet. (From Harris RD, Nyberg DA, Mack LA, et al: Anorectal atresia: Prenatal sonographic diagnosis. AJR 1987; 149:395–400. Used by permission.)

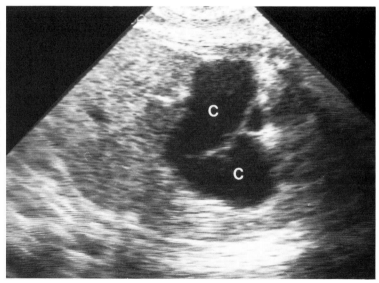

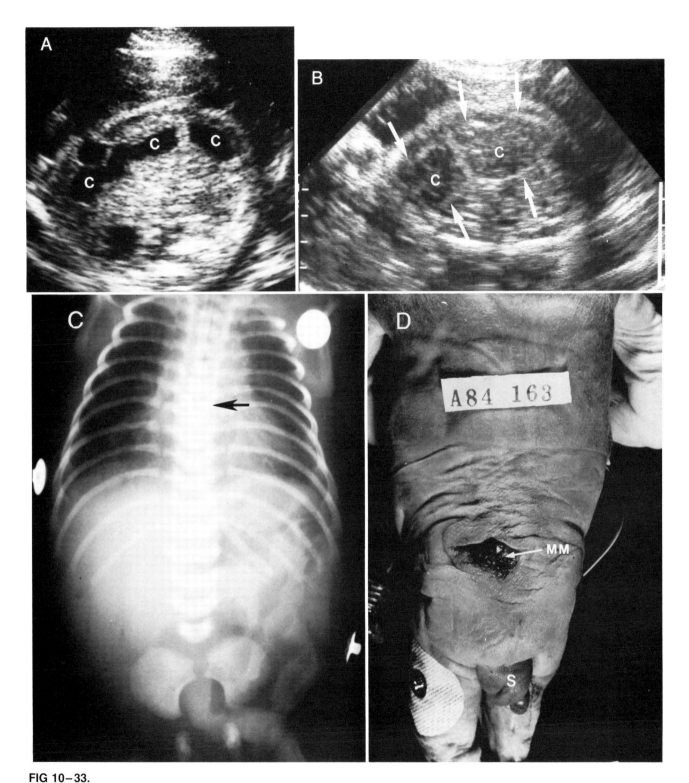

FIG 10-33.
Anorectal atresia. **A,** sonogram at 27 weeks shows minimally dilated colon *(C)* measuring 9 mm in diameter. **B,** repeated sonogram at 33 weeks shows progressive dilatation of colon *(C),* now measuring 27 mm in diameter *(arrows)* and filled with meconium. **C,** postnatal radiograph shows sacral agenesis and hemivertebrae *(arrow).* **D,** postmortem photograph in posterior view shows lumbar myelomeningocele *(MM)* and absence of the anus. Other anomalies included annular pancreas and renal dysplasia. *S* = scrotum. (Parts **A, B,** and **C** from Harris RD, Nyberg DA, Mack LA, et al: Anorectal atresia: Prenatal sonographic diagnosis. AJR 1987; 149:395-400. Used by permission.)

FIG 10–34.
Colon diameters from four fetuses with anorectal atresia *(dots)* compared with values obtained in 120 normal fetuses (mean ± 2 SD). One case (Fig 10–33) showed progressive dilatation from 27 to 33 weeks. (From Harris RD, Nyberg DA, Mack LA, et al: Anorectal atresia: Prenatal sonographic diagnosis. AJR 1987; 149:395–400. Used by permission.)

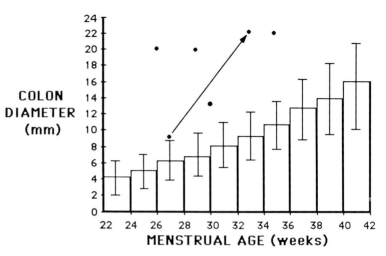

COLON DIAMETER (mm)

MENSTRUAL AGE (weeks)

Demonstration of this finding appears to be related to menstrual age, with the earliest age of diagnosis at 29 weeks (Fig 10–34).[114] Other unusual causes of large bowel dilatation include the meconium plug syndrome (see Fig 10–27) and Hirschsprung's disease. Since dilated small bowel can closely simulate large bowel, causes of small bowel dilatation should also be consid-

ered whenever large bowel dilatation is thought to be present (see Table 10–1).

It is presently unclear why a distal bowel obstruction should result in dilated colon if defecation does not occur antenatally. This observation supports other lines of evidence which suggest that, in fact, intestinal contents may normally pass to the amniotic fluid in

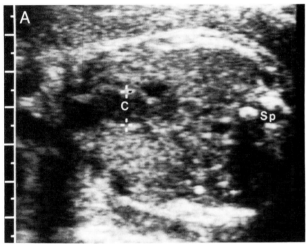

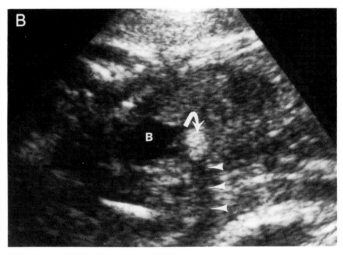

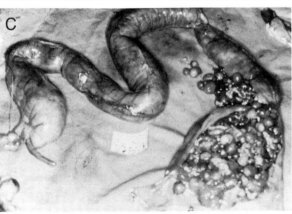

FIG 10–35.
Anorectal atresia with intraluminal meconium calcification. **A,** oblique scan at 28 weeks demonstrates a mildly prominent bowel loop thought to represent colon *(C)* in the lower abdomen. Marked oligohydramnios was present and fetal kidneys were not visualized. *Sp* = spine. **B,** longitudinal scan demonstrates an echogenic focus *(curved arrow)* with acoustic shadowing *(arrowheads)* just superior to the urinary bladder *(B)* that was thought to be located within the dilated colon. The infant died shortly after delivery at 42 weeks. Autopsy findings included anorectal atresia with dilated colon, single pelvic kidney, hypoplastic lungs, cardiac defect, and limb anomalies. **C,** pathologic specimen in another case of anorectal atresia detected prenatally shows multiple bean-like calcified meconium pellets within the dilated distal colon. (Part **C** from Shalev E, Weiner E, Zuckerman H: Prenatal ultrasound diagnosis of intestinal calcifications with imperforate anus. Acta Obstet Gynecol Scand 1983; 62:95–96. Used by permission.)

utero.[75] For example, intestinal microvillar enzymes are found in the amniotic fluid of normal fetuses, but are decreased in the amniotic fluid of fetuses with cystic fibrosis and are virtually undetectable in fetuses with anorectal atresia.[75] This data implies that normal fetuses pass some colon contents per rectum, that fetuses with cystic fibrosis are chronically "constipated" from inspissated meconium, and that anorectal atresia represents an absolute barrier to passage of colon contents.[75]

Calcified intraluminal meconium is another possible manifestation of anorectal atresia (Fig 10–35). This interesting finding has been most frequently reported in neonates with a supralevator atresia and also has been reported prenatally.[110, 117] The calcified meconium pellets can be found either proximal or distal to the site of obstruction. The cause of the intraluminal calcification is unknown, although it is presumably related to prolonged stasis. Other authors have proposed that alkaline urine from an colovesicle fistula may predispose to intraluminal meconium calcification, but this hypothesis has not been substantiated.

Amniotic fluid volume is either normal, or when associated with bilateral renal disorders, decreased in association with anorectal atresia. The presence of polyhydramnios should suggest either a diagnosis other than anorectal atresia or an additional anomaly such as esophageal atresia.[114]

Associated Anomalies

Additional malformations are present in up to 70% of neonates with anorectal atresia and in over 90% of fetuses detected prenatally. The genitourinary system is the most frequently involved organ system, which is not surprising in view of the common embryogenesis of the cloaca and urogenital sinus. Esophageal malformations and spinal abnormalities also are commonly present (Fig 10–36). The frequent concurrence of anorectal atresia and genitourinary malformations is reflected by two major groups of disorders: The VACTERL syndrome (vertebral, anal, cardiovascular, tracheoesophageal, renal, and limb malformations) and the caudal regression syndrome (renal agenesis or dysplasia, sacral agenesis, lower limb hypoplasia, and, in its severest form, sirenomelia).[113, 115, 118] Many malformations associated with anorectal atresia are random and do not necessarily fit into one of these syndromes. Specific malformations that may be associated with anorectal atresia include:

1. Genitourinary
    A. Renal agenesis or dysplasia
    B. Horseshoe kidney

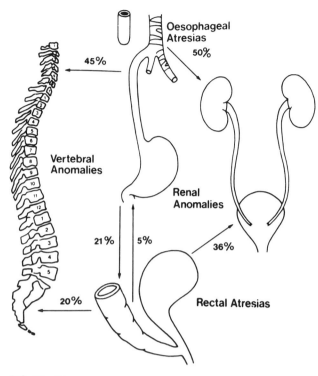

FIG 10–36.
Relationship between anorectal atresia, esophageal atresia, duodenal atresia, vertebral anomalies, and renal anomalies. These anomalies may be associated as part of the VACTERL syndrome (vertebral, anorectal, cardiac, tracheo-esophageal, renal, and limb anomalies). (From Atwell JD, Klidjian AM: J Pediatr Surg 1982; 17:237–240. Used by permission.)

    C. Uterine duplication abnormalities
2. Skeletal, vertebral
    A. Vertebral anomalies
    B. Sacral agenesis
    C. Sirenomelia
3. Gastrointestinal
    A. Tracheoesophageal atresia
4. Cardiovascular malformations
5. Central nervous system anomalies
6. Chromosomal abnormalities (trisomies 21 and 18)[111]

Prognosis

The prognosis for fetuses with anorectal atresia is poor due to the severity and high frequency of concurrent malformations. Bilateral renal agenesis or dysplasia is uniformly fatal, and cardiovascular or central nervous system malformations contribute to other deaths. Among survivors, bowel and bladder incontinence is common. Functional results appear to have improved with development of a surgical technique recently described by Pena and de Vries.[112, 116] In this technique, careful dissection from the posterior approach permits the bowel to be pulled through the levator muscle complex and improves bowel continence.[112, 116]

Persistent Cloaca (Cloacal Dysgenesis)

Clinical and Pathologic Findings

Persistent cloaca (cloacal dysgenesis) is a rare disorder resulting from failure of development of the urorectal septum (Fig 10–37).[121, 125] In simple terms, cloaca persistence can be considered as a severe type of anorectal atresia, with a common chamber shared by the distal gut (hindgut) and the genitourinary tract (urogenital sinus). This disorder is usually limited to females since males usually produce a distal fistula by the developing urethral folds.[125] Another malformation related embryologically to persistent cloaca is cloacal exstrophy in which breakdown of the cloacal membrane results in a low anterior abdominal wall defect (see Chapter 11).

Pathologic findings of persistent cloaca include confluence of the bladder, proximal urethra, upper two thirds of the vagina, and rectum with connection to the

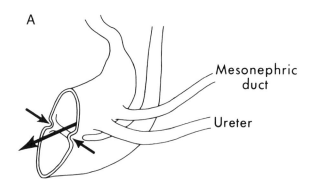

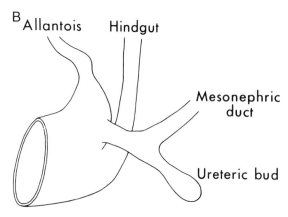

FIG 10–37.
A, diagramatic representation of normal separation of the cloaca into the rectum and urinary bladder. **B,** failure of normal development steps results in a persistent cloaca. (From Lande IM, Hamilton EF: The antenatal sonographic visualization of cloacal dysgenesis. J Ultrasound Med 1986; 5:275–278. Used by permission.)

perineum through a single common channel.[121, 125] Obstruction of the bladder, vagina, and intestine may result in dilated bowel, hydrocolpos, urethral obstruction, hydronephrosis, and oligohydramnios. Failure of the paired mullerian ducts to fuse also usually results in duplication of the uterus and vagina.

Sonographic Findings

Although rare, several cases of cloacal persistence have been reported on prenatal sonography.[120, 122–124] The typical sonographic appearance is a cystic pelvic mass (Fig 10–38), often septated, in association with oligohydramnios and impaired fetal growth.[120, 123, 124] Transient ascites was observed in two of three cases reported by Petrikovsky et al.[123] These authors suggest that transient ascites may represent urine that has escaped from the cloaca into the peritoneal cavity via the fallopian tubes. Later, chronic irritation by urine and meconium may occlude the tubes, leading to hydronephrosis and progressive enlargement of the pelvic mass (cloaca).

Associated Anomalies

Multiple associated anomalies are invariably present with persistent cloaca. In reviewing 56 cases of persistent cloaca, Bartholomew and Gonzales reported that 75% of children had anomalies of the upper urinary tract including renal agenesis, dysplasia, hydronephrosis, horseshoe kidney, and crossed renal ectopia.[119] Other anomalies that have been associated with persistent cloaca include vaginal and uterine duplication (40%), urachal remnants, tracheoesophageal fistual, duodenal atresia, and myelomeningocele.

Prognosis

The prognosis of persistent cloaca is directly related to the presence of associated anomalies. Excluding those cases associated with an abdominal wall defect (cloacal exstrophy), five of seven fetuses with persistent cloaca who were diagnosed on prenatal sonography subsequently died.[122, 123] However, two of the three fetuses diagnosed by Petrikovsky et al. lived following successful surgery after birth.[123]

Hirschsprung's Disease (Congenital Aganglionic Megacolon)

Clinical and Pathologic Findings

Hirschsprung's disease occurs in approximately 1 in 10,000 to 1 in 20,000 births.[126, 127] Males are affected three to four times more frequently than females. Caucasians are affected more frequently than blacks.[126]

Hirschsprung's disease is characterized by congen-

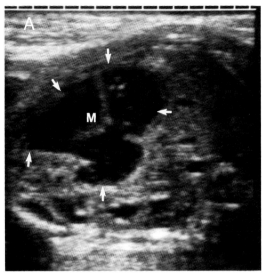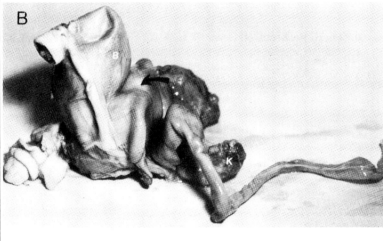

FIG 10–38.
Persistent cloaca. **A,** sonogram of pelvis at 27 weeks demonstrates a septated cystic mass *(M)* demarcated by arrows. No urinary bladder was identified, and marked oligohydramnios was present. Postmortem examination found anorectal atresia with a common chamber shared by the colon and urinary bladder. Other anomalies included absent urethra, absent seminal vesicles, absent phallus and bifid scrotum, pelvic right kidney with hydronephrosis, sacral meningocele, hypoplastic lungs, single umbilical artery, and deformation of the extremities and face. **B,** postmortem photograph of another fetus demonstrates a common chamber between the urinary bladder (B) and hindgut *(arrow).* K = kidney. (Part **B** from Lande IM, Hamilton EF: The antenatal sonographic visualization of cloacal dysgenesis. J Ultrasound Med 1986; 5:275–278. Used by permission.)

ital absence of the intramural myenteric parasympathetic nerve ganglia and sympathetic nerve plexus in a bowel segment. The rectum is invariably affected at the distal end, while the proximal extent of involvement is variable. Involvement is limited to the rectosigmoid in 74% of cases and distal to the splenic flexure in 90% of cases.[127, 131] The entire colon (total colonic aganglionosis) or distal ileum is involved in less than 10% of cases.[130]

It is generally accepted that aganglionosis results from failure of migrating ganglion cells originating from the neural crest to reach the affected bowel segment during embryologic development.[127, 132] Normal migration was previously thought to progress along vagal fibers in a cranial-caudal direction, reaching the proximal small bowel by 7 weeks and the rectosigmoid by 12 weeks.[127] However, Tam recently has shown that enteric innervation commences at both ends of the gut and proceeds toward the center in humans.[133]

Patients with Hirschsprung's disease present with symptoms of a bowel obstruction because the aganglionic bowel segment is unable to transmit a peristaltic wave. The bowel proximal to the site of aganglionosis develops hyperperistalsis, dilatation, and hypertrophy in response to the functional obstruction. Since this requires time to develop, bowel dilatation may not be present in utero or even at birth. In a survey of 1,196 patients treated in North America since 1955, only

8% of cases were diagnosed during the first month of life.[131] In a more recent review of 1,628 patients treated in Japan from 1978 to 1982, 49% of cases were diagnosed during the first month, and 70%–80% of patients were diagnosed during the neonatal period, reflecting a greater awareness of the disease in that country.[129]

The clinical diagnosis of Hirschsprung's disease previously required demonstration of absent ganglion cells on full-thickness rectal biopsies. Recently, accurate diagnoses have been made with anorectal manometry and staining of mucosal biopsies for acetylcholinesterase.[23, 128] Nerve fibers are abundantly present in the bowel wall of patients with Hirschsprung's disease, and these are rich in acetylcholinesterase.[128]

Sonographic Findings

Hirschsprung's disease rarely has been reported antenatally, even when specifically sought.[130] Wrobleski and Wesselhoeft reported a fetus with Hirschsprung's disease who demonstrated multiple segments of dilated small bowel and polyhydramnios at 33 weeks.[135] In this case, aganglionosis included the terminal ileum. Another case reported by Vermish et al. at 35 weeks demonstrated sonolucent areas that were interpreted as dilated bowel segments, although it is unclear whether these represented small bowel or large bowel.[134] Polyhydramnios also accompanied this case. Distinguishing Hirschsprung's disease from other causes of small bowel dilatation may be impossible.

Associated Anomalies

Hirschsprung's disease is usually sporadic. However, 4%–6% of cases are familial, and 2% are associated with a chromosomal disorder, usually trisomy 21.[126]

Prognosis

The major complication of Hirschsprung's disease is bowel perforation proximal to the site of obstruction. Meconium peritonitis develops in 10% of cases by the time of birth.[126] After birth, clinical symptoms include failure to pass meconium, bile-stained vomiting, and abdominal distention. Delay in the correct diagnosis can lead to necrotizing enterocolitis, bowel perforation, septicemia, and even death. The mortality rate during infancy is 20%.[126]

NON-BOWEL CYSTIC MASSES

A wide variety of cystic masses can be observed in the fetal abdomen (see Table 10–3). Excluding cystic masses arising from the urinary system (hydronephrosis, multicystic dysplastic kidneys, paranephric pseudocysts, hydroureter, distended urinary bladder) or dilated bowel (discussed above), the most common causes of intra-abdominal cystic mass include an ovarian cyst, meconium pseudocyst, enteric duplication cyst, or mesenteric cyst (lymphangioma).[186, 188] Less

common abdominal cysts that have been reported prenatally include choledochal cyst, liver or splenic cyst, hydrometrocolpos, urachal cyst, mesenchymal hamartoma, hemangioma, and varicocele dilatation of the umbilical vein.[181, 183, 184, 186, 187]

Awareness of the usual prevalence, location, and sonographic appearance of cystic malformation can help suggest the most likely diagnosis (see Table 10–3). For example, a cyst in the right upper quadrant is most likely to represent a choledochal cyst or, less likely, a hepatic cyst after excluding duodenal atresia. A cyst in the pelvis of a female fetus (Table 10–6) is most likely to be an ovarian cyst, hydrometrocolpos, or persistent cloaca (after excluding an enlarged urinary bladder). Specific types of non–urinary, non–bowel related cystic masses and the primary differential diagnoses are discussed further below.

Ovarian Cyst

Clinical and Pathologic Findings

Fetal ovarian cysts are the most common cause of an intra-abdominal cyst reported antenatally, excluding renal and bowel etiologies. These are benign, functional cysts which result from enlargement of otherwise normal follicles known to be present during the third trimester and early neonatal period.[136, 137, 139] De Sa found small follicular cysts in 34% (113 of 332) of newborns and infants who died within 28 days of life.[139] However, these cysts are usually too small (less than 1 mm) to visualize sonographically.

TABLE 10–6.

Differential Diagnosis of Pelvic Masses

Type of Anomaly	Sonographic Appearance	Amniotic Fluid	Associated Anomalies	Sex Involvement
Ovarian cyst	Usually solitary cyst, rounded margins, may have septations	Normal (increased in 10%)	Usually none—may be associated with fetal hypthyroidism, Rh sensitization	Females only
Hydrometrocolpos	Oval mass, may cause bulging of perineum	Normal	Genitourinary anomalies	Females only
Obstructive uropathy	Enlarged urinary bladder	Usually decreased	Renal dysplasia or hydronephrosis	Predominantly males
Megacystis-microcolon intestinal hypoperistalsis syndrome	Enlarged urinary bladder, hydroureters, hydronephrosis	Increased or normal	±Dilated bowel	Predominantly females
Anorectal atresia	Dilated distal colon—often U-shaped cystic mass	Decreased or normal	VACTERL syndrome, caudal regression syndrome, skeletal, CNS, gastrointestinal	Either
Persistent cloaca	Cystic mass, often septated	Decreased	Multiple anomalies— similar to anorectal atresia	Females
Urachal cyst	Smooth cystic mass	Normal	Rare	Either

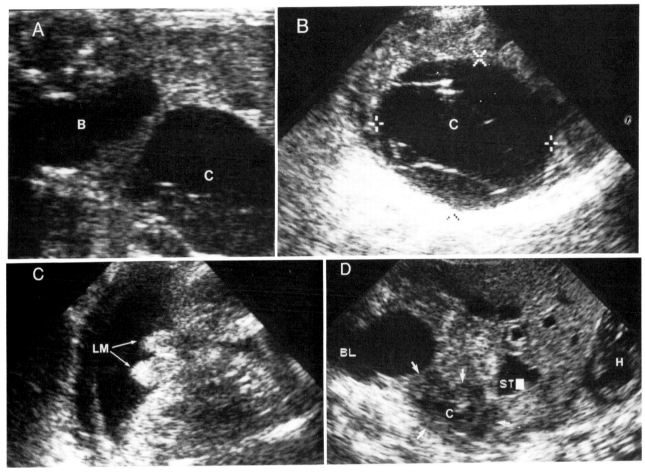

FIG 10–39.
Ovarian cyst. **A,** longitudinal sonogram at 33 weeks demonstrates a cystic mass *(C)* in the lower abdomen. *B* = urinary bladder. **B,** transverse view demonstrates smooth outer wall and several internal septations. **C,** transverse view of the perineum demonstrates female genitalia. *LM* = labia majora. **D,** follow-up sonogram 3 weeks later in coronal view demonstrates interval collapse of the cyst *(C)* outlined by arrows. Ovarian cysts usually resolve in utero or shortly after birth. *BL* = bladder; *ST* = stomach; *H* = heart.

Evidence suggests that ovarian cysts result from excessive stimulation of the fetal ovary by placental and maternal hormones. A higher prevalence of ovarian cysts has been noted in infants of mothers with diabetes, toxemia, or rhesus isoimmunization, presumably from excessive release of placental chorionic gonadotropins by the enlarged placenta. An association between ovarian cysts and fetal hypothyroidism has also been suggested on the basis of non–specific stimulation of pituitary glycoprotein hormone synthesis.[140, 142]

Sonographic Findings

Ovarian cysts frequently have been diagnosed on prenatal sonography (Figs 10–39 and 10–40). Individual case reports are common,[138, 144, 150, 152, 153] with several larger series reported by Nussbaum et al. (n=11), Lindeque et al. (n=7), Rizzo et al. (n=13), Iheda et al., and McKeener et al.[141, 143, 145, 147, 149, 150a, 152, 153] In no case has a fetal ovarian cyst been reported before the third trimester, even when an earlier sonogram was performed.[150] This fact probably reflects insufficient hormonal stimulation during early pregnancy.

The sonographic appearance of an ovarian cyst is variable depending on its size and complications of torsion or hemorrhage. An uncomplicated ovarian cyst appears as a unilocular cystic mass, occasionally with internal septations. Although usually localized to the pelvis or lower abdomen (see Fig 10–39),[151] some ovarian cysts can become very large (8–10 cm) and extend to the upper abdomen (see Figs 10–39 and 10–40). Most cysts are unilateral, although several cases of bilateral ovarian cysts have also been reported.[142, 143] Polyhydramnios has been reported in at least 10% of cases, probably secondary to extrinsic small bowel obstruction.[141, 150a]

When complicated by torsion or hemorrhage, ovar-

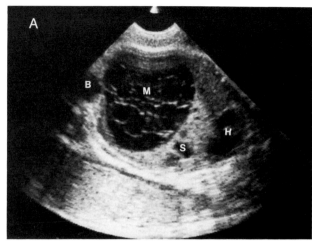

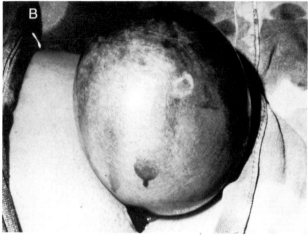

FIG 10–40.
Ovarian cyst. **A,** coronal sonogram at 35 weeks demonstrates a large septated mass *(M)* extending from the urinary bladder *(B)* to the inferior surface of the liver. *S* = stomach; *H* = heart. **B,** photograph of the specimen at the time of surgery demonstrates the smooth surface of this large ovarian cyst. (From Nguyen KT, Reid RL, Sauerbrei E: Antenatal sonographic detection of a fetal theca lutein cyst: A clue to maternal diabetes mellitus. J Ultrasound Med 1986; 5:665–667. Used by permission.)

ian cysts may appear complex or even solid.[149, 150a] Complicated ovarian cyst may also demonstrate a fluid-debris level, a retracting clot, and internal septa. The wall may be echogenic from dystrophic calcification associated with infarction. Ascites has been reported in association with ruptured ovarian cyst.[149]

The differential diagnoses for a cystic mass in the fetal pelvis or lower abdomen is shown in Table 10–6. A mesenteric or enteric duplication cyst may appear indistinguishable from an ovarian cyst.[149] Identification of male gender would exclude ovarian cyst or hydrometrocolpos and make persistent cloaca or megacystic-microcolon intestinal hypoperistalsis (MMIHS) highly unlikely. Other considerations in both sexes in-

clude urachal cyst, mesenteric cyst, or enteric duplication cyst. If the urinary bladder is not identified separate from the mass, other considerations for a cystic pelvic mass should include obstructive uropathy, MMIHS syndrome, and persistent cloaca. A complex or solid mass similar in appearance to a complicated ovarian cyst can also be differentiated from a meconium pseudocyst.

Associated Findings
Few other anomalies have been associated with a fetal ovarian cyst. As mentioned, fetal hypothyroidism has been observed.[142] Agenesis of the corpus callosum was reported in one fetus, but this probably was unrelated to the ovarian cyst.[151] Cystadenoma rarely has been reported in ovarian cysts during the first year of life, but has not been reported antenatally.[146]

Prognosis
The majority of ovarian cysts undergo spontaneous regression and involution following delivery or even in utero (see Fig 10–39). Birth dystocia and respiratory distress have been reported from very large cysts.[137] However, fetuses with cysts as large as 10 cm have been successfully delivered vaginally without complication. Some authors have recommended elective cesarean section if the cyst is large, whereas others have suggested a vaginal delivery unless dystocia develops. To avoid potential complications, such as torsion and hemorrhage, antenatal percutaneous aspiration of ovarian cysts has been proposed. Other authors suggest that fetal ovarian cysts should be managed conservatively by observation alone.[145]

Hydrometrocolpos

Clinical and Pathologic Findings
Congenital hydrometrocolpos is rare, occurring in less than 1 in 16,000 female births.[162] By contrast, hematometrocolpos that develops at puberty is relatively common with a prevalence of 1 in 1,000.[158]

Development of hydrometrocolpos requires two conditions: proximal hypersecretion of reproductive glands and vaginal obstruction.[156, 163] Glandular secretion responds to maternal hormonal stimulation, while vaginal obstruction results from abnormal recanalization of the cervix or vagina. Three types of obstruction are recognized:

1. Hymenal obstruction.
2. Midplane transverse septum.
3. Vaginal atresia.

Sonographic Findings

Hydrometrocolpos has been reported as a cystic (Fig 10–41) or solid mass (Fig 10–42) in the pelvis of a female fetus.[154, 155, 160] Like ovarian cysts, no case has been reported before the third trimester, probably because maternal hormonal stimulation is insufficient for glandular secretion before this age. Hydronephrosis may result from ureteral obstruction by the enlarged uterus. Peritoneal calcification has been observed in a single infant with hydrometrocolpos, presumably because aseptic peritonitis resulted from retrograde flow of uterine secretions through the fallopian tube.[189]

The primary differential considerations for a cystic pelvic mass in a female fetus include a bladder or ure-

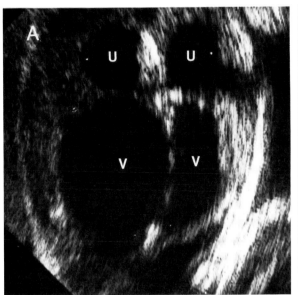

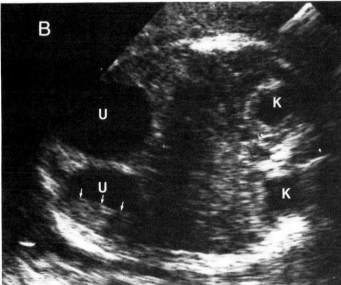

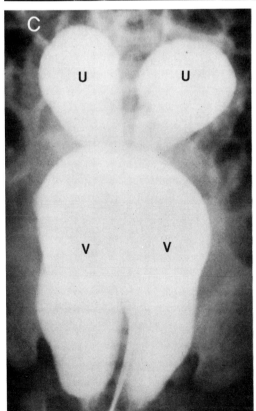

FIG 10–41.
Duplicated uterus and hydrometrocolpos. **A,** coronal sonogram at 35.5 weeks demonstrates distention and duplication of both the vagina *(V)* and uterus *(U)*. **B,** transverse scan through the upper pelvis demonstrates two dilated uterine cavities *(U)* and a fluid-debris level within the more dependent cavity *(small arrows)*. Moderate pelvocaliectasis is also noted of both kidneys *(K)*. **C,** hysterosalpingogram one day after birth confirms dilated and duplicated vagina *(V)* and uterus *(U)*. (From Russ PD, Zavitz WR, Pretorius DH, et al: Hydrometrocolpos, uterine didelphys, and septate vagina: An antenatal sonographic diagnosis. J Ultrasound Med 1986; 5:211–213. Used by permission.)

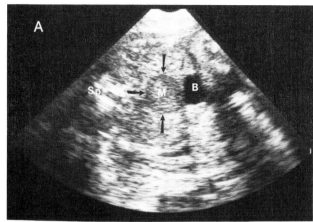

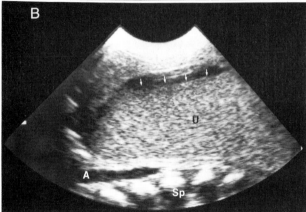

FIG 10–42.
Hydrometrocolpos. **A,** transverse sonogram at 30 weeks demonstrates a mass (*M,* delineated by arrows) just posterior to the urinary bladder *(B).* The differential diagnosis for such a mass includes meconium pseudocyst, hemorrhagic ovarian cyst, enteric duplication cyst, or bowel. *Sp* = spine. **B,** postnatal sonogram of the uterus in longitudinal plane demonstrates dilated uterus *(U)* and fluid-debris level *(small arrows).* Imperforate hymen was found with 50 ml of milky viscous material within the uterus. *A* = aorta; *Sp* = spine. (From Hill SJ, Hirsch JH: Sonographic detection of fetal hydrometrocolpos. J Ultrasound Med 1985; 4:323–325. Used by permission.)

teral abnormality, dilated bowel, ovarian cyst, or mesenteric or enteric cyst (see Tables 10–3 and 10–6). A specific diagnosis of hydrometrocolpos has been suggested when the mass bulges through the perineum.[154] Hydrometrocolpos also can be suggested when associated with uterine duplication anomalies (Fig 10–41).[160]

Associated Anomalies

Hydrometrocolpos is commonly associated with uterine duplication anomalies. Other malformations that may be associated with hydrometrocolpos include persistent urogenital sinus, anorectal atresia, renal agenesis, polycystic kidneys, esophageal atresia, duode-

nal atresia, and caudal regression. A triad of hydrometrocolpos, polydactyly, and congenital heart disease has been referred to as the McKusick-Kaufman syndrome and is inherited as an autosomal recessive trait.[157, 159] Associated anomalies are more likely when the site of obstruction is high (cervical or high vaginal).[162]

Prognosis

In a review of 44 infants with hydrometrocolpos, 8 died (18%).[161] The prognosis depends primarily on the presence and severity of associated disorders. An excellent outcome can be anticipated when abnormalities are confined to the uterus and vagina. Surgical intervention is necessary to relieve the obstruction.

Enteric Duplication Cyst

Clinical and Pathologic Findings

Enteric duplication cysts may develop anywhere along the course of the digestive tract, although the stomach is the least frequent site of involvement. Duplication cysts are located on the mesenteric side of the intestine and do not usually communicate with the normal gut. Males are affected twice as often as females.[62]

The two most accepted theories of embryogenesis regarding enteric duplications cysts involve (1) faulty recanalization of the gut lumen, and (2) failure of separation of the notochord from the endoderm. The latter theory presupposes transient attachment of the endodermal roof with the notochord during the fifth week. This idea is supported by the association of enteric duplication cysts with vertebral anomalies.[62]

Sonographic Findings

Duplication cysts of the stomach and ileum rarely have been reported on prenatal sonography as cystic intra-abdominal masses.[164, 165] The differential diagnoses for such a finding include mesenteric or omental cyst, ovarian cyst, urachal cyst, or hepatic cyst. Of course, renal cysts and dilated bowel segments should be excluded whenever an abdominal cystic mass is identified.

Associated Anomalies

Extra-intestinal anomalies are uncommonly associated with intra-abdominal enteric cysts, although vertebral defects may accompany esophageal duplication cysts.

Prognosis

About 85% of patients with enteric duplication cysts eventually become symptomatic from intussusception, pain, or bleeding.[62] Surgical resection is curative.

Mesenteric, Omental, and Retroperitoneal Cysts

Clinical and Pathologic Findings

The precise prevalence of mesenteric, omental, and retroperitoneal cysts is unknown, since they often are asymptomatic. These cysts usually represent abdominal lymphangiomas, although other etiologies have been identified.[170] The most common location is the small bowel mesentery, followed by the large bowel mesentery, omentum, and retroperitoneum. They typically are solitary, unilocular, or multilocular cysts lined by a layer of endothelial cells. The fluid may be serous, chylous, or even bloody.[169]

Sonographic Findings

The sonographic findings of mesenteric, omental, and retroperitoneal cysts are variable. They may be multiseptated or unilocular, small or large. Although typically sonolucent,[166] they may appear solid when hemorrhagic.[167] They are usually located in the mid-abdomen within the mesentery, omentum, or retroperitoneum, but unusual sites of involvement include the kidneys, spleen, liver, and other abdominal organs. Mesenteric and omental cysts are characteristically mobile, so they may fluctuate in position. An enteric duplication cyst or ovarian cyst may be indistinguishable from a mesenteric cyst.

Associated Anomalies

There are no significant anomalies associated with mesenteric cysts.

Prognosis

When symptomatic, these cysts should be surgically removed. Post-surgical recurrence is more likely for retroperitoneal cysts than for omental or mesenteric cysts.[168]

Choledochal Cyst

Clinical and Pathologic Findings

Choledochal cysts are rare.[170, 171] About one third of reported cases have been in Japanese people and, in this population, the female to male ratio is nearly equal. By comparison, females are affected four to five times more frequently than males among caucasians.[175]

Three types of choledochal cysts have been described (Fig 10–43).[175] Type I is a fusiform, sac-like

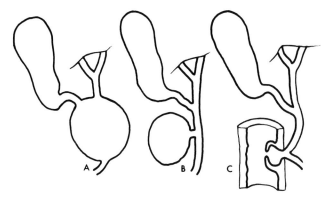

FIG 10–43.
Line drawing of types of choledochal cysts. Type I *(A)* is by far the most common and the type seen sonographically. (From Gray SW, Skandalakis JE: *Embryology for Surgeons*, Philadelphia, WB Saunders Co, 1972. Used by permission.)

dilatation of the common bile duct; type II is a diverticular dilatation of the common bile duct; and type III is a dilatation of the distal, intramural portion of the common bile duct (choledochocele).[171, 175] Other authors would add type IV as cystic dilatation of intrahepatic biliary ducts (Caroli's disease). Type I is by far the most common and the only type that has been reported on prenatal sonograms. Histologically, the cyst wall is thickened and fibrotic with dense connective tissue.

The pathogenesis of a choledochal cyst has remained speculative. Congenital weakness of the bile duct wall has been proposed. Dilatation due to obstruction also has been suggested, but this has not been widely accepted.[175] Recently, it has been shown that affected patients often have a long common channel of the biliary and main pancreatic ducts and that reflux of pancreatic juice into the biliary tree may be a causative factor.[179]

Sonographic Findings

A choledochal cyst can be identified as a simple, cystic mass in the upper abdomen or right upper quadrant (Fig 10–44)[172–174, 176, 178] Other considerations for a cystic mass in the upper abdomen include an enteric duplication cyst; congenital liver cyst; gallbladder duplication; situs inversus, in which case the "cyst" represents the fluid-filled stomach; and a distended duodenum from duodenal atresia. A definitive diagnosis of a choledochal cyst has been made prenatally by showing that biliary ducts lead to the cystic mass.[173] The earliest reported case to date was seen at 25 weeks.[176] In another case, the cyst was demonstrated at 31 weeks, but a sonogram 4–5 weeks earlier reportedly was normal.[176]

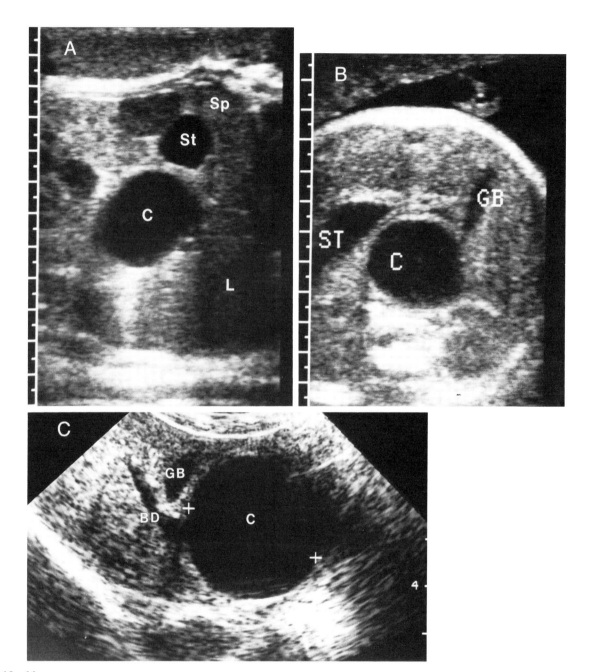

FIG 10–44.
Choledochal cyst. **A,** coronal sonogram at 36 weeks demonstrates a cyst *(C)* in the mid-upper abdomen that is separate from the stomach *(St)*. *Sp* = spleen; L = liver. **B,** transverse scan clearly shows separation of the cyst *(C)* from the stomach *(S)* and its location near the neck of the gallbladder *(GB)*. This appearance should be distinguished from duodenal atresia, in which case the cystic mass communicates with the stomach (see Figs 10–15 and 10–16). **C,** postnatal sonogram shows communication of the cyst *(C)* with the bile duct *(BD)* near the neck of the gallbladder *(GB)*.

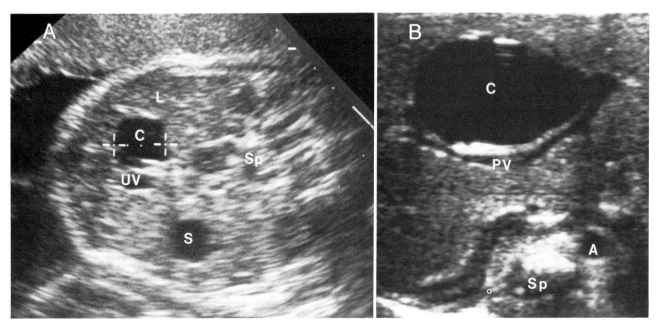

FIG 10–45.
Hepatic cyst. **A,** transverse sonogram at 36 weeks demonstrates a cyst *(C)* within the liver *(L)*. *S* = stomach; *UV* = umbilical vein; *Sp* = spine. **B,** postnatal transverse sonogram shows the location of the cyst *(C)* within the liver anterior to the right portal vein *(PV)*. No other abnormalities were identified in this infant. *Sp* = spine; *A* = aorta.

Associated Anomalies

Few other anomalies have been associated with a choledochal cyst, and these usually relate to abnormalities of the biliary tract.[175]

Prognosis

Unless correctly recognized and surgically removed following delivery, choledochal cysts can lead to complications of cholestasis, cholangitis, biliary cirrhosis, and portal hypertension. An increased incidence of bile duct cancer has also been noted. Clinical symptoms frequently are delayed until the second or third decade of life, at which time the mortality is high. The preferred surgical treatment is now total or subtotal resection of the cyst with Roux-en-Y hepaticojejunostomy.[180]

Liver Cyst

Clinical and Pathologic Findings

Congenital liver cyst is a rare disorder that possibly results from interruption of the intrahepatic biliary system.[181] Females are affected four times more frequently than males.[126] The cysts are most frequently located at the inferior margin of the right lobe. Histologically, they are lined with an inner layer of cuboidal epithelial cells or a dense fibrous layer.

Sonographic Findings

Several solitary liver cysts have been reported prenatally[4, 181] and these have been described as intrahepatic cystic masses (Fig 10–45). About 10% are multilocular.[175] Less likely considerations for a cystic mass located in the liver include cystic hepatoblastoma, mesenchymal hamartoma, hemangioendothelioma, and Caroli's disease. Splenic cysts have been identified even less frequently than liver cysts.[182, 217]

Associated Anomalies

There are no known associated anomalies with congenital solitary liver cysts.

Prognosis

Many liver cysts remain asymptomatic throughout life and are noted only as an incidental finding at autopsy. Infection, hemorrhage, and torsion of the cysts are potential complications.[126]

INTRA-ABDOMINAL CALCIFICATION

Intra-abdominal calcification or echogenic areas arise from a variety of sites (Table 10–7). These can be categorized by location as:

1. Peritoneal.
2. Intraluminal intestinal.

TABLE 10–7.

Causes of Echogenic Areas in the Fetal Abdomen

Calcification
    Peritoneal calcification
        Meconium peritonitis
        Hydrometrocolpos*
    Intraluminal meconium calcification
        Anorectal atresia
        Small bowel atresia
        Rarely isolated without bowel obstruction
    Parenchymal
        Liver
        Splenic
        Adrenal
        Complicated ovarian cyst (rare)
    Cholelithiasis—gallbladder
    Non-calcified
        Echogenic meconium

*Calcification from hydrometrocolpos not yet reported in utero.

---

3. Parenchymal (liver, splenic, adrenal, etc.).
4. Vascular.
5. Biliary.

It is important to distinguish calcification from simply areas of increased echogenicity which are frequently observed in the fetal abdomen (see Meconium ileus above). For this reason, acoustic shadowing should be demonstrated before calcification is reliably diagnosed. It is also important to define precisely the location of calcification and to search for other possible abnormalities.

Peritoneal calcification resulting from meconium peritonitis is probably the most common cause of intra-abdominal calcification. Due to its frequency and clinical importance, meconium peritonitis is discussed in detail below. Peritoneal calcification has also been reported in a neonate with vaginal obstruction and hydrometrocolpos,[189] although this has not been reported prenatally. Peritoneal and bladder wall calcification has also been described in association with obstruction of the urinary bladder related to posterior urethral valves.[191]

Meconium Peritonitis

Clinical and Pathologic Findings

Meconium peritonitis is a sterile chemical peritonitis resulting from in utero bowel perforation that nearly always involves the small bowel (Fig 10–46).[202] Neonatal studies suggest that the prevalence of meconium peritonitis is 1 in 30,000 live-births, although this probably underestimates its true prevalence in utero.

Approximately half the cases of meconium peritonitis are associated with an underlying bowel disorder, the most common being volvulus, atresia, or meconium ileus.[202] Bowel dilatation probably leads to vascular impairment of the bowel wall, necrosis, and perforation in these cases, although atresia may be a consequence rather than a cause of vascular ischemia. Those cases of meconium peritonitis without intestinal obstruction probably result from primary "idiopathic" vascular impairment.[209] Occlusion and thrombosis of mesenteric arteries are frequently demonstrated on pathologic examination in these cases.[202, 209] The bowel is particularly prone to ischemia in utero because any cause of fetal or neonatal hypoxia leads to a selective decrease in mesenteric blood flow.[199]

Whatever the underlying cause, meconium peritonitis is preceded by bowel perforation and extrusion of meconium and digestive enzymes into the peritoneal cavity where they incite an intense chemical peritonitis and secondary inflammatory response. Calcification may develop within days histologically, although radiographic evidence of calcification usually requires 1–2 weeks.[93, 200, 207] Over time, the inflammatory response may seal the perforation spontaneously.

Sonographic Findings

Prenatal sonographic findings of meconium peritonitis are variable depending on the extent of meconium leakage, the time interval since the bowel perforation, and the underlying bowel disorder. Peritoneal calcification is the most common and characteristic finding of meconium peritonitis on both prenatal sonography (Fig 10–47) and postnatal radiography.[203]

MECONIUM PERITONITIS

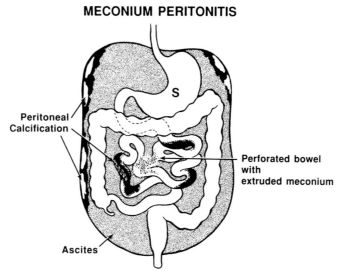

FIG 10–46.
Schematic drawing of meconium peritonitis. In utero bowel perforation results in extravasation of meconium. A chemical peritonitis stimulates development of peritoneal calcifications and, frequently, ascites.

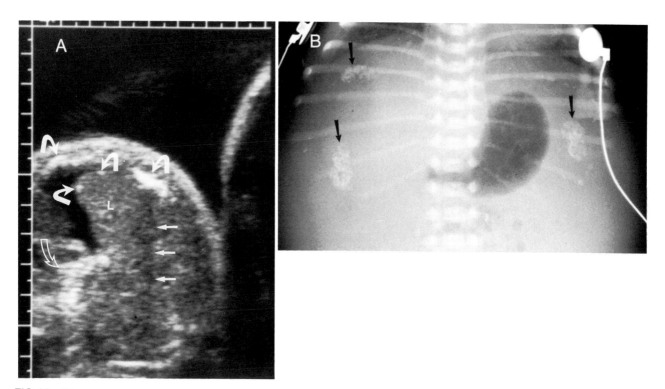

FIG 10–47.
Meconium peritonitis. **A,** transverse sonogram of the abdomen at 29 weeks demonstrates multiple calcific foci lining the visceral and parietal peritoneum *(curved arrows)* and centrally, near the root of the mesentery *(open arrow)*. Acoustic shadowing is seen from a large calcific deposit on the liver *(L)* margin. Also note polyhydramnios. **B,** postnatal radiograph shows multiple peritoneal calcifications *(arrows* indicate the largest foci). The infant did well and did not require surgery. (From Foster MA, Nyberg DA, Mahony BS, et al: Meconium peritonitis: Prenatal sonographic findings and their clinical significance. Radiology 1987; 165:661–665. Used by permission.)

Such calcification may occur in any part of the peritoneal cavity including the parietal peritoneum overlying the liver, the visceral peritoneum in the mesentery, or through the process vaginalis into the scrotum.[203, 211] Other sonographic findings of meconium peritonitis include meconium pseudocyst (14%), ascites (54%), and bowel dilatation (27%).[203] Polyhydramnios is present in the majority of cases (64%).

Peritoneal calcification of meconium peritonitis should be distinguished from intraluminal meconium calcification or inspissated meconium (see Figs 10–23 and 10–35).[192] Calcification of meconium peritonitis is usually linear in appearance and is often associated with ascites. By comparison, intraluminal meconium calcification appears as punctate foci that can be localized to the bowel lumen. Intra-abdominal calcifications should also be distinguished from simple echogenic "masses" in the fetal abdomen, which are thought to represent inspissated meconium. This finding is usually transient and is of no clinical significance, but it has occasionally been associated with other disorders including meconium ileus and cystic fibrosis (see Meconium Ileus above).

A meconium pseudocyst results from a contained bowel perforation (Fig 10–48).[201, 205, 210] The sonographic appearance is characteristic, with a hypoechoic mass (extra-luminal meconium) surrounded by an echogenic, calcified wall. Acoustic shadowing from the

echogenic wall may not be readily apparent. An evolving meconium pseudocyst may be difficult to distinguish from other intra-abdominal masses, including hemorrhagic ovarian cysts. An unusual presentation of meconium pseudocyst has been described as simulating a sacrococcygeal teratoma.[206]

Ascites is commonly demonstrated in association with meconium peritonitis, presumably reflecting the intense inflammatory response induced by the chemical peritonitis. The inflammatory response can also cause abdominal wall thickening and, in conjunction with ascites, mimic fetal hydrops.[198] Because it may be the primary or only sonographic abnormality, meconium peritonitis should be considered whenever fetal ascites is demonstrated. Echogenic ascites should suggest intraperitoneal meconium from a recent bowel perforation, in which case calcification may be absent (Fig 10–49).[203, 204] Serial sonograms may show development of characteristic peritoneal calcifications.[211]

The presence of bowel dilatation should suggest an associated bowel obstruction, most commonly from jejunoileal atresia, volvulus, or meconium ileus.[203] Approximately half of all cases of meconium peritonitis are associated with an underlying bowel obstruction.

Associated Anomalies

The underlying cause of meconium peritonitis can be divided into three major clinical categories:

1. Idiopathic.
2. Meconium ileus with cystic fibrosis.
3. Other causes of bowel obstruction, primarily jejunoileal atresia or volvulus.

As previously stated, approximately half the cases of meconium peritonitis are idiopathic in origin.

Meconium ileus with cystic fibrosis has been reported in 15% to 40% of infants diagnosed with meconium peritonitis in neonatal studies,[94] although this association is apparently less common in utero.[203] In their review of 35 fetuses with meconium peritonitis detected prenatally, Foster et al. noted that less than 10% of infants proved to have cystic fibrosis.[203] Furthermore, the presence of sonographically detectable peritoneal calcification was less frequently associated with cystic fibrosis (none of 31 cases) than was meconium peritonitis lacking detectable calcification (2 of 4 cases). However, another fetus with cystic fibrosis who was not included in this review demonstrated a meconium pseudocyst with a surrounding calcified wall.[201]

Some neonatal studies support the contention that radiographically visible calcifications are unlikely to be associated with cystic fibrosis, although the reason is

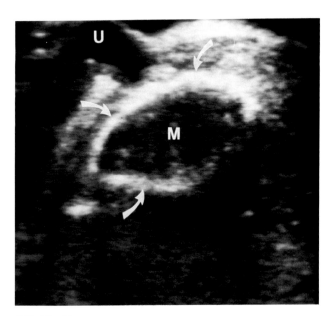

FIG 10–48.
Meconium pseudocyst. Longitudinal sonogram at 28 weeks demonstrates an oval mass *(M)* surrounded by a calcified wall *(arrows)*. A contained perforation with meconium pseudocyst from an ileal perforation was found at the time of surgery. *U* = umbilical cord insertion site into anterior abdominal wall.

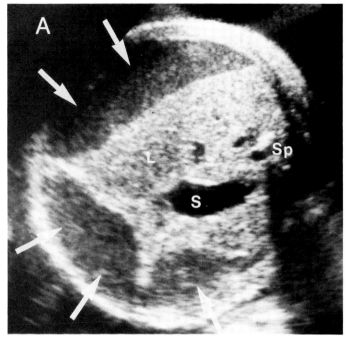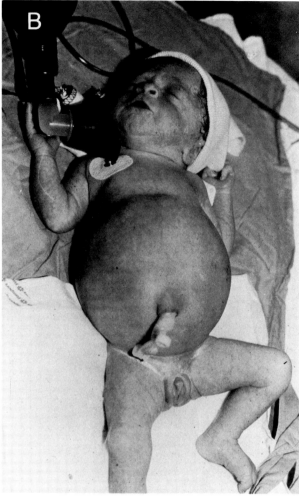

FIG 10–49.
Acute meconium peritonitis. **A,** transverse sonogram at 37 weeks shows echogenic ascites *(arrows)* compressing the liver *(L)* but no calcifications. Calcification may be absent when the time of perforation has been recent. *S* = stomach; *Sp* = spine. **B,** postnatal photograph shows marked distension of the abdomen. Ileal volvulus with acute perforation was found at the time of surgical correction. (From Foster MA, Nyberg DA, Mahony BS, et al: Meconium peritonitis: Prenatal sonographic findings and their clinical significance. Radiology 1987; 165:661–665. Used by permission.)

unclear.[200] Some authors have postulated that pancreatic enzymes, which are deficient in 80% of patients with cystic fibrosis, may be necessary for calcification to occur.[200] Another possibility is that the abnormally thick meconium which is so characteristic of meconium ileus is less likely to spill into the peritoneum following a bowel perforation. Therefore, a contained perforation secondary to meconium ileus might result in fewer peritoneal calcifications.[203]

Prognosis

The prognosis for fetuses with meconium peritonitis varies with the underlying etiology. In general, the prognosis is excellent following surgical resection of the perforated bowel segment. Some infants may not even require surgical intervention, presumably because the perforation seals spontaneously.[203]

On the other hand, those infants with meconium ileus and cystic fibrosis as the underlying etiology have a poor long-term prognosis, with complications of pancreatic insufficiency, multiple respiratory infections, chronic lung disease, and gastrointestinal disturbances.[94]

Sonographic findings occasionally may suggest the underlying etiology of meconium peritonitis (see Associated anomalies). However, until a specific biochemical or chromosomal marker for cystic fibrosis becomes available, attempting to distinguish meconium ileus from other causes of meconium peritonitis in individual cases undoubtedly will remain a troublesome clinical problem.

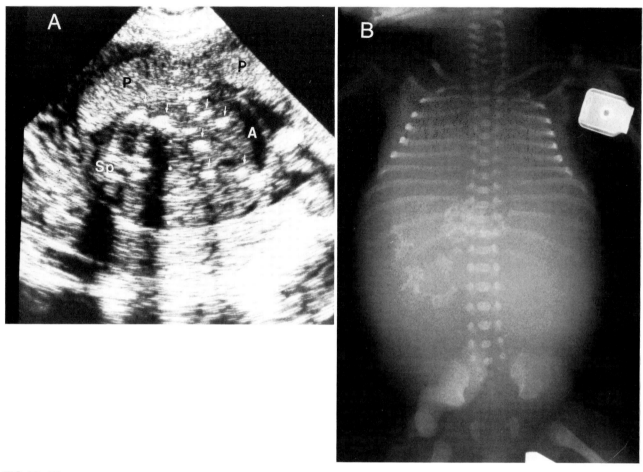

FIG 10–50.
Ischemic hepatic necrosis. **A,** transverse sonogram demonstrates multiple calcified foci *(small arrows)* throughout the liver. A small amount of ascites *(A)* is also noted. *Sp* = spine; *P* = placenta. **B,** postnatal radiograph shows multiple flocular calcifications throughout the liver. Ischemic hepatic necrosis was found at necropsy. This is a very unusual cause of intra-abdominal calcification. (From Nguyen DL, Leonard JC: Ischemic hepatic necrosis: A cause for fetal liver calcification. AJR 1986; 147:596–597. Used by permission.)

Other Causes of Abdominal Calcification

In addition to peritoneal calcification, intra-abdominal calcification may be located within the bowel, other abdominal organs, or within vascular structures. Intraluminal intestinal calcification is nearly always associated with bowel obstruction, (see Figs 10–23 and 10–35)[188, 190, 195] although exceptions have been reported.[192, 197] Possible causes of bowel obstruction include anorectal atresia (see Anorectal Atresia above), multiple bowel atresia, small bowel stenosis, volvulus, persistent cloaca, and total colonic aganglionosis.[188, 190, 195, 196] The calcification may be located either proximal or distal to the site of obstruction.

Parenchymal calcifications are primarily confined to the liver, although adrenal calcification potentially could result from infection or neuroblastoma. Widespread liver calcification should suggest a transplacental infection from varicella or the TORCH complex (toxoplasmosis, rubella, cytomegalovirus, or herpes simplex virus).[194] Liver calcifications also have been described in utero from ischemic hepatic necrosis (Fig 10–50).[193] A growing number of anecdotal reports suggest that small solitary liver calcification is not infrequently observed (Fig 10–51), and such a finding probably is of no clinical significance.[4]

LIVER, SPLEEN, AND BILIARY ABNORMALITIES

Liver and Spleen

Major malformations of the spleen and liver are uncommon compared to other abdominal organs. Suspected hepatomegaly and splenomegaly can be compared with normal measurements which have been reported (Table 10–8).[221, 224] Hepatomegaly and spleno-

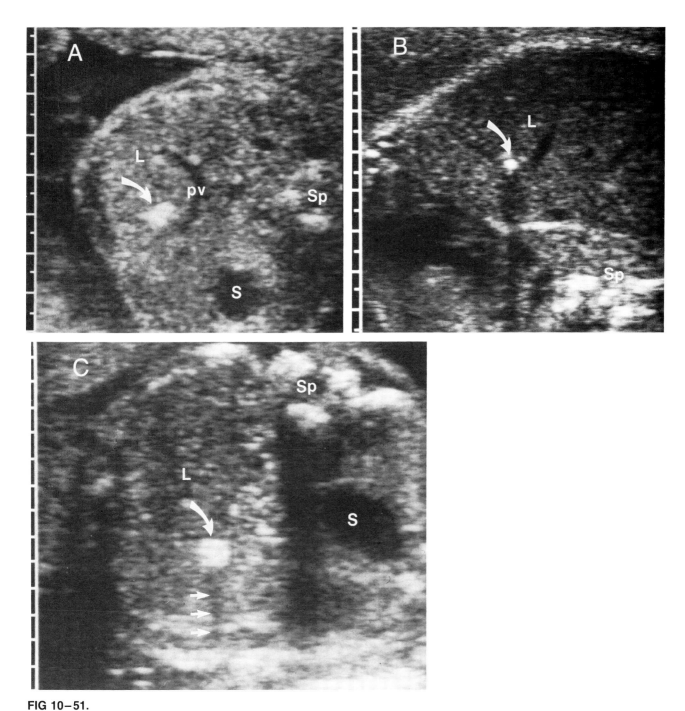

FIG 10–51.
Isolated liver calcification. **A,** transverse sonogram at 27 weeks demonstrates a single echogenic focus *(arrow)* within the liver *(L).* *Sp* = spine; *S* = stomach; *pv* = portal vein. **B,** another view shows slight acoustic shadowing *(small arrows)* emanating from the calcified focus *(curved arrow).* L = liver, S = stomach; Sp = spine. **C,** follow-up sonogram at 35 weeks, in oblique plane, shows persistence of the calcified focus *(arrow)* in the liver *(L).* No other abnormalities were identified on sonography or were found after birth. Such isolated liver calcifications appear to be of no clinical significance. *Sp* = spine.

TABLE 10–8.

Ultrasound Measurements* of the Fetal Liver From 20 Weeks' Gestation to Term†

Gestational Age (wk)	No. of Measurements	Arithmetic Mean (mm)	± 2 SD‡ (mm)
20	8	27.3	6.4
21	2	28.0	1.5
22	4	30.6	6.7
23	13	30.9	5.3
24	10	32.9	6.7
25	14	33.6	5.3
26	10	35.7	6.3
27	20	36.6	3.3
28	14	38.4	4.0
29	13	39.1	5.0
30	10	38.7	5.0
31	13	39.6	5.7
32	11	42.7	7.5
33	14	43.8	6.6
34	11	44.8	7.1
35	14	47.8	9.1
36	10	49.0	8.4
37	10	52.0	6.8
38	12	52.9	4.2
39	5	55.4	6.7
40	1	59.0	
41	2	49.3	2.4

*Mean length ± 2 SD.
†From Vintzileos AM, Neckles S, Campbell WA, et al: Fetal liver ultrasound measurements during normal pregnancy. *Obstet Gynecol* 1985; 66:477–480. Used by permission.
‡SD = standard deviation.

TABLE 10–10.

Causes of Fetal Splenomegaly

Immune hydrops
Non–immune hydrops
Infection
Inborn errors of metabolism
   Gaucher's
   Niemann-Pick's
   Wolman's
Leukemia

relatively rare. Both liver cysts and splenic cysts rarely have been detected in utero.[181, 217] Hemangioma of the liver is a congenital vascular malformation composed of innumerable capillary channels.[212] Hepatomegaly, anemia, and congestive heart failure may complicate large liver hemangiomas;[223] although histologically "benign", the mortality rate is high (81%) when congestive heart failure develops from arteriovenous shunting. The mortality rate can be reduced to 29% with medical, radiation, and surgical therapy.[212, 219] Several cases of cavernous hemangioma have been detected antenatally (Fig 10–53).[4, 218, 220] The sonographic appearance may be hyperechoic, hypoechoic, or mixed. Calcification occasionally may occur.

Tumors that may occur in the liver include heman-

megaly may be caused by a variety of disorders during the neonatal period (Tables 10–9 and 10–10), but have been infrequently recognized prenatally (Fig 10–52).[221, 224]

Causes of hepatosplenomegaly include immune or non-immune hydrops, hemolytic anemia, congenital infection (toxoplasmosis, cytomegalovirus, syphillis and rubella), and metabolic disorders (hypothyroidism).[215] Hepatomegaly is a constant feature of the Beckwith-Weidemann syndrome and cerebro-hepato-renal syndrome (Zellweger syndrome).[225] Extramedullary hematopoiesis occasionally has been reported to produce an enlarged, heterogeneous appearance of the liver.[4]

Liver and splenic masses in the neonatal period are

TABLE 10–9.

Causes of Fetal Hepatomegaly

Immune hydrops
Non–immune hydrops
Congenital infection
Hypothyroidism
Beckwith-Weidemann syndrome
Zellweger (cerebro-hepatorenal) syndrome

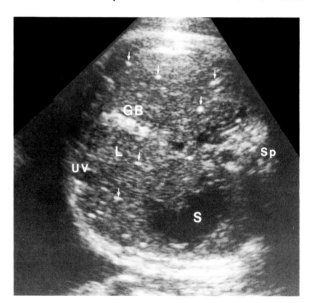

FIG 10–52.
Viral hepatitis. Transverse sonogram at 36 weeks shows an enlarged liver *(L)* that contains multiple echogenic foci ("starry sky"), an appearance that has been associated with hepatitis in adults. The gallbladder *(GB)* is also filled with echogenic material that was thought to represent sludge rather than stones. The fetus demonstrated an unusual intracranial appearance consistent with a destructive process on other views. At birth, a severe disseminated varicella infection was found. *S* = stomach, *SP* = spine; *UV* = umbilical vein.

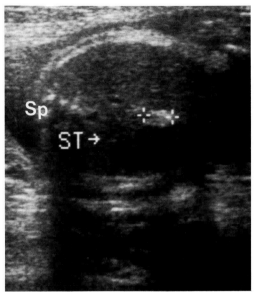

FIG 10–53.
Liver hemangioma. Transverse sonogram demonstrates an echogenic focus (outlined by graticules) within the liver reported to be a hemangioma. However, liver calcification could demonstrate a similar appearance. *ST* = stomach. *Sp* = spine. (From Hill LM. Sonographic detection of fetal gastrointestinal anomalies. Ultrasound Quarterly 1988: 6:35–37. Used by permission.)

gioendothelioma (Fig 10–54), mesenchymal hamartoma, and liver metastases.[213, 214, 222] Mesenchymal hamartoma is a developmental abnormality characterized by edematous, acellular connective tissue and fluid-filled spaces lacking a cellular lining; it is histologically similar to lymphangioma. On sonography, mesenchymal hamartoma typically appears as a multilobulated cystic mass, with most tumors diagnosed before 2 years of age.[216, 222]

Hepatoblastoma is the most common malignant tumor of the liver during the neonatal period and potentially is detectable by prenatal ultrasound.[213] Hepatoblastomas are extremely vascular, and rupture of the tumor may occur. They typically are solid and strongly echogenic on sonography. Calcifications may be demonstrated. Similar findings may be due to congenital neuroblastoma.[213] Hepatoblastomas are rarely cystic, and because of their highly vascular nature, demonstra-

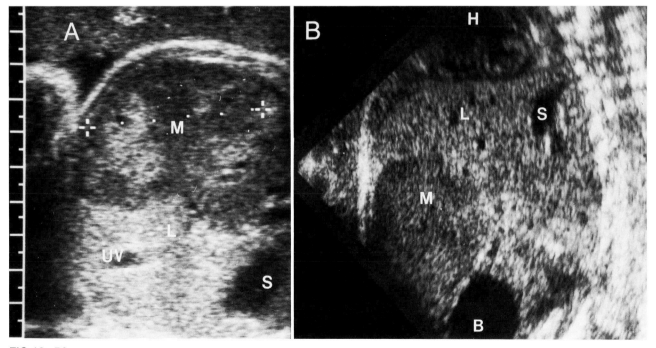

FIG 10–54.
Liver tumor. **A,** transverse cranial sonogram at 32 weeks shows a large hypoechoic mass *(M)* replacing much of the right lobe of the liver *(L)*. *UV* = umbilical vein; *S* = stomach. **B,** coronal scan of the same fetus demonstrates the mass *(M)* within the enlarged liver *(L)*. The mass proved to be a juvenile hemangioendothelioma. *S* = stomach; *B* = bladder; *H* = heart. (Courtesy of Fred N Hegge, MD, Emanuel Hospital, Portland, OR.)

FIG 10–55.
Normal gallbladder. Sonogram at 20 weeks demonstrates a large gallbladder *(GB)* relative to the stomach *(ST)*. This finding should not be mistaken for duodenal atresia, choledochal cyst, or other cystic mass.

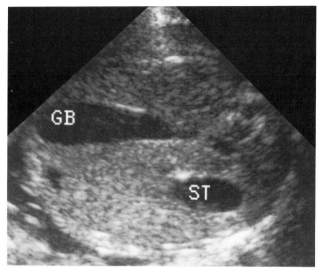

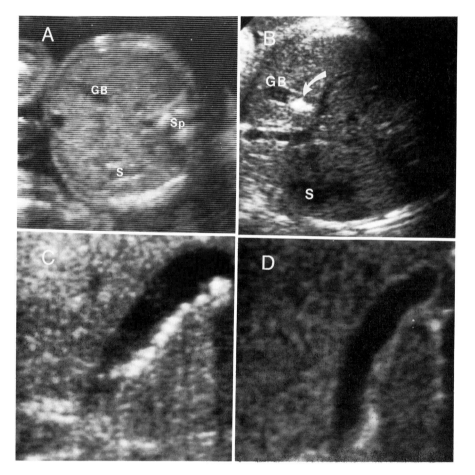

FIG 10–56.
Gallstones. **A,** transverse scan at 24 weeks shows a normal gallbladder *(GB)*. *Sp* = spine; *S* = stomach. **B,** repeat sonogram at 37 weeks shows echogenic foci *(arrow)* within the gallbladder *(GB)* consistent with gallstones. *S* = stomach. **C,** postnatal sonogram at 3 days of age demonstrates persistence of gallstones. **D,** follow-up examination at 43 days of age shows spontaneous resolution of gallstones. (From Klingensmith WC II, Cioffi-Ragan DT: Fetal gallstones. Radiology 1988; 167:143–144. Used by permission.)

tion of high arterial flow should be possible on Doppler studies.

Gallbladder Abnormalities

Agenesis of the gallbladder occurs in about 20% of patients with biliary atresia. Absence of the gallbladder also can occur in association with polysplenia and rare multiple anomaly syndromes. Failure to visualize the gallbladder in association with one of these disorders has not yet been specifically reported prenatally. On the other hand, the gallbladder may occasionally appear quite prominent and should not be mistaken for an abnormal cystic mass (Fig 10–55).

Several cases of fetal gallstones have been previously reported.[226, 229] Beretsky and Lankin observed typical findings of gallstones in a fetus at 36 weeks, and Klingensmith and Cioffi-Ragan reported identical findings at 37 weeks. (Fig 10–56)[226, 229] In both cases, gallstones were confirmed on postnatal sonograms, but spontaneously resolved by 1 to 2 months of age. In one case, an earlier sonogram at 24 weeks also was normal. Spontaneous resolution of idiopathic gallstones has also been observed among neonates.[227, 228]

Possible causes of gallstones in neonates include hemolytic disorders (spherocytosis, sickle cell anemia, thalassemia, and erythroblastosis fetalis) and non–hemolytic disorders (pancreatitis, cystic fibrosis, and hyperalimentation).[226] No underlying etiology has been reported in any case of the fetal gallstones, however. Because fetal gallstones resolve spontaneously and have not been reported to produce clinical symptoms, a conservative management of observation has been recommended.

It appears that biliary "sludge" may also develop in the fetal gallbladder; we have identified echogenic material consistent with sludge in several fetuses, including one with hepatitis (Fig 10–53). This observation is of interest, since sludge and a thickened gallbladder wall are commonly visualized in adults with hepatitis. Penzias and Treisman demonstrated a similar appearance of an echogenic gallbladder in association with maternal cholelithiasis and intrahepatic cholestasis.[230] The authors attributed the sonographic appearance to fetal gallstones, although postnatal scans were not obtained for confirmation.

SUMMARY

A wide variety of intra-abdominal abnormalities may be detected on prenatal sonography. Careful evaluation of the location, distribution, and sonographic appearance of the abnormality in conjunction with associated findings (amniotic fluid, ascites, calcification, and other anomalies) usually will suggest the correct diagnosis or a limited differential diagnosis. Familiarity with the underlying disease process, possible concurrent malformations, and the usual outcome are essential for determining the appropriate obstetric management of fetuses found to have an intra-abdominal abnormality.

REFERENCES

Normal Development and Overview

1. Abramovich DR: Fetal factors influencing the volume and composition of liquor amnii. J Obstet Gynaecol Br Commonw 1970; 77:865–877.
2. Bovicelli L, Rizzo N, Orsini LF, et al: Prenatal diagnosis and management of fetal gastrointestinal abnormalities. Semin Perinat 1983; 7:109–117.
3. Grelin ES: *Functional Anatomy of the Newborn.* New Haven, Yale University Press, 1973, pp 54–60.
4. Hill LH: Sonographic detection of fetal gastrointestinal anomalies. Ultrasound Quarterly 1988; 6:35–67.
5. Moore KL: *The Developing Human,* ed 4. Philadelphia, WB Saunders Co, 1988, pp 217–245.
6. Mukuno DH, Lee TG, Harnsberger HR, et al: Sonography of the fetal gastrointestinal system. Semin Ultrasound 1984; 5:194–209.
7. Nyberg DA, Mack LA, Patten RM, et al: Fetal bowel: Normal sonographic findings. J Ultrasound Med 1987; 6:3–6.
8. Pretorius DH, Gosink BB, Clautice-Engle T, et al: Sonographic evaluation of the fetal stomach: Significance of non–visualization. AJR 1988; 151:987–989.
9. Pritchard JA: Fetal swallowing and amniotic fluid volume. Obstet Gynecol 1966; 28:606–610.
10. Wigglesworth JS. Perinatal pathology, in *Major Problems in Pathology.* Philadelphia, WB Saunders Co, 1984, pp 289–329.
11. Zilanti M, Fernandez S: Correlation of ultrasonic images of fetal intestine with gestational age and fetal maturity. Obstet Gynecol 1983; 62:569–573.

Esophageal Atresia

12. Ashcraft KW, Goodwin C, Amoury RA, et al: Early recognition and aggressive treatment of gastroesophageal reflux following repair of esophageal atresia. J Pediatr Surg 1977; 12:317–321.
13. Barkin SZ, Pretorius DH, Beckett MK, et al: Severe polyhydramnios: Incidence of anomalies. AJR, 1987; 148:155–159.
14. Bishop PJ, Klein MD, Phillipart AL, et al: Transpleural repair of esophageal atresia without a primary

gastrostomy: 240 patients treated between 1951 and 1983. J Pediatr Surg 1985; 20:832–828.

15. Bowie JD, Clair MR: Fetal swallowing and regurgitation: Observation of normal and abnormal activity. Radiology 1982; 144:877–878.

16. Claiborne AK, Blocker SH, Martin CM, et al: Prenatal and postnatal sonographic delineation of gastrointestinal abnormalities in a case of the VATER syndrome. J Ultrasound Med 1986; 5:45–47.

17. Eyheremendy E, Pfister M: Antenatal real-time diagnosis of esophageal atresia. J Clin Ultrasound 1983; 11:395–397.

18. Farrant P: The antenatal diagnosis of oesophageal atresia by ultrasound. Br J Radiol 1980; 53:1202–1203.

19. Gray SW, Skandalakis JE: The esophagus, in *Embryology for Surgeons.* Philadelphia, WB Saunders Co, 1972, pp 63–100.

20. German JC, Mahour GH, Wooley MM: Esophageal atresia and associated anomalies. J Pediatr Surg 1976; 11:299–306.

21. Gross RE: *The Surgery of Infancy and Childhood.* Philadelphia, WB Saunders Co, 1953.

22. Hayden CK, Schwartz MZ, Davis M, Swischuk LE: Combined esophageal and duodenal atresia: Sonographic findings. AJR 1983; 140:225–226.

23. Hendren WH, Lillehei CW: Pediatric surgery. N Engl J Med 1988; 319:86–96.

24. Hobbins JC, Grannum PAT, Berkowitz RI, et al: Ultrasound in the diagnosis of congenital anomalies. Am J Obstet Gynecol 1979; 134:331–344.

25. Holder TM, Cloud DT, Lewis JE Jr, et al: Esophageal atresia and tracheoesophageal fistula. A survey of its members by the surgical section of the American Academy of Pediatrics. Pediatrics. 1964; 34:542–549.

26. Jolleys A: An examination of the birthweights of babies with some abnormalities of the alimentary tract. J Pediatr Surg 1981; 16:160–163.

27. Louhimo I, Lindahl H: Esophageal atresia: Primary results of 500 consecutively treated patients. J Pediat Surg 1983; 18:217–229.

28. Martin LW, Alexander F: Esophageal atresia. Surg Clin 1985; 65:1099–1113.

29. Pretorius DH, Meier PR, Johnson ML: Diagnosis of esophageal atresia in utero. J Ultrasound Med 1983; 2:475.

30. Pretorius DH, Drose JA, Dennis MA, et al: Tracheoesophageal fistula in utero. J Ultrasound Med 1987; 6:509–513.

31. Rabinowitz JG, Moseley JE, Mitty HA, et al: Trisomy 18, esophageal atresia, anomalies of the radius, and congenital hypoplastic thrombocytopenia. Radiology 1967; 89:488–491.

32. Rickham PP: Infants with esophageal atresia weighing under 3 pounds. J Pediatr Surg 1981; 16:595–598.

33. Waterson DJ, Bonham CRE, Aaberdeen E: Oesophageal atresia: tracheo-oesophageal fistula. Lancet 1962; 21:819–822.

34. Weinberg B, Diakoumakis EE: Three complex cases of foregut atresia: Prenatal sonographic diagnosis with radiographic correlation. J Clin Ultrasound 1985; 13:481–484.

35. Zemlyn M: Prenatal detection of esophageal atresia. J Clin Ultrasound 1981; 9:453–454.

The Stomach

36. Goldstein J, Reece AE, Yarkoni S, et al: Growth of the fetal stomach in normal pregnancies. Obstet Gynecol 1987; 70:641–644.

37. Fakhry J, Shapiro LR, Schechter A, et al: Fetal gastric pseudomasses. J Ultrasound Med 1987; 6:177–180.

38. Zimmerman HB: Prenatal demonstration of gastric and duodenal obstruction by ultrasound. J Can Assoc Radiol 1978; 29:138–141.

Situs Inversus

39. Adams R, Churchhill ED: Situs inversus, sinusitis and bronchiectasis. J Thor Surg 1937; 7:206–217.

40. Chitayat D, Lao A, Wilson D, et al: Prenatal diagnosis of asplenia/polysplenia syndrome. Am J Obstet Gynecol 1988; 158:1085–1087.

41. Garcia OL, Mehta AV, Pickoff AS, et al: Left isoinversion and complete atrio-ventricular block: A report of 6 cases. Am J Cardiol 1981; 48:1103.

42. Gray SW, Skandalakis JE: Body assymetry and splenic anomalies, in *Embryology for Surgeons,* Philadelphia, WB Saunders Co, 1972, pp 877–895.

43. Mayo CW, Rice RG: Situs inversus totalis; statistical review of data on seventy-six cases, with special reference to diseases of the biliary tract. Arch Surg 1949; 58:724–730.

44. Moller JH, Nakib A, Anderson RC, et al: Congenital cardiac disease associated with polysplenia. A developmental complex of bilateral "left-sidedness." Circulation 1967; 36:789–799.

45. Putschar WGJ, Manion WC: Congenital absence of the spleen and associated anomalies. Amer J Clin Path 1956; 26:429–470.

46. Stoker AF, Jonnes SV, Spence J: Ultrasound diagnosis of situs inversus in utero. S Afr Med J 1983; 64:832–834.

Duodenal Atresia

47. Atwell JD, Klidjian AM: Vertebral anomalies and duodenal atresia. J Pediatr Surg 1982; 17:237–240.

48. Boychuk RB, Lyons EA, Goodhand TK: Duodenal atresia diagnosed by ultrasound. Radiology 1978; 127:500.

49. Duenhoelter JH, Santos-Ramos R, Rosenfeld CR, et al: Prenatal diagnosis of gastrointestinal tract obstruction. Obstet Gynecol 1976; 47:618–620.

50. Fonkalsrud EW, deLorimier AA, Hays DM: Congenital atresia and stenosis of the duodenum. A review com-

piled from the members of the Surgical Section of the American Academy of Pediatrics. Pediatrics 1969; 43:79–83.

51. Gross BH, Filly RA: Potential for a normal fetal stomach to simulate the sonographic "double bubble" sign. J Can Assoc Radiol 1982; 33:39–40.

52. Houlton MCCC, Sutton M, Aitken J: Antenatal diagnosis of duodenal atresia. J Obstet Gynacecol Br Commonw 1974; 81:818–821.

53. Jouppila P, Kirkinen P: Ultrasonic and clinical aspects in the diagnosis and prognosis of congenital gastrointestinal anomalies. Ultrasound Med Biol 1984; 10:465–472.

54. Nelson LH, Clark CE, Fishburne JI, et al: Value of serial sonography in the utero detection of duodenal atresia. Obstet Gynecol 1982; 59:657–660.

55. Loveday BJ, Barr JA, Aitken J: The intra-uterine demonstration of duodenal atresia by ultrasound. Br J Radiol 1975; 48:1031–1032.

56. Romero R, Jeanty P, Gianluigi P, et al: The prenatal diagnosis of duodenal atresia. Does it make any difference? Obstet Gynecol 1988; 71:739–741.

Jejunoileal Atresia, Volvulus

57. Baxi LV, Yeh MN, Blanc WA, et al: Antepartum diagnosis and managment of in utero intestinal volvulus with perforation. N Engl J Med 1983; 308:1519–1521.

58. Bergmans MGM, Merkus JWWM, Baars AM: Obstetrical and neonatological aspects of a child with atresia of the small bowel. J Perinat Med 1984; 12:325–332.

59. De Lorimier AA, Fonkalsrud EW, Hays DM: Congenital atresia and stenosis of the jejunum and ileum. Surgery 1969; 65:819–827.

60. Dickson JAS: Apple peel small bowel: An uncommon variant of duodenal and jejunal atresia. J Pediatr Surg 1970; 5:595–600.

61. Fletman D, McQuown D, Kanchanapoom V, et al: "Apple peel" atresia of the small bowel: Prenatal diagnosis of the obstruction by ultrasound. Pediatr Radiol 1980; 9:118–119.

62. Gray SW, Skandalakis JE: The small intestines, in *Embryology for Surgeons.* Philadelphia, WB Saunders Co, 1972, pp 129–186.

63. Grosfeld JL, Ballantine TVN, Shoemaker R: Operative management of intestinal atresia and stenosis based on pathologic findings. J Pediatr Surg 1979; 14:368–375.

64. Kjoller M, Holm-Nielsen G, Meiland H, et al: Prenatal obstruction of the ileum diagnosed by ultrasound. Prenat Diagn 1985; 5:427–430.

65. Lyrenis S, Cnattingius S, Lingberg B: Fetal jejunal atresia and intrauterine volvulus—a case report. J Perinat Med 1982; 10:247–248.

66. Nikapota VLB, Loman C: Gray scale sonographic demonstration of fetal small-bowel atresia. J Clin Ultrasound 1979; 7:307–310.

67. Nixon HH, Tawes R: Etiology and treatment of small intestinal atresia: Analysis of a series of 127 jejunoileal

atresias and comparison with 62 duodenal atresia. Surgery 1971; 69:41–51.

68. Petrikovsky BM, Nochimson DJ, Campbell WA, et al: Fetal jejunoileal atresia with persistent omphalomesenteric duct. Am J Obstet Gynecol 1988; 158:173–175.

69. Ravitch MM, Barton BA: The need for pediatric surgeons as determined by the volume of work and the mode of delivery of surgical care. Surgery 1974; 76:754–763.

70. Samuel N, Dicker D, Feldberg D, et al: Ultrasound diagnosis and management of fetal intestinal obstruction and volvulus in utero. J Perinat Med 1984; 12:333–337.

71. Skoll AM, Marquette GP, Hamilton EF: Prenatal ultrasonic diagnosis of multiple bowel atresias. Am J Obstet Gynecol 1987; 156:472–73.

72. Touloukian RJ. Intestinal atresia. Clin Perinatology 1978; 5:3–18.

Meconium Ileus and Cystic Fibrosis

73. Benacerraf B, Chaudhury AK: Echogenic fetal bowel in the third trimester associated with meconium ileus secondary to cystic fibrosis. J Reprod Med 1989; 34(4):299–300.

74. Beaudet AL, Spence JE, Montes M, et al: Experience with new DNA markers for the diagnosis of cystic fibrosis. N Engl J Med 1988; 318:50–51.

75. Brock DJH: Prenatal diagnosis of cystic fibrosis, in Rodeck CH, Nicolaides KH (eds): *Prenatal Diagnosis.* New York, John Wiley & Sons, 1985, pp 159–175.

76. Brock DJH: Amniotic fluid alkaline phosphatase isoenzymes in early prenatal diagnosis of cystic fibrosis. Lancet 1984; ii:941–949.

77. Brock DJH: A comparative study of microvillar enzyme activities in the prenatal diagnosis of cystic fibrosis. Prenat Diagn 1985; 5:129–134.

78. Buchanan DJ, Rapoport S: Chemical comparison of normal meconium and meconium from a patient with meconium ileus. Pediatrics 1952; 9:304–310.

79. Caspi B, Elchalal U, Lancet U, et al: Prenatal diagnosis of cystic fibrosis: Ultrasonographic appearance of meconium ileus in the fetus. Prenat Diagn 1988; 8:379–382.

80. Fakhry J, Reiser M, Shapiro LR, et al: Increased echogenicity in the lower fetal abdomen: A common normal variant in the second trimester. J Ultrasound Med 1986; 5:489–492.

81. Gilbert F, Kwei-Lan T, Mendoza A, et al: Prenatal diagnostic options in cystic fibrosis. Am J Obstet Gynecol 1988; 158:947–952.

82. Gilbert F, Mulivor R: Personal communication.

83. Goldstein RB, Filly RA, Callen PW: Sonographic diagnosis of meconium ileus in utero. J Ultrasound Med 1987; 6:663–666.

84. Lince DM, Pretorius DH, Manco-Johnson ML et al: The clinical significance of increased echogenicity in the fetal abdomen. AJR 1985; 145:683.

85. Jassain MN, Gauderer WL, Fanaroff AA, et al: A perinatal approach to the diagnosis and management of gastrointestinal malformations. Obstet Gynecol 1982; 59:33–39.

86. Manco LG, Nunan FA Jr, Sohnen H, et al: Fetal small bowel simulating an abdominal mass at sonography. J Clin Ultrasound 1986; 14:404–407.

87. Meizner I: (Letter). J Clin Ultrasound 1987; 5:494.

88. Muller F, Frot JC, Aubry J, et al: Meconium ileus in cystic fibrosis fetuses. Lancet 1984; 2:223

89. Muller F, Aubry MC, Gasser B, et al: Prenatal diagnosis of cystic fibrosis. Prenat Diag 1986; 5:109–117.

90. Nugent CE, Gravius T, Green P, et al: Prenatal diagnosis of cystic fibrosis by chorionic villous sampling using 12 polymorphic desoxyribonecleic acid markers. Obstet Gynecol 1988; 71:213–215.

91. Nyberg DA, Hastrup W, Watts H, et al: Dilated bowel: A sonographic sign of cystic fibrosis. J Ultrasound Med 1987; 6:257–260.

92. Olsen MM, Luck SR, Lloyd-Still J, et al: The spectrum of meconium disease in infancy. J Pediatr Surg 1982; 17:479–481.

93. Tucker AS, Izant RJ: Problems with meconium. AJR 1971; 112:135–142.

94. Park RW, Grand RJ: Gastrointestinal manifestations of cystic fibrosis: A review. Gastroenterology 1981; 81:1143–61.

95. Wainwright BJ, Scambler PJ, Schmidtke J, et al: Localization of cystic fibrosis to human chromosome 7cen-q22. Nature 1985; 318:384–385.

96. White R, Woodward S, Leppert M, et al: A closely linked genetic marker for cystic fibrosis. Nature 1985; 318:382–384.

Non–obstructed Small Bowel Disorders

97. Berdon WE, Baker DH, Blanc, WA, et al: Megacystis-microcolon-intestinal hypoperistalsis syndrome: A new cause of intestinal obstruction in the newborn. Report of radiologic findings in five newborn girls. AJR 1976; 126:957–964.

98. Groli C, Zucca S, Cesaretti A: Congenital chloridorrhea: Antenatal ultrasonographic appearance. J Clin Ultrasound 1986; 14:293–295.

99. Kirkinen P, Jouppila P: Prenatal ultrasonic findings in congenital chloride diarrhoea. Prenat Diagn 1984; 4:457–461.

100. Krook PM: Megacystis-microcolon-intestinal hypoperistalsis syndrome in a male infant. Radiology 1980; 136:649.

101. Manco LG, Osterdahl P: The antenatal sonographic features of megacystis-microcolon-intestinal hypoperistalsis syndrome. J Clin Ultrasound 1984; 12:595–598.

102. Puri P, Lake BD, Gorman F, et al: Megacystis-microcolon-intestinal hypoperistalsis syndrome: A visceral myopathy. J Pediatr Surg 1983; 18:64–69.

103. Vezina WC, Morin FR, Winsberg F: Megacystic-

microcolon-intestinal hypoperistalsis syndrome: Antenatal ultrasound appearance. AJR 1979; 133:749–750.

104. Ventzileos AM, Eisenfeld LI, Herson VC, et al: Megacystis-microcolon-intestinal hypoperistalsis syndrome: Antenatal sonographic findings and review of the literature. Am J Perinatol 1986; 3:297–302.

Colon Atresia

105. Benson CD, Lofti MW, Brough AJ: Congenital atresia and stenosis of the colon. J Pediatr Surg 1968; 3:253–257.

106. Coran AG, Eraklis AJ: Atresia of the colon. Surgery 1969; 65:828–831.

107. Louw JH. Investigations into the etiology of congenital atresia of the colon. Dis Colon Rectum 1964; 7:471–478.

Anorectal Atresia

108. Barss VA, Benacerraf BR, Frigolotto FD: Antenatal sonographic diagnosis of fetal gastrointestinal malformation. Pediatrics 1985; 76:445–449.

109. Bean WJ, Calonge MA, Aprill CN, et al: Anal atresia: A prenatal ultrasound diagnosis. J Clin Ultrasound 1978; 6:111–112.

110. Berdon WE, Baker DH, Wigges HJ, et al: Calcified intraluminal meconium in newborn males with imperforate anus. AJR 1975; 125:449–455.

111. Boles ET Jr: Imperforate anus. Clin Perinatol 1978; 5:149–161.

112. deVries PA, Cox KL: Surgery of anorectal anomalies. Surg Clin North Am 1985; 65:1139–1169.

113. Duhamel B: From the mermaid to anal imperforation. The syndrome of caudal regression syndrome. Arch Dis Child 1961; 36:151–155.

114. Harris RD, Nyberg DA, Mack LA, et al: Anorectal atresia: Prenatal sonographic diagnosis. AJR 1987; 149:395–400.

115. Loewy JA, Richards DG, Toi A: In-utero diagnosis of the caudal regression syndrome: Report of three cases. J Clin Ultrasound 1987; 15:469–474.

116. Pena A: Surgical treatment of high imperforate anus. World J Surg 1985; 9:236–243.

117. Shalev E, Weiner E, Zuzherman H: Prenatal ultrasound diagnosis of intestinal calcifications with imperforate anus. Acta Obstet Gynecol Scand 1983; 62:95–96.

118. Temtamy SA, Miller JD: Extending the scope of the VATER association: Definition of the VATER syndrome. J Pediatr 1974; 85:345–349.

Persistent Cloaca

119. Bartholomew TH, Gonzales ET Jr: Urologic management in cloacal dysgenesis. Urology 1978; 11:549–557.

120. Holzgreve W: Brief clinical report: Prenatal diagnosis of persistent common cloaca with prune belly and anen-

cephaly in the second trimester. Am J Med Genet 1985; 20:729–732.

121. Kay R, Tank ES: Principles of management of the persistent cloaca in the female newborn. J Urology 1977; 117:102–104.

122. Lande IM, Hamilton EF: The antenatal sonographic visualization of cloacal dysgenesis. J Ultrasound Med 1986; 5:275–278.

123. Petrikovsky BM, Walzak MP Jr, D'Addaria PF: Fetal cloacal anomalies: Prenatal sonographic findings and differential diagnosis. Obstet Gynecol 1988; 72:464–469.

124. Shalev E, Feldman E, Weiner E, et al: Prenatal sonographic appearance of persistent cloaca. Acta Obstet Gynecol Scand 1986; 65:517–518.

125. Tank ES: The urologic complications of imperforate anus and cloacal dysgenesis. In Harrison JH, Gittes RF, Perlmutter AD, et al. (eds): *Campbell's Urology,* ed 4. Philadelphia, WB Saunders Co, 1979, pp 1889–1900.

Hirschsprung's Disease

126. Bergsma D: *Birth Defects Compendium,* ed 2. New York, Alan R. Liss, 1979.

127. Gray SW, Skandalakis JE: The colon and rectum, in *Embryology for Surgeons.* Philadelphia, WB Saunders Co, 1972, pp 187–216.

128. Ikawa H, Kim SH, Hendren WH, et al: Acetylcholinesterase and manometry in the diagnosis of the constipated child. Arch Surg 1986; 121:435–438.

129. Ideda K, Goto S: Diagnosis and treatment of Hirschsprung's disease in Japan: An analysis of 1628 patients. Ann Surg 1984; 199:400–405.

130. Jarmas AL, Weaver DD, Padilla LM, et al: Hirschsprung disease: Etiologic implications of unsuccessful prenatal diagnosis. Am J Med Genet 1983; 16:163–167.

131. Kleinhause S, Boley SJ, Sheran M, et al: Hirschsprung's disease: A survey of the members of the Surgical Section of the American Academy of Pediatrics. J Pediatr Surg 1979; 14:588–597.

132. Okamoto E, Ueda T: Embryogenesis of intramural ganglia of the gut and its relation to Hirschsprung's disease. J Pediatr Surg 1967; 2:437–443.

133. Tam PKH: An immunochemical study with neuron-specific-enolase and substance P of human enteric innervation—the normal developmental pattern and abnormal deviations in Hirschsprung's disease and pyloric stenosis. J Pediatr Surg 1986; 21:227–232.

134. Vermish M, Mayden KL, Confino E, et al: Prenatal sonographic diagnosis of Hirschsprung's disease. J Ultrasound Med 1986; 5:37–39.

135. Wrobleski D, Wesselhoeft: Ultrasonic diagnosis of prenatal intestinal obstruction. J. Pediatr Surg 1979; 14:598–600.

Ovarian Cyst

136. Bower R, Dehner LP, Ternberg JL: Bilateral ovarian cysts in the newborn. Am J Dis Child 1974; 128:731–733.

137. Carlson DH, Griscom NT: Ovarian cysts in the newborn. AJR 1972; 116:664–672.

138. Crade M, Gillooly M, Taylor KJW: In utero demonstration of an ovarian cystic mass by ultrasound. J Clin Ultrasound 1980; 8:251–252.

139. Desa DJ: Follicular ovarian cysts in stillbirths and neonates. Arch Dis Child 1975; 50:24–50.

140. Evers JL, Rolland R: Primary hypothyroidism and ovarian activity: Evidence for an overlap in the synthesis of pituitary glycoproteins. Br J Obstet Gynecol 1981; 88:195.

141. Ikeda K, Suita S, Nakano H: Management of ovarian cysts detected antenatally. J Pediatr Surg 1988; 23:432–435.

142. Jafri SZH, Bree RL, Silver TM, et al: Fetal ovarian cysts: Sonographic detection and association with hypothyroidism. Radiology 1984; 150:809–812.

143. Jouppila P, Kirkinen P, Tuononen S: Ultrasonic detection of bilateral ovarian cysts in the fetus. Eur J Obstet Gynecol Reprod Biol 1982; 13:87–92.

144. Lee TG, Blake SP: Prenatal fetal abdominal ultrasonography and diagnosis. Radiology 1977; 124:475–477.

145. Lindeque BG, du Toit JP, Muller LMM, et al: Ultrasonographic criteria for the conservative management of antenatally diagnosed fetal ovarian cysts. J Reprod Med 1988; 33:196–198.

146. Marshall JR: Ovarian enlargements in the first year of life. Ann Surg 1965; 161:372–377.

147. McKeener PA, Andrews H: Fetal ovarian cysts: A report of five cases. J Pediatr Surg 1988; 23:354–355.

148. Nguyen KT, Reid RL, Sauerbrei E: Antenatal sonographic detection of a fetal theca lutein cyst: A clue to maternal diabetes mellitus. J Ultrasound Med 1986; 5:665–667.

149. Nussbaum AR, Sanders RC, Hartman DS, et al: Neonatal ovarian cysts: Sonographic-pathologic correlation. Radiology 1988; 168:817–821.

150. O'Hagan DB, Pudifin J, Mickel RE, et al: Antenatal detection of a fetal ovarian cyst by real-time ultrasound. S Afr Med J 1985; 67:471–473.

150a. Rizzo N, Gabrielli S, Perolo A, et al: Prenatal diagnosis and management of fetal ovarian cysts. Prenat Diagn 1989; 9:97–104.

151. Sandler MA, Smith SJ, Pope SG, et al: Prenatal diagnosis of septated ovarian cysts. J Clin Ultrasound 1985; 13:55–57.

152. Tabsh KMA: Antenatal sonographic appearance of a fetal ovarian cyst. J Ultrasound Med 1982; 1:329–331.

153. Valenti C, Kassner EG, Yermakow V, et al: Antenatal diagnosis of a fetal ovarian cyst. Am J Obstet Gynecol 1975; 123:216–219.

Hydrometrocolpos

154. Davis GH, Wapner R, Kurtz AB et al: Antenatal diagnosis of hydrometrocolpos by ultrasound examination. J Ultrasound Med 1984; 3:371–374.

155. Hill SJ, Hirsch JH: Sonographic detection of fetal hydrometrocolpos. J Ultrasound Med 1985; 4:323–325.

156. Mahoney PJ, Chamberlain JW: Hydrometrocolpos in infancy. Congenital atresia of the vagina with abnormally abundant cervical secretions. J Pediatrics 1940; 17:772–780.

157. McKusick VA, Bauer RL, Koop CE, et al: Hydrometrocolpos as a simply inherited malformation. JAMA 1964; 189:813.

158. Radman H, Melvin, Askin J, et al: Hydrocolpos and hematocolpos. Surg Gynecol Obstet 1966; 27:2–6.

159. Robinow M, Shaw A: The McKusick-Kaufman syndrome: Recessively inherited vaginal atresia, hydrometrocolpos, uterovaginal duplications, anorectal anomalies, postaxial polydactyly and congenital heart disease. J Pediatr 1979; 94:776–778.

160. Russ PD, Zavitz WR, Pretorius DH, et al: Hydrometrocolpos, uterus didelphys and septate vagina: An antenatal sonographic diagnosis. J Ultrasound Med 1986; 5:211–213.

161. Spencer R, Levy DM: Hydrometrocolpos: Report of three cases and review of the literature. Ann Surg 1962; 155:558–571.

162. Westerhout FC, Hodgman JE, Anderson GV, et al: Congenital hydrocolpos. Am J Obstet Gynecol 1964; 89:957–961.

163. Wilson DA, Stacy TM, Smith EI: Ultrasound diagnosis of hydrocolpos and hydrometrocolpos. Radiology 1978; 128:451–454.

Enteric Duplication Cysts

164. Bidwell JK, Nelson A: Prenatal ultrasonic diagnosis of congenital duplication of the stomach. J Ultrasound Med 1986; 5:589–591.

165. van Dam LJ, de Groot CJ, Hazeborek FW, et al: Intrauterine demonstration of bowel duplication by ultrasound. Eur J Obster Gynecol Reprod Biol 1984; 18:229.

Mesenteric, Omental, and Retroperitoneal Cysts

166. Benacerraf BR, Figoletto FD: Prenatal sonographic diagnosis of isolated congenital cystic hygroma, unassociated with lymphedema or other morphologic abnormality. J Ultrasound Med 1987; 6:63–66.

167. Blumhagen JD, Wood BJ, Rosenbaum DM: Sonographic evaluation of abdominal lymphangiomas in children. J Ultrasound Med 1987; 6:487–495.

168. Kurtz RJ, Heimann Tomas M, Beck AR, et al: Mesenteric and retroperitoneal cysts. Ann Surg 1986; 203:109–112.

169. Vanek VW, Phillips AK: Retroperitoneal, mesenteric, and omental cysts. Arch Surg 1984; 119:838–842.

170. Walker AR, Putnam TC: Omental, mesenteric, and retroperitoneal cysts: A clinical study of 33 new cases. Ann Surg 1973; 178:13.

Choledochal Cyst

171. Alonso-Lej F, Rever WB Jr, Pessagno DJ: Collective review. Congenital choledochal cyst, with a report of 2, and an analysis of 94 cases. International Abstracts of Surgery. 1959; 108:1–30.

172. Dewbury KC, Aluwihare M, Birch SJ, et al: Prenatal ultrasound demonstration of a choledochal cyst. Br J Radiol 1980; 53:906–907.

173. Elrad H, Mayden KL, Ahart S, et al: Prenatal ultrasound diagnosis of choledochal cyst. J Ultrasound Med 1985; 4:553–555.

174. Frank JL, Hill MC, Chirathivat S, et al: Antenatal observation of a choledochal cyst by sonography. AJR 1981; 137:166–168.

175. Gray SW, Skandalakis JE: Extrahepatic biliary ducts and the gallbladder, in *Embryology for Surgeons.* Philadelphia, WB Saunders Co, 1972, pp 229–262.

176. Howel CG, Templeton JM, Weiner S, et al: Antenatal diagnosis and early surgery for choledochal cyst. J Pediatr Surg 1983; 18:387–393.

177. Mahour GH: Choledochal cyst in infants. Am J Dis Child 1973; 126:533–534.

178. Reuter K, Raptopoulos VD, Cantelmo N, et al: The diagnosis of choledochal cyst by ultrasound. Radiology 1980; 136:437–438.

179. Todani T, Watanabe Y, Fugii T, et al: Anomalous arrangement of the pancreatobiliary ductal system in patients with a choledochal cyst. Am J Surg 1984; 147:672–676.

180. Yamaguchi M: Congenital choledochal cyst: Analysis of 1,433 patients in the Japanese literature. Am J Surg 1980; 140:653–657.

Other Cystic Masses

181. Chung W-M: Antenatal detection of hepatic cyst. J Clin Ultrasound 1986; 14:217–219.

182. Dembner AG, Taylor KJW: Gray scale sonographic diagnosis: Multiple congenital splenic cysts. J Clin Ultrasound 1978; 6:173–174.

183. Fuster JS, Benasco C, Saad I: Giant dilatation of the umbilical vein. J Clin Ultrasound 1985; 13:363–365.

184. Hatijis CG, Philip AG, Anerson GG, et al: The in utero ultrasonic appearance of Klippel-Trenaunay-Weber syndrome. Am J Obstet Gynecol 1981; 139:872–974.

185. Jaffe R, Abramowicz J, Fejgin M, et al: Giant fetal abdominal cyst: Ultrasonic diagnosis and management. J Ultrasound Med 1987; 6:45–47.

186. Lewis BD, Doubilet PM, Heller VL, et al: Cutaneous and visceral hemangiomata in the Klippel-Trenaunay-Weber syndrome: Antenatal sonographic detection. AJR 1986; 147:598–600.

187. Persutte WH, Lenke RL, Kropp K, et al: Antenatal diagnosis of fetal patent urachus. J Ultrasound Med 1988; 7:399–403.

Intra-abdominal Calcification

188. Berdon WE, Baker DH, Wigges HJ, et al: Calcified intraluminal meconium in newborn males with imperforate anus. AJR 1975; 125:449–455.

189. Ceballos R, Hicks GM: Plastic peritonitis due to neonatal hydrometrocolpos: Radiologic and pathologic observations. J Pediatr Surg 1970; 5:63–70.

190. Hillcoat BL: Calcification of the meconium within the bowel of the newborn. Arch Dis Child 1962; 37:86–89.

191. Mahony BS, Callen PW, Filly RA: Fetal urethral obstruction: US evaluation. Radiology 1985; 157:221–224.

192. Miller JP, Smith SD, Newman B, et al: Neonatal Abdominal calcification: Is it always meconium peritonitis? J Pediatr Surg 1988; 23:555–556.

193. Nguyen DL, Leonard JC: Ischemic hepatic necrosis: A cause of fetal liver calcification. AJR 1986; 147:596–597.

194. Schackelford GD, Kirks DR: Neonatal hepatic calcification secondary to transplacental infection. Radiology 1977; 122:753–757.

195. Shalev E, Weiner E, Zuzherman H: Prenatal ultrasound diagnosis of intestinal calcifications with imperforate anus. Acta Obstet Gynecol Scand 1983; 62:95–96.

196. Skoll AM, Marquette GP, Hamilton EF: Prenatal ultrasonic diagnosis of multiple bowel atresias. Am J Obstet Gynecol 1987; 156:472–473.

197. Yousefzadeh DK, Jackson JH Jr., Smith WL, et al: Intraluminal meconium calcification without distal obstruction. Pediatr Radiol 1984; 14:23–27.

Meconium Peritonitis

198. Dillard JP, Edwards DU, Leopold GR: Meconium peritonitis masquerading as fetal hydrops. J Ultrasound Med 1987; 6:49–51.

199. Edelstone DI, Holzman IR: Regulation of perinatal intestinal oxygenation. Semin Perinatol 1984; 8:226–233.

200. Finkel LI, Slovis TL: Meconium peritonitis, intraperitoneal calcifications, and cystic fibrosis. Pediatr Radiol 1982; 12:92–93.

201. Fleischer AC, Davis RJ, Campbell L: Sonographic detection of a meconium-containing mass in a fetus: A case report. J Clin Ultrasound 1983; 11:103–105.

202. Forouhar F. Meconium peritonitis: Pathology, evolution, and diagnosis. Am J Clin Pathol 1982; 78:208–213.

203. Foster MA, Nyberg DA, Mahony BS, et al: Meconium peritonitis: Prenatal sonographic findings and clinical significance. Radiology 1987; 165:661–665.

204. Kurtz AB: AIUM film reading session. J Ultrasound Med 1986; 537.

205. Lauer JD, Cradock TV: Meconium pseudocyst: Prenatal sonographic and antenatal radiologic correlation. J Ultrasound Med 1982; 1:333–335.

206. Lockwood C, Ghidini A, Romero R, et al: Fetal bowel perforation simulating sacrococcygeal teratoma. J Ultrasound Med 1988; 7:227–229.

207. Neuhauser EB: The roentgen diagnosis of fetal meconium peritonitis. AJR 1944; 51:421–425.

208. Silverbach S: Antenatal real-time identification of meconium pseudocyst. J Clin Ultrasound 1983; 11:455–457.

209. Tibboel D, Gaillard JLJ, Molenaar JC: Importance of mesenteric vascular insufficiency in meconium peritonitis. Hum Pathol 1986; 17:411–416.

210. McGahan JP. Hanson F: Meconium peritonitis with accompanying pseudocyst: Prenatal sonographic diagnosis. Radiology 1983; 148:125–126.

211. Yankes JR, Bowie JD, Effman EI: Prenatal diagnosis of meconium peritonitis with inguinal hernias by ultrasonography. J Ultrasound Med 1988; 7:221–223.

Liver and Spleen Abnormalities

212. Berman B, Lim HW: Concurrent cutaneous and hepatic hemangioma in infancy: Report of a case and review of the literature. J Dermatol Surg Oncol 1978; 4:869–873.

213. Brunnelle F, Chaumont P: Hepatic tumors in children: Ultrasonic differentiation of malignant from benign lesions. Radiology 1984; 150:695–699.

214. Diakoumakis EE, Weinberg B, Seife B, et al: Infantile hemangioendothelioma of the liver. J Clin Ultrasound 1986; 14:137–139.

215. Eliezer S, Ester F, Ehud W, et al: Fetal splenomegaly, ultrasound diagnosis of cytomegalovirus infection: A case report. J Clin Ultrasound 1984; 12:520–521.

216. Foucar E, Wilhamson RA, Yin-Chin L, et al: Mesenchymal hamartoma of the liver identified by fetal sonography. AJR 1983; 140:970.

217. Lichman JP, Miller EI: Prenatal ultrasonic diagnosis of splenic cyst. J Ultrasound Med 1988; 7:637–638.

218. Nakamoto SK, Dreilinger A, Dattel B, et al: The sonographic appearance of hepatic hemangioma in-utero. J Ultrasound Med 1983; 2:239–241.

219. Nguyen L, Shardling B, Ein S et al: Hepatic hemangioma in childhood: Medical management or surgical management? J Pediatr Surg 1982; 17:576–579.

220. Platt LD, DeVore GR, Benner P, et al: Antenatal diagnosis of a fetal liver mass. J Ultrasound Med 1983; 2:521–522.

221. Schmidt W, Yarkoni S, Jeanty P, et al: Sonographic measurements of the fetal spleen: Clinical implications. J Ultrasound Med 1985; 4:667–672.

222. Stanley P, Hall TR, Woolley MM, et al: Mesenchymal hamartoma of the liver in childhood: Sonographic and CT findings. AJR 1986; 147:1035–1039.

223. Stone HH, Nielson IC: Haemangioma of the liver in the newborn. Arch Surg 1965; 90:319–322.

224. Vintzileos AM, Neckles S, Campbell WA, et al: Fetal liver ultrasound measurements during normal pregnancy. Obstet Gynecol 1985; 66:477–480.

225. Weinstein L, Anderson C: In-utero diagnosis of Beckwith-Wiedemann syndrome by ultrasound. Radiology 1980; 134:474.

Gallbladder Abnormalities

226. Beretsky I, Lanken DH: Diagnosis of fetal cholelithiasis using real-time high-resolution imaging employing digital detection. J Ultrasound Med 1983; 2:381–383.
227. Jacir NN, Anderson KD, Eichelberger M, et al: Chole-lithiasis in infancy: Resolution of gallstones in three of four infants. J Pediatr Surg 1986; 21:567–569.
228. Keller MS, Markle BM, Laffey PA, et al: Spontaneous resolution of cholelithiasis in infants. Radiology 1985; 157:345–348.
229. Klingensmith WC III, Ragan-Cioffi DT: Fetal gallstones. Radiology 1988; 167:143–144.
230. Penzias AS, Treisman O: Vitamin K-dependent clotting factor deficiency in pregnancy. Obstet Gynecol 1988; 72:452–454.

Abdominal Wall Defects

David A. Nyberg, M.D

Laurence A. Mack, M.D

Abdominal wall defects represent a common group of fetal anomalies, occurring in 1 in 2,000 live births. In conjunction with widespread maternal alpha-fetoprotein (AFP) screening, prenatal sonographic detection of abdominal wall defects has become increasingly common.[16, 40] When detected prior to fetal viability (approximately 24 menstrual weeks), knowledge of an abdominal wall defect provides the prospective parents the opportunity to make important decisions regarding the pregnancy.

Because excellent results can be expected following surgical correction of an isolated abdominal wall defect, parents may choose to continue the pregnancy when the defect represents gastroschisis or an omphalocele that is not associated with concurrent anomalies or chromosome abnormalities. On the other hand, pregnancy termination may be elected when the defect represents a complex malformation or when additional anomalies are present. These diverse options emphasize the importance of establishing the correct diagnosis and identifying major concurrent anomalies when an abdominal wall defect is detected prenatally. Detection of abdominal wall defects is also important in preparation for a planned delivery, so that pediatricians and surgeons can be notified and prompt treatment can be accomplished after birth.

This chapter discusses the pathogenesis, typical pathologic and sonographic findings, associated anomalies, and prognosis for both common and less common types of abdominal wall defects. Sonographic findings that are considered to be of diagnostic or prognostic importance are emphasized. A discussion of embryo-genesis and a general sonographic approach to abdominal wall defects precedes the discussion of individual malformations.

EMBRYOGENESIS

Development of the anterior abdominal wall occurs as the embryo folds in both cranial-caudal and lateral directions, changing the flat trilaminar embryonic disc into its curvilinear embryonic shape. With development of the cranial fold at the end of the third fetal week (menstrual week 5), the heart and pericardial cavity come to lie on the ventral surface of the embryo (Fig 11–1)[5] The heart later becomes incorporated into the central chest, with development of the lateral folds in the thoracic region. The heart is intimately connected with the septum transversum which will form the central tendon of the diaphragm.[5] As the primitive heart elongates and bends, it gradually invaginates into the pericardial cavity.

Lateral body walls (somatopleures) fold the sides of the embryo medially, changing the previously flattened embryonic disc to a roughly cylindrical form (see Fig 11–1).[5] As the lateral and ventral abdominal wall forms, part of the yolk sac is incorporated into the embryo as the midgut. Concurrently, the connection of the midgut with the yolk sac is reduced to a narrow yolk stalk, and there is relative constriction at the umbilicus. Coalescence of the body stalk with the yolk stalk forms the umbilical cord at 5–6 fetal weeks (7–8 menstrual weeks). As the umbilical cord forms, ventral

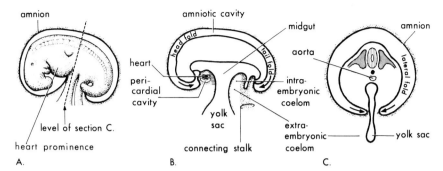

FIG 11–1.
Normal embryologic development at 40 menstrual days (26 fetal days) shows normal folding of the embryo. **A,** lateral view of the embryo. **B,** schematic longitudinal section shows head and tail folds. Note that the heart and pericardium lie on the ventral surface of the embryo at this age. Further folding incorporates the heart into the central chest. **C,** transverse section at the level shown in **A** shows the lateral folds. (From Moore KL: *The Developing Human,* ed 4. Philadelphia, WB Saunders Co. 1988. Used by permission.)

fusion of the lateral folds reduces the region of communication between the intraembryonic and extra-embryonic coeloms to a narrow communication that persists until about the tenth fetal week (12th menstrual week). Rapid expansion of the amniotic cavity obliterates the extra-embryonic coelom and forms the epithelial covering for the umbilical cord.

About 6 fetal weeks (8 menstrual weeks), rapid elongation of the midgut forms a midgut loop that herniates into the base of the umbilical cord (Fig 11–2).[5]

This physiologic bowel migration occurs because of the lack of intraabdominal space, which is filled primarily by the relatively large liver and kidneys. Within the umbilical cord, the midgut loop rotates 90 degrees counterclockwise around the axis of the superior mesenteric artery. During the tenth fetal week (12th menstrual week), the intestines return rapidly to the abdomen. As the large intestines return, they undergo a further 180-degree counterclockwise rotation.

A false-positive diagnosis of abdominal wall defect

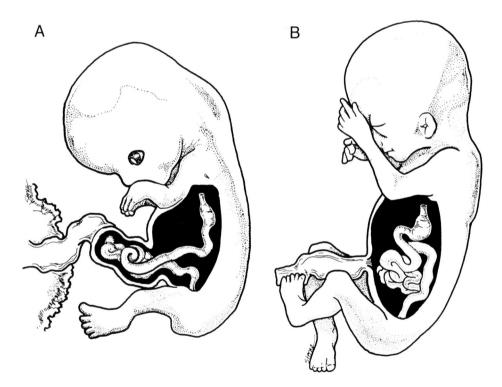

FIG 11–2.
Normal gut migration. **A,** bowel normally herniates into the base of the umbilical cord between 8 to 12 menstrual weeks (6 to 10 fetal weeks). **B,** bowel returns to the abdominal cavity by 12 menstrual weeks (10 fetal weeks). (From Cyr DR, Mack LA, Schoenecker SA, et al: Bowel migration in the normal fetus: US detection. Radiology 1986; 161:119–121. Used by permission.)

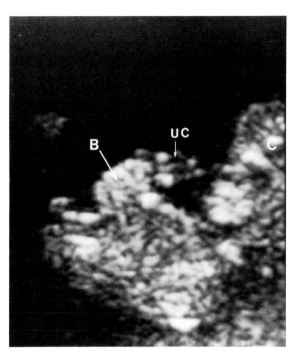

FIG 11–3.
Normal gut migration. Longitudinal sacn at 10 menstrual weeks shows herniation of echogenic bowel *(B)* into the base of the umbilical cord *(UC)*. Follow-up sonogram at 16 weeks shows normal umbilical cord insertion with return of the gut to the abdomen. *C* = cranium.

is possible between 6 to 12 weeks when the rapidly elongating midgut normally herniates into the base of the body stalk (umbilical cord) as part of normal gut migration (Fig 11–3).[1] Because this embryologic process can be readily observed sonographically, a reliable diagnosis of certain types of abdominal wall defects (gastroschisis and bowel-containing omphaloceles) may not be possible before 12 weeks.[1]

SONOGRAPHIC APPROACH TO ABDOMINAL WALL DEFECTS

Because abdominal wall defects occur early in embryologic development, it is theoretically possible to detect all major defects before the age of viability. In actual practice, small abdominal wall defects may be missed during routine obstetric scanning. This emphasizes the importance of routine views of the anterior abdominal wall and umbilical cord insertion site (Fig 11–4), as recommended by the guidelines adopted by the American Institute of Ultrasound in Medicine (see Chapter 1). Routine views of the urinary bladder and pelvis should also permit improved prenatal diagnosis of bladder and cloacal exstrophy.

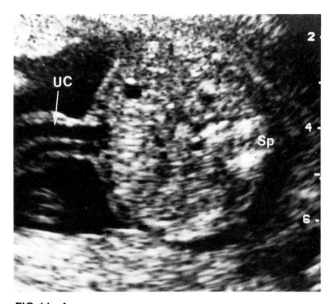

FIG 11–4.
Normal anterior abdominal wall. Transverse view of abdomen shows normal insertion of the umbilical cord *(UC)* into the anterior abdominal wall. This normal appearance excludes the vast majority of anterior abdominal wall defects. *Sp* = spine.

Once an abdominal wall defect is identified, it is important to categorize correctly the type of malformation (Tables 11–1 and 11–2). Gastroschisis and omphalocele are the two most common types of abdominal wall defects, reported with nearly equal frequency in 1 in 4,000 live-births. It is now well established that these two disorders differ markedly in their typical pathological findings, frequency of associated malformations, and prognosis. The sonographic findings are also distinctive enough that we believe a reliable diagnosis should be possible in nearly all cases (see Table 11–2). Using criteria outlined in Table 11–2, a correct diagnosis has been assigned in all but two cases of omphalocele or gastroschisis (n=48) seen at our institutions during the last 4 years. The two er-

TABLE 11–1.

Types of Abdominal Wall Defects

Common
  Gastroschisis
  Omphalocele
    Isolated
    Concurrent anomalies
    Beckwith-Wiedemann syndrome
    Chromosome abnormalities
Uncommon
  Ectopia cordis
  Limb-body wall complex
  Cloacal exstrophy
  Urachal (allantoic) cyst

TABLE 11-2.

Essential Pathologic and Clinical Features of Anterior Abdominal Wall Defects

	Gastroschisis	Omphalocele	LBWC*	Cloacal Exstrophy
Location	Right paraumbilical	Midline, cord insertion site	Lateral	Infraumbilical
Size defect	Small (2–4 cm)	Variable (2–10 cm)	Large	Variable
Membrane	–	+	+ (contiguous with placenta)	±
Liver involvement	–	Common	+	+
Ascites	–	Common	–	±
Bowel thickening	+	– (unless ruptured membrane)	–	±
Bowel complications	Common (15%)	–	–	–
Cardiac anomalies	Rare (ASD,PDA)	Common (complex)	Common	10–15%
Other anomalies	Rare	Common (50%–70%)	Always (scoliosis, cranial defects, limb defects)	Always (genitourinary spinal)
Chromosome abnormalities	–	common (30%–40%)	–	±

*LBWC = limb-body wall complex (body-stalk anomaly).

roneous diagnoses were both bowel-containing omphaloceles.

As an aid in distinguishing gastroschisis from omphalocele, we suggest answering a series of questions whenever an abdominal wall defect is identified prenatally. This approach should also permit recognition of less common, but more complex, types of abdominal wall defects including ectopia cordis, cloacal exstrophy, amniotic band syndrome, and the limb-body wall complex. Although occasional exceptions to this generalization invariably will occur, this approach should permit correct categorization of nearly all abdominal wall defects.

1. *Is a limiting membrane present?* Omphalocele is always covered by a "membrane" comprised of the peritoneum and the outer layer of the umbilical cord (amnion). By contrast, gastroschisis is characterized by a through-and-through defect not limited by a membrane.[26, 35] Sonographic identification of the membrane may actually be easier than clinical evaluation since the membrane may rupture during delivery but rarely ruptures in utero.[35, 43] Rupture of an omphalocele during delivery may explain why instances of chromosome abnormalities (trisomy 13 or 18) or externalized liver occasionally have been reported in neonatal series of "gastroschisis" but not in prenatal series.[32, 36] Umbilical

hernia can be distinguished from omphalocele because it is covered by skin and subcutaneous fat.

2. *What is the relation of the umbilical cord to the defect?* The abdominal wall defect of omphalocele is located at the umbilical cord insertion site, whereas the defect of gastroschisis is paraumbilical in location. Bladder and cloacal exstrophy defects are infraumbilical in location, and the defect of ectopia cordis is located cephalad to the umbilical cord insertion. The defect and membranes of the limb-body wall complex (LBWC) are intimately connected with the umbilical cord.

3. *What organs are eviscerated?* Identification of eviscerated organs can help determine the type of malformation present and can provide important prognostic information. For example, evisceration of the heart (ectopia cordis) carries a very grave prognosis, whether or not it is associated with an omphalocele. Eviscerated liver usually represents an omphalocele, although other complex defects (LBWC, pentalogy of Cantrell, and cloacal exstrophy) should also be considered. Eviscerated bowel alone usually represents gastroschisis but may also be seen from an omphalocele that contains only bowel (intracorporeal liver).

Bowel-containing omphaloceles are important to recognize since they tend to be small and they can be missed or misdiagnosed. Also, recent evidence suggests

A

B

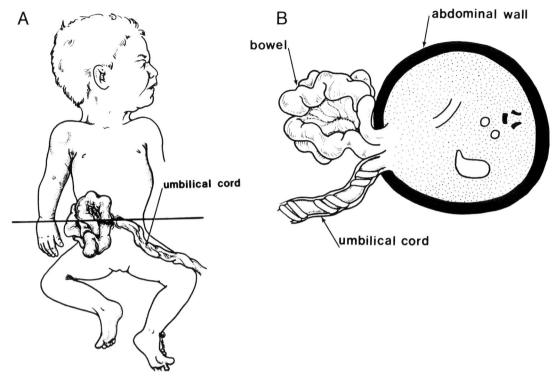

FIG 11-5.
Typical features of gastroschisis shown on external examination **(A)** and on cross-sectional view **(B)**. (Modified from Callen PW (ed): *Ultrasonography in Obstetrics and Gynecology*. Philadelphia, WB Saunders Co., 1988. Used by permission.)

that the absence of liver from the omphalocele sac carries a greater likelihood of an underlying chromosome malformation than omphaloceles that contain liver (see section on Omphalocele: Associated Anomalies below).[38]

4. *Is the bowel normal in appearance?* Near term, fetuses with gastroschisis commonly demonstrate mild bowel dilatation and bowel wall thickening, reflecting a chemical peritonitis caused by prolonged exposure of bowel to urine in the amniotic fluid.[7, 28] By contrast, the bowel in an omphalocele sac does not become directly exposed to amniotic fluid and demonstrates a more normal appearance. Marked bowel dilatation should suggest atresia or bowel infarction which frequently complicates gastroschisis but rarely is associated with omphalocele.[8, 42, 49]

5. *Are there additional malformations?* Omphalocele is commonly associated with concurrent malformations (50%–70%) and chromosome abnormalities (30%–40%), whereas other anomalies are rarely demonstrated with gastroschisis. An omphalocele seen in conjunction with severe scoliosis should suggest the diagnosis of the LBWC and an omphalocele associated a nondetectable urinary bladder should suggest the possibility of cloacal exstrophy. Demonstration of

other random defects (facial cleft, encephalocele) in combination with "gastroschisis" should suggest the amniotic band syndrome.

ABDOMINAL WALL MALFORMATIONS

Gastroschisis

Clinical and Pathologic Findings

Gastroschisis is a relatively small (2–4 cm) defect involving all layers of the abdominal wall (Fig 11–5). The defect is nearly always located just to the right of the umbilicus, although left-sided defects have been rarely described.[2] The most widely accepted etiology of gastroschisis, proposed by DeVries, suggests that the defect results from abnormal involution of the right umbilical vein which normally occurs 28–33 days post-conception (42–47 menstrual days).[2, 3] Other authors suggest that the defect is caused by disruption of the omphalomesenteric artery.[4]

The defect of gastroschisis is sporadic, and no genetic association or recurrence risks have been described. Maternal age is specifically not a risk factor. The reported incidence of gastroschisis has increased in recent years. This trend is thought to reflect both a

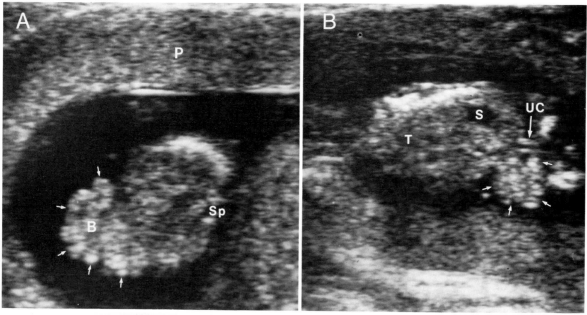

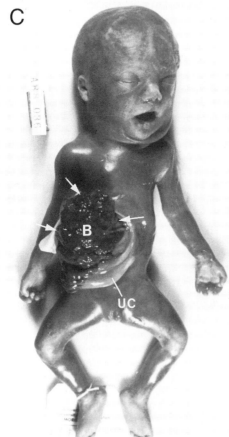

FIG 11–6.
Gastroschisis. **A,** transverse scan at 16 menstrual weeks in a woman referred for elevated MS-AFP demonstrates a relatively large amount of echogenic bowel *(B)*, delineated by arrows, eviscerated through the anterior abdominal wall. *SP* = spine; *P* = placenta. **B,** longitudinal scan demonstrates the bowel *(small arrows)* eviscerated through a defect adjacent to the umbilical cord insertion site *(UC)*, S = stomach; *T* = thorax. **C,** postnatal photograph shows bowel loops *(B)* demarcated by arrows eviscerated through an abdominal wall defect just to the right of the umbilical cord *(UC)*.

greater recognition of gastroschisis and a real increase in affected fetuses.[21, 36, 46] We have found a nearly equal frequency of omphalocele and gastroschisis with prenatal sonography.

The majority of fetuses with gastroschisis are now detected before 24 weeks with serum AFP screening and a targeted sonogram. Since eviscerated organs of gastroschisis come into direct contact with the amniotic fluid, AFP levels of gastroschisis tend to be higher than those associated with omphalocele.[40]

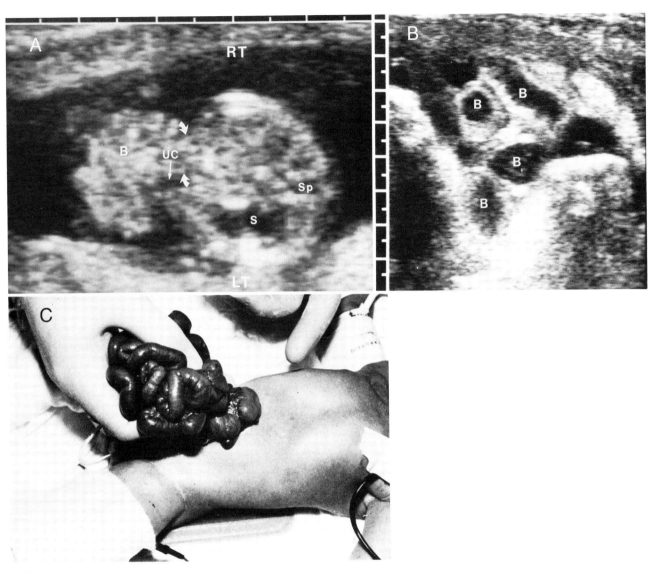

FIG 11–7.
Gastroschisis **A,** transverse scan at 13 menstrual weeks shows a large amount of bowel *(B)* eviscerated through an anterior abdominal wall defect. Note that the defect itself *(curved arrows)* is small in absolute terms (1 cm) and is located to the right of the umbilical cord insertion site *(UC)*. S = stomach; S = spine; *LT* = left; *RT,* = right. **B,** follow-up sonogram in the same fetus at 36 weeks shows eviscerated bowel loops *(B)* floating in the amniotic fluid. The abdominal wall defect and its relation with the cord insertion site are more difficult to visualize at this time, because of size and position of fetal structures. **C,** postnatal photograph shows normal appearance of fetal bowel. Mild dilatation of the bowel is typically present. This infant did well following surgical correction of the defect.

Sonographic Findings

The sonographic diagnosis of gastroschisis is highly reliable when the following characteristic findings are demonstrated: (1) the full-thickness abdominal wall defect is located just to the right of a normal umbilical cord insertion site; (2) a variable amount of bowel protrudes through the defect and floats in the surrounding amniotic fluid; and (3) eviscerated bowel may appear disproportionately large relative to the abdominal cavity, yet the defect itself is small, usually measuring less than 2 cm (Figs 11–6 and 11–7).[26] The abdominal cavity may be reduced in size, depending on the amount of eviscerated bowel.

Evaluation of eviscerated structures alone can usually suggest the correct diagnosis of gastroschisis.[1, 23, 43] Small bowel is always eviscerated, often accompanied by large bowel and, occasionally, the stomach or portions of the genitourinary system. Occasional reports have suggested that portions of the liver and the genitourinary system can also be eviscerated with gastroschisis, although this must be a very rare occurrence. In a large clinical series, liver was exposed in only three of 64 (5%) infants with gastroschisis,[33] whereas most prenatal studies and our own experience suggest that extracorporeal liver is never observed with true gastroschisis.[43] As a possible exception, Bair et al. reported one fetus with gastroschisis who showed extracorporeal liver on prenatal sonography.[7] However, the actual diagnosis is in doubt in this case because this series of omphalocele and gastroschisis also included anomalies that best fit the description of the limb-body wall complex.

When only bowel is eviscerated, other types of abdominal wall defects that should be considered include a bowel-containing omphalocele and the LBWC. Omphalocele can be distinguished by its characteristic location at the base of the umbilical cord and the presence of a limiting membrane. The LBWC usually demonstrates eviscerated liver, cranial and extremity defects, and scoliosis.[73]

Near term, eviscerated bowel exposed to amniotic fluid often appears slightly thickened and matted with gastroschisis (Fig 11–7).[7] This corresponds to its appearance at birth, when the bowel is covered by a fibrinous peel on its serosal surface and may look edematous and foreshortened. This appearance is thought to result from a chemical peritonitis induced by prolonged exposure of bowel to fetal urine in the amniotic fluid.[28] It is also the probable cause of the prolonged postoperative ileus experienced by many infants with gastroschisis, but not by infants with omphalocele. This fibrinous peel usually resolves by 4 weeks after birth.[51]

Mild dilatation of both the small and large bowel is also commonly seen when eviscerated bowel is exposed to amniotic fluid.[7] Development of marked bowel dilatation, however, should suggest bowel obstruction and/or ischemia (Fig 11–8).[8] Such bowel dilatation may be seen either external or internal to the abdominal cavity. Complications of gangrene, perforation, and meconium peritonitis may also occur (Fig 11–9).[6, 18] Bond et al. reported that 4 of 11 fetuses with gastroschisis in their series demonstrated bowel dilatation and wall nodularity, and all 4 infants showed complications of necrosis, atresias, or matted bowel after birth.[8] These authors suggest that early delivery should be considered in any fetus who demonstrates unusual bowel dilatation and mural thickening.

Polyhydraminos has been reported in the minority of cases of gastroschisis. When present, polyhydramnios should suggest the possibility of bowel obstruction or atresia (see Fig 11–9).

Associated Anomalies

Bowel-related abnormalities are both the most common and the most clinically important complications related to gastroschisis.[8, 18, 26, 27, 33, 42] By definition, the small bowel in gastroschisis is non–rotated and lacks secondary fixation to the dorsal abdominal wall. Intestinal atresia or stenosis is found in 7%–30% of fetuses secondary to intestinal and mesenteric ischemia that develops during embryologic development. Ischemia may result either from compression of the mesenteric vessels by the relatively small abdominal wall defect or from torsion of the eviscerated bowel around the mesenteric axis.[32, 33] Ischemia may also cause bowel perforations and meconium peritonitis (see Fig 11–9). The importance of bowel ischemia to the clinical outcome of gastroschisis is emphasized by two large neonatal series (n=170) in which half of the 23 infants with gastroschisis who presented with ischemia or gangrene subsequently died.[32, 33]

Anomalies other than bowel abnormalities rarely occur with gastroschisis. Hence, demonstration of extra-intestinal anomalies should suggest an alternative diagnosis. Cardiovascular malformations have been reported in 0%–8% of fetuses with gastroschisis but these tend to be minor and are not usually demonstrated on sonography.[36, 50]

Prognosis

The prognosis for fetuses identified with gastroschisis is generally excellent; the mortality rate has steadily and dramatically improved during the last three decades and is currently less than 10%.[32, 33, 36, 51] This remarkable achievement can be attributed to improved perinatal management including use of total parenteral nutrition and improved surgical technique. The greatest improvement has been shown in infants who weigh more than 2,500 grams. The major causes of neonatal death today are prematurity, sepsis, and intestinal complications related to bowel ischemia.[33, 50]

Management

Although the management of fetuses with gastroschisis will vary from institution to institution, we have adopted a standardized approach that we believe optimally treats the affected fetus.[18] The great majority of fetuses are now detected prior to 24 weeks with serum AFP screening and targeted sonograms.[16] Chromosomal analysis is not necessary following sonographic identification of gastroschisis, but can be performed if the diagnosis is in doubt or if amniocentesis is performed for other reasons (e.g., for confirmation of an abdominal wall defect by determination of amniotic fluid AFP). In-depth patient counseling should include discussions with a pediatric surgeon. If the pregnancy is continued, serial sonograms are performed to evaluate fetal growth and to detect possible bowel compli-

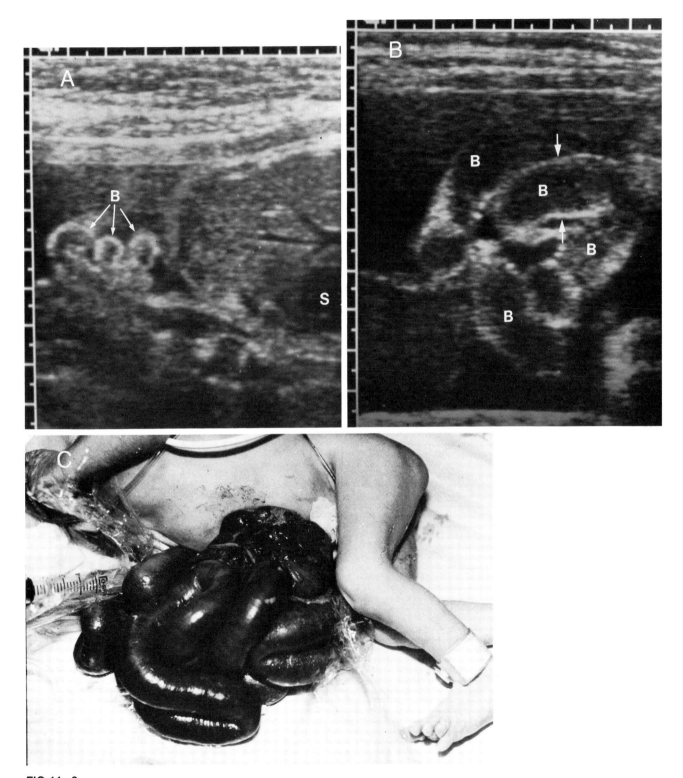

FIG 11–8.
Gastroschisis with bowel infarction. **A,** transverse scan at 28 weeks demonstrates bowel loops *(B)* floating in the amniotic fluid. *S* = stomach. **B,** follow-up sonogram at 34 weeks shows abnormal dilatation *(arrows)* of multiple small bowel loops *(B)*. **C,** postnatal photograph shows marked distension of small bowel loops from ischemia. Ninety percent of the small bowel was found to be infarcted.

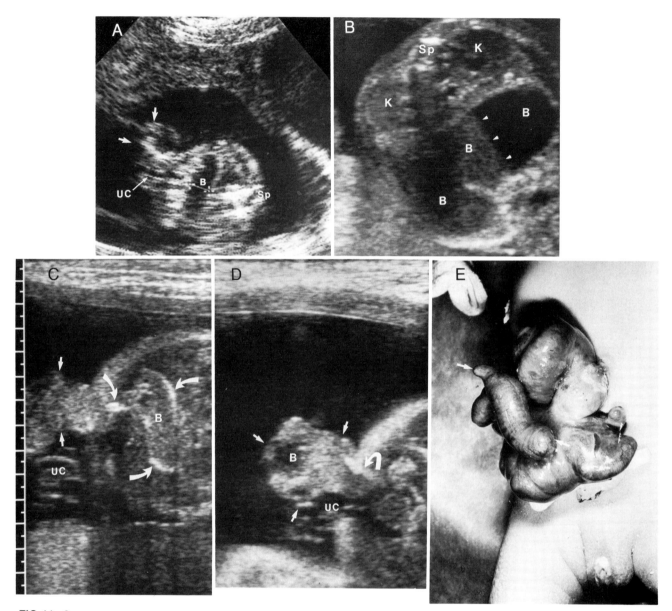

FIG 11–9.
Gastroschisis with bowel infarction and perforation. **A,** initial transverse scan at 18 weeks shows eviscerated bowel *(arrows)* just to the right of the umbilical cord insertion site *(UC).* An abnormally dilated loop of bowel *(B)* is identified coursing across the abdomen. *SP* = spine. **B,** follow-up sonogram at 27 weeks shows a markedly dilated bowel loop *(B)* within the abdominal cavity and a fluid-fluid level *(arrowheads)* within the dilated bowel loop. *SP* = spine; *K* = kidneys. **C,** follow-up scan 4 weeks later shows interval decompression of the the previously dilated bowel loop *(B).* Abnormally echogenic walls of the bowel *(curved arrows)* suggests development of meconium peritonitis. Eviscerated bowel is again noted adjacent to the umbilical cord insertion site *(UC).* **D,** eviscerated bowel *(B)* now appears abnormally confined and clumped *(arrows).* Linear echogenic areas *(curved arrow)* is noted extending across the abdominal wall defect, again suggesting meconium peritonitis. Also note development of polyhydramnios. *UC* = umbilical cord. **E,** postnatal photograph shows abnormally dilated and thickened bowel loops with meconium peritonitis on the serosal surface. Multiple sites of perforation and atresia *(arrows)* were identified. The infant has done poorly since surgery.

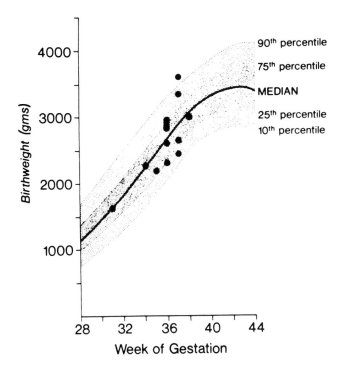

FIG 11-10.
Graph comparing birth weight with menstrual age in 16 infants with gastroschisis who were followed on prenatal sonography. An even distribution is shown about the median established for normal pregnancies. (From Fitzsimmons J, Nyberg DA, Cyr DR, et al: Perinatal management of gastroschisis. Obstet Gynecol 1988; 71:910–913. Used by permission.)

cations. Intrauterine growth retardation has been suggested as a possible complication in some neonatal-based studies of gastroschisis,[11, 32] although this has not been substantiated by a recent series of fetuses studied prenatally (Fig 11–10).[18]

Patients carrying a fetus with gastroschisis are delivered at, or near, a referral center staffed by experienced pediatric surgeons to facilitate prompt surgical correction of the abdominal defect. Some authorities recommend elective cesarean delivery to reduce the risk of bowel trauma and contamination.[18, 30] Others, however, have questioned the value of cesarean delivery to the eventual outcome.[22] Pre-term delivery at 36 weeks (following confirmation of lung maturity) has been suggested to minimize the risk of intrauterine bowel ischemia and possibly to decrease the time of postoperative ileus caused by prolonged exposure of bowel to amniotic fluid. However, Bond et al. suggest that early delivery be considered only in fetuses who show evidence of bowel dilatation and mural thickening on sonography.[8]

Primary closure of the abdominal wall defect is usually performed within 2 to 3 hours of delivery.[18] Prompt repair and closure of gastroschisis minimizes

problems of bacterial contamination, sepsis, hypothermia, and metabolic acidosis. Staged reduction and closure of the defect with a sialastic prosthesis is occasionally necessary for larger defects.[32] Following surgery, infants are treated with parenteral nutrition until normal bowel function resumes. The mean hospital stay is 20 days.[18]

Following corrective surgery, most patients can expect to lead a normal life. Potential complications are primarily related to the gastrointestinal tract and include recurrent bowel obstruction or esophageal reflux.[51] Subsequent bowel complications are more likely to develop in infants with bowel atresia and infants who required small bowel resection during the neonatal period.

Omphalocele

Clinical and Pathologic Findings

Omphalocele occurs in 1 in 4,000 births. An increased incidence of omphalocele has been observed with advancing maternal age, and infants born to older mothers are more likely to have an underlying chromosome abnormality.[19]

Pathologically, omphalocele is characterized by a midline defect of abdominal muscles, fascia, and skin that results in herniation of intra-abdominal structures into the base of the umbilical cord (Fig 11–11). Eviscerated abdominal structures are limited by a "membrane" which is actually comprised of two layers: the peritoneum and amnion.[2] While rupture of the membrane has been reported in 10%–20% of omphaloceles in clinical series, this complication rarely occurs in utero.[35, 43, 46] The limiting membrane presents a relative barrier to leakage of AFP into the amniotic fluid so that maternal serum AFP levels associated with omphalocele are generally lower and show a broader range than those observed with gastroschisis.[40]

Omphaloceles can be subcategorized pathologically either as (1) those that contain liver within the omphalocele sac (extracorporeal liver) or (2) those that contain a variable amount of bowel but no liver (intracorporeal liver) (Fig 11–12). This categorization is useful because each type produces a distinctive sonographic appearance and may also carry a different prognostic significance (see sections on Prognosis and Chromosomal Abnormalities below). Furthermore, the embryogenesis of each type may differ.[38, 47] Omphaloceles that contain only bowel may be considered simply as persistence of the primitive body stalk beyond 12 menstrual weeks.[3] However, since the liver is never found outside the abdominal cavity during normal embryologic development, omphaloceles with an extra-

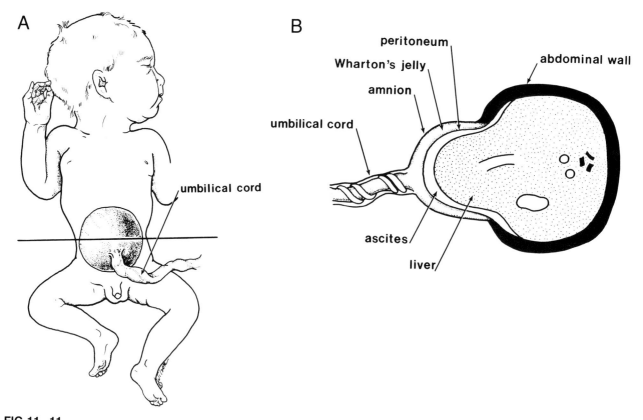

FIG 11–11.
Typical features of liver-containing omphalocele shown on external examination **(A)** and on cross-sectional view **(B)**. (Modified from Callen PW, (ed): *Ultrasonography in Obstetrics and Gynecology*. Philadelphia, WB Saunders Co, 1988. Used by permission.

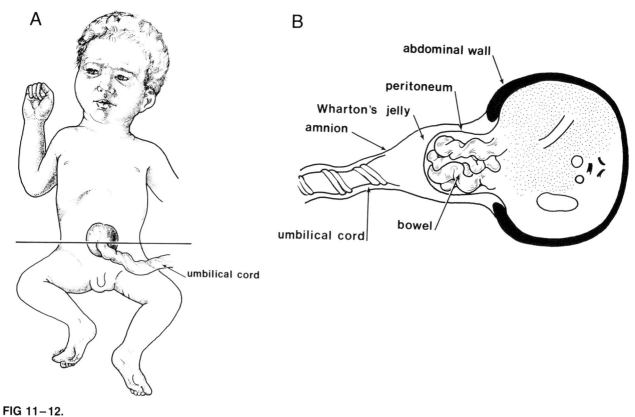

FIG 11–12.
Typical features of bowel-containing omphalocele (intracorporeal liver) shown on external examination **(A)** and on cross-sectional view **(B)**.

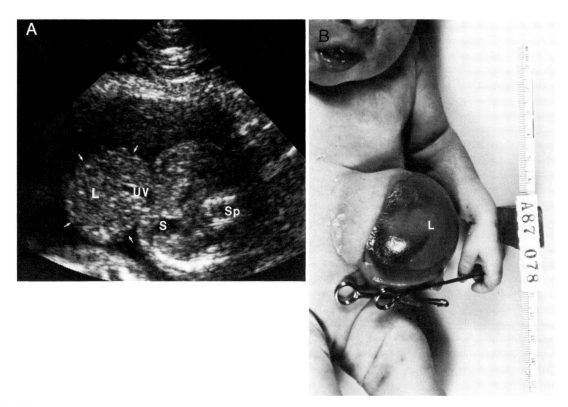

FIG 11–13.
Omphalocele. **A,** transverse sonogram at 20 weeks shows the liver *(L)* eviscerated through a relatively large, central abdominal wall defect. Note the intrahepatic portion of the umbilical vein *(UV)* courses directly through the defect. Also note that the surrounding membranes of peritoneum and amnion cannot be identified, although their presence is inferred by the compact eviscerated organs *(small arrows). S =* stomach; *Sp* = spine. **B,** photograph at necropsy, following spontaneous neonatal demise, shows externalized liver *(L)* covered by a translucent membrane. The clamp is attached to the umbilical cord insertion site. A ventricular septal defect was also present. The karyotype was a normal female.

corporeal liver may result from primary failure of body wall closure.[26, 47]

Sonographic Findings

Unlike gastroschisis, omphalocele may demonstrate a variable appearance depending on the size of the abdominal wall defect, type of eviscerated organs, presence of ascites, and associated anomalies (Figs 11–13 to 11–19).[10, 38, 45] Therefore, it is important to keep in mind those features that permit a reliable diagnosis of omphalocele and distinction from gastroschisis. Failure to observe these differences can lead to serious errors in interpretation and inappropriate management of affected fetuses.[20]

The central location of the abdominal wall defect at the base of the umbilical cord insertion site is a primary and diagnostic feature of omphalocele. However, since the umbilical cord inserts into the caudal-apical portion of the herniated sac, the relationship with the umbilical cord may be best visualized on sagittal or oblique scans rather than on transverse views alone. Demonstration of the intrahepatic umbilical vein

coursing through the defect is also evidence for the central location of the abdominal wall defect (see Fig 11–13).

The presence of a limiting membrane (amnion and peritoneum) is another essential feature of omphalocele (see Fig 11–15). However, the membrane itself may be difficult to visualize as a discrete structure when not outlined by ascites (see Fig 11–13). In this situation, the existence of a membrane is often inferred by showing that extracorporeal structures appear contained rather than floating freely in the amniotic fluid (see Fig 11–13). Amorphous material representing Wharton jelly may also be observed between the amnion and peritoneum (see Fig 11–15).

Ascites is commonly observed with omphalocele and its presence can provide supportive evidence for a limiting membrane.[7] A large amount of ascites, however, can be confused with amniotic fluid and may lead to an erroneous diagnosis of gastroschisis. As a distinguishing finding, the bowel contained within an omphalocele sac is not directly exposed to amniotic fluid and does not become thickened or dilated.[7]

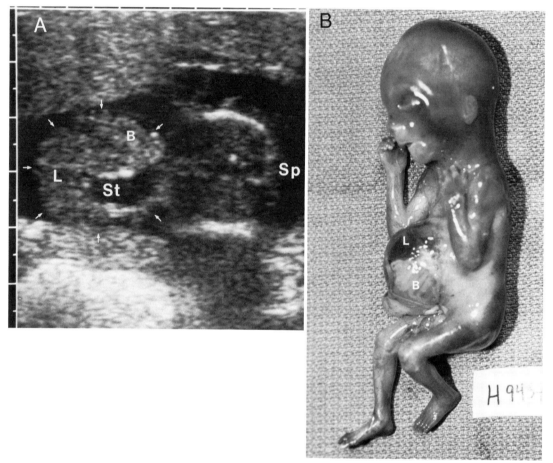

FIG 11–14.
Large omphalocele. **A,** transverse scan at 18 weeks shows a large omphalocele that contains liver *(L),* bowel *(B),* and stomach *(St).* Sp = spine. **B,** photograph at necropsy shows liver *(L)* and bowel *(B)* in the omphalocele sac. (From Hughes M, Nyberg DA, Mack LA, et al: Fetal omphalocele: Prenatal detection of concurrent anomalies and other predictors of outcome. Radiology, in press. Used by permission.)

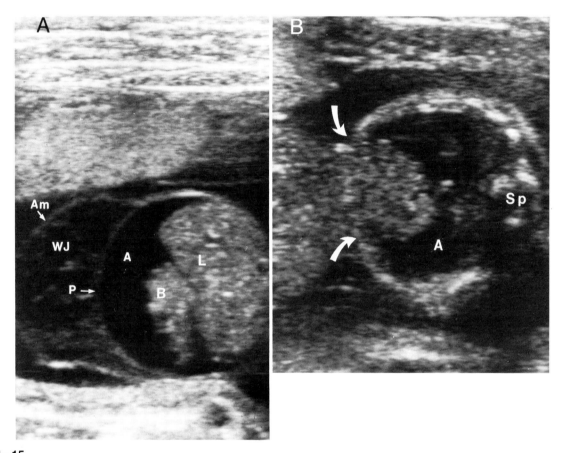

FIG 11–15.
Large omphalocele. **A,** transverse scan at 23 weeks shows eviscerated liver *(L)*, bowel *(B)*, and ascites *(A)* contained within an omphalocele sac. Note that the limiting membrane is comprised of both the peritoneum *(P)* and amnion *(Am)*, which are separated by Wharton jelly *(WJ)*. **B,** scan of the abdomen shows a large midline defect *(curved arrows)* with ascites *(A)* and relatively few organs within the abdominal cavity. *Sp* = spine.

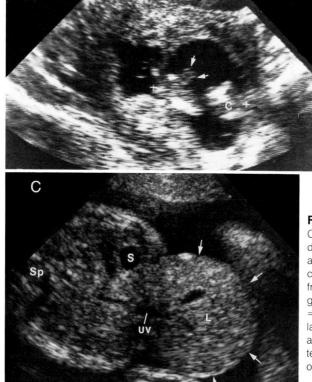
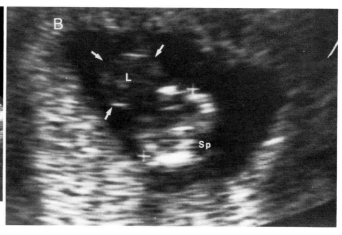

FIG 11–16.
Omphalocele at 12 weeks. **A,** longitudinal scan at 12 weeks demonstrates a soft tissue mass *(arrows)* protruding from the anterior abdomen. *C* = cranium. **B,** high-resolution, magnification scan in transverse plane confirms liver *(L)* protruding from the anterior abdominal wall. The size of eviscerated organs *(arrows)* is nearly equal to the abdominal diameter. *Sp* = spine. **C,** follow-up examination at 36 weeks shows the large omphalocele *(arrows)* containing liver *(L).* No other anomalies were detected on sonography or were present after birth, and the infant did well following surgical correction of the defect. *S* = stomach; *UV* = umbilical vein; *Sp* = spine.

As previously indicated, omphaloceles differ in their appearance by the presence or absence of liver from the omphalocele sac. Omphaloceles that contain only bowel comprised 50%–70% of omphaloceles in several large neonatal studies[33, 35] but the minority of omphaloceles in prenatal series (10%–25%).[7, 9, 43] A possible explanation for this discrepancy is that omphaloceles which contain only bowel tend to be small and can be missed with sonography; Mann et al. reported missing 6 of 7 small omphaloceles that presumably contained only bowel on prenatal sonography.[34] Alternatively, neonatal studies may have misdiagnosed some infants with a ruptured omphalocele as gastroschisis. Since the liver is never found outside the abdominal cavity during normal embryologic development,[5] demonstration of eviscerated liver should permit a reliable diagnosis of omphalocele at any age (see Fig 11–16).[15]

Omphaloceles that contain liver typically demonstrate a relatively large abdominal wall defect in comparison to the abdominal diameter (see Figs 11–13 to 11–16).[38] The liver can be identified by its homogeneous appearance and the presence of intrahepatic vessels. By comparison, omphaloceles that contain only bowel (intracorporeal liver) demonstrate a variable appearance, depending on the amount of bowel present

(see Figs 11–17 to 11–19). The bowel is characteristically more echogenic and irregular in appearance than the liver and does not contain intrahepatic vessels.[38]

When extracorporeal liver is demonstrated, it is important to distinguish omphalocele from the LBWC, a disorder that has been uniformly associated with a fatal outcome. The LBWC should be considered whenever marked scoliosis is demonstrated in association with omphalocele. Other typical findings of the LBWC include scoliosis, cranial defects, limb defects, abnormal cord attachment to the placental membranes, and abdominal wall defect.

A bowel-containing omphalocele should be distinguished from gastroschisis or umbilical hernia.[38] Gastroschisis can be readily distinguished by the absence of a limiting membrane, absent ascites, and its paraumbilical location.[39, 43] Distinguishing a small omphalocele from umbilical hernia may be more difficult, however, since both defects are located at the umbilical cord insertion site. However, the defect of omphalocele is limited only by a membrane, whereas the defect of umbilical hernia is covered by skin and subcutaneous fat.

Ultrasonographers should be aware of a potential false-positive diagnosis of omphalocele in normal fe-

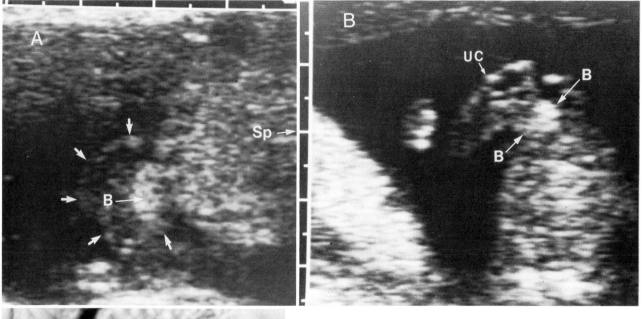

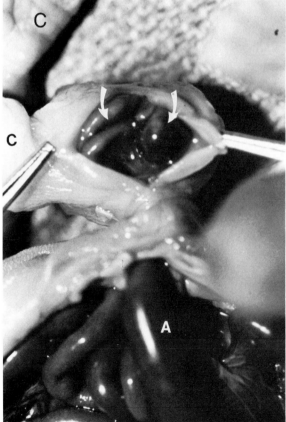

FIG 11–17.
Bowel-containing omphalocele. **A,** transverse sonogram at 15 weeks shows echogenic bowel *(B)* eviscerated through a small abdominal wall defect and surrounded by a "membrane" *(arrows)*. *Sp* = spine. **B,** another view of the same patient shows the echogenic bowel *(B)* herniated into the base of the umbilical cord *(UC)*. **C,** corresponding pathological specimen, following termination of pregnancy, shows bowel *(curved arrows)* herniated into the base of the umbilical cord *(C)*. Bowel within the abdominal cavity *(A)* has been exposed during autopsy. The only additional anomaly was Meckel diverticulum. The karyotype was trisomy 18. (From Nyberg DA, Fitzsimmons J, Mack LA, et al: Chromosome abnormalities in fetuses with omphalocele: Significance of omphalocele contents, J Ultrasound Med 1989; 8:299–308. Used by permission.)

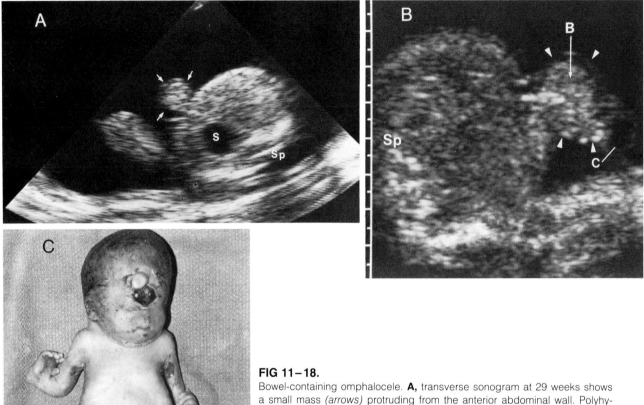

FIG 11–18.
Bowel-containing omphalocele. **A,** transverse sonogram at 29 weeks shows a small mass *(arrows)* protruding from the anterior abdominal wall. Polyhydramnios is also noted. *S* = stomach; *Sp* = spine. **B,** magnification view shows the mass represents bowel *(B)* herniated into the base of the umbilical cord *(C).* Other malformations identified on sonography included holoprosencephaly, cyclopia, and radial aplasia. *Sp* = spine. **C,** corresponding pathologic specimen confirms the sonographic findings and shows bowel herniated into a small omphalocele. The karyotype was a variant of trisomy 18. (Parts **B,C,** and **D** reprinted from Nyberg DA, Fitzsimmons J, Mack LA, et al: Chromosome abnormalities in fetuses with omphalocele: Significance of omphalocele contents. J Ultrasound Med 1989; 8:299–308. Used by permission.)

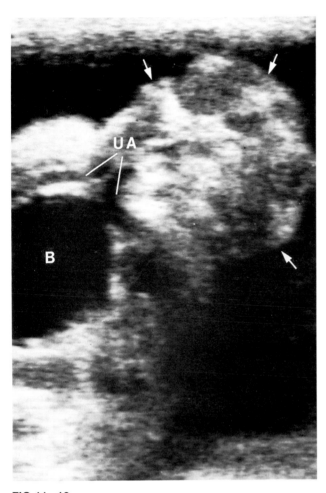

FIG 11–19.
Large bowel-containing omphalocele. Oblique scan of the lower abdomen at 32 weeks shows a large midline omphalocele *(arrows)* that appeared to contain only loops of bowel *(arrows)*. Trisomy 21 was found on chromosome analysis. *B* = urinary bladder; *UA* = umbilical arteries.

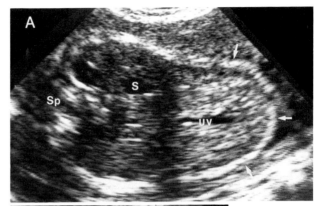

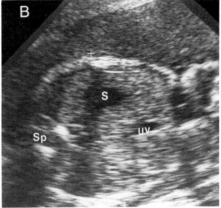

FIG 11–20.
Pseudo-omphalocele. **A,** transverse sonogram at 32 weeks shows distortion of the abdomen that could mistaken for an omphalocele. However, note that the subcutaneous fat *(arrows)* is intact. *S* = stomach; *UV* = umbilical vein; *Sp* = spine. **B,** scan a few minutes later with less compression shows a normal abdominal shape and no omphalocele. *S* = stomach; *UV* = umbilical vein; *Sp* = spine.

tuses (pseudo-omphalocele) by scanning in an oblique plane and/or by compressing the fetal abdomen (see Fig 11–20).[31, 44] Repeat scanning in a true transverse plane and using minimal compression should clarify any question of such a defect. A false-positive diagnosis of omphalocele has also been attributed to a thickened umbilical cord.[13]

Polyhydramnios has been noted in approximately one third of fetuses with omphalocele.[25] The etiology of polyhydramnios is not always clear. Nelson et al. suggest that polyhydramnios may indicate the presence of a high gastrointestinal obstruction such as midgut volvulus.[37] However, polyhydramnios might also result from a central nervous system anomaly, such as holoprosencephaly or a major chromosome disorder on the basis of decreased fetal swallowing. Whatever the mechanism, the presence of polyhydramnios may be

associated with a worse fetal outcome. In considering 22 fetuses with omphalocele who were not terminated, Hughes et al. observed deaths in 7 of 8 fetuses (88%) with abnormal amniotic fluid volume (polyhydramnios or oligohydramnios), compared to 3 of 12 fetuses (25%) with normal amniotic fluid volume.[25]

Associated Anomalies

Associated anomalies have been reported in 67%–88% of fetuses with omphalocele identified on prenatal sonography (Table 11–3),[7, 19, 25, 48] with a somewhat lower rate observed in large postnatal series (Table 11–4).[33, 36, 46] Cardiac anomalies are present in 30%–50% of fetuses with an omphalocele and are often complex. Central nervous system anomalies occur less frequently, but are easier to detect on prenatal sonography.[25] Genitourinary and gastrointestinal malformations are also relatively common. Compared to gastroschisis, however, small bowel atresia is uncommon with omphalocele, probably because the larger abdom-

TABLE 11–3.

Associated Malformations, Chromosome Abnormalities, and Mortality Rate in Fetuses Identified With Omphalocele in Selected Prenatal Studies

Author	Hughes[25]† (n=46)	Bair[7] (n=16)	Gilbert[19] (n=35)	Sermer[48] (n=17)
Overall anomaly rate	67%	88%	80%	71%
Cardiovascular malformations	35%	44%	47%	34%
Genitourinary anomalies	15%	38%	23%	47%
Gastrointestinal	15%	31%	NA*	29%
Small bowel atresia	4%	5%		
Anal atresia	4%	6%		
Esophageal atresia	4%			
Central nervous system	18%	–	17%	6%
Musculoskeletal	23%	38%	30%	29%
Facial cleft	5%	–	–	–
Beckwith-Wiedemann	5%	–	–	–
Chromosome abnormality	43% (13/30)	NA*	54% (19/35)	40% (4/10)
Uncorrected mortality rate	78%	75%	74%	59%

*NA = information not available.
†Percents reported for 40 cases, excluding 6 fetuses with inadequate followup or pathologic examination.

inal wall defect is less likely to compromise mesenteric blood flow.[49]

Other complex syndromes that may include omphalocele as a prominent feature include pentalogy of Cantrell (a "cephalic fold" defect) and cloacal exstrophy (a "caudal fold" defect).[11, 26] These more complex anomalies should be distinguished from typical omphaloceles (a "lateral fold" defect) because their pathogeneses, sonographic findings, associated anomalies, and prognoses differ markedly. Pentalogy of Cantrell is characterized by a large upper abdominal omphalocele, anterior diaphragmatic hernia, sternal cleft, ectopia cordis, and a variety of cardiovascular malformations. Cloacal exstrophy consists of a low abdominal wall defect associated with bladder or cloacal exstrophy and frequently other caudal anomalies (anal

TABLE 11–4.

Associated Malformations, Chromosome Abnormalities, and Mortality Rate in Infants With Omphalocele in Selected Postnatal Studies

Author	Mabogunje[33] (n=57)	Schwaitzenberg[46] (n=28)	Mayer[36] (n=28)
Overall anomaly rate	56%	72%	66%
Cardiovascular malformations	19%	41%	52%
Genitourinary anomalies	4%	15%	8%
Gastrointestinal			NA†
Small bowel atresia	9%	5%	
Anal atresia	4%	5%	
Esophageal atresia	4%	5%	
Central nervous system		5%	10%
Musculoskeletal	2%	10%	6%
Diaphragmatic hernia	7%	13%	8%
Cleft palate	2%		3%
Beckwith-Wiedemann	9%	10%	0
Chromosomal Abnormality	9% (5/57)	NA†	40%*
Uncorrected mortality rate	19%	26%	34%

*The actual number of chromosome anomalies was not reported.
†NA = information not available.

atresia, spinal abnormalities and/or meningomyelocele, and lower limb anomalies).

The Beckwith-Wiedemann syndrome is an autosomal dominant disorder characterized by gigantism, macroglossia and pancreatic hyperplasia (resulting in profound neonatal hypoglycemia).[29] It comprises 5%–10% of omphaloceles in postnatal series. Conversely, 12% of infants born with the Beckwith-Wiedemann syndrome have an omphalocele or umbilical hernia. Affected patients have an increased incidence of Wilms' tumor, renal anomalies, and hemihypertrophy. Minor chromosome aberrations have been identified in some cases.[41]

A specific sonographic diagnosis of Beckwith-Wiedemann syndrome has been made prenatally in several cases. One case was suggested by demonstration of an omphalocele in combination with a positive family history,[53] another was identified by detection of bilateral cystic kidneys and polyhydramnios in association with omphalocele,[54] and two others were diagnosed by demonstration of macroglossia without an associated omphalocele in conjunction with a positive family history.[12]

In addition to detection and evaluation of the omphalocele itself, sonography can help to determine the prognosis for an affected fetus by identification of major concurrent malformations.[25] Prenatal detection of any concurrent malformation significantly increases the likelihood of an underlying chromosome abnormality and subsequent death.[25] Because of the frequency of major cardiac defects, a careful fetal echocardiogram is recommended whenever an omphalocele is identified.[14]

Chromosome Abnormalities

Chromosome abnormalities have been reported in 10% to 40% of neonates with omphalocele, with a combined mean rate of 12%.[19, 24, 38] A higher frequency (40%) has been observed in most prenatal studies (see Tables 11–3 and 11–4), probably due to inclusion of more severely anomalous fetuses who die in utero or during the immediate neonatal period.[7, 19, 25, 48] Also, neonatal studies may have under reported the true prevalence of chromosome disorders since the number of infants who underwent chromosome analysis is not usually reported.

Trisomies 18 and 13 have been most commonly associated with omphalocele, followed by trisomy 21, 45 X (Turner syndrome), and triploidy.[19, 38] Conversely, approximately one third of fetuses with trisomy 13 and 10%–50% of fetuses with trisomy 18 will have an omphalocele.[29]

Awareness of risk factors associated with an underlying chromosome disorder in a fetus with a known omphalocele is potentially useful for patient counseling. In a series of 35 fetuses identified with omphalocele on prenatal sonography, Gilbert and Nicolaides recently reported that chromosome abnormalities were associated with advanced maternal age (≥33 years), male fetuses, and concurrent anomalies.[19] Compared to other series, however, this study reported an unusually high rate of chromosome abnormalities (54%), a preponderance of trisomy 18 (17 of 19 chromosome abnormalities), and a high (3 to 1) male-female involvement.

In another series of 26 fetuses with omphalocele and known karyotype, Nyberg et al. found that chromosome abnormalities were most significantly associated with absence of liver from the omphalocele sac (p < .0001, see Figs 11–17 to 11–19).[38] Statistical significance was also reached for advanced maternal age (p = .03), confirming the results of Gilbert and Nicolaides, but only a weak association was noted for the male sex (p = .23). Sonographic detection of concurrent malformations was also found to be statistically associated with an underlying chromosome abnormality in fetuses with omphalocele.[38] Malformations that were identified in such fetuses with chromosome abnormalities included holoprosencephaly, cerebellar hypoplasia, facial cleft, cystic hygroma, and cardiac malformations. Central nervous system anomalies were more readily detected than cardiac malformations in this series and correlated more strongly with abnormal karyotypes.

Prognosis

The prognosis for fetuses with omphalocele depends primarily on the presence and severity of concurrent anomalies.[21, 29, 33, 36] For this reason, the overall mortality rate for omphaloceles during the last two decades has not improved as much as for gastroschisis.[33] The presence of one or more concurrent malformations is associated with perinatal mortality of 80%, and the presence of a chromosome abnormality or a major cardiovascular malformation increases the mortality rate to nearly 100%.[25, 36] When no other anomalies are present, however, the mortality rate drops to nearly 10%, which is similar to that for gastroschisis.[29, 36, 50] In a prenatal series, Hughes et al. found that a relatively favorable prognosis could be expected in fetuses without chromosome abnormalities, sonographically detectable concurrent anomalies, or abnormal amounts of amniotic fluid volume (polyhydramnios or oligohydramnios).[25]

The possible contribution to fetal mortality of factors other than associated anomalies or chromosome abnormalities is unclear. Intuitively, a worse prognosis would be expected from large omphaloceles that contain a greater number of organs, assuming no difference in associated anomalies.[26, 52] Indeed, a worse outcome has been observed in "giant" omphaloceles due to respiratory insufficiency.[52] However, this contribution may be overshadowed by the greater importance of concurrent malformations and chromosome abnormalities.[38] Mayer reported that large omphaloceles (>5 cm) were associated with a greater neonatal mortality than small omphaloceles, whereas Mabogunje found that the size of the omphalocele was not significant.[33, 36] In the only prenatal study to evaluate this in detail, no statistical association was found between fetal mortality and either the absolute or relative size of the omphalocele.[25]

Schwaitzberg reported a higher perinatal mortality for neonates born with an extracorporeal liver (56% vs. 14%),[46] whereas Kirk and Wah observed a higher mortality rate for those with an intracorporeal liver (60% vs. 33%).[27] The largest neonatal series (n=57) found no significant difference between these two groups (21% vs. 18%).[33] The apparent disparity in these observations may be explained by the greater risk of chromosome abnormalities in fetuses with an intracorporeal liver.

Management

The appropriate mode of delivery for fetuses identified with an omphalocele is controversial.[11, 23, 27] Cesarean delivery has been suggested by some authorities to decrease the potential risk of infection and to avoid possible rupture of the sac during vaginal delivery. Others, however, have questioned the validity of this practice.[23, 27] Certainly, elective cesarean delivery may not be justifiable when major concurrent major malformations or chromosome abnormalities are present. Following delivery, infants should undergo a thorough clinical examination and fetal echocardiography. Those considered to be suitable surgical candidates then undergo surgical repair of their defect. In the absence of significant concurrent anomalies, prompt surgical repair has been reported to have a low perinatal mortality, with a prognosis approaching that of gastroschisis.[33]

Ectopia Cordis

Clinical and Pathologic Findings

Ectopia cordis is a rare malformation of the ventral wall that results in evisceration of the heart through the defect. Depending on its location, ectopia cordis has been classified into five categories: cervical, thora-

cocervical, thoracic, thoracoabdominal, and abdominal.[67] Ninety-five percent of cases are of the thoracic or thoracoabdominal types.

Thoracic ectopia cordis consists of a sternal defect, partially absent parietal pericardium, protrusion of all or part of the heart through the defect and, in most cases, an omphalocele. The less common thoracoabdominal ectopia cordis includes a diaphragmatic defect and, frequently, intrinsic cardiac defects. The combination of ectopia cordis, diaphragmatic defect, omphalocele or ventral abdominal wall defect, pericardial defect, and intracardiac malformation has been termed the pentalogy of Cantrell.[67, 70]

The pathogenesis of ectopia cordis is most commonly ascribed to failure of fusion of the lateral body folds in the thoracic region. Other authors suggest that ectopia cordis is a manifestation of the amniotic band syndrome since rupture of the chorion and/or yolk sac at 5 menstrual weeks might interfere with normal cardiac descent.[64] Ravitch suggests that the pentalogy of Cantrell results from aplasia of both the transverse septum that forms the anterior diaphragm and the associated pericardium between 14 and 18 days of embryonic life.[67]

Sonographic Findings

Ectopia cordis has been frequently diagnosed on prenatal sonography.* Demonstration of an extrathoracic heart is a dramatic finding which is, of course, diagnostic of ectopia cordia (Fig 11–21). However, only a portion of the heart may herniate through the defect, in which case the diagnosis is more difficult (Fig 11–22).[60, 68] Ectopia cordis and omphalocele may be missed in the face of oligohydramnios.[56]

Demonstration of both ectopia cordis and omphalocele should suggest a more specific diagnosis of pentalogy of Cantrell.[60] Although this diagnosis depends on the presence of an intracardiac malformation, the cardiac defect may be difficult to demonstrate due to distortion of cardiac structures. As a practical point, a dismal prognosis is associated with the combination of ectopia cordis and omphalocele, whether or not a cardiac defect is also present.

Associated Anomalies

Anomalies most frequently associated with ectopia cordis include omphalocele, cardiovascular malformations, and craniofacial defects.[55, 60, 62, 65] In a series of eight fetuses with ectopia cordis reported by Klingensmith et al., five 63% also had an omphalocele, and six (75%) fetuses also had structural cardiac defects (see

*References 55–57, 60, 62, 63, 65, 66, 68, 69, 71.

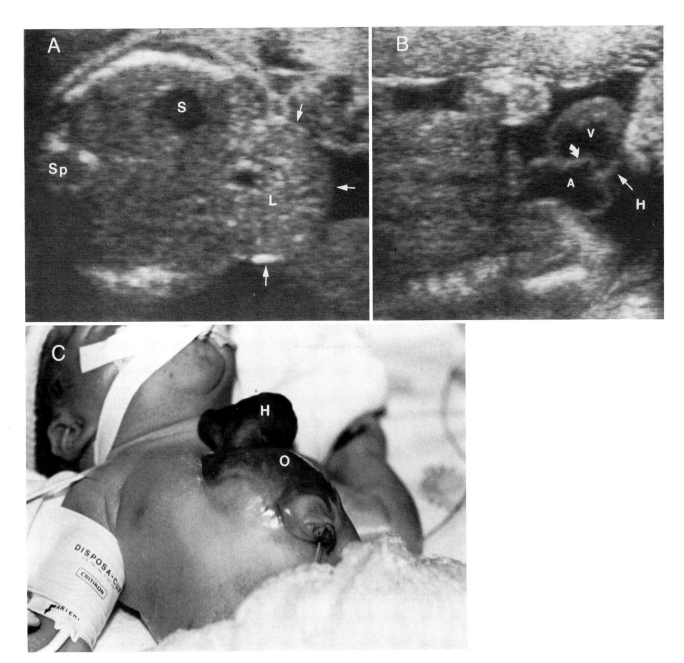

FIG 11–21.
Ectopia cordis with pentalogy of Cantrell. **A,** transverse scan at 24 weeks shows a supraumbilical omphalocele *(arrows)* containing liver *(L).* *S* = stomach; *Sp* = spine. **B,** scan at a more cephalic level demonstrates the heart *(H)* eviscerated into the amniotic fluid. An atrioventricular septal defect is identified with a single atrioventricular valve *(curved arrow)* separating a large atrial septal defect and ventricular septal defect. Other abnormalities found at necropsy included atrioventricular septal defect, double-outlet right ventricle, and pulmonic stenosis. *A* = atrium; *V* = ventricles. **C,** photograph prior to attempted surgical repair shows the externalized heart *(H)* and omphalocele *(O).*

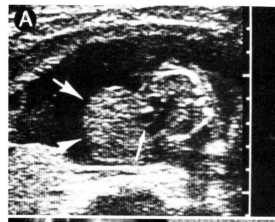

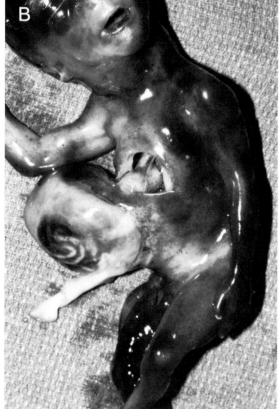

FIG 11–22.
Ectopia cordis. **A,** transverse sonogram at 18 weeks shows an omphalocele *(large arrows)* and a portion of the heart *(small arrow)* eviscerated through an anterior defect. **B,** photograph of pathologic specimen shows the omphalocele and partial evisceration of the heart. Note the relative cephalic location of this defect relative to the umbilical cord compared to typical omphaloceles. (From Seeds JW, Cefalo RC, Lies SC, et al: Early prenatal sonographic appearance of rare thoraco-abdominal eventration. Prenat Diag 1984; 4:437–441.)

Fig 11–21).[65] Cardiac defects usually include a ventricular septal defect with or without tetralogy of Fallot.[60, 65] Other possible anomalies include pulmonary hypoplasia, cranial defects, facial cleft, clubbed feet, and kyphoscoliosis.[60, 65] Interestingly, many of these

defects might be ascribed to the amniotic band syndrome.[64]

Chromosome abnormalities have been associated with ectopia cordis including one case of trisomy 18 reported by Klingensmith et al[65] and two cases of trisomy 18 among ten fetuses with the pentalogy of Cantrell reported by Ghidini et al.[60] Pentalogy of Cantrell has also been associated with trisomy 13 and 45,X (Turner syndrome) in postnatal reports.[59]

Prognosis

Ectopia cordis carries a very high mortality rate, with most infants dying within a few days of birth and few patients living more than a few months.[60] Surgical correction of the defect holds some promise, but the results have been disappointing, with few patients surviving the operation.[61, 70] Isolated ectopia cordis should have a somewhat better prognosis than that associated with an omphalocele,[58] although no survival has yet been reported of any fetus with ectopia cordis who was diagnosed prenatally.

Limb-Body Wall Complex

Clinical and Pathologic Findings

The limb-body wall complex (LBWC) is also referred to as the body-stalk anomaly or cyllosomas. It is a complex malformation that has no sex or familial predilection or known recurrence risk.[75, 76] Some cases of the LBWC have previously been misdiagnosed as omphalocele or gastroschisis. Whether or not the LBWC is embryologically distinct from the amniotic band syndrome (see below), we believe that recognition of the LBWC as a separate disorder is justified because of its severity of defects which are incompatible with extrauterine life.

Primary pathologic features of the LBWC include large cranial defects (exencephaly or encephalocele), facial clefts, a body-wall defect involving the thorax, abdomen, or both; and limb defects.[75, 76] Other common abnormalities include scoliosis and various internal malformations. A distinguishing pathologic feature is failure of fusion of the amnion and chorion. The amnion does not cover the umbilical cord normally, but rather extends as a sheet from the margin of the cord and is continuous with both the body wall and the placenta (Figs 11–23 and 11–24).[75]

Body defects are a constant feature of the LBWC. In a recent sonographic review of 13 fetuses with the LBWC who were evaluated by prenatal sonography, Patten et al. reported trunk defects in 12 cases (92%).[73] Similarly, in a larger autopsy series of 25 fetuses, Van Allen et al. found body defects in 96% of

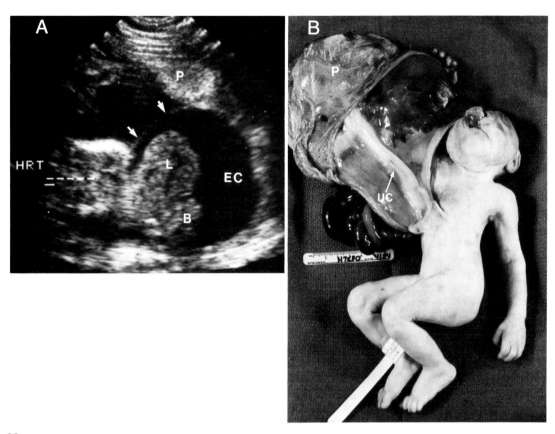

FIG 11–23.
Limb-body wall complex. **A,** transverse sonogram at level of thoracoabdominal junction demonstrates large anterior abdominal wall defect with liver *(L)* and bowel *(B)* herniated into extraembryonic coelom *(EC)*. Note continuity of the amniotic membrane *(arrows)* with the body wall and placenta *(P)*. *HRT* = heart. **B,** photograph of pathologic specimen shows the large abdominal wall defect. The umbilical cord *(UC)* is incorporated into the abnormal amniotic membrane, which is contiguous with the abdominal wall and the placenta *(P)*. Also note the presence of facial cleft and cranial defect. (From Patten RM, Van Allen M, Mack LA, et al: Limb-body wall complex: In utero sonographic diagnosis of a complicated fetal malformation. AJR 1986; 46:1019–1024. Used by permission.)

cases.[75] The body defects are generally large, involving both the thorax and abdomen in 64% of cases (see Fig 11–23). Left-sided body wall defects are three times more common than right-sided defects.[75] Typically, the eviscerated organs form a complex, bizarre-appearing mass entangled with membranes. Abdominal and thoracic contents herniate through this defect into the extraembryonic coelom.

The pathogenesis of the LBWC is uncertain. Some researchers have suggested that the primary defect involves body-stalk dysmorphogenesis. Smith and others have suggested that LBWC results from rupture of the amnion caused by vascular disruption or mechanical compression between the third and fifth weeks.[74, 75] A vascular etiology is supported by the predominance of disruptive defects and the high frequency of internal defects that can be attributed to vascular disruption.[75]

As previously suggested, some consider the LBWC simply to represent a severe form of the amniotic band syndrome. Indeed, amniotic bands are present in 40%

of cases of the LBWC, and some of the limb defects can be attributed to amniotic bands.[74] However, many of the other limb and structural defects found in association with the LBWC cannot be easily explained by amniotic bands. Van Allen suggests that the presence of amniotic bands is a consequence of early vascular disruption, but is not the primary abnormality itself.[74]

Sonographic Findings

Body defects are generally large, involving both the thorax and abdomen (see Figs 11–23 and 11–24). Typically, the eviscerated organs form a complex, bizarre-appearing mass entangled with membranes.[73] Fetal membranes are continuous with the body-wall or neural tube defect and the placenta (see Figs 11–23 and 11–24). If specifically sought, the umbilical cord can be seen to be short and adherent to placental membranes.

Spinal anomalies, including spinal dysraphic defects and/or scoliosis (usually severe), are present in

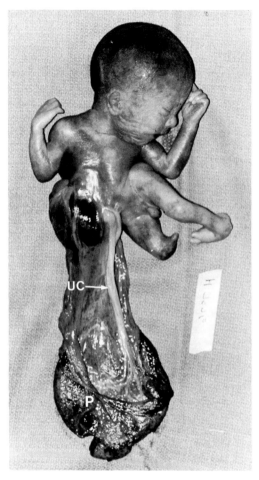

FIG 11–24.
Limb-body wall complex. Postmortem photograph of another fetus shows characteristic findings of the limb-body wall complex including a large thoracoabdominal defect. Note that the umbilical cord *(UC)* is incorporated into the abnormal amniotic membrane which is continuous with both the body wall defect and the placenta *(P)*. Also note marked scoliosis and extremity defects.

most cases of the LBWC (see Fig 11–24). Therefore, the combination of omphalocele and scoliosis should always suggest the diagnosis of the LBWC.[73] Distorted fetal position and the severity of the defects makes recognition of normal fetal parts difficult. Specific limb anomalies may be difficult to recognize, even though they are usually present on pathological examination. Cranial defects (anencephaly and encephalocele) were present in 6 of the 13 cases reported prenatally.[73]

Associated Anomalies

A variety of major structural defects accompany the LBWC. In the series of 25 fetuses with the LBWC reported by Van Allen et al., major anomalies included: limb defects (95%); marked scoliosis (77%); malformations of internal organs (95%); and craniofacial defects including facial cleft, and encephalocele or exen-

cephaly (56%).[75] Limb defects include clubfoot (32%), absent limbs or digits, arthrogryposis or web, polydactyly and syndactyly. Internal malformations, present in 95% of cases, include cardiac defects (56%), absent diaphragm (74%), bowel atresia (22%), and renal abnormalities including agenesis, hydronephrosis, or dysplasia (65%). Karyotypes have been reported to be normal in all cases.

Prognosis

The LBWC is invariably fatal.[73–76]

Amniotic Band Syndrome

Clinical and Pathologic Findings

The amniotic band syndrome is a group of malformations attributed to fibrous strands that entangle or trap various fetal parts.[80, 87, 88] Rupture of the amnion is thought to result in entanglement of fetal parts by the more "sticky" chorion. Torpin, who first proposed this hypothesis, also suggested that the amnion normally protects the fetus from contact with the amnion.[87, 88] Entrapment of fetal parts may cause amputation or slash defects in random sites, unrelated to embrological development. The estimated date of insult ranges from 6 menstrual weeks to 18 weeks.[80] The variable age of fetal entrapment can explain the spectrum of pathological findings seen with the amniotic band syndrome. Early entrapment (28 to 45 days post conception) can lead to severe craniofacial defects and internal malformations as seen with the LBWC, whereas late entrapment can lead to simple amputations or limb restrictions.[77, 78, 80, 84] Development of oligohydramnios could lead to deformation abnormalities including clubfoot.[81]

Similarities between the amniotic band syndrome and the LBWC are obvious. Whether they represent distinct disorders or a continuum is still open to question by some observers. Some authorities believe that the LBWC is due to a primary vascular abnormality that subsequently ruptures the amnion.[75]

Sonographic Findings

The amniotic band syndrome occasionally has been diagnosed on prenatal sonography.[79, 82, 83, 86] However, we have not yet encountered a documented case of amniotic band syndrome that produced an abdominal wall defect, excluding the LBWC or ectopia cordis (see Fig 11–21). This experience, and other evidence, supports the notion that the LBWC is a particularly severe form of amniotic band syndrome resulting from early amniotic rupture.

The diagnosis of amniotic band syndrome can be

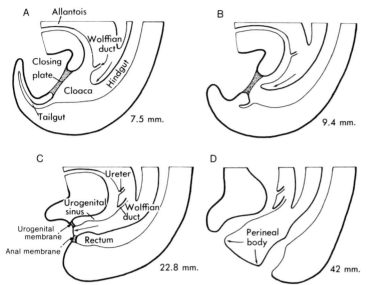

FIG 11–25.
Normal development of the cloaca and urinary bladder in the 7 mm to 42 mm embryo. The urorectal septum grows in a caudal direction to separate the cloaca into the hindgut posteriorly and the urogenital sinus (urinary bladder) anteriorly. The urorectal septum also divides the cloacal membrane into the urogenital membrane and anal membrane. Cloacal abnormalities resulting from failure of the urorectal septum to reach the cloacal membrane include persistent cloaca (see Chapter 12), bladder exstrophy, or cloacal exstrophy. (From Gray SW, Skandalakis JE: *Embryology for Surgeons*. Philadelphia, WB Saunders Co, 1972. Used by permission.)

suggested when multiple defects (abdominal wall defect, encephalocele, a facial cleft, or amputated fingers) are demonstrated or when fetal parts appear to be entrapped by the amniotic strands.[82] Craniofacial deformities are typically asymmetric and bizarre in location (see Chapter 6). Occasionally, adherent amniotic strands can be demonstrated (see Chapter 16).[82]

Associated Anomalies

A variety of malformations may be associated with the amniotic band syndrome including craniofacial defects, and limb defects.[80] Craniofacial deformities occur in about one third of cases and include asymmetric encephaloceles, microopthalmia, and bizarre facial clefts. Limb defects include constriction or amputation defects of the extremities. Clubfoot is found in up to one third of cases, possibly due to transient oligohydramnios resulting from ruptured membranes.[81] Like the LBWC, karyotypes of the amniotic band syndrome have been reported to be normal.

Prognosis

The prognosis for fetuses with the amniotic band syndrome varies, depending on the severity and distribution of anomalies. Few infants with severe craniofacial deformities survive.[85] In comparison, the prognosis is good and life expectancy is normal for mildly affected infants with isolated limb defects.

Cloacal and Bladder Exstrophy

Clinical and Pathologic Findings

Bladder exstrophy and cloacal exstrophy share a common embryologic origin in abnormal cloacal development, but differ in their severity and extent of involvement (Figs 11–25 to 11–27).[89, 105] Bladder exstrophy, occurring in 1 in 30,000 births, is characterized by a defect in the lower abdominal wall and anterior wall of the urinary bladder. As a result, the everted bladder becomes exposed on the lower abdominal wall (see Fig 11–26). The severity of bladder exstrophy can be clinically graded from mild to severe. In the mild form, exstrophy of the urethra and external bladder sphincter are present but diastasis of the pubic symphysis and rectus abdominus muscles is minimal. In the typical form, bladder exstrophy is accompanied by wide diastasis of the symphysis pubis.[90] The most severe form may be accompanied by omphalocele, inguinal hernia, undescended testis, ventrally located anal orifice, relaxed anal sphincter, and intermittent rectal prolapse.[89, 105]

Cloacal exstrophy is a rarer and more complex disorder than bladder exstrophy. It also occurs earlier in development and involves the primitive gut (see Fig 11–27). The incidence of cloacal exstrophy has been estimated as 1 in 200,000 births, but some cases have probably been misclassified as omphalocele. Cloacal exstrophy results in exstrophy of the bladder, in which there are two hemibladders (each with its ureteral orifice) separated by intestinal mucosa.[95, 105] The intestinal mucosa probably corresponds to the cecum since the ileum enters it as an ileal-vesicle fistula. Other common malformations include abdominal and pelvic defects, anorectal atresia, and spinal abnormalities. The combination of omphalocele, exstrophy of the bladder, imperforate anus, and spinal deformities has been referred to as the OEIS complex.[91] Cloacal exstrophy also is embryologically related to persistent cloaca, but the latter disorder does not have an abdominal wall defect (see Chapter 12).[96]

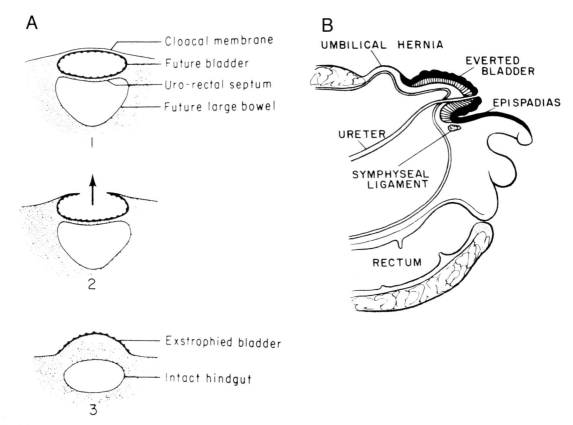

FIG 11-26.
Bladder exstrophy. **A,** events leading to bladder exstrophy. The anterior abdominal wall breaks down and results in eversion of the urinary bladder. **B,** schematic sagittal drawing shows typical findings of bladder exstrophy in a male. (From Muecke EC, in Walsh (ed): *Campbell's Urology,* ed 5. Philadelphia, WB Saunders Co, 1986, pp 1856–1880. Used by permission.)

Further understanding of bladder and cloacal exstrophy requires familiarity with normal embryologic development of the cloaca (see Fig 11–25).[92] During early pregnancy, the cloaca represents the distal confluence of (1) the hindgut, (2) the allantois (which forms the urinary bladder), and (3) the mesonephric ducts (which contribute to renal and genital development).[92] The cloacal membrane forms the anterior wall of the cloaca.[101] By the 8th menstrual week (6th fetal week), downward growth of the urorectal septum reaches the cloacal membrane, separating the cloaca into the urogenital sinus anteriorly and the hindgut posteriorly. The urorectal septum also subdivides the cloacal membrane into the urogenital membrane and the anal membrane. These membranes normally rupture by 11–12 menstrual weeks to produce patent urogenital and rectal tracts. Closure of the lower abdominal wall occurs at the same time the cloacal membrane retracts caudally. As the urorectal septum develops, the mesonephric ducts fuse into the cloaca laterally. These ducts form the seminal vesicles in the male but atrophy in the female. Induced by the mesonephric ducts, the paired paramesonephric ducts (mullerian ducts) fuse in the midline to form the uterovaginal cord, which in turn fuses with the urogenital sinus posteriorly. The sinovaginal bulbs then join and extend distally to form the vagina.[101]

If the urorectal septum fails to reach the cloacal membrane, then fusion of the mesodermal ridges and retraction of the cloacal membrane does not occur.[101] When the cloacal membrane regresses, both the bladder and rectum are exposed, resulting in cloacal exstrophy. The genitalia are duplicated, because the genital tubercles did not fuse. In bladder exstrophy, the urorectal septum successfully divides the cloaca, but the cloacal membrane does not retract normally so that the cloacal membrane becomes the anterior wall of the bladder. Regression of the cloacal membrane then results in direct exposure of the posterior bladder wall.

Sonographic Findings

Relatively few cases of bladder or cloacal exstrophy have been reported prenatally,[91, 93, 97, 99, 100, 102] although it is expected that more cases will be recognized with awareness of the typical sonographic find-

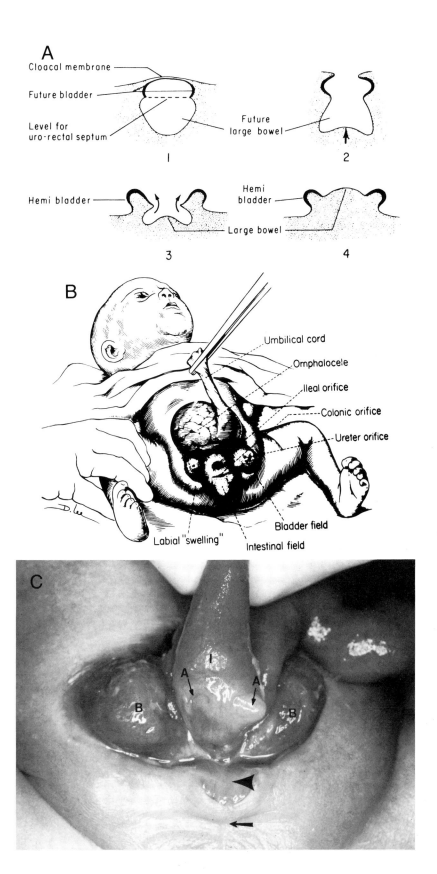

FIG 11–27.
Cloacal exstrophy. **A,** events leading to cloacal exstrophy. Both the anterior abdominal wall and urorectal septum break down. **B,** typical findings of cloacal exstrophy. Two hemibladders are separated by insertion of the bowel. A low omphalocele is also present. **C,** typical pathologic findings of cloacal exstrophy. The distal ileum (*I*) is prolapsed in this case. Note two hemibladders *(B),* two appendices *(A),* severe epispadius *(arrowhead),* and anal atresia *(arrow).* A small infraumbilical omphalocele was also present. (Part **A** from Mueck EC, in Walsh (ed): *Campbell's Urology,* ed 5. Philadelphia, WB Saunders Co, 1986, pp 1856–1880. Used by permission. Part **B** from Tank ES, in Walsh (ed) *Campbell's Urology,* ed 5. Philadelphia, WB Saunders Co, 1986, pp 1856–1880. Used by permission.)

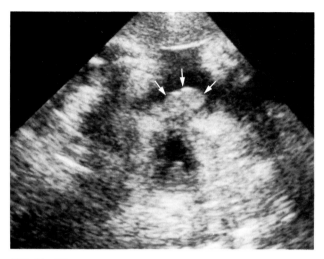

FIG 11–28.
Bladder exstrophy. Sonogram at 28 weeks shows a soft tissue area *(arrows)* representing heaped up bladder mucosa on the anterior surface of the lower abdominal wall. This finding was not prospectively recognized, however. Fetal hydrops developed on subsequent sonograms. At birth, bladder exstrophy and trisomy 21 were found. The infant survived with surgical correction of the defect.

ings. The primary finding in cases reported to date has been failure to visualize a normal urinary bladder (Fig 11–28).[91, 97, 100] A soft tissue mass, representing the exposed bladder mucosa, may also be demonstrated on the surface of the lower abdominal wall with bladder exstrophy (see Fig 11–28). The abdominal wall defect may be difficult to visualize due to its small size. Absence or splaying of the pubic rami and pelvic structures might be demonstrated, if sought. Other abnormalities that may be identified include abnormal genitalia and renal abnormalities such as hydronephrosis. Visualization of these findings is often difficult, particularly in the face of oligohydramnios caused by associated renal abnormalities.[93]

Demonstration of an anterior abdominal wall defect may be the primary sonographic finding of cloacal exstrophy (Figs 11–29 and 11–30), although the defect is relatively unimportant in comparison to the underlying complex. For this reason, cloacal exstrophy should be considered whenever an atypical abdominal wall defect is identified. The correct diagnosis of cloacal exstrophy can be suggested by failure to demonstrate the urinary bladder, together with more specific findings of cloacal exstrophy (low abdominal wall defect, soft tissue abdominal mass, and splaying of the pubic rami). Distinguishing the OEIS complex from LBWC may be more difficult, however, since both may demonstrate eviscerated liver and spinal abnormalities. As a distinguishing feature, the LBWC usually reveals craniofacial anomalies.

Failure to demonstrate a normal urinary bladder may also reflect other genitourinary disorders such as a persistent cloaca.[98, 102] This disorder typically shows a septated cystic mass in the pelvis and is not associated with an abdominal wall defect (see Chapter 12).[102, 105]

Associated Anomalies

Associated abnormalities of bladder exstrophy relate principally to the primary malformation and associated genitourinary anomalies. The severity of abnormalities is variable, although common findings in males include epispadias, incomplete descent of the testes, and bilateral inguinal hernias.[90, 103–105] Sex reassignment may be necessary in 1% to 2% of males if surgical correction does not result in an adequately functional penis. In females, cleft clitoris is common.

In comparison to bladder exstrophy, cloacal exstrophy is commonly associated with a variety of additional malformations.[89, 105] Genitourinary anomalies include didalphus (separation of the phallus), absence of the vagina, and renal anomalies. Other malformations may involve the gastrointestinal tract, cardiovascular system, or central nervous system.

The frequency of chromosome abnormalities associated with bladder or cloacal exstrophy is unknown. However, we have observed two fetuses with bladder exstrophy who had abnormal karyotypes, both with trisomy 21 (see Fig 11–28).

Prognosis

Bladder exstrophy can be surgically corrected with favorable results in most cases.[94] The major problems are the abdominal wall defect itself, urinary incontinence, and associated genital abnormalities. Divergent levator ani and puborectal muscles may result in rectal incontinence and anal prolapse. Surgical correction of the defect is necessary, since untreated patients with exstrophy of the bladder usually die of ascending pyelonephritis. Infertility is common, particularly among males. Uterine prolapse is a common complication among females. There is an increased frequency of malignant tumors involving the exstrophic bladder; bladder carcinoma occurred in 4% of 170 cases observed at the Mayo Clinic.[106]

Cloacal exstrophy has a very poor prognosis, with a 55% mortality rate.[95] This is due to the complexity of the malformation and the frequency of associated anomalies. Surgical correction requires a series of complex procedures including closure of the abdominal wall defect, functional bladder closure, anti-continence and anti-reflux procedures during early childhood. Surviving females usually undergo vaginal reconstruction at 14 to 18 years of age. Some authorities recom-

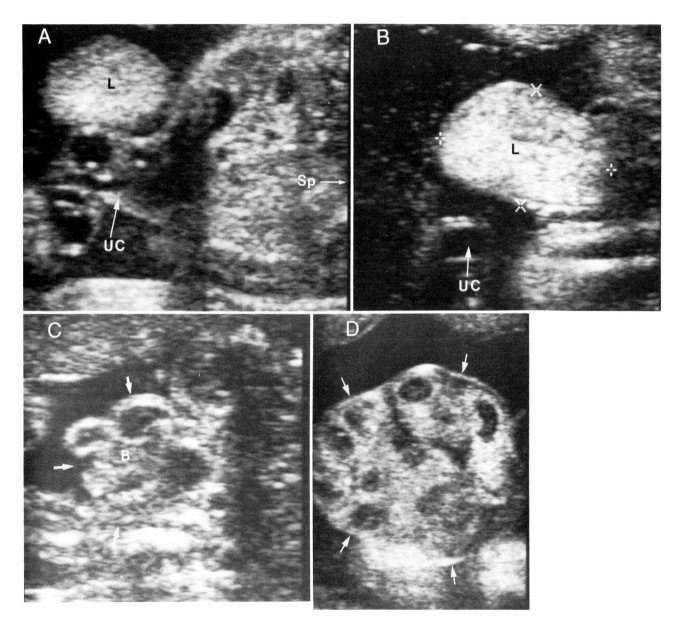

FIG 11–29.
Cloacal exstrophy. **A,** transverse scan at 24 weeks shows eviscerated liver *(L)* adjacent to a normal umbilical cord insertion site *(UC)*. Note that this pattern is not typical for either omphalocele or gastroschisis. *Sp* = spine. **B,** contiguous scan demonstrates a portion of the liver *(L)* eviscerated through the paraumbilical defect. *UC* = umbilical cord. **C,** scan at the same time shows a large amount of eviscerated bowel *(B),* marked by arrows. The urinary bladder was not identified, suggesting the diagnosis of cloacal exstrophy. **D,** repeat sonogram at 38 weeks shows a large amount of eviscerated bowel that now appears confined by a membrane *(arrows).* A complex cloacal exstrophy with infraumbilical omphalocele was present at birth.

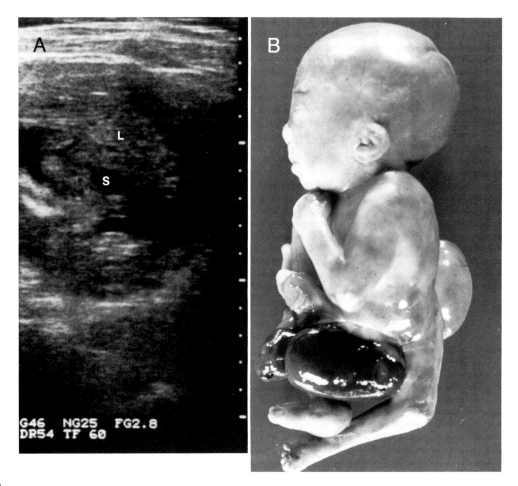

FIG 11–30.
Cloacal exstrophy. **A,** transerse sonogram at 20 weeks, performed because of an elevated MS-AFP level, shows a large anterior abdominal wall defect containing liver *(L)* and stomach *(S)*. Marked oligohydramnios is also present. **B,** photograph at postmortem examination shows the low infraumbilical omphalocele with ruptured membranes. A large myelomeningocele is also identified. Other abnormalities included anorectal atresia, absent external genitalia, multicystic dysplasia of a single kidney, and hypoplastic lungs. The karyotype was normal (46, XY). (From Kutzner DK, Wilson WG, Hogge WA: OEIS complex (cloacal exstrophy): Prenatal diagnosis in the second trimester. Prenat Diagn 1988; 8:247–253, Used by permission.)

mend routine conversion of males to females because of the poor results in attempting to create a functional penis.

Urachal/Allantoic Abnormalities

Clinical and Pathologic Findings

The allantois develops as an outpouching or diverticulum from that part of the yolk sac that eventually forms the cloaca (Fig 11–31).[101] In reptiles and birds this diverticulum projects outside the umbilical cord and serves as the source of oxygen exchange through the porous eggshell. Since the placenta assumes the function of oxygen exchange in mammals, the allantois obliterates and has no apparent function except for possible early hematopoesis. As the cloaca forms, the allantois remains connected to the urogenital sinus

through the urachus. The urachus extends from the umbilical cord to the ventral aspect of the urogenital sinus (urinary bladder). It narrows to a small fibrous band at or about the time of birth to become the median umbilical ligament.

While not a true abdominal wall defect, failure of the urachus to regress may result in complete or partial communication between the bladder and anterior abdominal wall. Urachal abnormalities (Fig 11–32) can be categorized into one of five groups (1) completely patent urachus, (2) urachal diverticulum, (3) urachal sinus, (4) urachal cyst, or (5) alternating sinus (cyst-like structure that can drain to either the bladder or the umbilicus).[108, 109, 111] In a review of 35 children with urachal abnormalities, Rich et al. reported that 19 had patent urachus, 12 had urachal cyst, and 4 had urachal sinus.[111]

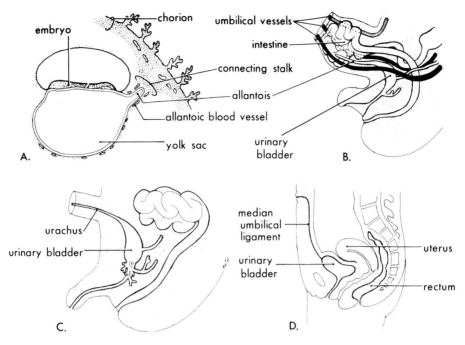

FIG 11–31.
Development of the allantois and urachus at **A,** 5 menstrual weeks (3 fetal weeks); **B,** 11 menstrual weeks; **C,** 14 weeks; and **D,** in the adult. (From Moore KL: *The Developing Human,* ed 4. Philadelphia, WB Saunders Co, 1988. Used by permission.)

Sonographic Findings

Persutte et al. demonstrated a patent urachus on prenatal sonography at 18 menstrual weeks (Fig 11–33).[110] The extra-abdominal component of the patent urachus appeared entirely cystic and communicated with the urinary bladder. The cystic mass subsequently resolved on serial sonograms, but a patent urachus was found after birth. Donnefeld et al. reported a nearly identical case.[107] Sachs et al. reported a transient tubular structure, possibly representing a urachal cyst, coursing from the bladder to the umbilicus in association with an allantoic cyst of the umbilical cord.[112]

The cystic appearance of a patent urachus or urachal cyst should be distinguished from an abdominal wall defect, particularly from cloacal or bladder exstrophy. In the latter case, the urinary bladder is ab-

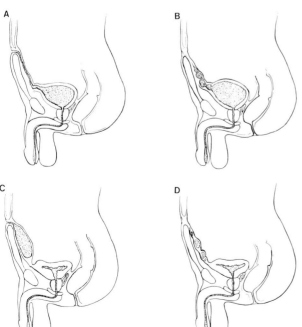

FIG 11–32.
Urachal anomalies. **(A)** patent urachus, **(B)** urachal diverticuli **(C)** urachal sinus, **(D)** multiple urachal cysts. (From Persutte WH, Lenke RR, Kropp K, et al: Antenatal diagnosis of fetal patent urachus. J Ultrasound Med 1988; 7:399–403, Used by permission.)

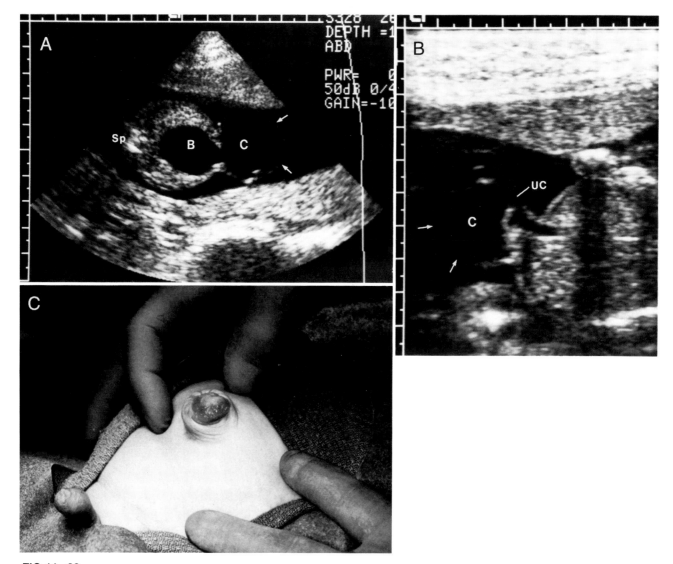

FIG 11–33.
Urachal cyst. **A,** transverse scan at 18 weeks shows a large *(arrows)* extra-abdominal cystic mass *(C)* contiguous with the urinary bladder *(B)*. *Sp* = spine. **B,** follow-up sonogram at 26 weeks shows the relation of the cystic mass *(C)* to the insertion of the umbilical cord *(UC)*. A subsequent scan at 30 weeks showed nearly complete interval decompression of the cyst. **C,** postnatal photograph shows patent urachus. (From Persutte WH, Lenke RR, Kropp K, et al: Antenatal diagnosis of fetal patent urachus. J Ultrasound Med 1988; 7:399–403. Used by permission.)

sent and bladder mucosa is demonstrated on the anterior abdominal wall. The persistent urachus may demonstrate a solid appearance (Fig 11–34) which may be difficult to distinguish from a small bowel-containing omphalocele or persistent omphalomesenteric duct.

Associated Anomalies

Rich et al. reported associated anomalies in 16 of 35 (46%) children with urachal abnormalities.[111] These included omphalocele, omphalomesenteric remnant, meningomyelocele, and various genitourinary anomalies (cryptorchidism, unilateral kidney, hydronephrosis, vaginal atresia).

Prognosis

The prognosis of urachal abnormalities depends on the presence of associated anomalies. In a neonatal series of 35 surgically corrected urachal abnormalities, Rich et al. reported only one death.[111]

SUMMARY

Sonography plays the primary role in the detection, evaluation, and follow-up of fetuses identified with an anterior abdominal wall defect. Gastroschisis typically is an isolated malformation that carries an ex-

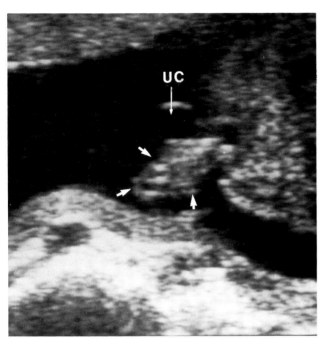

FIG 11–34.
Urachal cyst. Transverse scan of the abdomen demonstrates a small echogenic mass *(arrows)* adjacent to the umbilical cord *(UC)* insertion site. At delivery, this proved to be a persistent urachus protruding into the umbilicus in a fetus with Fryns syndrome. This appearance may be difficult to distinguish from small bowel-containing omphaloceles. (Courtesy of Dolores H Pretorius, MD.)

cellent prognosis. Omphalocele may also be isolated but is more frequently associated with concurrent malformations and/or chromosome anomalies and therefore carries a poor prognosis. Various syndromes may be associated with omphalocele including the pentalogy of Cantrell and Beckwith-Wiedemann syndrome. Sonographic findings should be able to distinguish correctly between gastroschisis and omphalocele in nearly all cases.

In addition to gastroschisis and omphalocele, other malformations that should be considered when an abdominal wall defect is identified include the LBWC, amniotic band syndrome, and cloacal exstrophy. Awareness of the typical pathologic findings seen with these disorders should permit their sonographic recognition.

REFERENCES

Embryogenesis

1. Cyr DR, Mack LA, Schoenecker SA, et al: Bowel migration in the normal fetus: US detection. Radiology 1986; 161:119–121.

2. DeVries PA: The pathogenesis of gastroschisis and omphalocele. J Pediatr Surg 1980; 15:245–251.

3. Duhamel B: Embryology of exomphalos and allied malformations. Arch Dis Child 1968; 38:142–147.

4. Hoyme HE, Higginbottom MC, Jones KL: The vascular pathogenesis of gastroschisis: Intrauterine interruption of the omphalomesenteric artery. J Pediatrics 1981; 98:228–231.

5. Moore KL: *The Developing Human,* ed 4. Philadelphia, WB Saunders Co, 1988, pp 65–86.

6. Tibboel D, Raine M, McNee M et al: Developmental aspects of gastroschisis. J Pediatr Surg 1986; 21:865–869.

Omphalocele and Gastroschisis

7. Bair JH, Russ PD, Pretorius DH, et al: Fetal omphalocele and gastroschisis: A review of 24 cases. AJR 1986; 147:1047–1051.

8. Bond SJ, Harrison MR, Filly RA, et al: Severity of intestinal damage in gastroschisis: Correlation with prenatal sonographic findings. J Pediatr Surg 1988; 23:520–525.

9. Brown BSJ: The prenatal ultrasonographic features of omphalocele: A study of 10 patients. J Can Assoc Radiol 1985; 36:312–316.

10. Cameron GM, McQuown DS, Modanlou HD, et al: Intrauterine diagnosis of an omphalocele by diagnostic ultrasonography. Am J Obstet Gynecol 1978; 131:821–822.

11. Carpenter MW, Curci MR, Dibbins AW, et al: Perinatal management of ventral wall defects. Obstet Gynecol 1984; 64:646–651.

12. Cobellis G, Iannoto P, Stabile M, et al: Prenatal ultrasound diagnosis of macroglossia in the Wiedemann-Beckwith syndrome. Prenat Diag 1988; 8:79–81.

13. Colley N, Knott PD, Gould SJ: Misdiagnosis of omphalocele associated with Edwards syndrome and congenital heart disease. Prenat Diagn 1987;7:377–381.

14. Crawford DC, Chapman MG, Allan LD: Echocardiography in the investigation of anterior abdominal wall defects in the fetus. Br J Obstet Gynecol 1985; 92:1034–1036.

15. Curtis JA, Watson L: Sonographic diagnosis of omphalocele in the first trimester of fetal gestation. J Ultrasound Med 1988; 7:97–100.

16. Dibbins AW, Curci MR, McCrann DJ Jr: Prenatal diagnosis of congenital anomalies requiring surgical correction. Am J Surg 1985; 149:528–533.

17. Fink IJ, Filly RA: Omphalocele associated with umbilical cord allantoic cyst: Sonographic evaluation in utero. Radiology 1983; 149:473–476.

18. Fitzsimmons J, Nyberg DA, Cyr DR, et al: Perinatal management of gastroschisis. Obstet Gynecol 1988; 71:910–913.

19. Gilbert WM, Nicolaides KH: Fetal omphalocele: Associated malformations and chromosomal defects. Obstet Gynecol 1987; 70:633–635.

20. Griffiths DM, Gough MH: Dilemmas after ultrasonic diagnosis of fetal abnormality. Lancet 1985; i:623–625.

21. Grosfeld JL, Dawes L, Weber TR: Congenital abdominal wall defects: Current management and survival. Surg Clin North Am 1981; 61:1037–1049.

22. Grundy H, Anderson RL, Goldberg JD, et al: Gastroschisis: Prenatal diagnosis and management. Presented to the Society of Perinatal Obstetricians, Las Vegas, NV, Feb. 3–6, 1988.

23. Hasan S, Hermansen: The prenatal diagnosis of ventral abdominal wall defects. Am J Obstet Gynecol 1986; 155:842–845.

24. Hauge M, Bugge M, Nielsen J: Early prenatal diagnosis of omphalocele constitutes indication for amniocentesis. Lancet 1983, ii:507.

25. Hughes MD, Nyberg DA, Mack LA, et al: Fetal omphalocele: Prenatal detection of concurrent anomalies and other predictors of outcome. Radiology, in press.

26. Hutchin P: Somatic anomalies of the umbilicus and anterior abdominal wall. Surg Gynecol Obstet 1965; 120:1075–1090.

27. Kirk EP, Wah R: Obstetric management of the fetus with omphalocele or gastroschisis: A review and report of one hundred twelve cases. Am J Obstet Gynecol 1983; 146:512–518.

28. Kluck P, Tibboel D, Van Der Kamp AWM, et al: The effect of fetal urine on the development of bowel in gastroschisis. J Pediatr Surg 1983; 18:47–50.

29. Knight PJ, Sommer A, Clatworthy HW: Omphalocele: A prognostic classification. J Pediatr Surg 1981; 16:599–604.

30. Lenke RR, Hatch EI: Fetal gastroschisis: A preliminary report advocating the use of cesarean section. Obstet Gynecol 1986; 67:395–398.

31. Lindfors KK, McGahan JP, Walter JP: Fetal omphalocele and gastroschisis: Pitfalls in sonographic diagnosis. AJR 1986; 147:797–800.

32. Luck SR, Sherman J, Raffensperger JG, et al: Gastroschisis in 106 consecutive newborn infants. Surgery 1985; 98:677–683.

33. Mabogunje OOA, Mahour GH: Omphalocele and gastroschsis: Trends in survival across two decades. Am J Surg 1984; 148:679–686.

34. Mann L, Ferguson-Smith MA, Desai M, Gibson AAM, et al: Prenatal assessment of anterior abdominal wall defects and their prognosis. Prenat Diagn 1984; 4:427–435.

35. Martin LW, Torres AM: Omphalocele and gastroschisis. Symposium on pediatric surgery. Surg Clin North Am 1985; 65:1235–1244.

36. Mayer T, Black R, Matlak ME, et al: Gastroschisis and omphalocele. Ann Surg 1980; 192:783–787.

37. Nelson PA, Bowie JD, Filston HC, et al: Sonographic diagnosis of omphalocele in utero. AJR 1981; 138:1178–1180.

38. Nyberg DA, Fitzsimmons J, Mack LA, et al: Chromosomal abnormalities in fetuses with omphalocele: Sig-

nificance of omphalocele contents. J Ultrasound Med 1989; 8:299–308.

39. Osborne J: Gastroschisis and omphalocele. Prenatal ultrasonic detection and its significance. Australas Radiol 1986; 30:113–116.

40. Palomaki GE, Hill LE, Knight GJ, et al: Second-trimester maternal serum alpha-fetoprotein levels in pregnancies associated with gastroschisis and omphalocele. Obstet Gynecol 1988; 71:906–90.

41. Pettenati MJ, Haines JL, Higgins RR, et al: Wiedemann-Beckwith syndrome: Presentation of clinical and cytogenetic data on 22 new cases and review of the literature. Hum Genet 1986; 74:143.

42. Pokorny WJ, Harberg FJ, McGill CW: Gastroschisis complicated by intestinal atresia. J Pediatr Surg 1981; 16:261–263.

43. Redford DH, McNay MB, Whittle MJ: Gastroschisis and exomphalos: Precise diagnosis by midpregnancy ultrasound. Br J Obstet Gynecol 1985; 92:54–59.

44. Salzman L, Kuligowska E, Semine A: Pseudoomphalocele: Pitfall in fetal sonography. AJR 1986; 146:1283–1285.

45. Schaffer RM, Barone C, Friedman AP: The ultrasonographic spectrum of fetal omphalocele. J Ultrasound Med 1983; 2:219–222.

46. Schwaitzenberg SD, Pokorny WJ, McGill CW, et al: Gastroschisis and omphalocele. Am J Surg 1982; 144:650–654.

47. Seashore JH: Congenital abdominal wall defects. Clin Perinatol 1978; 5:62–77.

48. Sermer M, Benzie RJ, Pitson L, et al: Prenatal diagnosis and management of congenital defects of the anterior abdominal wall. Am J Obstet Gynecol 1987; 156:308–312.

49. Shigemoto H, Horiya Y, Isomoto T, et al: Duodenal atresia secondary to intrauterine midgut strangulation by an omphalocele. J Pediatr Surg 1982; 17:420–421.

50. Stringel G, Filler RM: Prognostic factors in omphalocele and gastroschisis. J Pediatr Surg 1979; 14:515–519.

51. Swartz KR, Harrison MW, Campbell JR, et al: Long-term followup of patients with gastroschisis. Am J Surg 1986; 151:546–549.

52. Towne BH, Peters G, Cheng JHT: The problem of "giant" omphalocele. J Pediatr Surg 1980; 15:543–548.

53. Weinstein L, Anderson C: In utero diagnosis of Beckwith-Wiedemann syndrome by ultrasound. Radiology 1980; 134:474.

54. Winter SC, Curry CJR, Smith JC, et al. Prenatal diagnosis of the Beckwith-Wiedemann syndrome. Am J Med Genet 1986; 24:137–141.

Ectopia Cordis

55. Abu-Yousel MM, Wray AB, Williamson RA, et al: Antenatal ultrasound diagnosis of variant of pentalogy of Cantrell. J Ultrasound Med 1987; 6:535–538.

56. Baker ME, Rosenberg ER, Trofatter KF, et al: The in utero findings in twin pentalogy of Cantrell. J Ultrasound Med 1984; 3:525–527.

57. Carpenter MW, Curci MR, Dibbins AW, et al: Perinatal management of ventral wall defects. Obstet Gynecol 1984; 64:646–651.

58. Dobell ARC, Williams HB, Long RW: Staged repair of ectopia cordis. J Ped Surg 1982; 17:353.

59. Garson A, Hawkins EP, Mullins CE, et al: Thoracoabdominal ectopia cordis with mosaic Turner's syndrome: Report of a case. Pediatrics 1978; 62:218.

60. Ghidini A, Sirtori M, Romero R, et al: Prenatal diagnosis of pentalogy of Cantrell. J Ultrasound Med 1988; 7:567–472.

61. Greig DM: Cleft sternum and ectopia cordis. Edinbugh Med J 1926;33:480.

62. Haynor DR, Shuman WP, Brewer DR, et al: Imaging of fetal ectopic cordis: Role of sonography and computed tomography. J Ultrasound Med 1984; 3:25–28.

63. Harrison MR, Filly RA, Stanger P, et al: Prenatal diagnosis and management of omphalocele and ectopic cordis. J Pediatr Surg 1982; 17:64–66.

64. Kaplan LC, Matsuoka R, Gilbert EF, et al: Ectopia cordis and cleft sternum: Evidence of mechanical teratogenesis following rupture of the chorion or yolk sac. Am J Med Genet 1985; 21:187–199.

65. Klingensmith WC III, Cioffi-Ragan DT, Harvey DE: Diagnosis of ectopia cordis in the second trimester. J Clin Ultrasound 1988; 16:204–206.

66. Mercer LJ, Petres RE, Smeltzer JS: Ultrasonic diagnosis of ectopia cordis. Obstet Gynecol 1983; 61:523–525.

67. Ravitch MM: Cantrell's Pentalogy and notes on diverticulum of the left ventricle, in *Congenital Deformities of the Chest Wall and Their Operative Corrections.* Philadelphia, WB Saunders Co, 1977, pp 53–557.

68. Seeds JW, Cefalo RC, Lies SC, et al: Early prenatal sonographic appearance of rare thoraco-abdominal eventration. Prenat Diagn 1984; 4:437–441.

69. Todros T, Presbitero P, Montemurro D, et al: Prenatal diagnosis of ectopia cordis. J Ultrasound Med 1984; 3:429–431.

70. Toyama WM: Combined congenital defects of the anterior abdominal wall, sternum, diaphragm, pericardium, and heart: A case report and review of the literature. Pediatr 1872; 50:778–792.

71. Wicks JD, Levine MD, Mettler FA: Intrauterine sonography of thoracic ectopia cordis. AJR 1981; 137:619–622.

Limb-Body Wall Complex

72. Lockwood CJ, Scioscia AL, Hobbins JC: Congenital absence of the umbilical cord resulting from maldevelopment of embryonic body folding. Am J Obstet Gynecol 1986; 155:1049.

73. Patten RM, Van Allen M, Mack LA, et al: Limb-body wall complex: In utero sonographic diagnosis of a complicated fetal malformation. AJR 1986; 146:1019–1024.

74. Smith DW: *Recognizable Patterns of Human Malformation,* ed 3. Philadelphia, WB Saunders Co, 1981, 488–496.

75. Van Allen MI, Curry C, Gallagher: Limb body wall complex. I: Pathogenesis. Am J Med Genet 1987; 28:529–548.

76. Van Allen MI, Curry C, Walden L, et al: Limb-body wall complex. II: Limb and spine defects. Am J Med Genet 1987; 28:549–565.

Amniotic Band Syndrome

77. Ashkenazy M, Borenstein R, Katz Z, et al: Constriction of the umbilical cord by an amniotic band after midtrimester amniocentesis. Acta Obstet Gynecol Scand 1982; 61:89–91.

78. Baker CJ, Rudolph AJ: Congenital ring constrictions and intrauterine amputations. Am J Dis Child 1971; 212:393–400.

79. Fiske CE, Filly RA, Golbus MS: Prenatal ultrasound diagnosis of amniotic band syndrome. J Ultrasound Med. 1982; 1:45–47.

80. Higgenbottom MC, Jones KL, Hall BD, et al: The amniotic band disruption complex: Timing of amniotic rupture and variable spectra of consequent defects. J Pediatr 1979; 95:544–549.

81. Hunter AGW, Carpenter BF: Implications of malformations not due to amniotic bands in the amniotic band sequence. Am J Med Genet 1986; 24:691–700.

82. Mahony BS, Filly RA, Callen PW, et al: The amniotic band syndrome: Antenatal diagnosis and potential pitfalls. Am J Obstet Gynecol 1985; 152:63–68.

83. Lockwood C, Ghidini A, Romero R: Amniotic band syndrome in monozygotic twins: Prenatal diagnosis and pathogenesis. Obstet Gynecol 1988; 71:1012–1016.

84. Moessinger AC, Blanc WA, Byrne J, et al: Amniotic band syndrome associated with amniocentesis. Am J Obstet Gynecol 1981; 141:588–591.

85. Ossipoff V, Hall BD: Etiologic factors in the amniotic band syndrome: A study of 24 patients. Birth Defects 1977; 13:117–132.

86. Seeds JW, Cefalo RC, Herbert WNP: Amniotic band syndrome. Am J Obstet Gynecol 1982; 144:243–248.

87. Torpin R: Fetal malformations caused by amnion rupture during gestation. Springfield, IL, Charles C Thomas, 1968, pp 1–76.

88. Torpin R: Amniochorionic mesoblastic fibrous strings and amnionic bands. Am J Obstet Gynecol 1965; 91:65–75.

Cloacal and Bladder Exstrophy

89. Bartholomew TH, Gonzales ET Jr: Urologic management in cloacal dysgenesis. Urology 1978; 117:102.

90. Engel RME: Exstrophy of the bladder and associated anomalies. Birth Defects 1974; 10:146–149.

91. Gosden C, Brock DJH: Prenatal diagnosis of exstrophy of the cloaca. Am J Med Genet 1981; 8:95–109.

92. Gray SW, Skandalakis JE: *Embryology for Surgeons.* Philadelphia, WB Saunders Co, 1972.

93. Haygood VP, Wahbeh CJ: Prospects for the prenatal diagnosis and obstetric management of cloacal exstrophy. J Reprod Med 1983;28:807–812.

94. Hendren WH: Repair of cloacal anomalies: Current techniques. J Pediatr Surg 1986; 21:1159–1176.

95. Howell C, Caldamone A, Snyder H, et al: Optimal management of cloacal exstrophy. J Pediatr Surg 1983; 18:365–369.

96. Kay R, Tank ES: Principles of management of the persistent cloaca in the female newborn. J Urol 1977; 117:102–104.

97. Kutzner DK, Wilson WG, Hogge WA: OEIS complex (cloacal exstrophy): Prenatal diagnosis in the second trimester. Prenat Diagn 1988; 8:247–253.

98. Lande IM, Hamilton EF: The antenatal sonographic visualization of cloacal dysgenesis. J Ultrasound Med 1986; 5:275–278.

99. Meizner I, Bar-Ziv J: In utero prenatal ultrasonic diagnosis of a rare case of cloacal exstrophy. J Clin Ultrasound 1985; 13:500–502.

100. Mirk P, Calisti A, Fileni A: Prenatal sonographic diagnosis of bladder extrophy. J Ultrasound Med 1986; 5:291–293.

101. Moore KL: *The Developing Human,* ed 4. Philadelphia, WB Saunders Co, 1988, pp 217–285.

102. Petrikovsky BM, Walzak MP Jr, D'Addario PF: Fetal cloacal anomalies: Prenatal sonographic findings and differential diagnosis. Obstet Gynecol 1988; 72:464–469.

103. Soper RT, Kilger K: Vesico-intestinal fissure. J Urol 1964;92:490–501.

104. Tank ES, Lindenaner SM: Principles of management of exstrophy of the cloaca. Am J Surg 1970; 119:95–100.

105. Tank ES: Urologic complications of imperforate anus and cloacal dysgenesis, in *Campbell's Urology,* ed 4. Philadelphia, WB Saunders Co, 1986, pp 1889–2000.

106. Wattenberg A, Beare JB, Tormey AR Jr: Exstrophy of the urinary bladder complicated by adenocarcinoma. J Urol 1956; 76:583–594.

Urachal Abnormalities

107. Donnenfeld AE, Mennuti MT, Templeton JM, et al: Prenatal sonographic diagnosis of a vesico-allantoic abdominal wall defect. J Ultrasound Med 1989; 8:43–45.

108. Hinman F: Surgical disorders of the bladder and umbilicus of urachal origin. Surg Gynecol Obstet 1961; 113:605–614.

109. Perlmutter AD: Urachal disorders, in *Campbell's Urology,* ed 4. Philadelphia, WB Saunders Co, 1986, pp 1883–1888.

110. Persutte WH, Lenke RR, Kropp K, et al: Antenatal diagnosis of fetal patent urachus. J Ultrasound Med 1988; 7:399–403.

111. Rich RH, Hardy BE, Filler RM: Surgery for anomalies of the urachus. J Pediatr Surg 1983; 18:370–372.

112. Sachs L, Fourcroy JL, Wenzel DJ, et al: Prenatal detection of umbilical cord allantoic cyst. Radiology 1982; 145:445–446.

The Genitourinary Tract

Peter A. Grannum, M.D.

Antenatal sonography enables accurate identification and characterization of numerous anomalies of the fetal urinary tract. The information provided by ultrasound often dramatically influences obstetric and neonatal management.[2, 4, 5, 7–10] Therefore, every obstetric ultrasound during the second and third trimesters should include documentation of the fetal urinary bladder, evaluation of the fetal kidneys, and assessment of amniotic fluid volume.[6]

This chapter discusses the embryology and normal appearance of the urinary tract and focuses on major groups of malformations including renal agenesis, obstructive uropathy, and renal cystic disease. It concludes with a discussion of fetal gender and miscellaneous conditions affecting the fetal urinary tract.

EMBRYOLOGY

The ureteral bud arises as an outpouching of the mesonephric (wolffian) duct from the urogenital sinus at approximately 6 menstrual weeks (Fig 12–1).[16] The cloaca (the caudal portion of the urogenital sinus) narrows and elongates to form the neck of the bladder and the urethra several days later. The remainder of the urinary bladder derives from the allantois.

The ureteral bud gives rise to the ureter, renal pelvis, calyces, and collecting tubules via a dichotomous 15-generation branching pattern. Since the kidney will not develop without a ureteral bud, the ureteral bud also plays a crucial role in nephron induction via interaction with the metanephric blastema.[15] After 3–5 branchings of the ureteral bud, the nephrons begin to appear at approximately 10 menstrual weeks. Urine formation commences early in the second trimester of

pregnancy. Prior to 16 menstrual weeks the kidneys contribute little to amniotic fluid, but their role becomes increasingly important during the second half of gestation when fetal urination produces most of the amniotic fluid (see Chapter 4).

SONOGRAPHY OF THE NORMAL FETAL URINARY TRACT

Ultrasonography can examine the fetal kidneys and urinary bladder prenatally in a fair degree of detail. The fetal kidneys can be identified as early as 14–16 weeks, although accurate statements about their internal architecture usually cannot be made until approximately 16–18 weeks.[1, 3, 4] The fetal bladder can be identified as early as 10–12 weeks when urine production is thought to begin. Assessment of the amniotic fluid status represents an important aspect of the evaluation of the urinary tract, since many disorders associated with poor renal function result in the development of oligohydramnios.

On parasagittal or transverse scans at the level of the fetal lumbar spine, the kidneys appear as bilateral paraspinous structures with an elliptical or circular shape, respectively (Fig 12–2). They can be recognized as early as 12–14 weeks of gestation, although variations in fetal positioning and lack of contrast between the kidneys and surrounding tissues occasionally do not permit identification of both fetal kidneys. Furthermore, at this stage of gestation it is usually not possible to recognize the structures within the fetal kidney.

After 16 weeks of gestation more accurate statements concerning the internal structures of the fetal

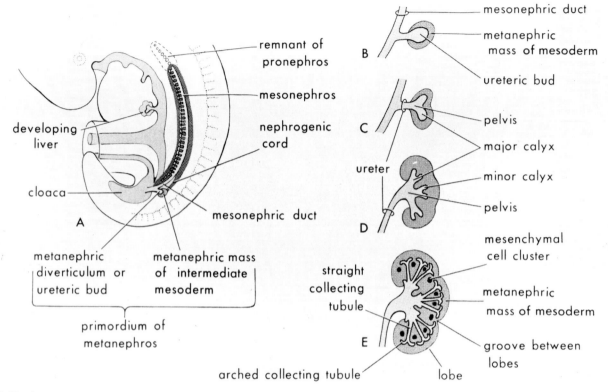

FIG 12–1.
Embryology of the kidney. **A,** lateral sketch of the 5-week embryo (7 menstrual weeks) shows the primordium of the metanephros or permanent kidney. **B** to **E,** these sketches show successive developmental stages of the metanephric diverticulum or ureteric bud into the ureter, renal pelvis, calyces, and collecting tubules between the fifth and eighth weeks. (From Moore KL: *The Developing Human: Clinically Oriented Embryology,* ed 4. Philadelphia, WB Saunders Co, 1988. Used by permission.)

kidney can be made, and sonography clearly defines at least 90% of fetal kidneys by approximately 20 menstrual weeks.[4] The renal sinus appears as a sonolucent "slit" within the central portion of the kidney. The hypoechoic medullae are arranged in anterior and posterior rows around the pelvic sinus. The medullae appear hypoechoic, probably because the tubules are thin-walled and fluid-filled. Early in gestation the renal cortex is extremely thin and difficult to discern.

As gestation progresses, echogenic retroperitoneal fat surrounding the kidneys clearly delineates their outlines, and the echogenic central sinus becomes more apparent.[12] The echogenic rim surrounding the kidney represents the renal capsule and perinephric fat. The relative hypoechogenicity of the medullae contrasts with the echotexture of the normal renal cortex, which usually approximates or may be even be slightly greater than that of the surrounding tissues. Recognition of this normal renal architecture is vital in distinguishing normal kidneys from those with cystic dysplasia.

The kidneys grow throughout gestation, and stan-

dard measurements for renal circumference, volume, thickness, width, and length have been reported as a function of menstrual age.[1, 11, 14] These reported measurements correspond with postnatal measurements of renal size obtained on stillborn fetuses. The ratio of kidney circumference to abdominal circumference remains constant at 0.27 to 0.30 throughout pregnancy (Table 12–1).[1] In the absence of ascites or other more rare causes of abdominal circumference enlargement, significant deviation from this pattern indicates renal enlargement. Diminution in renal size may be more difficult to discern. In general, however, the normal kidney length spans approximately 4–5 vertebral bodies (Figs 12–2 and 12–3).

Ultrasonography does not routinely visualize non–dilated fetal ureters. However, the fetal bladder can be seen as early as 10 weeks of gestation shortly after the commencement of fetal urine production. The normal bladder is an almost rectangularly shaped anechoic structure in the fetal pelvis. It has a very thin wall which may act as a specular reflector. The internal iliac arteries course along the lateral walls of the blad-

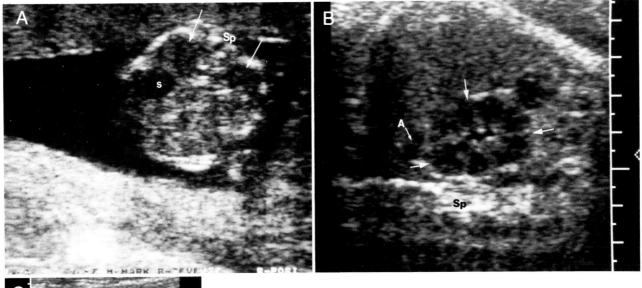

FIG 12–2.
Normal kidneys. **A,** transverse scan at the level of the fetal lumbar spine at 14 weeks shows bilateral paraspinous circular hypoechoic structures. At this stage of gestation, renal architecture is barely discernible. **B,** parasagittal scan of the left kidney at 22 weeks shows the elliptical shape of the paraspinous structure with the hypoechoic medullary pyramids arranged in anterior and posterior rows. **C,** parasagittal scan at 35 weeks shows the elliptical shape of the right kidney with a length spanning approximately 4 to 5 vertebral bodies. Note a small amount of fluid within the renal pelvis. This amount of fluid is frequently seen and typically not clinically significant. *Sp* = spine; *solid arrows* = kidneys; *A* = adrenal; *S* = stomach; *VB* = vertebral bodies; *P* = minimal pyelocaliectasis; *L* = liver.

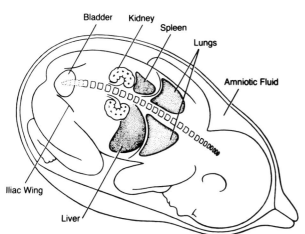

FIG 12–3.
Normal kidneys and normal amniotic fluid volume. The normal kidney spans approximately the length of 4 to 5 vertebral bodies in utero, as in the adult. Normal renal functions permit adequate amniotic fluid volume and lung development. (From Mahony BS: The genitourinary system, in Callen PW: *Ultrasonography in Obstetrics and Gynecology,* ed 2. Philadelphia, WB Saunders Co, 1988. Used by permission.)

TABLE 12–1.

Size of the Kidneys Relative to the Abdomen at Different Stages of Gestation*

Variable†	Gestational Age (wk)					
	<16 (n = 9)	17–20 (n = 18)	21–25 (n = 7)	26–30 (n = 11)	31–35 (n = 19)	>36 (n = 25)
Fetal kidney						
Anteriorposterior (cm)						
Mean	0.84	1.16	1.49	1.93	2.20	2.32
SD	0.24	0.24	0.37	0.19	0.32	0.32
Transverse (cm)						
Mean	0.86	1.13	1.64	2.00	2.34	2.63
SD	0.14	0.25	0.40	0.28	0.42	0.50
Circumference (cm)						
Mean	2.79	3.80	5.40	6.58	7.86	8.42
SD	0.64	0.72	0.68	0.67	0.86	1.39
Fetal abdomen						
Anteriorposterior (cm)						
Mean	2.92	3.73	5.12	6.74	8.50	8.88
SD	0.62	0.72	0.80	0.58	0.82	0.94
Transverse (cm)						
Mean	2.93	3.68	5.12	7.09	8.76	9.68
SD	0.59	0.56	0.49	0.61	0.89	1.44
Circumference (cm)						
Mean	9.66	12.37	17.36	22.03	28.11	30.45
SD	1.88	2.28	1.77	1.77	2.31	3.45
KC/AC ratio						
Mean	0.28	0.30	0.30	0.29	0.28	0.27
SD	0.02	0.03	0.02	0.02	0.03	0.04

*From Grannum P, Bracken M, Silverman R, et al: Assessment of fetal kidney size in normal gestation by comparison of ratio of kidney circumference to abdominal circumference. Am J Obstet Gynecol 1980; 136:249. Used by permission.
†Calculation of ratio (kidney circumference to abdominal circumference) used variables measured to eight decimal places.

der and should not be confused with bladder wall thickening (Fig 12–4). The fetus normally fills and empties the bladder every 20–30 minutes and produces an average of 25–30 ml/hr of urine near term (Fig 12–5).[13,17] Changes in bladder volume over time are quite evident with prolonged scanning and differentiate the urinary bladder from other cystic pelvic structures. Visualization of filling and emptying of the urinary bladder confirms that the fetus produces urine but does not indicate the quality of urine produced.

THE SONOGRAPHIC APPROACH TO URINARY TRACT ABNORMALITIES

A systematic approach to the abnormal urinary tract often permits accurate antenatal diagnosis. This approach includes (1) assessment of amniotic fluid volume, (2) location and characterization of urinary tract abnormalities, and (3) search for associated abnormalities. Fortunately, only a limited range of urinary tract anomalies manifest in utero and the overwhelming ma-

jority of these include the entities listed in Table 12–2.

The American Institute of Ultrasound in Medicine recommends that all second- and third-trimester ultrasounds include documentation of the fetal urinary bladder, evaluation of the fetal kidneys, and assessment of amniotic fluid volume.[6] It also indicates that suspicion of abnormalities may require a specialized evaluation.[6] Assessment of the following questions regarding these sonographic parameters assist in accurate prenatal diagnosis of many urinary tract abnormalities:

1. *Is oligohydramnios present without a history of ruptured membranes or evidence for intrauterine growth retardation? If so, urinary tract anomalies must be strongly suspected.*
2. *Is the urinary tract dilated? If so, what portions are affected and has the urinary tract spontaneously decompressed (ascites, urinoma, etc.)?*
3. *Are renal cysts present?*
4. *Are the kidneys abnormally echogenic or of abnormal size or shape?*

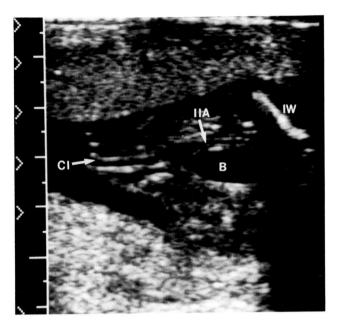

FIG 12–4.
Normal fetal bladder is almost rectangular-shaped and has a very thin wall. The internal iliac arteries course along the lateral aspects of the urinary bladder and should not be mistaken for bladder wall thickening. *B* = urinary bladder; *IW* = iliac wing; *CI* = umbilical cord insertion site; *IIA* = internal iliac artery.

5. *Are associated abnormalities present to indicate a syndrome?*

The initial step in the evaluation of the fetal urinary tract involves assessment of the quantity of amniotic fluid. A normal amount of amniotic fluid in the second half of gestation implies at least one functioning kidney, especially in the absence of anomalies that would otherwise produce polyhydramnios. Prior to 16 weeks, however, a normal amount of amniotic fluid may exist in the absence of renal function. On the other hand, decreased amniotic fluid volume at any time of gestation must alert the sonographer to search for urinary tract anomalies.

Oligohydramnios during the second trimester signifies a very poor prognosis.[19] A normal amount of amniotic fluid in the setting of a urinary tract abnormality, however, typically indicates a good prognosis.[27] Occasionally and paradoxically, polyhydramnios may occur in association with urinary tract anomalies, especially mesoblastic nephroma, unilateral obstructive uropathy, megacystis-microcolon-intestinal hypoplastic syndrome or other concomitant abnormalities of the central nervous system or gastrointestinal tract.[32, 63, 103, 229–231]

Localization and characterization of urinary tract abnormalities involve assessment of unilaterality or bilaterality of involvement. Unilateral disease occurs as a result of a defect at or proximal to the ureteral bud and typically has a good prognosis. Bilateral but asymmetric disease implies either a defect at the level of the cloaca (urethral level) or an asymmetric ureteral bud abnormality with obstruction or reflux. Bilateral symmetric disease often indicates a genetic abnormality (autosomal recessive polycystic kidney disease) or other severe abnormalities involving both ureteral bud systems (renal agenesis or bilateral multicystic dysplastic kidney).

In cases with urinary tract dilatation, determination of distribution and degree of dilatation helps to lo-

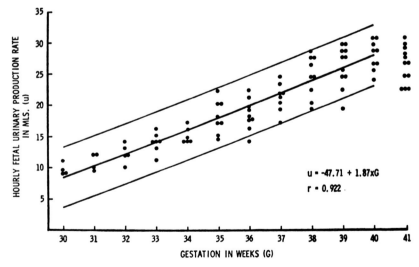

$$u = -47.71 + 1.87 \times G$$
$$r = 0.922$$

FIG 12–5.
Normal hourly third-trimester fetal urinary production rate, 92 cases. This graph shows the relationship between the hourly fetal urinary production rate and the menstrual age between 30 and 41 weeks in normal pregnancy. (From Wladimiroff JW, Campbell S: Fetal urine-production rates in normal and complicated pregnancy. Lancet 1974; 1:151. Used by permission.)

TABLE 12–2.

Urinary Tract Abnormalities

1. Renal agenesis or severe hypoplasia[35-50]
2. Crossed renal ectopia and pelvic kidney[51, 52]
3. Obstructive uropathy or urinary tract dilatation
   a. Ureteropelvic junction (UPJ) obstruction[53-66]
   b. Ureterovesical junction (UVJ) obstruction and megaureter[67-82]
   c. Urethral level obstruction or megacystis[83-105]
4. Renal cystic disease[108-115]
   a. Cystic renal dysplasia[116-122]
   b. Multicystic dysplastic kidney disease[123-135]
   c. Autosomal recessive (infantile) polycystic kidney disease[136-146]
   d. Autosomal dominant (adult) polycystic kidney disease[147-158]
   e. Syndromes associated with renal cysts[159-228]
5. Renal tumors[229-233]
6. Ambiguous genitalia[253-255]

calize and assess the severity of involvement (Tables 12–3 and 12–4)[18, 25] Obstruction of the fetal urinary tract occurs at the ureteropelvic junction (UPJ), ureterovesical junction (UVJ), or urethra. Although a fetus can have obstructive uropathy in the absence of urinary tract dilatation, dilatation of the urinary tract frequently (but not necessarily) signifies obstruction.[18, 20, 25, 33] Detection of urinary tract dilatation pre-

natally warrants postnatal evaluation. Optimally, the postnatal assessment should occur after 48–72 hours to avoid confusion introduced by the dehydration typically present in the first 48 hours of life.[31] Urinary tract dilatation may also occur with reflux, non–obstructive megacystis, and other causes but implies an intrinsic genitourinary abnormality in over 95% of cases and indicates an increased incidence of extra-urinary anomalies (Table 12–5).[25, 64, 103, 164] Hydrocolpos, intrapelvic sacrococcygeal teratoma, or other pelvic masses extrinsic to the urinary tract represent rare causes for urinary tract obstruction and dilatation.[22, 28, 34] Features indicative of obstructive uropathy often occur in the absence of urinary tract dilatation and may dominate the sonographic findings. In addition to oligohydramnios, these associated features include cystic renal dysplasia and evidence for spontaneous urinary tract rupture or decompression (ascites, paranephric urinoma, or dystrophic bladder wall calcification) (Figs 12–6 to 12–8).[96, 121]

Several sonographic and physiologic criteria per-

TABLE 12–3.

Prenatal Grading of Fetal Hydronephrosis After 20 Weeks' Gestation*

Grade	Calyceal Dilatation	Size of Pelvis
I	Physiological	< 1 cm
II	Normal calyces	1–1.5 cm
III	Slight dilatation	> 1.5 cm
IV	Moderate dilatation	> 1.5 cm
V	Severe dilatation + atrophic cortex	> 1.5 cm

*Modified from Grignon A, Filion R, Filiatrault D, et al: Urinary tract dilatation in utero: Classification and clinical applications. Radiology 1986; 160:645.

TABLE 12–4.

Postnatal Outcome of 70 Cases in Which Kidneys Were Suspected to Have Hydronephrosis on Antenatal Sonography*

Antenatal		Postnatal		
Grade†	Number of Kidneys	Normal	Medical Management	Surgical Management
I	29	28 (97%)	1 (3%)	0
II	31	15 (48%)	4 (13%)	12 (39%)
III	16	2 (13%)	4 (25%)	10 (62%)
IV	14	0	0	14 (100%)
V	2	0	0	2 (100%)

*Modified from Grignon A, Filion R, Filiatrault E, et al: Urinary tract dilatation in utero: Classification and clinical applications. Radiology 1986; 160:645.
†Grade refers to the degree of pyelocaliectal dilatation after 20 weeks' gestation.

TABLE 12–5.

Hydroureteronephrosis in Newborns: 146 Cases*

N	Category	% of Total Affected Newborns	% Males	% With Ipsilateral or Contralateral Dysplasia	% With Other Urinary Structural Anomalies	% With Extra-urinary Anomalies
32	UPJ† obstruction	22	56	22	28	19
27	Posterior urethral valves	18.5	100	0	1	22
20	Ectopic ureterocele	13.7	55	10	5	15
18	Deficient abdominal muscles	12.3	100	33	—	33
11	Lower ureteral and UVJ† obstruction	7.5	73	9	54	36
8	Infection without reflux or obstruction	5.5	75	12	37	62
7	Reflux without obstruction	5	57	28	28	43
7	Neurogenic hydronephrosis	5	28	0	0	0
5	Bladder diverticulum or septation	3.4	80	20	40	40
4	Hydronephrosis of questionable cause	2.7	100	0	25	75
3	Obstruction of non–duplicated ectopic ureter	2	67	67	0	100
2	Simple ureterocele	1.3	50	50	0	0
2	Other urethral lesions	1.3	100	0	100	0

*Modified from Lebowitz RL, Griscom NT: Neonatal hydronephrosis. 146 cases. Radiol Clin N Am 1977; 15:49–59.
†UPJ = ureteropelvic junction; UVJ = ureterovesical junction.

mit assessment of renal function in utero and may assist in selection of fetuses who may potentially benefit from in utero surgery.[21, 26] In cases with obstructive uropathy, detection of cystic renal dysplasia, either on the basis of cortical cysts or intense cortical echogenicity, correlates with poor renal function.[121] However, not all dysplastic fetal kidneys have sonographically visible cysts or increased echogenicity.[121]

Other means of assessing the fetal renal function require interventive procedures. Percutaneous drainage of the fetal bladder with documentation of reaccumulation of urine indicates the presence of urine formation but does not provide information regarding the quality of urine formation. Absence of urine reaccumulation, however, correlates with a poor prognosis. Determination of fetal urine electrolytes via an indwelling catheter within the fetal bladder provides an additional means of determining fetal urine function (Fig 12–9).[23] The presence of abnormally increased concentrations of sodium and chloride with increased urine osmolality correspond with the presence of cystic dysplasia and poor renal function at birth or autopsy (see

Chapter 20). Grannum et al. have also found an excellent correlation between urine electrolyte determinations and neonatal outcome in 12 cases.[24]

Some fetuses with severe or progressive urinary tract dilatation as an isolated abnormality but with normal renal function may benefit from in utero decompression of the urinary tract via surgery or an indwelling shunt catheter.[21, 26] In such cases, results from the International Fetal Surgery Registry concerning 62 continuing pregnancies with in utero shunts in place indicate an overall survival rate of 48%.[30]

Detection of urinary tract abnormalities may indicate the presence of other anomalies or a syndrome and warrants a search for associated anomalies. For example, bilateral renal cystic disease with encephalocele indicates the Meckel-Gruber syndrome, and renal cysts in a dwarf with a small thorax provide strong evidence of asphyxiating thoracic dysplasia (Jeune's syndrome). In such cases, the associated anomalies often determine the prognosis to a much greater degree than do the renal abnormalities and may preclude in utero therapy.

FIG 12–6.
Urine ascites. Transverse scan of the fetal abdomen shows a large amount of ascites. A small fluid collection is also noted in the retroperitoneum, indicating evidence for decompression of the urinary tract into the peritoneal cavity secondary to obstructive uropathy. *A* = ascites; *open arrow* = spine; *small arrow* = retroperitoneal fluid collection.

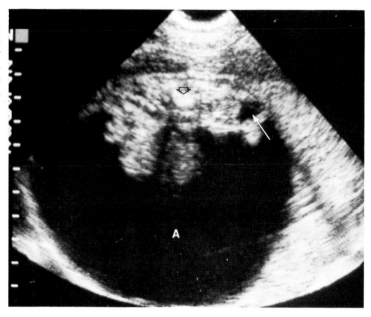

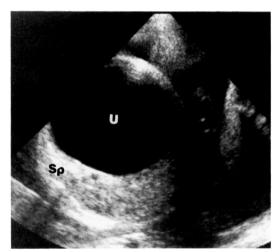

FIG 12–7.
Paranephric urinoma. A large unilocular paraspinous fluid-filled mass frequently indicates the presence of a paranephric urinoma, as this transverse scan of the fetal abdomen demonstrates. *U* = urinoma; *Sp* = fetal spine.

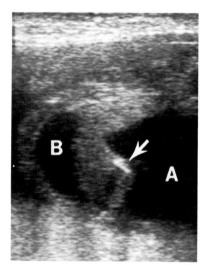

FIG 12–8.
Dystrophic bladder wall calcification at the site of bladder perforation secondary to posterior urethral valvular obstruction. Oblique scan of the pelvis and lower abdomen at 23 weeks shows a high-amplitude echo with posterior acoustical shadowing arising from the thickened urinary bladder wall. Urinary ascites also is present. Autopsy confirmed the presence of dystrophic bladder wall calcification at the site of bladder perforation. *Arrow* = dystrophic bladder wall calcification; *B* = thick-walled urinary bladder; *A* = urinary ascites. (From Mahony BS, Callen PW, Filly RA: Fetal urethral obstruction: US evaluation. Radiology 1985; 157:221–224. Used by permission.)

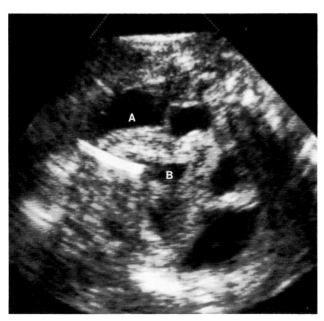

FIG 12–9.
Catheter within the fetal urinary bladder. Catheterization of the fetal bladder may provide information regarding quantity and quality of urine production and may decompress a dilated bladder. *B* = bladder; *A* = amniotic fluid.

Renal Agenesis

Clinical and Pathologic Findings

Bilateral renal agenesis occurs in approximately 1 in 3,000 to 1 in 10,000 births.[38, 43, 49] It seems to be transmitted in a polygenic pattern with a recurrence rate of 2%–5%.[46, 47] Some cases have a possible X-linked, autosomal recessive or autosomal dominant inheritance.[42, 44] Potter suggested that the term renal agenesis be reserved for those cases in which both kidneys and ureters are absent, whereas renal aplasia indicates absence only of the kidneys.[43] Bilateral renal agenesis probably results from failure of metanephros development with failure of the ureteric bud to induce differentiation of the metanephric blastema into renal parenchyma. This may result from lack of development of the ureteric bud itself.

Potter described a syndrome found in bilateral renal agenesis exemplified by pulmonary hypoplasia, limb deformities, and typical facies (Fig 12–10).[43] In pulmonary hypoplasia, the lungs weigh less than half the expected weight and have reduced numbers of alveoli and conducting airways.[35, 49] The limb deformities include abnormal hand and foot positioning, bowed legs, clubbed feet, and hip dislocation. Typical facies in Potter's syndrome include low-set ears, redundant skin, parrot beak nose, receding chin, and a prominent fold arising at the inner canthus of each eye.

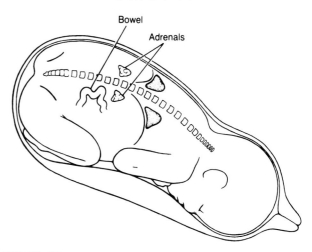

FIG 12–10.
Renal agenesis. Bilateral renal agenesis or severe hypoplasia causes anhydramnios and the Potter sequence. In the absence of kidneys in the renal fossae, the adrenal glands may assume an oval shape and should not be mistaken for kidneys. In addition, hypoechoic bowel within the renal fossae may also mimic kidneys. (From Mahony BS: The genitourinary system, in Callen PW (ed): *Ultrasonography in Obstetrics and Gynecology*. Philadelphia, WB Saunders Co, 1988. Used by permission.)

Most of these findings probably result from the severe oligohydramnios that ensues, although the relationship with low-set ears has not been established. Similar findings occur in the setting of severe oligohydramnios arising from a variety of causes.[48]

Oligohydramnios has been reported in pregnancies with bilateral renal agenesis as early as the 14th week of gestation.[47] Although the fetal kidneys begin to produce urine after the tenth week of gestation, they do not become a major source of urine production until the 14th–16th week. Hence, a normal amount of amniotic fluid at 10–14 weeks of gestation does not preclude the diagnosis of bilateral renal agenesis.

Although the incidence of unilateral renal agenesis has not been definitively determined, it probably occurs approximately 4–20 times more commonly than does bilateral renal agenesis.[36, 45] Approximately 4%–5% of cases have a family history of bilateral renal agenesis, bilateral severe renal dysgenesis, or agenesis of the kidney with dysgenesis of the other.[45] Unilateral renal agenesis may be a very difficult diagnosis to confirm antenatally because the adrenal or bowel in the renal fossa may simulate the kidney (Fig 12–11). Unlike bilateral renal agenesis, however, fetuses with unilateral renal agenesis would be expected to fill and empty their bladders normally, have a normal amount of amniotic fluid, and have a good prognosis.

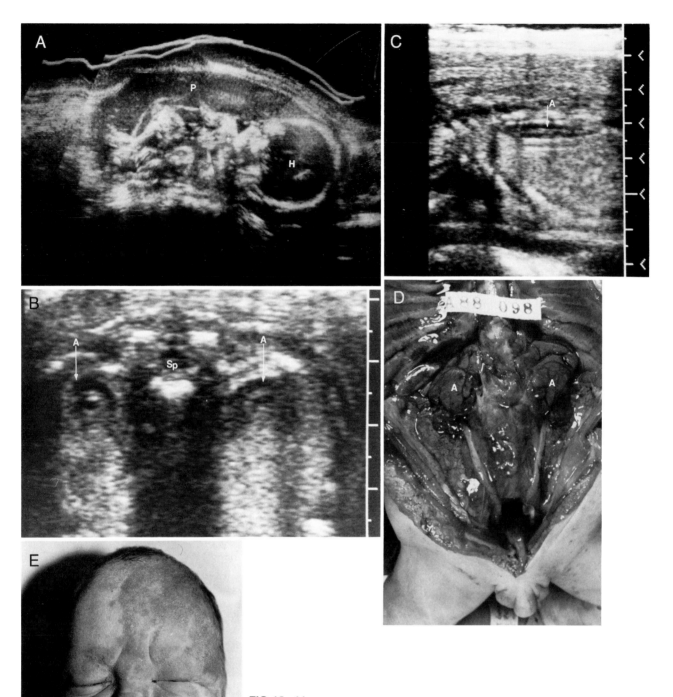

FIG 12–11.
Bilateral renal agenesis. **A,** longitudinal scan of the uterus shows fetal crowding and absence of amniotic fluid. **B,** transverse scan at the level of the fetal lumbar spine shows bilateral, paraspinous, hypoechoic structures superficially resembling kidneys. However, the bladder was not visualized during the examination. **C,** parasagittal scan shows an oval paraspinous structure in the renal fossa. This is the adrenal, not the kidney. Note the absence of amniotic fluid. **D,** postmortem photograph of the abdomen shows the oval adrenals but absence of the kidneys. **E,** postmortem photograph of a similar neonate with bilateral renal agenesis shows the typical Potter facies. H = head; P = placenta; SP = spine; A = adrenal glands.

Sonographic Findings

The lack of urine production associated with bilateral renal agenesis results in severe oligohydramnios and absence of a demonstrable urinary bladder (Fig 12–11). These are the only constant sonographic features of this uniformly lethal disorder. As mentioned earlier, the normal fetus voids at least once an hour but never completely empties the bladder, and the bladder normally should be visualized after the 13th week of gestation.[35, 37] Identification of a normal bladder excludes the diagnosis of bilateral renal agenesis. Although a small midline urachal diverticulum may resemble the bladder, its lack of filling and emptying distinguishes it from the bladder.

If the bladder is not seen initially, the examination should be carried out for 60–90 minutes before stating its absence. Visualization of the bladder can be hampered by the severe oligohydramnios and breech position. In cases with severe oligohydramnios, a single intravenous administration of furosemide (20–60 mg) to the mother has been used in an attempt to induce fetal diuresis within 15–45 minutes after administration.[50] Fluid in the bladder following furosemide administration indicates the presence of at least one functioning kidney. However, absence of urine in the bladder following furosemide challenge is not a reliable indicator of bilateral renal agenesis. Several reports document the failure of this test to distinguish between bilateral renal agenesis and intrauterine renal failure from severe intrauterine growth retardation.[40, 41, 46] Other causes may also result in non–visualization of the bladder (Table 12–6).

Non–visualization of the urinary bladder is more significant than apparent visualization of the kidneys. In bilateral renal agenesis, the adrenal glands often assume a discoid, oval, or reniform shape which can create confusion in distinguishing between the kidneys and adrenals (see Fig 12–11). The most reliable feature that discriminates the kidney from an adrenal gland is identification of the hypoechoic renal medullae. Sonographic visualization of anatomic detail may be quite limited by the lack of amniotic fluid and fetal flexion associated with the oligohydramnios. In some cases, therefore, intra-amniotic instillation of warmed isotonic saline may improve visualization. This is rarely warranted, however, since the diagnosis depends upon absence of bladder visualization, and severe second-trimester oligohydramnios for any reason has a dismal prognosis.

Associated Anomalies

Approximately 14% of fetuses with bilateral renal agenesis have associated cardiovascular anomalies including tetralogy of Fallot, ventriculoseptal defect, atrioseptal defect, hypoplastic left ventricle, coarctation of the aorta, transposition of the great vessels, and hypoplastic aorta.[49] Approximately 40% of affected fetuses have musculoskeletal malformations (sirenomelia, absent radius and fibula, digital anomalies, sacral agenesis, diaphragmatic hernia, and cleft palate (Figs 12–12 and 12–13).[49] Central nervous system malformations (hydrocephaly, meningocele, cephalocele, holoprosencephaly, anencephaly, and microcephaly) and gastrointestinal malformations (duodenal atresia, imperforate anus, tracheoesophageal fistula, malrotation, and omphalocele) have also been reported.[49] Ten percent of cases with multicystic dysplastic kidney disease have contralateral renal agenesis, a lethal combination.

CROSSED RENAL ECTOPIA AND PELVIC KIDNEY

Clinical and Pathologic Findings

Crossed renal ectopia occurs in approximately 1 in 7,000 births and may mimic unilateral renal agenesis.[51] The ectopic kidney in crossed, fused ectopia is abnormally large and bi-lobed, unlike the contralateral kidney in unilateral renal agenesis.[51] Renal ectopia may cause obstructive uropathy or reflux and occur in conjunction with other cardiovascular or gastrointestinal abnormalities.[51]

Pelvic kidney occurs in approximately 1 in 1,200 necropsies and may also mimic unilateral renal agenesis.[52] Ectopic kidney has an increased association with multiple congenital anomalies involving the skeletal, cardiovascular, gastrointestinal, and gynecologic systems.[52]

TABLE 12–6.

Causes for Non–visualization of the Fetal Urinary Bladder

1. Bilateral renal agenesis.
2. Bilateral multicystic dysplastic kidney.
3. Unilateral renal agenesis with contralateral multicystic dysplastic kidney.
4. Unilateral renal agenesis or multicystic dysplastic kidney with contralateral severe obstruction or dysplasia.
5. Severe bilateral obstruction or dysplasia.
6. Severe infantile (autosomal recessive) polycystic kidney disease.
7. Severe intrauterine growth retardation.
8. Persistent cloaca.
9. Bladder or cloacal exstrophy.

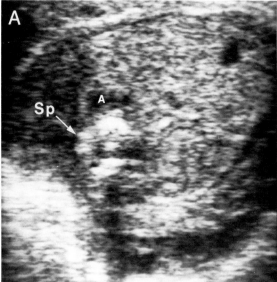

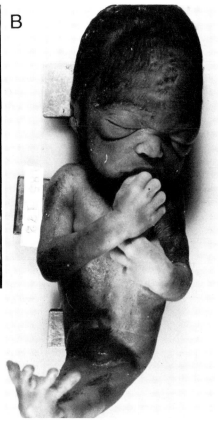

FIG 12–12.
Bilateral renal agenesis with sirenomelia. **A,** transverse scan of the fetal abdomen at the level of the lumbar spine demonstrates anhydramnios and absence of visualization of the kidneys. The urinary bladder was not seen during the examination. Note the relatively prominent adrenal gland. **B,** postmortem photograph of the fetus shows the sirenomelia. *Sp* = spine; *A* = adrenal.

Sonographic Findings

Greenblatt et al. described a case of crossed, fused renal ectopia in one twin at 36 weeks.[51] No kidney was evident in the right renal fossa, but an enlarged and bilobed kidney filled the left renal fossa. No other anomalies were evident.

Hill et al. reported two cases of pelvic kidneys at 34–36 weeks' gestation (Fig 12–14).[52] One case occurred in a twin with a large midline encephalocele. The right kidney was normal, but the left kidney was small and located in the pelvis. The co-twin was normal. In the second case, a singleton fetus had a sacral meningomyelocele, hydrocephalus, and a right pelvic kidney. The right adrenal gland remained in its anatomically correct position but assumed an ovoid shape. The normal left kidney was seen in the left renal fossa.

URETEROPELVIC JUNCTION (UPJ) OBSTRUCTION

Clinical and Pathologic Findings

UPJ obstruction represents the most common cause of neonatal hydronephrosis and constitutes 20%–50% of all congenital urologic disorders diagnosed in utero.[59, 64] It occurs more commonly in

males, usually as a sporadic phenomenon, although familial cases have been reported.[53, 55, 62, 65] Since 85%–90% of affected neonates appear entirely normal on physical examination, and only 55% are diagnosed by age 5 years, antenatal detection of UPJ obstruction permits early therapy of a correctable anomaly that may otherwise remain unrecognized for years.[2, 66] UPJ obstruction resolved spontaneously in 3%–10% of cases during the neonatal period, but 90% of patients requiring postnatal surgery have significant reduction of pelvicaliceal distension and normal renal function.[2, 18, 59]

The etiology of UPJ obstruction includes kinks, fibrous adhesions, ureteral valves, or unusual shapes of the pyeloureteral outlet.[60] Occasionally, UPJ obstruction can be inherited as a dominant trait.[56] The ureteropelvic junction is an important site for the propulsion of urine, and both circular and longitudinal muscularis layers are critical in this function. An absent longitudinal muscularis layer of the ureteropelvic junction was noted in 69 representative cases with UPJ obstruction in one series.[54]

Sonographic Findings

A dilated renal pelvis is essential for the diagnosis of UPJ obstruction (Figs 12–15 and 12–16). The degree of dilatation varies depending upon the severity of

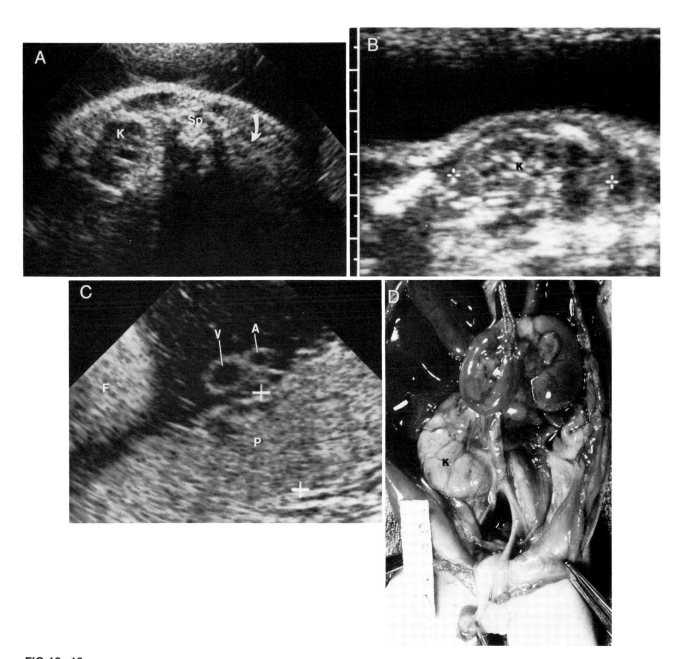

FIG 12–13.
Unilateral renal agenesis with single umbilical artery. **A,** transverse scan at the level of the lumbar spine shows the right kidney but absence of the left kidney. **B,** right parasagittal scan shows the right kidney. **C,** transverse scan of the umbilical cord demonstrates only one umbilical artery with the umbilical vein. **D,** postmortem photograph of a different fetus with unilateral renal agenesis shows the absence of the left kidney. This fetus also had a meningomyelocele and a single umbilical artery. *K* = kidney; *Sp* = spine; *curved arrow* = empty left renal fossa; *A* = single umbilical artery; *V* = umbilical vein; *P* = placenta; *F* = fetus.

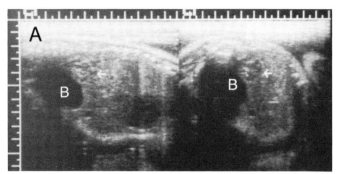

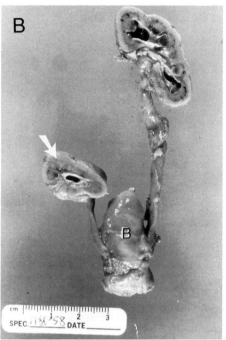

FIG 12–14.
Pelvic kidney. **A,** dual-image scan at 34 weeks shows the small left pelvic kidney. On the longitudinal scan *(left),* the kidney is near the bladder. On the transverse scan *(right),* the pelvic kidney is to the left of the bladder. This twin also had a large midline occipital encephalocele. **B,** autopsy specimen photographed from behind shows the ectopic left kidney and normal right kidney with hydroureter. *B* = bladder; *arrow* = left pelvic kidney. (From Hill LM, Peterson CS: Antenatal diagnosis of fetal pelvic kidneys. J Ultrasound Med 1987; 6:393–396. Used by permission.)

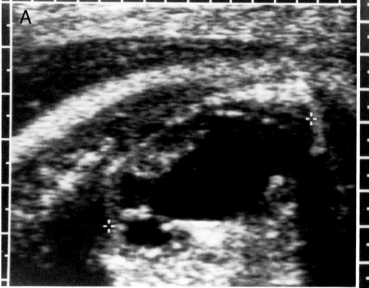

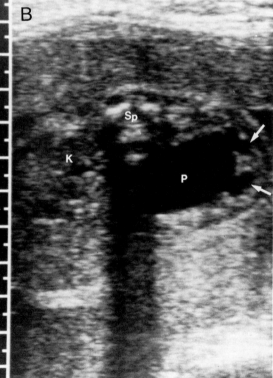

FIG 12–15.
Unilateral ureteropelvic junction obstruction. **A,** parasagittal scan of the right kidney shows dilatation of the renal pelvis and calyces. **B,** transverse scan of the kidneys shows the dilated right renal pelvis and calyces. The renal pelvic diameter/kidney diameter ratio is approximately 67%, and the renal pelvic diameter is approximately 20 mm. Both of these parameters indicate evidence for significant pyelocaliectasis that frequently requires postnatal surgical management. The contralateral kidney is normal. This fetus also has a cleft palate and an imperforate anus. *P* = renal pelvis; *arrows* = dilated calyces; *K* = normal left kidney; *Sp* = spine.

URETEROPELVIC JUNCTION OBSTRUCTION

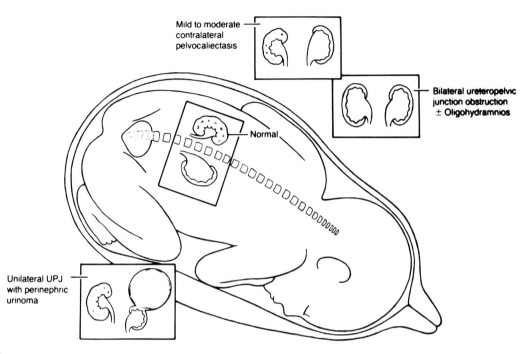

FIG 12–16.
Ureteropelvic junction (UPJ) obstruction. The degree of obstruction and dilatation varies. UPJ obstruction occurs bilaterally in approximately 10%–30% of cases. Severe UPJ obstruction can cause marked thinning of the renal parenchyma or rupture of the kidney with a resultant urinoma. Unilateral UPJ obstruction occasionally has concomitant polyhydramnios, but bilateral severe UPJ obstruction results in oligohydramnios. (From Mahony BS: The genitourinary system, in Callen PW (ed): *Ultrasonography in Obstetrics and Gynecology*. Philadelphia, WB Saunders Co, 1988. Used by permission.)

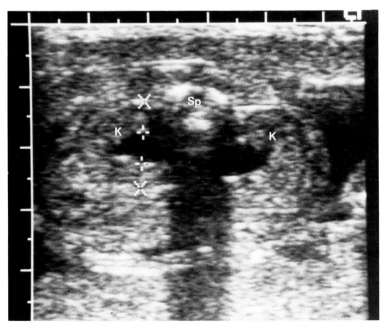

FIG 12–17.
Minimal renal pyelocaliectasis. Transverse scan at the level of the lumbar spine demonstrates minimal bilateral pyelocaliectasis at 20 menstrual weeks. The pelvis measures approximately 5 mm in diameter bilaterally, and the renal pelvic diameter-kidney diameter ratio is approximately 33% bilaterally. This degree of pyelocaliectasis is seen frequently and typically is not clinically significant. In this fetus, it had resolved on a follow-up scan at 31 weeks. *Sp* = spine; + = renal pelvic diameter; *x* = renal diameter; *K* = kidney.

obstruction. Measurements of the anteroposterior diameter of the renal pelvis and kidney, as well as assessment of the amount of calicectasis after 19 weeks, provide useful information regarding the degree of dilatation. A pelvic diameter of less than 10 mm and a ratio between the pelvic diameter and kidney diameter of less than 50% in the absence of rounded calyces probably is physiologic and rarely progresses (Fig 12–17).[2, 25, 29] On the other hand, a pelvic diameter of more than 10–15 mm and a ratio between the pelvic diameter and kidney diameter of more than 50% with rounded calyces indicates significant pyelocaliectasis that frequently requires surgical management (Table 12–4).[25] Even when the ratio between the pelvic diameter and kidney diameter is less than 50%, rounded calyces usually indicate hydronephrosis.[63] Occasionally, infundibulopelvic stenosis produces megacalyces in the absence of pyelocaliectasis.[167]

Since most UPJ obstructions are unilateral, a normal functioning contralateral kidney produces a normal amount of amniotic fluid and a visible urinary bladder. Paradoxically, polyhydramnios may occasionally occur with incomplete UPJ obstruction, presumably as a result of impaired renal concentrating ability and increased renal output (Fig 12–18).[32, 63] Severe UPJ obstruction in the setting of a contralateral non–functioning or absent kidney produces severe oligohydramnios and absence of bladder visualization. A normal amount of amniotic fluid in the setting of bilateral UPJ obstruction may indicate an incomplete obstruction,

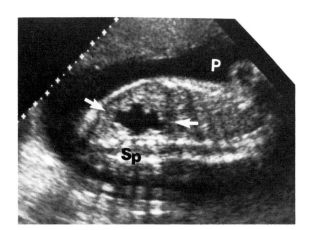

FIG 12–18.
Unilateral UPJ obstruction with mild polyhydramnios. Parasagittal scan demonstrates a dilated renal pelvis and calyces without ureterectasis. The contralateral kidney and bladder were unremarkable. The amniotic fluid volume is mildly increased. Additional scans showed other large pockets of amniotic fluid. Occasionally, unilateral renal disease may be associated with polyhydramnios, possibly secondary to increased renal output of the contralateral kidney. *Sp* = spine; *P* = polyhydramnios; *arrows* = kidney.

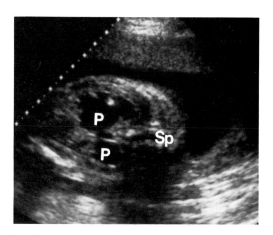

FIG 12–19.
Bilateral UPJ obstruction. Oblique scan through the fetal abdomen at the level of the lumbar spine demonstrates dilatation of the renal pelvis and calyces bilaterally. The degree of dilatation is asymmetric, and the amniotic fluid volume is normal, indicating the obstructions are not complete. *P* = dilated renal pelvis and calyces bilaterally; *Sp* = spine.

an obstruction of recent onset, or a concomitant cause for excessive amniotic fluid production (Fig 12–19).

Unilateral UPJ obstruction usually does not require prenatal intervention, if the contralateral kidney functions normally with normal egress of amniotic fluid.[27, 59] Rarely, the renal pelvis in UPJ obstruction may dilate to an enormous size, distend the abdomen, and compress the thorax; such cases may require prenatal decompression to prevent dystocia and permit lung development.[58] Fortunately, bilateral severe UPJ obstruction is quite rare. In general, quantification of the amniotic fluid volume represents an indirect assessment of residual renal function. Since severe oligohydramnios prior to 26 weeks of gestation correlates with an increased probability of developing pulmonary hypoplasia, management of bilateral UPJ obstruction depends upon the gestational age, amniotic fluid volume, and renal function.

Associated Anomalies

Unilateral UPJ obstruction may occur with contralateral renal agenesis or multicystic dysplasia, both of which may produce profound oligohydramnios if the UPJ obstruction is severe. Visualization of a paranephric urinoma or urinary ascites from rupture of the collecting system correlates with severe obstruction and low probability of residual renal function.[57, 83] A paranephric urinoma creates a large unilocular cystic flank mass that touches the fetal spine (see Fig 12–7).[57] UPJ obstruction has also been associated with Hirschsprung's disease, cardiovascular abnormalities, neural tube defects, esophageal atresia, imperforate anus, congenital hip dislocation, and the adrenogenital syndrome.[54, 64]

URETEROVESICAL JUNCTION (UVJ) OBSTRUCTION AND MEGAURETER

Clinical and Pathologic Findings

Megaureter refers to a dilated ureter. It is more common in males and usually occurs sporadically, although familial cases of primary vesicoureteral reflux have been reported.[69, 72, 73, 77, 82] Vesicoureteral reflux has been reported in 26%–34% of asymptomatic siblings of patients with reflux.[67, 71]

Megaureter may be caused by obstruction to the flow of urine, vesicoureteral reflux, or other conditions in which neither obstruction nor reflux occur. Primary megaureter refers to a dilated ureter caused by an intrinsic ureteral defect, whereas secondary megaureter refers to a dilated ureter resulting from vesicoureteric reflux secondary to an obstruction at another level. In obstructive primary megaureter, the obstruction occurs at the level of or just above the ureterovesical

junction. The obstruction may result from stenosis of the ureteral valves or from fibrosis or abnormal musculature of a narrow segment of a ureter just proximal to the ureterovesical junction.[68, 79, 80] In refluxing primary megaureter, a loss of anti-reflux mechanism at the UVJ produces a dilated ureter. The cause for the ureteral dilatation remains idiopathic in conditions for which neither an obstructive nor reflux etiology can be found.

Duplication of the renal collecting system occurs in up to 4% of the population and represents the most common major urinary tract anomaly.[70] The lower pole moiety characteristically refluxes, and the upper pole moiety obstructs in an ectopic ureterocele associated with duplication of the ureters. Ectopic ureterocele occurs bilaterally in approximately 15% of cases and frequently requires postnatal surgery.

Sonographic Findings

Megaureter usually appears as a tortuous, fluid-filled structure that often can be traced from the bladder to the kidney.[81] However, the ureteral tortuosity frequently prevents visualization of the ureter through-

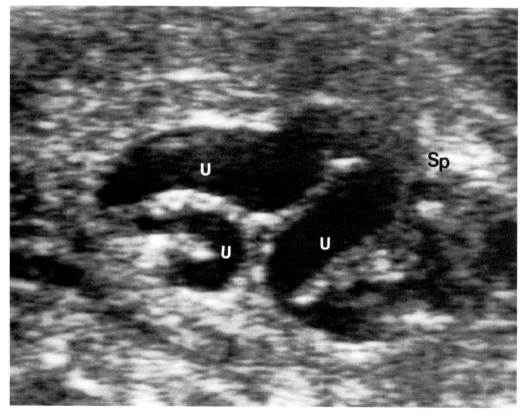

FIG 12–20.
Tortuous dilated ureter. Right parasagittal scan of the fetal abdomen demonstrates a markedly tortuous fluid-filled structure, a portion of which touches the fetal spine. This indicates that it is a retroperitoneal structure and most likely genitourinary in origin. This fetus has ureterectasis secondary to reflux associated with posterior urethral valvular obstruction. *Sp* = spine; *U* = dilated, tortuous ureter.

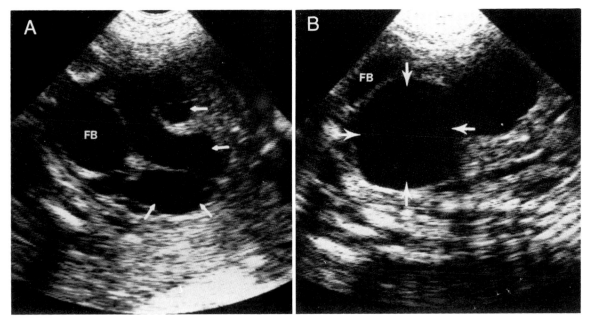

FIG 12–21.
Ureteral stenosis at 24–28 weeks. **A,** scan of the pelvis and lower abdomen at 24 weeks shows a large, serpentine fluid-filled structure posterior to the urinary bladder. **B,** similar scan at 28 weeks demonstrates that the enlarged retrovesicular mass compresses and displaces the urinary bladder. Autopsy confirmed the presence of a blind left ureteral pouch with atresia of the distal ureter, massive left ureteral dilation, and renal dysplasia. *FB* = fetal urinary bladder; *arrows* = dilated left ureter. (From Montana SA, Cyr DR, Lenke RR, et al: Sonographic detection of fetal ureteral obstruction. AJR 1985; 145:595. Used by permission.)

out its entire course (Fig 12–20). Documentation that the serpentine fluid-filled structure touches the fetal spine, originates from the renal pelvis, and extends into the retrovesicular position distinguishes a dilated ureter from fluid-filled bowel.[74]

The size of a dilated ureter varies from a small structure to an enormous serpentine structure measuring several centimeters in diameter. A huge megaureter often, but not necessarily indicates a secondarily dilated ureter. The diagnosis of UVJ obstruction can be made when a megaureter is seen in the absence of megacystis. However, megacystis with megaureters secondary to reflux can occur in the absence of bladder outlet obstruction.[33] The presence of pyelocaliectasis in UVJ obstruction depends upon the severity of obstruction in most cases. Complete UVJ obstruction typically produces severe pyelocaliectasis with destruction of kidney tissue or cystic dysplasia (Fig 12–21). Incomplete UVJ obstruction or reflux megaureter typically produces mild to moderate pyelocaliectasis without cystic dysplasia.

A dilated upper pole moiety with a normal lower pole intrarenal collecting system indicates an obstructed duplex collecting system (Figs 12–22 to 12–24). A dilated and enlarged upper pole moiety may displace the non–dilated lower pole of the kidney inferiorly and laterally. In cases with a duplex collecting

system associated with an ectopic ureterocele, the related thin-walled and fluid-filled ureterocele within the bladder may be difficult to detect in utero, as is detection of the two distinct ureters and collecting systems.[75]

No specific prenatal intervention usually is necessary in unilateral megaureter. In bilateral megaureter with a normal amount of amniotic fluid, expectant management is recommended. The presence of a normal amount of amniotic fluid suggests normal renal function.

Associated Anomalies
Megaureter occurs with an increased incidence of associated contralateral renal agenesis, complete or incomplete duplex system, contralateral cystic dysplastic kidney, and Hirschsprung's disease.[76, 78, 82]

DISTAL URINARY TRACT OBSTRUCTION AND MEGACYSTIS

Clinical and Pathologic Findings
Obstruction distal to the ureterovesical junction most commonly results from posterior urethral valves. Urethral obstruction from posterior urethral valves almost exclusively affects the male fetus and usually oc-

ECTOPIC URETEROCELE

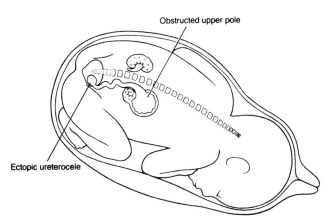

FIG 12–22.
Ectopic ureterocele. The obstructed upper pole moiety associated with an ectopic ureterocele may enlarge and displace the non–dilated lower pole moiety. However, the lower pole moiety may become dilated, often secondary to reflux. The thin-walled ectopic ureterocele may occasionally be visible within the urinary bladder. (From Mahony BS: The genitourinary system, in Callen PW (ed): *Ultrasonography in Obstetrics and Gynecology,* ed 2. Philadelphia, WB Saunders Co, 1988. Used by permission.)

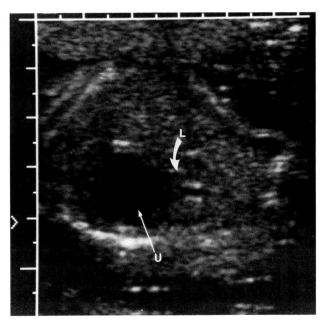

FIG 12–23.
Duplex collecting system with obstructed upper pole moiety. Parasagittal scan of the right kidney shows the fluid-filled obstructed upper pole moiety of a duplex kidney displacing the lower pole moiety inferiorly. *U* = upper pole obstructed moiety; *L* = displaced lower pole moiety.

curs as a sporadic condition but can occur in families or twins.[85, 92] Young et al. described three types of urethral valves.[105] In type I, folds distal to the verumontanum insert into the lateral wall of the urethra. In type II, folds arising in the verumontanum pass proximal to the bladder neck, where they divide into finger-like membranes. In type III, valves consisting of a diaphragm-like structure with a small perforation arise distal to the verumontanum but do not attach to it. Only the types I and II posterior urethral valves cause obstruction of clinical significance.

Following the commencement of fetal urine production, obstruction of the urethra leads to megacystis, megaureter, and hydronephrosis with or without the presence of cystic dysplasia and/or evidence for urinary tract rupture. Distention of the bladder may distort and shorten the intravesicular portion of the ureters and lead to vesicoureteral reflux and hydronephrosis. The reflux and concomitant severity of kidney damage often is not symmetrical, and the kidney spared from reflux has a better functioning capacity following delivery than does the affected kidney.[64, 89, 91, 104] The renal damage probably results from increased intraluminal pressure within the urinary tract during nephrogenesis which may produce renal dysplasia (see subsequent section on Cystic Renal Dysplasia).

Table 12–7 lists other less common causes for urethral level obstruction or megacystis. In obstructive uropathy, the degree of megacystis, hydronephrosis, renal dysplasia, and oligohydramnios correlates with the

severity of obstruction. Urethral stricture typically occurs in the region of the prostatic urethra and mimics posterior urethral valves with variable degrees of obstructive uropathy. Urethral agenesis, on the other hand, typically produces massive bladder enlargement with severe hydronephrosis, cystic renal dysplasia, severe oligohydramnios, and pulmonary hypoplasia. The bladder may enlarge to the extent that it causes dystocia. In fetuses with persistence of the cloaca, the urinary bladder is incompletely separated from the rectum and frequently results in a large pouch into which the intestinal, urinary, and reproductive tracts enter (see Chapter 11). Affected fetuses typically have an imperforate anus and urethral abnormalities ranging from agenesis to stenosis.

Rarely, the urinary bladder may enlarge in the absence of obstruction with the megacystis-microcolon-

TABLE 12–7.
Causes of an Enlarged Fetal Urinary Bladder

1. Posterior urethral valves.
2. Urethral stricture.
3. Urethral agenesis.
4. Persistent cloaca with associated urethral agenesis or stenosis.
5. Megacystis-microcolon-intestinal hypoperistalsis syndrome.

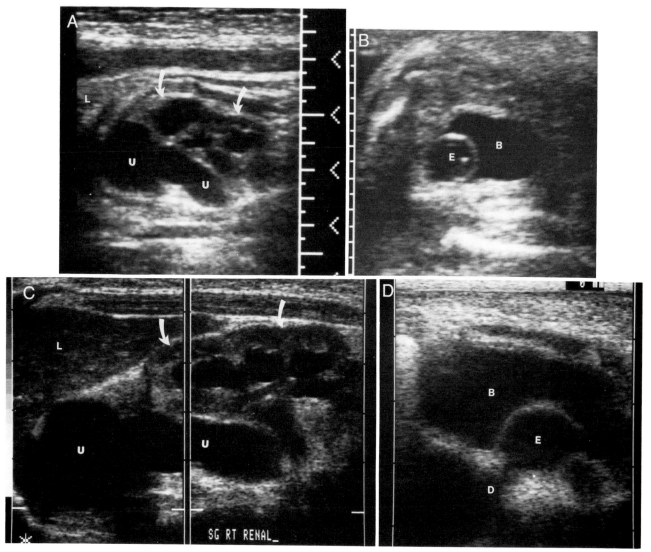

FIG 12–24.
Duplex collecting system with ectopic ureterocele. **A,** parasagittal scan of the right fetal kidney demonstrates a severely dilated upper pole moiety leading into a dilated ureter. The lower pole moiety is displaced inferiorly and exhibits moderate pyelocaliectasis. **B,** the thin-walled ectopic ureterocele is noted within the urinary bladder on this scan of the fetal pelvis. **C,** postnatal sagittal dual-image scan of the right kidney confirms the prenatal findings. **D,** postnatal parasagittal scan of the right pelvis shows the ectopic ureterocele within the bladder. *U* = upper pole obstructed moiety extending into dilated ureter; *L* = displaced lower pole moiety with moderate pyelocaliectasis; *E* = ectopic ureterocele; *B* = urinary bladder; *D* = dilated distal right ureter; *L* = liver.

URETHRAL LEVEL OBSTRUCTION

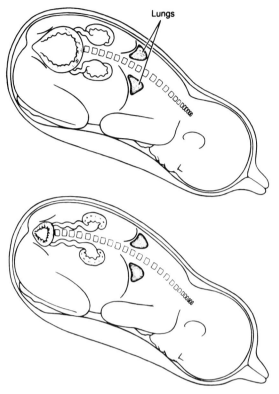

FIG 12–25.
Urethral level obstruction. The sonographic features of urethral obstruction vary, but the cardinal signs are a thick-walled dilated bladder and a dilated proximal urethra. The degree of megacystis, ureterectasis, and pyelocaliectasis varies and may be mild. Concomitant oligohydramnios correlates with a poor prognosis secondary to pulmonary hypoplasia. (From Mahony BS: The genitourinary system, in Callen PW (ed): *Ultrasonography in Obstetrics and Gynecology.* Philadelphia, WB Saunders Co, 1988. Used by permission.)

intestinal hypoperistalsis syndrome.[97, 99, 102, 103] This rare syndrome of unknown etiology typically affects females and produces abdominal distention secondary to the enlarged non–obstructed bladder, shortened and dilated proximal small bowel, malrotated microcolon, and absent or ineffective peristalsis. Unlike in Hirschsprung's disease, the bowel has normal or increased numbers of ganglion cells. Although the urinary tract findings may mimic urethral level obstruction, the amniotic fluid volume in the megacystis-microcolon-intestinal hypoperistalsis syndrome is typically increased or normal rather than decreased.

Sonographic Findings

Distal urinary tract obstruction produces a broad spectrum of sonographic features antenatally, depending on the degree and duration of obstruction (Figs 12–25 to 12–30 and Table 12–8). The cardinal signs of urethral level obstruction include persistent dilatation of the urinary bladder and proximal urethra and thickening of the urinary bladder wall in the setting of oligohydramnios (see Figs 12–25 and 12–26). An obstructed urinary bladder assumes a fusiform or pear-shaped appearance, with the neck of the pear representing the bladder neck and the dilated upper portion of the urethra. A completely obstructed and massively dilated bladder assumes a spherical shape and fills almost the entire fetal abdomen. A massively dilated fluid-filled structure arising from the fetal pelvis in the presence of severe oligohydramnios indicates strong evidence for megacystis from complete bladder obstruction.

Visualization of the dilated proximal urethra in this setting confirms the diagnosis of urethral obstruction but is not always demonstrable because of fetal positioning. Decompression of the urinary bladder, either spontaneously or following needle or shunt placement, demonstrates the bladder wall thickening secondary to its hypertrophied detrusor muscle. If spontaneous decompression of the bladder has occurred, the presence of a thick-walled bladder suggests that an obstruction was present previously, although it may be difficult to determine whether the obstruction was complete or incomplete. The bladder wall characteristically thickens to approximately 10–15 mm in fetuses with urethral obstruction but a non–dilated bladder. Rarely, the dilated urinary bladder may prolapse through the perineum (see Fig 12–30).

Other features indicative of urinary tract obstruction assist in the diagnosis of urethral level obstruction, but they do not occur uniformly, and their absence should not preclude the diagnosis.[87, 96, 98] Oligohydramnios occurs in approximately 50% of fetuses with urethral level obstruction, and 40% of affected fetuses have ureterectasis or hydronephrosis (see Table 12–8).[96] Severe oligohydramnios frequently occurs in complete bladder outlet obstruction, especially after 16 weeks of gestation. Dilated ureters secondary to vesicoureteral reflux typically are quite tortuous and often massively dilated. The pyelocaliectasis associated with distal urinary tract obstruction resembles that associated with more proximal obstructions but tends to be bilateral and asymmetric. Spontaneous decompression of the bladder, ureter, or renal pelvis may cause extravasation of urine and result in urinary ascites or a paranephric urinoma; it often indicates a poor prognosis (see Figs 12–6 and 12–8).[83, 96]

Detection of renal cortical cysts in the setting of distal urinary tract obstruction accurately indicates the presence of renal dysplasia (see Fig 12–29).[121] Hyper

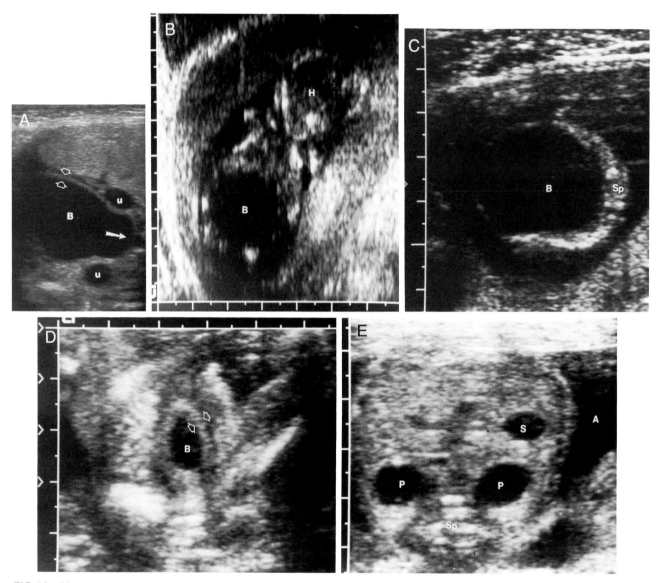

FIG 12–26.
Variable degrees of urinary bladder dilatation with urethral level obstruction. **A,** coronal scan of the pelvis and abdomen at 25 weeks shows marked dilatation of the urinary bladder and proximal urethra as well as dilated distal ureters. Note the anhydramnios and mildly thickened bladder wall. **B** and **C,** coronal **(B)** and transverse abdominal **(C)** scans of another fetus at 14 weeks shows marked dilatation of the bladder, filling virtually the entire abdomen. Oligohydramnios is present. Massive dilatation of the urinary bladder with severe oligohydramnios presents strong evidence of complete urethral obstruction. **D** and **E,** transverse scan of the pelvis **(D)** in another fetus at 17 weeks demonstrates a non–dilated but thick-walled urinary bladder. Transverse scan of the kidneys **(E)** demonstrates moderate bilateral pyelocaliectasis. Note the low normal amniotic fluid volume. *B* = bladder; *U* = ureterectasis; *open arrows* = thickened wall of the urinary bladder; *straight arrow* = dilated proximal urethra; *Sp* = spine; *P* = dilater renal pelves; *S* = stomach; *A* = amniotic fluid. (Part **A** from Mahony BS, Callen PW, Filly RA: Fetal urethral obstruction: US evaluation. Radiology 1985; 157:221. Used by permission.)

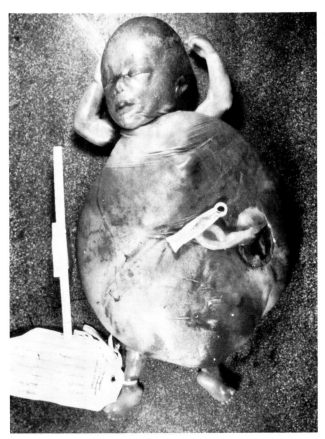

FIG 12–27.
Prune-belly syndrome. Postmortem photograph of a fetus with urethral obstruction demonstrates the marked distention of the abdomen associated with the prune-belly syndrome.

echogenicity of the renal parenchyma also correlates with a high probability for renal dysplasia, but assessment of renal echogenicity is quite subjective, and not all echogenic kidneys are dysplastic (Figs 12–31 and 12–32).[121] Table 12–9 demonstrates the sensitivities and specificities of these two sonographic criteria in the diagnosis of renal dysplasia.[121] The size of the kidneys and the presence or absence of pelvocaliectasis do not appear to be useful in the assessment of renal dysplasia secondary to urethral level obstruction. Dysplastic kidneys may be abnormally small or large, and some hydronephrotic kidneys are dysplastic, whereas others are not. Poor prognostic indicators in urethral level obstruction include oligohydramnios, a large amount of urine ascites, and/or dystrophic bladder wall or peritoneal calcification (Table 12–8).[121]

The sonographic features of a megacystis-microcolon-intestinal hypoperistalsis syndrome closely mimic those of urethral level obstruction with the exception of the amniotic fluid volume (Fig 12–33). Although urethral level obstruction typically produces oligohydramnios, oligohydramnios has not been reported with the megacystis-microcolon-intestinal hypoperistalsis syndrome, and most cases with this syndrome have increased amniotic fluid volume.[103] All cases reported

prenatally have been detected at 31–36 weeks on the basis of massive distention of the fetal bladder, which did not empty completely and exhibited only small changes in volume over 1-hour observation periods. Approximately 25% of reported cases also demonstrated thickening of the bladder wall, and most cases had pyelocaliectasis and ureterectasis. No gastric or intestinal abnormalities have been identified prenatally.

Associated Anomalies

Other anomalies of the genitourinary system have been described in 20%–25% of patients with posterior urethral valve obstruction. These include duplication of the urethra, megalourethra, cryptorchidism, and hypospadias.[64, 86, 93–95] Other associated anomalies include patent ductus arteriosus, tracheal hypoplasia, mitral stenosis, total anomalous pulmonary vein drainage, scoliosis, and imperforate anus.[64] Chromosomal abnormalities, including trisomies 18 and 13, del 2q, and 69XXY, have been reported.[100]

When considering the diagnosis of distal urinary tract obstruction, the sonographer should examine the fetal perineum to determine the sex. Visualization of male external genitalia provides strong evidence that the obstruction results from posterior urethral valves.

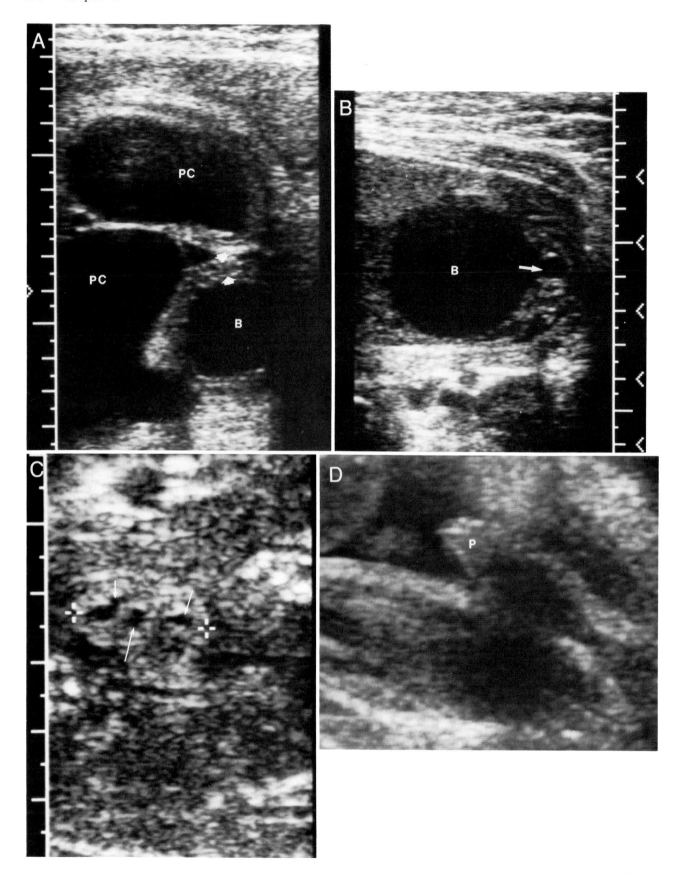

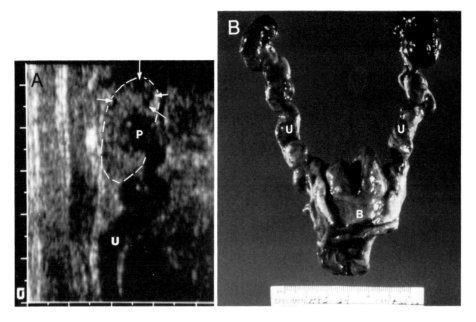

FIG 12–29.
Urethral obstruction with cystic dysplasia. **A,** coronal sonogram demonstrates a small echogenic kidney with numerous cortical cysts. Mild pyelocaliectasis is present without caliecectasis. Ureterectasis is also noted. **B,** autopsy specimen in a similar case demonstrates small kidneys with bilateral ureterectasis and a thick-walled bladder. *Dotted line* = renal outlines; *P* = renal pelvis; *U* = ureter; *small arrows* = cortical cysts.

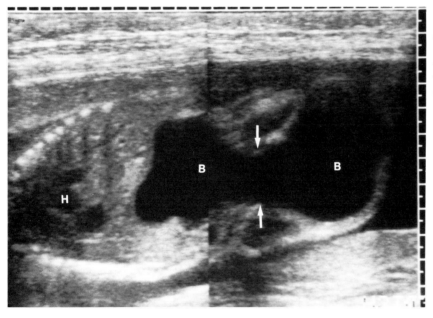

FIG 12–30.
Dilated urinary bladder with prolapse through the perineum. This longitudinal dual-image scan shows an unusual case of dilatation of the urinary bladder with prolapse of the bladder through the perineum. *B* = bladder; *arrows* = expected level of perineum; *H* = heart.

←**FIG 12–28.**
Variable degrees of pyelocaliectasis and ureterectasis with urethral level obstruction. **A,** oblique scan of the fetal abdomen demonstrates marked bilateral pyelocaliectasis with extreme thinning of the renal parenchyma. The urinary bladder is mildly dilated, but thick-walled, with the bladder wall measuring 7 mm in thickness. Marked oligohydramnios is present. **B,** coronal scan of the pelvis of another fetus demonstrates dilatation of the bladder and proximal urethra as well as severe oligohydramnios. **C,** scan of the kidney of the fetus in Figure 12–28,B shows a small echogenic kidney with cortical cysts but no pyelocaliectasis. **D,** demonstration of the penis in this clinical setting yields strong evidence for urethral level obstruction secondary to posterior urethral valves. *PC* = severe bilateral pyelocaliectasis; *B* = bladder; *arrowheads* = thickened bladder wall; *graticules* = small echogenic kidney containing numerous small cysts; *small arrows* = small cysts within echogenic kidney; *P* = penis.

TABLE 12–8.

Antenatal Sonographic Features of Fetuses With Urethral Obstruction*

	Subsequent Demise (n = 25)	Survival (n = 15)	Total (n = 40)
Menstrual weeks at presentation			
14–20	32%	7%	22.5%
21–29	56%	60%	57.5%
30–35	12%	33%	20%
Amniotic fluid volume			
Decreased	80%	7%	52.5%
Low normal or borderline decreased	8%	33%	17.5%
Normal	12%	53%	27.5%
Increased	0	7%	2.5%
Dilated posterior urethra	48%	47%	47.5%
Dilated urinary bladder	88%	93%	90%
Thickened bladder wall	92%	93%	92.5%
Ureterectasis	44%	33%	40%
Calicectasis			
None or mild	80%	27%	60%
Moderate or marked	20%	73%	40%
Intraperitoneal fluid (urine ascites)			
None	76%	73%	75%
Small	4%	20%	10%
Large	20%	7%	15%
Paranephric pseudocyst (urinoma)	8%	7%	7.5%
Dystrophic bladder wall or peritoneal calcification	20%	0	12.5%

*Modified from Mahony BS, Callen PW, Filly RA: Fetal urethral obstruction: US evaluation. Radiology 1985; 157:221–224.

In fetuses with massive distention of the urinary bladder, one must also consider the megacystis-intestinal hypoperistalsis syndrome, the caudal regression anomaly, or urethral atresia. Each of these entities occurs in fetuses of either gender, but the megacystis-intestinal hypoperistalsis syndrome occurs more commonly in females.[97, 99, 102, 103] Fetuses with this syndrome typically have polyhydramnios or a normal amniotic fluid volume; approximately 7% of reported cases have had an omphalocele.[103]

BLADDER OR CLOACAL EXSTROPHY

Clinical and Pathologic Findings

Bladder exstrophy occurs in approximately 1 in 25,000 to 1 in 40,000 births, more commonly in males than females. It probably results from failure of mesoderm to contribute to the allantoic extension of the cloaca during early embryogenesis.[107] This results in exteriorization of the pelvic viscera on the abdominal surface.

TABLE 12–9.

Value of Sonographic Criteria in the Prediction of Renal Dysplasia in Obstructive Uropathy*

	Sensitivity (%)	Specificity (%)	(+) Predictive Value (%)	(−) Predictive Value (%)
Renal cysts	44	100	100	44
Increased renal echogenicity	73	80	89	57
Pyelocaliectasis	41	73	78	35

*Modified from Mahony BS, Filly RA, Callen PW, et al: Fetal renal dysplasia: Sonographic evaluation. Radiology 1984; 152:143.

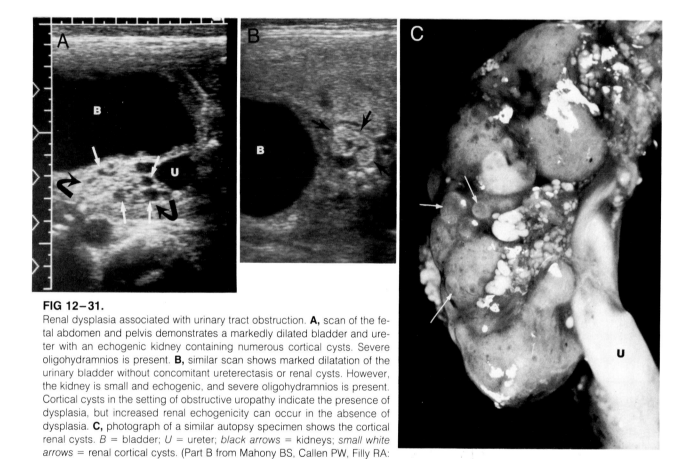

FIG 12–31.
Renal dysplasia associated with urinary tract obstruction. **A,** scan of the fetal abdomen and pelvis demonstrates a markedly dilated bladder and ureter with an echogenic kidney containing numerous cortical cysts. Severe oligohydramnios is present. **B,** similar scan shows marked dilatation of the urinary bladder without concomitant ureterectasis or renal cysts. However, the kidney is small and echogenic, and severe oligohydramnios is present. Cortical cysts in the setting of obstructive uropathy indicate the presence of dysplasia, but increased renal echogenicity can occur in the absence of dysplasia. **C,** photograph of a similar autopsy specimen shows the cortical renal cysts. *B* = bladder; *U* = ureter; *black arrows* = kidneys; *small white arrows* = renal cortical cysts. (Part B from Mahony BS, Callen PW, Filly RA: Fetal urethral obstruction: US evaluation. Radiology 1985; 157:221–224. Used by permission.)

RENAL PARENCHYMAL RESPONSES TO OBSTRUCTION

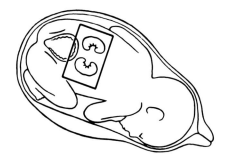
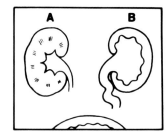

A. Normal
B. Thinned, normal echogenicity, no cysts

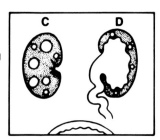
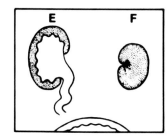

C. Increased echogenicity with cysts ≡ dsyplasia
D. Thinned, increased echogenicity with cysts ≡ dysplasia

E. Thinned, increased echogenicity, no cysts-probable dysplasia
F. Small, increased echogenicity, no cysts-probable dysplasia

FIG 12–32.
Renal parenchymal responses to obstruction. **A,** in distal urinary tract obstruction without reflux the kidney may remain normal. **B,** pyelo-caliectasis may thin the renal parenchyma. **C,** cystic dysplasia may occur with renal cysts, fibrosis (increased echogenicity), and poor function (lack of pyelocaliectasis). **D,** cystic dysplasia may occur with persistent pyelocaliectasis. **E,** increased renal echogenicity without visible cysts suggests, but is not diagnostic of dysplasia. **F,** a small echogenic kidney without pyelocaliectasis is also suggestive, but not diagnostic of dysplasia. (From Mahony BS: The genitourinary system, in Callen PW (ed): *Ultrasonography in Obstetrics and Gynecology,* ed 2. Philadelphia, WB Saunders Co, 1988. Used by permission.)

Cloacal exstrophy is estimated to occur in 1 in 200,000 to 1 in 250,000 live births, with both sexes being equally affected.[106] It also probably arises from a defect in the early development of the mesoderm but results in a more complex anomaly than bladder exstrophy. It is a lethal anomaly in its most severe form, but milder, correctable forms exist. The dominant manifestations include (1) persistence of a common cloaca into which the ureters, ilium, and hindgut open; (2) complete breakdown of the cloacal membrane with exstrophy of pelvic viscera and often an omphalocele; and (3) lumbosacral meningomyelocele.

Sonographic Findings
Bladder exstrophy, cloacal exstrophy, and persistent cloaca each result in an abnormal or absent bladder but normal amniotic fluid volume (see Chapter 10). Mirk et al. described a fetus with bladder exstrophy at 36 weeks who had absence of a bladder within the pelvis in association with a 4.7 cm solid mass protruding from the abdominal wall immediately superior to the genitalia.[107] This mass represented the inverted exstrophied bladder. Meizner et al. suggested cloacal

exstrophy at 31 weeks in a fetus with an omphalocele, lumbosacral meningomyelocele, clubfeet, narrow chest, and a normal amount of amniotic fluid.[106]

RENAL CYSTIC DISEASE

The majority of fetuses with renal cysts have an obstructive uropathy resulting in either renal dysplasia (Potter type IV) or multicystic dysplastic kidney disease (Potter type II).[108–115] Numerous syndromes or diseases (infantile or adult polycystic kidney diseases, Meckel-Gruber syndrome, Zellweger syndrome, Jeune's syndrome, trisomy 13, or 18, etc.) may also produce renal cysts at varying rates and warrant careful search for associated anomalies, especially in the absence of features indicative of urinary tract obstruction. Other rare possibilities include a simple renal cyst, lymphangiectasia, liquefaction of a renal tumor, or hematoma. Occasionally, dilated calyces without pyelocaliectasis may mimic cortical cysts, as may a small paranephric urinoma. Table 12–10 delineates the criteria for classification of cystic kidney diseases.

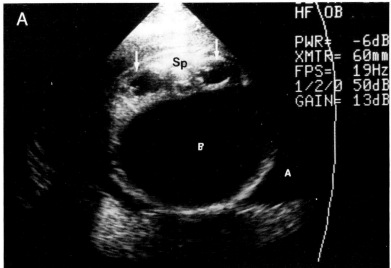

FIG 12–33.

Megacystis-microcolon-intestinal hypoperistalsis syndrome. **A,** transverse scan at the level of the lumbar spine demonstrates marked urinary bladder dilatation with mild to moderate bilateral pyelocaliectasis. The amniotic fluid volume is normal. **B,** postnatal upper gastrointestinal tract series in a similar case demonstrates severe dilatation of the stomach and proximal duodenum. Peristalsis was diminished. Microcolon is still evident from previous barium enema, indicating hypoperistalsis affecting the entire bowel. *B* = bladder; *Sp* = spine; *arrows* = bilateral pyelocaliectasis; *A* = amniotic fluid; *S* = stomach; *D* = duodenum; *C* = microcolon. (Part **A** courtesy of Harris J Finberg MD, Phoenix, AZ. Part **B** from Manco LG, Osderdahl P: The antenatal sonographic features of megacystis-microcolon-intestinal hypoperistalsis syndrome. J Clin Ultrasound 1984; 12:595. Used by permission.)

Cystic Renal Dyplasia (Potter Type IV)

Clinical and Pathologic Findings

Urinary tract obstruction may produce increased intraluminal pressure within the urinary tract during nephrogenesis and lead to renal dysplasia.[116, 117] The type and severity of dysplasia probably depends predominantly upon the time in fetal life that the obstruction develops. According to the Potter classification, type II multicystic dysplastic kidney results from an early developmental obstruction, whereas type IV cystic renal dysplasia results from an obstructive phenomenon developing later in fetal life as a result of posterior urethral valves.[120, 122] Beck et al. demonstrated in the fetal lamb that ureteral obstruction occurring prior to the 70th day of gestation (term, 147–150 days) resulted in renal dysplasia (i.e., large amount of undifferentiated mesenchymal stroma, parenchymal disorganization, cystic dilatation of Bowman spaces, and marked fibrosis).[116] On the other hand, obstruction occurring after 80 days of gestation resulted in hydronephrosis but no cystic dysplasia. Harrison et al. have reported similar findings and have demonstrated that early prenatal relief of the obstruction may prevent the development of cystic dysplasia.[116, 118, 119]

Cystic renal dysplasia occurs most frequently in humans affected with urethral level obstruction but may also occur secondary to UPJ or UVJ obstruction. The severity of renal dysplasia varies, but extensive dysplasia indicates irreversible renal damage with significantly reduced renal functional capacity.[23, 117]

Sonographic Findings

Demonstration of renal cortical cysts in the setting of obstructive uropathy effectively indicates the presence of cystic renal dysplasia as early as 21 menstrual weeks (see Figs 12–29, 12–32, 12–33).[121] However, the absence of visible cysts does not permit accurate prediction of the absence of dysplasia, since not all dysplastic kidneys have cysts or the size of the cysts may be too small to resolve (Table 12–9). Dysplastic kidneys also tend to have greatly increased echogenicity but may be of normal echogenicity.[121] Renal size and presence or absence of pyelocaliectasis are not accurate indicators of renal dysplasia.

TABLE 12–10.

Criteria for Classification of Cystic Kidney Diseases*

	Autosomal Recessive	Autosomal Dominant	Cystic Dysplasia
Synonyms	Infantile polycystic kidney disease	Adult polycystic kidney disease	Potter type IIA (enlarged) multicystic kidneys (enlarged)
	Potter type I	Potter type III	Potter type IIB (hypoplastic)
Kidney lesion as part of syndrome	No	Often as Potter type III changes (see below)	Frequent (see below)
Incidence	About 1 in 40,000	About 1 in 1,000	Including all types about 1 in 1000?
Pathology of kidney			
Macroscopic shape	Reniform	Reniform	Usually loss of reniform shape
Size	Enlarged, only normal at the beginning	Enlarged, only normal at the beginning	Ranging from hyperplastic to hypoplastic kidneys
Symmetry	Symmetrical	Symmetrical, at the beginning asymmetrical even over a period of years	Often asymmetrical, symmetrical involvement often in case of Potter sequence
Microscopic location of cysts	Dilated collecting ducts	Cysts in all parts of nephron including collecting ducts	Usually complete loss of kidney architecture
Pathology of urinary tract	No other malformations (90% or more in perinatal group, ~60% in neonatal group; ~25% in infantile group; 10% in juvenile group), usually no glomerular cysts	No other malformations	Additional malformations, frequent ureteral obstruction
Diameter of cysts	At onset up to 2 mm, with longer survival up to several cm	At onset small, later very different, up to several cm	Different, up to several cm
Connective tissue	Usually not increased	Usually not increased, in later stages slight increase	Increased
Primitive ducts	None	None	Present
Cartilage	None	None	Nearly pathognomonic but not always present
Liver changes	Congenital hepatic fibrosis	In about one third of adult cases "cystic liver", rare in children	None
Associated symptoms	Cystic pancreas (rare)	Berry aneurysms	Very often different associated malformations
Main clinical manifestations	Neonatal period: respiratory distress. With prolonged survival renal insufficiency and portal hypertension (highly variable)	Usual onset 3rd–5th decade, sometimes in children, very rare in newborns with respiratory distress and renal insufficiency. Pain and enlargement of kidneys, proteinuria, haematuria, hypertension, nephrolithiasis, urinary infection, cerebral haemorrhage	Variable: latent (unilateral involvement) or Potter sequence. Frequently symptoms from additional malformations
Risk for siblings	25%	50% (in extremely rare cases of spontaneous mutation no risk)	Unknown, usually below 10%. (in rare cases autosomal recessive, autosomal dominant or X-linked inheritance
Risk for children	Below 1% (unless non-affected parent is not related to the affected person, or no case in her/his family)	50%	Usually below 10% (in rare cases of autosomal inheritance up to 50%)
Manifestation in affected family members	Often similar course in siblings	Variable, often similar within the same family. Recurrence of early manifestations possible	Variable, in same family renal agenesis, dysplasia, cortical cysts and hydronephrosis possible

Parental kidneys	No alterations	Demonstration of one affected parent (unless parents are too young to demonstrate cystic changes in ultrasound). Rare cases of spontaneous mutation	Unilateral agenesis or dysplasia in up to about 10% in one parent
Prenatal diagnosis	By ultrasound: increased echogenicity, enlargement, oligohydramnios. Often visible only in the second half of pregnancy. Biochemical methods not confirmed	In rare cases by ultrasound with cystic echogenic kidneys but normal amniotic fluid volume. In informative families by linkage analyses (reliability 95%)	Possible early in pregnancy
Potter sequence	Rare	Rare	Present in bilateral cases

*Modified from Zerres K: Genetics of cystic kidney disease: Criteria for classification and genetic counseling. Pediatr Nephrol 1987; 1:397–404. Used by permission.

Multicystic Dysplastic Kidney Disease (Potter Type II)

Clinical and Pathologic Findings

Multicystic dysplastic kidney disease is characterized by the formation of renal cysts resulting from dilated collecting tubules.[124] It can be unilateral, bilateral, or segmental and probably results from atresia of the ureteral bud system during embryogenesis. Unilateral atresia of the ureteral bud system at the level of the upper third of the ureter, with concomitant atresia of the renal pelvis and infundibula, produces unilateral multicystic dysplastic kidney disease. Segmental atresia of the proximal third of the ureter without atresia of the renal pelvis and infundibulum results in the hydronephrotic type of multicystic dysplastic kidney.[126] Segmental multicystic dysplastic kidney occurs following ureteral atresia of the collecting system supplied by the atretic ureter in a duplex kidney.[125, 131]

The atresia of the ureteral bud system resulting in a multicystic dysplastic kidney prevents the metanephric blastema from inducing formation of nephrons. Therefore, the affected kidney characteristically has no normal renal parenchyma proximal to the atretic segment. The collecting tubules within the anomalous kidney become cystically enlarged to varying degrees without macroscopic intercommunication. Although a multicystic dysplastic kidney effectively represents a functionless kidney, the drastic reduction in nephron formation is seldom absolute, and an affected kidney may exhibit minimal residual urine formation.[128] This minimal residual urine formation may result in a change in size or appearance of the affected kidney as gestation progresses.[128]

In bilateral multicystic dysplastic kidney disease, the prognosis is uniformly fatal. Unilateral multicystic dysplastic kidney disease has a good prognosis, if the contralateral kidney is normal. In this setting, most urologists suggest follow-up with close observation after delivery rather than prophylactic nephrectomy.[134]

Sonographic Findings

Multicystic dysplastic kidney disease creates a paraspinous flank mass characterized by numerous cysts resembling a cluster of grapes involving the entire kidney (Figs 12–34 to 12–36).[124, 129, 134, 135] The cysts are of various sizes without identifiable communication or anatomic arrangement. Except in cases with segmental multicystic dysplastic kidney disease, no normal renal parenchyma exists in the affected kidney, and the large cysts frequently distort the contour of the mass. The sonographic findings correlate well with the pathologic appearance.[128]

The amount of amniotic fluid and the presence or absence of urinary bladder visualization depends upon the contralateral kidney. Unilateral multicystic dysplastic kidney disease with a normal contralateral kidney produces a normal amniotic fluid volume and normal bladder (Fig 12–37). Bilateral multicystic dysplastic kidney disease produces profound oligohydramnios and absence of fetal urinary bladder filling (see Fig 12–36).

One classification of multicystic dysplastic kidney disease differentiates between enlarged kidneys (type IIA) from kidneys that are small or of normal size (type IIB).[124] Because the type IIB variety can present with small or normal-sized kidneys, kidney size alone should not be utilized as a criterion for diagnosis of multicystic dysplastic kidney disease. A multicystic dysplastic kidney may enlarge or diminish in size and may disappear resulting in a picture similar to renal agenesis (Fig 12–38).[128, 132]

MULTICYSTIC DYSPLASTIC KIDNEYS

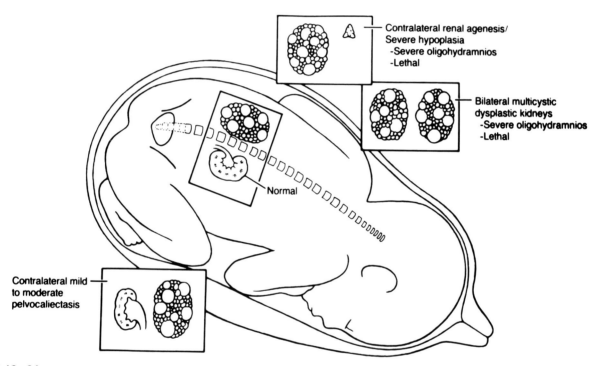

Contralateral renal agenesis/
Severe hypoplasia
-Severe oligohydramnios
-Lethal

Bilateral multicystic
dysplastic kidneys
-Severe oligohydramnios
-Lethal

Normal

Contralateral mild
to moderate
pelvocaliectasis

FIG 12-34.
Multicystic dysplastic kidney disease may be unilateral, bilateral, or associated with contralateral renal agenesis. Although the affected kidney typically produces very little urine, it may change in size throughout gestation. Since the contralateral kidney is the only potentially functional kidney, it must be examined carefully. (From Mahony BS: The genitourinary system, in Callen PW (ed): *Ultrasonography in Obstetrics and Gynecology,* ed 2. Philadelphia, WB Saunders Co, 1988. Used by permission.)

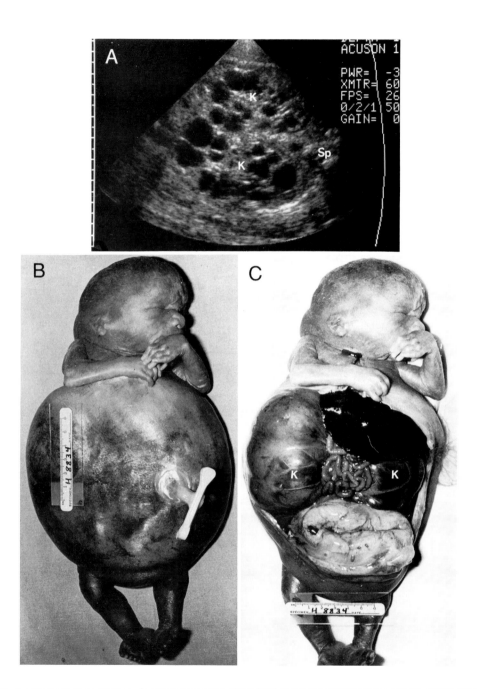

FIG 12–35.
Bilateral multicystic dysplastic kidney disease. **A,** transverse scan of the fetal abdomen demonstrates severe oligohydramnios and multiple bilateral cysts of varying sizes without detectable intercommunication or anatomic arrangement. The enlarged cystic kidneys distend the fetal abdomen. **B** and **C,** photographs of a similar autopsy specimen demonstrate marked abdominal wall distension secondary to the enlarged multicystic dysplastic kidneys. *Sp* = spine; *K* = kidneys.

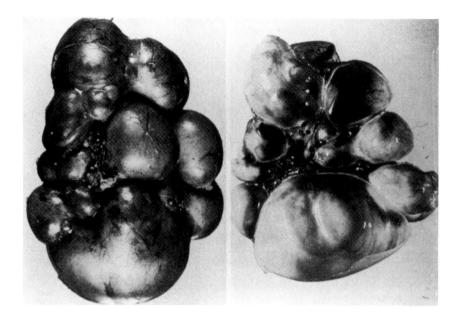

FIG 12–36.
Multicystic dysplastic kidney disease. Whole *(left)* and cut *(right)* autopsy specimens of a multicystic dysplastic kidney illustrate the numerous variable sized cysts without detectable intercommunication or normal renal parenchyma. Microscopic intercommunication may be present. (From Zerres K, Volpel M-C, Weib H: Cystic kidneys: Genetics, pathologic anatomy, clinical picture, and prenatal diagnosis. Hum Genet 1984; 68:104–135. Used by permission.)

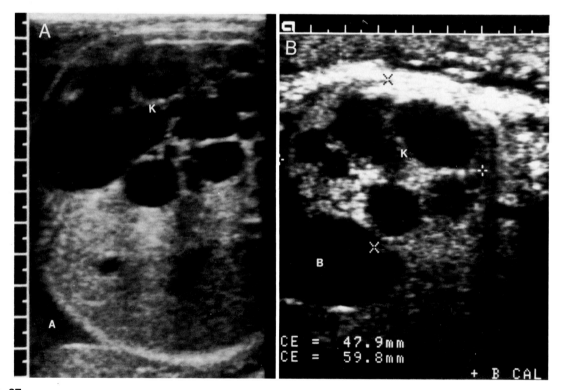

FIG 12–37.
Unilateral multicystic dysplastic kidney disease. **A,** transverse scan of the abdomen shows multicystic dysplastic kidney but a normal amount of amniotic fluid. The normal amniotic fluid volume indicates the presence of a functioning contralateral kidney. **B,** parasagittal scan shows the multicystic dysplastic kidney and also fluid within the urinary bladder. The urine within the bladder also indicates a functioning contralateral kidney. *K* = multicystic dysplastic kidney; *A* = amniotic fluid; *B* = bladder.

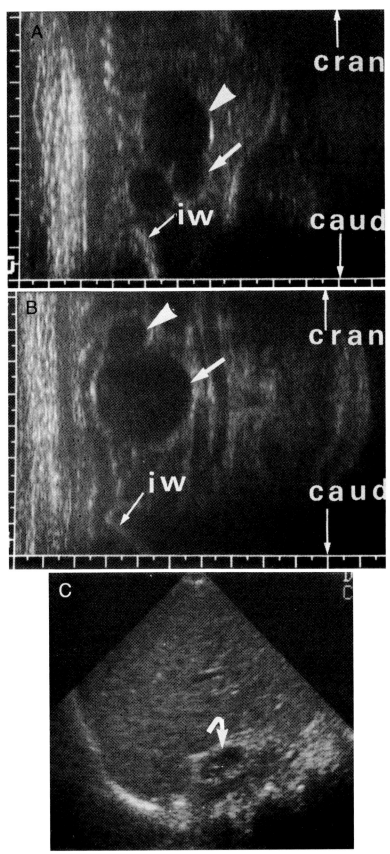

FIG 12–38.
Changing appearance of multicystic dysplastic kidney. **A,** coronal scan at 27 weeks shows a right multicystic dysplastic kidney. **B,** follow-up prenatal scan demonstrates that the previous largest cyst has decreased in size, and the current largest cyst is in the caudal aspect of the kidney. **C,** postnatal scan at 6 months shows that the right kidney has diminished drastically in size. *IW* = iliac wing; *cran* = cranial; *caud* = caudal; *arrowhead* = dominant cyst of the cranial aspect of kidney; *arrow* = dominant cyst of caudal aspect of kidney; *curved arrow* = small kidney postnatally. (From Hashimoto BE, Filly RA, Callen PW: Multicystic dysplastic kidney in utero: Changing appearance on US. Radiology 1986; 159:107–109. Used by permission.)

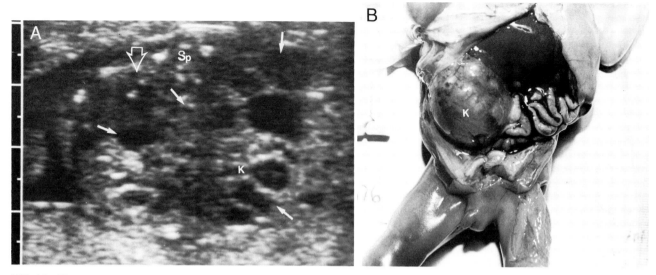

FIG 12-39.
Unilateral multicystic kidney disease with contralateral renal agenesis. **A,** transverse scan at the level of the lumbar spine demonstrates unilateral multicystic dysplastic left kidney. No right kidney was evident, and severe oligohydramnios was present. The dysplastic left kidney fills the right abdomen and extends partially into the left abdomen. **B,** similar autopsy specimen demonstrates the enlarged multicystic dysplastic right kidney with absent left kidney. *K and small arrows* = multicystic dysplastic left kidney; *Sp* = spine; *open arrow* = right renal fossa with right renal agenesis.

Associated Anomalies

Multicystic dysplastic kidney disease may occur in association with anomalies of the cardiovascular system, hydrocephaly, microcephaly, spina bifida, diaphragmatic hernia, cleft palate, duodenal stenosis, imperforate anus, sirenomelia, and tracheoesophageal fistula with bilateral absence of the radius and thumb (see Fig 12-40).[124] Chromosomal anomalies also can be present. Similar anomalies have been associated with unilateral multicystic dysplastic kidney disease.[123, 127]

Contralateral renal anomalies occur in approximately 40% of fetuses with multicystic dysplastic kidney disease (Figs 12-35, 12-39, 12-40).[129] Bilateral multicystic dysplasia occurs in 20% of cases, and contralateral renal agenesis occurs in 10% of cases. Approximately 10% of fetuses with unilateral multicystic dysplastic kidney disease have contralateral hydronephrosis, usually from UPJ obstruction. The degree of obstruction in such cases determines the amount of amniotic fluid and warrants close follow-up to watch for progression of dilatation or diminution of amniotic fluid. Minimal contralateral renal pelvic distension occurs frequently and lacks clinical significance.[129]

Autosomal Recessive (Infantile) Polycystic Kidney Disease (Potter Type I)

Clinical and Pathologic Findings

Autosomal recessive (infantile) polycystic kidney disease (Potter type I) occurs in approximately 1 in 40,000 to 1 in 60,000 newborns but recurs in 25% of cases. Symmetric enlargement of both kidneys characterizes the condition and results from a primary defect of the collecting tubules. Bilateral medullary ectasia produces innumerable 1-2 mm cysts involving non-obstructed renal collecting tubules. The calyces, papillae, and renal pelvis are normal.[15] Infantile polycystic kidney disease has a variable presentation and expressivity depending upon the degree of renal involvement. Although it may be visible pathologically as early as 48-50 days of gestation, the severity of disease correlates inversely with the degree of proliferation of the bile ducts and hepatic fibrosis.[139, 140, 146]

Infantile polycystic kidney disease has been categorized into four groups, based upon the age at which the disease process manifests clinically (Fig 12-41).[136] Some authors indicate that when the disease process occurs in a subsequent pregnancy it tends to be group specific, although others disagree.[113, 136, 138] The perinatal variety produces massively enlarged kidneys in 90% of cases and renal failure in utero or at birth. This variety is the most common form of infantile polycystic kidney disease and typically produces death from pulmonary hypoplasia.[137] In the neonatal variety, the kidneys are not as enlarged as in the perinatal variety in 60% of cases, but the disease onset occurs within the first month after birth and death occurs within 1 year. These cases have mild associated hepatic fibrosis. Cases that present later during the first year of life or between 1 and 5 years of age show progressively less re-

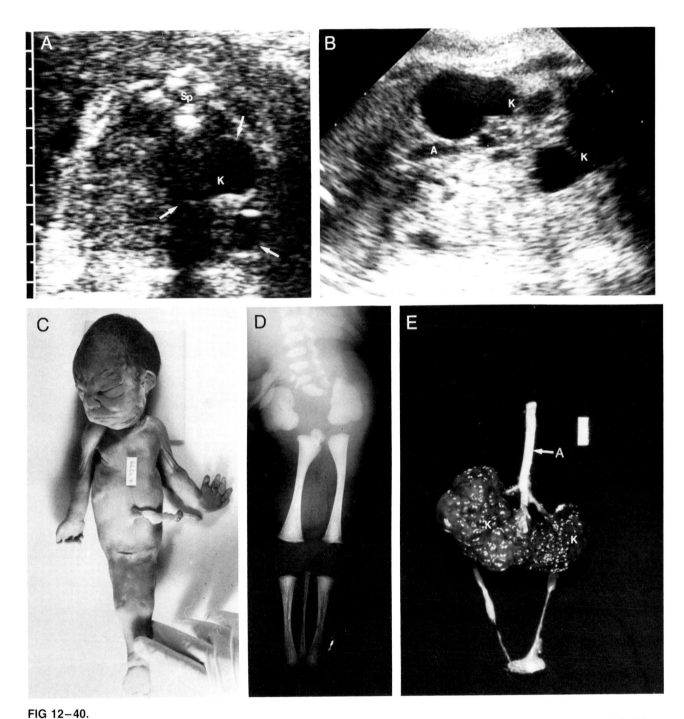

FIG 12–40.
Bilateral multicystic dyplastic kidney with sirenomelia. **A,** transverse scan of the abdomen demonstrates a multicystic dyplastic right kidney. The contralateral kidney was not visualized, but severe oligohydramnios was present. **B,** because the contralateral kidney was not visualized, transvaginal ultrasound was performed demonstrating bilateral multiple cysts adjacent to the descending aorta. On this basis the diagnosis of bilateral multicystic dysplastic kidney was made. Because of the severe oligohydramnios, sirenomelia was not appreciated. **C** and **D,** postnatal photograph and radiograph demonstrate the sirenomelia. Note that the abdomen is not distended by the multicystic dysplastic kidneys. **E,** autopsy specimen of a similar case with small, multicystic dysplastic kidneys shows the innumerable variable-sized cysts without normal parenchyma in kidneys which are normal to mildly enlarged. *K* = multicystic dysplastic kidneys; *Sp* = spine; *A* = aorta.

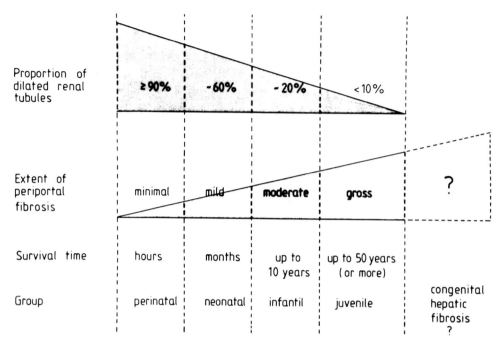

FIG 12-41.
Manifestations of autosomal recessive polycystic kidney disease, according to the subclassification of Blythe and Ockenden. (From Zerres K, Volpel M-C, Weib H: Cystic kidneys: Genetics, pathologic anatomy, clinical picture, and prenatal diagnosis. Hum Genet 1984; 68:104–135. Used by permission.)

nal involvement but more hepatic fibrosis and hepatosplenomegaly. The disease course in these cases depends more upon the development of portal hypertension and esophageal varices than on renal failure.

Sonographic Findings

Especially in a fetus at familial risk for infantile polycystic kidney disease, the diagnosis of this disorder can be made as early as 16 menstrual weeks on the basis of oligohydramnios and characteristic renal findings. Infantile polycystic kidney disease typically produces bilaterally enlarged fetal kidneys that maintain their reniform shape but have abnormally increased echogenicity (Figs 12–42 and 12–43). The renal cortex may appear echogenic with the medullae hypoechoic early in pregnancy, but this pattern reverses later in pregnancy when a peripheral rim of hypoechoic cortex surrounds the echogenic medullae. The multiple interfaces produced by the numerous tiny cysts result in the characteristic increased renal echogenicity. Occasionally, the cysts achieve adequate size so that they are visible sonographically (see Fig 12–43). The kidneys may be so enlarged that they produce dystocia.[139]

As mentioned previously, the kidney circumference-abdominal circumference ratio assists in assessment of renal size.[1] In the normal fetus this ratio remains constant at 0.27–0.30 throughout gestation (see Table 12–1).[1] Enlargement of the fetal kidneys is not the sole criterion for the diagnosis of infantile

polycystic kidney disease, however, since enlarged kidneys alone have been reported with a normal outcome.[142, 145] The increased renal echogenicity, oligohydramnios, and decreased or absent amounts of urine within the bladder are crucial to the diagnosis.

INFANTILE POLYCYSTIC KIDNEYS

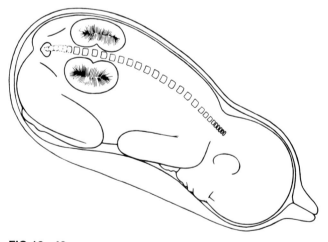

FIG 12-42.
Autosomal recessive (infantile) polycystic kidney disease typically produces enlarged fetal kidneys that maintain their reniform shape but exhibit increased echogenicity, often with oligohydramnios. (From Mahony BS: The genitourinary system, in Callen PW (ed): *Ultrasonography in Obstetrics and Gynecology*. Philadelphia, WB Saunders Co, 1988. Used by permission.)

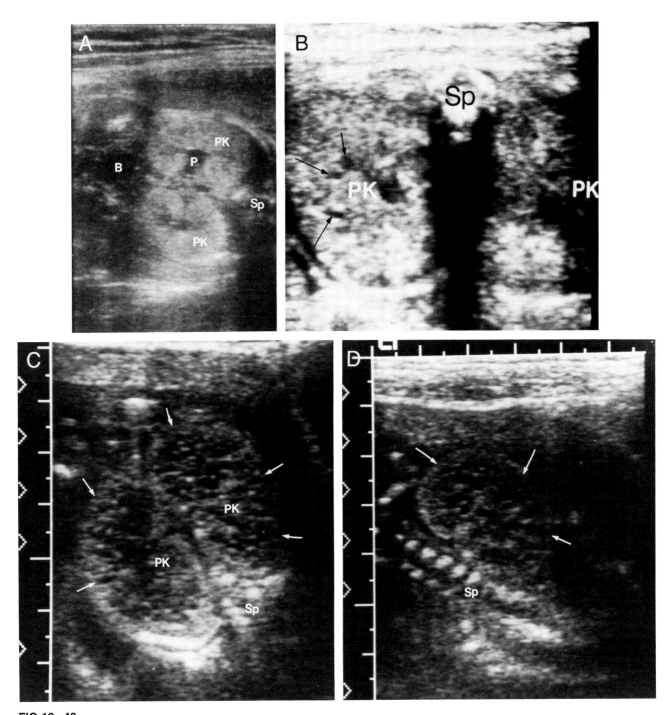

FIG 12–43.
Variable appearance of autosomal recessive polycystic kidney disease. **A,** sagittal scan of the kidneys shows them to be enlarged and echogenic bilaterally without visible cortical cysts. The kidneys almost fill the entire abdomen. Severe oligohydramnios is present, but a small amount of urine is present within the renal pelvis and bladder. **B,** transverse scan at the level of the lumbar spine shows bilaterally enlarged and echogenic kidneys. Several small cysts are visible within the kidneys. Severe oligohydramnios is present. **C** and **D,** transverse and parasagittal scans, respectively, show marked bilateral enlargement of the kidneys with innumerable very small cysts in the setting of severe oligohydramnios. Note that the enlarged kidneys almost completely fill the abdomen and span a length of 9–10 vertebral bodies. *PK* = polycystic kidneys; *Sp* = spine; *P* = renal pelvis; *B* = bladder; *small arrows* = visible cysts.

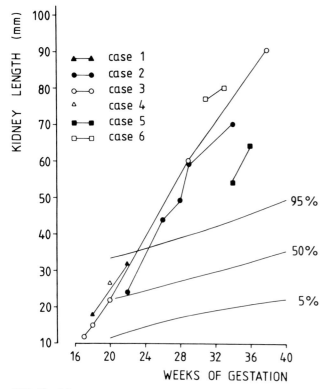

FIG 12–44.
Renal lengths vs. gestational age in six cases of autosomal recessive polycystic kidney disease. Early in gestation the renal size may be normal in autosomal polycystic kidney disease, but the kidneys typically become abnormally enlarged later in gestation. (From Zerres K, Hansmann M, Mallmann R, et al: Autosomal recessive polycystic kidney disease. Problems of prenatal diagnosis. Prenat Diagn 1988; 8:215–229. Used by permission.)

In general, the prenatal diagnosis of infantile polycystic kidney disease is limited to the mid-second trimester and beyond (Fig 12–44). A normal sonogram of a fetus at risk for infantile polycystic kidney disease does not ensure absence of the disease.[139, 140] The sonogram usually, but not always, shows evidence for recurrence by approximately 24 menstrual weeks, but it may not be possible to make a definitive diagnosis or an accurate statement about recurrence prenatally in the less severe forms.[143] Progression of the disease can occur in utero with the development of oligohydramnios and abnormal kidneys.[139, 140, 143, 145] The 25% recurrence risk warrants early attempts at prenatal diagnosis in subsequent pregnancies.

Associated Anomalies

Fetuses with infantile polycystic kidney disease do not appear to have an increased risk for associated malformations.[113, 144] In patients whose infantile polycystic kidney disease manifests postnatally, cystic changes can be found in the liver, with portal and interlobular fibrosis accompanied by biliary duct hyperplasia, biliary dilatation, and portal hypertension.

Autosomal Dominant (Adult) Polycystic Kidney Disease (Potter Type III)

Clinical and Pathologic Findings

Autosomal dominant (adult) polycystic kidney disease is a common genetic disorder of unknown etiology characterized by multiple renal parenchymal cysts. It results from dilatation of the collecting tubules and other tubular segments of the nephrons. The autosomal dominance signifies a 50% recurrence risk, but the penetrance of the gene is virtually 100%. However, the expressivity of the gene varies from a severe form presenting with neonatal death to a mild form detected incidentally at autopsy in adults.[147] The disease process usually presents clinically during the fourth decade of life, although neonatal and infantile cases have been reported.[148–152, 156]

In autosomal dominant (adult) polycystic kidney disease the defect apparently occurs at the level of the ampulla but differs from multicystic dysplastic kidney disease in that the renal involvement is not universal. Considerable variation in the degree of renal involvement occurs in patients of the same age. Macroscopically, affected kidneys usually are enlarged bilaterally, with variable-sized cysts ranging up to several centimeters in diameter.

Sonographic Findings

The prenatal diagnosis of autosomal dominant (adult) polycystic kidney disease had been reported as early as 23½ weeks of gestation.[152–155, 157, 158] The condition should be suspected when cystic echogenic kidneys are detected with a normal amount of amniotic fluid in a fetus with a family history for the disorder. The positive family history is a critical element in making the diagnosis (Fig 12–45).[154] In one report, the kidneys were normal in the mid-trimester but became abnormal on serial examinations.[152] One kidney may be more severely affected than the other.[112, 152] Evaluation of the kidneys of both parents assists in confirmation of the diagnosis in the fetus or neonate. Chorionic villus sampling using a highly polymorphic probe genetically linked to the locus of the mutant gene has been used in prenatal diagnosis.[155]

Pretorius et al. reviewed the follow-up of seven cases of autosomal dominant (adult) polycystic kidney disease detected in utero or shortly after birth.[154] One of the seven cases was terminated at 23½ weeks, and one died in the neonatal period. Four of the remaining five cases had normal renal function, and three of these

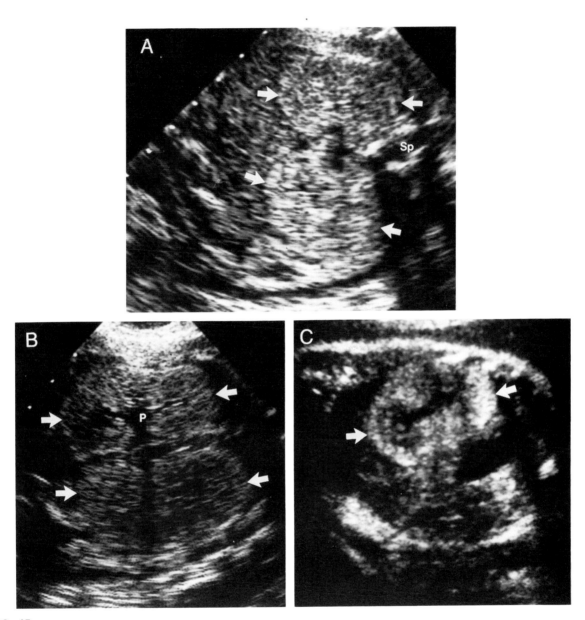

FIG 12–45.
Autosomal dominant (adult) polycystic kidney disease. **A** and **B,** transverse **(A)** and longitudinal **(B)** scans through the fetal kidneys at 23½ weeks' gestation shows enlarged and echogenic kidneys. No cysts were evident. **C,** longitudinal scan through the right kidney at 31 weeks' gestation in a different fetus shows enlarged and echogenic kidneys without visible cysts. A positive family history of autosomal dominant (adult) polycystic kidney disease is a critical element in making the diagnosis of this disorder prenatally. *Arrows* = kidneys; *P* = renal pelvis; *Sp* = spine. (From Pretorius DH, Lee ME, Manco-Johnson ML, et al: Diagnosis of autosomal dominant polycystic kidney disease in utero and in the young infant. J Ultrasound Med 1987; 6:249. Used by permission.)

TABLE 12–11.

Syndromes Associated With Cystic Kidneys*

Syndrome	Inheritance	Kidney Involvement
Meckel syndrome	ar	(Nearly) always
Asphyxiating thoracic dystrophy	ar	Frequent
Zellweger syndrome	ar	Frequent
Chromosomal disorders (different)	—	35%
VATER association	nh(ar)	50%
Ehlers-Danlos syndromes	different	More frequent
Prune-belly syndrome	(ar)	Frequent
Dandy-Walker syndrome	(ar)	Single cases
Oral-facial-digital syndrome I	X-linked dominant	Single cases
Laurence-Moon-Bardet-Biedl syndrome	ar	More frequent
Short rib-polydactyly syndrome		
Type 1: Saldino-Noonan	ar	?
Type 2: Majewski	ar	−20%
Type 3:	ar	?
Kaufman-McKusick syndrome	ar	Frequent
Hypothalamic hamartoma syndrome	nh?	Frequent
Lissencephaly syndrome	?	Single cases?
Tuberous sclerosis	ad	Rare
v.Hippel-Lindau syndrome	ad	More frequent
Retina-renal dysplasia syndromes	ar	Always
Ivemark's syndrome	ar	Always
Branchio-oto-renal syndrome	ad	Frequent
Robert's syndrome	ar	Rare?
Fryns syndrome	ar	More frequent
Hepatic fibrosis, polycystic kidney, colobomata, and encephalopathy syndrome	ar	Single case
Acro-renal-mandibular syndrome	ar	Rare?
Apert syndrome	ad	Single cases
Goldenhar syndrome	nh (ar) (ad?)	Single cases
DiGeorge	nh (ar?) (ad?)	Single cases
Marden-Walker syndrome	ar?	Rare
Beckwith-Wiedemann syndrome	nh (ad?)	Rare
Congenital hemihypertrophy	nh	Rare
Smith-Lemli-Opitz syndrome	ar	Rare
Glutaric aciduria, type II	ar	Single cases?

*Modified from Zerres K, Volpel M-C, Weif H: Cystic kidneys. Genetics pathologic anatomy, clinical picture, and prenatal diagnosis. Hum Genet 1984; 68:104–135. Used by permission.
ad = autosomal dominant; ar = autosomal recessive; nh = not inheritable; ( ) = single cases; ar? = questionable recessive.

had normal blood pressure up until 4 years of age. The variability of outcome indicates that prenatal counseling will continue to be difficult.

Associated Anomalies

Autosomal dominant (adult) polycystic kidney disease has been associated primarily with cystic lesions in the liver, but cysts have also been seen in the pancreas, spleen, lungs, testes, ovaries, and epididymis. The reports of prenatal sonographic detection of this disease have not described cysts in extra-renal locations.

SYNDROMES ASSOCIATED WITH RENAL CYSTS

Renal cysts often occur as a manifestation of a variety of syndromes.[159–228] Therefore, detection of renal cysts warrants careful search for associated anomalies

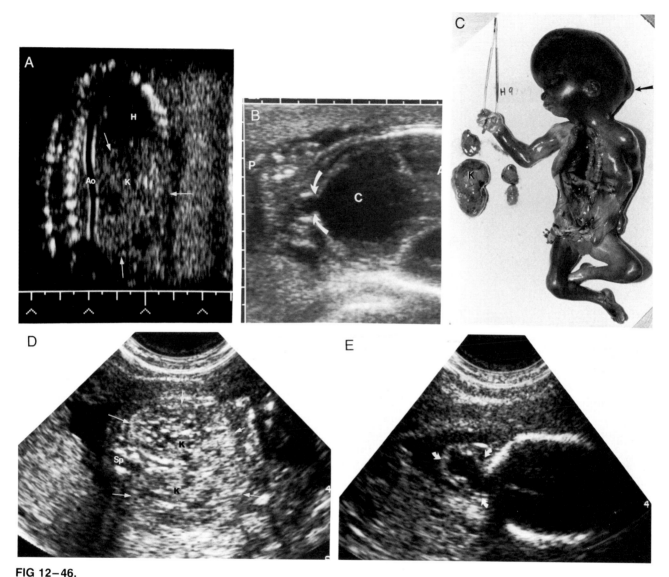

FIG 12–46.
Meckel-Gruber syndrome. **A,** parasagittal scan of the trunk shows an enlarged and echogenic kidney almost completely filling the abdomen. Severe oligohydramnios was also present. **B,** axial scan of the posterior fossa shows a small cephalocele. This fetus also had Dandy-Walker malformation. **C,** postmortem examination confirmed the prenatal findings. Polydactyly also was present. **D** and **E,** in a subsequent pregnancy, similar prenatal findings were present. The transverse scan of the fetal abdomen **(D)** shows the enlarged and echogenic kidneys with numerous small cysts. On the axial scan of the posterior fossa **(E),** an encephalocele is noted. Other scans showed a Dandy-Walker malformation and cleft lip. *K and small arrows* = echogenic kidneys containing numerous small cysts; *Ao* = aorta; *arrows* = cephalocele; *C* = posterior fossa cyst; *Sp* = spine; *P* = posterior; *A* = anterior; *H* = heart.

indicative of a syndrome, especially in the absence of urinary tract dilatation. Table 12–11 lists the causes for the overwhelming majority of fetal renal cysts.

Non–obstructive cystic renal dysplasia occurs in approximately 95% of cases with the Meckel-Gruber syndrome. This rare, lethal autosomal recessive disorder often produces enlarged, echogenic kidneys with numerous small cysts and oligohydramnios (Figs 12–46 and 12–47). Approximately 80% of cases also have an encephalocele. Other common findings include polydactyly and cleft lip and palate. The 25% re-

currence risk mandates a careful search for these findings in subsequent pregnancies. Even in the absence of familial risk, detection of cystic renal dysplasia warrants search for an encephalocele, and identification of an encephalocele calls for careful evaluation of the fetal kidneys.

Renal cortical cysts also occur in a variety of other inherited syndromes, especially autosomal recessive asphyxiating thoracic dysplasia (Jeune's syndrome), cerebro-hepatorenal (Zellweger) syndrome, and short rib-polydactyly syndrome. Asphyxiating thoracic dysplasia

FIG 12–47.
Cystic kidneys in Meckel-Gruber syndrome. Whole *(left)* and cut *(right)* autopsy specimens of a kidney affected with the Meckel-Gruber syndrome show multiple small cysts scattered throughout the entire renal parenchyma. (From Zerres K, Volpel M-C, Weib H: Cystic kidneys: Genetics, pathologic anatomy, clinical picture, and prenatal diagnosis. Hum Genet 1984; 68:104–135. Used by permission.)

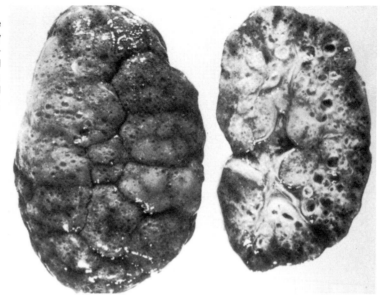

also typically produces mild to moderate rhizomelic limb shortening and a small thorax, whereas the short rib-polydactyly syndrome causes obvious micromelia, short ribs, narrow thorax, and polydactyly with frequent cardiovascular anomalies. In such cases, the associated findings dominate the sonographic picture and prognosis (see Chapter 13). In fetuses with the cerebro-hepatorenal syndrome, on the other hand, relatively subtle ultrasound findings may occur including lissencephaly, micropolygyria, hypertelorism, hepatomelay, hypotonia, and stippled epiphysis. Although these findings may be difficult to detect in the absence of familial risk, careful evaluation of fetuses at risk may detect recurrence.

Renal cysts may also occur in fetuses with serious chromosomal abnormalities. For example, approximately 33% of fetuses with trisomy 13 have renal cysts indicative of a multicystic dysplastic kidney (Fig

12–48).[160, 169] Affected fetuses also often have holoprosencephaly, intrauterine growth retardation, and extremity abnormalities (see chapters 5 and 13). Approximately 10% of fetuses with trisomy 18 also have renal cysts among other findings. Therefore, detection of renal cysts, especially in the absence of evidence for urinary tract obstruction, mandates a careful search for associated anomalies and consideration for prenatal karyotyping in fetuses with findings suggestive of trisomy.

PITFALLS AND RARE CAUSES FOR RENAL CYSTS

Several other rare conditions may produce renal cysts. A macroscopic simple renal cyst may rarely manifest antenatally as an incidental finding.[221] Other tu-

FIG 12–48.
Trisomy 13 with large echogenic cystic kidneys. Longitudinal scan of the kidney at 31 weeks shows innumerable cysts in the enlarged echogenic kidney. Other scans showed alobar holoprosencephaly, hypotelorism, and omphalocele. *K* = kidney. (From Nyberg DA, Mack LA, Bronstein A, et al: Holoprosencephaly: Prenatal sonographic diagnosis. AJR 1987; 149:151. Used by permission.)

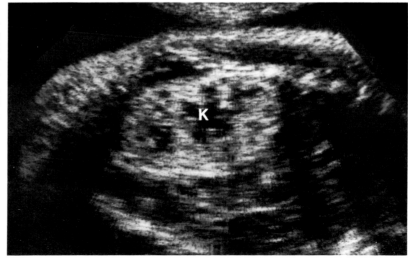

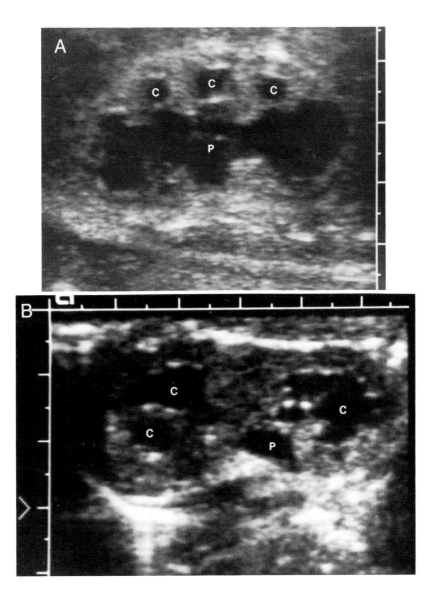

FIG 12–49.
Dilated calyces resembling cortical renal cysts. **A,** longitudinal scan of the kidney shows several fluid-filled structures apparently within the renal cortex. Slight changes in transducer angulation show these to intercommunicate with the remainder of the dilated infundibulae and pelvis, indicating that they are dilated calyces rather than cortical cysts. **B,** longitudinal scan of a fetus with stenosis of the infundibulae shows the dilated calyces aligned around the renal pelvis. Their anatomic arrangement suggests that they are dilated calyces rather than cortical cysts. *C* = dilated calyces resembling cortical cysts; *P* = renal pelvis.

FIG 12–50.

Mesoblastic nephroma is the most common congenital renal neoplasm. It is a predominantly solid hamartoma with a usually benign course. Polyhydramnios frequently occurs in association with mesoblastic nephroma. (From Mahony BS: The genitourinary system, in Callen PW (ed): *Ultrasonography in Obstetrics and Gynecology,* ed 2. Philadelphia, WB Saunders Co. 1988. Used by permission.)

MESOBLASTIC NEPHROMA WITH POLYHYDRAMNIOS

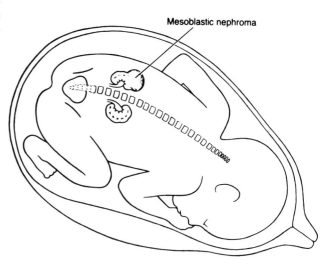

Mesoblastic nephroma

mors conceivably could resemble a renal cyst. For example, lymphangiectasis may rarely affect the kidneys. A mesoblastic nephroma typically is solid but could become necrotic with a cystic center. A fetus with severe thrombocytopenia might develop a spontaneous renal hematoma that evolves into a cystic lesion. Each of these conditions is rare.

A variety of conditions may create a false impression that renal cysts exist. A small paranephric urinoma adjacent to the renal capsule may mimic a cortical cyst, but the elliptical shape of the urinoma usually distinguishes it from a cortical cyst. This distinction is of little clinical significance, however, since most cases with a paranephric urinoma also have renal dysplasia.[57, 83] Rarely, infundibulopelvic stenosis occurs and results in isolated dilatation of the calyces, which resemble cysts (Fig 12–49).[199] Documentation that these "cysts" align in anterior and posterior rows symmetrically around the renal pelvis and are of similar sizes avoids confusion between isolated calycectasis and cortical cysts. Similarly, the medullary pyramids may appear quite hypoechoic, but their

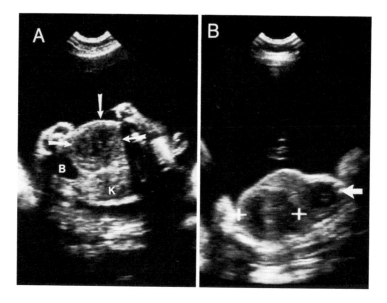

FIG 12–51.

Mesoblastic nephroma. **A,** oblique scan of the fetal abdomen at 34 weeks shows the large solid right renal mass. The left kidney is normal. Polyhydramnios is present. *Arrows* = mesoblastic nephroma; *K* = normal left kidney; *B* = bladder. **B,** parasagittal scan shows the solid right renal tumor distorting the abdominal contour and extending slightly to the left of midline. Polyhydramnios again is noted. *Calipers* = right mesoblastic nephroma; *arrow* = heart. (From Guilian BB: Prenatal ultrasonographic diagnosis of fetal renal tumors. Radiology 1984; 152:69–70. Used by permission.)

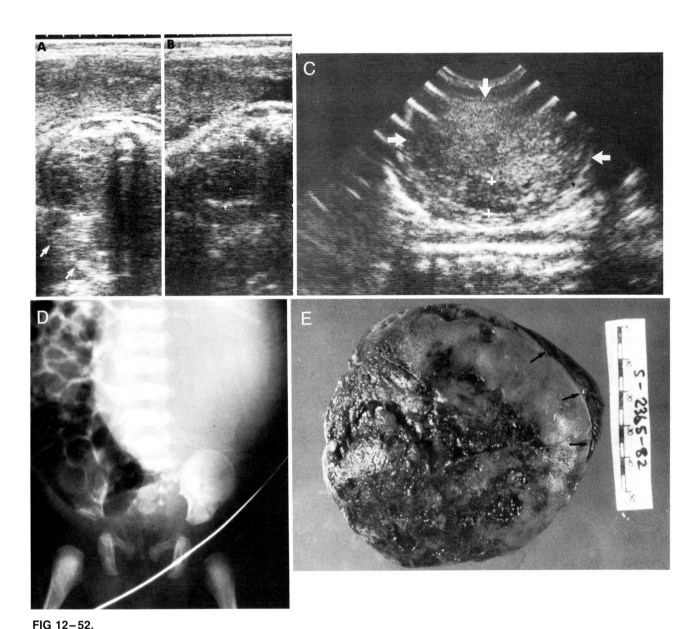

FIG 12–52.
Mesoblastic nephroma. **A** and **B,** transverse **(A)** and parasagittal **(B)** scans at the level of the left kidney at 35 weeks show a well-circumscribed 4 cm solid mass. *Graticles* + = solid renal mass; *arrows* = anterior abdominal wall. **C,** postnatal left parasagittal sonogram demonstrates a 7-cm solid mass with residual renal parenchyma posteriorly. *Arrows* = mass; *graticles* = residual renal parenchyma. **D,** postnatal supine radiograph shows the large left-sided abdominal mass displacing bowel to the right. **E,** cut nephrectomy section illustrates the solid mesoblastic nephroma almost completely replacing renal tissue. The tumor contains numerous areas of hemorrhagic necrosis. *Arrows* = rim of remaining renal tissue. (From Ehman RL, Nicholson SF, Mackin GA: Prenatal sonographic detection of congenital mesoblastic nephroma in a monozygotic twin pregnancy. J Ultrasound Med 1983; 2:555–557. Used by permission.)

symmetric size and orientation surrounding the renal pelvis should produce little confusion.

MESOBLASTIC NEPHROMA AND OTHER RARE RENAL TUMORS

Clinical and Pathologic Findings

Tumors of the fetal kidneys rarely occur, and most fetal renal neoplasms are mesoblastic nephroma.[229-231] A mesoblastic nephroma is a solitary hamartoma. Curative therapy usually consists of nephrectomy postnatally, although rare reports exist of recurrence after nephrectomy. Wilms' tumor or other renal tumors are exceedingly rare in the fetus and neonate. However, focal renal dysplasia may produce a focal area of increased renal echogenicity which grows at a faster rate than the remainder of the kidney and mimics a solid neoplasm.[232, 233]

Sonographic Findings

Mesoblastic nephroma produces a large, solitary, predominantly solid mass arising from the kidney (Figs 12–50 to 12–52).[229-231] The adjacent kidney is normal, but the mesoblastic nephroma does not have a well-defined capsule. Polyhydramnios frequently occurs in association with mesoblastic nephroma. The

reason for this association remains unclear, but detection of a predominantly solid fetal renal mass in the presence of polyhydramnios provides convincing evidence for a mesoblastic nephroma. Differentiation between a solid renal neoplasm and focal renal dysplasia may be very difficult without postnatal renal biopsy, unless a dilated ureter can be traced from the segmental renal dysplasia.[232, 233]

ADRENAL NEUROBLASTOMA

Clinical and Pathologic Findings

Adrenal neuroblastoma is the most common neonatal abdominal tumor and accounts for 12%–25% of all perinatal neoplasms.[235, 241, 244, 246, 247, 251] The incidence varies from 1 in 7,100 to 1 in 10,000 live births. Adrenal neuroblastoma usually is unilateral, and 50% of affected neonates have metastasis. The most common sites for metastasis prenatally include the liver, subcutaneous tissue, and placenta.[234, 238]

Sonographic Findings

The normal adrenal gland appears as a disc-shaped hypoechoic structure superior to the kidneys.[243] It has a hyperechoic border and a central hyperechoic line and may be seen as early as 9–10 weeks. Adrenal neuro-

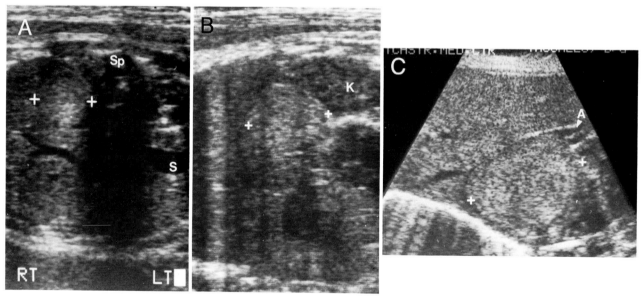

FIG 12–53.
Neuroblastoma. **A,** transverse scan of the upper abdomen at 35 weeks shows an echogenic solid mass in the right upper quadrant of the abdomen. **B,** parasagittal scan of the right upper quadrant demonstrates the echogenic mass to be superior to and separate from the compressed right kidney. **C,** postnatal right parasagittal scan shows the solid adrenal mass with a small amount of residual normal adrenal tissue. *Graticules* = neuroblastoma; *K* = kidney; *A* = adrenal; *Sp* = spine; *S* = stomach; *Rt* = right; *Lt* = left. (From Ferraro EM, Fakhry J, Aruny JE, et al: Prenatal adrenal neuroblastoma: Case report with review of the literature. J Ultrasound Med 1988; 7:275–278. Used by permission.)

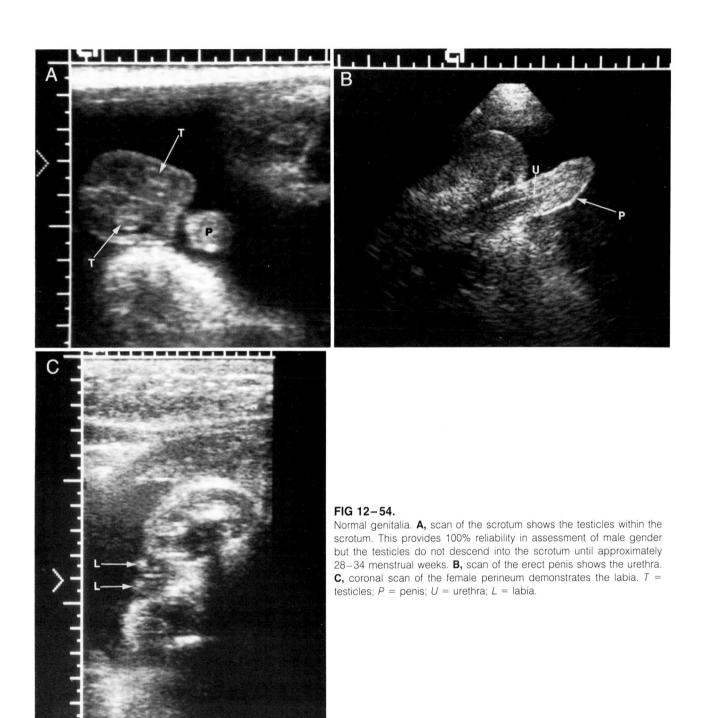

FIG 12–54.
Normal genitalia. **A,** scan of the scrotum shows the testicles within the scrotum. This provides 100% reliability in assessment of male gender but the testicles do not descend into the scrotum until approximately 28–34 menstrual weeks. **B,** scan of the erect penis shows the urethra. **C,** coronal scan of the female perineum demonstrates the labia. *T* = testicles; *P* = penis; *U* = urethra; *L* = labia.

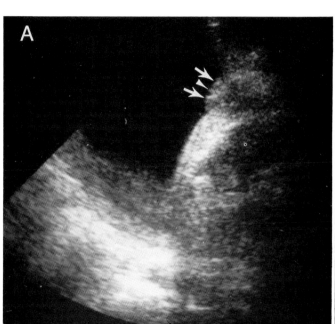

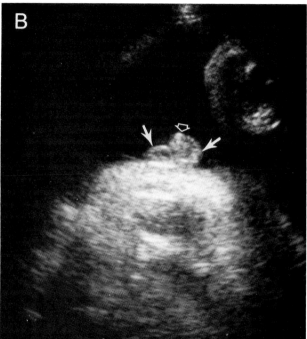

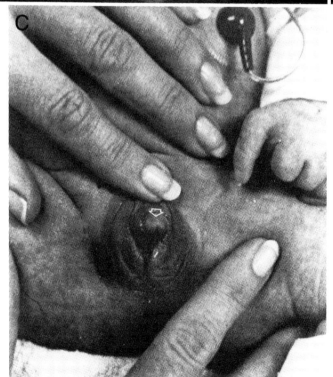

FIG 12–55.
Ambiguous genitalia, 34 weeks. **A,** scan of the fetal perineum shows a small midline cleft separating two rounded structures. This appearance suggests either labia majora or scrotal sacs. No testicles are evident. **B,** scan obtained at a slightly more cephalad level displays a small midline structure projecting between the two rounded structures. **C,** postnatal photograph shows the cleft empty scrotal sac and hypospadius resembling labia with clitoral enlargement. This is a genotypic male. *Arrowhead* = small midline cleft; *solid arrows* = empty scrotal sacs; *open arrow* = small penis. (From Cooper C, Mahony BS, Bowie JD, et al: Prenatal ultrasound diagnosis of ambiguous genitalia. J Ultrasound Med 1985; 4:433. Used by permission.)

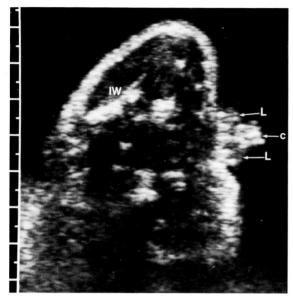

FIG 12–56.
Ambiguous genitalia, enlarged clitoris. Scan of the fetal perineum shows a prominent clitoris projecting between the labia. Differentiation between a prominent clitoris and a relatively small penis may be very subtle. *C* = clitoris; *L* = labia; *IW* = iliac wing. (Courtesy of Frederick N Hegge, MD, Emanuel Hospital, Portland, OR.)

blastoma produces a retroperitoneal mass separate from the liver and superior to the kidney (Fig 12–53). The mass often is hyperechoic but may have a mixed echotexture with solid and cystic components.[238–240, 242] Hepatic or placental metastasis may occur.[234, 238] Distinction between a neuroblastoma and an adrenal hem-

orrhage may be very difficult unless follow-up examination shows liquefaction of the adrenal mass; however, fetal adrenal hemorrhage is rare. Intra-abdominal pulmonary sequestration should also be considered (see Chapter 8).

Occasionally, maternal symptoms secondary to in-

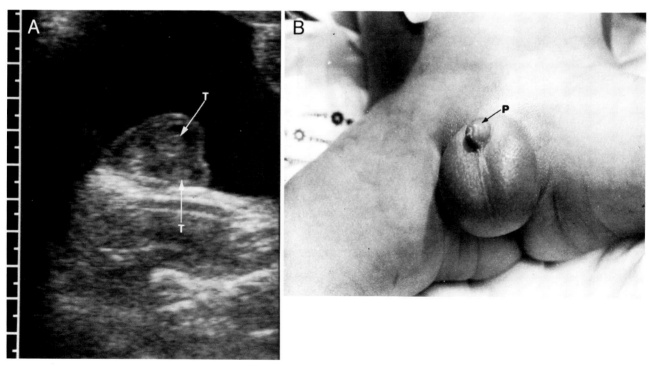

FIG 12–57.
Ambiguous genitalia, micropenis. **A,** scan of the fetal perineum shows the scrotum containing testicles. No penis was identified prenatally, and fetal urination was visualized coming from the superior region of the scrotum. Documentation of the testicles within the scrotum confirmed male gender, even though a penis was not visualized. **B,** postnatal photograph shows the normal scrotum but small penis. *T* = testicles; *P* = penis.

creased catecholamines produced by disseminated neuroblastoma and crossing the placenta into the maternal circulation herald the presence of the neuroblastoma.[234, 245, 248, 249] Affected pregnancies often have maternal tachycardia and nausea and vomiting during the third trimester in association with non–immune hydrops fetalis.

FETAL GENDER

Clinical and Pathologic Findings

Attempts to document fetal gender serve numerous important purposes. Careful analysis of the fetal perineum may detect ambiguous genitalia.[253] Cases with discrepant sonographic and amniocentesis data regarding fetal sex may indicate the presence of an intersex state such as testicular feminization with male karyotype but female external genitalia.[255] In twin pregnancies, documentation of different genders permits accurate assessment of dizygoticity and confirms that both sacs have been sampled in amniocenteses. Among fetuses at risk for severe X-linked disorders, identification of a female fetus excludes the possibility of the disorder. For each of these reasons and because of the parents' frequent desire to know the fetal sex prenatally, the sonologist should be familiar with the accuracy and limitations of sonographic assessment of fetal sex.[254]

Sonographic Findings

The testicles normally descend into the scrotum between 28 and 34 menstrual weeks.[252] Documentation of the testicles within the scrotum provides 100% reliability in gender assessment (Fig 12–54). Other means of assessing fetal gender are less accurate. Inopportune fetal positioning precludes perineal visualization in approximately 30% of fetuses, dependent upon gestational age.[252, 254] Ultrasonography incorrectly assigns fetal gender in approximately 3% of cases, even after adequate perineal visualization. In a review by Elejalde et al., genitalia were not seen in 1,223 of 3,891 (31.4%) cases, and gender was incorrectly assigned in 113 of 3,891 (2.9%) cases.[254] Among the 113 fetuses whose gender was incorrectly assigned, 39 (34.5%) were male and 74 (65.5%) female.[254]

Accurate sonographic assessment of fetal gender requires unequivocal distinction between the labia and scrotum (see Fig 12–54). Although identification of a penis provides evidence suggestive of a male fetus, lack of penile visualization should not alter the assessment when testicles are seen within the scrotum. Further-

more, the clitoris may be quite prominent or the penis quite small resulting in errors in gender assessment. However, based upon visualization of the fetal perineum, the diagnosis of ambiguous genitalia can be made prenatally (Figs 12–55 to 12–57).[253]

SUMMARY

Congenital malformations of the urinary tract occur with high frequency. The sonographer plays a crucial role in the evaluation of the fetal urinary tract and detects a variety of abnormalities that dramatically change obstetric and perinatal management. Detection, localization, and characterization of anomalies provide useful prognostic information to optimize perinatal management.

REFERENCES

Introduction/Overview

1. Grannum, P, Bracken M, Silverman R, et al: Assessment of fetal kidney size in normal gestation by comparison of ratio of kidney circumference to abdominal circumference. Am J Obstet Gynecol 1980; 136:249–254.
2. Grignon A, Filiatrault D, Homsy Y, et al: Ureteropelvic junction stenosis: Antenatal ultrasonographic diagnosis, postnatal investigation, and follow-up. Radiology 1986; 160:649–651.
3. Hadlock FP, Deter RL, Carpenter R, et al: Sonography of fetal urinary tract anomalies. AJR 1981; 137:261–267.
4. King LR, Coughlin PWF, Bloch EC, et al: The case for immediate pyeloplasty in the neonate with ureteropelvic junction obstruction. J Urol 1984; 132:725–728.
5. Lawson TL, Foley WD, Berland LL, et al: Ultrasonic evaluation of fetal kidneys: Analysis of normal size and frequency of visualization as related to stage of pregnancy. Radiology 1981; 138:153–156.
6. Leopold GR: Antepartum obstetric ultrasound examination guidelines. J Ultrasound Med 1986; 5:241–242.
7. Mandell J, Kinard HW, Middlestaedt CA, et al: Prenatal diagnosis of unilateral hydronephrosis with early postnatal reconstruction. J Urol 1984; 132:303–307.
8. Schwoebel MG, Sacher P, Bucher HU, et al: Prenatal diagnosis improves the prognosis in children with obstructive uropathy. J Pediatr Surg 1984; 19:187–190.
9. Spirnak JP, Mahoney S, Resnick MI, et al: Incidental fetal hydronephrosis: Clinical implication. Urology 1984; 24:105–108.
10. Thorup J, Mortensen T, Diemer H, et al: The prognosis of surgically treated congenital hydronephrosis after diagnosis in utero. J Urol 1985; 134:914–917.

Normal Development

11. Bertagnoli L, Lalatta F, Gallicchio MD, et al: Quantitative characterization of the growth of the fetal kidney. J Clin Ultrasound 1983; 11:349–356.

12. Bowie JD, Rosenberg ER, Andreotti MD, et al: The changing sonographic appearance of fetal kidneys during pregnancy. J Ultrasound Med 1983; 2:505–507.

13. Campbell S, Wladimiroff JW, Dewhurst CJ: The antenatal measurement of fetal urine production. Br J Obstet Gynaecol 1973; 80:680–686.

14. Jeanty P, Dramaix-Wilmet M, Elkhazen N: Measurement of fetal kidney growth on ultrasound. Radiology 1982; 144:159–162.

15. Mellins HZ: Cystic dilatations of the upper urinary tract: A radiologist's developmental model. Radiology 1984; 153:291–301.

16. Moore KL: The urogenital system, in *The Developing Human: Clinically Oriented Embryology,* ed. 4. Philadelphia, WB Saunders Co, 1988, pp 246–285.

17. Wladimiroff JW, Campbell S: Fetal urine-production rates in normal and complicated pregnancy. Lancet 1974; 1:151–154.

The Sonographic Approach to Urinary Tract Abnormalities

18. Arger PH, Coleman BG, Mintz MC, et al: Routine fetal genitourinary tract screening. Radiology 1985; 156:485–489.

19. Barss VA, Benacerraf BR, Frigoletto FD: Second trimester oligohydramnios, a predictor of poor fetal outcome. Obstet Gynecol 1984; 64:608–610.

20. Blane CE, Koff SA, Baverman RA, et al: Non–obstructive hydronephrosis: Sonographic recognition and therapeutic implications. Radiology 1983; 147:95–99.

21. Crombleholme TM, Harrison MR, Langer JC, et al: Early experience with open fetal surgery for congenital hydronephrosis. J Pediatr Surg 1988; 23:1114–1121.

22. Davis GH, Wapner RJ, Kurtz AB, et al: Antenatal diagnosis of hydrometrocolpos by ultrasound examination. J Ultrasound Med 1984; 3:371–374.

23. Glick PL, Harrison MR, Golbus MS, et al: Management of the fetus with congenital hydronephrosis. II: Prognostic criteria and selection for treatment. J Pediatr Surg 1985; 20:376–387.

24. Grannum PA, Ghidini A, Scioscia AL: The assessment of fetal renal reserve in low level obstructive uropathy. Lancet, submitted for publication.

25. Grignon A, Filion R, Filiatrault D, et al: Urinary tract dilatation in utero: Classification and clinical applications. Radiology 1986; 160:645–647.

26. Harrison MR, Golbus MS, Filly FA, et al: Fetal surgery for congenital hydronephrosis. N Engl J Med 1982; 306:591–593.

27. Hellstrom WJG, Kogan BA, Jeffrey RB, et al: The natural history of prenatal hydronephrosis with normal amounts of amniotic fluid. J Urol 1984; 132:947–950.

28. Hill SJ, Hirsch JH: Sonographic detection of fetal hydrometrocolpos. J Ultrasound Med 1985; 4:323–325.

29. Hoddick WK, Filly RA, Mahony BS, et al: Minimal fetal renal pyelectasis. J Ultrasound Med 1985; 4:85–89.

30. International Fetal Registry.

31. Laing FC, Burke VD, Wing VW, et al: Postpartum evaluation of fetal hydronephrosis: Optimal timing for follow-up sonography. Radiology 1984; 152:423–424.

32. Ray D, Berger N, Ensor R: Hydramnios in association with unilateral fetal hydronephrosis. J Clin Ultrasound 1982; 10:82–84.

33. Reuter KL, Lebowitz RL: Massive vesicoureteral reflux mimicking posterior urethral valves in a fetus. J Clin Ultrasound 1985; 13:584–587.

34. Russ PD, Zavitz WR, Pretorius DH, et al: Hydrometrocolpos, uterus didelphys, and septate vagina: An antenatal sonographic diagnosis. J Ultrasound Med 1986; 5:211–213.

Renal Agenesis

35. Alcorn D, Adamson TM, Lambert TF, et al: Morphological effects of chronic tracheal ligation and drainage in the fetal lamb lung. J Anat 1977; 123:649–660.

36. Austin CW, Brown JM, Friday RO: Unilateral renal agenesis presenting as a pseudomass in utero. J Ultrasound Med 1984; 3:177–179.

37. Campbell S: The antenatal detection of fetal abnormality by ultrasonic diagnosis, in *Birth Defects* [Proceedings]. Vienna, IV International Conference, 1973.

38. Carter CO, Evans K: Birth frequency of bilateral renal agenesis. J Med Genet 1981; 18:158.

39. Dubbins PA, Kurtz AB, Wapner RJ, et al: Renal agenesis: Spectrum of in utero findings. J Clin Ultrasound 1981; 9:189–193.

40. Goldenberg RL, Davis RO, Brumfield CG: Transient fetal anuria of unknown etiology: A case report. Am J Obstet Gynecol 1984; 149:87.

41. Harman CR: Maternal furosemide may not provoke urine production in the compromised fetus. Am J Obstet Gynecol 1984; 150:322–323.

42. McPherson E, Carey J, Kramer A, et al: Dominantly inherited renal adysplasia. Am J Med Genet 1987; 26:863–872.

43. Potter EL. Bilateral absence of ureters and kidneys: A report of 50 cases. Obstet Gynecol 1965; 25:3–12.

44. Romero R, Cullen M, Grannum P, et al: Antenatal diagnosis of renal anomalies with ultrasound. III: Bilateral renal agenesis. Am J Obstet Gynecol 1985; 151:38–43.

45. Roodhooft AM, Birnholz JC, Holmes LB: Familial nature of congenital absence and severe dysplasia of both kidneys. N Engl J Med 1984; 310:1341–1345.

46. Rosenberg ER, Bowie JD: Failure of furosemide to induce diuresis in a growth-retarded fetus. AJR 1984; 142:485–486.

47. Schmidt W, Kubli F: Early diagnosis of severe congenital malformations by ultrasonography. J Perinat Med 1982; 10:233–241.
48. Thomas IT, Smith DW: Oligohydramnios: Cause of the non–renal features of Potter's syndrome, including pulmonary hypoplasia. J Pediatr 1974; 84:811–814.
49. Wilson RD, Baird PA: Renal agenesis in British Columbia. Am J Med Genet 1985; 21:153–169.
50. Wladimiroff JW: Effect of furosemide on fetal urine production. Br J Obstet Gynaecol 1975; 82:221–224.

Renal Ectopia

51. Greenblatt AM, Beretsky I, Lankin DH, et al: In utero diagnosis of crossed renal ectopia using high-resolution real-time ultrasound. J Ultrasound Med 1985; 4:105–107.
52. Hill LM, Peterson CS: Antenatal diagnosis of fetal pelvic kidneys. J Ultrasound Med 1987; 6:393–396.

Ureteropelvic Junction Obstruction

53. Ahmed S, Savage JP: Surgery of pelviureteric obstruction in the first year of life. Aust NZ J Surg 1985; 55:253–261.
54. Antonakopoulos GN, Fuggle WJ, Newman J, et al: Idiopathic hydronephrosis. Arch Pathol Lab Med 1985; 109:1097–1101.
55. Atwell JD: Familial pelviureteric junction hydronephrosis and its association with a duplex pelvicaliceal system and vesicoureteric reflux. A family study. Br J Urol 1985; 57:365–369.
56. Buscemi M, Shanske A, Mallet E, et al: Dominantly inherited ureteropelvic junction obstruction. Urology 1985; 24:568–571.
57. Callen PW, Bolding D, Filly RA, et al: Ultrasonographic evaluation of fetal paranephric pseudocysts. J Ultrasound Med 1983; 2:309–312.
58. Drake DP, Stevens PS, Eckstein HB: Hydronephrosis secondary to ureteropelvic obstruction in children: A review of 14 years of experience. J Urol 1978; 119:649–651.
59. Guys JM, Borella F, Monfort G: Ureteropelvic junction obstructions: Prenatal diagnosis and neonatal surgery in 47 cases. J Pediatr Surg 1988; 23:156–158.
60. Hanna MK, Jeffs RD, Sturgess JM, et al: Ureteral structure and ultrastructure. Part II: Congenital ureteropelvic junction obstruction and primary obstructive megaureter. J Urol 1976; 116:725–730.
61. Jaffe R, Abramowicz J, Fejgin M, et al: Giant fetal abdominal cyst: Ultrasonic diagnosis and management. J Ultrasound Med 1987; 6:45–47.
62. Johnston JH, Evans JP, Glassberg KI, et al: Pelvic hydronephrosis in children: A review of 219 personal cases. J Urol 1977; 117:97–101.
63. Kleiner B, Callen PW, Filly RA: Sonographic analysis of

the fetus with ureteropelvic junction obstruction. AJR 1987; 148:359–363.
64. Lebowitz RL, Griscom NT: Neonatal hydronephrosis: 147 cases. Radiol Clin N Am 1977; 15:49–59.
65. Raffle RB: Familial hydronephrosis. Br Med J 1955; 1:580.
66. Snyder HM, Lebowitz RL, Colodny AH, et al: Ureteropelvic junction obstruction in children. Urol Clin N Am 1980; 7:273–290.

Ureterovesical Obstruction and Megaureter

67. Dwoskin JY: Siblins uropathology. J Urol 1976; 115:726–727.
68. Gosling JA, Dixon JS: Functional obstruction of the ureter and renal pelvis. A histological and electron microscopic study. Br J Urol 1978; 50:145–152.
69. Hanna MK, Jeffs RD: Primary obstructive megaureter in children. Urology 1975; 6:419–427.
70. Jeffrey RB, Laing FC, Wing VW, et al: Sonography of the fetal duplex kidney. Radiology 1984; 153:123–124.
71. Jerkins GR, Noe HN: Familial vesicoureteral reflux: A prospective study. J Urol 1982; 128:774–778.
72. Mebust WK, Forest JD: Vesicoureteral reflux in identical twins. J Urol 1972; 108:635–636.
73. Mogg RA: Familial and adult reflux. Birth Defects 1977; 8:365–366.
74. Montana MA, Cyr DR, Lenke RR, et al: Sonographic detection of fetal ureteral obstruction. AJR 1985; 145:595–596.
75. Nussbaum AR, Dorst JP, Jeffs RD, et al: Ectopic ureter and ureterocele: Their varied sonographic manifestations. Radiology 1986; 159:227–235.
76. Sant GR, Barbalias GA, Klauber GT: Congenital ureteral valves—An abnormality of ureteral embryogenesis. J Urol 1985; 133:427–431.
77. Stevens FD, Joske RA, Simmons RT: Megaureter with vesicoureteric reflux in twins. Aust NZ J Surg 1955; 24:192.
78. Swenson O, MacMahon E, Jaques WE, et al: A new concept of the etiology of megaloureters. N Engl J Med 1952; 246:41.
79. Tokunaka S, Koyanagi T: Morphologic study of primary nonreflux megaureters with particular emphasis on the role of urethral sheath and ureteral dysplasia. J Urol 1982; 128:399–402.
80. Tokunaka S, Koyanagi T, Tsuji I: Two infantile cases of primary megaloureter with uncommon pathological findings: Ultrastructural study and its clinical implication. J Urol 1980; 123:214–217.
81. Val Dunn V, Glasier CM: Ultrasonographic antenatal demonstration of primary megaureters. J Ultrasound Med 1985; 4:101–103.
82. Wood BP, Ben-Ami T, Teele RL, et al: Ureterovesicle obstruction and megaloureter: Diagnosis by real-time ultrasound. Radiology 1985; 156:79–81.

Distal Urinary Tract Obstruction and Megacystis

83. Avni EF, Thoua Y, Van Gansbeke, et al: Development of the hypodysplastic kidney: Contribution of antenatal US diagnosis. Radiology 1987; 164:123–125.

84. Beck AD: The effect of intrauterine urinary obstruction upon the development of the fetal kidney. J Urol 1971; 105:784–789.

85. Doraiswamy NV, Al Badr MSK: Posterior urethral valves in siblings. Br J Urol 1983; 55:448–449.

86. Fernbach SK, Maizels M: Posterior urethral valves causing urinary retention in an infant with duplication of the urethra. J Urol 1984; 132:353–355.

87. Glazer GM, Filly RA, Callen PW: The varied sonographic appearance of the urinary tract in the fetus and newborn with urethral obstruction. Radiology 1982; 144:563–568.

88. Glick PL, Harrison MR, Adzick NS, et al: Correction of congenital hydronephrosis in utero. IV: In utero decompression prevents renal dysplasia. J Pediatr Surg 1984; 19:649–657.

89. Greenfield SP, Hensle TW, Berdon WE: Urinary extravasation in the newborn male with posterior urethral valves. J Pediatr Surg 1982; 17:751–756.

90. Henneberry MO, Stephens FD: Renal hypoplasia and dysplasia in infants with posterior urethral valves. J Urol 1980; 123:912–915.

91. Johnston JH: Vesicoureteric reflux with urethral valves. Br J Urol 1979; 51:100–104.

92. Kjellberg SR, Ericsson NO, Rudhe U: Urethral valves, in *The Lower Urinary Tract in Childhood. Some Correlated Clinical and Roentgenologic Observations.* Stockholm, Almqvist & Wiksell, 1957, pp 203–254.

93. Krueger RP, Churchill BM: Megalourethra with posterior urethral valves. Urology 1981; 18:279–281.

94. Krueger RP, Hardy BE, Churchill BM: Cryptorchidism in boys with posterior urethral valves. J Urol 1980; 124:101–102.

95. Lorenzo RL, Turner WR, Bradford BF, et al: Duplication of the male urethra with posterior urethral valves. Pediatr Radiol 1981; 11:39–41.

96. Mahony BS, Callen PW, Filly RA: Fetal urethral obstruction: US evaluation. Radiology 1985; 157:221–224.

97. Manco LH, Osterdahl P: The antenatal sonographic features of megacystismicrocolon-intestinal hypoperistalsis syndrome. J Clin Ultrasound 1984; 12:595–598.

98. Meizner I, Bar-Ziv J, Katz M: Prenatal ultrasonic diagnosis of the extreme form of prune belly syndrome. J Clin Ultrasound 1985; 13:581–583.

99. Nelson LH, Reiff RH: Megacystis-microcolon-intestinal hypoperistalsis syndrome and anechoic areas in the fetal abdomen. Am J Obstet Gynecol 1982; 144:464–467.

100. Nicolaides KH, Rodeck CH, Gosden CM: Rapid karyotyping in non–lethal fetal malformations. Lancet 1986; 1:283–288.

101. Schwartz RD, Stephens FD, Cussen LJ: The pathogenesis of renal dysplasia. II: The significance of lateral and medial ectopy of the ureteric orifice. III: Complete and incomplete urinary obstruction. Invest Urol 1981; 19:97–103.

102. Vezina WC, Morin FR, Winsberg R: Megacystic-microcolon-intestinal hypoperistalsis syndrome: Antenatal ultrasound appearance. Am J Roentgenol 1979; 133:749–750.

103. Vintzileos AM, Eisenfeld LI, Herson VC, et al: Megacystis-microcolon-intestinal hypoperistalsis syndrome: Prenatal sonographic findings and review of the literature. Am J Perinatol 1986; 3:297–302.

104. Warshaw BL, Hymes LC, Trulock TS, et al: Prognostic features in infants with obstructive uropathy due to posterior urethral valves. J Urol 1985; 133:240–243.

105. Young HH, Frontz WA, Baldwin JC: Congenital obstruction of the posterior urethra. J Urol 1919; 3:289.

Bladder or Cloacal Exstrophy and Persistent Cloaca

106. Meizner I, Bar-Ziv J: In utero prenatal ultrasonic diagnosis of a rare case of cloacal exstrophy. J Clin Ultrasound 1985; 13:500–502.

107. Mirk P, Calisti A, Fileni A: Prenatal sonographic diagnosis of bladder extrophy. J Ultrasound Med 1986; 5:291–293.

Renal Cysts

108. Bernstein J: The morphogenesis of renal parenchymal maldevelopment (renal dysplasia). Pediatr Clin N Am 1971; 18:395–407.

109. Bernstein J: A classification of renal cysts, in Gardner KD Jr (ed): *Cystic Diseases of the Kidney.* New York, John Wiley & Sons, 1976, pp 7–30.

110. Fong KW, Rohmani MR, Rose TH, et al: Fetal renal cystic disease. AJR 1986; 146:767–773.

111. Kissane JM: The morphology of renal cystic disease, in Gardner KD Jr (ed): *Cystic Diseases of the Kidney.* New York, John Wiley & Sons, 1976, pp 31–63.

112. Madewell JE, Hartman DS, Lichtenstein JE: Radiologic-pathologic correlations in cystic disease of the kidney. Radiol Clin N Am 1979; 17:261–279.

113. Resnik J, Vernier RL: Cystic disease of the kidney in the newborn infant. Clin Perinatol 1981; 8:375–390.

114. Risdon RA: Renal dysplasia. J Clin Path 1971; 24:57–71.

115. Zerres K: Genetics of cystic kidney disease. Criteria for classification and genetic counseling. Pediatr Nephrol 1987; 1:397–404.

Cystic Renal Dysplasia

116. Beck D: The effect of intra-uterine urinary obstruction upon the development of the fetal kidney. J Urol 1971; 105:784–789.

117. Bernstein J: Renal hypoplasia and dysplasia, in Edel-

mann CM (ed): *Pediatric Kidney Disease,* vol II. Boston, Little, Brown & Co, 1978, pp 547–554.

118. Glick PL, Harrison MR, Adzick NS, et al: Correction of congenital hydronephrosis in utero. IV: In utero decompression prevents renal dysplasia. J Pediatr Surg 1984; 19:649–657.

119. Glick PL, Harrison MR, Noall RA, et al: Correction of congenital hydronephrosis in utero. III: Early midtrimester ureteral obstruction produces renal dysplasia. J Pediatr Surg 1983; 18:681–687.

120. Henneberry MO, Stephens FD: Renal hypoplasia and dysplasia in infants with posterior urethral valves. J Urol 1980; 123:912–915.

121. Mahony BS, Filly RA, Callen PW: Fetal renal dysplasia: Sonographic evaluation. Radiology 1984; 152:143–146.

122. Schwarz RD, Stephens FD, Cussen LJ: The pathogenesis of renal dysplasia. I: Quantification of hypoplasia and dysplasia. Invest Urol 1981; 19:94–97.

Multicystic Dysplastic Kidney Disease

123. Bearman DB, Hine PL, Sanders RC: Multicystic kidney: A sonographic pattern. Radiology 1976; 118:685–688.

124. D'Alton M, Romero R, Grannum P, et al: Antenatal diagnosis of renal anomalies with ultrasound. IV: Bilateral multicystic kidney disease. Am J Obstet Gynecol 1986; 54:532–537.

125. Diard F, LeDosseur P, Cadier L, et al: Multicystic dysplasia in the upper component of the complete duplex kidney. Pediatr Radiol 1984; 14:310–313.

126. Felson B, Cussen LJ: The hydronephrotic type of unilateral congenital multicystic disease of the kidney. Semin Roentgenol 1975; 10:113–123.

127. Greene LF, Feinzaig W, Dahlin DC: Multicystic dysplasia of the kidney: With special reference to the contralateral kidney. J Urol 1971; 103:482–487.

128. Hashimoto BE, Filly RA, Callen PW: Multicystic dysplastic kidney in utero: Changing appearance on US. Radiology 1986; 159:107–110.

129. Kleiner B, Filly RA, Mack L, et al: Multicystic dysplastic kidney: Observations of contralateral disease in the fetal population. Radiology 1986; 161:27–29.

130. Mackie GG, Stephens FD: Duplex kidneys: A correlation of renal dysplasia with position of the ureteral orifice. J Urol 1975; 114:274–280.

131. Newman LB, McAllister WH, Kissane J: Segmental renal dysplasia associated with ectopic ureteroceles in childhood. Urology 1974; 3:23–26.

132. Pedicelli G, Jequier S, Bowen A, et al: Multicystic dysplastic kidneys: Spontaneous regression demonstrated with US. Radiology 1986; 160:23–26.

133. Potter EL. Type II cystic kidney: Early ampullary inhibition, in *Normal and Abnormal Development of the Kidney.* Chicago, Year Book Medical Publishers, Inc, 1972, pp 154–181.

134. Sanders RC, Hartman DS: The sonographic distinction between neonatal multicystic kidney and hydronephrosis. Radiology 1984; 151:621–625.

135. Stuck KJ, Koff SA, Silver TM: Ultrasonic features of multicystic dysplastic kidney: Expanded criteria. Radiology 1982; 143:217–221.

Autosomal Recessive (Infantile) Polycystic Kidney Disease

136. Blyth H, Ockenden BG: Polycystic disease of kidneys and liver presenting in childhood. J Med Genet 1971; 8:257–284.

137. Bosniak MA, Ambos MA: Polycystic kidney disease. Semin Roentgenol 1975; 10:133–143.

138. Chilton SJ, Cremin BJ: The spectrum of polycystic disease in children. Pediatr Radiol 1981; 11:9–15.

139. Luthy DA, Hirsch JH: Infantile polycystic kidney disease: Observations from attempts at prenatal diagnosis. Am J Med Genet 1985; 20:505–517.

140. Mahony BS, Callen PW, Filly RA, et al: Progression of infantile polycystic kidney disease in early pregnancy. J Ultrasound Med 1984; 3:277–279.

141. Potter EL: Type I cystic kidney: Tubular gigantism, in *Normal and Abnormal Development of the Kidney.* Chicago, Year Book Medical Publishers, Inc, 1972, pp 141–153.

142. Romero R, Cullen M, Jeanty P, et al: The diagnosis of congenital renal anomalies with ultrasound. II: Infantile polycustic kidney disease. Am J Obstet Gynecol 1984; 150:259–262.

143. Simpson JL, Sabbagha RE, Elias S, et al: Failure to detect polycystic kidneys in utero by second trimester ultrasonography. Human Genetics 1982; 60:295.

144. Spence HM, Singleton R: Cysts and cystic disorders of the kidney: Types, diagnosis, treatment. Urol Surv 1972; 22:131.

145. Stapleton FB, Hilton S, Wilcox J: Transient nephromegaly simulating infantile polycystic disease of the kidneys. Pediatrics 1981; 67:554–559.

146. Vinaixa F, Gotzens VJ, Tejedo-Mateu A: Tubular gigantism of the kidney in a 41 mm, Streeter's 23rd horizon, human fetus with a comparative study of renal structures in normal human fetuses at a similar stage of development. Eur Urol 1984; 10:331–335.

Autosomal Dominant (Adult) Polycystic Kidney Disease

147. Dalgaard OZ: Bilateral polycystic disease of the kidney: A follow-up of two hundred eighty-four patients and their families. Acta Med Scand [Suppl] 1957; 328.

148. Eulderink F, Hogewind BL: Renal cysts in premature children. Arch Pathol Lab Med 1978; 102:592–595.

149. Fellows RA, Leonidas JC, Beatty EC Jr: Radiologic features of "adult type" polycystic kidney disease in the neonate. Pediat Radiol 1976; 4:87–92.

150. Kaye C, Lewy PR: Congenital appearance of adult-type

(autosomal dominant) polycystic kidney disease. J Pediatr 1974; 85:807–810.

151. Loh JP, Haller JO, Kassner EG, et al: Dominantly inherited polycystic kidneys in infants: Association with hypertrophic pyloric stenosis. Pediatr Radiol 1977; 6:27–31.

152. Main D, Mennuti MT, Cornfeld D, et al: Prenatal diagnosis of adult polycystic kidney disease. Lancet 1983; 2:337–338.

153. Milutinovic J, Fialkow PJ, Phillips LA, et al: Autosomal dominant polycystic kidney disease: Early diagnosis and data for genetic counselling. Lancet 1980; 1:1203–1206.

154. Pretorius DH, Lee ME, Manco-Johnson ML, et al: Diagnosis of autosomal dominant polycystic kidney disease in utero and in the young infant. J Ultrasound Med 1987; 6:249–255.

155. Reeders ST, Zerres K, Ga IA, et al: Prenatal diagnosis of autosomal dominant polycystic kidney disease with a DNA probe. Lancet 1986; 2:6–8.

156. Shokeir MH: Expression of "adult" polycystic renal disease in the fetus and newborn. Clin Genet 1978; 14:61–72.

157. Zerres K, Weiss H, Bulla M: Prenatal diagnosis of an early manifestation of autosomal dominant adult-type polycystic kidney disease. Lancet 1982; 2:988.

158. Zerres K, Hansmann M, Knopfle G, et al: Clinical case reports. Prenatal diagnosis of genetically determined early manifestation of autosomal dominant polycystic kidney disease. Human Genet 1985; 71:368–369.

Syndromes and Rare Causes for Renal Cysts

159. Bartman J, Barraclough G: Cystic dysplasia of the kidneys studied by microdissection in a case of 13-15 trisomy. J Pathol Bacteriol 1965; 89:233–238.

160. Bernstein J, Crough AJ, McAdams AJ: The renal lesion in syndromes of multiple congenital malformations. Birth Defects 1974; 10:35–43.

161. Chen H, Yang SS, Gonzalez E, et al: Short rib polydactyly syndrome. Majewski type. Am J Med Genet 1980; 7:215–222.

162. Chevalier RL, Garland TA, Buschi AJ: The neonate with adult-type autosomal dominant polycystic kidney disease. Int J Pediatr Nephrol 1981; 2:73–77.

163. Conley ME, Beckwith JB, Mancer JFK, et al: The spectrum of the DiGeorge syndrome. J Pediatr 1979; 94:883–890.

164. Cote GB: Potter's syndrome and chromosomal anomalies. Hum Genet 1981; 58:220.

165. Crawfurd MA: Renal dysplasia and asplenia in two sibs. Clin Genet 1978; 14:338–344.

166. Danks DM, Tippett P, Adams C, et al: Cerebro-hepato-renal syndrome of Zellweger. J Pediatr 1975; 86:382–387.

167. Dieker H, Edwards RH, ZuRhein G, et al: The lissencephaly syndrome. Birth Defects 1969; 5:53–64.

168. Dieterich E, Straub E: Familial juvenile nephronophthisis with hepatic fibrosis and neurocutaneous dysplasia. Helv Paediatr Acta 1980; 35:261–267.

169. Doege TC, Thuline HC, Priest JH, et al: Studies of a family with the oral-facial-digital syndrome. N Engl J Med 1964; 271:1073–1078.

170. Egli F, Stadler G: Malformations of kidney and urinary tract in common chromosomal aberrations. Humangenetik 1973; 18:1–15.

171. Fraser FC, Lytwyn A: Spectrum of anomalies in the Meckel syndrome, or "Maybe there is a malformation syndrome with at least one constant anomaly". Am J Med Genet 1981; 9:67–73.

172. Freeman MV, Williams DW, Schimke RN: The Roberts syndrome. Clin Genet 1974; 5:1–16.

173. Fried K, Liban E, Lurie M, et al: Polycystic kidneys associated with malformations of the brain, polydactyly and other birth defects in newborn sibs. J Med Genet 1971; 8:285–290.

174. Friedrich U, Brogard Hansen K, Hauge M, et al: Prenatal diagnosis of polycystic kidneys and encephalocele (Meckel syndrome). Clin Genet 1979; 15:278–286.

175. Frimodt-Moller PC, Nissen HM, Dyreborg U: Polycystic kidneys as the renal lesion in Lindau's disease. J Urol 1981; 125:868–870.

176. Frydman M, Magenis RE, Mohandas TK: Chromosome abnormalities in infants with prune belly anomaly: Association with trisomy 18. Am J Med Genet 1983; 15:145–148.

177. Garcia CJ, Taylor KJW, Weiss RM: Congenital megacalyces: Ultrasound appearance. J Ultrasound Med 1987; 6:163–165.

178. Gardner KD Jr: Juvenile nephronophthisis and renal medullary cystic disease, in Gardner KD Jr (ed): *Cystic Diseases of the Kidney.* New York, John Wiley & Sons, 1976, p 173.

179. Gorlin RJ, Jue KL, Jacobsen U: Oculoauriculovertebral dysplasia. J Pediatr 1963; 63:991–999.

180. Grote W, Weisner D, Janig U: Prenatal diagnosis of a short-rib polydactyly syndrome type Saldino-Noonan at 17 weeks' gestation. Eur J Pediatr 1983; 140:63–66.

181. Gruskin AB, Baluarte HJ, Cote ML: The renal disease of thoracic asphyxiating dystrophy. Birth Defects 1974; 10:44–50.

182. Halal F, Desgranges MF, Leduc B: Acrorenal-mandibular syndrome. Am J Med Genet 1980; 5:277–284.

183. Hall JG, Pallister PD, Clarren SK: Congenital hypothalamic hamartoblastoma, hypopituitarism, imperforate anus, and postaxial polydactyly—a new syndrome? Part I: Clinical, causal, and pathogenic considerations. Am J Med Genet 1980; 7:47–74.

184. Harris RE, Fuchs EF, Kaempf MJ: Medullary sponge kidney and congenital hemihypertrophy: Case report and literature review. J Urol 1981; 126:676–678.

185. Harrison AR, Williams JP: Medullary sponge kidney and congenital hemihypertrophy. Br J Urol 1971; 43:552–561.

186. Harrod MJE, Stokes J, Peede LF: Polycystic kidney disease in a patient with the oral-facial-digital syndrome-type I. Clin Genet 1976; 9:183–186.

187. Herdman RC, Langer LO: The thoracic asphyxiant dystrophy and renal disease. Am J Dis Child 1968; 116:192–201.

188. Hunter AGW, Rothman SJ, Hwang WS: Hepatic fibrosis, polycystic kidney, colobomata, and encephalopathy in siblings. Clin Genet 1974; 6:82–89.

189. Hurley RM, Dery P, Nogrady MB: The renal lesion of the Laurence-Moon-Beidl syndrome. J Pediatr 1975; 87:206–209.

190. Ivemark BJ, Oldfelt V, Zetterstrom R: Familial dysplasia of kidneys, liver and pancreas. A probable genetically determined syndrome. Acta Paediatr Scand 1959; 48:1–11.

191. Jaatoul NY, Haddad NE, Khoury LA: Brief clinical report and review: The Marden-Walker syndrome. Am J Med Genet 1982; 11:259–271.

192. Jan JE, Hardwick DF, Lowry RB, et al: Cerebro-hepato-renal syndrome of Zellweger. Am J Dis Child 1970; 119:274–277.

193. Johnson VP: Smith-Lemli-Opitz syndrome: Review and report of two affected siblings. Z Kinderheilkd 1975; 119:221–234.

194. Johnson VP, Petersen LP, Holzwarth DR, et al: Mid-trimester prenatal diagnosis of short-limb dwarfism (Saldino-Noonan syndrome). Birth Defects 1982; 18:133–141.

195. Juberg RC, Gilbert EF, Salisbury RS: Trisomy C in an infant with polycystic kidneys and other malformations. J Pediatr 1970; 76:598–603.

196. Karjalainen O, Aula P, Seppala M, et al: Prenatal diagnosis of the Meckel syndrome. Obstet Gynecol 1981; 57:13S–15S.

197. Kurnit DM, Steele MW, Pinsky L, et al: Autosomal dominant transmission of a syndrome of anal, ear, renal, and radial congenital malformations. J Pediatr 1978; 93:270–273.

198. Landing BH, Gwinn JL, Lieberman E: Cystic diseases of the kidney in children, in Gardner KD Jr. (ed): *Cystic Diseases of the Kidney.* New York, John Wiley & Sons, 1976, p 187.

199. Lucaya J, Enriquez G, Delgado R, et al: Infundibulopelvic stenosis in children. AJR 1984; 142:471–474.

200. Lee KR, Wulfsberg E, Kepes JJ: Some important radiological aspects of the kidney in Hippel-Lindau syndrome: The value of prospective study in an affected family. Radiology 1977; 122:649–653.

201. Lehnert W, Wendel U, Lindenmaier S, et al: Multiple acyl-CoA dehydrogenation deficiency (glutaric aciduria type II), congenital polycystic kidneys, and symmetric warty dysplasia of the cerebral cortex in two brothers. I: Clinical, metabolic and biochemical findings. Eur J Pediatr 1982; 139:56–59.

202. Lubinsky M, Severn C, Rapoport JM: Fryns syndrome: A new variable multiple congenital anomaly (MCA) syndrome. Am J Med Genet 1983; 14:461–466.

203. Mauseth R, Lieberman E, Heuser ET: Infantile polycystic disease of the kidneys and Ehlers-Danlos syndrome in an 11-year-old patient. J Pediatr 1977; 90:81–83.

204. Melnick M, Hodes ME, Nance WE, et al: Branchio-oto-renal dysplasia and branchio-oto dysplasia: Two distinct autosomal dominant disorders. Clin Genet 1978; 13:425–442.

205. Mitnick JS, Bosniak MA, Hilton S, et al: Cystic renal disease in tuberous sclerosis. Radiology 1983; 147:85–87.

206. Moerman PH, Verbeken E, Fryns JP, et al: The Meckel syndrome. Pathological and cytogenetic observations in eight cases. Hum Genet 1982; 62:240–245.

207. Mottet NK, Jensen H: The anomalous embryonic development associated with trisomy 13-15. Am J Clin Pathol 1965; 43:334–347.

208. Nadjmi B, Flanagan MJ, Christian JR: Laurence-Moon-Biedl syndrome. Am J Dis Child 1969; 117:352–356.

209. O'Callaghan TJ, Edwards JA, Tobin M, et al: Tuberous sclerosis with striking renal involvement in a family. Arch Intern Med 1975; 135:1082–1087.

210. Pardes JG, Engel IA, Blomquist K, et al: Ultrasonography of intrauterine Meckel's syndrome. J Ultrasound Med 1984; 3:33–35.

211. Passarge E, McAdams AJ: Cerebro-hepato-renal syndrome: A newly recognized hereditary disorder of multiple congenital defects, including sudanophilic leukodystrophy, cirrhosis of the liver, polycystic kidneys. J Pediatr 1967; 71:691–702.

212. Pettersen JC: Gross anatominal studies of a newborn with the Meckel syndrome. Teratology 1983; 28:157–164.

213. Poznanski AK, Nosanchuk JS, Baublis J, et al: The cerebro-hepato-renal syndrome (CHRS); (Zellweger's syndrome). Am J Roentgenol Radium Ther Necl Med 1970; 109:313–322.

214. Rehder H, Labbe F: Prenatal morphology in Meckel's syndrome. Prenat Diagn 1981; 1:161–171.

215. Rohde RA, Hodgman JE, Cleland RS: Multiple congenital anomalies in the E-trisomy group (group 16–18) syndrome. Pediatrics 1964; 33:258–270.

216. Rosenberg JC, Bernstein J, Rosenberg B: Renal cystic disease associated with tuberous sclerosis complex: Renal failure treated by cadaveric kidney transplantation. Clin Nephrol 1975; 4:109–112.

217. Shah KJ: Renal lesion in Jeune's syndrome. Br J Radiol 1980; 53:432–436.

218. Shokeir MH, Houston CS, Awen CF: Asphyxiating thoracic chondrodystrophy: Association with renal disease and evidence for possible heterozygous expression. J Med Genet 1971; 8:107–112.

219. Smith DW, Opitz JM, Inhorn SL: A syndrome of multiple developmental defects including polycystic kidneys and intrahepatic biliary dysgenesis in two siblings. J Pediatr 1965; 67:617–624.

220. Spranger J, Grimm B, Weller M, et al: Short-rib-polydactyly (SRP) syndromes, types Majewski and Saldino-Noonan. Z Kinderheikd 1974; 116:73–94.

221. Steinhardt GF, Slovis TL, Perlmutter AD: Simple renal cysts in infants. Radiology 1985; 155:349–350.
222. Taylor AI: Autosomal trisomy syndromes: A detailed study of 27 cases of Edward's syndrome and 27 cases of Patau's syndrome. J Med Genet 1968; 5:227–252.
223. Waldherr R, Lennert T, Weber HP, et al: The nephronophthisis complex. Virchows Arch (Pathol Anat) 1982; 394:235–254.
224. Wapner RJ, Kurtz AB, Ross RD, et al: Ultrasonographic parameters in the prenatal diagnosis of Meckel syndrome. Obstet Gynecol 1981; 57:388–392.
225. Warkany J, Passarge E: Congenital malformations in autosomal trisomy syndromes. Am J Dis Child 1966; 112:502–517.
226. Wigger HJ, Blanc WA: The prune belly syndrome. Pathol Annu 1977; 12:17–39.
227. Zerres K, Weicker H: "Adulte" Form der polyzystischen Nierenerkrankung (Typ III nach Potter) bei Kindern. poster session, 17. Tagung der Gesettschaft fur Anthropologie und Humangenetic, Gottingen 1981; 23.
228. Zerres K, Volpel MC, Weiss H: Cystic kidneys. Genetics, pathologic anatomy, clinical picture, and prenatal diagnosis. Human Genet 1984; 68:104–135.

Renal Tumors

229. Ehman RL, Nicholson SF, Machin GA: Prenatal sonographic detection of congenital mesoblastic nephroma in a monozygotic twin pregnancy. J Ultrasound Med 1983; 2:555–557.
230. Geirrson RT, Ricketts NEM, Taylor DJ, et al: Prenatal appearance of a mesoblastic nephroma associated with polyhydramnios. J Clin Ultrasound 1985; 13:488–490.
231. Guilian BB: Prenatal ultrasonographic diagnosis of fetal renal tumors. Radiology 1984; 152:69–70.
232. Sanders RC, Nussbaum AR, Solez K: Renal dysplasia: Sonographic findings. Radiology 1988; 167:623–626.
233. Gordillo R, Vilaro M, Sherman NH, et al: Circumscribed renal mass in dysplastic kidney: Pseudomass vs. tumor. J Ultrasound Med 1987; 6:613–617.

Neuroblastoma

234. Anders D, Kindermann G, Pfeifer U: Metastasizing fetal neuroblastoma with involvement of the placenta simulating fetal erythroblastosis. Report of two cases. J Pediatr 1973; 82:50–53.
235. Becker JM, Schneider KM, Krasna IH: Neonatal neuroblastoma. Prog Clin Cancer 1970; 4:382–386.
236. Birner WF: Neuroblastoma as a cause of antenatal death. Am J Obstet Gynecol 1961; 82:1388–1391.
237. Chatten J, Voorhees ML: Familial neuroblastoma. N Engl J Med 1967; 277:1230–1236.

238. Ferraro EM, Fakhry J, Aruny JE, et al: Prenatal adrenal neuroblastoma. J Ultrasound Med 1988; 7:275–278.
239. Fowlie F, Giacomantonia M, McKenzie E, et al: Antenatal sonographic diagnosis of adrenal neuroblastoma. J Can Assoc Radiol 1987; 37:50.
240. Guillian BB, Chang CCN, Yoss BS: Prenatal ultrasonographic diagnosis of fetal neuroblastoma. J Clin Ultrasound 1986; 14:225–227.
241. Isaacs H Jr: Perinatal (congenital and neonatal) neoplasms: A report of 110 cases. Pediatr Pathol 1985; 3:165–216.
242. Janetschek G, Weitzel D, Stein W, et al: Prenatal diagnosis of neuroblastoma by sonography. Urology 1984; 24:397–402.
243. Lewis E, Kurtz AB, Dubbins PA, et al: Real-time ultrasonographic evaluation of normal fetal adrenal glands. J Ultrasound Med 1982; 1:265–270.
244. Johnson CC, Spitz MR: Neuroblastoma: Case-control analysis of birth characteristics. J Natl Cancer Inst 1985; 74:789–792.
245. Moss TJ, Kaplan L: Association of hydrops fetalis with congenital neuroblastoma. Am J Obstet Gynecol 1978; 132:905–906.
246. Schneider KM, Becker JM, Krasna IH: Neonatal neuroblastoma. Pediatrics 1965; 36:359–366.
247. Schwischuk LE: *Radiology of the Newborn and Young Infant,* ed 2. Baltimore, Williams & Wilkins, 1980, pp 602–609.
248. Van der Slikke JW, Balk AG: Hydramnios with hydrops fetalis and disseminated fetal neuroblastoma. Obstet Gynecol 1980; 55:250–253.
249. Voute PA, Wadman SK, Van Putten WJ: Congenital neuroblastoma. Symptoms in the mother during pregnancy. Clin Pediatr 1970; 9:206–207.
250. White SJ, Stuck KJ, Blane CE, et al: Sonography of neuroblastoma. AJR 1983; 141:465–468.
251. Young JL Jr, Miller RW: Incidence of malignant tumors in US children. J Pediatr 1975; 86:254–258.

Fetal Gender

252. Birnholz JC: Determination of fetal sex. N Engl J Med 1983; 309:942–944.
253. Cooper C, Mahony BS, Bowie JD, et al: Prenatal ultrasound diagnosis of ambiguous genitalia. J Ultrasound Med 1985; 4:433–436.
254. Elejalde BR, de Elejalde MM, Ketiman T: Visualization of the fetal genitalia by ultrasonography: A review of the literature and analysis of its accuracy and ethical implications. J Ultrasound Med 1985; 4:633–639.
255. Stephens JD: Prenatal diagnosis of testicular feminization. Lancet 1984; 2:1038.

13

The Extremities

Barry S. Mahony, M.D.

Fetal extremity abnormalities are neither rare nor esoteric.[14, 72, 77] As a group, extremity malformations are among the most amenable to sonographic diagnosis during the second trimester of pregnancy. This permits the sonologist to play a central role in the antenatal diagnosis and subsequent management of affected pregnancies. Other methods for confirming or elucidating extremity abnormalities prenatally (i.e., fetoscopy, amniography, radiography, amniocentesis, umbilical blood sampling) may provide adjunct information in some cases, but in most cases yield less information than the sonogram.[74] Therefore, sonography has become the primary, most sensitive, and most accurate prenatal method for detecting extremity malformations.

Although documentation of each fetal bone is neither necessary nor practical in the vast majority of obstetric sonograms, numerous structures of the fetal musculoskeletal system can be seen clearly.[11] The relatively simple maneuver of measuring the fetal femur will lead to the accurate identification of most fetal skeletal abnormalities, especially the lethal syndromes.[72] Measurement of the femur length, therefore, must be a routine documented part of the obstetrical examination.[1]

Occasionally, the amount of amniotic fluid and fetal positioning dictate which portions of the extremities can be well imaged. Restriction of fetal motion by oligohydramnios, for example, may limit the evaluation of one or more extremities. Conversely, extreme polyhydramnios may make detailed extremity survey difficult and time consuming because of increased distance from the transducer surface and frequent fetal movements. Practice, patience, and persistence, however, usually permit adequate visualization in order to predict the presence or absence of many extremity abnormalities.

This chapter provides a comprehensive, but not exhaustive review and reference source of the fetal extremities for the practicing sonologist. It also provides an approach to categorize and minimize the number of diagnostic possibilities when confronted by one of the numerous and varied extremity malformations. Although prenatal ultrasound may not always permit an exact diagnosis, thorough evaluation usually limits the diagnostic possibilities to one of several entities and provides useful prognostic information for pregnancy management.

EMBRYOGENESIS

By the end of the embryonic period (10 menstrual weeks) the extremity bones, joints, and musculature have differentiated into structures with relative position and form identical to those of an adult.[26] Endochondral ossification begins toward the end of the embryonic period, when the midshaft of the long bones converts from a cartilaginous model into bone.[30] Limb joint structures and musculature also develop during embryogenesis. By the middle to end of the embryonic period all large joints have complete joint cavities, and muscular activity has begun.[8, 22–25, 27–29, 31] Since ultimate joint structure and function depend upon extremity movement in utero, failure of extremity motion during development may result in a variety of malformations and postural deformities.[252, 256–258] Therefore, attention to extremity motion may prove useful in predicting ultimate limb function.

Ossification of the clavicle and mandible begins at 8 menstrual weeks, and all of the appendicular long bones, phalanges, ilium, and scapula have begun to os-

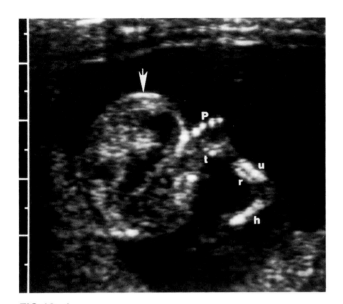

FIG 13–1.
Normal 12-week upper extremity. The extremity bones become visible sonographically at approximately the time ossification commences. This sonogram of a fetus at 12 menstrual weeks clearly illustrates the highly echogenic ossification of the humerus, radius, ulna, phalanges, and thumb. Note that the calvarium rostral to the orbits has not yet begun to ossify. *h* = humerus; *r* = radius; *u* = ulna; *p* = phalanges; *t* = thumb; *arrow* = specular echo arising from the fetal head (not from ossification).

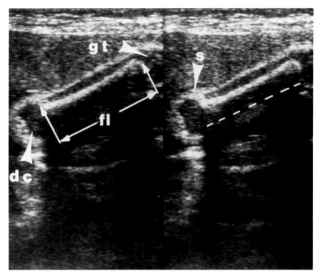

FIG 13–2.
Normal femur. Dual-image scan of the femur demonstrates that the sonographic femur length measures only the ossified femoral diaphysis and does not include the nonossified cartilages of the distal epiphysis or greater tuberosity. In addition, the measurements do not include the specular reflection arising from the surface of the distal epiphyseal cartilage. The femur appears to curve slightly as the ossified diaphysis joins the larger epiphyseal cartilage. The shadowing from the ossified diaphysis makes the femur look narrower than it is; the broken line indicates the approximate location of the medial margin of this femur. *fl* = femur length; *dc* = distal epiphysis; *gt* = greater tuberosity; *s* = specular echo from surface of distal epiphyseal cartilage. (From Mahony BS, Filly RA: High-resolution sonographic assessment of the fetal extremities. J Ultrasound Med 1984; 3:489–498. Used by permission.)

sify by the end of the first trimester (Fig 13–1). Between 12 and 16 weeks the metacarpals and metatarsals ossify, and during the fifth and sixth months the pubis, talus, and calcaneus ossify. Ossification of all of the carpal bones and the remaining tarsals does not occur until after birth. The secondary ossification centers within the epiphyseal cartilages of the distal femur, proximal tibia, and occasionally the proximal humerus appear prenatally.[35, 50, 52, 58] The remaining secondary epiphyseal ossification centers do not ossify until after birth.

NORMAL SONOGRAPHIC FINDINGS

Antenatal sonography clearly defines details of the fetal extremities.[11] In the lower extremities, the echopenic femoral head epiphyseal cartilage resides between the ossified ischium and femoral diaphysis. The proximal and distal ends of the ossified femoral diaphysis flare slightly to join the larger epiphyseal cartilages and give the femur a slightly bowed appearance especially evident medially.[33] Acoustic shadowing caused by the diaphyseal ossification produces a false impression that the diaphysis is too thin for the width of the epiphyseal cartilages, but the width of the epi-

physeal cartilage enables extrapolation of the true diaphyseal width (Fig 13–2).[11]

The echogenic material in and about the knee clearly defines the echopenic cartilages of the patella, distal femur, and proximal tibia and fibula (Fig 13–3).[11] During the third trimester, the secondary epiphyseal ossification centers of the distal femur and then of the proximal tibia become visible centrally positioned within their respective cartilages.[35, 51, 52, 69] These secondary epiphyseal ossification centers enlarge centrifugally as gestation progresses.[51, 57] Since the proximal tibial epiphyseal ossification center grows more rapidly than does the distal femoral epiphyseal ossification center, their sizes are approximately equal near term.[57] The tibia and fibula begin and end at approximately the same level proximally and distally. The cartilaginous tips of the bones create echopenic gaps between the ossified diaphyses of these bones as well as of the ossified metatarsals and phalanges (Fig 13–4).

The clavicle and scapula define the shoulder girdle. The scapula imaged in long axis coronally has a characteristic shape resembling a "Y" with the supraspinatus,

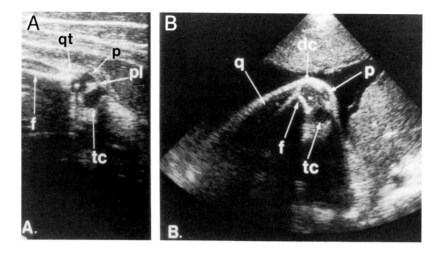

FIG 13–3.
Normal third-trimester knee. **A,** sagittal scan of the extended knee shows the femoral diaphysis, quadriceps tendon, patella, patellar ligament, and proximal tibial epiphyseal cartilage. **B,** scan of the flexed knee demonstrates the distal end of the ossified diaphysis, the quadriceps muscle group, the patella, and the epiphyseal cartilages of the distal femur and proximal tibia. Note the small, echogenic, secondary epiphyseal ossification center within the distal femoral epiphyseal cartilage. *f* = femoral diaphysis; *qt* = quadriceps tendon; *p* = patella; *pl* = patellar ligament; *tc* = proximal tibial epiphyseal cartilage; *q* = quadriceps muscle; *dc* = distal femoral epiphyseal cartilage. (From Mahony BS, Filly RA: High-resolution sonographic assessment of the fetal extremities. J Ultrasound Med 1984; 3:489–498. Used by permission.)

subscapularis, and infraspinatus muscles in their respective fossae. The scapula has a triangular shape when imaged posteriorly (Fig 13–5). The clavicles can be seen if not obscured by flexion of the fetal head. They grow at a linear rate of approximately 1 mm per week reaching a length of 20 mm at 20 weeks and 40 mm at 40 weeks (see Appendix).[68]

The humeral head epiphyseal cartilage resides between the ossified distal clavicle, scapula, and proximal humeral diaphysis (Fig 13–6).[51] At the elbow, the non–ossified coronoid fossa delineates the medial and lateral humeral epicondyles. The more proximal extent of the ulna at the elbow distinguishes it from the radius. Demonstration of the ulna and radius ending at

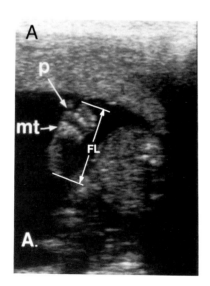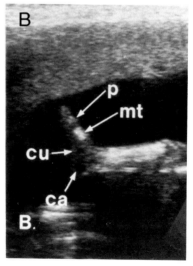

FIG 13–4.
Normal foot at 19.5 weeks. **A,** plantar scan of the foot clearly shows the ossified metatarsals and phalanges. The foot length is measured from the heel to the tip of the first or second toe. **B,** sagittal scan of the same foot shows that the calcaneus, cuboid, and other tarsal bones are not yet ossified. *mt* = metatarsals; *p* = phalanges; *ca* = calcaneus; *cu* = cuboid. (From Mahony BS, Filly RA: High-resolution sonographic assessment of the fetal extremities. J Ultrasound Med 1984; 3:489–498. Used by permission.)

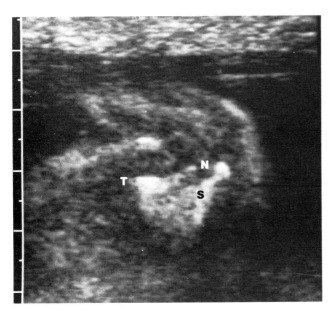

FIG 13–5.
Normal scapula. This oblique scan through the fetal shoulder clearly shows the scapula. *t* = scapular tip; *n* = scapular notch; *s* = scapular spine.

the same level at the wrist effectively excludes many radial ray defects (Fig 13–7). The non–ossified carpals produce a conglomerate zone of gray echoes antenatally, but the ossified metacarpal and phalanges are readily visualized if the fetus extends the hand.

The epiphyseal ossification centers of the knee and shoulder appear and enlarge at variable rates but in a predictable sequence. The epiphyseal ossification center of the distal femur appears at 28–35 weeks, followed 2–3 weeks later by the proximal tibial center, then by the proximal humeral epiphyseal ossification center at greater than 38 weeks.[35, 51, 52] Intrauterine

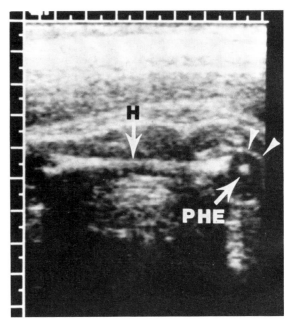

FIG 13–6.
Normal humerus and proximal humeral epiphyseal ossification center. Scan of the humerus shows the secondary ossification center of the proximal humeral epiphysis, which appears near term centrally within the epiphyseal cartilage. *H* = humerus; *PHE* = proximal humeral epiphyseal ossification center; *arrow heads* = epiphyseal cartilage. (From Mahony BS, Bowie JD, Killam AP, et al: Epiphyseal ossification centers in the assesssment of fetal maturity: Sonographic correlation with the amniocentesis lung profile. Radiology 1986; 159:521–524. Used by permission.)

growth retardation may delay this sequence.[69] Since the size of these epiphyseal ossification centers correlates with the amniotic fluid lecithin/sphingomyelin ratio, their identification and measurement may provide useful information regarding fetal lung maturation.[51, 64] Furthermore, since virtually all fetuses born at greater

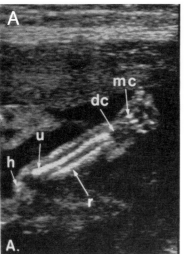
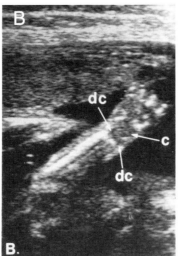

FIG 13–7.
Normal forearm at 24 weeks. **A,** the cartilage between the proximal ulna and the distal humerus is clearly seen on this longitudinal scan of the forearm. The more proximal extent of the ulna at the elbow distinguishes it from the radius. The ulna and radius end at the same level at the wrist. **B,** the cartilaginous carpal bones create a conglomerate area of midrange echoes distal to the radial and ulnar cartilages. *u* = ulna; *h* = humerus; *r* = radius; *c* = carpus; *dc* = distal cartilaginous ends of the radius and ulna; *mc* = metacarpals. (From Mahony BS, Filly RA: High-resolution sonographic assessment of the fetal extremities. J Ultrasound Med 1984; 3:489–498. Used by permission.)

than 38 weeks have mature lungs, identification of the proximal humeral epiphyseal ossification center provides useful information regarding lung maturity, although not all fetuses with mature lungs have a visible proximal humeral epiphyseal ossification center (see Fig 13−6).[51]

EXTREMITY MEASUREMENTS

Many biometric studies correlate the length of the ossified femoral diaphysis with menstrual age and yield consistent and well-defined results.[4, 36, 40−47, 54, 56, 59−67] Assessment of femur length also assists in prediction of disturbances of fetal growth. Few studies report lengths of limb bones other than the femur (Table 13−1).[4, 44, 46, 47, 54]

Attention to technical detail maximizes reproducibility and minimizes measurement error.[32, 39, 43, 48]

Published measurements of femoral length correspond only to measurement of the ossified diaphyses and exclude the epiphyseal cartilages (see Fig 13−2).[11] Since the ossified diaphysis may be artifactually foreshortened by scanning obliquely through the shaft, the longest measurement showing both proximal and distal epiphyseal cartilages simultaneously usually is the most accurate. Conversely, one may overestimate the diaphyseal length by including in the measurement a portion of the bone width at the end of the diaphysis if the bone orients obliquely through the scan plane.[11] The specular echo arising from the edge of the epiphyseal cartilage should not be included in diaphyseal measurement.[39] As recommended by Deter et al. estimation of menstrual age based on extremity length should use menstrual age as the independent variable.[4, 36] On the other hand, prediction of a short-limbed bone dysplasia should compare extremity measurements with other growth parameters.

TABLE 13−1.

Normal Extremity Long Bone Lengths and Biparietal Diameter at Different Menstrual Ages*†

Menstrual Age (weeks)	Biparietal Diameter	Femur	Tibia	Fibula	Humerus	Radius	Ulna
13	2.3(0.3)	1.1(0.2)	0.9(0.2)	0.8(0.2)	1.0(0.2)	0.6(0.2)	0.8(0.3)
14	2.7(0.3)	1.3(0.2)	1.0(0.2)	0.9(0.3)	1.2(0.2)	0.8(0.2)	1.0(0.2)
15	3.0(0.1)	1.5(0.2)	1.3(0.2)	1.2(0.2)	1.4(0.2)	1.1(0.1)	1.2(0.1)
16	3.3(0.2)	1.9(0.3)	1.6(0.3)	1.5(0.3)	1.7(0.2)	1.4(0.3)	1.6(0.3)
17	3.7(0.3)	2.2(0.3)	1.8(0.3)	1.7(0.2)	2.0(0.4)	1.5(0.3)	1.7(0.3)
18	4.2(0.5)	2.5(0.3)	2.2(0.3)	2.1(0.3)	2.3(0.3)	1.9(0.2)	2.2(0.3)
19	4.4(0.4)	2.8(0.3)	2.5(0.3)	2.3(0.3)	2.6(0.3)	2.1(0.3)	2.4(0.3)
20	4.7(0.4)	3.1(0.3)	2.7(0.2)	2.6(0.2)	2.9(0.3)	2.4(0.2)	2.7(0.3)
21	5.0(0.5)	3.5(0.4)	3.0(0.4)	2.9(0.4)	3.2(0.4)	2.7(0.4)	3.0(0.4)
22	5.5(0.5)	3.6(0.3)	3.2(0.3)	3.1(0.3)	3.3(0.3)	2.8(0.5)	3.1(0.4)
23	5.8(0.5)	4.0(0.4)	3.6(0.2)	3.4(0.2)	3.7(0.3)	3.1(0.4)	3.5(0.2)
24	6.1(0.5)	4.2(0.3)	3.7(0.3)	3.6(0.3)	3.8(0.4)	3.3(0.4)	3.6(0.4)
25	6.4(0.5)	4.6(0.3)	4.0(0.3)	3.9(0.4)	4.2(0.4)	3.5(0.3)	3.9(0.4)
26	6.8(0.5)	4.8(0.4)	4.2(0.3)	4.0(0.3)	4.3(0.3)	3.6(0.4)	4.0(0.3)
27	7.0(0.3)	4.9(0.3)	4.4(0.3)	4.2(0.3)	4.5(0.2)	3.7(0.3)	4.1(0.2)
28	7.3(0.5)	5.3(0.5)	4.5(0.4)	4.4(0.3)	4.7(0.4)	3.9(0.4)	4.4(0.5)
29	7.6(0.5)	5.3(0.5)	4.6(0.3)	4.5(0.3)	4.8(0.4)	4.0(0.5)	4.5(0.4)
30	7.7(0.6)	5.6(0.3)	4.8(0.5)	4.7(0.3)	5.0(0.5)	4.1(0.6)	4.7(0.3)
31	8.2(0.7)	6.0(0.6)	5.1(0.3)	4.9(0.5)	5.3(0.4)	4.2(0.3)	4.9(0.4)
32	8.5(0.6)	6.1(0.6)	5.2(0.4)	5.1(0.4)	5.4(0.4)	4.4(0.6)	5.0(0.6)
33	8.6(0.4)	6.4(0.5)	5.4(0.5)	5.3(0.3)	5.6(0.5)	4.5(0.5)	5.2(0.3)
34	8.9(0.5)	6.6(0.6)	5.7(0.5)	5.5(0.4)	5.8(0.5)	4.7(0.5)	5.4(0.5)
35	8.9(0.7)	6.7(0.6)	5.8(0.4)	5.6(0.4)	5.9(0.6)	4.8(0.6)	5.4(0.4)
36	9.1(0.7)	7.0(0.7)	6.0(0.6)	5.6(0.5)	6.0(0.6)	4.9(0.5)	5.5(0.3)
37	9.3(0.9)	7.2(0.4)	6.1(0.4)	6.0(0.4)	6.1(0.4)	5.1(0.3)	5.6(0.4)
38	9.5(0.6)	7.4(0.6)	6.2(0.3)	6.0(0.4)	6.4(0.3)	5.1(0.5)	5.8(0.6)
39	9.5(0.6)	7.6(0.8)	6.4(0.7)	6.1(0.6)	6.5(0.6)	5.3(0.5)	6.0(0.6)
40	9.9(0.8)	7.7(0.4)	6.5(0.3)	6.2(0.1)	6.6(0.4)	5.3(0.3)	6.0(0.5)
41	9.7(0.6)	7.7(0.4)	6.6(0.4)	6.3(0.5)	6.6(0.4)	5.6(0.4)	6.3(0.5)
42	10.0(0.5)	7.8(0.7)	6.8(0.5)	6.7(0.7)	6.8(0.7)	5.7(0.5)	6.5(0.5)

*From Merz E, Mi-Sook KK, Pehl S: Ultrasonic mensuration of fetal limb bones in the second and third trimesters. J Clin Ultrasound 1987; 15:175−183. Used by permission.
†Mean values (cm); value of 2 SD in parentheses.

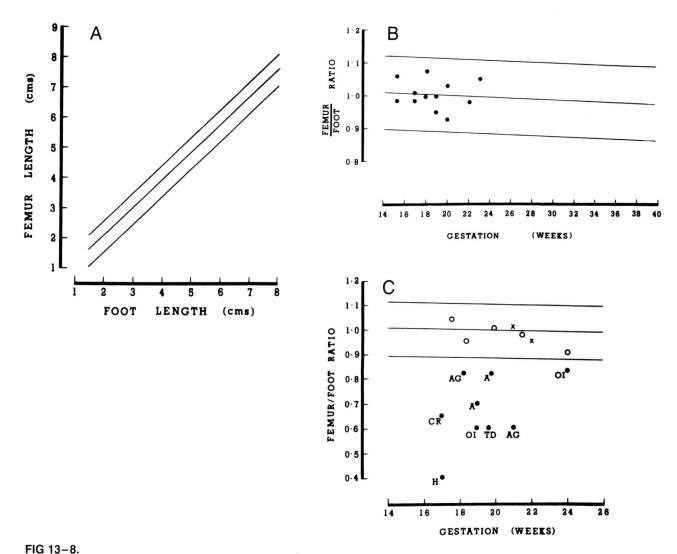

FIG 13–8.
Foot length correlated with femur length. **A,** graph shows the normal relationship between the femur length and the foot length between 14 and 40 weeks, with the 5th and 95th percentile limits. **B,** graph demonstrates the fifth and 95th percentile confidence intervals of the normal femur-foot length ratio from 14 to 40 weeks. The dots indicate the femur-foot length ratio of 12 specimens plotted on the ultrasound nomogram. **C,** this graph illustrates that the femur-foot length ratio remains normal for normal small fetuses or growth-retarded fetuses but is abnormally low for fetuses affected by skeletal dysplasia. *Open circles* = normal small fetuses; *crosses* = growth-retarded fetuses; *closed circles* = skeletal dysplasia; *A* = achondroplasia; *AG* = achondrogenesis; *OI* = osteogenesis imperfecta; *TD* = thanatophoric dysplasia; *CR* = caudal regression; *H* = hypophosphatasia. (From Cambell J, Henderson A, Cambell S: The fetal femur-foot length ratio: A new parameter to assess dysplastic limb reduction. Obstet Gynecol 1988; 72:181–184. Used by permission.)

The foot length, which can be accurately measured during the second and third trimesters, is nearly equal to the femur length, so that the normal femur length/foot length ratio remains near unity (Fig 13–8; also see Appendix).[34, 53, 57] These observations may prove useful in distinguishing fetuses with dwarfism from those that are constitutionally small or symmetrically growth retarded.[34]

PREVALENCE OF ANOMALIES AND ACCURACY OF SONOGRAPHIC DIAGNOSIS

Data compiled from seven series confirm the accuracy of sonographic diagnosis for evaluation of the fetal extremities.[71–74, 76–78] Among these series, four studies evaluated a total of 173 fetuses at risk for skeletal dysplasia based upon a positive family history of a recurrent disorder, two studies screened a total of approximately 19,000 obstetrical patients for fetal extremity abnormalities, and one study reviewed the experience of a university hospital.

Sonographic screening for extremity abnormalities has detected dwarfism in 0.075%–0.1% of pregnancies, and dwarfs represent approximately 1%–3.5% of fetuses with sonographically detectable abnormalities.[72, 77] The prenatal prevalence of skeletal dysplasias probably exceeds the prevalence at birth because many fetuses with skeletal dysplasia do not survive (Table 13–2).[70, 75]

A formidable number of deformities may affect the

TABLE 13–2.

Approximate Birth Prevalence of Skeletal Dysplasias

Dysplasia	Approximate Birth Prevalence
Lethal	
Thanatophoric dysplasia	1/10,000
Achondrogenesis	1/40,000
Osteogenesis imperfecta, type II	1/60,000
Congenital hypophosphatasia	1/100,000
Chondrodysplasia punctata, rhizomelic type	1/110,000
Campomelic dysplasia	1/150,000
Others	1/200,000 or less
Nonlethal	
Heterozygous achondroplasia	1/30,000
Osteogenesis imperfecta, type I	1/30,000
Asphyxiating thoracic dysplasia	1/70,000
Others	1/200,000 or less
Total	1/4,000
Total detected by prenatal ultrasound	1/1,000

TABLE 13–3.

Nomenclature Regarding Most Limb Abnormalities

Bone shortening	
Acromelia	Shortening of distal segments
Mesomelia	Shortening of middle segments
Micromelia	Shortened extremities
Rhizomelia	Shortening of proximal segments
Focal absence	
Acheiria	Absence of the hands
Acheiropodia	Absence of the hands and feet
Adactyly	Absence of the fingers or toes
Amelia	Absence of an extremity
Apodia	Absence of the feet
Hemimelia	Absence of extremity below the knee or elbow
Phocomelia	Absent or deficient development of middle segment of an extremity with preservation of proximal and distal segments
Sirenomelia	Fusion of the legs
Contractures and postural deformities	
Arthrogryposis	Extremity contractures
Cavus	Hollow foot (exaggeration of arch)
Equinus	Extension of the foot
Talipes	Clubfoot
Valgus	Bent outward
Varus	Bent inward
Subtle hand and foot deformities	
Clinodactyly	Overlapping digits
Polydactyly	Extra digits
Syndactyly	Fused digits

fetal extremities (Tables 13–3 and 13–4).[2, 16, 18] However, the list of abnormalities usually recognized prenatally is much more manageable. For example, the above-mentioned 7 series describe 16 different diagnoses among the 55 cases detected prenatally, but over half had 1 of 4 diagnoses: Thanatophoric dysplasia (n=10 cases), osteogenesis imperfecta (n=8 cases), achondrogenesis (n=7 cases), and achondroplasia (n=5 cases).

Among the four prenatal series which studied 173 fetuses at risk for extremity malformations, 25 fetuses (14.5%) had a recurrent dwarfism detected by second-trimester ultrasound and nearly half of these were osteogenesis imperfecta, achondrogenesis, or achondroplasia.[71, 73, 74, 78] In the retrospective review of a university hospital between 1981 and 1984, Pretorius et al. reported 13 lethal cases of fetal dwarfism seen at 19.5–36 weeks.[76] Dwarfism was correctly diagnosed in 11 (85%) cases, and the specific type of dwarfism was diagnosed in 7 (54%) cases (thanatophoric dysplasia, achondrogenesis, and osteogenesis imperfecta).

Many fetuses with lethal extremity abnormalities present with severe manifestations readily apparent on

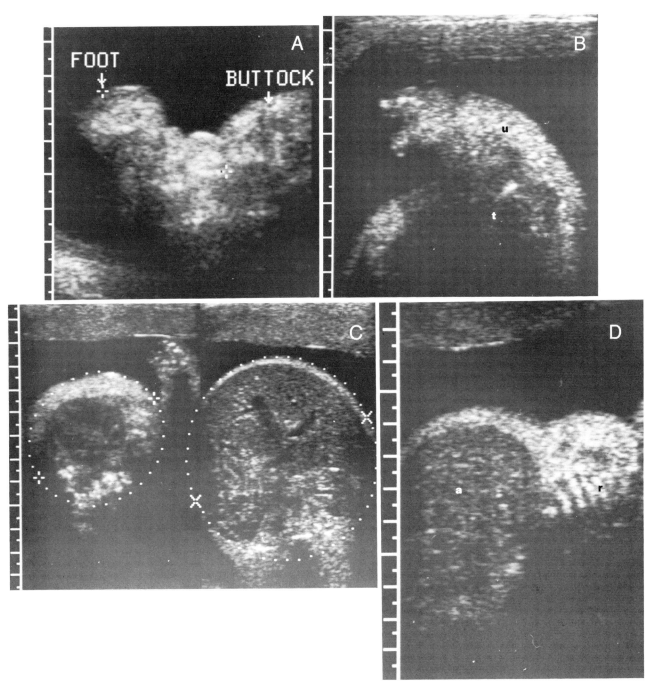

FIG 13–9.
Severe micromelia and small thorax at 34 weeks, highly indicative of a lethal skeletal dysplasia. Diagnosis: Thanatophoric dysplasia. **A,** from the buttock to the foot measures only approximately 4.5 cm on this sagittal scan of the lower extremity. **B,** the upper extremity is so short that it orients at almost a right angle with the thorax. **C,** the thoracic circumference *(left)* measured at the level of the four chamber view of the heart is unmistakably small relative to the abdominal circumference *(right).* **D,** the short ribs demarcate a very small thorax on this sagittal scan of the abdomen and thorax. *(Continued.)*

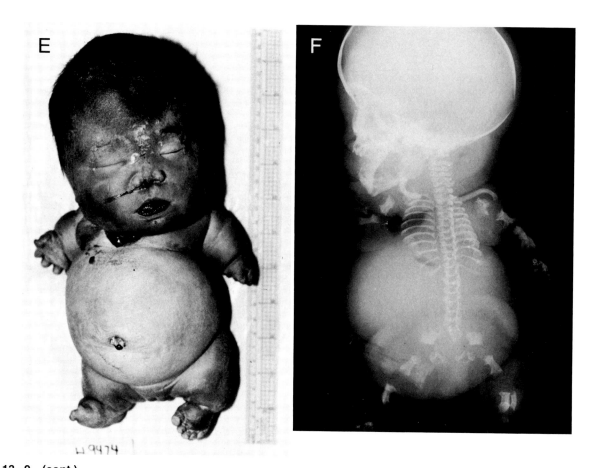

FIG 13–9 (cont.).
E and **F,** postnatal photograph and radiograph confirm the prenatal findings. *U* = upper extremity; *t* = thorax; *a* = abdomen; *r* = ribs.

the prenatal ultrasound (Fig 13–9). Because the nonlethal syndromes typically manifest with milder manifestations, the sensitivity and specificity of ultrasound detection of these syndromes would be expected to be lower than for the lethal syndromes, especially in the absence of genetic risk. None of the above series reports any false-positive diagnoses of extremity abnormalities, and to our knowledge, no false-positive diagnosis of a fetal skeletal dysplasia has been reported. However, false-positive interpretation of relatively subtle hand and foot deformities as well as missed diagnoses occur.[12, 72, 285]

SONOGRAPHIC APPROACH TO EXTREMITY ABNORMALITIES

Since many extremity abnormalities occur in a sporadic or autosomal recessive pattern, the sonologist is usually the first to detect an unexpected problem. However, most extremity abnormalities occur in the setting of polyhydramnios, concomitant fetal structural anomalies, or a positive family history for a recurrent syndrome. Each of these signals the sonologist to examine the extremities.[19, 20, 72] In the vast majority of reported cases, including the screening series by Hegge et al., extremity malformations were detected in conjunction with one or more of these risk factors.[72] Therefore, pedigree analysis, assessment of amniotic fluid volume, and fetal survey are essential for prenatal detection of and distinction among the various abnormalities involving the musculoskeletal system.

Assessment of the following questions assists in prenatal diagnosis of many abnormalities of the fetal extremities:

1. *Are the extremity bones abnormally short or focally absent?*
   a. Shortening of the extremity bones indicates the presence of skeletal dysplasia.
   b. Focal absence of extremity bones usually indicates amputation, radial ray defect, or sirenomelia.
2. *Are the extremities anomalously postured or immobile?*
   a. Anomalous posturing or immobility suggests the presence of contractures.
3. *Are subtle hand and foot deformities present?*
   a. Polydactyly, syndactyly, etc. often occur in the setting of other severe and more obvious abnormalities.

Following the detection of an extremity disorder, evaluation of the distribution and severity of the abnormality as well as of associated findings may help to determine a specific diagnosis. Although the sonologist need not memorize the names and specific features of each of the recognizable deformities, awareness of several principles and familiarity with specific features for which to search facilitate accurate diagnosis.

Skeletal Dysplasia

A shortened bone length confirms the presence of skeletal dysplasia, although some bone dysplasias (especially heterozygous achondroplasia) do not produce shortened bone lengths early in gestation.[183, 186] A fe-

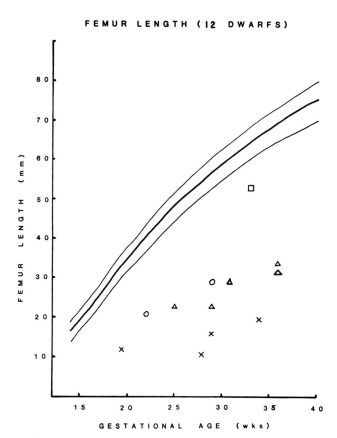

FIG 13–10.
Micromelia in lethal skeletal dysplasias, The lethal skeletal dysplasias tend to cause marked extremity shortening, with the femur length measuring many standard deviations below the mean, as indicated by this graph correlating femur length with gestational age. *Curves* = mean ±2 standard deviations; X = achondrogenesis; O = osteogenesis imperfecta; *square* = campomelic dwarfism; *triangles* = thanatophoric dwarfism. (From Pretorius DH, Rumack CM, Manco-Johnson ML, et al: Specific skeletal dysplasia in utero: Sonographic diagnosis. Radiology 1986; 159:237–242. Used by permission.)

tus whose bones measure greater than 2 SD below the mean for a known menstrual age should be considered at risk for dwarfism, and many dwarf syndromes cause the extremity bones to measure significantly shorter than 2 SD below the mean by 22 weeks (Fig 13–10). Occasionally, limb shortening can be recognized as early as 12–13 weeks when sonography can first measure the femur length reliably.

Following the detection of shortened extremity bones, evaluation of the following sonographic parameters and questions permits accurate prenatal diagnosis of many skeletal dysplasias:

1. *What is the degree of bone shortening (see Table 13–4)?*

   The severity of bone shortening varies from extreme (many standard deviations below the mean, with the limbs oriented at approximately right angles to the fetal trunk) to mild-to-moderate (with a more normal orientation of the limbs to the fetal trunk).

TABLE 13–4.

Short-limbed Skeletal Dysplasias Identifiable at Birth, Categorized by Degree of Bone Shortening

Severe shortening
  Common
    Thanatophoric dysplasia
    Achondrogenesis
    Osteogenesis imperfecta, type II
  Uncommon or rare
    Chondrodysplasia punctata, rhizomelic type
    Diastrophic dysplasia
    Homozygous dominant achondroplasia
    Mesomelic dysplasias
    Short-rib polydactyly syndrome
    Other rare dysplasias (atelosteogenesis, boomerang
      dysplasia, de la Chapelle dysplasia,
      dyssegmental dysplasia, fibrochondrogenesis,
      etc.)
Mild-to-moderate shortening
  Common
    Asphyxiating thoracic dysplasia
    Heterozygous achondroplasia
    Osteogenesis imperfecta, type III
  Uncommon to rare
    Campomelic dysplasia
    Chondroectodermal dysplasia
    Congenital hypophosphatasia
    Other rare dysplasias (acromesomelic dysplasia,
      Kniest dysplasia, metatropic dysplasia,
      spondyloepiphyseal dysplasia congenita, etc)

2. *What is the distribution of involvement (Table 13–5)?*

   Rhizomelic, mesomelic, or acromelic bone shortening occurs with different dysplasias.

TABLE 13–5.

Short-limbed Dwarfisms Identifiable at Birth, Categorized by Distribution of Shortening

Diffuse shortening
  Common
    Achondrogenesis
    Thanatophoric dysplasia
    Osteogenesis imperfecta, types II, III
  Uncommon to rare
    Campomelic dysplasia
    Diastrophic dysplasia
    Homozygous achondroplasia
    Hypophosphatasia
    Metatropic dysplasia
    Short-rib polydactyly syndrome
    Other rare dysplasias
Rhizomelia
  Common
    Asphyxiating thoracic dysplasia
    Heterozygous achondroplasia
  Uncommon to rare
    Chondrodysplasia punctata, rhizomelic type
    Chondroectodermal dysplasia
    Spondyloepiphyseal dysplasia
Mesomelia
  Acromesomelic dysplasias
  Mesomelic dysplasias

3. *Are bone fractures or extremity bowing present (Table 13–6)?*
   a. Fractures usually indicate osteogenesis imperfecta.
   b. Extremity bowing may indicate the presence of fracture, campomelic dysplasia, or a rare dysplasia.

TABLE 13–6.

Causes for Bowing of Extremity Bones

Common
  Achondrogenesis
  Campomelic dysplasia
  Hypophosphatasia
  Osteogenesis imperfecta, type II
  Thanatophoric dysplasia
Rare
  Acromesomelic dysplasia
  Boomerang dysplasia
  Chondroectodermal dysplasia
  Diastrophic dysplasia
  Dyssegmental dysplasia
  Fibrochondrogenesis
  Larsen's syndrome
  Mesomelic dysplasias
  Oto-palato-digital syndrome
  Roberts' syndrome
  Spondyloepiphyseal dysplasia congenita

TABLE 13–7.

Causes for Hypomineralization of Bone

Osteogenesis imperfecta
Hypophosphatasia
Achondrogenesis

c. Thanatophoric dysplasia may produce a "telephone receiver" appearance of the extremity bones.
4. *What is the degree and distribution of ossification (Table 13–7)?*
   a. Diffuse hypomineralization usually indicates osteogenesis imperfecta or hypophosphatasia.
   b. Focal hypomineralization of the spine indicates achondrogenesis.
5. *What is the calvarial configuration?*
   Cloverleaf skull deformity with micromelia indicates thanatophoric dysplasia.
6. *What is the thoracic size?*
   a. A small thorax indicates a high probability of pulmonary hypoplasia, but the thoracic shape often does not assist in rendering a specific diagnosis.
   b. Rib fractures with concavity of the thoracic cage usually indicate osteogenesis imperfecta.
7. *Is polydactyly present (Table 13–8)?*
   a. Polydactyly with skeletal dysplasia usually indicates short-rib polydactyly syndrome, chondrodysplasia punctata, or asphyxiating thoracic dysplasia.

Even in the absence of a family history for a recurrent skeletal dysplasia, careful assessment of these criteria permits accurate diagnosis of a specific skeletal dysplasia in over 50% of cases on the basis of sonography alone and enables accurate assessment of prognosis in approximately 85% of lethal dwarfs.[76]

Focal Loss of Extremity Bone

Focal absence of an extremity bone varies markedly in severity ranging from loss of a single bone or segment of bone to loss of an entire extremity. The loss of bone contrasts with dysplasias in which the bones may be extremely foreshortened but are

TABLE 13–8.

Short-limbed Skeletal
Dysplasias With Polydactyly

Short-rib polydactyly syndrome
Chondroectodermal dysplasia
Asphyxiating thoracic dysplasia

present. The following questions may be helpful in the evaluation of a fetus with focal limb loss:
1. *What is the distribution of limb loss?*
   a. Asymmetric amputations in non–embryologic distributions indicate the amniotic band syndrome or limb-body wall complex.
   b. Symmetric limb loss with preservation of distal components often suggests the Roberts' syndrome.
   c. Fusion of the entire lower extremity indicates sirenomelia.
2. *Is the hand oriented at an acute angle to the wrist?*
   a. Sharp radial angulation of the hand at the wrist with absence of the distal radius indicates a radial ray deformity.

Anomalous Posture or Hand and Foot Deformities

Extremity contractures often occur in conjunction with other severe anomalies which limit fetal mobility and dominate the sonographic picture. In some affected cases, fetal contractures and persistent lack of mobility are so striking that they are unmistakable with real-time ultrasound. In other cases, however, the contractures may be quite subtle and require meticulous attention to fetal positioning and limb motion in order to be detected.

Clinodactyly, polydactyly, syndactyly, and other subtle hand and foot deformities also often occur as a manifestation of a syndrome. Their detection requires meticulous attention to detail. Prenatal detection of these deformities may facilitate diagnosis of a lethal syndrome or permit proper parental counseling and early neonatal treatment.

Prediction of Outcome

The prognosis varies widely among the numerous extremity abnormalities amenable to prenatal sonographic diagnosis. Some entities have an invariably lethal prognosis while others have a variable or good prognosis but one which is certainly not uniformly lethal in early infancy. The most crucial dwarf syndromes for the sonologist to identify at any time in gestation, but especially after 24 weeks, include those for which the fetus has little or no chance for survival. The accurate assessment of prognosis in these cases will obviate heroic procedures to save the fetus.

Lethal short-limbed dysplasias typically are manifest on the antenatal sonogram before 24 weeks, with striking micromelia or other severe manifestations of characteristic features which permit accurate distinc-

TABLE 13–9.

Helpful Sonographic Features in the Differential Diagnosis of the More Common Lethal Skeletal Dysplasias That May Present Prenatally, Listed in Approximate Order of Prevalence.

Dysplasia	Helpful Sonographic Features
Thanatophoric dysplasia	Cloverleaf skull (14% cases); narrow spine; platyspondyly
Achondrogenesis	± absent vertebral body and sacral ossification
Osteogenesis imperfecta, type II	Multiple fractures; rib fractures; ± decreased bone echogenicity or "thick" bones
Congenital hypophosphatasia	Thin, delicate bones; ± fractures; ± decreased bone echogenicity
Campomelic dysplasia	Anterior bowing of femur, tibia, fibula, but of overall normal length
Chondrodysplasia punctata, rhizomelic type	Stippled epiphyses; rhizomelic shortening; contractures; dorsal and ventral ossification of vertebral bodies
Homozygous dominant achondroplasia	Both parents achondroplastic dwarfs; ± cloverleaf skull
Short-rib polydactyly syndrome	Polydactyly; ± cleft lip, renal cysts

tion from nonlethal syndromes (Table 13–9 and Fig 13–9). Some of the dysplasias which are not invariably lethal exhibit variable expressivity of phenotype. As a general rule (and with inevitable exceptions), however, those dysplasias that manifest later and with less severe features have a better prognosis than do the lethal syndromes (Table 13–10).

In general, the prognosis for fetuses with focal limb loss or extremity contractures also tends to obey this rule. For example, the Roberts' syndrome and the pseudo-thalidomide syndrome may represent variations in phenotypic expression of the same entity. Severely affected fetuses have a high perinatal mortality rate, unlike those with mild manifestations of the syn-

TABLE 13–10.

Helpful Sonographic Features in the Differential Diagnosis of the More Common Skeletal Dysplasias With a Variable or Good Prognosis That May Present Prenatally. Dysplasias Are Listed in Approximate Order of Prevalence

Dysplasia	Helpful Sonographic Features	Prognosis
Heterozygous achondroplasia	Progressive rhizomelic shortening in late second or early third trimester	Good
Osteogenesis imperfecta, types I, IV	Normal extremity bone lengths ± isolated fractures	Good
Asphyxiating thoracic dysplasia	Rhizomelic shortening ± narrow thorax, polydactyly, renal cysts	Variable
Chondroectodermal dysplasia	Polydactyly; large atrial septal defect	Variable
Acromesomelic dysplasia	Shortened and bowed middle and distal segments	Variable
Cleidocranial dysplasia	Normal extremity bone lengths; partial or total absence of clavicles; brachycephaly	Good
Diastrophic dysplasia	"Hitchhiker" thumb; multiple contractures	Variable
Kniest dysplasia	Kyphoscoliosis; metaphyseal flaring; short trunk and broad thorax with platyspondyly	Good
Larsen's syndrome	Normal extremity bone lengths; contractures; hypertelorism; double or triple calcaneal ossification center	Good
Mesomelic dysplasia	Mesomelic shortening	Good
Metatropic dysplasia	Marked metaphyseal flaring; kyphoscoliosis	Variable
Osteopetrosis	Normal extremity bone lengths; hepatosplenomegaly	Variable
Oto-palato-digital syndrome	Normal extremity bone lengths; mild femoral bowing; hypoplasia of proximal radius	Variable
Spondyloepiphyseal dysplasia congenita	Shortened, mildly bowed femurs; short trunk; micrognathia	Variable

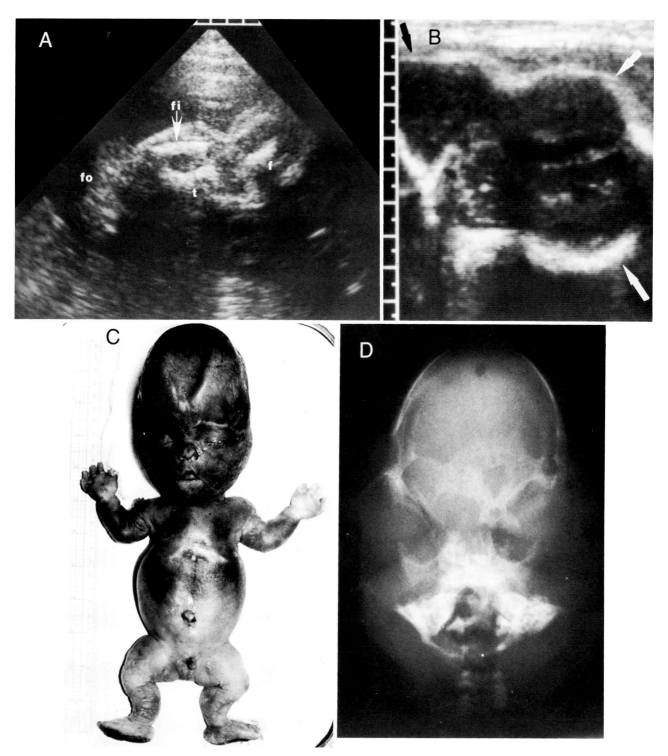

FIG 13–11.
Thanatophoric dysplasia with cloverleaf skull deformity at 26 weeks. **A,** sagittal scan of one lower extremity shows micromelia. **B,** the cloverleaf deformity of the skull *(arrows)* exhibits a tri-lobed appearance which renders head measurements inaccurate. The intact calvarium distinguishes the cloverleaf skull from encephalocele. The combination of severe dwarfism and cloverleaf skull deformity provides convincing prenatal evidence for thanatophoric dysplasia. **C,** postnatal photograph shows the limb shortening, small thorax, and skull deformity. **D,** postnatal skull radiograph of another fetus with thanatophoric dysplasia shows the characteristic tri-lobed appearance of the skull. *f* = femur; *t* = tibia; *fi* = fibula; *fo* = foot; *arrows* = cloverleaf skull.

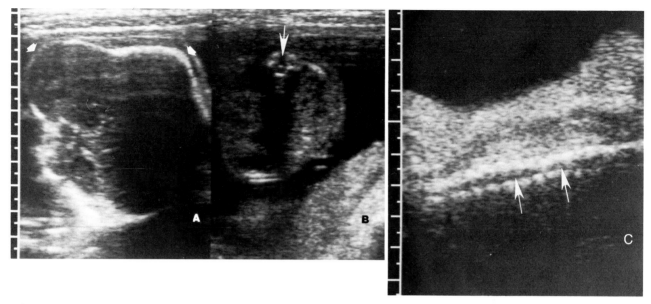

FIG 13–12.
Thanatophoric dysplasia with cloverleaf skull and narrow spinal canal. **A,** oblique scan of the head shows the typical tri-lobed cloverleaf deformity of the skull *(arrowheads).* Although the cloverleaf skull deformity may be present in a variety of syndromes and occurs in only a minority of fetuses with thanatophoric dysplasia, the combination of cloverleaf skull and dwarfism without familial risk indicates thanatophoric dysplasia. **B** and **C,** the spinal canal *(arrows)* of this fetus also appeared narrow on these axial **(B)** and coronal **(C)** views of the thoracolumbar spine, as described by Elaljede et al.[86] Platyspondyly (vertebral body flattening) is pathognomonic of thanatophoric dysplasia.

drome. On the other hand, the degree of subtlety created by hand and foot deformities does not correlate with the prognosis in many cases.

LETHAL DYSPLASIAS

Prior to the initial report of thanatophoric dysplasia in 1967, very little was known about the lethal skeletal dysplasias. With the exception of achondrogenesis, the dysplasias were erroneously categorized merely as achondroplasia or chondrodystrophy. Since that time, numerous disorders have been recognized and categorized, and many more remain unclassified. Thanatophoric dysplasia, achondrogenesis, and osteogenesis imperfecta account for the vast majority of cases with lethal short-limbed dysplasia seen prenatally. The remaining lethal cases occur only rarely, and new syndromes are frequently being described.

Thanatophoric Dysplasia

Clinical and Pathologic Findings

Thanatophoric dysplasia, probably the most common lethal dysplasia, occurs in approximately 1 in 4,000 to 1 in 15,000 births.[70, 75, 77, 93, 94] The term derives from the Greek, meaning "death bearing".[92] With few exceptions, reported cases of thanatophoric dys-

plasia have occurred sporadically, in which case the sonologist will be the first to detect the unexpected deformity.[18, 89]

Sonographic Findings

Approximately 50% of cases with thanatophoric dysplasia present with large-for-dates measurements secondary to polyhydramnios.[89] The most striking sonographic features, however, include marked extremity shortening and the cloverleaf skull deformity (Fig 13–11).[72, 76, 84, 86, 89, 91, 94, 98] The micromelia predominantly involves the proximal portions (rhizomelia), but the extremities are all markedly foreshortened. The cloverleaf skull (Kleeblattschadel) deformity results from premature craniosynostosis and creates a distinctive tri-lobed appearance. Hydrocephaly and cranial enlargement often accompany the cloverleaf skull deformity.[86, 97] The absence of calvarial defect distinguishes the cloverleaf skull deformity from encephalocele.[87, 91] Other features of thanatophoric dysplasia include bowed limbs with soft tissue redundancy, a narrow thorax, and flattened vertebral bodies (platyspondylisis) with a narrow spinal canal (Fig 13–12).[18, 76, 91] Although the platyspondylisis is a characteristic feature of thanatophoric dysplasia, it usually requires radiography for confirmation.[76]

Among 25 reported cases of thanatophoric dysplasia detected by prenatal sonography, all occurred spo-

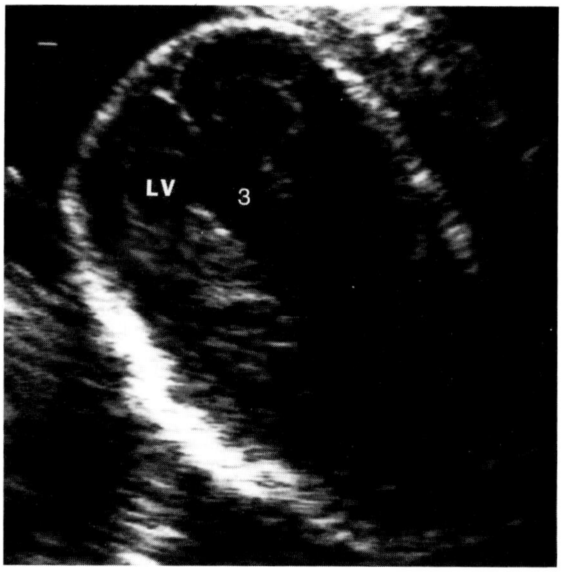

FIG 13–13.
Thanatophoric dysplasia with agenesis of the corpus callosum. Approximately 25% of thanatophoric dwarfs with cloverleaf skull deformity also have agenesis of the corpus callosum, as this coronal scan of the head shows at 25 weeks.[76, 97] *LV* = lateral cerebral ventricle; *3* = third cerebral ventricle. (From Pretorius DH, Rumack CM, Manco-Johnson ML, et al: Specific skeletal dysplasias in utero: Sonographic diagnosis. Radiology 1986; 159:237–242. Used by permission.)

radically and were detected between 16 and 36 menstrual weeks with severe micromelia.* Because of the absence of familial risk, most cases were scanned for obstetrical reasons, usually large-for-dates measurements during the third trimester of pregnancy. Six cases were detected during the second trimester, however, implying that screening ultrasonography can detect this abnormality at or prior to 24 weeks' gestation.[77, 79, 81, 82, 86, 97] Sixteen (64%) had a cloverleaf skull deformity, 16 (64%) had polyhydramnios, 5 (20%) had an unmistakably small thorax, and 4 (16%) had soft tissue redundancy. Four cases with the cloverleaf skull deformity also had agenesis of the corpus callosum (Fig 13–13).[76, 97] One case also described a narrow spinal canal with hypoplastic vertebrae[86]; we have seen a similar case and believe this feature may be a useful diagnostic finding.

The most useful finding that enables accurate prenatal diagnosis of thanatophoric dysplasia in the setting of severe micromelia is the presence of the cloverleaf skull deformity. Although this deformity only occurs in approximately 14% of cases with thanatophoric dysplasia and may occur with a variety of other non–dwarf syndromes, it occurs only in short-limbed dwarfs who have either thanatophoric dysplasia or homozygous achondroplasia.[80, 91] Since the parents of a fetus with homozygous achondroplasia are readily recognizable as achondroplastic dwarfs, whereas those of a thanatophoric are typically of normal stature, no confusion should exist between these two lethal syndromes.[90, 91] Detection of the cloverleaf skull deformity in a micromelic dwarf, therefore, permits accurate prenatal diagnosis of thanatophoric dysplasia.[91] This finding is also important because some authors suggest that thanatophoric dwarfism with the cloverleaf skull deformity may be transmitted in an autosomal recessive pattern, unlike the sporadic transmission of the dysplasia without the skull deformity.[86, 95]

In the absence of these characteristic features, other very rare lethal short-limbed dysplasias (fibrochondrogenesis, schneckenbecken dysplasia, atelosteogenesis, Torrance dysplasia, San Diego dysplasia, etc.) may mimic thanatophoric dysplasia and require postnatal radiographic and histologic evaluation for diagnosis.[88, 167, 174, 180] Nevertheless, the general rule holds true that severe micromelia carries a dire prognosis.

Achondrogenesis

Clinical and Pathologic Findings

Achondrogenesis occurs in approximately 1 in 40,000 births and represents probably the second most common lethal short-limbed dwarfism, although the exact incidence is not known.[70, 75, 108] Unlike the vast majority of cases with thanatophoric dysplasia, achondrogenesis is inherited as an autosomal recessive trait.[17, 18] Parents with a prior affected child, therefore, have a 25% chance of recurrence. However, the rarity of the syndrome dictates that most cases detected by the sonographer will probably not have a positive family history.

Disorganization of cartilage causes absence of normal bony architecture in achondrogenesis and results in the characteristic severely retarded or absent skeletal ossification with profound limb length reduction of all extremity tubular bones.[107] Vertebral body and sacral ossification is also typically absent or severely delayed, so that the fetus develops a short trunk and thorax.[107] The absence of vertebral body ossification permits unusually clear sonographic visualization of the relatively lucent spinal column on longitudinal scans even as early as the middle of the second trimester. Only two vertebral ossification centers per spinal segment are visible on cross-section scans of the spine.[76, 106]

Two types of achondrogenesis exist: Type I (Parenti-Fraccaro) and type II (Langer-Saldino).[17, 100] Three distinct prototypes of type II achondrogenesis

*72, 76, 77, 79, 81, 82, 84–87, 89, 91, 94, 96–98.

TABLE 13–11.

Classification and Sonographic Features of Achondrogenesis

Type	Prototype	% of Cases	Degree of Extremity Shortening	Rib Fractures	Calvarial Ossification	Vertebral Body Ossification
I		20	Severe	Yes	Poor	Poor
II						
	II	20	Severe	No	Good	Poor
	III	40	Moderate to severe	No	Good	Poor
	IV	20	Moderate	No	Good	Good

also occur (Table 13–11).[109] Approximately 80% of achondrogenesis is type II, and half of these cases are of one of the three prototypes.[109] Degrees of ossification vary among the different types and prototypes of achondrogenesis.[15, 109] For example, all type II achondrogenesis have normal calvarial ossification, but type I may have diminished calvarial mineralization.[15, 109] On the other hand, virtual absence of vertebral body ossification occurs in all types except prototype IV, in which the vertebral bodies may only be underdeveloped. In other words: All cases of achondrogenesis have diminished or absent vertebral body ossification except prototype IV (approximately 20% of cases); all cases of type II achondrogenesis (approximately 80% of cases) have normal calvarial ossification; and prototypes II and III (approximately 60% of achondrogenesis cases) have normal calvarial ossification but severely diminished or absent vertebral body ossification. Only prototype IV may have both normal calvarial and vertebral body ossification.

Although variable underdevelopment of the vertebral bodies may occur in other lethal dysplasias (thanatophoric dysplasia, homozygous achondroplasia, short-rib polydactyly), none of these have concomitant calvarial underossification.[15, 17] Furthermore, severe hypophosphatasia may also have severe delay in calvarial and spinal ossification (similar to type I achondrogenesis), but severe hypophosphatasia typically has diffuse underossification, in contrast to the more focal lack of ossification in achondrogenesis.[15, 17] Therefore, even though not all fetuses with achondrogenesis have absent vertebral body ossification and normal calvarial ossification, the combination of these two features serves to differentiate achondrogenesis from other lethal short-limbed dwarfs (Fig 13–14).[106]

Sonographic Findings

Among 15 reported cases of achondrogenesis detected with prenatal ultrasound to date, all had striking micromelia, and six (40%) were detected at 15–19

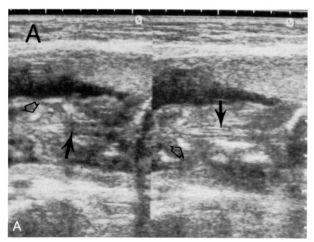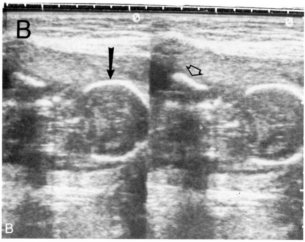

FIG 13–14.

Achondrogenesis at 19 weeks. **A,** absence of spinal ossification permits abnormally clear visualization of the spinal column on these dual-image coronal scans of the trunk. *Solid arrows* = spinal column; *open arrows* = ossified iliac ala. **B,** the calvarial ossification is normal, but the extremity bones are shortened on this dual-image scan of the head, upper arm, and thorax. Although not all fetuses with achondrogenesis have each of these features (absent spinal ossification, normal calvarial ossification, and micromelia), this combination of findings distinguishes achondrogenesis. *Solid arrow* = calvarium; *open arrow* = humerus. (From Mahony BS, Filly RA, Cooperberg PL: Antenatal sonographic diagnosis of achondrogenesis. J Ultrasound Med 1984; 3:333–335. Used by permission.)

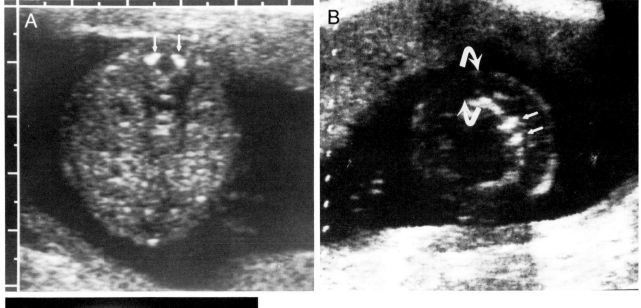

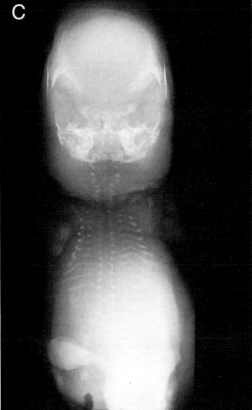

FIG 13–15.
Achondrogenesis with absent vertebral body ossification. **A** and **B,** these axial scans through the abdomen and pelvis in two different fetuses show ossification of the posterior elements but complete absence of vertebral body ossification. **C,** postmortem radiograph confirms the prenatal findings. *Straight arrows* = posterior element ossification; *curved arrows* = soft tissue redundancy. (Parts B and C from Pretorius DH, Rumack CM, Manco-Johnson ML, et al: Specific skeletal dysplasias in utero: Sonographic diagnosis. Radiology 1986; 159:237–242. Used by permission.)

TABLE 13-12.

Classification and Sonographic Features of Osteogenesis Imperfecta

Type	Usual Inheritance Pattern	Typical Prenatal Sonographic Features			Usual Outcome
		Bone Shortening	Fractures	Bone Echogenicity	
I	Autosomal dominant	No	Isolated in 5% of cases; otherwise none	Normal	Good; deafness in 35%
IIA	Autosomal dominant; many new mutations	Severe	Innumerable	± Decreased	Lethal
IIB	Autosomal recessive	Moderate of femur only	Numerous	Normal	Lethal
IIC	Autosomal recessive	Moderate of all extremity bones	Numerous	Normal	Lethal
III	Autosomal recessive	Moderate of femur only	Numerous	± Decreased	Severe handicaps
IV	Autosomal dominant	No	Occasional, isolated	Normal	Good

weeks on the basis of sonographic findings obtained because of a positive family history for the disorder.* In 13 (87%) cases vertebral body ossification was noted to be decreased or absent, and in 3 of these cases the calvarial ossification was noted to be normal, whereas 5 other cases had decreased calvarial ossification and 1 had both normal calvarial and vertebral ossification (Fig 13-15). In the 6 remaining cases the calvarial ossification was not noted. Additional findings included a narrow thorax (6 cases; 40%), deformed extremity bones (5 cases; 33%), polyhydramnios (7 cases; 47%), and hydrops fetalis (5 cases; 33%). As with thanatophoric dysplasia and other lethal dysplasias with severe micromelia, soft tissue redundancy may erroneously produce the appearance of subcutaneous edema in the absence of true hydrops fetalis.[106]

Osteogenesis Imperfecta

Clinical and Pathologic Findings

Osteogenesis imperfecta encompasses a group of clinically and genetically heterogeneous disorders involving defective collagen and predominantly characterized by repeated fractures of brittle bones.[111, 112, 133-135] Although the classification of osteogenesis imperfecta frequently changes, the Sillence classification, first proposed in 1979 with subsequent modifications, is probably the most widely accepted (Table 13-12).[111, 133] Among the four main groups, this classification recognizes two severe or lethal types (II and III) and two relatively mild forms (I and IV).

Types I and IV are further divided into A and B subtypes, based upon the presence or absence of dentinogenesis imperfecta, and type II is also divided into subtypes A, B, and C. Type III may only represent a heterogeneous subtype of type IIB.[132, 133]

Type II osteogenesis imperfecta accounts for the majority of cases of osteogenesis imperfecta detected with prenatal ultrasound. Among 33 sonographic reports of osteogenesis imperfecta detected prenatally to date, 20 (61%) had type II.* Although not specifically stated, the majority (approximately 80%) of these reported cases probably involved type IIA. Type IIA osteogenesis imperfecta, the classical subtype with innumerable fractures, severe extremity shortening ("accordian" or "telescoped" bones), and decreased bone echogenicity occurs with a frequency of approximately 1 in 60,000 births, with most cases arising as a new mutation and only occasional autosomal dominant or rare autosomal recessive recurrences (Fig 13-16).[128, 133]

Most cases (14 of 20 or 70%) of type II osteogenesis imperfecta have been detected in the absence of familial risk for recurrence. This is especially true of type IIA in which only two (10%) cases had a stated positive family history.[116, 136] Other stated findings or reasons for scanning included small-for-dates with intrauterine growth retardation (six cases), large-for-dates with polyhydramnios (three cases), screening ultrasonography (three cases), and premature rupture of membranes (one case). The diagnosis of lethal osteogen-

*19, 74, 76, 101, 104, 105, 106, 108.

*76, 77, 111, 114, 116, 117, 119-121, 124-126, 131, 135, 136, 139, 140.

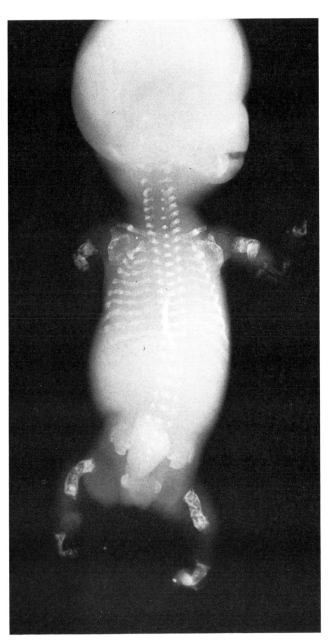

FIG 13–16.
Osteogenesis imperfecta, type IIA. Representative postmortem photograph of osteogenesis imperfecta type IIA illustrates the innumerable fractures with limb shortening ("accordian effect") and angulation. Also note the irregular contour of the ribs secondary to the numerous fractures.

esis imperfecta was suggested as early as 13.5 weeks and made definitively as early as 15 weeks.[111, 136] Since many cases were scanned for obstetrical reasons, however, the diagnosis frequently was not rendered until the third trimester or during labor. As expected, none of these fetuses survived.

The features of type IIB osteogenesis imperfecta include moderately shortened femurs with visible iso-

lated fractures. This is a severe, but not necessarily lethal syndrome. The sonographic distinction between type IIB and IIC osteogenesis imperfecta is quite subtle, but the lethal type IIC has shortening of all limbs, unlike the isolated femoral shortening of type IIB (Fig 13–17).[133] Furthermore, the distinction between type IIB and type III also is quite subtle.

Sonographic Findings

The classical sonographic features of type IIA osteogenesis imperfecta include the following (Figs 13–18 to 13–21):

1. Severe micromelia with deformity (sharp angulation or bowing) and apparent thickening of the limb bones, probably secondary to numerous fractures with the exuberant callus formation typical of this disorder. Because of the exuberant callus, one rarely visualizes the fracture lines.

2. Diffuse hypomineralization characterized by decreased echogenicity of the skeleton with abnormally increased transmission of the ultrasound beam through the skeleton indicative of diffuse hypomineralization. Skull hypomineralization permits abnormally clear visualization of the brain and ventricular system because of the absence of reverberation artifact as the sound beam penetrates the fetal head and may lead to the impression of "pseudo-hydrocephalus." The calvarium also may be abnormally compressible.

3. Multiple rib fractures with collapse of the thoracic cage.

Based upon reported or described sonographic findings, only four fetuses identified with type II osteogenesis imperfecta probably had subtype B or C detected, and in each case a positive family history signaled the sonologist to examine the extremities in detail.[111, 119, 126] This is not surprising, given the fact that the prenatal manifestations of types IIB and IIC are much less obvious than are those of type IIA. Three of the four cases of type IIB reported to date were diagnosed prior to 24 weeks, and the fourth was not examined until 29 weeks; each case was electively terminated based upon the sonographic findings and familial history.

Although the distinctions between type IIB and type III osteogenesis imperfecta are quite subtle, three of four sonographic reports of type III osteogenesis imperfecta describe decreased echogenicity of the extremity bones, unlike the normal echogenicity of type IIB.[110, 111, 119, 129] Three cases of recurrent type III osteogenesis imperfecta were diagnosed at 15–19 weeks on the basis of extremity shortening with isolated frac-

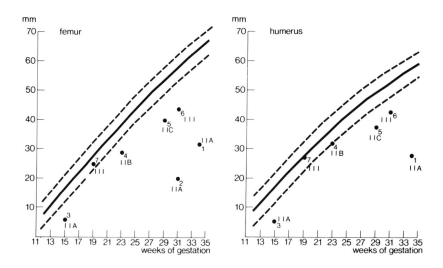

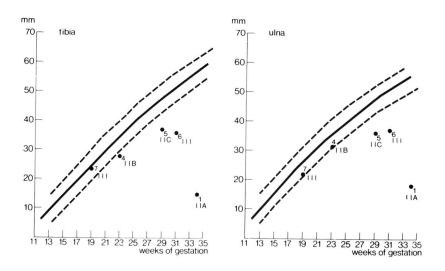

FIG 13–17.

Variations of the degree of extremity bone shortening among the different types of osteogenesis imperfecta. These graphs correlate the lengths of the femur, humerus, tibia, and ulna with gestational age and show that fetuses with types IIB, IIC, and III tend to have mild-to-moderate extremity bone shortening, whereas type IIA typically has severe micromelia. (From Brons JTJ, van der Harten HJ, Wladimiroff JW, et al: Prenatal ultrasonographic diagnosis of osteogenesis imperfecta. Am J Obstet Gynecol 1988; 159:176–181. Used by permission.)

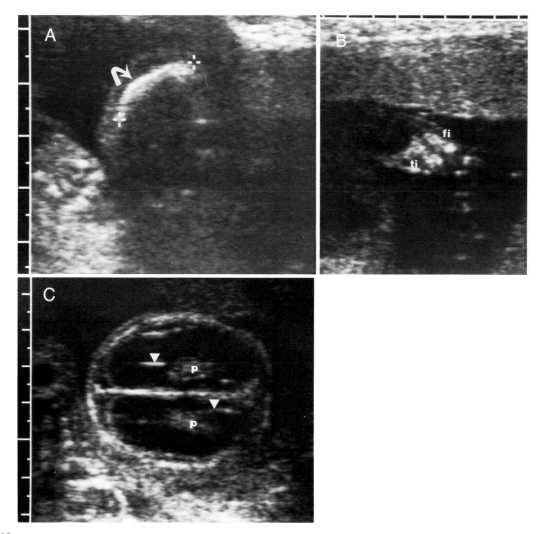

FIG 13–18.
Osteogenesis imperfecta, type IIA, at 19 weeks. **A,** the femur *(curved arrow)* is short and curved. **B,** the tibia and fibula are also short, relatively thickened, and of decreased echogenicity on this coronal scan of the lower leg. *ti* = tibia; *fi* = fibula. **C,** poor calvarial mineralization produces "pseudohydrocephalus", but documentation that the choroid plexus fills the bodies of the lateral ventricles confirms the absence of ventricular dilatation. *P* = choroid plexus; *arrowheads* = lateral ventricular walls. *(Continued.)*

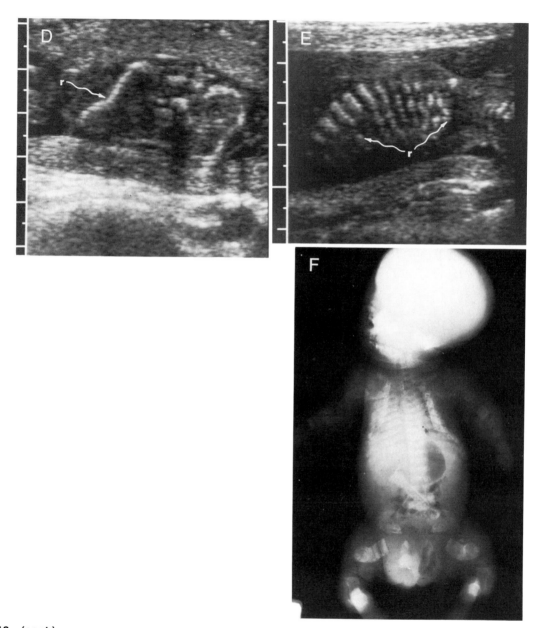

FIG 13–18   (cont.).
D, axial scan of the thorax demonstrates characteristic concavity of the rib cage from multiple rib fractures. *r* = rib. **E,** sagittal scan of the thorax also shows multiple rib deformities with decreased rib echogenicity indicating multiple fractures. *r* = ribs. **F,** postnatal radiograph confirms the prenatal findings.

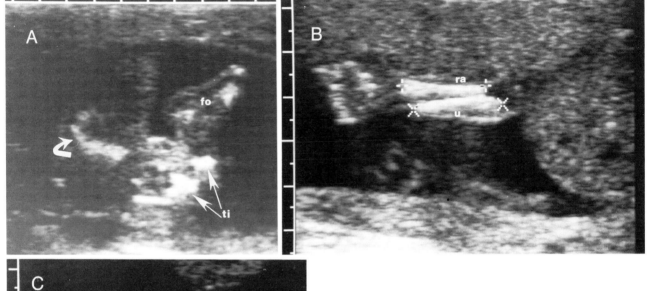

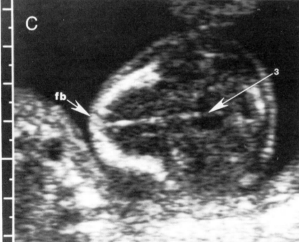

FIG 13–19.
Osteogenesis imperfecta, type IIA, at 18 weeks with some bones appearing relatively normal. **A,** this longitudinal scan of the lower extremity shows that the femur and tibia are short, angulated and relatively thickened. A displaced tibial fracture results in gross deformity. *Curved arrow* = femur; *ti* = tibia; *fo* = foot. **B,** the radius and ulna appear normal on this scan of the forearm. *ra* = radius; *u* = ulna. **C,** only the frontal bone is ossified on this axial scan of the head. *fb* = frontal bone; *3* = non–dilated third ventricle.
(Continued.)

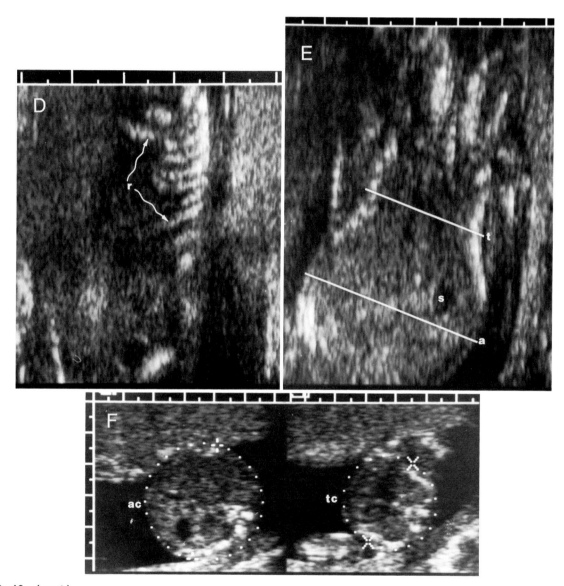

FIG 13–19 (cont.).
D, the ribs are poorly ossified with multiple fracture deformities demonstrated on this sagittal scan of the thorax. *r* = ribs. **E,** the thorax is small, as shown in this coronal scan of the anterior thorax and trunk. *t* = thoracic diameter; *a* = abdominal diameter; *s* = stomach. **F,** this dual-image scan confirms that the thoracic circumference (9 cm) is small relative to the abdominal circumference (12.1 cm); *tc* = thoracic circumference; *ac* = abdominal circumference.

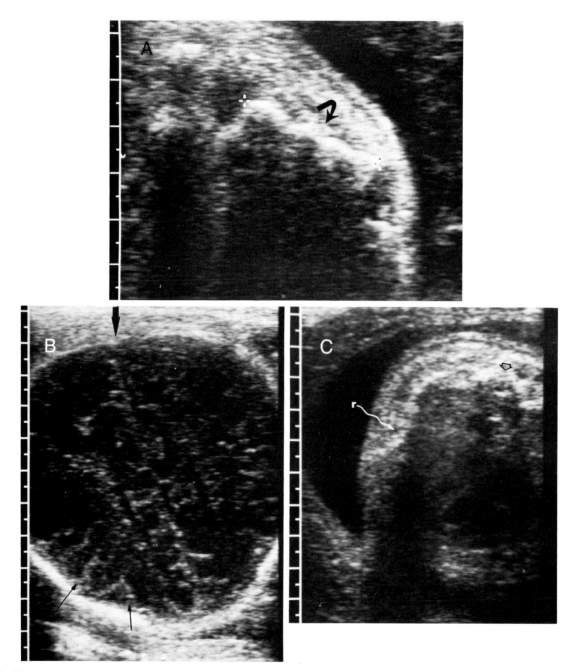

FIG 13–20.
Osteogenesis imperfecta, type IIA, during the third trimester. **A,** the femur *(curved arrow)* is short, relatively thick, and has a wavy appearance, probably secondary to the "accordian" effect of numerous fractures with exuberant callus formation. No discrete fractures are evident. **B,** the poor calvarial ossification permits abnormally clear visualization of the peripheral sulci and gyri of the brain *(small arrows)*. Also the calvarium may be compressible by gentle external pressure *(large arrow)*. **C,** concavity of the thoracic rib cage is a characterisitc feature of this disorder. *r* = rib; *open arrow* = spine.

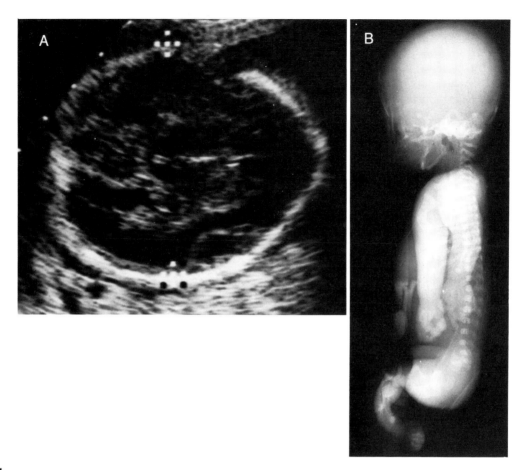

FIG 13–21.
Osteogenesis imperfecta with apparently normal calvarial ossification at 22 weeks. **A,** prenatal axial sonogram of the head at the level of the biparietal diameter *(graticules)* shows apparently normal ossification. **B,** however, postnatal radiograph shows almost complete absence of calvarial ossification. One cannot exclude poor ossification in osteogenesis imperfecta, since the degree of ossification necessary to produce a normal-appearing sonogram is not determined. (From Pretorius DH, Rumack CM, Manco-Johnson ML et al: Specific skeletal dysplasias in utero: Sonographic diagnosis. Radiology 1986; 159:237–242. Used by permission.)

tures, and two of these also described decreased extremity bone echogenicity[110, 111]. Each of these was electively terminated. The fourth case of type III osteogenesis imperfecta did not have a family history of the disorder and was not evaluated until 31 weeks but also showed decreased bone echogenicity, extremity shortening, and isolated fractures but normal ribs.[111] Although this fetus died at birth, type III osteogenesis imperfecta is described as having a severe, but not necessarily lethal prognosis.

Other Lethal Short-Limbed Dwarf Syndromes

Especially in the presence of a positive family history for a recurrent dysplasia, prenatal sonography also can detect a variety of other rare, lethal short-limbed dwarf syndromes. In the absence of familial risk, sonographic features of these syndromes often would be ex-

pected to be detectable but probably not distinctive enough in most cases to permit a specific antenatal diagnosis.

Campomelic Syndrome

Clinical and Pathologic Findings

The campomelic syndrome occurs with a frequency of approximately 1 in 150,000 births and probably recurs as an autosomal recessive trait, although most cases occur sporadically.[70, 75, 144] Like many other skeletal dysplasias, it probably includes a heterogeneous group of disorders, with some cases being more severely affected than others.[143–145] The campomelic syndrome has been considered to be uniformly lethal, but in a review of 97 reported cases Houston et al. described 6 patients who survived beyond 1 month of age and 3 documented to be alive beyond 1 year, with

1 case alive at 17 years.[18, 144] The non-survivors tended to have more severe manifestations of the syndrome than the survivors.

The characteristic features of campomelic ("bent bone") dysplasia include ventral bowing of shortened tibiae and femora with severe talipes equinovarus, absent or hypoplastic fibulae, hypoplastic pedicles of the thoracic vertebrae, and extremely small scapulae.[2, 17, 18, 143, 144] The ventral bowing of the tibiae and femora probably results from a primary shortness of the calf and hamstring musculature which, in turn, leads to the talipes equinovarus deformity.[144, 146] Especially in the setting of familial risk, the long bone changes and scapular hypoplasia should be visible prenatally. Affected fetuses also frequently have midthoracic scoliosis, cleft palate, cerebral ventricular dilatation, pyelocaliectasis, and congenital heart disease but die of complications from laryngotracheomalacia.[144]

Sonographic Findings

Among eight cases of campomelic syndrome seen with prenatal ultrasound to date, three were evaluated at 17–22 weeks because of familial risk, and recurrence was documented prior to elective termination (Fig 13–22).[73, 76, 141, 142, 144, 147] The described sonographic features in these cases included ventral bowing of shortened tibiae and femora with predominant involvement of the tibiae. One case had absent fibulae and another had hydrocephaly.[142, 147] None of these reports described the characteristic scapular or foot changes. Among the remaining five cases, none occurred in the setting of familial risk, and in each case the diagnosis was not made until postmortem examination. The non-diagnostic findings in these cases included polyhydramnios (four cases), oligohydramnios (one case), shortened femurs (two cases), decreased vertebral body ossification (one case), and bowed lower extremity bones (one case; subtle at 22 weeks but obvious at 36 weeks).

Chondrodysplasia Punctata—Rhizomelic Type

Clinical and Pathologic Findings

The rhizomelic type of chondrodysplasia punctata occurs in approximately 1 in 110,000 births and results in neonatal death or severe mental retardation with death in early childhood.[70, 148] It usually is inherited in an autosomal recessive manner.[18, 149, 150]

Sonographic Findings

Certain features of the rhizomelic form of chondrodysplasia punctata may manifest on the prenatal sonogram and permit confident antenatal diagnosis in a fetus at risk for recurrence.[2, 17, 18] The syndrome results in severe micromelia, especially of the humeri but also of the femora with multiple joint contractures. In the absence of familial risk, the severity of the symmetric rhizomelic shortening helps to distinguish this entity from others with less severe rhizomelia and a variable prognosis (i.e., heterozygous achondroplasia and asphyxiating thoracic dystrophy). Furthermore, late in the third trimester the characteristic stippling of the humeral and femoral cartilaginous epiphyses may be visible, although epiphyseal stippling is not present in all cases (Fig 13–23).[148] The vertebral bodies in chondrodysplasia punctata (rhizomelic type) have distinctive ventral and dorsal ossification centers separated by a bar of cartilage which might be detectable sonographically.[17]

Congenital Hypophosphatasia

Clinical and Pathologic Findings

Congenital (lethal) hypophosphatasia, which recurs in an autosomal recessive manner probably with more than one allele, is a rare inborn error of metabolism characterized by abnormal bone mineralization with a deficiency of alkaline phosphatase.[151, 153, 155] The incidence is approximately 1 in 100,000 births.[153, 154]

Sonographic Findings

Among reported cases of congenital hypophosphatasia detected with prenatal sonography to date, all occurred in fetuses with a 25% recurrence risk.[74, 151, 153, 155, 157] Five of six cases were detected on initial sonography at 14–16 weeks with subsequent elective termination and, one was not seen until 36 weeks' gestation but died at birth. Two other cases at risk had normal sonograms at 14–18 weeks and subsequently delivered normal newborns.[152, 153]

The sonographic features of congenital hypophosphatasia include moderate to severe micromelia and diffuse hypomineralization, the degree of which may resemble that in osteogenesis imperfecta IIA. However, in contrast to the thickened bones of osteogenesis imperfecta IIA, the extremity bones in congenital hypophosphatasia tend to be delicate or may even be absent. Early sonographic reports described the inability of ultrasound to define the fetal head in congenital hypophosphatasia.[151, 153] Improved resolution and real-time scanning should show the fetal head to be present but with an absent or thin and poorly echogenic calvarium which is easily compressible. One case also showed concomitant oligohydramnios and arthrogryposis at 16 weeks.[157]

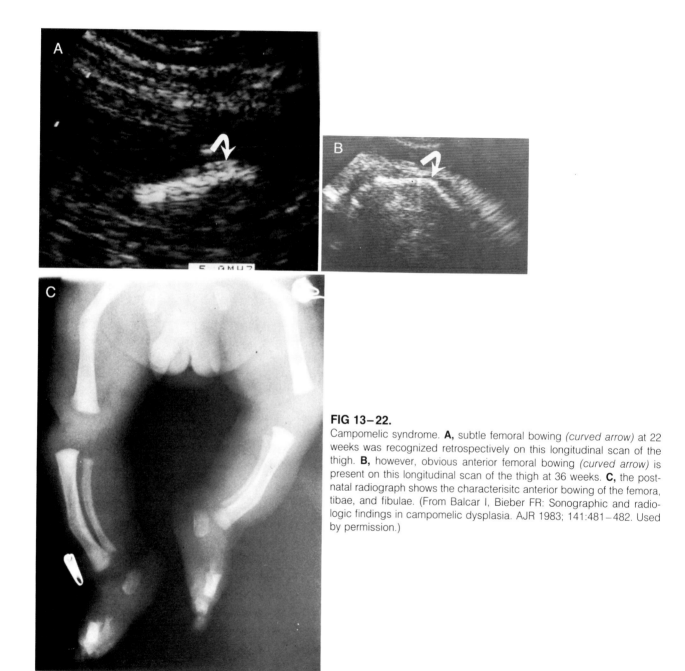

FIG 13–22.
Campomelic syndrome. **A,** subtle femoral bowing *(curved arrow)* at 22 weeks was recognized retrospectively on this longitudinal scan of the thigh. **B,** however, obvious anterior femoral bowing *(curved arrow)* is present on this longitudinal scan of the thigh at 36 weeks. **C,** the post-natal radiograph shows the characterisitc anterior bowing of the femora, tibae, and fibulae. (From Balcar I, Bieber FR: Sonographic and radio-logic findings in campomelic dysplasia. AJR 1983; 141:481–482. Used by permission.)

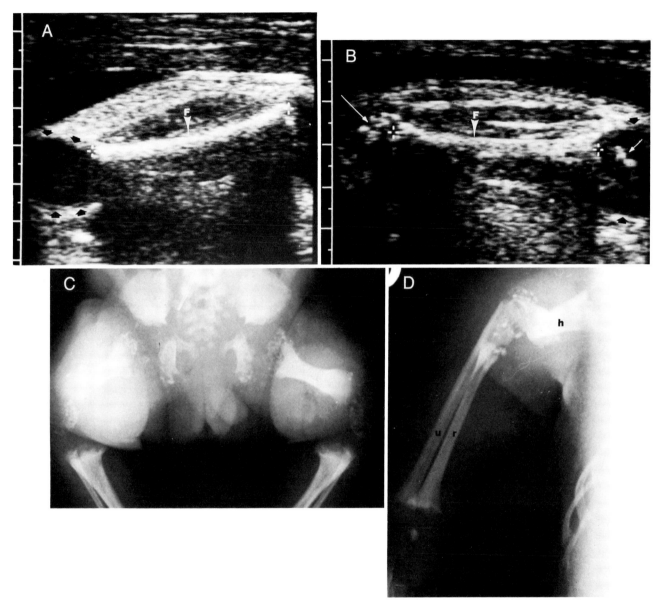

FIG 13–23.
Chondrodysplasia punctata, rhizomelic form, at 37 weeks. **A** and **B,** longitudinal scans of the femur show large epiphyseal cartilages *(black arrows)* with stippled calcification *(white arrows)*. The femora measured 51 mm in length (mean for 27 wks). The humeri measured only 30 mm (mean for 20 wks) and also showed similar epiphyseal findings. Other extremity bone lengths were normal. *F* = femur. **C** and **D,** postnatal radiographs of the lower limbs **(C)** and upper limb **(D)** confirm the prenatal findings. *r* = radius; *u* = ulna; *h* = humerus.

Homozygous Dominant Achondroplasia

Homozygous dominant achondroplasia may manifest many of the same features as thanatophoric dysplasia including severe micromelia and cloverleaf skull.[90, 158] Since it occurs only in the setting of at least one parent (and usually both parents) being affected with heterozygous achondroplasia, homozygous achondroplasia is rare and should be readily distinguishable from thanatophoric dysplasia.[90, 158] The micromelia of homozygous achondroplasia occurs earlier in gestation and to a much more severe degree than with heterozygous achondroplasia. One case seen at approximately 18 weeks already had micromelia.[158]

Short-Rib Polydactyly Syndrome

Clinical and Pathologic Findings

Short-rib polydactyly syndrome, another rare and lethal skeletal dysplasia with several different types is probably inherited in an autosomal recessive manner.[159, 164, 166] Characteristic features include micromelia, short ribs with a narrow thorax, and polydactyly with frequent cardiovascular or genitourinary anomalies, especially cystic renal dysplasia.[159, 164, 166] Three different types have been recognized with additional variants.[163] The distinguishing features among the three types are as follows: The Saldino-Noonan type has narrow metaphyses; the Majewski type has cleft lip/cleft palate and disproportionately shortened tibiae; and the Naumoff-type has wide metaphyses with spurs.[163, 165]

These distinctions, while real, are of little clinical utility to the sonographer since in most cases a positive family history will signal a careful search for recurrence. In the absence of familial risk, the features may not be sufficiently outstanding to permit distinction among the types of the syndrome. Nevertheless, the severity and distribution of abnormalities help to distinguish the short-rib polydactyly syndrome from other entities.[159, 163, 166] For example, the micromelia and narrow chest resemble thanatophoric dysplasia, but polydactyly is not a feature of thanatophoric dwarfism. On the other hand, chondroectodermal dysplasia exhibits limb shortening, a small thorax, and polydactly, but the severity of involvement is much less severe than in short-rib polydactyly.[163] Similarly, asphyxiating thoracic dysplasia may resemble chondroectodermal dysplasia, but the limb shortening is only mild-to-moderate and occurs in only 60% of cases, and polydactyly occurs in only 14% of cases.[164]

Sonographic Findings

Among reported cases of short-rib polydactyly detected prenatally to date, all but one were recurrences detected at 16–23 weeks prior to elective termination or fetal demise in pregnancies at risk for the disorder.[78, 160, 161–163, 165, 166] Two cases of recurrent Saldino-Noonan type had severe oligohydramnios which precluded adequate extremity visualization, whereas three cases of Majewski type each had severe micromelia and a very narrow thorax. Polydactyly was seen in one of the cases of Majewski type and polyhydramnios in another. One case without familial risk for recurrence showed marked micromelia with flared metaphyses, narrow chest, and polydactyly (Fig 13–24).[163] On the basis of these sonographic findings the diagnosis of Naumoff-type short-rib polydactyly was made and confirmed on postmortem examination. This fetus also had hydrops fetalis and hypoplastic vertebral bodies detected prenatally.

Other Very Rare Lethal Dysplasias

Numerous other rare lethal dysplasias may occur prenatally. The following discussion lists several of these, especially those seen sonographically. It is not meant to be a comprehensive list but provides an indication of the magnitude and diversity of rare possibilities. Numerous cases of lethal dwarfism remain unclassified, and many more dysplasias undoubtedly will be described.[174] Although affected cases exhibit severe manifestations readily apparent sonographically that indicate a severe problem, definitive diagnosis usually is made at postmortem examination.

Atelosteogenesis[168, 176].—This generalized chondrodysplasia affects endochondral bone formation and mineralization and results in severe micromelia, especially involving the rhizomelic portions. One case at 31 weeks documented severe micromelia with visualization of only one bone in each lower extremity and none in the upper extremities in a fetus with a frontal cephalocele and polyhydramnios.[168] Atelosteogenesis was diagnosed on postmortem examination.

Boomerang dysplasia[175].—Three cases of this rare dysplasia have been reported, all males with normal siblings. Ultrasound at 28 weeks in one case showed a possible achondrogenesis syndrome. Postmortem examination showed diffuse hypomineralization and only two extremity long bones, both of which were bowed like a boomerang.

De la Chapelle dysplasia[181].—Three cases in one family and one additional sporadic case had this lethal entity, characterized by micromelia, short thorax, equinovarus deformity, and cleft palate. It has not been detected with prenatal ultrasound. However, Elejalde

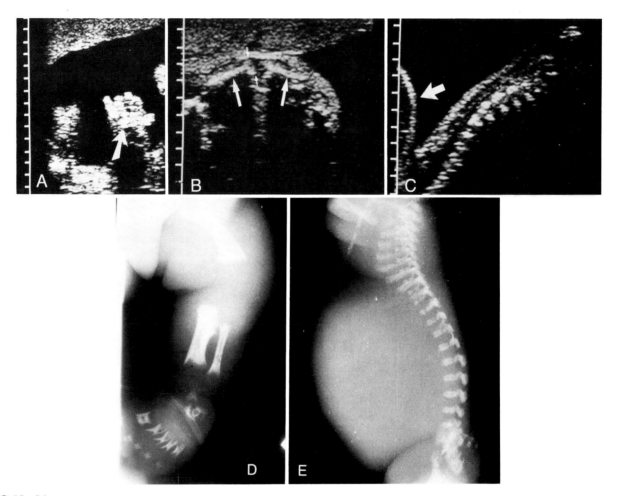

FIG 13–24.
Naumoff-type short-rib polydactyly syndrome. **A,** scan of the hand shows polydactyly. The arrow points to the folded sixth finger. **B,** this scan shows severe micromelia with widened metaphyses, and marginal spurs. Other scans showed polyhydramnios, small thorax, hyperextension of the neck, hypoplastic vertebral bodies, and hydrops. *Large arrows* = femur (left) and tibia (right); *small arrows* = widened distal femoral metaphysis with marginal spurs. **C,** sagittal scan of the thoracic and cervical spine shows hyperextension of the neck and hypoplastic vertebral bodies. Other scans showed a small thorax, polyhydramnios hypoplastic vertebral bodies and hydrops. *Arrow* = occiput. **D,** postmortem radiograph of the lower extremity displays the micromelia with widened metaphyses and marginal spurs. **E,** postmortem radiograph of the spine demonstrates hypoplastic vertebral bodies and short ribs. (From Meizner I, Bar-Ziv J: Prenatal ultrasonic diagnosis of short-rib polydactyly syndrome (SRPD) type III: A case report and a proposed approach to the diagnosis of SRPD and related conditions. J Clin Ultrasound 1985; 13:284–287. Used by permission.)

et al. suggest that the Weyers' syndrome may represent the same entity as de la Chapelle dysplasia.[169] They describe a case at 19 weeks of a fetus at genetic risk for the Weyers' syndrome with sonographically detected micromelia, especially involving the ulnae and fibulae, small thorax, and bilateral hydronephrosis with oligohydramnios.

Dyssegmental dysplasia[171, 173].—This rare, lethal entity is characterized by micromelic, thick, and bowed extremity bones and marked disorganization of the vertebral bodies with segmentation defects. A case with autosomal recessive recurrence examined at 18 weeks showed marked micromelia, with decreased echogenicity of extremity bones and vertebral bodies

as well as angulation of the spine and irregular narrowing of the spinal canal prior to elective termination.[173]

Fibrochondrogenesis[170, 180].—This rare, lethal autosomal recessive entity has not been reported on prenatal ultrasound. Its sonographic features would be expected to resemble thanatophoric dysplasia.

Jarcho-Levin syndrome[178, 179].—Spondylothoracic dysostosis type I is a rare autosomal recessive entity characterized by multiple vertebral and rib defects resulting in a constricted, short thorax and respiratory death in infancy. Since extremity lengths are normal, it is not a short-limbed dwarfism. The characteristic "crab-like" configuration of the trunk has permitted prenatal sonographic diagnosis at 17–20 weeks in two cases at risk for recurrence and in an additional sporadic case at 23 weeks.[178, 179] Each of these pregnancies was electively terminated. However, sonography did not detect the features of Jarco-Levin syndrome in a recurrent case examined at 10, 18, 30, and 38 weeks' gestation that died at birth.[177]

Schneckenbecken dysplasia[167].—This lethal dysplasia resembles thanatophoric dysplasia in degree of severity but has a characteristic snail-like radiographic appearance of the pelvis. It has not been detected with prenatal ultrasound.

DYSPLASIAS WITHOUT A UNIFORMLY LETHAL PROGNOSIS

With inevitable exceptions, the dysplasias with a variable or good prognosis (or at least one which is not almost uniformly lethal in early infancy) tend to present later in gestation and with milder features than the uniformly lethal syndromes. For this reason, the sensitivity and specificity of sonography for detection of many of the nonlethal dysplasias would be expected to be quite low, especially in the absence of familial risk and before 24 weeks, when many parents request accurate diagnosis. Probably for these reasons (and, perhaps, reporting bias), far fewer reports of sonographic detection of nonlethal dysplasias exist than of lethal dysplasias.

Nevertheless, many dysplasias with a relatively good prognosis potentially create sonographic findings prior to the third trimester, and some of these might exhibit distinctive characteristics to enable definitive diagnosis, even in the absence of familial risk. The following discussion concerns the expected sonographic features of these osteochondrodysplasias (see Table 13–10).

Heterozygous Achondroplasia

Clinical and Pathologic Findings

Heterozygous achondroplasia is a relatively common dysplasia caused by retardation of endochondral bone formation and is compatible with normal life span and mentation.[17, 186] Its exact prevalence is difficult to ascertain, because in the past many short-limbed dysplasias were erroneously categorized as heterozygous achondroplasia, but heterozygous achodroplasia probably occurs in approximately 1 in 30,000 births.[70, 77] Approximately 80% of cases result

from a spontaneous mutation, with the remainder being inherited in an autosomal dominant mode.[18] The cardinal signs of heterozygous achondroplasia postnatally include moderate rhizomelic shortening, a large calvarium but small skull base, saddle-nose deformity, thoracolumbar kyphosis with lack of normal increase in interpedicular distance caudally, squared-off iliac wings, and relatively short proximal and middle phalanges (trident hands).[2, 17, 18]

Sonographic Findings

A surprising paucity of reports documents the sonographic appearance of heterozygous achondroplasia prenatally.[72, 183, 186, 187] The prenatal reports concentrate on the discrepancy between head size and femur length, which becomes progressively more apparent during the third trimester (Fig 13–25).

In seven affected fetuses scanned during the second and third trimesters because one parent was affected by heterozygous achondroplasia, the fetal femur lengths became progressively more disproportionately shortened relative to the biparietal diameter.[186] Affected fetuses had a normal femur length relative to bi-

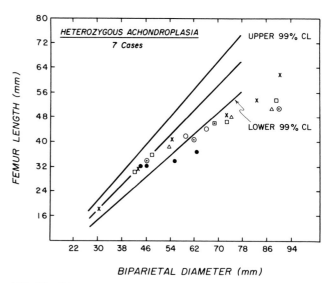

FIG 13–25.
Femur length vs. biparietal diameter in recurrent heterozygous achodroplasia. Graph compares the femur length and biparietal diameter in seven cases of recurrent heterozygous achondroplasia and illustrates the characteristic progressive shortening of the femur length relative to the biparietal diameter during the second and third trimesters. The femur length falls below the 99% confidence limit *(CL)* by the time the biparietal diameter corresponds with approximately 27 menstrual weeks. The symbols on the graph indicate individual cases seen at advancing stages of gestation. (From Kurtz AB, Filly RA, Wapner RJ, et al: In utero analysis of heterozygous achondroplasia: Variable time of onset as detected by femur length measurements. J Ultrasound Med 1986; 5:137–140. Used by permission.)

parietal diameter when initially scanned, but in all affected fetuses the femur length fell below the 99% confidence limit for a biparietal diameter corresponding to approximately 27 weeks. Although not specifically stated as such, this progressive discrepancy during the third trimester presumably resulted from less than anticipated femoral growth rather than from abnormal head enlargement. No other findings were apparent. The absence of this discrepant growth pattern helps to exclude recurrence, but one cannot exclude heterozygous achondroplasia on the basis of a normal femur length prior to approximately 27 weeks.[77, 182, 183, 186]

We have also seen two additional cases of heterozygous achondroplasia that fit this growth pattern, one of which was a recurrent case and the other was a spontaneous mutation with clearly defined saddle-nose deformity. In the absence of an affected parent with heterozygous achondroplasia, on the other hand, other cases have shown this same growth pattern. One case proved to be asphyxiating thoracic dysplasia, and another had short stature in the absence of classical heterozygous achondroplasia. Therefore, although the correlation between biparietal diameter and femur length provides reliable evidence for presence or absence of recurrent heterozygous achondroplasia when the fetus carries a 50% chance of being affected, in the absence of this recurrence risk we caution against the relative lack of specificity of the biparietal diameter-femur length graph. We speculate that some of these cases may represent hypochondroplasia or pseudo-achondroplasia, which resemble achondroplasia but with milder features.[184, 185, 188, 190, 191] In one reported case of hypochondroplasia detected prenatally of a fetus at risk for recurrence, the femur lengths were normal during the mid-second trimester but unequivocally abnormal by the end of the second trimester.[189]

Asphyxiating Thoracic Dysplasia

Clinical and Pathologic Findings

Asphyxiating thoracic dysplasia (Jeune's syndrome) occurs with a prevalence of approximately 1 in 70,000 births and recurs by autosomal recessive transmission, but the phenotype manifests with variable expressivity.[17, 18, 70] Consequently, the clinical manifestations vary widely from perinatal death from respiratory failure to latent phenotypes without respiratory symptoms and a good prognosis.[18] The characteristic features include mild-to-moderate rhizomelic limb shortening, small thorax, and renal dysplasia.[17, 18, 166] Approximately 14% of cases also have polydactyly.[164] In cases with a positive family history, the 25% recurrence risk alerts the sonologist to search for these features.

Sonographic Findings

Among five cases of asphyxiating thoracic dysplasia detected with prenatal ultrasound to date, four were detected at 16–23 weeks in fetuses at 25% risk for the disorder based upon family history.[193, 195–198] Each of these affected pregnancies was electively terminated following detection of mild-to-moderate limb shortening with rhizomelic predominance. In three cases a narrow chest was detected prenatally, and one case also had severe oligohydramnios, probably from renal dysplasia.[197] Two affected fetuses scanned sequentially during the second trimester both had borderline short femora at 16–17 weeks, but the femoral lengths fell progressively below the 99% confidence limit relative to the biparietal diameter at 19–23 weeks.[195, 196] One additional case with probable asphyxiating thoracic dysplasia or chondroectodermal dysplasia but without reported familial risk had moderate rhizomelic shortening, a narrow chest, and polyhydramnios at 34 weeks' gestation.[198] This fetus died at birth.

We have followed an additional case of asphyxiating thoracic dysplasia without familial risk from 19–38 weeks (Fig 13–26). At 19 weeks the femur length was approximately 1 SD below the mean, and mild dilatation of the lateral cerebral ventricles was evident, but no other abnormalities were apparent. By 25 weeks the ventricular dilatation had resolved, but the femur length had fallen beyond the 99% confidence limit, and mild polyhydramnios had developed. This pattern persisted and displayed the similarity in growth pattern between heterozygous achondroplasia and asphyxiating thoracic dysplasia. Furthermore, a profile view of the face indicated absence of the nasal bridge, suggestive of heterozygous achondroplasia. Even in retrospect, the thoracic size of this fetus was not noticeably small.

Although some authors report that the key factor leading to the diagnosis of asphyxiating thoracic dysplasia is an abnormally small thorax, unfortunately the normal sonographic relationship between thoracic size and menstrual age is not fully defined and varies among different series.[4, 192, 194] Furthermore, since many of the osteochondrodysplasias (and all those reported in one series) had a small thorax, this feature does not help distinguish asphyxiating thoracic dysplasia from other entities.[76] Nevertheless, it may be a helpful sign to search for and, when unmistakably severe, may help to predict a poor prognosis secondary to pulmonary hypoplasia.

FIG 13–26.
Asphyxiating thoracic dysplasia at 30 weeks. **A,** profile view of the face shows absence of the nasal bridge *(arrow).* **B,** coronal view of the trunk fails to show obvious thoracic hypoplasia. Based upon the absence of obvious thoracic dysplasia and progressive shortening of the femur length relative to the biparietal diameter since 18 weeks, the most likely diagnosis prenatally was heterozygous achondroplasia. *n* = nose; *f* = forehead; *t* = thoracic diameter; *a* = abdominal diameter; *s* = stomach.

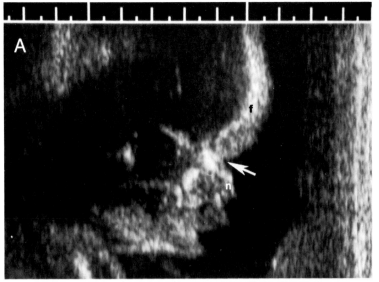

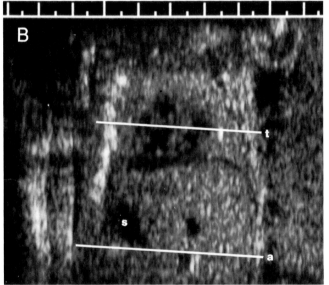

Chondroectodermal Dysplasia

Clinical and Pathologic Findings

Chondroectodermal dysplasia (Ellis-van Creveld syndrome) occurs in approximately 1 in 200,000 births with a high prevalence among an Amish community and recurs as an autosomal recessive trait.[16, 70] It resembles asphyxiating thoracic dysplasia closely, except that almost all cases of chondroectodermal dysplasia have polydactyly.[199, 200] The manifestations of chondroectodermal dysplasia are much less severe than in the short-rib polydactyly syndrome corresponding with a better prognosis.[159, 163, 165] The predominant features of chondroectodermal dysplasia include mild-to-moderate limb shortening and post-axial polydactyly. Approximately 50% of cases also have congenital heart disease, mainly atrial septal defect.[18]

Sonographic Findings

Among five reported cases of fetuses with chondroectodermal dysplasia seen with prenatal ultrasound to date, four had a positive family history for the disorder and were examined at 17–21 weeks.[71, 72, 77, 199, 200] Three of these cases had moderate rhizomelic shortening, and one also had visible polydactyly, but one only demonstrated equivocal evidence for short ribs. One additional case reported from a screening program in Sweden showed micromelia but a "normal thorax" at 13 weeks in the absence of familial risk.[77]

Diastrophic Dysplasia

Clinical and Pathologic Findings

Diastrophic ("distorted") dysplasia is a rare autosomal recessive disorder with variable expression of phenotype ranging from severe to mild.[202-204] Severely affected cases typically have micromelia, flexion limitations of finger joints (resulting in the characteristic fixed lateral positioning of the thumb, termed the "hitchhiker thumb"), extension limitations of the elbows and hips, club feet, progressive scoliosis, micrognathia, and cleft palate.[16, 18, 203] Diastrophic dysplasia causes increased infant mortality, but affected cases who survive infancy have normal intellectual development and a normal expected life span if the progressive kyphoscoliosis does not compromise cardiac and pulmonary function.[17, 203] For this reason, diastrophic dysplasia is included among dysplasias without a lethal prognosis, recognizing that the general rule holds that severe manifestations of dysplasia signify a poor prognosis, even in syndromes with variable phenotypes.

Sonographic Findings

Among six cases of diastrophic dysplasia detected with prenatal ultrasound to date, all occurred in severely affected fetuses with a 25% autosomal recessive risk for having the disorder.[73, 78, 201, 203-205] Each was examined at 16–20 weeks and displayed severe micromelia prior to elective termination. Two cases also showed bowing of extremity bones, and in two cases the characteristic "hitchhiker thumb" deformity was documented. In the absence of familial risk for diastrophic dysplasia, detection of the "hitchhiker thumb" deformity in a fetus with micromelia might enable prenatal diagnosis of this rare dysplasia.

Osteogenesis Imperfecta, Types I and IV

Clinical and Pathologic Findings

Type I osteogenesis imperfecta is probably the most common type of osteogenesis imperfecta, occurring in approximately 1 in 28,500 births.[133] Since this recurs by autosomal dominant transmission and only rarely by spontaneous mutation, most affected cases of this type will have an affected parent.[133] Although affected fetuses have overall normal limb lengths and only approximately 5% of cases have a bone fracture at birth, extremity bone bowing with fracture and diminished echogenicity may occur later in gestation.[115, 123, 133] Type IV osteogenesis imperfecta resembles type I except it does not produce deafness or blue sclerae.

Sonographic Findings

Among five cases of probable type I osteogenesis imperfecta detected with prenatal ultrasound to date, four had an affected parent.[73, 74, 115, 123, 130] Initial ultrasound prior to approximately 20 weeks was normal in

three cases, but subsequent scans showed bowed or fractured femora with the fracture healing during the third trimester.[73, 115, 123] One case demonstrated normal ossification, even on postnatal radiograph, whereas another case showed decreased extremity ossification during the third trimester.[73, 115]

We have also seen a case of recurrent type I osteogenesis imperfecta which had a normal ultrasound at 14 weeks. At 31 weeks the extremity lengths were appropriate with normal echogenicity, but femoral and tibial fractures were present (Fig 13–27). Three weeks later the tibial fracture had healed, but radial and bilateral femoral fractures were present. To our knowledge, type IV osteogenesis imperfecta has not been detected prenatally but would be expected to demonstrate findings similar to type I.

Other Rare Nonlethal Dysplasias

The Second International Nomenclature of Constitutional Diseases of Bone also lists the following rare defects of growth of tubular bones and/or spine identifiable at birth and, therefore, potentially detectable at least in the latter stages of gestation.[9] Prenatal ultrasound rarely detects any of the following, and the sonographic features may be very subtle.

Acromesomelic Dysplasia

As the name implies, acromesomelic dysplasia involves shortened middle and distal segments of the extremities. Inherited as an autosomal recessive trait, the predominant extremity features include bowed and shortened radius, distal ulnar hypoplasia, and very short hand and feet bones.[16, 18]

Cleidocranial Dysplasia

Cleidocranial dysplasia occurs as an autosomal dominant trait with highly variable expression in most cases but as a spontaneous mutation in one third of cases.[17, 18] Its cardinal features, which might be manifest sonographically, include partial or total aplasia of the clavicles and brachycephaly with increased biparietal diameter.

Kniest Dysplasia

This dysplasia is probably inherited as an autosomal dominant trait and shows mild-to-moderate limb shortening with progressive kyphoscoliosis and platyspondyly resulting in a short trunk and broad thorax.[17, 18] The extremity bones have a dumbbell appearance from metaphyseal and epiphyseal splaying, and the epiphyses are irregular and punctate.[18]

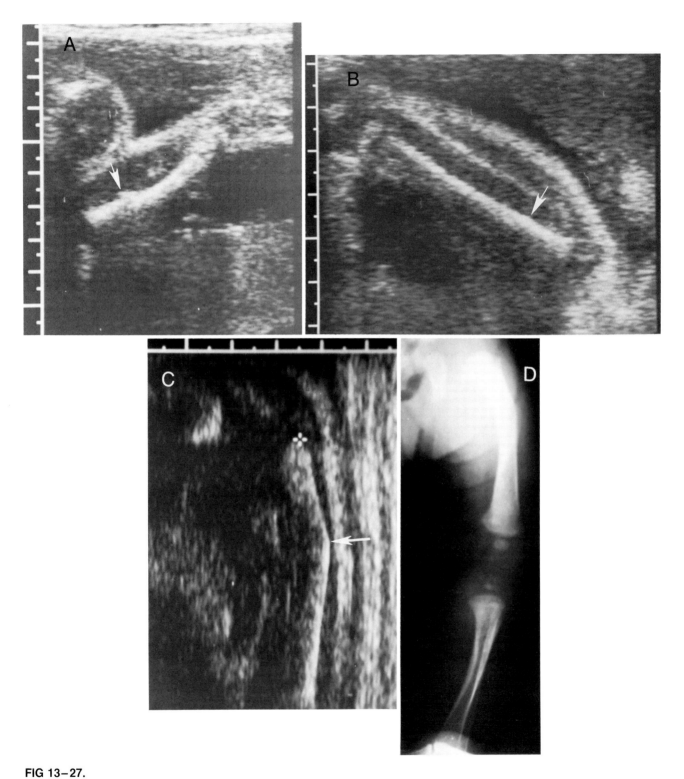

FIG 13–27.
Osteogenesis imperfecta, type I, with isolated healing extremity fractures during the third trimester. **A,** longitudinal scan of the tibia at 31 weeks shows a mid-shaft fracture with some callus formation *(arrow)*. **B,** 3 weeks later the tibial fracture has healed *(arrow = site of prior fracture)*. **C,** however, angulation deformity of the proximal femur is now present *(arrow)* on this longitudinal scan of the thigh. **D,** postnatal radiograph of the lower extremity shows the angulation deformity of the healed proximal femoral fracture. No tibial fracture was evident.

Larsen's Syndrome

This occurs sporadically and has a variable prognosis. Multiple joint dislocations of large joints, clubfoot, hypertelorism, depressed nasal bridge, flattened frontal bone with prominent forehead, micrognathia, and abnormal vertebral segmentation with kyphoscoliosis characterize the syndrome.[17, 18] The extremities attain overall normal length but the metatarsals, metacarpals, and distal phalanges are short. A double or triple calcaneal ossification center may be present.[18]

Mesomelic Dysplasias

The mesomelic dysplasias are a heterogeneous group of entities characterized by disproportionate shortening of the middle segments (radius, ulna, tibia, fibula) of the extremities.[16, 18] Although severe shortening of these segments may occur, the distribution of shortening helps distinguish these entities with a good prognosis.

The types of mesomelic dysplasias detectable at birth recur by autosomal dominant transmission with the exception of the Langer type, which is autosomal recessive.[18] *Langer* type has proximal hypoplasia of the radius, fibula, and tibia, and distal hypoplasia of the ulna with ulnar deviation of the hands. Mandibular hypoplasia is also present. *Neivergelt* type produces rhomboid-shaped middle segments with proximal radial dislocation, elbow contracture, and talipes. *Rienhart-Pfeiffer* type has curved radii with proximal radial dislocation and distal ulnar hypoplasia resulting in bowing of the forearm and ulnar deviation of the hands. Proximal hypoplasia and curvature of the fibula also occur. *Robinow* type causes distal ulnar hypoplasia and proximal radial dislocation as well as craniofacial dysmorphic features and hypoplastic external genitalia. *Werner* type results in very small tibiae, proximal fibular dislocation, thumb aplasia, and polydactyly.

Metatropic Dysplasia

Metatropic dysplasia probably recurs as an autosomal recessive trait.[18] It causes shortened extremity bones with marked metaphyseal flaring, a narrow thorax but a relatively long trunk, progressive kyphoscoliosis, and may produce a characteristic tail-like appendage over the sacrum.[17, 18] We detected a case characterized by marked metaphyseal flaring (Fig 13–28).

Osteopetrosis Congenita

Osteopetrosis congenita is a rare autosomal recessive disorder characterized in infants by hepatosplenomegaly and dense bones.[18] Overall extremity bone lengths tend to be normal. It has not been diagnosed with prenatal ultrasound to our knowledge and probably requires radiographic diagnosis.

Oto-Palato-Digital Syndrome

This rare syndrome may manifest in males at birth with short thumbs and great toes, mild lateral bowing of the femora, radial head dislocation, and cleft palate.[17, 18] It is probably transmitted via an autosomal dominant or X-linked recessive trait in males and X-linked recessive trait in females.

Spondyloepiphyseal Dysplasia Congenita

The congenital form of spondyloepiphyseal dysplasia occurs by autosomal dominant transmission with variable expression of the phenotype.[17, 18] It tends to produce subtle manifestations at birth, including a short trunk, barrel-shaped thorax, and mildly bowed and shortened femora. However, a lethal phenotypic expression may occur with dysplastic or absent vertebrae, short ribs, bell-shaped thorax, and lack of ossification of the pubis, ischia, talus, calcaneus, distal femoral epiphysis, and proximal tibial epiphysis.[18] A lethal case detected at 24 weeks showed polyhydramnios, short extremity bones, micrognathia, and a small thorax.[5]

FOCAL LIMB LOSS OR ABNORMALITY

Several entities are manifest on the prenatal sonogram either as fusion of the limbs or as focal absence of an extremity bone, segment, or entire limb. These do not represent bone dysplasias. Since their manifestations may be striking and severe but with a variable or good prognosis dependent upon distribution of abnormalities, occasional cases may represent exceptions to the general guideline that severe micromelia signifies a poor prognosis. In general, however, the guideline holds true. Furthermore, in the lethal skeletal dysplasias small bones are evident, whereas the affected segments of limb contain no bone in phocomelias or limb loss deformities.

Amniotic Band Syndrome

Clinical and Pathologic Findings

Both the amniotic band syndrome and the limb-body wall complex often produce variable, but frequently striking abnormalities of the fetal extremities. The amniotic band syndrome occurs sporadically with an incidence of as high as 1 in 1,200 births and 1 in 56 spontaneous abortions.[213, 219, 220]

Although the etiology of the syndrome remains in dispute, most authors ascribe to the hypothesis eluci-

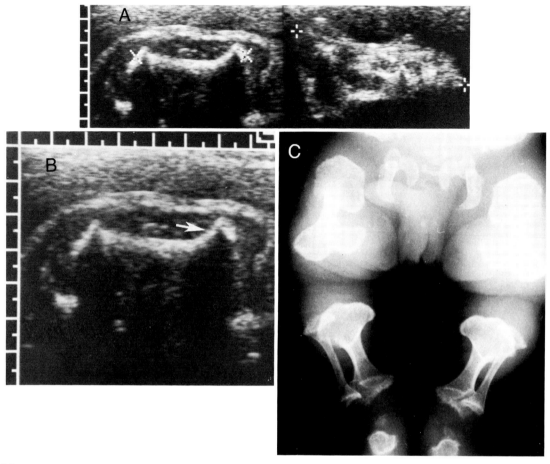

FIG 13–28.
Metatropic dwarfism at term. **A,** this dual-image scan shows a short femur (left portion of scan) measuring only 45 mm in length (mean for 24.5 weeks). Other extremity long bones were also proportionately short. However, the foot length of 75 mm (right portion of scan) was near mean for term. Therefore, the femur length/foot length ratio was abnormally decreased at 60%.[34] **B,** this longitudinal scan of the femur shows that the femoral metaphyses flare far more than normal *(arrow).* **C,** postnatal radiograph confirms the lower extremity findings.

dated by Torpin, who asserted that rupture of the amnion leads to transient oligohydramnios and subsequent entanglement of embryonic or fetal tissue by fibrous bands emanating from the chorionic side of the amnion (Fig 13–29).[221] Depending upon the time of rupture and the distribution and orientation of the bands slashing across the developing fetus, deformities occur ranging from subtle amputation or lymphedema to amputation of large portions of the fetus. Torpin also suggested that, following disruption of the amnion, the fetus may adhere to and fuse with the chorion producing maldevelopment of the subjacent fetal tissue.[221]

Based upon the observation that the amniotic band syndrome seems to occur far more commonly in monozygotic twins than in dyzygotic twins, some authors now assert that the syndrome may result from a teratogenic event since monozygotic, but not dizygotic, twinning may result from a teratogenic insult.[207, 208, 214]

Alternatively, it may arise from a multifactorial or polygenic cause.

Whatever its underlying mechanism, the amniotic band syndrome causes variable patterns of deformity but a proclivity for certain anomalies including constriction rings, extremity amputation or lymphedema, facial clefts in bizarre and non–embryologic distributions, large abdominal wall or chest wall defects, and encephaloceles occurring in locations other than the midline.[215, 220]

Although extremity amputations may result from teratogenic or genetic causes, several distinguishing features help identify amputations related to the amniotic band syndrome.[215, 221] Identification of a band of tissue within a constriction ring with distal lymphedema or protrusion of uncovered bone distal to the soft tissue at the site of an amputation represent convincing evidence for the amniotic band syndrome.

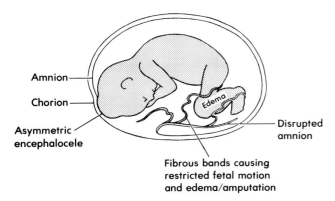

Amnion
Chorion
Asymmetric encephalocele
Edema
Disrupted amnion
Fibrous bands causing restricted fetal motion and edema/amputation

FIG 13–29.
Amniotic band syndrome. The amniotic band syndrome is postulated to result from rupture of the amnion with subsequent formation of fibrous bands which may entangle the fetus and lead to extremity amputations or lymphedema, asymmetric encephalocele, bizarre facial clefts, and large thoraco-abdominal wall defects. (From Randal SB, Filly RA, Callen PW et al: Amniotic sheets. Radiology 1988; 166:633–636. Used by permission.)

Constriction ring defects occur in most, if not all, unequivocal examples of the amniotic band syndrome (Fig 13–30).[220] Furthermore, amputations resulting from this syndrome typically occur asymmetrically, unlike the characteristic bilaterally symmetrical genetic or teratogenic amputations (Fig 13–31).

Sonographic Findings
Among 18 reported cases of the amniotic band syndrome between 16 and 31 weeks, detected abnormalities included extremity anomalies (ten cases; 56%), asymmetric encephalocele or discordant anencephaly (eight cases; 45%), large body wall defects, (seven cases; 39%), amniotic bands (seven cases; 39%), facial cleft (four cases; 22%), scoliosis (three cases; 17%), and one case each of oligohydramnios, polyhydramnios, and micrognathia.* Four cases occurred in twin pregnancies.[207, 214, 215, 224] It is possible that the three cases with severe scoliosis represented examples of the limb-body wall complex.[72]

Limb-Body Wall Complex

Clinical and Pathologic Findings
The limb-body wall complex produces a lethal set of invariably severe fetal malformations similar to the amniotic band syndrome, with the exception of marked scoliosis and a high incidence of defects involving the internal organs not frequently apparent in the amniotic band syndrome.[217, 222, 223] The limb-body

*72, 206, 207, 209, 211, 212, 214–216, 224, 225.

wall complex occurs sporadically with an incidence of approximately 1 in 4,000 births.[222] Van Allen et al. reviewed 25 cases of the limb-body wall complex and found limb abnormalities in 95%, internal organ defects in 95%, marked scoliosis in 77%, thoracoabdominal schisis in 64%, neural tube defects in 60%, and facial clefts in 40%.[222, 223] Only 40% had amniotic bands.

Although most authors believe that the limb-body wall complex results from rupture of the amnion between the third and fifth weeks of embryogenesis, recent data argue that the complex results from systemic alteration of embryonic blood supply in the majority of cases and amniotic bands or compression defects in the minority of cases.[217, 222, 223] The marked scoliosis probably results from decreased or absent paraspinous or thoracolumbar musculature on the same side as the body-wall defect.[223]

Sonographic Findings
Among 15 cases of the limb-body wall complex at 15–34 weeks reported to date, all fetuses died (five cases) or were electively terminated (ten cases).[210, 217] Sonography detected 14 of 15 (93%) body wall defects, 11 of 12 (92%) cases with scoliosis, 7 of 8 (88%) cases with neural tube defects, and 7 of 9 (78%) cases with amniotic bands. However, prenatal sonography detected only 5 of 14 (36%) cases with extremity abnormalities including only 4 of 12 (33%) with absent or hypoplastic limbs. The detected limb deformities included absent extremities, bilateral clubfeet or positional abnormalities, discrepant femur lengths, and syndactyly.

Roberts' Syndrome

Clinical and Pathologic Findings
Considerable confusion exists whether or not the Roberts' syndrome and the pseudo-thalidomide syndrome represent separate conditions or variations in phenotypic expression of one rare, autosomal recessive disorder.[2, 231] Severely affected patients with extreme manifestations have the Roberts' syndrome with a high perinatal mortality, whereas those with a significantly less severe phenotype have the pseudo-thalidomide syndrome and a better prognosis.[2, 229]

The characteristic features of the Roberts' syndrome include tetraphocomelia, bilateral cleft lip and palate, hypertelorism, microcephaly, and growth retardation.[2, 18, 226] The phocomelia typically occurs symmetrically and involves the upper extremities more severely than the lower limbs. In severe cases, a three-digit hand attaches to the shoulder, with an absence of

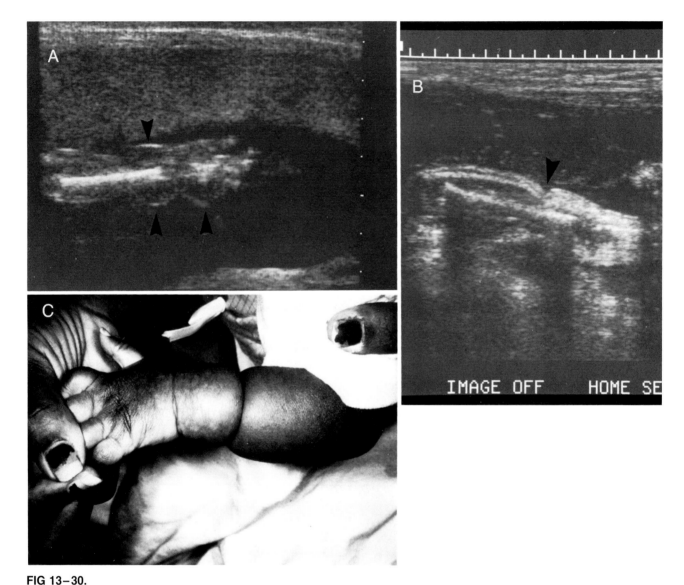

FIG 13–30.
Amniotic band constrictions. **A,** scan of the left arm at 18.6 weeks shows subcutaneous edema of the hand and forearm *(arrows).* **B,** scan of the left arm at 38.6 weeks clearly defines the point of constriction in the forearm *(arrow).* **C,** photograph of the left arm at 6 weeks of age demonstrates the constriction band. (From Hill LM, Kislak S, Jones N: Prenatal ultrasound diagnosis of a forearm constriction band. J Ultrasound Med 1988; 7:293–295. Used by permission.)

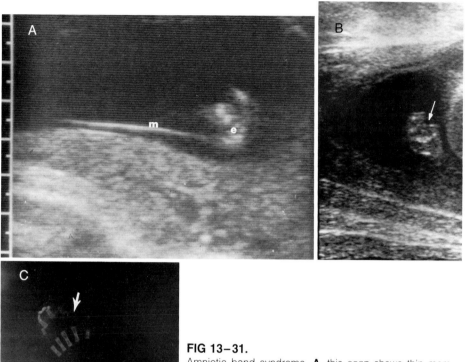

FIG 13–31.
Amniotic band syndrome. **A,** this scan shows thin membranes attached to a fetal extremity. **B,** scan of the hand shows absence of the distal phalanx of the thumb and second finger with distal syndactyly. **C,** postnatal radiograph confirms the prenatal hand findings. *m* = membrane; *e* =extremity; *arrow* = amputation site.

the humerus, radius, and ulna. Bowing of the legs, flexion contractures, clubfoot, and syndactyly also occur. Cytogenetic findings of amniocytes from affected pregnancies often show characteristic centromeric separation and puffing.[231]

Sonographic Findings

Two case reports describe phocomelia at 19 and 22 weeks in pregnancies at 25% risk for recurrence of the Roberts' syndrome.[73] One case had tetraphocomelia and oligohydramnios with renal agenesis, and the other had femoral shortening, a claw deformity of the distal extremities, and a premaxillary protuberance. A third case occurred in a polyhydramniotic pregnancy without described familial risk at 32 weeks with short humeri and cerebral ventricular dilation.[228] A fourth case, probably representing the Roberts' syndrome, described phocomelia at 27 weeks.[72]

We have also seen two cases of the Roberts' syndrome in the absence of genetic risk during the second trimester. One case at 20 weeks showed: normal femur lengths; radial, ulnar, fibular, and thumb aplasia; syndactyly; clubfeet; mild polyhydramnios; and mild dilatation of the lateral cerebral ventricles (Fig 13–32). Postnatal fibroblast culture confirmed the presence of abnormal centromeric separation and puffing. The other case at 25 weeks showed severe upper extremity phocomelia and a single deformed lower extremity (Fig 13–33).

The extremity malformations of the Roberts' syndrome resemble those of the thalidomide syndrome and the femur-fibula-ulna syndrome. One report documents the sonographic detection of the thalidomide syndrome at 17 weeks in the fetus of a woman with leprosy receiving adjuvant treatment with thalidomide.[227] The sonogram detected severe phocomelia of the upper extremities with only a residual spicule at the shoulder as well as bilateral aplasia of the tibia and fibula with attachment of the feet to the thigh. One report

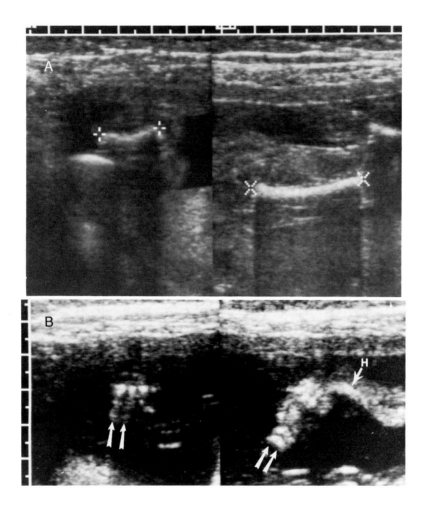

FIG 13–32.
Roberts' syndrome at 20 weeks. **A,** this dual-image scan of the humerus (left portion of the scan) and femur (right portion of the scan) demonstrates the short humerus. The humeral length is approxiamtely 4 SD below the mean. The femur is of normal length. Normally, at 20 week's gestation the humeral and femoral lengths are nearly equal. **B,** this dual-image scan shows fused fingers (left portion of the scan) and absence of the radius and ulna, with the hand attached at a right angle to the upper arm (right portion of the scan). Throughout the entire course of the examination two of the fingers *(arrows)* remained fused bilaterally, indicative of syndactyly. Other scans showed shortened tibiae but absent fibulae, mild polyhydramnios, and mild dilatation of the lateral cerebral ventricles. *H* = humerus.

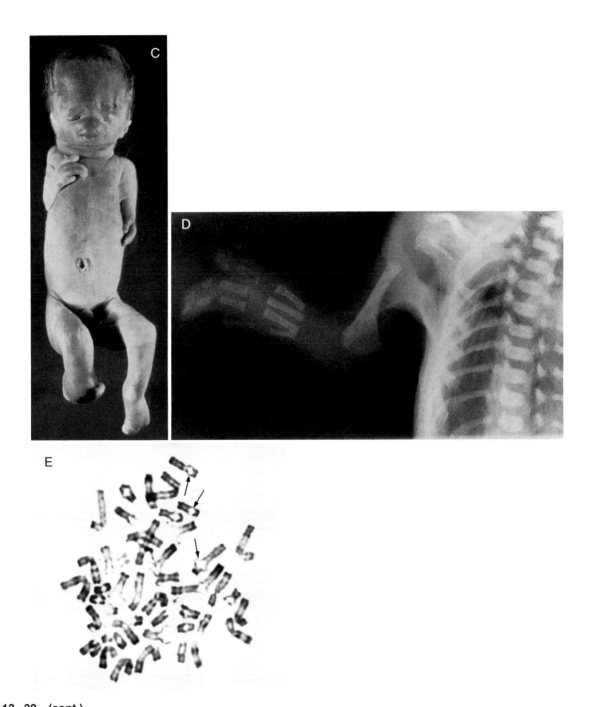

FIG 13–32   (cont.).
C and **D,** postmortem photograph and x-ray confirm the prenatal findings. **E,** C-banded chromosomes from cultured fibroblasts postnatally exhibit the extreme centromere separation *(arrows)* indicative of the Roberts' syndrome. (Chromosomal analysis performed by Children's Hospital Cytogenetics Laboratory, Seattle, WA.)

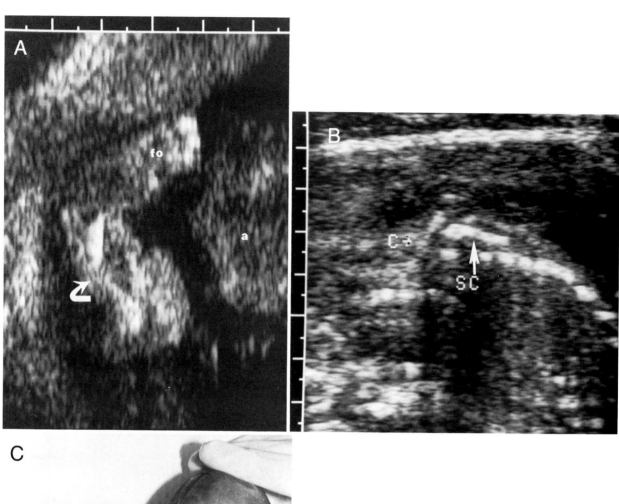

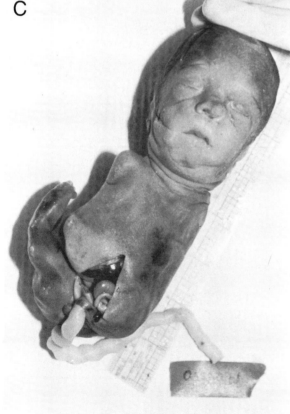

FIG 13–33.
Roberts' syndrome at 25 weeks. **A,** scan of the lower extremity shows a single deformed lower extremity. **B,** scan of the shoulder demonstrates absence of the upper extremity. **C,** photograph at autopsy confirms the prenatal findings. *a* = lower abdomen; *curved arrow* = femur; *fo* = foot; *c* = clavicle; *sc* = scapula.

of the femur-fibula-ulna syndrome at 35 weeks describes a short femur, absent fibula, and two absent fingers.[230]

Radial Ray Defects

A wide variety of entities may result in aplasia or hypoplasia of the radius and thumb, including (but not limited to) the Holt-Oram syndrome, thrombocytopenia and absent radius syndrome, the acro-renal syndrome, Nager's acrofacial dysostosis, the VACTERL (vertebral defects, anal atresia, cardiac defects, tracheo-esophageal atresia, renal and limb anomalies) association, Fanconi's syndrome, trisomy 18 and 13, Poland's sequence, and de Lange's syndrome.[2, 5, 16, 18, 240]

Reports of six cases document that prenatal ultrasound can detect radial ray defects during the second trimester of pregnancy but all second-trimester reported diagnoses occurred in fetuses with a 25%–50% risk for having the disorder.[73, 233, 234, 236–239] The characteristic sonographic features of a radial ray defect are sharp radial deviation of the hand and absence of visualization of the distal radius at the same level as the ulna (Fig 13–34).

Holt-Oram Syndrome

Clinical and Pathologic Findings

The Holt-Oram syndrome consists of skeletal abnormalities (ranging from severe phocomelia to minor abnormalities evident only on radiography) and a wide range of cardiac abnormalities. The skeletal manifestations tend to involve the left upper extremity more than the right and often include radial ray defects (Fig 13–35). Since complete penetrance occurs in transmission of the Holt-Oram syndrome, the recurrence risk is 50%, although the phenotype shows variable expression.[233, 239]

Sonographic Findings

Among three reported cases of the Holt-Oram syndrome detected with prenatal ultrasound, each represented a recurrent case, and two were detected at 14–22 weeks.[233, 239] One of these had a documented ventriculoseptal defect, bilateral absence of the radius, and two digits absent on both hands.[239] The other also had a documented ventriculoseptal defect but only borderline left radial shortening, not confirmed radiographically at term.[233] The third case was not evaluated until 34 weeks, at which time ventriculoseptal defect, polyhydramnios, absent radii, sharp angulation of

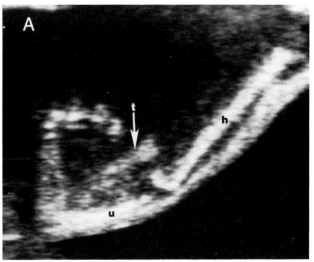

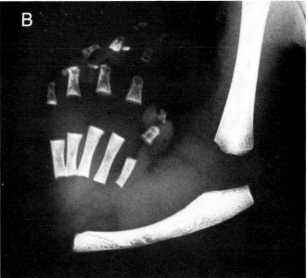

FIG 13–34.
Absent radius at 27 weeks. **A,** sonogram of the upper extremity shows absence of the radius but presence of the thumb. *B,* postnatal photograph confirms the prenatal findings. *U* = ulna; *h* = humerus; *t* = thumb.

the hands at the wrist, two absent fingers on the left, and one absent finger on the right were evident.

Thrombocytopenia and Absent Radius Syndrome

Clinical and Pathologic Findings

The thrombocytopenia and absent radius syndrome recurs by autosomal recessive inheritance.[235] All cases have bilateral absence of the radius and, in contrast to other conditions characterized by radial absence, in this syndrome the thumb is always present.[235] The ulna and humerus may also be shortened or ab-

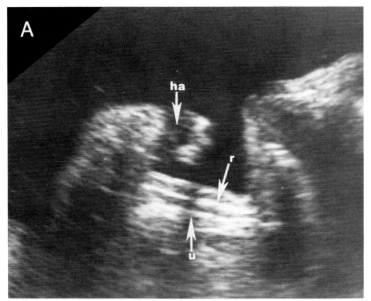

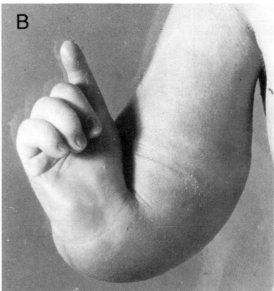

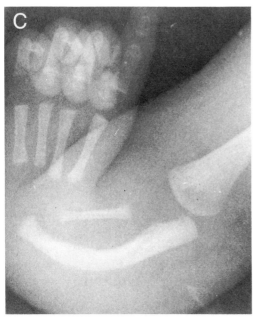

FIG 13–35.

Holt-Oram syndrome at 32 weeks. **A,** the sonogram at 32 weeks obtained because of size greater than dates measurements demonstrates polyhydramnios and a shortened right upper extremity with the hand oriented at a right angle to the fore-arm. No thumb was present. The radius was present but short. On this scan the distal portion of the ulna was shadowed by the hand. Other scans showed severe levoposition of the heart with absence of stomach in the abdomen, indicating an unusual right-sided diaphragmatic hernia. **B** and **C,** autopsy and postnatal radio-graph confirmed the above findings. *ha* = hand; *r* = radius; *u* = ulna.

sent, in which case the five-fingered hand attaches at the shoulder.[235] Approximately 30% of cases have cardiac anomalies, predominantly tetralogy of Fallot.[235]

Sonographic Findings

Among three cases of thrombocytopenia and absent radius syndrome detected with prenatal ultrasound, all were detected during the second trimester in fetuses at risk for the disorder.[73, 235, 236, 237] Each report documented absent radii prenatally, and two reports documented the hand positioned at a right angle to the forearm.

Other Radial Ray Defects

The two other prenatal sonographic reports of radial ray defects occurred in recurrent *Acro-renal syndrome* at 18 weeks and sporadic *Nager's acrofacial dysostosis* at 30 weeks.[232, 238] Both of these syndromes are very rare. The acro-renal syndrome, which exhibits dominant transmission from father to son, demonstrated crossed renal ectopia, absence of the radius and thumb with sharp lateral deviation of the hand at the wrist, and bowing of a shortened ulna.[238] Nager's acrofacial dysostosis at 30 weeks demonstrated polyhydramnios, micrognathia, malformed external ear, and very shortened upper extremities with only four shortened digits on the right hand.[232]

In the absence of familial risk for a radial ray defect, most cases detected prenatally (like the reported case of Nager's acrofacial dysostosis) will probably have more obvious concomitant anomalies which signal a careful search for an extremity abnormality. However, serendipitous detection of a radial ray defect probably warrants search for other manifestations of the VACTERL syndrome and chromosomal analysis. Detection during the third trimester probably justifies fetal umbilical blood sampling to assess platelet count.

Proximal Focal Femoral Deficiency

Congenital proximal focal femoral deficiency occurs in approximately 1 in 50,000 births, usually sporadically but with an increased incidence in infants of diabetic mothers.[241] It produces shortening or absence of the femur and has been documented on the basis of an isolated finding of an abnormally shortened femur with mid-diaphyseal angulation at 33 weeks in a pregnancy complicated by poorly controlled juvenile-onset insulin-dependent diabetes mellitus.[241]

Sirenomelia

Clinical and Pathologic Findings

The "mermaid syndrome" of lower extremity fusion, a severe manifestation of the caudal regression syndrome, occurs in approximately 1 in 60,000 births.[242, 244] It frequently occurs in the setting of severe oligohydramnios, usually from lethal bilateral renal agenesis or multicystic dysplasia. The lower extremity fusion ranges from a membrane fusing the thighs but separate lower legs to total fusion of the lower legs with one midline femur and fibula. Intermediate between these two extremes is soft tissue fusion with two femora but one midline fibula.

Sonographic Findings

The extreme oligohydramnios with resultant limitation of fetal motion and of extremity visualization limit the sensitivity of ultrasound in the prenatal detection of sirenomelia (Fig 13–36).[243–245] Approximately 50% of reported cases evaluated with prenatal ultrasound were not diagnosed as sirenomelia until after birth because of the concomitant severe oligohydramnios. In the setting of bilateral renal agenesis or multicystic dysplastic kidneys with severe oligohydramnios, however, demonstration of a single lower extremity

or femora consistently held in a side-by-side relationship enables prenatal diagnosis of sirenomelia (Fig 13–37).[243–245]

Associated Findings

Bilateral renal agenesis or multicystic dysplastic kidneys, oligohydramnios, intrauterine growth retardation, imperforate anus, ambiguous genitalia, and a single umbilical artery occur in virtually all reported cases of sirenomelia.[243–245] Other findings that occur commonly in association with sirenomelia include other skeletal deformities (90%), severe scoliosis (45%), heart defects (36%), and anterior abdominal wall defects (36%).[245]

CONTRACTURES AND POSTURAL DEFORMITIES

Normal embryonic and fetal development requires extremity movement as early as 7–8 menstrual weeks.[8] Extremity contractures or deformity develop in the absence of normal prenatal joint movement from severe oligohydramnios, extrinsic compression, or inherent inability of the embryo or fetus to move.[253, 267] Consequently, several extremity abnormalities create abnormal fetal posture or absent limb movement. Unfortunately, the terminology referring to the myriad of entities characterized by extremity contractures is quite confusing, but review of four terms aids in clarification: Arthrogryposis multiplex congenita; fetal akinesia deformation sequence; pterygium syndromes; and Pena-Shokeir phenotype.

Arthrogryposis Multiplex Congenita

Arthrogryposis multiplex congenita describes a fetus with multiple extremity contractures and encompasses a wide spectrum of heterogeneous disorders characterized by decreased fetal movement.[255] The outcome and recurrence risks for arthrogryposis multiplex congenita vary widely, depending upon the underlying etiology of the movement disorder as well as the concomitant anomalies. The four major causes of decreased fetal movement include (1) structural limitation of fetal movement (oligohydramnios, multiple gestation, extrauterine pregnancy, bicornuate uterus, etc.); (2) abnormalities of fetal nerve function or innervation; (3) intrinsic abnormalities of fetal musculature; or (4) defective fetal connective tissue.

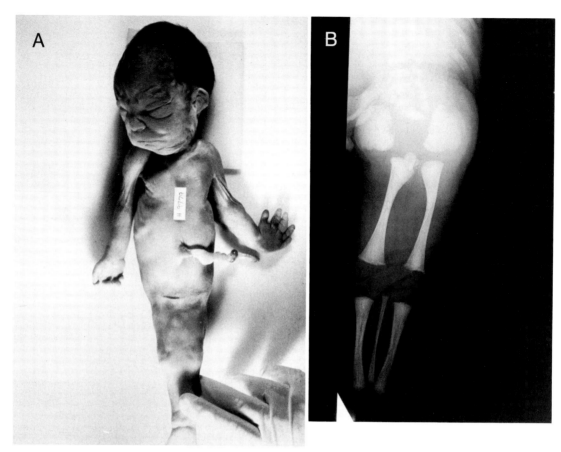

FIG 13–36.
Sirenomelia at 27 weeks. **A,** and **B,** postmortem photograph and radiograph of a fetus with sirenomelia show two femora and tibiae but a single midline fibula and soft tissue fusion. This breech fetus had anhydramnios and bilateral multicystic dysplastic kidneys at 27 weeks. These limitations precluded prenatal visualization of sirenomelia. The constant side-by-side relationship of the femora may suggest this finding prenatally.

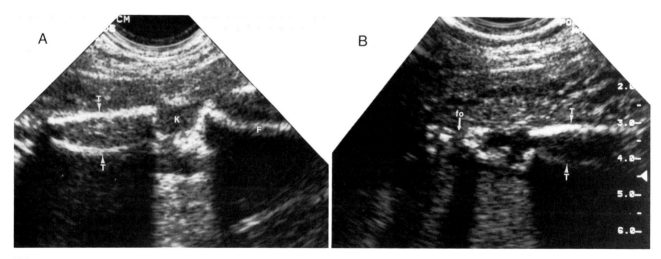

FIG 13–37.
Sirenomelia at 25 weeks. **A,** longitudinal scan of the lower thigh, knee, and leg demonstrates a single femur attached to two tibiae. The leg is extended, and severe oligohydramnios is present. **B,** longitudinal scan of the distal tibiae shows the two tibiae but only one foot. Additional scans showed one dysplastic kidney and contralateral renal agenesis. *F* = femur; *K* = knee; *T* = tibiae; *fo* = foot.

Fetal Akinesia Deformation Sequence

Abnormalities of any of the above systems leading to decreased fetal movement may result in the fetal akinesia deformation sequence.[253, 267] This sequence leads to deformations that closely resemble those characteristic of Potter's syndrome with extreme oligohydramnios secondary to bilateral renal agenesis. However, oligohydramnios need not exist to produce the fetal akinesia deformation sequence. For example, similar abnormalities occur in the Pena-Shokeir phenotype in the absence of oligohydramnios, and paralysis with curare during the latter half of fetal development in an animal model produces this phenotype.[253, 267] The phenotype is characterized by intrauterine growth retardation, micrognathia, depressed nasal tip, limb anomalies, pulmonary hypoplasia, short umbilical cord, and polyhydramnios.[259] Limb anomalies include limitation of joint movement, abnormal shape and position, and deficient bone growth and calcification. These anomalies all imply that normal fetal bone growth, ossification, and position each require normal extremity function.[259] The shortness of the umbilical cord indicates that its growth occurs in response to tensile forces affected by availability of intrauterine space and fetal movement during early development.[265]

Pterygium Syndromes

Pterygium is a descriptive term referring to webbing of the skin across a joint.[257] Limb pterygia at birth signify reduced intrauterine mobility of the webbed joints, probably occurring in the first trimester as a sequela of the fetal akinesia deformation sequence.[253, 257] Numerous limb pterygium syndromes exist of varying severity, prognosis, and inheritance pattern.[257] Hall et al. describe 15 different syndromes associated with limb pterygia and review 350 infants with arthrogryposis.[257] Eleven of these infants had limb pterygia, seven with the autosomal recessive multiple pterygium syndrome, three with a lethal variant of the autosomal recessive multiple pterygium syndrome, and one with a sporadic form of lethal popliteal pterygium syndrome.

The popliteal pterygium syndrome is the most common dominantly inherited limb pterygium syndrome, although most cases occur sporadically.[257] Predominant manifestations include cleft lip and palate, popliteal pterygium, syndactyly, and equinovarus foot deformity. Multiple pterygium syndrome is the most common recessively inherited disorder having limb pterygia.[257] At least three forms of lethal multiple pterygium syndrome exist, and all three forms consistently have cystic hygroma of the neck, hydrops, and hypoplastic lungs in association with the multiple pterygia across large joints.[253] Most cases also have polyhydramnios.[258]

Pena-Shokeir Phenotype

The Pena-Shokeir phenotype describes a set of malformations produced by the fetal akinesia deformation sequence and characterized by arthrogryposis multiplex congenita.[259] Approximately 20% of cases also have limb pterygia.[262] It is neither a diagnosis nor a syndrome, but its severe and lethal manifestations also include polyhydramnios, intrauterine growth retardation, pulmonary hypoplasia, short umbilical cord, and facial deformities correlating with the phenotype produced by the fetal akinesia deformation sequence.[259] Many patients with the Pena-Shokeir phenotype also have thin, underossified bones which fracture easily.[259] The *Neu-Laxova syndrome* and *restrictive dermopathy,* both very rare lethal autosomal recessive disorders, also result in a similar phenotype.[268, 273] This underscores the viewpoint that normal extremity development requires normal fetal limb function.

Sonographic Findings

The confusing and variable terminology in the literature regarding prenatal sonographic reports of extremity contractures limits somewhat the utility of analysis of these reports regarding specific diagnosis and outcome. Many of the reports concern cases detected on the basis of deformities seen of fetuses with a positive family history for a recurrent disorder. In the absence of familial risk, however, the sonographic features are not sufficiently distinctive to permit differentiation among a wide variety of syndromes with similar phenotypes. For example, recurrent autosomal dominant distal arthrogryposis was detected at 18 weeks on the basis of flexed wrists and overriding, clenched fingers, but overriding fingers may also occur in a variety of other entities, including trisomy 13 or 18 syndromes (Figs 13–38 and 13–39).[16, 18, 247]

Nevertheless, reports of a total of 36 cases document that prenatal sonography can detect a wide variety of fetuses with arthrogryposis multiplex congenita or the fetal akinesia deformation sequence phenotype, especially in the setting of familial risk (Fig 13–40 and Table 13–13). Approximately 70% of the cases occurred in the setting of a familial risk for recurrence of the disorder. In the absence of familial risk, the accuracy of prenatal sonography in detection of these fetuses may be much lower, especially if the manifestations are subtle. However, detection of the "full-blown" fetal akinesia deformation phenotype signifies a dismal

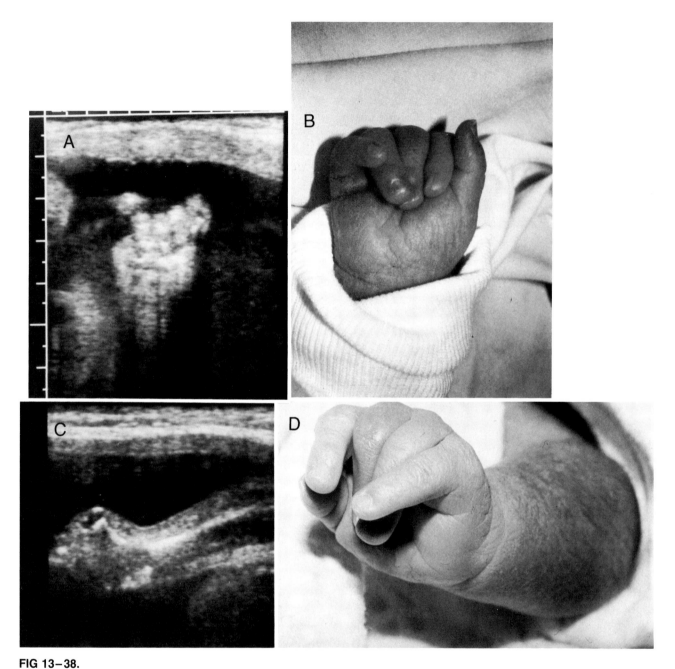

FIG 13–38.
Distal arthrogryposis, type I (autosomal dominant). **A,** sonogram of the right hand at 29 weeks shows persistent fisting of the hand with overriding fingers. In this entity, hand contractures typically result in a tight fist with overlapping fingers and thumb adduction. The overlapping fingers closely resemble the hand positioning frequently seen in trisomy 13. **B,** postnatal photograph at 37 weeks confirms the prenatal findings. **C,** sonogram of the left forearm, wrist, and hand at 29 weeks displays persistent fisting with extension of the wrist. **D,** postnatal photograph confirms the findings. (From Baty BJ, Cubberley D, Morris C, et al: Prenatal diagnosis of distal arthrogryposis. Am J Med Genet 1988; 29:501–510. Used by permission.)

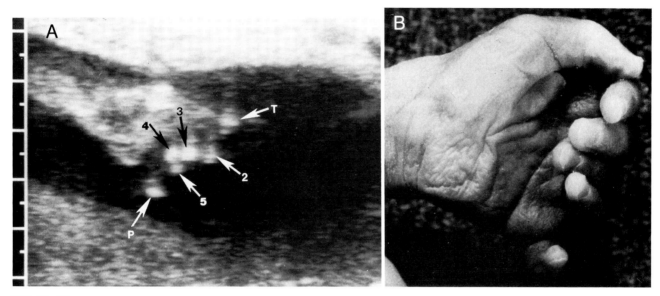

FIG 13-39.
Trisomy 13 with overlapping digits. **A,** sonogram shows the hand findings. The hand of this fetus remained persistently fisted with overlapping of the fifth digit onto the fourth. Polydactyly also was noted. On the basis of these findings and associated multicystic dysplastic kidney, a prenatal karyotype was performed confirming trisomy 13. **B,** corresponding postnatal photograph confirms the prenatal findings. *T* = thumb; *2–5* = digits; *P* = polydactyly.

prognosis. The case reports state information regarding survival in 33 of the 36 cases. Thirteen of the 36 cases underwent elective termination of pregnancy, and only one of the remaining 23 reported cases survived. The sole survivor has autosomal dominant type I distal arthrogryposis.[247]

OTHER HAND AND FOOT DEFORMITIES

As the previous discussion attests, prenatal ultrasound can detect numerous deformities of the hands and feet, especially during a targeted examination of these structures because of familial risk for deformity or based upon identification of concomitant anomalies.[72, 287] In the absence of these predisposing factors, the yield for screening ultrasound of the hands and feet would be expected to be low.[72]

Talipes
Clubfoot (talipes) is a common foot deformity which occurs in approximately 1 in 250 to 1 in 1,000 births.[283] Talipes typically occurs with syndromes characterized by multiple congenital anomalies, especially those resulting from the fetal akinesia deformation sequence, although it may occasionally occur as an isolated entity.[284, 285] Most cases of talipes have the equinovarus deformity in which the foot is plantar-flexed and inverted, but a variety of other talipes deformities may occur (Fig 13–41).[290]

The sonographic features of talipes depend upon the type of deformity present. In talipes equinovarus, for example, the foot deviates medially at the ankle and remains fixed at a right angle to the distal tibia and fibula so that the long axis of the foot resides in the same longitudinal plane of section as the tibia and fibula. Normally, in this plane of section the ankle and foot are seen in short axis (Fig 13–42).[285, 287] Among four sonographic series regarding 36 cases of talipes detected prenatally with ultrasound, 32 (89%) occurred in conjunction with other deformities which signaled the sonologist to examine the feet carefully.[278, 279, 283, 285, 287] The four cases without other detected anomalies had isolated clubfoot deformity at birth.[278, 285]

The prenatal detection of clubfoot, therefore, provides useful information to the parents and alerts the sonologist to search for other subtle deformities but probably does not significantly alter perinatal management in the vast majority of cases (Figs 13–43 to 13–45). Furthermore, one must exercise caution in making the diagnosis of isolated clubfoot, since the fetus may hold the foot in a position suggesting talipes in the absence of structural deformity at birth (Fig 13–46).[285]

Clinodactyly and Overlapping Digits
Contractures of the hands and feet may also occur, as discussed previously, resulting in abnormally fisted or overlapping digits with clinodactyly in a wide variety of syndromes. Taybi lists 37 causes for clinodactyly,

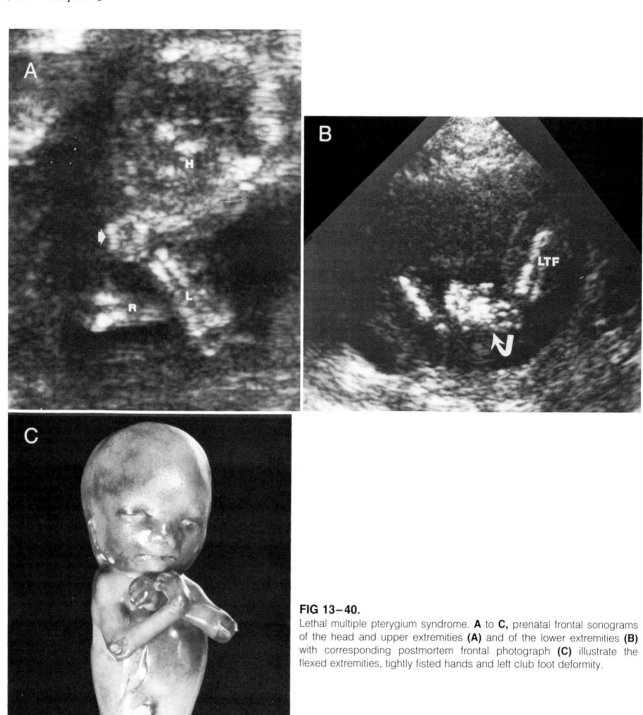

FIG 13–40.
Lethal multiple pterygium syndrome. **A** to **C,** prenatal frontal sonograms of the head and upper extremities **(A)** and of the lower extremities **(B)** with corresponding postmortem frontal photograph **(C)** illustrate the flexed extremities, tightly fisted hands and left club foot deformity.

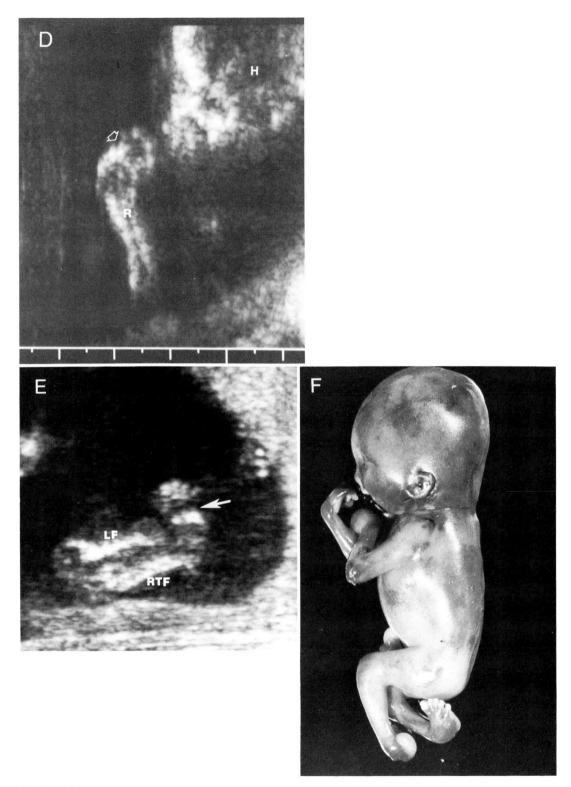

FIG 13–40   (cont.).
D to **F,** corresponding lateral images of the same fetus indicate similar findings. This fetus remained motionless throughout the entire course of the sonographic examination. *H* = head; *L* = left forearm; *solid arrow head* = fisted left hand; *R* = portion of right forearm; *open arrow head* = fisted right hand; *LTF* = left tibia/fibula; *curved arrow* = left talipes equinovarus; *LF* = left femur; *RTF* = right tibia/fibula; *straight arrow* = right talipes equinovarus.

TABLE 13–13.

Extremity Contractures Detected With Prenatal Ultrasound

Case	Sonographic Findings	Reference
I. Arthrogryposis		
1	Overriding, clenched fingers; flexed hands at 18 weeks	247
2–4	Fisted hands; IUGR (2 cases); clubfoot, polyhydramnios, diaphragmatic hernia, cerebral ventricular dilatation (1 case each) at 20–32 weeks.	280
5	Flexed knees, hip, elbows, hand without motion; hydrops; short extremities at 28 weeks.	255
6	Upper extremity contractures, bilateral clubfoot; cystic hygroma colli with hydrops at 19 weeks.	285
7	Arthrogryposis; clinodactyly; unilateral clubfoot at 23.5 weeks.	285
8	Rigid hands; clubfoot; short limbs at 18 weeks.	287
9	Arthrogryposis; clubfoot; polyhydramnios at 23 weeks.	287
10	Extended knees; flexed hips, ankles, elbows, hands; polyhydramnios; edema without serous effusions at 38 weeks.	256
11	Normal at 18 weeks but no movement at 23–25 weeks; polyhydramnios at 35 weeks.	266
12	Arthrogryposis of knees, elbows; short, bowed extremities with decreased echogenicity; oligohydramnios at 16 weeks.	157
II. Pterygium Syndromes		
13	Flexed, short limbs, polyhydramnios, cystic hygroma colli at 19 weeks.	251
14	Motionless, short limbs; clubfeet; hydrops at 18 weeks.	277
15	Motionless, short limbs; cystic hygroma colli with hydrops at 22 weeks.	277
16	Motionless, flexed extremities, clubfoot, hydrops, cystic hygroma colli at 19 weeks.	263
III. Pena-Shokeir		
17	Flexed, motionless legs; retrognathia; polyhydramnios; soft-tissue edema at 32 weeks.	250
18	Normal at 13, 23 weeks; contractures of wrists, ankles at 29.5 weeks with hydrops.	249
19	Decreased movement, hydrops at 31 weeks.	249
20–27	8–12 weeks normal; 15–20 weeks absent movement and edema; 29 weeks decreased movement, edema, polyhydramnios.	261
28	No movement, polyhydramnios, small thorax at 28 weeks.	262
29	Flexed wrists, ankles; claw-like campodactyly; rocker-bottom feet; scalp edema; small thorax at 31 weeks.	268
30	Polyhydramnios at 24 weeks; decreased movement at 27–39 weeks with extended knees and flexed elbows at 39 weeks.	270
31	26 weeks: ulnar deviation of hand, knees flexed, flexed fingers, rocker-bottom feet, micrognathia, polyhydramnios, IUGR, depressed nasal tip, no breathing. 36 weeks: campodactyly, small thorax, clubfoot, deformed ear.	274
32	Decreased movement, scoliosis, clubfoot, polyhydramnios, ventricular dilatation at 18.5 weeks.	271
IV. Restrictive Dermopathy		
33	Normal at 17, 21 weeks; contractures at 32 weeks.	275
34	Normal at 11, 13 weeks; flexion contractures, small thorax, polyhydramnios, thick placenta, small and open mouth at 32 weeks.	276
V. Neu-Laxova		
35	Flexion deformities, rocker-bottom feet, hypoechoic bones, IUGR, polyhydramnios, edema, microcephaly at 28–37 weeks.	269
VI. Humero-Radial Synostosis		
36	Flexed elbows at 17–20 weeks.	272

IUGR = intrauterine growth retardation

and Smith lists 36 causes (Figs 13–38 and 13–39).[16,18] Although detection of overlapping digits or clinodactyly may suggest the presence of a trisomy 13, 18, or 21, it is certainly not pathognomonic for a chromosomal aberration, and other more obvious anomalies typically dominate the sonographic picture in these syndromes. Nevertheless, detection of this persistent deformity should also alert the sonologist to search diligently for other anomalies and consider amniocentesis for karyotyping.[280–282]

Polydactyly and Syndactyly

Detection of polydactyly or syndactyly typically occurs in the setting of multiple, more obvious anoma-

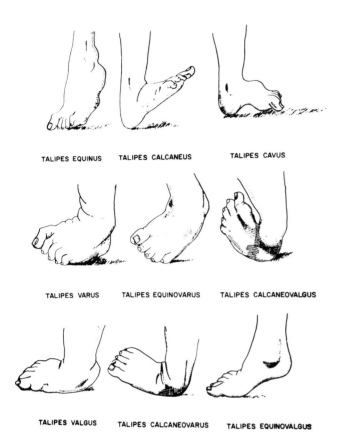

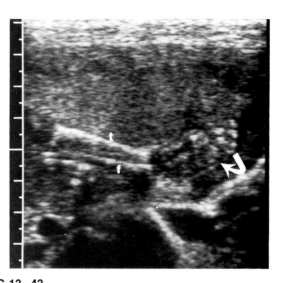

FIG 13–43.
Talipes equinovarus with oligohydramnios. This sonogram shows the long axis of the foot *(curved arrow)* in the same longitudinal plane as the tibia and fibula in this case with severe oligohydramnios. The varus angulation of the foot in this case is not as severe as in many with talipes equinovarus. *t* = tibia; *f* = fibula.

FIG 13–41.
Types of clubfoot (talipes). (From Sucheston ME, Cannon MS (eds): Congenital Malformations. Philadelphia, FA Davis Co, 1973. Used by permission.)

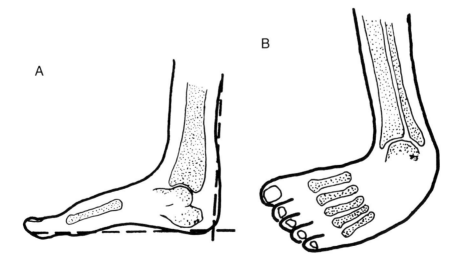

FIG 13–42.
Normal foot vs. talipes. **A,** sagittal drawing of the lower leg and foot shows the normal relationships. **B,** coronal drawing of the lower leg shows the abnormal relationships of talipes in which the metatarsals are visible in the same plane of section as the tibia and fibula but orient roughly perpendicularly to these two long bones. (From Jeanty P, Romero R, D'Alton M, et al: In utero sonographic detection of hand and foot deformities. J Ultrasound Med 1985; 4:595–601. Used by permission.)

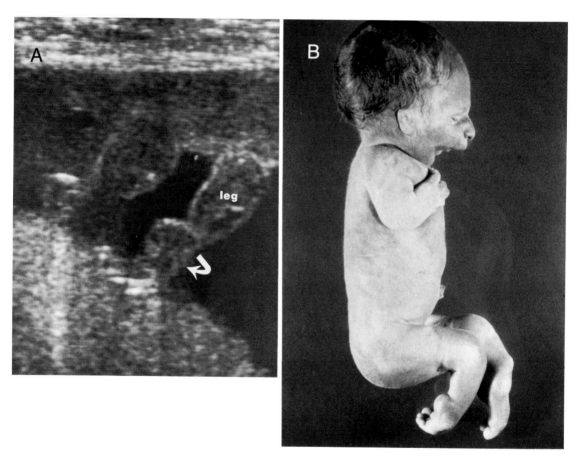

FIG 13–44.
Talipes equinus with the Roberts' syndrome. **A,** this longitudinal scan of the leg and foot displays talipes equinus in a polyhydramniotic pregnancy. Additional scans showed shortened tibia and humerus, absent fibula, radius, ulna and thumbs, syndactyly, mild polyhydramnios, and mild dilation of the lateral cerebral ventricles (see Fig 13–32). **B,** postmortem photograph confirms the talipes equinus. *Leg =* lower leg; *curved arrow =* foot.

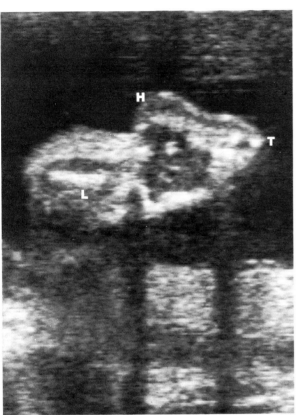

FIG 13–45.
Talipes equinus with polyhydramnios. Longitudinal scan of the leg and foot displays equinus deformity in a polyhydramniotic pregnancy. This fetus also had severe micromelia. Many cases of talipes occur in the absence of oligohydramnios. *L* = leg; *H* = heel; *T* = toes.

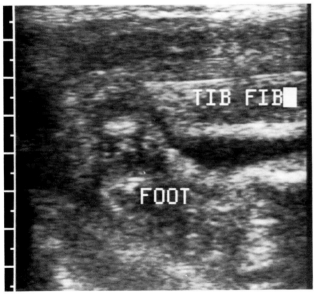

FIG 13–46.
False-positive diagnosis of talipes equinovarus at 34 weeks. This fetus held the foot in an equinovarus position throughout the course of the sonographic evaluation but was normal at birth, indicating the possibility of a false-positive prenatal diagnosis of talipes. *TIB FIB* = tibia and fibula imaged in long axis simultaneous to long axis imaging of the sharply inverted foot.

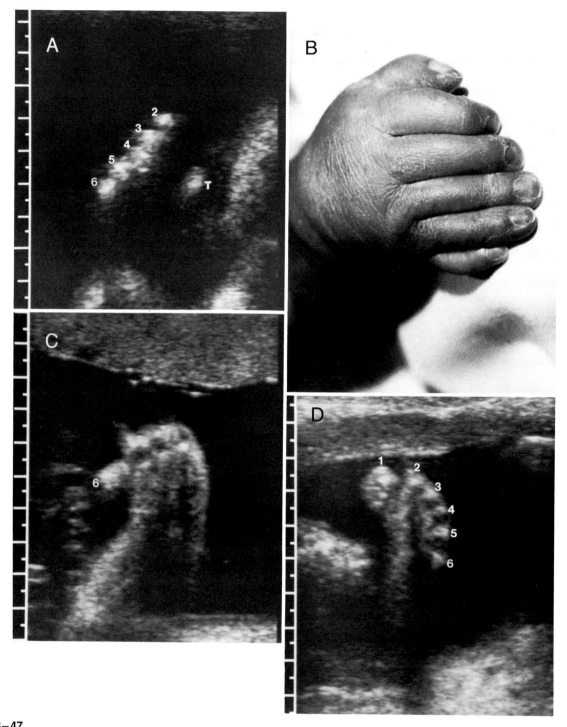

FIG 13–47.
Polydactyly associated with the Smith-Lemli-Opitz type II syndrome. **A,** and **B,** section through the right hand and corresponding postnatal photograph shows the six digits (1–6). **C,** the left hand had a rudimentary sixth digit (6) projecting off the ulnar side and **D** and **E,** scans of a foot and corresponding postnatal photograph also show polydactyly. Both feet were similar. Additional scans showed massive hydrocephalus with the Dandy-Walker malformation, polyhydramnios, and micropenis. *T* = thumb; *6* = sixth digit.

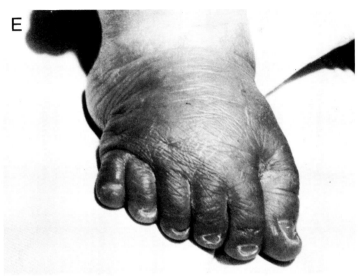

E

FIG 13–47   (cont.).

lies or a positive family history (Figs 13–32, 13–47, and 13–48).[72, 286] In such cases, delineation of the hand anomaly may help differentiate among several diagnoses. For example, detection of polydactyly in a fetus with micromelia and a small thorax implies the short-rib polydactyly syndrome rather than thanatophoric dysplasia. In a fetus with moderate limb shortening and a small thorax, polydactyly suggests chondroectodermal dysplasia instead of asphyxiating thoracic dysplasia.[163, 164, 167] Detection of isolated poly-

dactyly alerts the sonologist to search for other findings. A false-positive diagnosis of polydactyly can occur (Fig 13–49).

Syndactyly may be suspected when the digits remain persistently together, but syndactyly occurring as an isolated anomaly would be expected to be very difficult to confirm (see Fig 13–32). One can exclude the presence of syndactyly only if the fetus splays open the digits or interdigitates the fingers. Subtle phalangeal hypoplasias have been detected when specifically sought

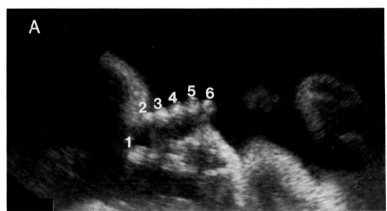

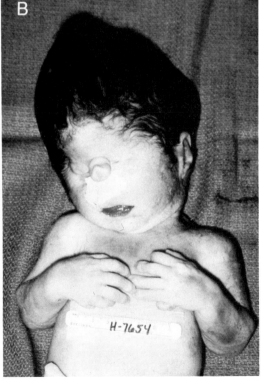

FIG 13–48.
Polydactyly with holoprosencephaly in trisomy 13. **A,** sonogram of the hand shows the six digits (1–6). Additional scans showed cebocephaly and holoprosencephaly. **B,** corresponding postnatal photograph confirms the prenatal findings. (From Nyberg DA, Mack LA, Hirsch J, et al: Fetal hydrocephalus: Sonographic detection and clinical significance of associated anomalies. Radiology 1987; 163:187–191. Used by permission.)

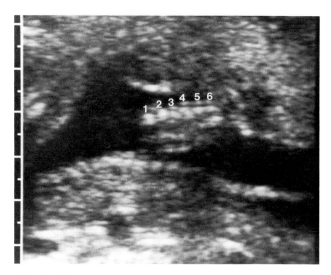

FIG 13-49.
False diagnosis of polydactyly at 19 weeks. Sonogram demonstrates apparent polydactyly as an incidental and isolated finding. The other hand and other fetal parts were not adjacent to the hand. A normal neonate was born at term. Although the fetus may conceivably have held its hand with one finger flexed and crossed over another, the reason for this misinterpretation remains undetermined. *1-6* = phalanges.

based upon a known genetic risk, but routine search for these deformities would be exceedingly time-consuming and non-productive.[281]

EXTREMITY ENLARGEMENT OR MASSES

Rarely, the sonologist may detect abnormal enlargement of the extremities. Typically the enlargement represents a manifestation of readily apparent concomitant deformities, such as edema from hydrops fetalis or constriction bands with distal lymphedema from the amniotic band syndrome (Fig 13-50).[212] Other causes for extremity enlargement are rare but have been reported on the basis of prenatal sonography. For example, the Marfan syndrome was correctly diagnosed at 23-24 weeks on the basis of unmistakably long extremity bones in a fetus whose mother had this autosomal dominant disorder.[292, 295] Asymmetric limb hypertrophy may occur with the Klippel-Trenaunay-Weber syndrome of cutaneous hemangiomata or lymphangiomata with arteriovenous fistulae and has been detected with prenatal ultrasound.[291, 294, 296, 297]

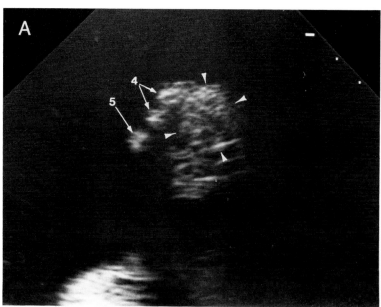
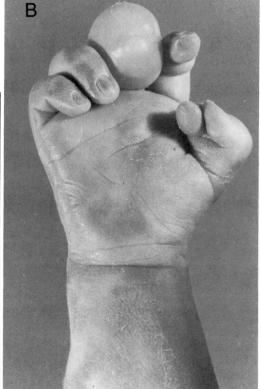

FIG 13-50.
Focal extremity enlargement. **A,** oblique sonogram of the hand shows focal enlargement of the third digit, probably secondary to constriction relative to an amniotic band. **B,** postnatal photograph confirms the prenatal findings and also shows a bifid thumb which was not detected prenatally. *Arrowheads* = enlarged third digit; *4* = middle and distal phalanges of fourth digit; *5* = fifth digit.

The hemangiomata typically create multiloculated cystic areas of the soft tissues of the extremities as well as elsewhere. Hegge et al. reported a case of trisomy 18 with a spherical mass replacing the left forearm.[72]

Undoubtedly, other rare extremity neoplasms or causes for enlargement will be reported in the future. For example, in the setting of polyhydramnios, visceromegaly, large-for-dates measurements and macroglossia, detection of unilateral limb enlargement may imply the presence of the Beckwith-Wiedemann syndrome, especially if a familial risk for the disorder exists.

CONCLUSION

Sonography has become the most sensitive and accurate method for detection of extremity malformations. It displays the fetal extremities without distortion and permits accurate antenatal diagnosis and prognosis in a wide variety of syndromes involving the extremities.

REFERENCES

Overview

1. American Institute of Ultrasound in Medicine: *Official Guidelines and Statements on Obstetrical Ultrasound.* Oct, 1985.
2. Bergsma D (ed): *Birth Defects Compendium,* ed 2. New York, Alan R Liss, Inc, 1979.
3. Cremin BJ, Beighton P: Dwarfism in the newborn: The nomenclature, radiological features and genetic significance. Br J Radiol 1974; 47:77–93.
4. Deter RL: Evaluation of studies of normal growth, in Deter RL, Harrist RB, Birnholz JC, et al (eds): *Quantitative Obstetrical Ultrasonography.* New York, John Wiley & Sons, 1986, pp 65–111.
5. Donnenfeld AE, Mennuti MT: Second trimester diagnosis of fetal skeletal dysplasias. Obstet Gynecol Surv 1987; 42:199–217.
6. Entin MA: Patterns of deformities in congenital anomalies of the upper limb and their relation to the classification. Birth Defects 1977; 13:231–241.
7. Grannum PA, Hobbins JC: Prenatal diagnosis of fetal skeletal dysplasias. Semin Perinatol 1983; 7:125–137.
8. Hill LM, Breckle R, Wolfgram KR: An ultrasonic view of the developing fetus. Obstet Gynecol Surv 1983; 38:375–398.
9. International nomenclature of constitutional diseases of bone: Am J Radiol 1978; 131:352–354.
10. Jeanty P, Romero R: Fetal limbs: Normal anatomy and congenital malformations. Semin Ultrasound, CT, and MR 1984; 5:253–268.
11. Mahony BS, Filly RA: High-resolution sonographic assessment of the fetal extremities. J Ultrasound Med 1984; 3:489–498.
12. Manchester DK, Pretorius DH, Avery C, et al: Accuracy of ultrasound diagnoses in pregnancies complicated by suspected fetal anomalies. Prenat Diagn 1988; 8:109–117.
13. McGuire J, Manning F, Lange I, et al: Antenatal diagnosis of skeletal dysplasia using ultrasound. Birth Defects 1987; 23:367–384.
14. Poznanski AK: Bone dysplasias: Not so rare, definitely important. AJR 1984; 142:427–428.
15. Sillence DO, Rimoin DL, Lachman R: Neonatal dwarfism. Pediatr Clin North Am 1978; 25:453–483.
16. Smith DW: *Recognizable Patterns of Human Malformation,* ed 3. Philadelphia, WB Saunders Co, 1982.
17. Spranger JW, Langer LO, Weidemann HR: *Bone Dysplasias: An Atlas of Constitutional Disorders of Skeletal Development.* Philadelphia, WB Saunders Co, 1974.
18. Taybi H: *Radiology of Syndromes and Metabolic Disorders,* ed 2. Chicago, Year Book Medical Publishers, Inc, 1983.
19. Thomas RL, Hess LW, Johnson TRB: Prepartum diagnosis of limb-shortening defects with associated hydramnios. Am J Perinatol 1987; 4:293–299.
20. Wong WS, Filly RA: Polyhydramnios associated with fetal limb abnormalities. AJR 1983; 140:1001–1003.
21. Zador IE, Bottoms SF, Tse GM, et al: Nomograms for ultrasound visualization of fetal organs. Soc Perinatal Obstet, Feb. 1987.

Embryology

22. Gardner E, Gray DJ: Prenatal development of the human hip joint. Am J Anat 1950; 87:163–212.
23. Gardner E, Gray DJ: Prenatal development of the human shoulder and acromioclavicular joints. Am J Anat 1953; 92:219–259.
24. Gardner E, Gray DJ, O'Rahilly R. The prenatal development of the skeleton and joints of the human foot. J Bone Joint Surg 1959; 41-A:847–876.
25. Gardner E, O'Rahilly, R: The early development of the knee joint in staged human embryos. J Anat 1968; 102:289–299.
26. Garn SM, Burdi AR, Babler WJ, et al: Early prenatal attainment of adult metacarpal-phalangeal rankings and proportions. Am J Phys Anthropol 1975; 43:327–332.
27. Gray DJ, Gardner E: Prenatal development of the human knee and superior tibiofibular joints. Am J Anat 1950; 86:235–288.
28. Gray DJ, Gardner E: Prenatal development of the human elbow joint. Am J Anat 1951; 88:429–470.
29. Gray DJ, Gardner E, O'Rahilly R: The prenatal development of the skeleton and joints of the human hand. Am J Anat 1957; 101:169–223.
30. O'Rahilly R, Gardner E: The initial appearance of ossification in staged human embryos. Am J Anat 1972; 134:291–308.
31. Sledge CB: Developmental anatomy of joints, in

Resnick D, Niwayama G (eds): *Diagnosis of Bone and Joint Disorders,* vol 1. Philadelphia, WB Saunders Co, 1981, pp 2–20.

Extremity Measurements

32. Abramowicz J, Jaffe R: Comparison between lateral and axial ultrasonic measurements of the fetal femur. Obstet Gynecol 1988; 159:921–922.

33. Abrams SL, Filly RA: Curvature of the fetal femur: A normal sonographic finding. Radiology 1985; 156:490.

34. Campbell J, Henderson A, Campbell S: The fetal femur/foot length ratio: A new parameter to assess dysplastic limb reduction. Obstet Gynecol 1988; 72:181–184.

35. Chinn DH, Bolding DB, Callen PW, et al. Ultrasonographic identification of fetal lower extremity epiphyseal ossification centers. Radiology 1983; 147:815–818.

36. Deter RL, Rossavik IK, Hill RM, et al: Longitudinal studies of femur growth in normal fetuses. J Clin Ultrasound 1987; 15:299–305.

37. Goldstein I, Lockwood CJ, Reece A, et al: Sonographic assessment of the distal femoral and proximal tibial ossification centers in the prediction of pulmonic maturity in normal women and women with diabetes. Am J Obstet Gynecol 1988; 159:72–76.

38. Goldstein I, Reece A, Hobbins JC: Sonographic appearance of the fetal heel ossification centers and foot length measurements provide independent markers for gestational age assessment. Am J Obstet Gynecol 1988; 159:923–926.

39. Goldstein RB, Filly RA, Simpson G: Pitfalls in femur length measurements. J Ultrasound Med 1987; 6:203–207.

40. Hadlock FP, Harrist RB, Deter RJ, et al: Fetal femur length as a predictor of menstrual age: Sonographically measured. AJR 1982; 138:875–878.

41. Hadlock FA, Harrist RB, Fearneyhough TC, et al: Use of femur length/abdominal circumference ratio in detecting the macrosomic fetus. Radiology 1985; 154:503–505.

42. Hill LM, Breckle R, Gehrking WC, et al: Use of femur length in estimation of fetal weight. Am J Obstet Gynecol 1985; 152:847–852.

43. Jeanty P, Beck GJ, Chervenak FA, et al. A comparison of sector and linear array scanners for the measurement of fetal femur. J Ultrasound Med 1985; 4:525–530.

44. Jeanty P: Letter. Radiology 1983; 147:602.

45. Jeanty P, Rodesch F, Delbeke D, et al: Estimation of gestational age from measurements of fetal long bones. J Ultrasound Med 1984; 3:75–79.

46. Jeanty P, Kirkpatrick C, Dramaix-Wilmet D, et al: Ultrasonic evaluation of fetal limb growth. Radiology 1981; 140:165–168.

47. Jeanty P, Dramaix-Wilmet M, van Kerkem J, et al: Ultrasonic evaluation of fetal limb growth II. Radiology 1982; 143:751–754.

48. Krook PM, Wawrukiewicz AS, Hackethorn JC: Caveats in the sonographic determination of fetal femur length for estimation of gestational age. Radiology 1985; 154:823–824.

49. Lockwood C, Benacerraf B, Krinsky A, et al: A sonographic screening method for Down syndrome. Am J Obstet Gynecol 1987; 157:803–808.

50. Mahony BS, Callen PW, Filly RA: The distal femoral epiphyseal ossification center in the assessment of third trimester age: Sonographic identification and measurement. Radiology 1985; 155:201–204.

51. Mahony BS, Bowie JD, Killam AP, et al: Epiphyseal ossification centers in the assessment of fetal maturity: Sonographic correlation with the amniocentesis lung profile. Radiology 1986; 159:521–524.

52. McLeary RD, Kuhns LR: Sonographic evaluation of the distal femoral epiphyseal ossification center. J Ultrasound Med 1983; 2:437–438.

53. Mercer BM, Sklar S, Shariatmadar A: Fetal foot length as a predictor of gestational age. Am J Obstet Gynecol 1987; 156:350–355.

54. Merz E, Kim-Kern M-S, Pehl S: Ultrasonic mensuration of fetal limb bones in the second and third trimester. J Clin Ultrasound 1987; 15:175–183.

55. Munsick RA: Human fetal extremity lengths in the interval from 9 to 21 menstrual weeks of pregnancy. Am J Obstet Gynecol 1984; 149:883–887.

56. Ott WJ: Fetal femur length, neonatal crown-heel length, and screening for intrauterine growth retardation. Obstet Gynecol 1985; 65:460–464.

57. Platt LD, Medearis AL, DeVore GR, et al: Fetal foot length: Relationship to menstrual age and fetal measurements in the second trimester. Obstet Gynecol 1988; 71:526–531.

58. Pyle SI, Hoerr NL: *A Radiographic Standard of Reference for the Growing Knee.* Springfield, Charles C Thomas, 1969, p 38.

59. Quinlan RW, Allen G, Cruz AC: Clinical utility of the relationship between fetal femur length and biparietal diameter. J Reprod Med 1984; 29:323–326.

60. Roopnarinesingh S, Ramsewak S: Decreased birth weight and femur length in fetuses of patients with the sickle-cell trait. Obstet Gynecol 1986; 68:46–48.

61. Ruvolo KA, Filly RA, Callen PW: Evaluation of fetal femur length for prediction of gestational age in a racially mixed obstetric population. J Ultrasound Med 1987; 6:417–419.

62. Seeds JW, Cefalo RC, Bowes WA: Femur length in the estimation of fetal weight less than 1500 grams. Am J Obstet Gynecol 1984; 149:233–235.

63. Shalev E, Feldman E, Weiner E, et al: Assessment of gestational age by ultrasonic measurement of the femur length. Acta Obstet Gynecol Scand 1985; 64:71–74.

64. Tabsh KMA: Correlation of ultrasonic epiphyseal centers and the lecithin: sphingomyelin ratio. Obstet Gynecol 1984; 64:92–96.

65. Tse CH, Lee KW: A comparison of the fetal femur

length and biparietal diameter in predicting gestational age in the third trimester. Aust NZ J Obstet Gynaec 1984; 24:186–188.

66. Vintzeleos AM, Campbell WA, Neckles S, et al: The ultrasound femur length as a predictor of fetal length. Obstet Gynecol 1984; 64:779–782.

67. Warda AH, Deter RL, Rossavik IK, et al: Fetal femur length: A critical reevaluation of the relationship to menstrual age. Obstet Gynecol 1985; 66:69–75.

68. Yarkoni S, Schmidt W, Jeanty P. et al: Clavicular measurement: A new biometric parameter for fetal evaluation. J Ultrasound Med 1985; 4:467–470.

69. Zilianti M, Fernandez S, Azuaga A, et al: Ultrasound evaluation of the distal femoral epiphyseal ossification center as a screening test for intrauterine growth retardation. Obstet Gynecol 1987; 70:361–364.

Prevalence of Anomalies and Accuracy of Sonographic Diagnosis

70. Camera G, Mastroiacovo P: Birth prevalence of skeletal dysplasias in the Italian multicentric monitoring system for birth defects, in Papadatos CJ, Bartsocas CS (eds): *Skeletal Dysplasias*. New York, Alan R Liss, 1982, pp 441–449.

71. Filly RA, Golbus MS, Carey JC, et al: Short-limbed dwarfism: Ultrasonographic diagnosis by mensuration of fetal femoral length. Radiology 1981; 138:653–656.

72. Hegge FN, Prescott GH, Watson PT: Utility of a screening examination of the fetal extremities during obstetrical sonography. J Ultrasound Med 1986; 5:639–645.

73. Hobbins JC, Bracken MB, Mahoney MJ: Diagnosis of fetal skeletal dysplasias with ultrasound. Am J Obstet Gynecol 1982; 142:306–312.

74. Kurtz AB, Wapner RJ: Ultrasonographic diagnosis of second-trimester skeletal dysplasia: A prospective analysis in a high-risk population. J Ultrasound Med 1983; 2:99–106.

75. Oriole IM, Castilla EE, Barbosa JG: Birth prevalence rates of skeletal dysplasias. J Med Genet 1986; 23:328–332.

76. Pretorius DH, Rumack CM, Manco-Johnson ML, et al: Specific skeletal dysplasias in utero: Sonographic diagnosis. Radiology 1986; 159:237–242.

77. Weldner B-M, Persson P-H, Ivarsson SA: Prenatal diagnosis of dwarfism by ultrasound screening. Arch Dis Child 1985; 60:1070–1072.

78. Wladimiroff JW, Niermeijer MF, Laar J, et al: Prenatal diagnosis of skeletal dysplasia by real-time ultrasound. Obstet Gynecol 1984; 63:360–364.

Lethal Dysplasias

Thanatophoric Dysplasia

79. Beetham FGT, Reeves JS: Early ultrasound diagnosis of thanatophoric dwarfism. J Clin Ultrasound 1984; 12:43–44.

80. Brahmam S, Jenna R, Wittenauer HJ: Sonographic in utero appearance of Kleeblattschadel syndrome. J Clin Ultrasound 1979; 7:481–484.

81. Burrows PE, Stannard MW, Pearrow J, et al: Early antenatal sonographic recognition of thanatophoric dysplasia with cloverleaf skull deformity. AJR 1984; 143:841–843.

82. Camera G, Dodero D, de Pascale S: Prenatal diagnosis of thanatophoric dysplasia at 24 weeks. Am J Med Genet 1984; 18:39–43.

83. Campbell RE: Thanatophoric dwarfism in utero: A case report. AJR 1971; 112:198–201.

84. Chervenak FA, Blakemore KJ, Isaacson G, et al: Antenatal sonographic findings of thanatophoric dysplasia with cloverleaf skull. Am J Obstet Gynecol 1983; 146:894–895.

85. Cremin BJ, Shaff MI: Ultrasonic diagnosis of thanatophoric dwarfism in utero. Radiology 1977; 124:479–480.

86. Elejalde BR, de Elejalde MM: Thanatophoric dysplasia: Fetal manifestations and prenatal diagnosis. Am J Med Genet 1985; 22:669–683.

87. Fink IJ, Filly RA, Callen PW, et al: Sonographic diagnosis of thanatophoric dwarfism in utero. J Ultrasound Med 1982; 1:337–339.

88. Horton WA, Rimoin DL, Hollister DW, et al: Further heterogeneity within lethal neonatal short-limbed dwarfism: The platyspondylic types. J Pediatr 1979; 94:736–742.

89. Isaacson G, Blakemore KJ, Chervenak FA: Thanatophoric dysplasia with cloverleaf skull. Am J Dis Child 1983; 137:396–398.

90. Langer LO, Spranger JW, Greinacher I, et al: Thanatophoric dwarfism: A condition confused with achondroplasia in the neonate, with brief comments on achondrogenesis and homozygous achondroplasia. Radiology 1969; 92:285–303.

91. Mahony BS, Filly RA, Callen PW, et al: Thanatophoric dwarfism with the cloverleaf skull: A specific antenatal sonographic diagnosis. J Ultrasound Med 1985; 4:151–154.

92. Maroteaux P, Lamy M, Robert JM: Le nasisme thanatophore. Presse Med 1967; 75:2519–2524.

93. Maroteaux P, Stanescu V, Stanescu R: The lethal chondrodysplasias. Clin Orthoped 1976; 114:31–45.

94. Moore QS, Banik S: Ultrasound scanning in a case of thanatophoric dwarfism with cloverleaf skull. Br J Radiol 1980; 53:241–245.

95. Partington MW, Gonzales-Crussi F, Khakee SG, et al: Cloverleaf skull and thanatophoric dwarfism. Arch Dis Child 1971; 46:656–664.

96. Shaff MI, Fleischer AC, Battino R, et al: Antenatal sonographic diagnosis of thanatophoric dysplasia. J Clin Ultrasound 1980; 8:363–365.

97. Stamm ER, Pretorius DH, Rumack CM, et al: Kleeblattschadel anomaly: In utero sonographic appearance. J Ultrasound Med 1987; 6:319–324.

98. Weib H, Rosseck U, Zerres K, et al: Ultrasonographic

findings and human genetic aspects in the prenatal diagnosis of a case of thanatophoric dwarfism with cloverleaf skull. Geburtshilfe Frauenheilkd 1984; 44:525–528.

99. Young RS, Pochaczevsky R, Leonidas JC, et al: Thanatophoric dwarfism and cloverleaf skull ("Kleeblattschadel"). Radiology 1973; 106:401–405.

Achondrogenesis

100. Andersen PE: Achondrogenesis type II in twins. Br J Radiol 1981; 54:61–65.

101. Benacerraf B, Osathanondth R, Bieber FR: Achondrogenesis type I: Ultrasound diagnosis in utero. J Clin Ultrasound 1984; 12:357–359.

102. Chen H, Liu CT, Yang SS: Achondrogenesis: A review with special consideration of achondrogenesis type II (Langer-Saldino). Am J Med Genet 1981; 10:379–394.

103. Golbus MS, Hall BD, Filly RA, et al: Prenatal diagnosis of achondrogenesis. J Pediatr 1977; 91:464–466.

104. Graham D, Tracey J, Winn K, et al: Early second trimester sonographic diagnosis of achondrogenesis. J Clin Ultrasound 1983; 11:336–338.

105. Johnson VP, Yiu-Chiu VS, Wierda DR, et al: Midtrimester prenatal diagnosis of achondrogenesis. J Ultrasound Med 1984; 3:223–226.

106. Mahony BS, Filly RA, Cooperberg PL: Antenatal sonographic diagnosis of achondrogenesis. J Ultrasound Med 1984; 3:333–335.

107. Saldino RM: Lethal short-limbed dwarfism: Achondrogenesis and thanatophoric dwarfism. AJR 1971; 112:185–197.

108. Smith WL, Breitweiser TD, Dinno N: In utero diagnosis of achondrogenesis, type I. Clin Genet 1981; 19:51–54.

109. Whitley CB, Gorlin RJ: Achondrogenesis: New nosology with evidence of genetic heterogeneity. Radiology 1983; 148:693–698.

Osteogenesis Imperfecta

110. Aylsworth AS, Seeds JW, Guilford WB, et al: Prenatal diagnosis of a severe deforming type of osteogenesis imperfecta. Am J Med Genet 1984; 19:707–714.

111. Brons JTJ, Van der Harten HJ, Wladimiroff JW, et al: Prenatal ultrasonographic diagnosis of osteogenesis imperfecta. Am J Obstet Gynecol 1988; 159:176–181.

112. Byers PH, Bonadio JF, Steinmann B: Osteogenesis imperfecta: Update and perspective. Am J Med Genet 1984; 17:429–435.

113. Byers PH, Tsipouras P, Bonadio JF, et al: Perinatal lethal osteogenesis imperfecta (OI type II): A biochemically heterogeneous disorder usually due to new mutations in the genes for type I collagen. Am J Hum Genet 1988; 42:237–248.

114. Carpenter MW, Abuelo D, Neave C: Midtrimester diagnosis of severe deforming osteogenesis imperfecta with autosomal dominant inheritance. Am J Perinatol 1986; 3:80–83.

115. Chervenak FA, Romero R, Berkowitz RL, et al: Antenatal sonographic findings of osteogenesis imperfecta. Am J Obstet Gynecol 1982; 143:228–230.

116. Dinno ND, Yacoub UA, Kadlec JF, et al: Midtrimester diagnosis or osteogenesis imperfecta, Type II. Birth Defects 1982; 18(3A):125–132.

117. Elejalde BR, de Elejalde MM: Prenatal diagnosis of perinatally lethal osteogenesis imperfecta. Am J Med Genet 1983; 14:353–359.

118. Elias S, Simpson JL, Griffin LP: Intrauterine growth retardation in osteogenesis imperfecta. JAMA 1978; 239:23.

119. Ghosh A, Woo JSK, Wan CW, et al: Simple ultrasonic diagnosis of osteogenesis imperfecta type II in early second trimester. Prenat Diagn 1984; 4:235–240.

120. Griffin ER, Webster JC, Almario VP: Ultrasonic and radiological features of osteogenesis imperfecta congenita: Case report. Milit Med 1983; 148:157–158.

121. Heller RH, Winn KJ, Heller RM: The prenatal diagnosis of osteogenesis imperfecta congenita. Am J Obstet Gynecol 1975; 121:572–573.

122. Key TC, Horger EO: Osteogenesis imperfecta as a complication of pregnancy. Obstet Gynecol 1978; 51:67–71.

123. Kuller J, Bellantoni J, Dorst J, et al: Obstetric management of a fetus with nonlethal osteogenesis imperfecta. Obstet Gynecol 1988; 74:477–479.

124. Merz E, Goldhofer W: Sonographic diagnosis of lethal osteogenesis imperfecta in the second trimester: Case report and review. J Clin Ultrasound 1986; 14:380–383.

125. Milsom I, Mattsson L-A, Dahlen-Nilsson I: Antenatal diagnosis of osteogenesis imperfecta by real-time ultrasound: Two case reports. Br J Radiol 1982; 55:310–312.

126. Patel ZM, Shah HL, Madon PF, et al: Prenatal diagnosis of lethal osteogenesis imperfecta (OI) by ultrasonography. Prenat Diagn 1983; 3:261–263.

127. Pokoly TB, Kiumehr M: Monitoring of fetus with osteogenesis imperfecta and severe anemia. Am J Obstet Gynecol 1978; 131:818.

128. Pope FM, Cheah KSE, Nicholls AC, et al: Lethal osteogenesis imperfecta congenita and a 300 base pair gene deletion for an alpha(1)-like collagen. Br Med J 1984; 288:431–434.

129. Robinson LP, Worthen NJ, Lachman RS, et al: Prenatal diagnosis of osteogenesis imperfecta type II. Prenat Diagn 1987; 7:7–15.

130. Rumack CM, Johnson ML, Zunkel D: Antenatal diagnosis. Clin Diagn Ultrasound 1981; 8:210–230.

131. Shapiro JE, Phillips JA, Byers PH, et al: Prenatal diagnosis of lethal perinatal osteogenesis imperfecta (OI type II). J Pediatr 1982; 100:127–133.

132. Sillence DO, Barlow KK, Garber AP, et al: Osteogenesis imperfecta type II: Delineation of the phenotype with

reference to genetic heterogeneity. Am J Med Genet 1984; 17:407–423.

133. Sillence DO, Senn A, Danks DM: Genetic heterogeneity in osteogenesis imperfecta. J Med Genet 1979; 16:101–116.

134. Spranger J: Osteogenesis imperfecta: A pasture for splitters and lumpers. Am J Med Genet 1984; 17:425–428.

135. Spranger J, Cremin B, Beighton P: Osteogenesis imperfecta congenita. Pediatr Radiol 1982; 12:21–27.

136. Stephens JD, Filly RA, Callen PW, et al: Prenatal diagnosis of osteogenesis imperfecta type II by real-time ultrasound. Hum Genet 1983; 64:191–193.

137. St J Brown B: The prenatal ultrasonographic diagnosis of osteogenesis imperfecta lethalis. J Can Assoc Radiol 1984; 35:63–66.

138. Van der Rest M, Hayes A, Marie P, et al: Lethal osteogenesis imperfecta with amniotic band lesions: Collagen studies. Am J Med Genet 1986; 24:433–446.

139. Woo JSK, Ghosh A, Liang S-T, et al: Ultrasonic evaluation of osteogenesis imperfecta congenita in utero. J Clin Ultrasound 1983; 11:42–44.

140. Zervoudakis IA, Strongin MJ, Schrotenboer KA, et al: Diagnosis and management of fetal osteogenesis imperfecta congenita in labor. Am J Obstet Gynecol 1978; 131:116–117.

Campomelia

141. Balcar I, Bieber FR: Sonographic and radiologic findings in campomelia dysplasia. AJR 1983; 141:481–482.

142. Fryns JP, Van den Berghe K, Van Assche A, et al: Prenatal diagnosis of campomelia dwarfism. Clin Genet 1981; 19:199–201.

143. Hall BD, Spranger JW: Campomelia dysplasia: Further elucidation of a distinct entity. Am J Dis Child 1980; 134:285–289.

144. Houston CS, Opitz JM, Spranger JW, et al: The campomelic syndrome: Review, report of 17 cases, and follow-up on the currently 17 year old boy first reported by Maroteaux et al in 1971. Am J Med Genet 1983; 15:3–28.

145. Khajavi AR, Lackman D, Rimoin R, et al: Heterogeneity in the camptomelic syndromes. Radiology 1976; 120:641–647.

146. Lazjuk GI, Shved IA, Cherstvoy ED, et al: Campomelic syndrome: Concepts of the bowing and shortening in the lower limbs. Teratology 1987; 35:1–8.

147. Winter R, Rosenkranz W, Hofmann H, et al: Prenatal diagnosis of campomelic dysplasia by ultrasonography. Prenat Diagn 1985; 5:1–8.

Chondrodysplasia Punctata—Rhizomelic Type

148. Curry CJR, Magenis RE, Brown M, et al: Inherited chondrodysplasia punctata due to a deletion of the terminal short arm of an X chromosome. N Engl J Med 1984; 311:1010–1015.

149. Gilbert EF, Opitz JM, Spranger JW, et al: Chondrodysplasia punctata—rhizomelic form: Pathologic and radiologic studies of three infants. Eur J Pediatr 1976; 123:89–109.

150. Happle R: X-linked dominant chondrodysplasia punctata: Review of literature and report of a case. Hum Genet 1979; 56:65–73.

Hypophosphatasia

151. Benzie R, Doran TA, Escoffery W, et al: Prenatal diagnosis of hypophosphatasia. Birth Defects 1976; 16:271–282.

152. Kousseff BG, Mulivor RA: Prenatal diagnosis of hypophosphatasia. Obstet Gynecol 1981; 57:9S–12S.

153. Mulivor RA, Mennuti M, Zackai EH, et al: Prenatal diagnosis of hypophosphatasia: Genetic, biochemical, and clinical studies. Am J Hum Genet 1978; 30:271–282.

154. Rattenbury JM, Blau K, Sandler M, et al: Prenatal diagnosis of hypophosphatasia. Lancet 1976; 1:306.

155. Rudd NL, Miskin M, Hoar DI, et al: Prenatal diagnosis of hypophosphatasia. N Engl J Med 1976; 295:146–148.

156. Weingast GR, Hopper KD, Gottesfeld SA, et al: Congenital lymphangiectasia with fetal cystic hygroma: Report of two cases with coexistent Down's syndrome. J Clin Ultrasound 1988; 16:663–668.

157. Wladimiroff JW, Niermeijer MF, Van der Harten JJ, et al: Early prenatal diagnosis of congenital hypophosphatasia: Case report. Prenat Diagn 1985; 5:47–52.

Homozygous Achondroplasia

158. Filly RA, Golbus MS: Ultrasonography of the normal and pathologic fetal spine. Radiol Clin North Am 1982; 20:311–323.

Short-Rib Polydactyly

159. Cooper CP, Hall CM: Lethal short-rib polydactyly syndrome of the Majewski type: A report of three cases. Radiology 1982; 144:513–517.

160. Gembruch U, Hansmann M, Fodisch HJ: Early prenatal diagnosis of short-rib polydactyly (SRP) syndrome Type I (Majewski) by ultrasound in a case at risk. Prenat Diagn 1985; 5:357–362.

161. Grote W, Weismer D, Jaenig U, et al: Prenatal diagnosis of short-rib polydactyly syndrome type Saldino-Noonan at 17 weeks gestation. Eur J Pediatr 1983; 140:63.

162. Johnson VP, Petersen LP, Holzwarth DR, et al: Midtrimester prenatal diagnosis of short-limb dwarfism (Saldino-Noonan syndrome). Birth Defects 1982; 18:133–141.

163. Meizner I, Bar-Ziv J: Prenatal ultrasonic diagnosis of short-rib polydactyly syndrome (SRPS) type III: A case report and a proposed approach to the diagnosis of

SRPS and related conditions. J Clin Ultrasound 1985; 13:284–287.

164. Naumoff P, Young LW, Mazer J, et al: Short-rib polydactyly syndrome type 3. Radiology 1977; 122:443–447.

165. Richardson MM, Beaudet AL, Wagner ML, et al: Prenatal diagnosis of recurrence of Saldino-Noonan dwarfism. J Pediatr 1977; 91:467–471.

166. Thomson GSM, Reynolds CP, Cruickshank J: Antenatal detection of recurrence of Majewski dwarf (short-rib polydactyly syndrome type II Majewski). Clin Radiol 1982; 33:509–517.

Very Rare Lethal Dysplasias

167. Borochowitz Z, Jones KL, Silbey R, et al: A distinct lethal neonatal chondrodysplasia with snail-like pelvis: Schneckenbecken dysplasia. Am J Med Genet 1986; 25:47–59.

168. Chervenak FA, Isaacson G, Rosenberg JC, et al: Antenatal diagnosis of frontal cephalocele in a fetus with atelosteogenesis. J Ultrasound Med 1986; 5:111–113.

169. Elejalde BR, de Elejalde MM, Booth C, et al: Prenatal diagnosis of Weyers syndrome (Deficient ulnar and fibular rays with bilateral hydronephrosis). Am J Med Genet 1985; 21:439–444.

170. Eteson DJ, Adomian GE, Ornay A, et al: Fibrochondrogenesis: Radiologic and histologic studies. Am J Med Genet 1984; 19:277–290.

171. Gruhn JG, Gorlin RJ, Langer LO: Dyssegmental dwarfism: A lethal anisospondylic camptomicromelic dwarfism. Am J Dis Child 1978; 132:382–386.

172. Handmaker SD, Campbell JA, Robinson LD, et al: Dyssegmental dwarfism: A new syndrome of lethal dwarfism. Birth Defects 1977; 13(3D):79–90.

173. Kim HJ, Costales F, Wallach RC: Prenatal diagnosis of dyssegmental dwarfism. Prenat Diagn 1986; 6:143–150.

174. Knowles S, Winter R, Rimoin D: A new category of lethal short-limbed dwarfism. Am J Med Genet 1986; 25:41–46.

175. Kozlowski K, Sillence D, Cortis-Jones R, et al: Boomerang dysplasia. Br J Radiol 1985; 58:369–371.

176. Maroteaux P, Spranger J, Stanescu V, et al: Atelosteogenesis. Am J Med Genet 1982; 13:15–25.

177. Poor MA, Alberti O, Griscom T, et al: Nonskeletal malformations in one of three siblings with Jarcho-Levin syndrome of vertebral anomalies. J Pediatr 1983; 103:270–272.

178. Romero R, Ghidini A, Eswara MS, et al: Prenatal findings in a case of spondylocostal dysplasia type I (Jarcho-Levin syndrome). Obstet Gynecol 1988; 71:988–991.

179. Tolmie JL, Whittle MJ, McNay MB, et al: Second trimester prenatal diagnosis of the Jarcho-Levin syndrome. Prenat Diagn 1987; 7:129–134.

180. Whitley CB, Langer LO, Ophoven J, et al: Fibrochondrogenesis: Lethal, autosomal recessive chondrodysplasia with distinctive cartilage histopathology. Am J Med Genet 1984; 19:265–275.

181. Whitley CB, Burke BA, Granroth G, et al: de le Chapelle dysplasia. Am J Med Genet 1986; 25:29–39.

Dysplasias Without Uniformly Lethal Prognosis

Heterozygous Achondroplasia

182. Elejalde BR, de Elejalde MM, Hamilton PR, et al: Prenatal diagnosis in two pregnancies of an achondroplastic woman. Am J Med Genet 1983; 15:437–439.

183. Filly RA, Golbus MS, Carey JC, et al: Short-limbed dwarfism: Ultrasonographic diagnosis by mensuration of fetal femoral length. Radiology 1981; 138:653–656.

184. Hall BD, Spranger J: Hypochondroplasia: Clinical and radiological aspects in 39 cases. Radiology 1979; 133:95–100.

185. Heselson NG, Cremin BJ, Beighton P: Pseudoachondroplasia, a report of 13 cases. Br J Radiol 1977; 50:473–482.

186. Kurtz AB, Filly RA, Wapner RJ, et al: In utero analysis of heterozygous achondroplasia: Variable time of onset as detected by femur length measurements. J Ultrasound Med 1986; 5:137–140.

187. Leonard CO, Sanders RC, Lau HL: Prenatal diagnosis of the Turner syndrome, a familial chromosomal rearrangement and achondroplasia by amniocentesis and ultrasonography. Johns Hopkins Med J 1979; 145:25–27.

188. Sommer A, Young-Wee T, Frye T: Achondroplasia-Hypochondroplasia complex. Am J Med Genet 1987; 26:949–957.

189. Stoll C, Manini P, Bloch P, et al: Prenatal diagnosis of hypochondroplasia. Prenat Diagn 1985; 5:423–426.

190. Wynne-Davies R, Walsh WK, Gormley J: Achondroplasia and hypochondroplasia. J Bone Joint Surg 1981; 63-B:508–515.

191. Wynne-Davies R, Hall CM, Young ID: Pseudoachondroplasia: Clinical diagnosis at different ages and comparison of autosomal dominant and recessive types. A review of 32 patients (26 kindreds). J Med Genet 1986; 23:425–434.

Asphyxiating Thoracic Dysplasia

192. Callan NA, Colmorgen GHC, Weiner S: Lung hypoplasia and prolonged preterm ruptured membranes: A case report with implications for possible prenatal ultrasonic diagnosis. Am J Obstet Gynecol 1985; 151:756–757.

193. Elejalde BR, de Elejalde MM, Pausch D: Prenatal diagnosis of Jeune syndrome. Am J Med Genet 1985; 21:433–438.

194. Fong K, Ohlsson A, Zalev A: Fetal thoracic circumference: A prospective cross-sectional study with real-time ultrasound. Am J Obstet Gynecol 1988; 158:1154–1160.

195. Lipson ML, Rice J, Adomian G, et al: Prenatal diagnosis of asphyxiating thoracic dysplasia. Am J Med Genet 1984; 18:273–277.
196. Schinzel A, Savoldelli G, Briner J, et al: Prenatal sonographic diagnosis of Jeune syndrome. Radiology 1985; 154:777–778.
197. Skiptunas SM, Weiner S: Early prenatal diagnosis of asphyxiating thoracic dysplasia (Jeune's syndrome): Value of fetal thoracic measurement. J Ultrasound Med 1987; 6:41–43.
198. Zimmer EZ, Weinraub Z, Raijman A, et al: Antenatal diagnosis of a fetus with an extremely narrow thorax and short-rib dwarfism. J Clin Ultrasound 1984; 12:112–114.

Chondroectodermal Dysplasia

199. Bui T-H, Marsk L, Eklof O: Prenatal diagnosis of chondroectodermal dysplasia with fetoscopy. Prenat Diagn 1984; 4:155–159.
200. Mahoney MJ, Hobbins JC: Prenatal diagnosis of chondroectodermal dysplasia (Ellis-van Creveld syndrome) with fetoscopy and ultrasound. N Engl J Med 1977; 297:258–260.

Diastrophic Dysplasia

201. Gollop RR, Eigier A: Prenatal ultrasound diagnosis of diastrophic dysplasia at 16 weeks. Am J Med Genet 1987; 27:321–324.
202. Horton WA, Rimoin DL, Lachman RS, et al: The phenotypic variability of diastrophic dysplasia. J Pediatr 1978; 93:609–613.
203. Kaitila I, Ammala P, Karjalainen D, et al: Early prenatal detection of diastrophic dysplasia. Prenat Diagn 1983; 3:237–244.
204. Mantagos S, Weiss RR, Mahoney M: Prenatal diagnosis of diastrophic dwarfism. Am J Obstet Gynecol 1981; 139:111–113.
205. O'Brien GD, Rodeck C, Queenan JT: Early prenatal diagnosis of diastrophic dwarfism by ultrasound. Br Med J 1980; 280:1300.

Osteogenesis Imperfecta, Types I and IV
(See Osteogenesis Imperfecta under Lethal Dysplasias).

Focal Limb Loss or Abnormality

Amniotic Band Syndrome

206. Borlum K-G: Amniotic band syndrome in second trimester associated with fetal malformations. Prenat Diagn 1984; 4:311–314.
207. Donnenfeld AE, Dunn LK, Rose NC: Discordant amniotic band sequence in monozygotic twins. Am J Med Genet 1985; 20:685–694.
208. Fiedler JM, Phelan JP: The amniotic band syndrome in monozygotic twins. Am J Obstet Gynecol 1983; 146:863–864.
209. Fiske CE, Filly RA, Golbus MS: Prenatal ultrasound diagnosis of amniotic band syndrome. J Ultrasound Med 1982; 1:45–47.
210. Fried AW, Woodring JH, Shier RW, et al: Omphalocele in limb/body wall deficiency syndrome: Atypical sonographic appearance. J Clin Ultrasound 1982; 10:400–402.
211. Herbert WNP, Seeds JW, Cefalo RC, et al: Prenatal detection of intra-amniotic bands: Implications and management. Obstet Gynecol 1985; 65:36S–38S.
212. Hill LM, Kislak S, Jones N: Prenatal ultrasound diagnosis of a forearm constriction band. J Ultrasound Med 1988; 7:293–295.
213. Kalousek DK, Bamforth S: Amnion rupture sequence in previable fetuses. Am J Med Genet 1988; 31:63–73.
214. Lockwood C, Ghidini A, Romero R: Amniotic band syndrome in monozygotic twins: Prenatal diagnosis and pathogenesis. Obstet Gynecol 1988; 71:1012–1016.
215. Mahony BS, Filly RA, Callen PW, et al: The amniotic band syndrome: Antenatal diagnosis and potential pitfalls. Am J Obstet Gynecol 1985; 152:63–68.
216. Malinger G, Rosen N, Achiron R, et al: Pierre Robin sequence associated with amniotic band syndrome: Ultrasonographic diagnosis and pathogenesis. Prenat Diagn 1987; 7:455–459.
217. Patten RM, Allen MV, Mack LA, et al: Limb-body wall complex: In utero sonographic diagnosis of a complicated fetal malformation. AJR 1986; 146:1019–1024.
218. Randel SB, Filly RA, Callen PW, et al: Amniotic sheets. Radiology 1988; 166:633–636.
219. Rushton DI: Amniotic band syndrome. Br Med J 1983; 286:919–920.
220. Seeds JW, Cefalo RC, Herbert WNP: Amniotic band syndrome. Am J Obstet Gynecol 1982; 144:243–248.
221. Torpin R: *Fetal Malformations Caused by Amnion Rupture During Gestation.* Springfield, IL, Charles C Thomas, 1968, pp 1–76.
222. Van Allen MI, Curry C, Gallagher L: Limb body wall complex: I. Pathogenesis. Am J Med Genet 1987; 28:529–548.
223. Van Allen MI, Walden CE, Gallagher L, et al: Limb-body wall complex: II. Limb and spine defects. Am J Med Genet 1987; 28:549–565.
224. Worthen NJ, Lawrence D, Bustillo M: Amniotic band syndrome: Antenatal ultrasonic diagnosis of discordant anencephaly. J Clin Ultrasound 1980; 8:453–455.
225. Yamaguchi M, Yasuda H, Kuroki T, et al: Early prenatal diagnosis of amniotic band syndrome. Am J Perinatol 1988; 5:5–8.

Roberts' Syndrome

226. Freeman MVR, Williams DW, Schimke RN, et al: The Roberts syndrome. Clin Genet 1974; 5:1–16.
227. Gollop TR, Eigier A, Neto JG: Prenatal diagnosis of thalidomide syndrome. Prenat Diagn 1987; 7:295–298.

228. Grundy HO, Burlbaw J, Walton S, et al: Roberts syndrome: Antenatal ultrasound—A case report. J Perinat Med 1988; 16:71.

229. Herrmann J, Feingold M, Tuffli GA, et al: A familial dysmorphogenetic syndrome of limb deformities, characteristic facial appearance and associated anomalies: The "pseudothalidomide" or "SC-syndrome". Birth Defects 1969; 5(3):81–89.

230. Hirose K, Koyanagi T, Hara K, et al: Antenatal ultrasound diagnosis of the femur-fibula-ulna syndrome. J Clin Ultrasound 1988; 16:199–203.

231. Tomkins D, Hunter A, Roberts M: Cytogenetic findings in Roberts-SC phocomelia syndrome(s). Am J Med Genet 1979; 4:17–26.

Radial Ray Defects

232. Benson CB, Pober BR, Hirsch MP, et al: Sonography of Nager acrofacial dysostosis syndrome in utero. J Ultrasound Med 1988; 7:163–167.

233. Brons JTJ, Van Geijn HP, Wladimiroff JW, et al: Prenatal ultrasound diagnosis of the Holt-Oram syndrome. Prenat Diagn 1988; 8:175–181.

234. Filkins K, Russo J, Bilinki I, et al: Prenatal diagnosis of thrombocytopenia absent radius syndrome using ultrasound and fetoscopy. Prenat Diagn 1984; 4:139–142.

235. Hall JG: Thrombocytopenia and absent radius (TAR) syndrome. J Med Genet 1987; 24:79–83.

236. Luthy DA, Hall JG, Graham CB: Prenatal diagnosis of thrombocytopenia with absent radius. Clin Genet 1979; 15:495–499.

237. Luthy DA, Mack L, Hirsch J, et al: Prenatal ultrasound diagnosis of thrombocytopenia with absent radii. Am J Obstet Gynecol 1981; 141:350–351.

238. Meizner I, Bar-Ziv J, Barki Y, et al: Prenatal ultrasonic diagnosis of radial-ray aplasia and renal anomalies (acro-renal syndrome). Prenat Diagn 1986; 6:223–225.

239. Muller LM, de Jong G, Van Heerden KMM: The antenatal ultrasonographic detection of the Holt-Oram syndrome. S Afr Med J 1985; 68:313–315.

240. Rabinowitz JG, Moseley JE, Mitty HA, et al: Trisomy 18, esophageal atresia, anomalies of the radius, and congenital hypoplastic thrombocytopenia. Radiology 1967; 89:488–491.

Focal Femoral Deficiency

241. Graham M: Congenital short femur: Prenatal sonographic diagnosis. J Ultrasound Med 1985; 4:361–363.

Sirenomelia

242. Duhamel B: From the mermaid to anal imperfection: The syndrome of caudal regression. Arch Dis Child 1961; 36:152–155.

243. Honda N, Shimokawa H, Yamaguchi Y, et al: Antenatal diagnosis of sirenomelia (sympus apus). J Clin Ultrasound 1988; 16:675–677.

244. Raabe RD, Harnsberger HR, Lee TG, et al: Ultrasonographic antenatal diagnosis of "Mermaid syndrome": Fusion of fetal lower extremities. J Ultrasound Med 1983; 2:463–464.

245. Sirtori M, Ghidini A, Romero R, et al: Prenatal diagnosis of sirenomelia. J Ultrasound Med 1989; 8:83–88.

246. Von Lennep E, El Khazen N, DePierreux G, et al: A case of partial sirenomelia and possible vitamin A teratogenesis. Prenat Diagn 1985; 5:35–40.

Contractures and Postural Deformities

247. Baty BJ, Cubberley D, Morris C, et al: Prenatal diagnosis of distal arthrogryposis. Am J Med Genet 1988; 29:501–510.

248. Bendon R, Dignon P, Siddiqi T: Prenatal diagnosis of arthrogryposis multiplex congenita. J Pediatr 1987; 111:942–947.

249. Cardwell MS: Pena-Shokeir syndrome: Prenatal diagnosis by ultrasonography. J Ultrasound Med 1987; 6:619–621.

250. Chen H, Bhimberg B, Immken L, et al: The Pena-Shokeir syndrome: Report of five cases and further delineation of the syndrome. Am J Med Genet 1983; 16:213–224.

251. Chen H, Immken L, Lachmen R, et al: Syndrome of multiple pterygia, camptodactyly, facial anomalies, hypoplastic lungs and heart, cystic hygroma, and skeletal anomalies: Delineation of a new entity and review of lethal forms of multiple pterygium syndrome. Am J Med Genet 1984; 17:809–826.

252. Christianson AL, Nelson MM: Four cases of trisomy 18 syndrome with limb reduction malformations. J Med Genet 1984; 21:293–294.

253. Davis JE, Kalousek DK: Fetal akinesia deformation sequence in previable fetuses. Am J Med Genet 1988; 29:77–87.

254. Emerson DS, Brown DL, Mabie BC: Prenatal sonographic diagnosis of hip dislocation. J Ultrasound Med 1988; 7:687–689.

255. Goldberg JD, Chervenak FA, Lipman RA, et al: Antenatal sonographic diagnosis of arthrogryposis multiplex congenita. Prenat Diagn 1986; 6:45–49.

256. Merz E, Goldofer W: Sonographic image of arthrogryposis multiplex congenita. Geburtshilfe Frauenheilkd 1985; 45:406–409.

257. Hall JG, Reed SD, Rosenbaum KN, et al: Limb pterygium syndromes: A review and report of eleven patients. Am J Med Genet 1982; 12:377–409.

258. Hall JG: The lethal multiple pterygium syndromes (editorial comment). Am J Med Genet 1984; 17:803–807.

259. Hall JG: Invited editorial comment: Analysis of Pena-Shokeir phenotype. Am J Med Genet 1986; 25:99–117.

260. Herva R, Conradi NG, Kalimo H, et al: A syndrome of multiple congenital contractures: Neuropathological

analysis of five fetal cases. Am J Med Genet 1988; 29:67–76.

261. Kirkinen P, Herva R, Leisti J: Early prenatal diagnosis of a lethal syndrome of multiple congenital contractures. Prenat Diagn 1987; 7:189–196.

262. Lindhout D, Hageman G, Beemer FA, et al: The Pena-Shokeir syndrome: Report of nine Dutch cases. Am J Med Genet 1985; 21:655–668.

263. Lockwood C, Irons M, Troiani J, et al: The prenatal sonographic diagnosis of lethal multiple pterygium syndrome: A heritable cause of recurrent abortion. Am J Obstet Gynecol 1988; 159:474–476.

264. MacMillan RH, Harbert GM, Davis WD, et al: Prenatal diagnosis of Pena-Shokeir syndrome type I. Am J Med Genet 1985; 21:279–284.

265. Miller ME, Higginbottom M, Smith DW: Short umbilical cord: Its origin and relevance. Pediatrics 1981; 67:618–621.

266. Miskin M, Rothberg R, Rudd NL, et al: Arthrogryposis multiplex congenita—Prenatal assessment with diagnostic ultrasound and fetoscopy. J Pediatr 1979; 95:463–464.

267. Moessinger AC: Fetal akinesia deformation sequence: An animal model. Pediatrics 1983; 72:857–863.

268. Muller LM, de Jong G: Prenatal ultrasonographic features of the Pena-Shokeir I syndrome and the Trisomy 18 syndrome. Am J Med Genet 1986: 25:119–129.

269. Muller LM, de Jong G, Mouton SCE, et al: A case of the Neu-Laxova syndrome: Prenatal ultrasonographic monitoring in the third trimester and the histopathological findings. Am J Med Genet 1987; 26:421–429.

270. Ohlsson A, Fong KW, Rose TH, et al: Prenatal sonographic diagnosis of Pena-Shokeir syndrome type I, or fetal akinesia deformation sequence. Am J Med Genet 1988; 29:59–65.

271. Pursutte WH, Lenke RR, Kurezynski TW, et al: Antenatal diagnosis of Pena-Shokeir syndrome (type I) with ultrasonography and magnetic resonance imaging. Obstet Gynecol 1988; 72:472–475.

272. Savoldelli G, Schinzel A: Prenatal ultrasound detection of humeral-radial synostosis in a case of Antley-Bixler syndrome. Prenat Diagn 1982; 2:219–223.

273. Scott CI, Louro JM, Laurence KM, et al: Letter to the editor: Comments on the Neu-Laxova syndrome and CAD complex. Am J Med Genet 1981; 9:165–175.

274. Shenker L, Reed K, Anderson C, et al: Syndrome of camptodactyly, ankyloses, facial anomalies, and pulmonary hypoplasia (Pena-Shokeir syndrome): Obstetric and ultrasound aspects. Am J Obstet Gynecol 1985; 152:303–307.

275. Toriello HV: Restrictive dermopathy and report of another case (editorial comment). Am J Med Genet 1986; 24:625–629.

276. Witt DR, Hayden MR, Holbrook KA, et al: Restrictive dermopathy: A newly recognized autosomal recessive skin dysplasia. Am J Med Genet 1986; 24:631–648.

277. Zeitune M, Fejgin MD, Abramowicz J, et al: Prenatal diagnosis of the pterygium syndrome. Prenat Diagn 1988; 8:145–149.

Other Hand and Foot Deformities

278. Benacerraf BR, Frigoletto FD: Prenatal ultrasound diagnosis of clubfoot. Radiology 1985; 155:211–213.

279. Benacerraf BR: Antenatal sonographic diagnosis of congenital clubfoot: A possible indication for amniocentesis. J Clin Ultrasound 1986; 14:703–706.

280. Benacerraf BR, Frigoletto FD, Greene MF: Abnormal facial features and extremities in human trisomy syndromes: Prenatal ultrasonographic appearance. Radiology 1986; 159:243–246.

281. Benacerraf BR, Osathanondh, Frigoletto FD: Sonographic demonstration of hypoplasia of the middle phalanx of the fifth digit: A finding associated with Down syndrome. Am J Obstet Gynecol 1988; 159:181–183.

282. Bundy AL, Saltzman DH, Pober B, et al: Antenatal sonographic findings in trisomy 18. J Ultrasound Med 1986; 5:361–364.

283. Chervenak FA, Tortora M, Hobbins JC: Antenatal sonographic diagnosis of clubfoot. J Ultrasound Med 1985; 4:49–50.

284. Cowell HR, Wein BK: Genetic aspects of clubfoot. J Bone Joint Surg 1980; 62:1381–1384.

285. Hashimoto BE, Filly RA, Callen PW: Sonographic diagnosis of clubfoot in utero. J Ultrasound Med 1986; 5:81–83.

286. Iaccarino M, Lonardo F, Giugliano M, et al: Prenatal diagnosis of Mohr syndrome by ultrasonography. Prenat Diagn 1985; 5:415–418.

287. Jeanty P, Romero R, d'Alton M, et al: In utero sonographic detection of hand and foot deformities. J Ultrasound Med 1985; 4:595–601.

288. Nyberg DA, Mack LA, Hirsch JH, et al: Fetal hydrocephalus: Sonographic detection and clinical significance of associated anomalies. Radiology 1987; 163:187–191.

289. Sauerbrei EE: The split-image artifact in pelvic ultrasonography. The anatomy and physics. J Ultrasound Med 1985; 4:29–34.

290. Sucheston ME, Cannon MS (eds): *Congenital Malformations.* Philadelphia, FA Davis Co, 1973.

Enlargement, Masses, or Abnormal Echogenicity

291. Hatjis CG, Philip AG, Anderson GG, et al: The in utero ultrasonographic appearance of Klippel-Trenaunay-Weber syndrome. Am J Obstet Gynecol 1981; 139:972–974.

292. Koenigsberg M, Factor S, Cho S, et al: Fetal Marfan syndrome: Prenatal ultrasound diagnosis with pathological confirmation of skeletal and aortic lesions. Prenat Diagn 1981; 1:241–247.

293. Lamminen A, Jaaskelainen J, Rapola J, et al: High-frequency ultrasonography of skeletal muscle in chil-

dren with neuromuscular disease. J Ultrasound Med 1988; 7:505–509.

294. Lewis BD, Doubilet PM, Heller VL, et al: Cutaneous and visceral hemangiomata in the Klippel-Trenaunay-Weber syndrome: Antenatal sonographic detection. AJR 1986; 147:598–600.

295. Pyeritz RE: Maternal and fetal complications of pregnancy in the Marfan syndrome. Am J Med 1981; 71:784–790.

296. Shah KD, Chervenak FA, Marchevsky AM, et al: Fetal giant hemangiolymphangioma: Report of a case. Am J Perinatol 1987; 4:212–214.

297. Shalev E, Romero S, Nseir T, et al: Klippel-Trenaunay-Weber syndrome: Ultrasonic prenatal diagnosis. J Clin Ultrasound 1988; 16:268–270.

298. Warhit JM, Goldman MA, Sachs L, et al: Klippel-Trenaunay-Weber syndrome: Appearance in utero. J Ultrasound Med 1983; 2:515–518.

Hydrops and Ascites

Yogesh P. Shah, M.D.

Frank P. Hadlock, M.D.

Fetal hydrops, defined as an excess of fetal body water, is generally categorized by the underlying etiology into immune and non-immune types. Ascites is usually associated with both immune and non-immune hydrops, although it may also be seen as an isolated finding. Whenever possible, isolated ascites should be distinguished from generalized hydrops, because of inherent differences in the etiology, prognosis, and management of affected pregnancies.

Prenatal ultrasound has assumed a primary role in detecting, monitoring, and guiding fetal therapy of affected pregnancies with fetal hydrops and ascites. This chapter discusses fetal hydrops due to immune and non–immune causes separately followed by a discussion of isolated ascites.

IMMUNE HYDROPS

The clinical approach to immune hydrops has significantly changed over the last 20 years, parallel with prophylaxis against isoimmunization, routine screening for atypical antibodies, availability of intrauterine therapy, and improvements in prenatal sonography. Although non–immune hydrops is now more common than immune hydrops, recognition and treatment of immune hydrops remains an important clinical problem.

Immune hydrops is primarily due to incompatibility of maternal antibodies with rhesus (Rh) antigens on fetal red blood cells. The Rh blood group was first discovered in 1940 by Landsteiner and Weiner, and distinct antigens (D, C, and E) were subsequently identified.[24] Rh isoimmunization can potentially occur when the mother is Rh negative and the fetus is Rh positive. In the United States, approximately 15% of whites and 8% of blacks are Rh negative.[16]

Rh(D) isoimmunization initially accounted for 98% of all cases of immune hydrops, and this is still the most common type. With widespread prophylaxis against Rh(D) antibodies, however, isoimmunization against other blood group antigens now comprises a greater proportion of immune hydrops (Table 14–1). These include antigens in the Rh system (E and C), Kell system, and Duffy system.

Pathogenesis

A maternal immune (antibody) response develops when the mother is exposed to red blood cell antigens different from her own. Fetal red blood cells do not normally cross the placental barrier, so that exposure of fetal cells to the maternal circulation typically occurs at the time of delivery of a previous pregnancy and/or previous abortion (spontaneous or therapeutic). Other events that can sensitize maternal antibodies include spontaneous fetal/maternal hemorrhage within the placenta from a placental abruption or intervillous hemorrhage, amniocentesis, or transfusion of mismatched blood.

Unlike red blood cells, maternal antibodies (IgG) freely cross the placental/fetal barrier. Fetal hemolysis results from binding of maternal antibodies to antigens on the surface of fetal red blood cells. Subsequently, fetal anemia stimulates erythropoiesis in extramedullary sites, especially in the liver and spleen. Depending on the severity of erythropoiesis, hepatomegaly and alter-

TABLE 14–1.

Hemolytic Disease Resulting From Irregular Antibodies*

Blood Group System	Antigens Related to Hemolytic Disease	Severity of Hemolytic Disease	Proposed Management
Lewis	Not a proved cause of hemolytic disease of the newborn.		
I	Not a proved cause of hemolytic disease of the newborn.		
Kell	K	Mild to severe with hydrops fetalis	Amniotic fluid bilirubin studies
	k	Mild	Expectant
	Ko	Mild	Expectant
	Kp^a	Mild	Expectant
	Kp$_b$	Mild	Expectant
	Js^a	Mild	Expectant
	Js^b	Mild	Expectant
Duffy	Fy^a	Mild to severe with hydrops fetalis	Amniotic fluid bilirubin studies
	Fy^b	Not a cause of hemolytic disease of the newborn.	
	Fy^3	Mild	Expectant
Kidd	Jk^a	Mild to severe	Amniotic fluid bilirubin studies
	Jk^b	Mild	Expectant
	Jk^3	Mild	Expectant
MNSs	M	Mild to Severe	Amniotic fluid bilirubin studies
	N	Mild	Expectant
	S	Mild to severe	Amniotic fluid bilirubin studies
	s	Mild to severe	Amniotic fluid bilirubin studies
	U	Mild to severe	Amniotic fluid bilirubin studies
	Mi^a	Moderate	Amniotic fluid bilirubin studies
	Mt^a	Moderate	Amniotic fluid bilirubin studies
	Vw	Mild	Expectant
	Mur	Mild	Expectant
	Hil	Mild	Expectant
	Hut	Mild	Expectant
Lutheran	Lu^a	Mild	Expectant
	Lu^b	Mild	Expectant
Diego	Di^a	Mild to severe	Amniotic fluid bilirubin studies
	Di^b	Mild to severe	Amniotic fluid bilirubin studies
Xg	Xg^a	Mild	Expectant
p	PP$_1$^{pk}(Tj^a)	Mild to severe	Amniotic fluid bilirubin studies
Public antigens	Yt^a	Moderate to severe	Amniotic fluid bilirubin studies
	Yt^b	Mild	Expectant
	Lan	Mild	Expectant
	En^a	Moderate	Amniotic fluid bilirubin studies
	Ge	Mild	Expectant
	Jr^a	Mild	Expectant
	Co^a	Severe	Amniotic fluid bilirubin studies
	Co^{a-b-}	Mild	Expectant
Private antigens	Batty	Mild	Expectant
	Becker	Mild	Expectant
	Berrens	Mild	Expectant
	Biles	Moderate	Amniotic fluid bilirubin studies
	Evans	Mild	Expectant
	Gonzales	Mild	Expectant
	Good	Severe	Amniotic fluid bilirubin studies
	Heibel	Moderate	Amniotic fluid bilirubin studies
	Hunt	Mild	Expectant
	Jobbins	Mild	Expectant
	Radin	Moderate	Amniotic fluid bilirubin studies
	Rm	Mild	Expectant
	Ven	Mild	Expectant
	Wright^a	Severe	Amniotic fluid bilirubin studies
	Wright^b	Mild	Expectant
	Zd	Moderate	Amniotic fluid bilirubin studies

*From Weinstein L: Irregular antibodies causing hemolytic disease of the newborn: A continuing problem. Clin Obstet Gynecol 1982; 25(2):321–332. Used by permission.

ations in the liver may result in portal and umbilical venous hypertension which, in turn, may result in fetal ascites and placental edema. Hypoproteinemia may result from decreased protein synthesis by the abnormal liver and impaired placental perfusion of amino acids.[2, 6] The end result, fetal hydrops, is thought to result from a combination of anemia, portal hypertension, hepatic dysfunction, hypoproteinemia, and low oncotic pressure.[6] High-output cardiac failure may also contribute to fetal hydrops, however this does not appear to be a predominant factor since fetuses with immune hydrops generally have normal blood volume.[6, 28]

While the sequence of events outlined above is widely accepted, the interaction of contributing factors is complex, so that clinical manifestations of fetal hydrops are not always predictable.[6, 9, 30] Nevertheless, this process provides a basis for understanding and interpreting sonographic findings of immune hydrops, as well as some types of non-immune hydrops.

Clinical Approach

A clinical approach to immune hydrops is outlined in Figure 14–1. If the screening antibody screen is positive, antibodies are subsequently identified and quantified and the father's blood is tested for the corresponding antigen. Women found to have Rh antibodies are then followed with serial antibody titers until a "critical" level is reached (1:8 to 1:16 or greater).[6, 16, 31] Fetuses considered to be at risk for developing hydrops are then monitored with amniotic fluid analysis and prenatal sonography.[31]

In general, the risk of fetal hydrops is related to the severity of hemolysis. Determination of amniotic fluid Δ OD 450 gives an indirect measure of bilirubin, and therefore the degree of hemolysis during the third trimester.[6, 25] These results are evaluated using Liley's three-zone chart (Fig 14–2), which plots normal range values for Δ OD 450 against gestational age from 26 weeks to term. Zone II may be further divided into upper and lower subzones (IIa and IIb). The closer the value falls to zone III, the higher the risk of fetal hydrops and the more closely the pregnancy is monitored.[31] When the value for a single determination falls in zone I, subsequent amniocentesis can usually be deferred for an additional 2–3 weeks. The trend in serial Δ OD 450 values is also important in assessing the frequency of fetal monitoring.

Multiple amniocenteses frequently are required for determination of Δ OD 450, and ultimately for evaluation of fetal lung maturity. Ultrasound guidance is generally used during amniocentesis to avoid the placenta and minimize the risk of further maternal sensitization and antibody production.[19]

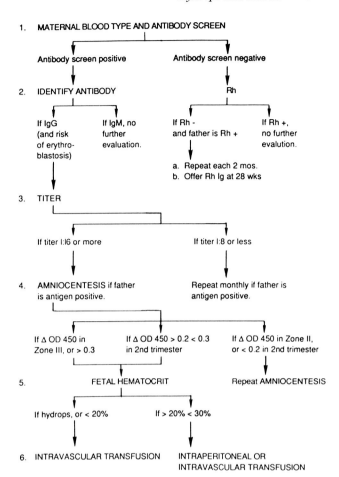

FIG 14–1.
General guidelines for evaluation and treatment of Rh isoimmunization. (From Parer JT: Severe Rh immunization—current methods of in utero diagnosis and treatment. Am J Obstet Gynecol 1988; 58:1323–1327. Used by permission.)

The limitations as well as the benefits of amniotic fluid evaluation should be recognized. Falsely evaluated results may be obtained if the amniotic fluid sample is contaminated with meconium or blood or if the gestational age is not known with certainty.[8, 25, 30] More importantly, extrapolating the Liley curves to the second trimester has been found to be a poor predictor of the severity of fetal hemolysis.[18, 30] Nicolaides et al. found that sonographic evidence of hydrops was associated with low, rather than elevated values of Δ OD 450 during the second trimester, probably due to the dilutional effect in excess fluid.[30] Other authors have also found extrapolated Liley curves to be inaccurate during the second trimester.[6, 16]

Cordocentesis represents a more direct method for evaluating fetal anemia than does amniotic fluid analysis.[5, 11, 12, 17, 36] This method requires sonographically guided aspiration of fetal blood from the umbilical vessels, usually the umbilical vein near its insertion into

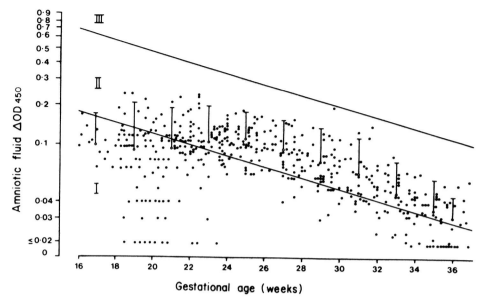

FIG 14–2.
Normal Liley curves extrapolated to the second trimester compares amniotic fluid Δ OD 450 with gestational age. *Dots* indicate values from 497 normal pregnancies not complicated by fetal hemolysis. (From Nicolaides KH, Rodeck CH, Misbashan RS: Have Liley charts outlived their usefulness? Am J Obstet Gynecol 1986; 155:90–94. Used by permission.)

the placenta. Although cordocentesis is an invasive technique, it avoids potential false-positive and false-negative results that may accompany amniotic fluid analysis. It also provides an opportunity for simultaneous therapy with intravascular fetal transfusion.

Parer recommends fetal hematocrit evaluation by cordocentesis when the Δ OD 450 is greater than 0.2 and advocates intrauterine transfusion when the Δ OD 450 is greater than 0.3.[31] However, according to the data of Nicolaides et al., a Δ OD 450 cutoff level of 0.2 would identify only 90% of fetuses with severe hemolysis (hemoglobin < 6 gm/ml) and would also include 54% of fetuses with mild hemolysis (hemoglobin 6–9.7 gm/ml) during the second trimester.[30] Therefore, Nicolaides et al. suggest that cordocentesis is the only reliable means of assessing the severity of hemolysis during the second trimester.[30]

Sonographic Findings

Classic sonographic features of fetal hydrops include serous cavity effusions (ascites, pleural and/or pericardial effusions), polyhydramnios, placental edema, and skin edema (anasarca).[9, 52] Other sonographic findings of fetal hydrops may include hepatosplenomegaly and alterations in fetal or umbilical vessels. The diagnosis of fetal hydrops is readily made when all of these findings are demonstrated. However, these findings may occur alone or in combination, depending on the duration and severity of the process.

Sonographic evidence of hydrops generally reflects the severity of fetal hemolysis, although this relationship is inconsistent. Hydropic fetuses usually have a hematocrit less than 15% and total protein levels below 3 gm/dl.[9, 16] However, the converse is not always true. For example, Chitkara et al. observed serous cavity effusions in only five of eight fetuses with a hematocrit less than 15%.[9]

Ascites typically is one of the earliest manifestations of hydrops (Fig 14–3), whereas pleural and/or pericardial effusions are characteristic of more severe hydrops.[3, 9, 14] Of five fetuses with evidence of hydrops reported by Chitkara et al., two had ascites only, one had ascites with pleural and pericardial effusion, one had ascites and pleural effusion, and one had ascites and pericardial effusion. In no case was pericardial effusion seen in the absence of ascites.[9]

Early development of ascites supports the importance attributed to portal hypertension in the pathogenesis of immune hydrops.[6] Ascites that accompanies fetal hydrops should be distinguished from isolated ascites (discussed later in this chapter), since the latter usually is associated with different etiologies and a more favorable prognosis. However, this distinction is occasionally difficult, particularly when hydrops is mild and other manifestations are absent. Hence, isolated ascites frequently is included in the discussion of fetal hydrops.

A small amount of ascites is identified on sonography as fluid between bowel loops, along the abdominal flanks, or within the pelvis.[3, 45, 54] Care should be taken

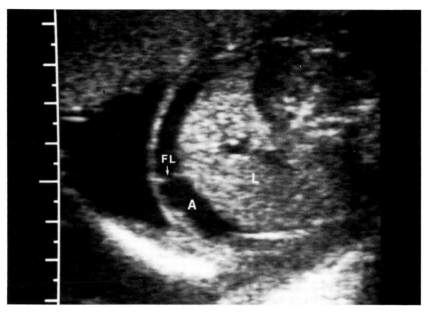

FIG 14–3.
Immune hydrops and ascites. Transverse scan of the abdomen at 28 weeks' gestation in a fetus with immune hydrops demonstrates a small amount of ascites *(A)* surrounding the liver *(L)* and falciform ligament *(FL)*. Mild polyhydramnios is also present. Hydrops resolved after intravascular transfusion.

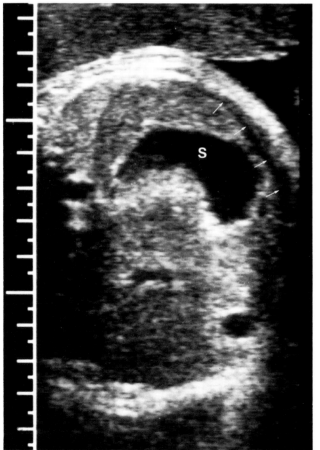

FIG 14–4.
Pseudoascites. Transverse scan demonstrates a hypoechoic rim *(arrows)* surrounding the abdomen that represents abdominal wall musculature. This should not be confused with true ascites. *S* = stomach.

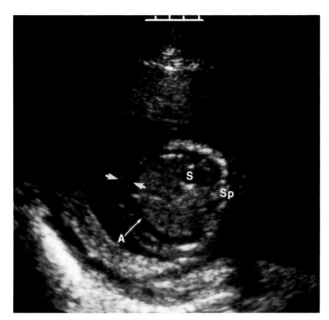

FIG 14–5.
Anasarca and immune hydrops. Transverse scan of the abdomen at 21 weeks shows ascites *(A)* and marked skin and subcutaneous thickening *(arrows)*. S = stomach; Sp = spine.

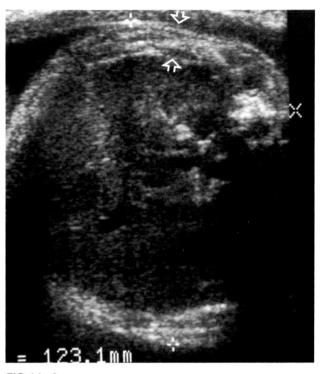

FIG 14–6.
Macrosomia. Transverse scan of the abdomen shows increased subcutaneous fat *(open arrows)* in a macrosomic fetus. This subcutaneous fat should not be confused with subcutaneous edema.

to distinguish true ascites from "pseudoascites", which is observed as a hypoechoic band surrounding the fetal abdomen and represents normal abdominal wall musculature (Fig 14–4).[113, 120] Care also should be taken to distinguish pericardial effusion from the normally hypoechoic fetal myocardium.

Polyhydramnios usually accompanies fetal hydrops, although oligohydramnios may also be present. Chitkara et al. suggest that polyhydramnios is one of the earliest sonographic signs of fetal hydrops before other abnormalities develop.[9] Either subjective or semiquantitative methods can be used for evaluation of polyhydramnios (see Chapter 3), although the present authors prefer a subjective evaluation.

Placental edema can be recognized on sonography as increased placental thickness. Hoddick et al. found that placental thickness normally increases with gestational age but it also is dependent on the surface area of the placenta within the uterus.[22] In general, however, the placenta normally measures less than 4 cm in thickness.[22] Chitkara et al. found that the placenta was abnormally thickened (greater than 4 cm) in 50% of fetuses with severe immune hydrops (hematocrit less than 15%) and in 14% of cases with moderate hydrops (hematocrit 16%–20%).[9] Severe polyhydramnios may appear to compress the placenta and result in normal placental thickness.

Edema of the skin and subcutaneous tissues (anasarca) is generally defined as a skin thickness greater than 5 mm (Fig 14–5). However, mild edema may be difficult to distinguish from the normal integument. Also the integument may be thickened in association with other conditions including macrosomia (Fig 14–6). Furthermore, skin edema is considered a relatively late manifestation of fetal hydrops.[9, 38] For these reasons, evaluation of anasarca is often difficult.

Hepatosplenomegaly is a pathologic hallmark of immune hydrops (Fig 14–7). Since extramedullary hematopoiesis and hepatomegaly are considered to be early events in the process leading to immune hydrops, quantifying liver size is potentially useful. By measuring the sagittal length of the right lobe on serial sonograms, Vintzileos et al. found that the liver grew more than 5 mm per week in all fetuses with severe immune hydrops who required transfusion or delivery within 2 weeks of the sonogram.[37] By contrast, Nicolaides et al. found that evaluation of liver size was of no value in predicting the severity of anemia.[29] Measurement of the fetal liver also may be technically difficult.

Alterations in fetal and umbilical vessels have been evaluated as a means for monitoring both immune and non–immune hydrops (Fig 14–8). DeVore et al. suggest that the umbilical vein diameter increases before other manifestations of hydrops in Rh hemolytic anemia.[13] Measuring the umbilical vein diameter within

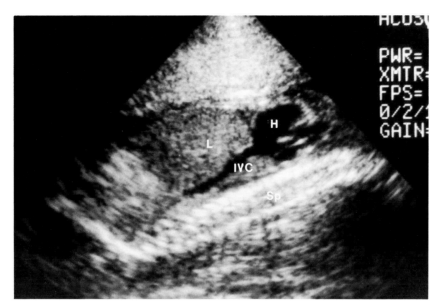

FIG 14–7.
Hepatomegaly and dilated inferior vena cava in Rh isoimmunization. Sagittal sonogram of a fetus with Rh immune hydrops demonstrates enlargement of the liver *(L)* with extension of the right lobe to the lower abdomen. Also note prominence of the inferior vena cava *(IVC)*. *SP* = spine; *H* = heart.

both the amniotic fluid as well as within the liver, they found that an increased diameter (> 1 cm) may precede other signs of hydrops.[13] Similar findings have been made by some investigators,[23, 27] but have not been confirmed by others.[9, 29, 39]

The ductus venosus, which is not easily visualized in normal fetuses, may also become more prominent with developing portal hypertension (Figs 14–8 and 14–9). This observation can be explained by increased blood flow through the ductus venosus, thereby circumventing passage through the liver parenchyma. However, no formal study of this observation has been performed.

A possible relationship between Doppler studies

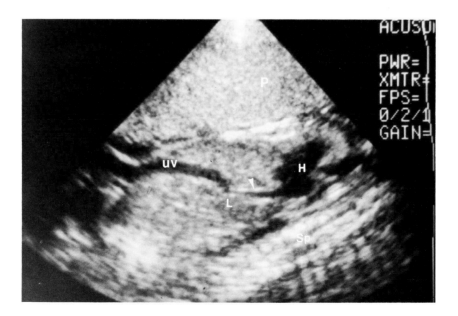

FIG 14–8.
Prominent ductus venosus in Rh isoimmunization. Sagittal scan in a fetus with Rh sensitization (same fetus as Fig 14–7) shows prominence of the ductus venosus *(arrowhead)* as it continues cephalically from the intrahepatic portion of the umbilical vein *(UV)*. Also note mild thickening of the placenta *(P)*. These findings preceded other evidence of hydrops in this case. *H* = heart; *Sp* = spine.

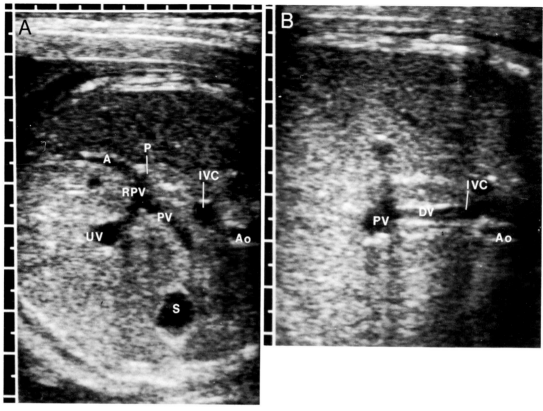

FIG 14–9.
Prominent ductus venosus and immune hydrops. **A,** transverse scan of the abdomen at 32 weeks in a fetus with rhesus isoimmunization that shows normal vasculature. Mild fetal hydrops was noted on other images. *UV* = umbilical portion of left portal vein; *RPV* = main right portal vein; *A* = anterior division of right portal vein; *P* = posterior division of right portal vein; *PV* = main portal vein; *IVC* = inferior vena cava; *Ao* = aorta; *S* = stomach. **B,** scan angled toward the fetal head shows the ductus venosus *(DV)* coursing from the undivided portal vein *(PV)* to the inferior vena cava *(IVC)*. The ductus venosus usually is difficult to visualize in normal fetuses but appears to enlarge with fetal hydrops. *Ao* = aorta.

and fetal hematocrit has been examined by several investigators.[16] Kirkenen et al. observed increased umbilical venous velocity in fetuses with Rh-isoimmunized hydrops,[23] whereas others have found that Doppler studies are of no value in the prediction of fetal hematocrit.[16] In summary, the clinical utility of evaluating fetal and umbilical vessels to predict immune hydrops remains uncertain.

Prognosis

The prognosis for pregnancies affected with Rh-immune hydrops varies with the onset and severity of hydrops. Approximately 20%–25% of affected fetuses become hydropic, and 20% die without intervention.[6] A history of Rh-related hydrops or stillbirth in a previous affected pregnancy increases the risk of hydropic death in the current pregnancy to 90% without treatment.[6]

With early surveillance and aggressive management, the prognosis of immune hydrops can be significantly improved. The reported prognosis varies between centers, however, depending on selection criteria, gestational age at the time of treatment, and the type of treatment. Harman et al. reported an overall survival rate of 92% for sensitized fetuses, including a survival rate of 100% for non–hydropic fetuses and 75% for hydropic fetuses.[19] Using intravascular transfusion in 47 fetuses with Rh sensitization (including 32 with hydrops), Grannum and Copel reported an overall survival rate of 79%, including 60% for fetuses with a gestational age less than 26 weeks and 100% for fetuses greater than 26 weeks.[16]

Management

Major advances have been made in the management of women with Rh isoimmunization, the most important of which has been widespread and effective prophylaxis against Rh sensitization. With routine administration of Rh immunoglobulin (RhoGAM) to Rh negative women at the time of their potential sensitization to the Rh antigen, the incidence of sensitization has been reduced approximately four-fold.[8] However, despite Rh prophylaxis, sonographers will continue to encounter immune hydrops because of instances of unsuccessful prophylaxis and because of isoimmunization to non-Rh(D) antigens.

Management of pregnancies with fetal hemolysis from Rh sensitization includes serial amniocentesis and/or cordocentesis to determine the severity of hemolysis, fetal transfusion via intraperitoneal transfusion or intravascular (umbilical venous) transfusion, and pre-term delivery at a time when the risks of continued hemolysis are balanced against the risks of prematurity. Other management options that have been proposed, but which are rarely utilized, include maternal plasmapheresis and maternal immunosuppressive therapy.[16]

Intrauterine fetal transfusion was initially described by Liley in 1963 using fluoroscopic guidance and intra-amniotic injection of radiopaque dye which is swallowed by the fetus.[26] This made it possible for the first time to directly treat fetuses suffering from Rh-immune hydrops. However, intraperitoneal transfusion (IPT) originally carried a high fetal mortality and morbidity, in large part due to the difficulty in directing needle placement in the fetal abdomen.

Ultrasound guidance was proposed by Hansman in 1972[18] and subsequently by others.[11, 21] Real-time ultrasound guidance was first used by Cooperberg and Carpenter in 1977.[11] Real-time sonographic guidance now permits very precise placement of the needle into the fetal peritoneal cavity where the blood is infused and subsequently resorbed by the fetus.[1, 4, 10, 11] Precise control of intrauterine transfusion has also re-

duced the procedural-related mortality from 51% to less than 5%.[19]

The optimal time for fetal transfusion is when fetal hemolysis has progressed to the point of moderate anemia but before development of hydrops. Intrauterine transfusion usually is not performed after 32 weeks because of the excellent survival rate of delivery after this age.[35] The amount of blood (packed, group O, Rh negative) instilled into the peritoneal cavity varies with gestational age and can be approximated by the formula: volume = (menstrual age in weeks − 20) × 10 ml.[6] Fetal heart rate is monitored throughout the transfusion; development of bradycardia is an indication for termination of the procedure.

After intraperitoneal transfusion, sonographic evaluation is useful for monitoring absorption of intraperitoneal fluid and for monitoring changes in hydrops. Hashimoto et al. found that peritoneal fluid was absorbed in all non-hydropic fetuses between 8–12 days following intraperitoneal transfusion, depending on the quantity of blood infused.[20] However, intraperitoneal fluid was seen as long as 24 days after intraperitoneal transfusion in hydropic fetuses. Persistent intraperitoneal fluid could reflect slow absorption of red blood cells or reaccumulation of fetal ascites.

Cordocentesis has rapidly become a widely accepted method for obtaining samples of fetal blood and for accomplishing direct intravascular transfusion as early as 17 weeks' gestation (Fig 14–10).[5, 12, 17, 34–36] Originally proposed by Rodeck et al. using fetoscopy,[34]

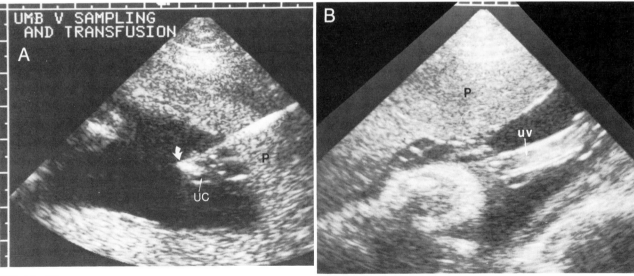

FIG 14–10.
Cordocentesis and umbilical vein transfusion at 22 weeks. **A,** under sonographic guidance, the needle tip *(curved arrow)* is placed into the umbilical cord *(UC)* near its insertion with the placenta *(P)*. Umbilical vein sampling confirmed fetal anemia prior to hydrops in this fetus with Rh sensitization. **B,** injection of blood displays the lumen of the umbilical vein *(UV)* with echogenic blood products and microbubbles. *P* = placenta. (Courtesy of Harris Finberg, MD, Phoenix, AZ.)

cordocentesis is now performed under ultrasound guidance.[17] Precise sonographic guidance permits puncture of the umbilical cord, usually near its insertion site into the placenta.

Because of the technical skill required for successful cordocentesis, this procedure is usually limited to high-risk referral centers. Even then, successful cordocentesis may be difficult in the second trimester when the umbilical cord is small. Increased placental thickness and fetal mobility due to polyhydramnios may present additional obstacles to successful cordocentesis. Potential complications of cordocentesis include umbilical vein thrombosis and acute fetal distress.[31]

Intravascular transfusion provides a rapid and effective method for fetal transfusion. In contrast, intraperitoneally transfused blood may be absorbed erratically, especially in the presence of ascites.[16] Reversal of significant improvement in fetal hydrops usually can be demonstrated in fetuses with mild to moderate hydrops following intravascular transfusion. Grannum and Copel found that of 25 surviving fetuses that were initially seen with mild to moderate hydrops, reversal of hydrops was demonstrated in 14 after one treatment, 6 after two treatments, and 2 after three or more treatments.[16]

NON-IMMUNE HYDROPS

Non-immune hydrops fetalis (NIHF) was first distinguished from immune hydrops by Potter in 1943.[88] When first described, NIHF represented less than 20% of all cases of fetal hydrops. However, with effective prophylaxis against Rh immunization, NIHF now comprises 90% of cases of fetal hydrops.[38]

The reported prevalence of NIHF is 1 in 2,500 to 3,500 births, although this estimate varies with the definition of NIHF. For example, some authors require demonstration of edema, ascites, and pleural effusions for the diagnosis of NIHF, while others have included cases in which an isolated fluid collection (ascites or pleural effusion) is observed.[52, 59]

Pathogenesis

Unlike immune hydrops, NIHF is a heterogeneous disorder resulting from a wide variety of underlying etiologies.[56, 70, 78, 86] The success in identifying an underlying cause depends both on the criteria for inclusion of hydrops and the effort in establishing a diagnosis. Earlier studies reported that an underlying cause could be identified in only 40% of cases of NIHF, although more recent studies suggest that careful prenatal and postnatal investigation may identify an etiologic

TABLE 14–2.

Pathophysiologic Classification of Hydrops Fetalis*

1. Primary myocardial failure
   Arrhythmia (e.g., paroxysmal atrial tachycardia, familial heart block)
   Severe anemia (e.g., glucose-6-phosphatase dehydrogenase deficiency, thalassemia)
   Twin-twin transfusion syndrome
   Myocarditis (e.g., coxsackievirus, TORCH)
   Cardiac malformation
2. High-output failure
   Severe anemia (e.g., thalassemia, Gaucher's disease)
   Arteriovenous shunt
3. Obstruction of venous return
   Congenital neoplasm/other space-occupying lesions (e.g., neuroblastoma, retroperitoneal fibroids, vena caval thrombosis)
4. Decreased plasma oncotic pressure
   Decreased albumin formation (e.g., congenital cirrhosis, hepatitis)
   Increased albumin excretion (e.g., congenital nephrotic syndrome of Finnish type)
5. Increased capillary permeability
   Anoxia (e.g., congenital infection, placental edema)
6. Obstruction of lymph flow (e.g., Turner's syndrome)

*Modified from Giacoia GP: Hydrops fetalis. Clin Pediatr 1980; 19:334.

factor in up to 84% of cases.[70] The word "cause" is used with some caution in this context, however, because an understandable cause and effect relationship with the fetal anomaly may be lacking. It may be more proper, therefore, to classify some of these relationships as associations.

Theoretically, development of edema can be attributed to one of six principal factors (1) primary myocardial failure; (2) high-output cardiac failure; (3) decreased plasma oncotic pressure; (4) increased capillary permeability; (5) obstruction of venous return; or (6) obstruction of lymphatic flow (Table 14–2).[74] In individual cases, one or more of these mechanisms may be responsible.

Table 14–3 outlines a partial list of possible causes of NIHF categorized by the general site of involvement.[70] In many cases, the pathophysiologic mechanism leading to fetal hydrops can be explained, although in other cases the etiology of hydrops is uncertain. Disorders that may result in high-output cardiac failure include vascular malformations of the cranium (vein of Galen aneurysm), placenta (chorioangioma), umbilical cord (hemangioma), liver (hemangioendothelioma), or coccyx (sacrococcygeal teratoma). Obstruction of venous or lymphatic flow may result from chylothorax, thoracic or cardiac tumors, cystic adenomatoid malformation of the lung, diaphragmatic hernia, or

TABLE 14–3.

Conditions Associated With NIHF*

Categories	Individual Conditions
Cardiovascular	Arrhythmias (tachyarrhythmia, complex dysrhythmia, heart block)
	Anatomic defects (hypoplastic left heart, Ebstein's anomaly, aortic or pulmonic stenosis, aortic or pulmonic atresia, cardiosplenic syndromes, valvular insufficiency, atrioventricular canal defect, single ventricle, tetralogy of Fallot, premature closure of the foramen ovale or ductus anteriosus)
	Coronary artery embolus
	Cardiomyopathy
	Endocardial fibroelastosis
	Myocarditis (coxsackievirus, CMV)
	Tumor (rhabdomyoma, hemangioma, teratoma)
Pulmonary	Diaphragmatic hernia
	Cystic adenomatoid malformation of the lung
	Pulmonary sequestration
	Pulmonary lymphangiectasia
	Chylothorax
	Pulmonary hypoplasia
	Tumors (hamartoma, hemangioma, sarcoma)
Chromosomal	Trisomy 21
	Other trisomies (18,13)
	Turner's syndrome (45X)
	XX/XY mosaicism
	Triploidy
Hematological	α-thalassemia
	Arteriovenous shunts (e.g., vascular tumors)
	Fetal Kasabach-Merritt syndrome
	Hemorrhage
	Vena cava, portal vein, or femoral obstruction (e.g. thrombosis)
	G_6PD deficiency
Twin Pregnancy	Twin-twin transfusion syndrome
Infections	CMV
	Toxoplasmosis
	Parvovirus
	Syphilis
	Congenital hepatitis
	Herpes simplex, type I
	Rubella
	Leptospirosis
	Chagas' disease
	Coxsackievirus
	Respiratory syncytial virus
Neoplastic	Neuroblastoma
	Teratoma (sacrococcygeal, mediastinal)
	Congenital leukemia
	Hemangioendothelioma of the liver
	Pulmonary leiomyosarcoma
	Tuberous sclerosis (rhabdomyoma)
Liver	Hepatic fibrosis
	Cholestasis
	Polycystic disease of the liver
	Biliary atresia
	Hepatic vascular malformation
	Familial cirrhosis
	Giant cell hepatitis
	Hepatic necrosis
	Metabolic disorders (Gaucher's disease, sialidosis, gangliosidosis GM_1, mucopolysaccharidosis)
	Tumors (hemangioendothelioma)

(Continued.)

TABLE 14–3   (cont.).

Categories	Individual Conditions
Cranial	Vein of Galen aneurysm
Skeletal	Achondroplasia
	Achondrogenesis
	Osteogenesis imperfecta
	Thanatophanic dwarfism
	Short-rib polydactyly syndrome (Saldino-Noonan, Majewski types)
	Asphyxiating thoracic dysplasia
	Conradi's disease
Malformation	Pena-Shokeir, type I
Syndromes	Lethal multiple pterygium syndrome
	Noonan syndrome with congenital heart defect
	Arthrogryposis multiplex congenita
	Hypophosphatasia
	Neu-Laxova syndrome
	Francois syndrome, type III
	Recessive cystic hygroma
	Idiopathic
Metabolic	Gaucher's disease
Disorders	Gangliosidosis
	Hurler's syndrome
	Mucolipidosis
Placenta and	Chorioangioma
Umbilical	Chorionic vein thrombosis
Cord	Feto-maternal transfusion
	Placental and umbilical vein thrombosis
	Umbilical cord torsion
	True cord knots
	Angiomyxoma of the umbilical cord
	Aneurysm of the umbilical artery
Maternal	Severe diabetes mellitus
	Severe anemia
	Hypoproteinemia
Miscellaneous	Congenital lymphedema
	Antepartum indomethacin (causing fetal ductus closure and secondary NIHF)

*Adapted from Holzgreve W, Holzgreve B, Cruz JR: Non-immune hydrops fetalis: Diagnosis and management. Semin Perinatol 1985; 9:52.
CMV = cytomegalovirus; NIHF = non-immune hydrops fetalis.

venous thrombosis. Fetal anemia resulting from decreased production of red blood cells, defective hemoglobin, fetal hemorrhage, or increased hemolysis may lead to hydrops by stimulating a sequence of events similar to that proposed for immune hydrops.

In a review of 50 cases of NIHF, Holzgreve et al. reported the following causes and associations with NIHF: cardiac abnormalities, 22%; chromosome abnormalities, 14%; multiple anomaly syndromes, 12%; α-thalassemia, 10%; twin-twin transfusion, 8%; pulmonary abnormalities, 6%; and renal, gastrointestinal, and other abnormalities, 8%.[70]

Clinical Approach

Unlike immune hydrops, there is no single laboratory test to screen pregnancies at risk for NIHF. In the great majority of patients, therefore, prenatal sonography represents the sole means for detecting NIHF. In

these cases, size-dates discrepancy resulting from polyhydramnios is a common reason for referral to sonography.[70] Hutchinson et al. stated that when polyhydramnios, maternal anemia, and hypertension were used as clinical indications for sonographic evaluation, approximately 80% of fetuses with NIHF or more would be detected after 28 weeks' gestation.[73]

The diagnostic approach to NIHF is outlined in Table 14–4.[56, 59, 64] Immune hydrops can be excluded by the indirect Coombs' test. Clinical history and laboratory studies of maternal serum may identify other maternal causes for NIHF including thalassemia, metabolic disease, anemia, and certain intrauterine infections. Most cases, however, require more invasive methods including amniocentesis or cordocentesis. Cordocentesis provides the most rapid and direct means for evaluating hematologic disorders, serum protein, metabolic abnormalities, and the fetal karyotype.[72]

TABLE 14–4.

Diagnostic Approach in Prenatal Evaluation of NIHF*

	Diagnostic	Possible Etiology of NIHF
Maternal Evaluation	Antibody screening (Indirect Coombs' test)	Immunological causes of hydrops (Rh and other incompatibilities)
	Maternal CBC and indices	Thalassemia carrier state
	Maternal blood chemistry studies	G_6PD deficiency and pyruvate kinase deficiency carrier state
	Kleihauer-Betke test	Fetal-maternal transfusion
	TORCH screen	Congenital intrauterine infections
	History	Pertinent history for hereditary diseases, metabolic diseases, infections, diabetes, anemia, and medications
Invasive Fetal Evaluation	Amniocentesis	Fetal karyotype, amniotic fluid culture, CMV, alpha-fetoprotein, metabolic test, restriction endonuclease test (thalassemia), L/S ratio (obstetrical management)
	Fetal blood aspiration	Rapid karyotype and metabolic tests (chromosomal or metabolic abnormalities)
		Hemoglobin chain analysis (thalassemias)
		Fetal plasma analysis for specific IgM (intrauterine infection)
		Fetal plasma albumin (hypoalbuminemia)
Non–invasive Fetal Evaluation	Fetal monitoring	Evaluation of fetal well-being, need for intervention and timing as well as mode of delivery
	Sonography	(Refer to Table 14–5.)

*Modified from Holzgreve W, Holzgreve B, Curry JR: Non-immune hydrops fetalis: Diagnosis and management. Semin Perinatol 1985; 9:52.
CMV = cytomegalovirus; NIHF = Non-immune hydrops fetalis.

Sonographic Findings

Sonographic findings of NIHF are generally indistinguishable from those of immune hydrops. However, the sonographic appearance among individual fetuses is highly variable. One or more findings of ascites, pleural effusions, pericarial effusion, anasarca, polyhydramnios, and placental edema may occur together or in isolation.[59, 60, 73, 78] For example, ascites is frequently an early and prominent manifestation of NIHF, but occasionally it may be absent even in association with severe hydrops.

Because the manifestations of NIHF are diverse, reported sonographic criteria for inclusion of NIHF also vary widely. We concur with others who suggest that the diagnosis of NIHF should be reserved to more than one serous cavity effusion (ascites, pleural effusion, or pericardial effusion), or a serous effusion in conjunction with anasarca.[52] While some studies have included isolated fluid collections (ascites or pleural effusions) as NIHF, this is often due to other causes that may carry a more favorable prognosis. For example, isolated ascites usually is caused by intra-abdominal abnormalities, primarily urinary obstruction, or intestinal disorders[58, 95] (see section on Ascites in this chapter).

The sonographic approach to the fetus with NIHF should reflect the diversity of causes and associations previously described. Structural abnormalities, which may involve nearly any organ system, can be identified in up to 25% to 40% of fetuses with NIHF.[51, 74] Therefore, a systematic approach to the fetus with NIHF is necessary (Table 14–5). Specific disorders that are most commonly associated with NIHF are discussed further below.

Prognosis

The overall prognosis of NIHF is poor, with mortality rates ranging from 50%–98% and most authors reporting a perinatal mortality rate greater than 90%.[58, 73, 74, 78] This rate approaches 100% when a fetal structural abnormality is identified sonographically.[51, 74] As previously noted, generalized lymphangiectasia is universally fatal.

The prognosis may be more favorable for some types of disorders resulting in NIHF. These include gastrointestinal or genitourinary causes of isolated ascites and unusual causes of isolated pleural effusions.

Management

At present, optimal obstetric management of NIHF relies on early prenatal diagnosis, pre-term delivery before development of gross serous cavity effusions, and prompt postpartum management of the infant in a

TABLE 14–5.

Possible Sonographic Findings in the Evaluation of Non-Immune Hydrops*

	Sonographic Findings	Possible Diagnosis
Head	Intracranial mass	Vein of Galen aneurysm
	Cystic intracranial mass	Porencephalic cyst
	Intracranial bleeding	Thrombocytopenia
	Microcephaly	CMV, toxoplasmosis
	Cranial defect with mass	Encephalocele
Neck	Mass	Cystic hygroma, paratracheal hemangioma, hemangioendothelioma
	Nuchal thickening	Chromosomal abnormality (trisomy 21)
Thorax	Small thorax	Pulmonary hypoplasia, dwarfism, Pena-Shokeir syndrome
	Chest mass	Cystic adenomatoid malformation, pulmonary leiomyosarcoma, extra-lobar pulmonary sequestration, diaphragmatic hernia
Heart	Mass	Tumor
	Poorly contracting heart	Heart failure
	Irregular heart rhythm	Cardiac dysrhythmia
	Structural cardiac abnormalities	Congenital cardiac malformation
	Pericardial effusion with mass	Pericardial teratoma
	Pericardial calcification	Intrauterine infections
Abdomen	Dilated bowel loops	Gastrointestinal obstruction, atresia, volvulus
	Calcification	Meconium peritonitis
	Hepatic mass	Hemangioma, hemangioendothelioma, hepatoblastoma
	Hepatosplenomegaly	Intrauterine infection, extramedullary hematopoiesis
Genitourinary	Retroperitoneal mass	Neuroblastoma
	Hydronephrosis	Obstructive uropathy
	Echogenic kidneys	Cystic kidney disease
	Thickened urinary bladder wall	Obstructive uropathy
Extremities	Short extremities	Dwarfism
	Fractures	Osteogenesis imperfecta
	Contractures	Arthrogryposis
Placenta	Thick	Intrauterine infections, extramedullary hematopoiesis, anemia
	Mass	Chorioangioma
Amniotic Cavity	Umbilical cord abnormalities	Torsion knot, angiomyxoma, hemangioma, umbilical artery aneurysm
	Twin gestation with discordant growth	Twin-twin transfusion

*Modified from Fleischer AC, Killam AP, Boehm FH, et al: Radiology 1981; 141:163–168.
CMV = cytomegalovirus.

high-risk perinatal center. Occasionally, specific therapy can be administered in utero, for example, anti-arrhythmic therapy for fetal tachycardia.

CONDITIONS ASSOCIATED WITH NON-IMMUNE HYDROPS

Cardiac Anomalies

Cardiac anomalies are among the most common causes of non-immune hydrops in white populations, accounting for 22%–40% of cases.[38, 40, 76, 84, 96] Cardiac dysrhythmias may lead to non-immune hydrops and these may either be tachyarrhythmias or bradyarrhythmias (Figs 14–11, 14–12).[68] Tachyarrhythmia is

particularly important to detect because it is one of the few treatable causes of non-immune hydrops with pharmacologic therapy (see Fig 14–11).[69, 76]

Structural cardiac anomalies that may lead to non-immune hydrops are associated with a poor prognosis.[93] In addition to valvular and septal defects and complex anomalies (see Chapter 8), cardiac tumors such as atrial hemangioma, rhabdomyoma, or intrapericardial teratoma (Fig 14–13) may also cause non-immune hydrops by obstructing blood flow.[56, 73, 87, 90] Extracardiac anomalies and chromosome abnormalities should be considered when cardiac anomalies are demonstrated.[55]

Sonographic findings of non-immune hydrops due to cardiac anomalies are generally indistinguishable

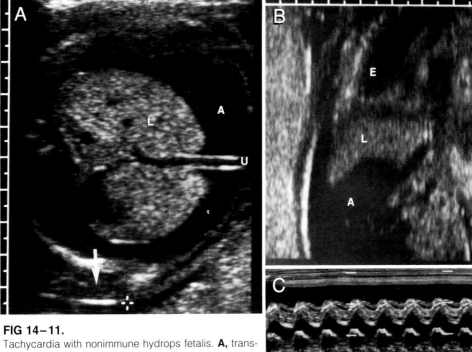

FIG 14–11.
Tachycardia with nonimmune hydrops fetalis. **A,** transverse scan of the abdomen shows marked ascites *(A)* and subcutaneous edema *(arrow)* in a fetus with supraventricular tachycardia. *L* = liver; *U* = umbilical vein. **B,** sagittal scan of the thorax shows large ascites *(A)* and pleural effusions *(E)*. *L* = liver. **C,** M-mode echocardiogram shows supraventricular tachycardia. Sinus rhythm was restored with maternal pharmacologic therapy.

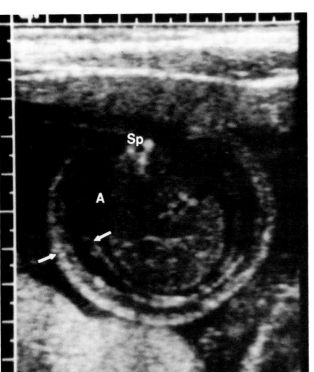

FIG 14–12.
Third degree heart block with hydrops fetalis. Transverse scan of the abdomen shows ascites *(A)* and marked subcutaneous edema *(arrows)* in a fetus with third degree heart block. *A* = ascites; *Sp* = spine.

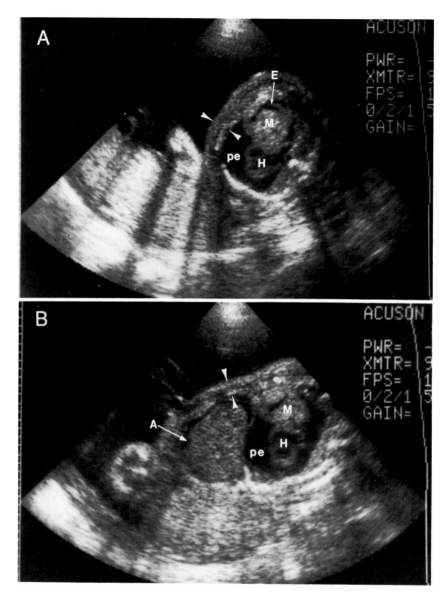

FIG 14–13.
Pericardial teratoma with hydrops fetalis. **A,** transverse scan through the thorax demonstrates pericardial effusion *(pe)*, pleural effusion *(E)*, subcutaneous edema *(arrowheads)* and polyhydramnios. An echogenic mass *(M)* representing a pericardial teratoma displaces the heart *(H)* to the right. **B,** sagittal view demonstrates echogenic mass *(M)*, pericardial effusion *(PE)*, subcutaneous edema *(arrowheads)* and ascites *(A)*. *H* = heart.

from other causes of hydrops. DeVore has suggested that isolated pericardial effusion is the earliest sonographic finding of developing hydrops in fetuses with structural cardiac anomalies,[15] although this observation has not been confirmed by others.

Anemia and Hematologic Disorders

Hematologic disorders may account for up to 10% of cases of non-immune hydrops.[70] The pathogenesis of hydrops from these disorders is thought to be similar to immune hydrops, with fetal anemia as the common factor. Fetal anemia may result from a variety of causes

including fetal hemorrhage, defective red blood cell production, production of abnormal hemoglobin (thalassemia), or increased hemolysis.[82, 85] Intrauterine infections, for example, from parvovirus, may also lead to fetal hydrops by producing red blood cell hemolysis.[41, 48, 79]

Homozygous α-thalassemia is inherited as an autosomal recessive disorder with a 25% recurrence rate for subsequent pregnancies. It is the major cause of non-immune hydrops among patients from Southeast Asia.[67, 97] In this disorder, the inability to produce α-hemoglobin chains results in abnormal hemoglobin (Bart hemoglobin) rather than fetal or adult hemoglobin. Hypoxia and high-output cardiac failure develop because of the difficulty of Bart's hemoglobin in releasing oxygen to fetal tissues.

Non-immune hydrops due to homozygous α-thalassemia is universally fatal to the fetus and it is also associated with significant maternal morbidity. Women carrying a fetus affected with homozygous α-thalassemia frequently experience preeclampsia, microcytic anemia, and size-dates discrepancy. The carrier state of thalassemia can be diagnosed by red blood cell indices and hemoglobin electrophoresis. If both parents are carriers, an affected fetus can be diagnosed by DNA analysis of cultured cells and by umbilical cord sampling.

Hsieh et al. suggest that fetuses with α-thalassemia show a larger umbilical vein diameter and greater velocity through the umbilical vein on Doppler examination compared to fetuses with other causes of non–immune hydrops.[71] These observations are similar to those of Kirkenen et al. in studying fetuses with severe Rh-isoimmunized hydrops.[23] Proposed explanations for these findings include (1) increased blood volume in an attempt to compensate for insufficient tissue oxygenation; or (2) decrease in blood viscosity resulting from severe anemia. The validity and clinical utility of these observations require further study.

Twin-Twin Transfusion

The twin-twin transfusion syndrome, which is unique to monozygotic twin pregnancies, may account for up to 8% of cases of non-immune hydrops (Fig 14–14).[70] The recipient twin is plethoric, macrosomic, and hydropic due to volume overload. The donor twin usually shows signs of intrauterine growth retardation but may also become hydropic secondary to severe anemia.[58, 78] Diagnosis of the twin-twin transfusion syndrome should be suspected when the smaller twin weighs less than 20% of the larger twin or when evidence of hydrops develops in either twin.[93] Discrepancy in amniotic fluid volume with polyhydramnios developing in the larger twin is the single most common finding of the twin-twin transfusion syndrome.[49] One should recall, however, that discrepancies in amniotic fluid volume or hydrops may be secondary to congenital anomalies which are also increased in frequency among monozygotic twins. The twin-twin transfusion syndrome is further discussed in Chapter 15.

Chromosome Abnormalities

Chromosome abnormalities are a relatively common cause of non-immune hydrops, accounting for up to 14% of cases.[70] The most common chromosome abnormalities associated with hydrops include trisomy 13, 18, and 21; triploidy; and Turner's syndrome.[70, 73, 93] The etiologic mechanism of hydrops may vary from case to case, but congestive heart failure and lymphatic obstruction are most commonly implicated. Because of the association of chromosome abnormalities with non-immune hydrops, fetuses with otherwise unexplained causes of hydrops should be considered for chromosome analysis by amniocentesis or cordocentesis prior to delivery.

Generalized fetal hydrops that is associated with cystic hygromata is commonly referred to as lymphangiectasia (Fig 14–15). This appearance should probably be distinguished from other types of non-immune hydrops since these fetuses have a universally fatal outcome and are more frequently associated with chromosome abnormalities (see Chapters 7 and 17). Amniotic fluid volume may be normal or decreased when the cystic hygroma replaces the amniotic fluid space.[91]

Hereditary and Metabolic Disorders

Hereditary and metabolic disorders may account for up to 12% of cases of non-immune hydrops.[70] These include the Pena-Shokeir syndrome, arthrogryposis multiplex congenita, Neu-Laxova syndrome, and the Saldino-Noonan syndrome.[50, 70] However, these syndromes rarely are diagnosed with certainty on the basis of prenatal sonographic findings.

Various metabolic disorders also have been associated with non–immune hydrops, although it is uncertain how many of these present with isolated ascites that may be induced by hepatomegaly and liver dysfunction. These include Gaucher's disease, gangliosidosis, Hurler's syndrome, and mucolipidosis. Prenatal diagnosis of such metabolic disorders may be possible by enzymatic assay analysis in cultured fibroblasts.

Thoracic Abnormalities

Thoracic abnormalities account for about 6% of cases of NIHF.[70] These include cystic adenomatoid malformation of the lung, pulmonary sequestration, diaphragmatic hernia, and neoplasms (cardiac, pericardial, mediastinal, or rare lung neoplasms).[43, 62, 65, 99, 100] The probable pathogenesis of hydrops in these cases is obstruction of venous or lymphatic flow. Interference of amniotic fluid exchange through the lungs might also contribute to NIHF.

While pleural effusion is a common manifestation of severe hydrops, isolated hydrothorax (chylothorax) may also be an isolated finding. Like isolated ascites,

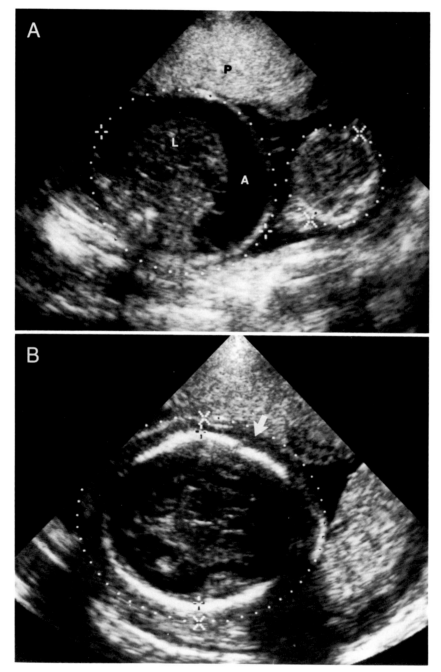

FIG 14–14.
Twin transfusion syndrome. **A,** transverse scan through the abdomens of both twins shows marked discrepancy in size of the twins, with the twin depicted on the right being significantly small and the twin depicted on the left being significantly large with a quantity of ascites. *L* = liver; *A* = ascites; *P* = placenta. **B,** axial scan of the hydropic twin shows scalp edema *(arrow).*

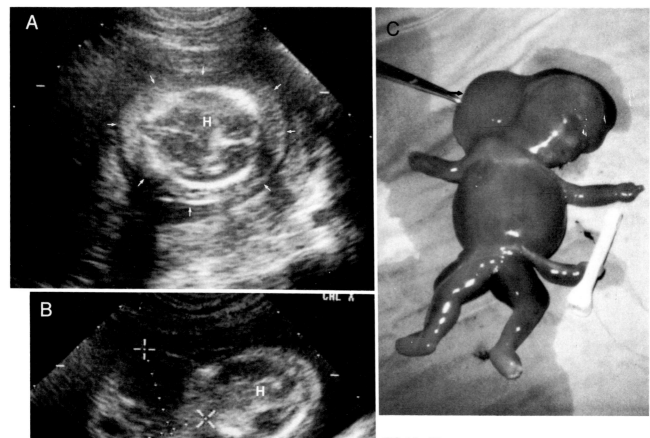

FIG 14–15.
Lymphangiectasia associated with Turner's syndrome
(X). **A,** axial scan of the head *(H)* shows marked scalp
edema *(arrows).* **B,** scan angled through the neck
shows nuchal cystic hygromas *(graticules)* at the occiput. *H* = head. **C,** postmortem photograph confirms
the diffuse lymphangiectasia and cystic hygroma
(curved arrow) in this fetus with Turner's syndrome
(45X).

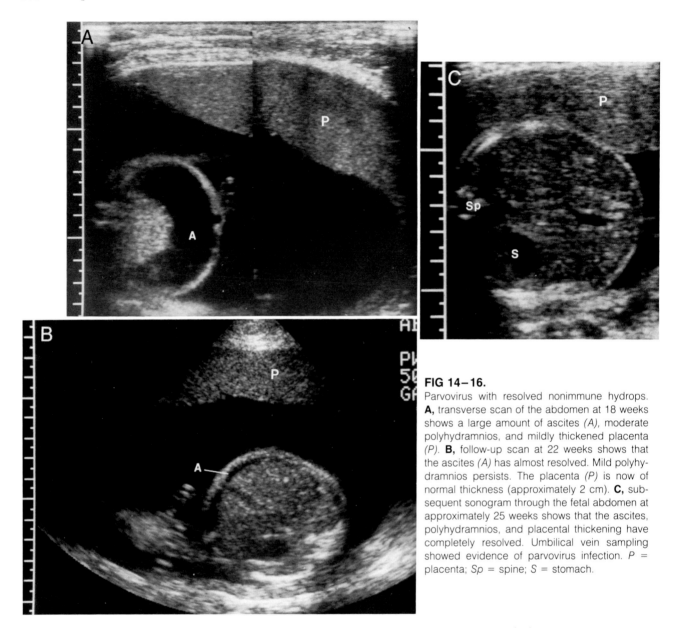

FIG 14–16.
Parvovirus with resolved nonimmune hydrops. **A,** transverse scan of the abdomen at 18 weeks shows a large amount of ascites *(A)*, moderate polyhydramnios, and mildly thickened placenta *(P)*. **B,** follow-up scan at 22 weeks shows that the ascites *(A)* has almost resolved. Mild polyhydramnios persists. The placenta *(P)* is now of normal thickness (approximately 2 cm). **C,** subsequent sonogram through the fetal abdomen at approximately 25 weeks shows that the ascites, polyhydramnios, and placental thickening have completely resolved. Umbilical vein sampling showed evidence of parvovirus infection. *P* = placenta; *Sp* = spine; *S* = stomach.

isolated hydrothorax should be distinguished from generalized hydrops whenever possible. Fetuses with hydrothorax may be managed with in utero aspiration or by placement of a pleuroamniotic shunt.[47]

Infections

A variety of infectious agents have been associated with NIHF and ascites. These include toxoplasmosis, parvovirus, syphilis, cytomegalovirus (CMV), and coxsackievirus.[41, 42, 70, 78, 79, 89, 103, 124] Infectious causes are undoubtedly responsible for some of the cases of NIHF that have been observed to resolve spontaneously (Fig 14–16).[75, 116, 119]

Parvovirus appears to cause NIHF by stimulating hemolysis of red blood cells.[41, 48] This agent has a well-known predilection for the hematopoietic system and may even cause aplastic crisis in patients with sickle-cell anemia. Rodis and associates suggest that up to 38% of women who are exposed and infected by human parvovirus during pregnancy have adverse outcomes including spontaneous abortions, intrauterine fetal death, and congenital anomalies.[92] The diagnosis of in utero parvovirus can be established by findings of positive antibodies in the maternal serum and the presence of the viral agent in fetal blood or fetal organs. Fetal anemia and increased number of nucleated red blood cells may be seen in the fetal blood obtained by cordocentesis.[48]

In most cases, infectious causes of NIHF are indis-

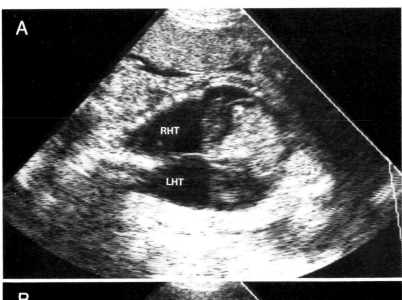

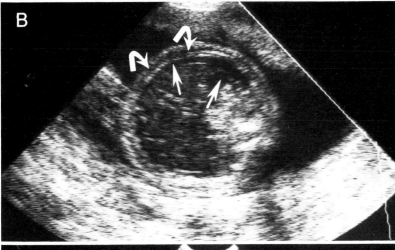

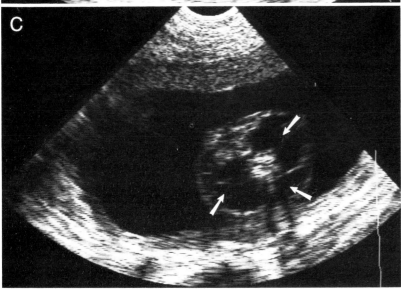

FIG 14–17.
Paratracheal hemangioma with hydrops at 33 weeks. **A,** coronal scan of the thorax shows large bilateral pleural effusions. *LHT* = left hemithorax; *RHT* = right hemithorax. **B,** transverse scan of the abdomen demonstrates subcutaneous edema *(curved arrows)* and ascites *(straight arrows)*. **C,** transverse scan of the fetal neck shows multiple cystic masses bilaterally *(arrows)*. Paratracheal hemangioma was found at autopsy. (From Lenke RR, Cyr DR, Mack LA, et al: Fetal hydrops secondary to a paratracheal hemangiomatous malformation. J Ultrasound Med 1986; 5:223–225. Used by permission.)

tinguishable from other causes. Occasionally, however, unusual calcifications in the pericardium, liver, or brain may suggest the correct diagnosis.

Neoplasms

Various neoplasms or masses may be associated with NIHF including neuroblastoma, sacrococcygeal teratoma, congenital leukemia, hemangioendothelioma of the liver or neck, and cardiac or pericardial tumors (Fig 14–17).[55, 63, 76, 81, 87, 90] Possible pathogenic mechanisms include high-output cardiac failure from shunting through vascular tumors, vascular compression, or development of anemia by intra-tumor hemorrhage. Most fetal tumors should be identified on sonography from an anatomic survey of the fetus.

Miscellaneous Conditions

Various skeletal disorders and dwarfing syndromes have been associated with NIHF. These include achondroplasia, achondrogenesis, osteogenesis imperfecta, thanatophoric dwarfism, asphyxiating thoracic dysplasia, and short-rib polydactyly syndrome.[70, 93, 98] The pathogenesis leading to hydrops is unclear in these cases. Perhaps the hypoplastic thorax is a contributing factor by interfering with amniotic fluid transfer through the lung.

Abnormalities of the placenta or umbilical cord may occasionally result in NIHF. Placental abnormalities that have been associated with NIHF include chorioangioma (Fig 14–18) and placental vein thrombosis. Cord abnormalities may include torsion, knots, or thrombosis, which may impede vascular flow.

Various gastrointestinal and genitourinary abnormalities have been associated with "hydrops".[57, 95] Careful review of the sonographic findings in these cases, however, usually indicates the presence of isolated ascites rather than a generalized condition. Occasionally, however, ascites due to a gastrointestinal or genitourinary cause may be associated with other evidence of hydrops, particularly thickening of the abdominal wall.[57] In this situation, the latter finding may represent a localized inflammatory reaction.

ASCITES

Fetal ascites usually is seen in association with fetal hydrops and is one of the earliest manifestations of hy-

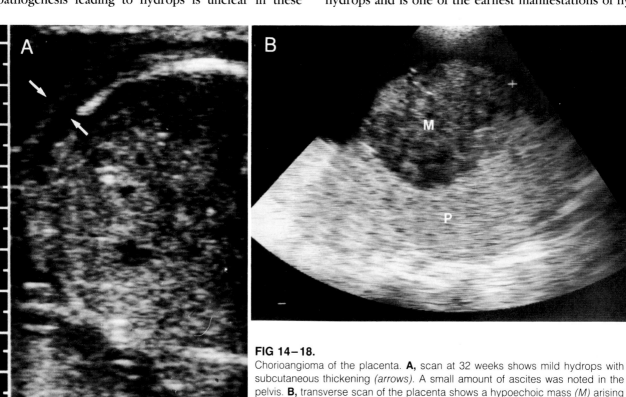

FIG 14–18.
Chorioangioma of the placenta. **A,** scan at 32 weeks shows mild hydrops with subcutaneous thickening *(arrows).* A small amount of ascites was noted in the pelvis. **B,** transverse scan of the placenta shows a hypoechoic mass *(M)* arising from the fetal surface of the placenta *(P).* This was confirmed to be a chorioangioma.

dropic decompensation. However, when ascites occurs in isolation, it is usually secondary to an intra-abdominal disorder rather than to a generalized condition. Because of inherent differences in etiology, prognosis, and management, isolated ascites should be distinguished from generalized hydrops whenever possible. Nevertheless, the distinction between these two groups of disorders is sometimes unclear, and previous studies have frequently classified isolated ascites as fetal hydrops.

Pathogenesis

As noted, isolated fetal ascites usually can be attributed to structural or functional abnormalities within the fetal abdomen (Table 14–6). Genitourinary or gastrointestinal anomalies account for approximately 60%–70% of all cases, with obstructive uropathy as the most frequently cited cause of the genitourinary system anomaly.[115, 117, 121, 123] In this situation, urinary ascites develops from transudation or leakage of urine into the peritoneal cavity. Other genitourinary anomalies that may be associated with isolated ascites include renal hypoplasia, polycystic kidneys, hydrometrocol-

TABLE 14–6.

Causes of Ascites

Immune hydrops
Non-immune hydrops (see Table 14–3)
Genitourinary (urinary ascites)
    Urethrovesical obstruction (most
        common)
    UPJ obstruction
    Renal hypoplasia
    Cystic dysplastic kidney
    Congenital nephrotic syndrome
    Hydrometrocolpos
    Cloacal anomalies
    Ovarian cyst with torsion
Gastrointestinal
    Meconium peritonitis
    Midgut volvulus
    Jejunoileal atresia
    Diaphragmatic hernia
Liver
    Hepatitis
    Fibrosis
    Biliary atresia
    Hepatic necrosis
    Tumors
Metabolic storage disease
    Wolman disease
    Gaucher's disease
    GM gangliosidosis
    Sialidosis

UPJ = ureteropelvic junction.

pos, cloacal anomalies, and congenital nephrotic syndrome.[70, 78, 118]

Gastrointestinal causes of ascites include midgut volvulus, small bowel atresia, and meconium peritonitis.[57, 95, 104, 106, 108] Development of ascites is probably due to inflammation of serosal surfaces or venous and lymphatic obstruction with transudation of fluid into the abdominal cavity.

Various liver disorders may cause isolated ascites including hepatitis, fibrosis, or liver masses. These probably cause ascites in a manner similar to adults with obstruction of venous flow through the liver. Arteriovenous shunting probably is also a factor in the case of certain liver masses, such as cavernous hemangiomas.

Metabolic storage diseases are important causes of ascites to consider, since they are inheritable disorders. These include Wolman disease, Gaucher's disease, GM_1 gangliosidosis, and sialidosis. The cause of ascites in these cases in uncertain, but is possibly related to hypoproteinemia or sinusoidal obstruction by Kupffer's cells that become swollen with storage material.

Sonographic Findings

The sonographic diagnosis of fetal ascites usually is obvious, with fluid seen surrounding the liver and spleen, bowel, extrahepatic portion of the umbilical vein, and the falciform ligament.[105, 111, 114] However, a small amount of ascites is more difficult to detect and the absolute quantity of fluid detected is related to fetal size. In a retrospective review, as little as 12–14 ml of fluid was seen easily in fetuses at 18–20 weeks, while 30–40 ml of fluid was necessary for detection in fetuses greater than 30 weeks.[112] As previously cautioned, sonographers should not confuse "pseudoascites" for small amounts of true ascites (see section on Immune Hydrops above).

If signs of generalized hydrops are absent and isoimmunization has been excluded by appropriate clinical and laboratory tests, sonographic findings may be useful in establishing the underlying diagnosis of ascites. The genitourinary and gastrointestinal tracts should be given special attention in this evaluation.

Among genitourinary causes of ascites, the kidneys should be carefully evaluated to exclude hydronephrosis, cystic dysplasia, or neoplasm. However, even a normal appearance of the kidneys does not exclude the possibility of urinary ascites. In the case of urethral level obstruction, the urinary bladder wall usually is thickened and may occasionally show bladder wall calcification (Fig 14–19).[115] The pelvis should be examined for masses including ovarian cysts or hydrometrocolpos.

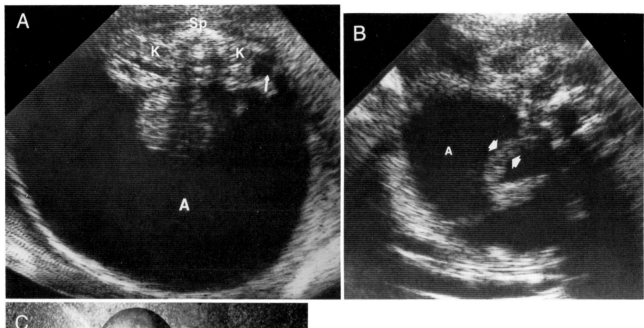

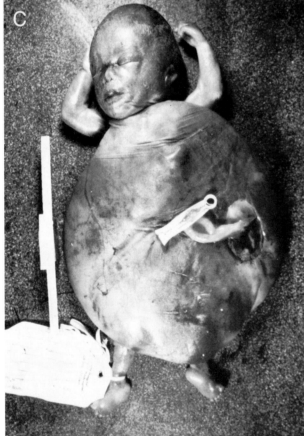

FIG 14–19.
Urinary ascites secondary to posterior urethral valves. **A,** transverse scan through the abdomen demonstrates a large amount of ascites *(A).* A small amount of fluid *(arrow)* is also identified adjacent to the left kidney. The kidneys appear normal without hydronephrosis. *K =* kidney; *S =* spine. **B,** Transverse scan of the pelvis shows a thickened urinary bladder wall *(arrows). A =* ascites. **C,** Postmortem photograph shows prune-belly syndrome with marked abdominal distension due to urinary ascites.

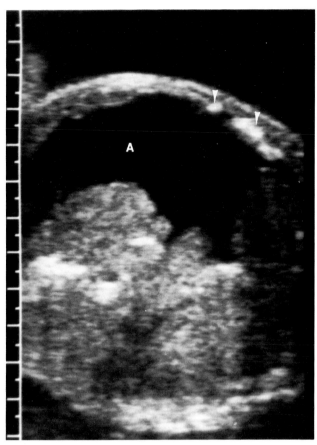

FIG 14–20.
Ascites secondary to meconium peritonitis. Oblique scan of the abdomen shows large ascites *(A)*. Also note peritoneal calcifications *(arrowheads)* that are characteristic of meconium peritonitis.

Among gastrointestinal abnormalities of ascites, meconium peritonitis is most frequently cited. Meconium peritonitis can usually be suspected by demonstrating echogenic meconium plaques on the peritoneal surface (Fig 14–20).[104, 106] However, peritoneal calcification may be subtle and can be overlooked.[57, 108] Occasionally the peritoneal inflammation can also cause thickening of the abdominal wall, thereby mimicking generalized hydrops.[57]

Other gastrointestinal causes of ascites may also be recognized on prenatal sonography. For example, volvulus or jejunoileal atresia may be suggested by proximal bowel dilatation. Although metabolic storage diseases have not been identified on sonography to our knowledge, demonstration of hepatomegaly might be a possible finding. In utero infection might be suggested by demonstrating unusual calcifications.

Management

If the underlying cause of ascites is not determined by sonography, further evaluation may include amnio-

centesis or paracentesis. In the case of urinary ascites, urea and creatinine can be quantified, and in the case of meconium peritonitis, ascites can be analyzed for granulocytes, leukocytes, lanugo hairs, and meconium.[121, 122]

Metabolic storage diseases may be identified by finding evacuolated lymphocytes in the peripheral blood and excretion of oligosaccharides in the urine.[109] The specific diagnosis is established by a specific lysosomal enzyme assay and peripheral blood leukocytes or cultured fibroblasts. Thin-layer chromatography of the oligosaccharides in amniotic fluid may be indicated when a diagnosis of persistent fetal ascites has been established.[109]

In cases with rapidly accumulating ascites or pleural effusions, in utero paracentesis or thoracentesis may be performed for therapeutic purposes. This is especially important to avoid abdominal dystocia if vaginal delivery is contemplated. The present authors favor a conservative approach, however, because ascites is often self-limiting or transitory, and the prognosis may be favorable.

SUMMARY

Fetal hydrops and ascites are frequently observed abnormalities on prenatal sonography. Sonographic evaluation is extremely helpful in monitoring affected pregnancies and in assessing the prognosis. The underlying disorder may also be identified. Isolated fluid collections (ascites or pleural effusions) should be distinguished from generalized hydrops whenever possible because of differences in etiology, prognosis, and management. Careful evaluation of intra-abdominal organs may identify the cause of isolated ascites.

REFERENCES

Immune Hydrops

1. Acker D, Frigoletto F, Birnholz J, et al: Ultrasound facilitated intrauterine transfusions. Am J Obstet Gynecol 1980; 138:1200–1204.
2. Barnes SE: Hydrops fetalis. Molecular aspects of medicine 1977; 1:244.
3. Benacerraf B, Frigoletto FD: Sonographic sign for the detection of early fetal ascites in the management of severe isoimmune disease without intrauterine transfusion. Am J Obstet Gynecol 1985; 152:1039–1041.
4. Berkowitz RL, Hobbins JC: Intrauterine transfusion utilizing ultrasound. Obstet Gynecol 1981; 57:33–36.
5. Berkowitz RL, Chitkara U, Goldberg JD, et al: Intrauter-

ine intravascular transfusion for severe red blood cell isoimmunization. Ultrasound-guided percutaneous approach. Am J Obstet Gynecol 1986; 155:574–581.

6. Bowman JM: The management of Rh isoimmunization. Obstet Gynecol 1978; 52:1–16.

7. Bowman JM: Suppression of Rh-isoimmunization. Obstet Gynecol 1978; 52:385–393.

8. Bowman JM: Rhesus hemolytic disease, in Vald N (ed). *Antenatal and Neonatal Screening*, New York, Oxford University Press, 1984, pp 314.

9. Chitkara U, Wilkins I, Lynch L, et al: The role of sonography in assessing severity of fetal anemia in Rh and Kell isoimmunized pregnancies. Obstet Gynecol 1988; 71:393–398.

10. Clewell WH, Dunne MG, Johnson ML: Fetal transfusion with real time ultrasound guidance. Obstet Gynecol 1981; 57:516–520.

11. Cooperberg PL, Carpenter CW: Ultrasound as an aid to intrauterine transfusion. Am J Obstet Gynecol 1977; 128:239–241.

12. Daffos F, Capella-Pavlovsky M, Forestier F: Fetal blood sampling during pregnancy with the use of a needle guided by ultrasound. A study of 606 consecutive cases. Am J Obstet Gynecol 1985; 153:655–660.

13. DeVore GR, Mayden K, Tortora, et al: Dilatation of fetal umbilical vein in rhesus hemolytic anemia: A predictor of severe disease. Am J Obstet Gynecol 1981; 141:464–466.

14. DeVore G, Donnerstein R, Kleinman C, et al: Fetal echocardiography. II: The diagnosis and significance of pericardial effusion in the fetus using real-time directed m-mode ultrasound. Am J Obstet Gynecol 1982; 144–693.

15. Frigoletto FD, Umansky I, Birnholz J, et al: Intrauterine fetal transfusion in 365 fetuses during 15 years. Am J Obstet Gynecol 1981; 139:781–790.

16. Grannum PAT, Copel JA: Prevention of Rh isoimmunization and treatment of the compromised fetus. Semin Perinatol 1988; 12:324–335.

17. Grannum PAT, Copel JA, Plaxe SC, et al: In utero exchange transfusion by direct intravascular injection in severe erythroblastosis fetalis. N Engl J Med 1986; 314:1431–1434.

18. Hansman M, Lang N: Intrauterine transfusion unter Ultrashall kontrolle. Klin Wochenscher 1972; 50:930.

19. Harman CR, Manning FA, Bowman JM, et al: Severe Rh disease: Poor outcome is not inevitable. Am J Obstet Gynecol 1983; 145:823–829.

20. Hashimoto B, Filly RA, Callen PW, et al: Absorption of fetal intraperitoneal blood after intrauterine transfusion. J Ultrasound Med 1987; 6:421–423.

21. Hobbins JC, Davis ED, Webster J: A new technique utilizing ultrasound to aid in IUT. J Clin Ultrasound 1979; 4:135–137.

22. Hoddick WK, Mahony BS, Callen PW, et al: Placental thickness. J Ultrasound Med 1985; 4:479–482.

23. Kirkenen P, Jouppila P, Eik-Nes S: Umbilical vein blood flow in rhesus isoimmunization. Br J Obstet Gynaecol 1983; 90:640–643.

24. Landsteiner K, Weiner AS: Agglutinable factor in human blood recognized by immune serum for rhesus blood. Proc Soc Exper Biol Med 1940; 43:223.

25. Liley AW: Liquor amnii analysis in the management of pregnancy complicated by rhesus sensitization. Am J Obstet Gynecol 1961; 82:1359–1370.

26. Liley AW: Intrauterine transfusion of fetus in hemolytic disease. Br Med J 1963; 2:1107–1109.

27. Mayden K: The umbilical vein diameter in Rh isoimmunization. Med Ultrasound 1980; 4:119–125.

28. Nicolaides KH, Clevell WH, Rodeck CA: Measurement of human fetoplacental blood volume in erythroblastosis fetalis. Am J Obstet Gynecol 1987; 157:50–53.

29. Nicolaides KH, Fontanarosa M, Gabbe SG, et al: Failure of ultrasonographic parameters to predict the severity of fetal anemia in rhesus isoimmunization. Am J Obstet Gynecol 1988; 158:920–926.

30. Nicolaides KH, Rodeck CH, Mibashan RD, et al: Have Liley charts outlived their usefulness? Am J Obstet Gynecol 1986; 155:90–94.

31. Parer JT: Severe Rh isoimmunization—Current methods of in utero diagnosis and treatment. Am J Obstet Gynecol 1988; 158:1323–1327.

32. Pielet BW, Socol ML, MacGregor SN, et al: Cordocentesis: An appraisal of risks. Am J Obstet Gynecol 1988; 159:1497–1500.

33. Robertson JG: Evaluation of the reported methods of interpreting spectrophotometric tracings of amniotic fluid in rhesus isoimmunization. Am J Obstet Gynecol 1966; 95:120–126.

34. Rodeck CH, Holman CA, Karnicki J, et al: Direct intravascular fetal blood transfusion by fetoscopy in severe rhesus isoimmunization. Lancet 1981; i:625–627.

35. Scott JR, Kochenour NH, Larkin RM, et al: Changes in the management of severely Rh-immunized patients. Am J Obstet Gynecol 1984; 149:336–341.

36. Socol ML, MacGragor SN, Pieset BW, et al: Percutaneous umbilical transfusion in severe rhesus isoimmunization: Resolution of fetal hydrops. Am J Obstet Gynecol 1987; 157:1369–1375.

37. Vintzileos A, Campbell W, et al: Fetal liver ultrasound measurements in isoimmunized pregnancies. Obstet Gynecol 1986; 68:162–167.

38. Warsof SL, Nicolaides KH, Rodeck KC: Immune and non-immune hydrops. Clin Obstet Gynecol 1986; 29:533.

39. Witter FR, Graham D: The utility of ultrasonically measured umbilical vein diameter in isoimmunized pregnancies. Am J Obstet Gynecol 1983; 146:225–226.

Non-Immune Hydrops

40. Allan LD, Crawford DC, Sheridan R, et al: Etiology of non-immune hydrops: The value of echocardiography. Br J Obstet Gynecol 1986; 93:223–225.

41. Anand A, Gray E. Brown T, et al: Human parvovirus infection in pregnancy and hydrops fetalis. N Engl J Med 1987; 316:183–186.

42. Bates HR: Coxsackie virus B3 calcified pancarditis and hydrops fetalis. Am J Obstet Gynecol 1970; 106:629–630.

43. Benacerraf BR, Frigoletto FD: In utero treatment of a fetus with diaphragmatic hernia complicated by hydrops. Am J Obstet Gynecol 1986; 155:817–818.

44. Benacerraf BR, Greene MR, Holmes LB: The prenatal sonographic features of Noonan's syndrome. J Ultrasound Med 1989; 8:59–63.

45. Blott M, Nicolaides K, Greenough A: Pleuroamniotic shunting for decompression of fetal pleural effusions. Obstet Gynecol 1988; 71:798–800.

46. Blumenthal DH, Rushovich AM, Williams RK, et al: Prenatal sonographic findings of meconium peritonitis with pathologic correlation. J Clin Ultrasound 1982; 10:350–352.

47. Bose C: Hydrops fetalis and in utero intracranial hemorrhage. J Pediatr 1978; 93:1023–1024.

48. Brown T, Anard A, Ritchie LD, et al: Intrauterine parvovirus infection associated with hydrops fetalis. Lancet 1989; ii:1033–1034.

49. Brown DL, Benson CB, Driscoll SG, et al: Twin-twin transfusion syndrome: Sonographic findings. Radiology 1989; 170:61–63.

50. Cardwell MS: Pena Shokeir syndrome. Prenatal diagnosis by ultrasonography. J Ultrasound Med 1987; 6:619–621.

51. Castillo RA, DeVore GD, Hadi HA, et al: Non-immune hydrops fetalis. Clinical experience and factors related to poor outcome. Am J Obstet Gynecol 1986; 155:812–816.

52. Chinn DH: Ultrasound evaluation of hydrops fetalis, in Callen PW (ed): *Ultrasonography in Obstetrics and Gynecology*, ed 2. Philadelphia, WB Saunders Co, 1988, pp 277–296.

53. Chinn DH, Filly RA, Callen PW, et al: Congenital diaphragmatic hernia diagnosed prenatally by ultrasound. Radiology 1983; 148:119–123.

54. Crawford DC, Chita SK, Allan LD: Prenatal detection of congenital heart disease: Factors affecting obstetric management and survival. Am J Obstet Gynecol 1988; 159:352–356.

55. Cyr DR, Guntheroth WG, Nyberg DA, et al: Prenatal diagnosis of an intrapericardial teratoma: A cause of non-immune hydrops. J Ultrasound Med 1988; 7:87–90.

56. Davis CL: Diagnosis and management of non-immune hydrops fetalis. J Reprod Med 1982; 27:594–600.

57. Dillard JP, Edwards DU, Leopold GR: Meconium peritonitis masquerading as fetal hydrops. J Ultrasound Med 1987; 6:49–57.

58. Etches PC, Lemons JA: Non-immune hydrops fetalis: Report of 22 cases including three siblings. J Pediatr 1979; 64:326–332.

59. Fleischer AC, Killam AP, Boehm FH, et al: Hydrops fetalis: Sonographic evaluation and clinical implications. Radiology 1981; 141:163–168.

60. Ghorashi B, Gottesfeld KR: Recognition of the hydropic fetus by gray-scale ultrasound. J Clin Ultrasound 1976; 4:193.

61. Giacoia GP: Hydrops fetalis. Clin Pediatr 1980; 19:334.

62. Gilsanz V, Emons D, Hansmann M, et al: Hydrothorax, ascites and right diaphragmatic hernia. Radiology 1986; 158:243.

63. Gonen R, Fong K, Chiasson DA: Prenatal sonographic diagnosis of hepatic hemangioendothelioma with secondary non-immune hydrops fetalis. Obstet Gynecol 1989; 73:485–487.

64. Gough JD, Keeling JW, Castle B, et al: The obstetric management of non–immunological hydrops. Br J Obstet Gynecol 1986; 93:226.

65. Graham D, Winn K, Dex W, et al: Prenatal diagnosis of cystic adenomatoid malformation of the lung. J Ultrasound Med 1982; 1:9–12.

66. Graves GR, Boshett, TF: Non-immune hydrops fetalis. Antenatal diagnosis and management. Am J Obstet Gynecol 1987; 148:563–565.

67. Guy G, Coady D, Jansen V, et al: Alpha-thalassemia hydrops fetalis: Clinical and ultrasonographic considerations. Am J Obstet Gynecol 1985; 153:500–504.

68. Hardy JD, Soloman S, Banswell GS, et al: Congenital complete heart block in newborn associated with maternal systemic lupus erythematosus and other connective tissue disorders. Arch Dis Child 1979; 54:7.

69. Harrington JT, Kangos JJ, Sikka A, et al: Successful treatment of fetal congestive heart failure secondary to tachycardia. N Engl J Med 1981; 304:1527–1529.

70. Holzgreve W, Curry CJR, Golbus MS, et al: Investigation of nonimmune hydrops fetalis. Am J Obstet Gynecol 1984; 150:805–812.

71. Hsieh FJ, Chang F-M, Huang H-C, et al: Umbilical vein blood flow measurement in nonimmune hydrops fetalis. Obstet Gynecol 1988; 71:188–191.

72. Hsieh FJ, Chang F-M, Koi T-M, et al: Percutaneous ultrasound-guided fetal blood sampling in the management of non-immune hydrops fetalis. Am J Obstet Gynecol 1987; 157:44–49.

73. Hutchinson AA, Drew JH, Yu VYH, et al: Nonimmunologic hydrops fetalis: A review of 61 cases. Obstet Gynecol 1982; 59:347–352.

74. Im SS, Rizos N, Joutsi P, et al: Nonimmunologic hydrops fetalis. Am J Obstet Gynecol 1984; 148:566–569.

75. Kirkenen P, Jouppila P, Leisti J: Transient fetal ascites and hydrops with a favorable outcome. J Reprod Med 1987; 32:379.

76. Kleinman C, Donnerstein R, DeVore G, et al: Fetal echocardiography for evaluation of in utero congestive heart failure. N Engl J Med 1982; 306:568–575.

77. Lenke RR, Cyr DR, Mack, LA, et al: Fetal hydrops sec-

ondary to paratracheal hemangiomatous malformation. J Ultrasound Med 1986; 5:223–225.

78. Mahony BS, Filly RA, Callen PW, et al: Severe nonimmune hydrops fetalis: Sonographic evaluation. Radiology 1984; 151:757–767.

79. Maeda H, Shinohawa H, Satoh S, et al: Nonimmunologic hydrops fetalis resulting from intrauterine human parvovirus B-19 infection: Report of two cases. Obstet Gynecol 1988; 72:482–485.

80. Maidman JE, Yeager C, Anderson V, et al: Prenatal diagnosis and management of nonimmunologic hydrops fetalis. Obstet Gynecol 1980; 56:571–576.

81. McGahan JP, Schneider JM: Fetal neck hemangioendothelioma with secondary hydrops fetalis: Sonographic diagnosis. J Clin Ultrasound 1986; 14:384–388.

82. Mentzer WC, Collier E: Hydrops fetalis associated with erythrocyte G-6 PD deficiency and maternal ingestion of fava beans and ascorbic acid. J Pediatr 1975; 86:565–567.

83. Naides SJ, Weiner CP: Antenatal diagnosis and palliative treatment of nonimmune hydrops fetalis secondary to parvovirus B19 infection. Prenat Diagn 1989; 9:105–114.

84. Olson R, Nishibatake M, Arya S, et al: Nonimmunologic hydrops fetalis due to intrauterine closure of fetal foramen ovale. Birth Defects 1987; 23:433–442.

85. Perkins RP: Hydrops fetalis and stillbirth in a male glucose—6 phosphate dehydrogenase deficient fetuses possibly due to maternal ingestion of sulfisaxazole: A case report. Am J Obstet Gynecol 1971; 111:379–381.

86. Perlin BM, Pomerance JJ, Schifrin BS: Nonimmunologic hydrops fetalis. Obstet Gynecol 1981; 57:584–588.

87. Platt LD, Geierman CA, Turkel SB, et al: Atrial hemangioma and hydrops fetalis. Am J Obstet Gynecol 1981; 141:107–109.

88. Potter EL: Universal edema of fetus unassociated with erythroblastosis. Am J Obstet Gynecol 1943; 46:130–134.

89. Price JM, Fisch AE, Jacobson J: Ultrasonic findings in fetal cytomegalovirus infection. J Clin Ultrasound 1978; 6:268.

90. Rasmussen SL, Hwang WS, Harder J, et al: Intrapericardial teratoma. Ultrasonic and pathologic features. J Ultrasound Med 1987; 6:159–162.

91. Robinow M, Spisso K, Buschi A, et al: Turner syndrome: Sonography showing fetal hydrops simulating hydramnios. AJR 1980; 135:846–848.

92. Rodis JF, Hovick T Jr, Quinn DT, et al: Human parvovirus infection in pregnancy. Obstet Gynecol 1988; 72:733–738.

93. Romero R, Pilu G, Jeanty P, et al: *Prenatal Diagnosis of Congenital Anomalies.* Norwalk, Connecticut, Appleton and Lange, 1988, pp 414–423.

94. Seifer DB, Ferguson JE II, Behrens CM, et al: Nonimmune hydrops fetalis in association with hemangioma of the umbilical cord. Obstet Gynecol 1985; 66:283–286.

95. Seward JF, Zusman J: Hydrops fetalis associated with small bowel volvulus. Lancet 1978; 2:52–53.

96. Silverman NH, Kleinman CS, Rudolph AM, et al. Fetal atrioventricular valve insufficiency associated with nonimmune hydrops. A two dimensional echocardiographic and pulsed Doppler ultrasound. Circulation 1985; 72:825–832.

97. Stein J, Berg C, Jones JA, et al: A screening protocol for prenatal population at risk for hemoglobin disorders: Results of its application to a group of Southeast Asians and blacks. Am J Obstet Gynecol 1984; 150:333–341.

98. Straub W, Zarabi M, Mazer JL: Fetal ascites associated with Conradi's disease (chondrodysplasia punctata). Report of a case. J Clin Ultrasound 1983; 11:234–236.

99. Thomas CS, Leopold GR, Hilton S, et al: Fetal hydrops associated with extralobar pulmonary sequestration. J Ultrasound Med 1986; 5:668–671.

100. Weiner C, Warner M, Pringle K, et al: Antenatal diagnosis and palliative treatment of nonimmune hydrops fetalis secondary to pulmonary extralobar sequestration. Obstet Gynecol 1986; 68:275–280.

101. Whittle MJ, Gilmore DH, McNay MB, et al: Diaphragmatic hernia presenting in utero as a unilateral hydrothorax. Prenat Diagn 1989; 9:115–118.

Ascites

102. Bair JH, Russ PD, Pretorius DH, et al: Fetal omphalocele and gastroschisis: A review of 24 cases. AJR 1986; 147:1047–1051.

103. Binder ND, Buckmaster JW, Benda GI: Outcome for fetus with ascites and cytomegalovirus infection. Pediatr 1988; 82:100–103.

104. Blumenthal DH, Rushovich AM, Williams RK, et al: Prenatal sonographic findings of meconium peritonitis with pathologic correlation. J Clin Ultrasound 1982; 10:350–352.

105. Cederqvist LL, Williams LR, Symchych, et al: Prenatal diagnosis of fetal ascites by ultrasound. Am J Obstet Gynecol 1977; 128:229–230.

106. Foster MA, Nyberg DA, Mahony BS, et al: Meconium peritonitis: Prenatal sonographic findings and their clinical significance. Radiology 1987; 165:661–665.

107. France NE, Back EH: Neonatal ascites associated with urethral obstruction. Arch Dis Child 1954; 29:565–568.

108. Garb M, Rad FF, Roseborough J: Meconium peritonitis presenting as fetal ascites on ultrasound. Br J Radiol 1980; 53:602–604.

109. Gillan JE, Lowden JA, Gaskin K, et al: Congenital ascites as a presenting sign of lysosomal storage disease. J Pediatr 1984; 104:225–231.

110. Griscom NT, Colodny AH, Rosenberg HK, et al: Diagnostic aspects of neonatal ascites: Report of 27 cases. AJR 1977; 128:961–970.

111. Hadlock FP, Deter RL, Garcia-Pratt J, et al: Fetal ascites not associated with Rh incompatibility: Recognition

and management with sonography. AJR 1980; 134:1225–1230.

112. Hashimoto B, Filly RA, Callen PW: Sonographic detection of fetal intraperitoneal fluid. J Ultrasound Med 1986; 5:203–204.

113. Hashimoto B, Filly RA, Callen PW: Fetal pseudoascites. Further anatomic observations. J Ultrasound Med 1986; 5:151–152.

114. Johnson T, Graham DM, Sanders RC: Ultrasound-detected paracentesis of massive fetal ascites. J Clin Ultrasound 1982; 10:140–142.

115. Mahony BS, Callen PW, Filly RA: Fetal urethral obstruction: US evaluation. Radiology 1985; 157:221–224.

116. Mueller-Heubach E, Mazer J: Sonographically documented disappearance of fetal ascites. Obstet Gynecol 1983; 61:253–257.

117. Persutte WH, Lenke RL, Kropp KA, et al: Atypical presentation of fetal obstructive uropathy. J Diag Med Sonog 1989; 1:12–15.

118. Petrovsky BM, Walzak MP Jr, D'Addario PF: Fetal cloacal anomalies: Prenatal sonographic findings and differential diagnosis. Obstet Gynecol 1988; 72(3):464–469.

119. Platt LD, Collea JV, Joseph DM: Transitory fetal ascites. An ultrasound diagnosis. Am J Obstet Gynecol 1978; 132:906–908.

120. Rosenthal SJ, Filly RA, Callen PW: Fetal pseudoascites. Radiology 1979; 131:195–197.

121. Shalev J, Ben-Rafael Z, Goldman B, et al: Mid-trimester diagnosis of bladder neck obstruction by ultrasound and paracentesis. J Med Genet 1983; 20:223–230.

122. Shimokawa H, Matsuyama T, Maeda H, et al: Cytology of fetal ascites and antenatal diagnosis of meconium peritonitis. Asia Oceania J Obstet Gynaecol 1986; 12:513–516.

123. Shweni PM, Kamberan SR, Ramdial K: Fetal ascites. A report of 6 cases. S Afr Med J 1984; 66:616–618.

124. Szeifert G, Gsecsei K, Toth Z, et al: Prenatal diagnosis of ascites caused by cytomegalovirus hepatitis. Acta Paediatr Hung 1985; 26:311–316.

Twin Gestations

Dolores H. Pretorius, M.D.

Barry S. Mahony, M.D.

Twin gestations are common high-risk pregnancies that cause increased rates of perinatal complications and mortality.[2, 5] Depending upon the type of twinning, the adverse effects to fetuses that are common in or specific to plural gestations include co-twin demise, prematurity, intrauterine growth retardation (IUGR), traumatic delivery, polyhydramnios or oligohydramnios, twin transfusion syndrome, acardiac twinning, conjoined twins, and fetal anomalies.[1, 2] Furthermore, twin pregnancies also have adverse maternal effects including an increased incidence of hypertension (15%), preeclampsia (5%–25%), abruption (2%–6%), and postpartum hemorrhage (6%–22%).[11, 15]

This chapter discusses the incidence, embryology, and associated fetal risks of twin gestations. It then explores the sonographic approach to the evaluation of twins and the many potential fetal hazards surrounding these high-risk pregnancies.

PREVALENCE

Twin gestations occur with an overall prevalence of approximately 1 in 80 live births. Twins are either dizygotic (two zygotes) or monozygotic (one zygote). Whereas the incidence of dizygotic twins varies on the basis of maternal age, race, and parity, the prevalence of monozygotic twins is relatively constant at 1 in 250 births in all maternal age groups and races (Table 15–1).[3, 4] The differences in dizygotic twinning rates probably result from differences in gonadotropin production; the father has little influence upon the rate of twinning.[9]

The true prevalence of multiple fetuses may be as high as 5%, depending on inclusion of the increasing numbers of patients undergoing ovulation induction and of those felt to have a "vanishing" twin.[5, 7, 28–30] The prevalence of twinning has been reported to be 6.8% to 17% after treatment with clomiphene citrate and 18% to 53.5% after treatment with gonadotropins.[8]

EMBRYOLOGY

The type of twinning depends upon the number of fertilized ova (zygotes) and the timing of zygotic division.[2, 3, 6] Approximately two thirds of twin pregnancies are dizygotic and one third are monozygotic. Fertilization of two ova results in dizygotic twins who are no more genetically similar than siblings, whereas fertilization of a single ovum which subsequently divides produces monozygotic twins with identical genotype. Each dizygotic twin has its own placenta and set of membranes.

If initial division of the morula occurs during the first 4 days following monozygotic fertilization, each twin has its own complete placenta and set of membranes (Fig 15–1). This situation occurs in approximately one third of monozygotic twin gestations. If the blastocyst does not separate until later in the first week following fertilization (after implantation but before formation of the amniotic cavity), the twins share a single placenta but develop in separate amnionic cavities. This situation occurs in approximately two thirds of monozygotic twin gestations. Failure of the blastocyst

TABLE 15–1.

Rates of Twinning by Type of Zygosity in Different Geographic Locations*

Location	Monozygotic	Dizygotic
Nigeria	5.0%	49%
United States		
Afro-American	4.7%	11.1%
White	4.2%	7.1%
England/Wales	3.5%	8.8%
Calcutta, India	3.3%	8.1%
Japan	3.0%	1.3%

*Modified from MacGillivray I: Epidemiology of twin pregnancy. Semin Perinatol 1986; 10:4–8.

to separate until the second week of gestation (following formation of the amnion) results in twins who develop in a single amnionic cavity, and initial division of the embryonic tissue after 13 days of gestation results in conjoined twins. Fortunately, both of these situations occur in only approximately 1%–3% of twin pregnancies, with conjoined twinning being the rarest form.

AMNIONICITY AND CHORIONICITY

Determination of amnionicity and chorionicity is important in the prenatal evaluation of twins as well as in possible medical applications after birth (e.g., skin

grafts, organ transplants, etc). Table 15–2 lists helpful features in the prenatal prediction of amnionicity, chorionicity, and zygosity.

Since dizygotic twins invariably each have their own complete placenta and set of membranes, all dizygotic twins are diamnionic and dichorionic (i.e., two amnionic cavities and two placentae). The placentas may be separate or fused, but no vascular anastomoses exist between them generally.[1] Documentation that the twins are of different sexes confirms dizygosity. Since dizygous twins need not be of different genders; however, documentation of dizygosity in twins of the same sex may be very difficult even following birth. The number of placentae provides little assistance in this regard, since in both dizygous and monozygous twinning the placentae may be either widely separated or immediately adjacent to each other. The separate placentae and amnionic cavities protect dizygous twins from many of the prenatal hazards encountered by twins who share these structures.

As mentioned above, monozygotic twins may have separate amnionic cavities and placentae (diamnionic-dichorionic), separate amnionic cavities but one fused placenta (diamnionic-monochorionic), or one amnionic cavity and one fused placenta (monoamnionic-monochorionic).[1] All dichorionic gestations are also diamnionic; two layers of chorion and two layers of amnion separate the twins. Monochorionic twin pregnancies are all monozygotic and either have only two

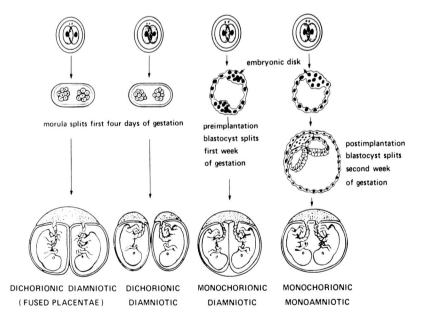

FIG 15–1.
Relationship among amnionicity, chorionicity, and timing of separation of the morula or blastocyst in dizygotic twin gestations. A morula that splits during the first 4 days of gestation results in a diamnionic-dichorionic pregnancy with fused or unfused placentae. A blastocyst that splits prior to implantation produces a diamnionic-monochorionic pregnancy, whereas a blastocyst that splits following implantation results in a monoamnionic-monochorionic pregnancy. (From Fox H: *Pathology of the Placenta.* Philadelphia, WB Saunders Co, 1988. Used by permission.)

TABLE 15–2.

Helpful features in the Antenatal Sonographic Prediction of Amnionicity, Chorionicity and Zygosity in Twin Pregnancies*

Sonographic Feature	Diamnionic Dichorionic Dizygotic (67%)	Diamnionic Dichorionic Monozygotic (11%)	Diamnionic Monochorionic Monozygotic (22%)	Monoamnionic Monochorionic Monozygotic (1%)
Number of placental sites				
Either one or two	X	X		
One only			X	X
Membrane separating the twins				
Thick	X^A	X^A		
Thin			X^A	
Not present			B	X
Fetal gender				
Concordant		X	X	X
Concordant or discordant	X			
Other features				
"Stuck twin"		(unusual)	X	
Twin transfusion syndrome			X	X
Acardiac twin	(rare)	(rare)	X	X
Entangled cords				X
Conjoined twins				X

*Numbers in parentheses refer to approximate percentage of all twins in the United States.
A = predictive value may decrease with advancing gestation; B = may be difficult to detect in the first trimester and in "stuck twins."

layers of amnion separating the twins or a single amniotic cavity, but virtually all monochorionic twin pregnancies have placental vascular anastomoses including artery-to-artery, artery-to-vein, and vein-to-vein.[1] Therefore, all these fetuses are at risk for the twin transfusion syndrome, poor outcome of a surviving twin after its co-twin's death, acardiac twinning, umbilical cord entanglement, or conjoined twinning. For these reasons, monochorionic pregnancy significantly increases perinatal morbidity and mortality. Obviously, a membrane separating the twins excludes umbilical cord entanglement and conjoined twinning. Monoamnionic twins (all of whom are also monochorionic and monozygotic), on the other hand, are at unique risk for both these problems, each of which markedly increases perinatal morbidity and mortality.

PERINATAL MORBIDITY AND MORTALITY

Because of the numerous potential fetal hazards that twins encounter, twin perinatal mortality is approximately 4–10 times greater than for singletons (Table 15–3).[13–17] For example, in one series twins had a perinatal mortality rate of 13.9% compared with the singleton perinatal mortality rate of 3.3%.[14] Fur-

thermore, the mortality rate associated with delivery of the second twin approximately doubles that of the first twin.[12]

Perinatal mortality rates in most series are approximately 10% for diamnionic-dichorionic twins, 25% for

TABLE 15–3.

Approximate Frequency of Obstetric Complications Associated With Twin Gestation

Complication	Frequency (%)
Malpresentation	40–50
Pre-term delivery (<37 weeks)	25–55
"Vanishing twin"	20–50
Maternal hypertension	15
Intrauterine growth retardation	15–30
Postpartum hemorrhage	6–22
Preeclampsia	5–25
Premature rupture of membranes	5–15
Polyhydramnios	6–12
Severe oligohydramnios	8
Congenital anomalies	6–10
Cord accidents	2–10
Abruption	2–6
Co-twin demise (second or third trimester)	0.5–7
Twin transfusion syndrome	1–2
Acardiac twinning	<1
Conjoined twinning	<1

diamnionic-monochorionic twins, and 50% for monoamnionic-monochorionic twins.[1, 10] The increased perinatal mortality for diamnionic-dichorionic twins relative to singleton pregnancies results from the increased incidence of prematurity, intrauterine growth retardation (IUGR), traumatic delivery, aberrations of amniotic fluid volume, and possibly from fetal anomalies as well as from problems of the maternal-placental unit (preeclampsia, placental infarcts, amnionitis, etc).[11, 15]

The increased perinatal mortality rates for monochorionic pregnancies results from these potential problems in addition to the placental vascular anastomoses that may lead to the twin transfusion syndrome or acardiac twins. The very high mortality rates for monoamnionic twins relates to each of the above potential complications as well as the potential for umbilical cord entanglement or conjoined twinning; approximately 30%–40% of monoamnionic twins die from umbilical cord entanglement, and the majority of conjoined twins are stillborn.

THE SONOGRAPHIC APPROACH

Detection of a multiple gestation provides many benefits regarding obstetrical management. For example, detection of a twin pregnancy enables increased antepartum surveillance, including serial nonstress testing and sonography for detection of IUGR, fetal anomalies, and determination of the optimal mode of delivery.[11, 20] Some authors justify routine obstetrical sonography purely on the basis of detection of twin gestations.[13] When sonography was not routine but was readily available, only 47% of twins were diagnosed before the 24th week of pregnancy.[13] Routine sonography prior to 20 weeks' gestation in a large series in Sweden, however, improved early twin detection to 95%.[16]

Assessment of Amnionicity and Chorionicity

An assessment of amnionicity and chorionicity constitutes the initial step in the prenatal sonographic evaluation of a twin pregnancy. This can be accomplished in many cases by addressing the following (Table 15–2):

1. *Is a membrane present separating the fetuses?* Visualization of the separating membrane indicates a diamnionic pregnancy (Fig 15–2). Lack of visualization of the separating membrane indicates that the pregnancy remains at risk for monoamnionicity and its

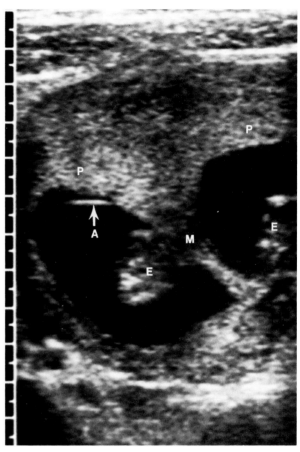

FIG 15–2.
Diamnionic-dichorionic twin pregnancy at 7 menstrual weeks. Transverse scan of the uterus shows twin living embryos separated by a thick membrane indicative of diamnionicity and dichorionicity. The thin amnion of one of the twins is only visible where it orients perpendicular to the ultasound beam and creates a specular echo. E = embryos; M = separating membrane; A = amnion; P = developing placentae.

common inherent complications, such as entangled umbilical cords and conjoined twinning (Figs 15–3, 15–4). Non–visualization of a separating membrane, however, is not sufficient evidence for a monoamnionic gestation.

2. *Are two separate placentae present?* Identification of two distinctly separate placentae indicates a diamnionic-dichorionic pregnancy, which excludes the twin transfusion syndrome and parabiotic twinning (Fig 15–5). On the other hand, identification of only one placental site does not reliably predict a monochorionic pregnancy.

3. *Is the sex of the co-twins discordant?* A male and female co-twin pair indicates dizygotic fertilization, in which case placentation must be diamnionic and dichorionic. Identification of same sex co-twins, however, does not reliably predict monozygosity, monochorionicity, or monoamnionicity.

FIG 15–3.
Entangled umbilical cords in monoamnionic-monochorionic twins. Transverse scan of a twin pregnancy shows a single placenta and intertwining segments of the umbilical cord from both twins. This finding in the absence of a separating membrane indicates monoamnionicity. P = placenta; *arrows* = intertwined segments of umbilical cords. (Also see Fig 16–52.)

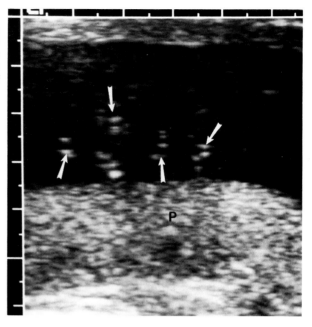

4. If a separating membrane is present, is it thin or thick? In a diamnionic-dichorionic gestation the separating membrane is comprised of four layers (two amnions and two chorions), whereas the membrane of a diamnionic-monochorionic gestation is composed of only two layers (two amnions). Therefore, the separating membrane in a dichorionic pregnancy tends to be thicker than in a monochorionic gestation (Fig 15–6). A thin membrane indicative of monochorionic placentation appears hair-like and wispy; it is often difficult to see and is generally identified only over a short length or where it is perpendicular to the insonation beam and creates a specular echo. The thick membrane is easily seen in the first trimester, whereas a thin mem-

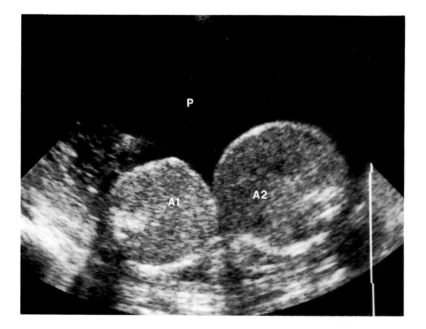

FIG 15–4.
Monoamnionic-monochorionic twins with polyhydramnios. Transverse scan through the abdomen of both monoamnionic-monochorionic twins shows no separating membrane. With variations in maternal position, both twins sank into the dependent portions of the single polyhydramniotic sac and no separating membrane could be seen. Note that the abdomen of one twin is unmistakably smaller than the other twin, indicative of intrauterine growth retardation of the smaller twin. The larger twin is large for dates but not edematous. *A1* = abdomen of smaller twin; *A2* = abdomen of larger twin; *P* = polyhydramnios.

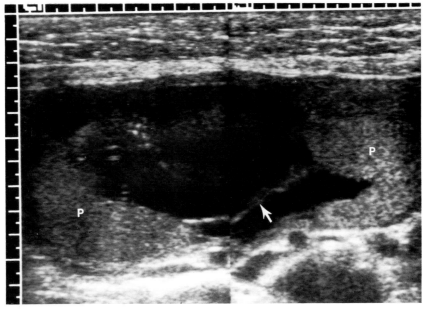

FIG 15–5.
Two separate placentae in a diamnionic-dichorionic pregnancy. Dual-image scan demonstrates the two separate placentae indicative of dichorionicity. The separating membrane extends from the edge of one placenta diagonally to the opposite edge of the other placenta. Two placentae are most frequently the result of a dizygotic gestation but about 10% of cases result from a monozygotic gestation. *P* = placentae; *arrow* = separating membrane.

brane often is not visible until the second trimester (Fig 15–2).[18]

Various authors have used one or more of the above criteria for determining the amnionicity and chorionicity of twin gestations. Barss et al. correctly identified the amnionicity and chorionicity in 33 of 34 cases (23 diamnionic-dichorionic and 11 diamnionic-monochorionic) by evaluating the number of placentae (separate or single mass) and thickness of the separating membrane in each case.[18] Eleven of 23 dichorionic pregnancies had distinctly separate placentae, and the

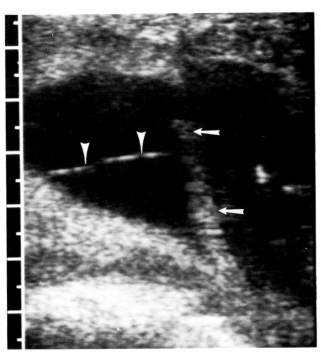

FIG 15–6.
Triplet pregnancy at 8 weeks with one thin membrane and one thick membrane. Transverse scan of a triplet pregnancy during the first trimester illustrates the difference in membrane thickness between a thick (dichorionic) membrane and a thin (monochorionic) membrane. In this case the thin membrane is especially well seen because it orients perpendicular to the ultrasound beam. The thick membrane is clearly visible even though it orients parallel to the ultrasound beam. *Arrowheads* = thin membrane; *arrows* = thick membrane.

separating membrane appeared thick in all dichorionic pregnancies. Only one monochorionic case was misclassified as dichorionic.

In a retrospective study of 55 cases, Hertzberg et al. reported that identification of a thick membrane accurately indicated a dichorionic gestation in 38 of 42 (90%) cases.[21] Among the 13 monochorionic pregnancies (one of which was also monoamnionic), a thin membrane accurately predicted monochorionicity, but in nine of these cases no membrane was seen, and in one case the thickness of the membrane was indeterminant. Their success rate in identifying thick membranes in dichorionic gestations decreased from 100% in the first trimester to 89% in the second trimester and 36% in the third trimester. In cases of thin membranes seen with diamnionic-monochorionic gestations, their success rate was 0% in the first trimester, 25% in the second trimester, and 17% in the third trimester.

Townsend et al. reviewed 75 twin gestations and found that thick membranes had a predictive value of 83% for dichorionicity and thin membranes had a predictive value of 83% for diamnionic-monochorionic pregnancy.[24] They also confirmed that in most cases thick membranes appeared progressively thinner throughout pregnancy (Fig 15–7). One technical limitation Townsend et al. observed was artifactual thick-

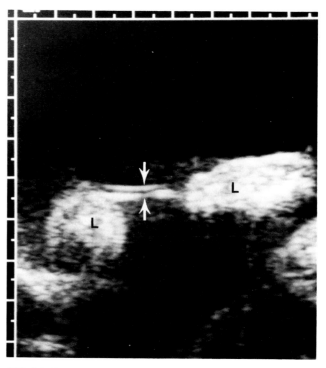

FIG 15–8.
Two layers of a diamnionic-monochorionic pregnancy. This scan demonstrates the two adjacent amnions of a diamnionic-dichorionic gestation. *Arrows* = two layers of separating membrane; *L* = limbs of one twin.

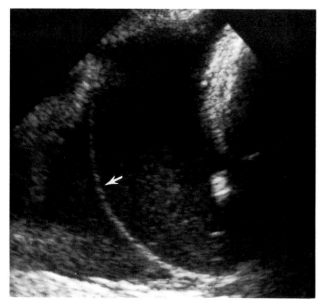

FIG 15–7.
Separating membrane during the third trimester. The thick membrane of a diamnionic-dichorionic pregnancy appears progressively thinner throughout pregnancy and may resemble a thin membrane of a diamnionic-monochorionic pregnancy during the third trimester, as this scan of a "thick" separating membrane shows. *Arrow* = separating membrane.

ening of a diamnionic-monochorionic membrane, and they postulated that in such cases the apparent membrane thickening results from specular reflection when the membrane orients directly perpendicular to the sound beam.

D'Alton et al. also have noted that high resolution, magnified ultrasound may identify the individual layers of the separating membrane in twin pregnancies.[20] Four layers of the membrane indicate a diamnionic-dichorionic gestation, whereas two layers signify a diamnionic-monochorionic pregnancy (Fig 15–8). It is important not to misinterpret sections of the umbilical cord as membrane. Although D'Alton et al. have reported success in seeing the layers of the membrane, this has not been verified in the literature by other investigators.

Although lack of membrane visualization suggests monoamnionic-monochorionic placentation, one must beware of several potential pitfalls in this regard. Mahony et al. reported that of 11 cases in which no membrane was seen, only one was monoamnionic-monochorionic.[22] Visualization of the thin separating membrane of a diamnionic-monochorionic pregnancy may be especially difficult in the first trimester, early second trimester, or in the third trimester (Fig 15–9).

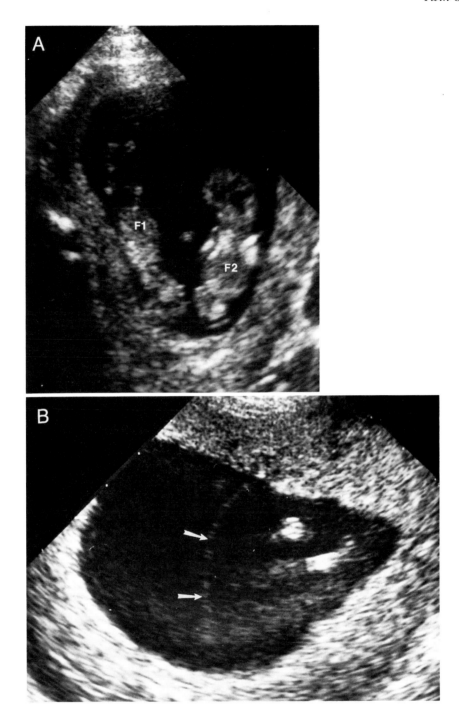

FIG 15–9.
Thin separating membrane of a diamnionic-monochorionic pregnancy at 10 weeks. **A,** transabdominal scan of the uterus shows two fetuses but no visible separating membrane. **B,** transvaginal scan of the uterus demonstrates the thin separating membrane. *F1* = one twin; *F2* = second twin; *arrows* = separating membrane.

Examination of the fetuses with the mother in different positions (supine, decubitus, and erect) often assists in this assessment. In a diamnionic pregnancy, unlike in the rare monoamnionic gestation, the twins do not both sink freely into all dependent portions of the uterus with changes in maternal position. In addition, changes in maternal position often cause reorientation of the membrane so that it becomes visible.

Occasionally, one twin may reside within a very oligohydramniotic sac adjacent to the uterine wall and appear constantly "stuck" to the uterus despite variations in maternal position (Fig 15–10).[22] In the setting

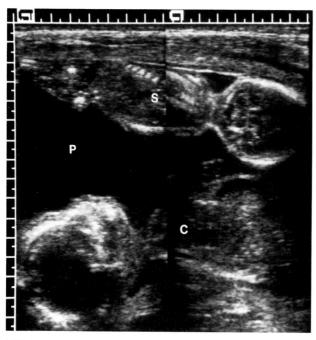

FIG 15–10.
Lack of visualization of separating membrane adjacent to a "stuck" twin. Longitudinal dual-image scan at 20 weeks shows one twin adjacent to the uterine wall with the co-twin in the dependent portions of a polyhydramniotic sac. Although a separating membrane is not evident on this scan, its presence can be inferred by the absence of mobility of the "stuck" twin with changes in maternal positioning. Careful scanning often demonstrates portions of the separating membrane adjacent to the "stuck" twin. *S* = "stuck" twin; *C* = co-twin in polyhydramniotic sac; *P* = polyhydramnios.

of a "stuck" twin, the examiner must carefully examine the region adjacent to the affected twin to identify the thin membrane. Whenever the separating membrane cannot be documented, the possibility of monoamnionicity persists; the umbilical cord for both twins should be examined for potential entanglement, and both fetuses should be assessed for shared fetal parts indicative of conjoined twins.[19, 23, 25] Clearly, in some cases, the examiner feels more confident in the assessment of amnionicity and chorionicity than in other cases. In equivocal cases reporting confidence levels may be appropriate.

COMMON PROBLEMS IN TWIN GESTATIONS

Following the assessment of amnionicity and chorionicity, the sonographic evaluation of a twin gestation includes the parameters delineated in Chapter 2 for high-risk pregnancies. As mentioned previously and discussed separately below, the common problems which may be assessed with ultrasound include: Co-twin demise, prematurity, IUGR, traumatic delivery,

oligohydramnios or polyhydramnios, the "stuck" twin phenomenon, twin transfusion syndrome, acardiac twins, conjoined twinning, and fetal anomalies (Table 15–3).

Co-Twin Demise

Clinical and Pathologic Findings

Because of the many potential hazards encountered by twins, these pregnancies have an increased co-twin mortality rate. The reported frequency of single fetal death in plural gestations ranges from 0.5% to 6.8%, with the more recent reports indicating the higher incidence rates.[26] Approximately 70%–75% of cases of antenatal co-twin death occur in monochorionic pregnancies. At least one of monoamniotic twins frequently dies from umbilical cord entanglement or from the effects of conjoined twinning. However, the incidence of diamniotic-monochorionic co-twin fetal demise exceeds that of dichorionic pregnancies which, in turn, exceeds that of singleton pregnancies for many of the reasons listed above.[26] At least in the second half of pregnancy, co-twin demise renders the surviving twin at increased risk for anomalies of a variety of or-

TABLE 15–4.

Structural Defects and Malformations Seen in Monozygous Twins*

Structural defects in survivor of monozygotic twin pair
  Central nervous system defects
    Cerebellar necrosis
    Hydranencephaly
    Hydrocephalus
    Microcephaly
    Multicystic encephalomalacia
    Porencephaly
    Spinal cord transection
  Gastrointestinal defects
    Appendiceal atresia
    Colonic atresia
    Small bowel atresia
  Renal defects
    Congenital renal cortical necrosis
    Horseshoe kidney
  Hemifacial microsomia
  Terminal limb defects
  Aplasia cutis congenita
Associated malformations
  Anencephaly
  Holoprosencephaly
  Cloacal exstrophy
  Sirenomelia
  VACTERL association

*Modified from Jones KL, Benirschke K: The developmental pathogenesis of structural defects: The contribution of monozygotic twins. Semin Perinatol 1983; 7:239–243.

gan systems secondary to thromboembolic vascular occlusion from the dead co-twin via placental anastomoses (Table 15–4).[26, 27, 32, 85, 89]

Sonographic Findings

Co-twin demise that occurs during the latter stages of embryogenesis or early in the fetal period may result in the "vanishing" twin phenomenon. Although controversy exists regarding the concept of the "vanishing twin," histologic evidence verifies its existence in some cases.[33] The "vanishing" phenomenon occurs during the latter half of the first trimester or the early part of the second trimester of pregnancy and apparently carries no significant risk to the living co-twin.[28, 29]

Various reports cite the incidence of vanishing twin to range widely from 0% to 78%.[26, 29, 30] Landy et al. found that 21.2% of twins verified to be alive with real-time sonography disappeared subsequently (Fig 15–11).[30] The disappearance rate increased to 48% among gestations with a second empty or abnormal sac but one in which a living embryo was not confirmed. Since first trimester vaginal bleeding is the only clinical sign of this phenomenon, however, at least some of the empty or abnormal "sacs" probably represent small extrachorionic hematomas rather than a resorbing or blighted "vanishing" twin.[28, 29] On the other hand, characteristic perivillous fibrin deposition of the placenta or embryonic remnants provides postpartum histologic evidence of the vanishing twin phenomenon in

approximately 50% of cases, and this same focal degenerative change of the placenta occurs in 25% of uncomplicated term pregnancies.[28] Therefore, the incidence of the vanishing twin phenomenon may indeed be high.

Co-twin demise that occurs during the middle stages of gestation with pregnancy continuation of the remaining single living fetus results in fetus papyraceous. A small but recognizable non–viable fetus is present at delivery. The dead fetus has undergone flattening, necrosis, atrophy, and sometimes mummification.[17] Fetus papyraceous is thought to occur in approximately 1 per 12,000 live births or in 1 per 184 twin births.[29] Sonography identifies a single living fetus with a second smaller, non–living fetus within a smaller gestational sac near the uterine wall (Figs 15–12 and 15–13).

Numerous anomalies may occur in the survivor of a monozygotic twin pair after death of the co-twin (Table 15–4).[83, 87] Many of these anomalies may be explained by the release from the dead twin of thromboplastic material which crosses through placental anastomoses to the live twin.[1] The anomalies postulated to occur secondary to embolization following death of a co-twin predominantly involve the head and other well-perfused fetal organ systems. For example, multicystic encephalomalacia causes significant brain damage and may result in mental retardation, seizure disorders, and spasticity.[31, 34] Detection of co-twin de-

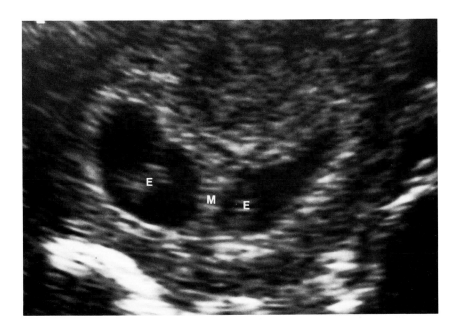

FIG 15–11.
"Vanishing" twin. Sonogram of the uterus at 7 weeks shows a twin living diamnionic-dichorionic pregnancy. Real-time ultrasound clearly demonstrated the normal heartbeat of both embryos. A follow-up ultrasound at 16 weeks showed a single live pregnancy with no evidence for the prior co-twin. *E* = embryos; *M* = separating membrane.

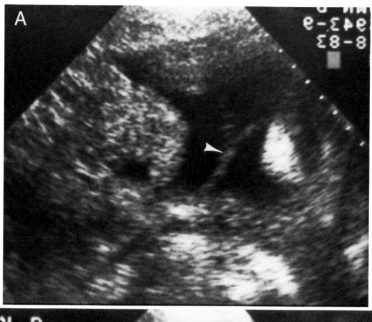

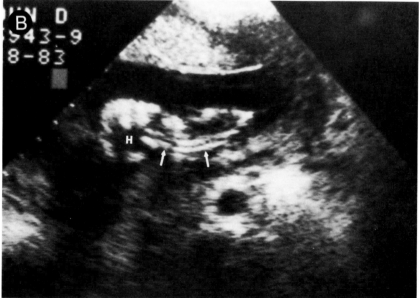

FIG 15–12.
Fetus papyraceous at 35 weeks. **A,** sonogram shows fetal parts on both sides of a membrane and a normal 35-week fetus. **B,** with the patient in the decubitus position a small nonliving fetus is visible with a crown rump length compatible with 13 weeks. *Arrowhead* = membrane separating the twins; *arrows* = spine of fetus papyraceous; *H* = head of fetus papyraceous.

mise, therefore, mandates a careful survey of the living twin for possible sequelae of thromboembolism.

Prematurity

Clinical and Pathologic Findings

Approximately 25%–55% of twins are delivered prior to term.[12, 15, 36] This accounts in great part for the increased mortality rate of twins relative to singletons and undoubtedly results from one of several or a combination of factors including uterine distension, polyhydramnios, fetal distress, and preeclampsia.[2]

Sonographic Findings

Ultrasound provides useful information for obstetrical management of these pregnancies by (1) assessment of menstrual age on the basis of growth parameters, especially when performed in the first half of pregnancy; (2) amniocentesis guidance for assessment of lung maturity; and (3) documentation of potential fetal

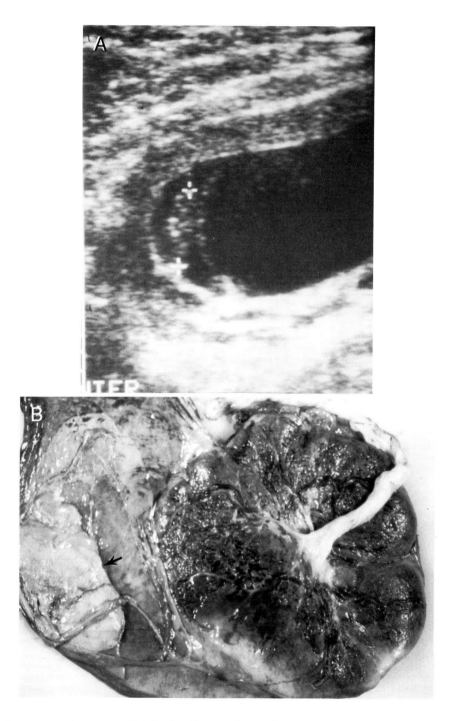

FIG 15–13.
Fetus papyraceous. **A,** sonogram shows a small fetal pole without cardiac motion and a crown rump length (distance between graticules) consistent with 8 weeks' gestational age. A second normal 20-week fetus with cardiac motion was also identified. **B,** pathological specimen of the placenta at term shows the normal placenta on the right and a sac with a fetus papyraceous of approximately 8 weeks on the left *(arrow)*.

anomalies that may preclude heroic measures when delivery is imminent.

Intrauterine Growth Retardation

Clinical and Pathologic Findings

Intrauterine growth retardation (IUGR) affects approximately 15% to 30% of twin pregnancies.[12, 15, 43] Various definitions for IUGR exist, but the two used most commonly include infants weighing less than the 10th percentile of expected singleton weight for gestational age or a birth weight difference of greater than 20% between twins.[37, 43] IUGR usually affects one twin but occasionally affects both twins.

Sonographic Findings

Given the observation that IUGR occurs with increased frequency in twins compared with singletons, the appropriate method for sonographic assessment of twin growth patterns remains controversial. Various investigators have suggested the use of different growth charts for twins than for singletons, since beginning at around 30 weeks twin fetuses as a group tend to have a slower growth rate than singletons, and mean weight for twins at term is approximately 10% lower than for singletons.[39, 40, 41] Twin growth charts may be skewed, however, by the much higher incidence of IUGR among twins compared with singletons, and utilization of twin growth charts may diminish the sensitivity of ultrasound for predicting abnormal growth.

More recent sonographic investigations of twin growth show a decreased rate of growth in biparietal diameter (after 31 to 32 weeks of gestation) and abdominal circumference (after 32 to 33 weeks of gestation) relative to singletons.[38, 44] Since postnatal measurements showed normal head size, the decreased biparietal diameter growth rate probably resulted from dolichocephaly related to intrauterine compression.[44] The reduced abdominal circumference reflects the significantly reduced mean birth weight of twins compared with singletons.[44] Because the abdominal circumference correlates far more strongly with fetal weight than with third-trimester gestational age, diminished rates of growth of the abdominal circumference in twins do not justify the use of specific twin growth charts to assess third-trimester gestational age. On the other hand, charts developed for singleton pregnancies are useful in the evaluation of multigestational pregnancies, since size and weight of fetuses are the most important factors in formulating an optimal treatment plan.

Several investigators have advocated the use of different sonographic standards to diagnose IUGR in twin pregnancies than those utilized for singletons. For example, Houlton reported that 40% of the smaller co-twins were small for gestational age (SGA) when a 3–5mm difference in biparietal diameter existed, whereas 71% of the twins were SGA when the difference was 6 mm or more.[40] Haney et al. also found that a difference in biparietal diameter between twins of greater than 6 mm resulted in a poor neonatal outcome.[39] However, most of these publications appeared over 10 years ago, prior to the use of multiple parameters to assess IUGR. Furthermore, given the fact that most twin pregnancies are dizygotic and therefore genotypically distinct, it is not surprising to find that co-twin growth patterns may differ in the third trimester, even in the absence of IUGR. This is especially true if the sonogram documents dizygosity by visualizing fetuses of differing gender. Discordancy of twin size is not a risk factor at term if the lighter twin weighs at least 2,500 grams.[35]

Utilizing multiple biometric parameters, Chitkara et al. found that the highest overall accuracy for diagnosing an IUGR twin at birth was obtained from an estimation of fetal weight and femur length.[37] As expected, the most sensitive measurement in diagnosing IUGR was the abdominal circumference. Doppler sonography also may be extremely helpful in evaluating twin pregnancies for IUGR (see below).

We believe that the growth status of each twin should be evaluated individually using the same sonographic parameters throughout gestation as for singleton pregnancies: Biparietal diameter, head circumference, femur length, abdominal circumference, and amniotic fluid volume (Fig 15–14). This involves an independent assessment of amniotic fluid volume in the amniotic cavity of each twin. These parameters then should be compared with prior sonograms of the same twin to assess appropriateness of interval growth and to evaluate for co-twin growth discrepancy. We assess significant growth discordance when one twin meets the criteria for IUGR and the other does not.

Traumatic Delivery

In approximately 50% of twin pregnancies, one or both of the twins is breech, and ultrasound reliably predicts the malpresentation.[11] Approximately 90% of such cases undergo cesarean delivery to minimize birth trauma and the possibility of umbilical cord prolapse.[11, 36] When one or both twins are not in vertex presentation, cesarean delivery virtually eliminates the differential in morbidity and mortality for the second twin compared with the first twin.[36]

Because of the high mortality rate from umbilical

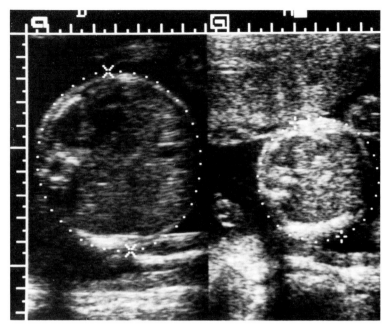

FIG 15–14.
Intrauterine growth retardation of one twin at 29 weeks. Dual-image sonogram shows a normal abdominal circumference of the twin depicted on the left, but the abdominal circumference for the co-twin is only mean for 20–21 weeks, indicative of intrauterine growth retardation of the co-twin. *x graticules* = abdominal circumference of normal twin; + *graticules* = abdominal circumference of growth-retarded twin.

cord entanglement in monoamniotic pregnancies, early cesarean delivery of monoamniotic twins minimizes the likelihood of cord entanglement and eliminates the risk of fetal interlocking during vaginal delivery.[42] The timing of optimal delivery in such cases remains undetermined, however, since the presence of a mature amniocentesis lung profile does not assure lung maturity of both twins in the same amniotic cavity.

Polyhydramnios and Oligohydramnios

Clinical and Pathologic Findings

Polyhydramnios occurs in approximately 6%–12% of twin pregnancies, an incidence figure that is 4–30 times that of singleton pregnancies. Reports of associated perinatal mortality rates range from 23% to 87%.[2, 7, 57] Two fetuses normally produce more amniotic fluid than a single fetus, however, and borderline or mild polyhydramnios during the mid-trimester frequently occurs in the absence of detectable fetal or maternal cause.

Reports suggest that 30%–70% of twin pregnancies with polyhydramnios have fetal abnormalities.[50, 51] As is true with singleton pregnancies, increasing severity of polyhydramnios in twin pregnancies correlates directly with the likelihood of determining the underlying etiology and inversely with the prognosis (see Chapter 3). Polyhydramnios also leads to pre-term delivery in approximately 44% of cases, with important consequences for perinatal morbidity and mortality.[50] Polyhydramnios in one sac with oligohydramnios in the other sac has been reported to have a perinatal

mortality rate of 71%, despite a variety of intervention procedures including serial removal of fluid from the polyhydramniotic cavity, selective feticide, and injection of saline into the oligohydramniotic cavity.[47]

Sonographic Findings

Detection of oligohydramnios and/or polyhydramnios in twin gestations warrants a careful search for structural abnormalities associated with either of these findings (see Chapter 3). In addition to the common causes for oligohydramnios (decreased urine output, ruptured membranes, IUGR, etc.) or for polyhydramnios (neural tube defect, upper gastrointestinal obstruction, hydrops, etc), one must also consider the common etiologies unique to multiple gestations such as the "stuck" twin phenomenon or the twin transfusion syndrome (Table 15–5).[22]

TABLE 15–5.

Causes for Disparity of Amniotic Fluid Volume in Diamniotic Twin Gestations

Common
Stuck twin phenomenon
(approximately 2/3 twin transfusion syndrome)
Uncommon
Oligohydramniotic twin
Decreased urine output
Ruptured amnion
Growth retardation
Polyhydramniotic twin
Neural tube defect
Upper gastrointestinal tract obstruction
Hydrops (other than twin transfusion syndrome)
Etc. (see Chapter 3)

The 'Stuck' Twin Phenomenon

Clinical and Pathologic Findings

The term "stuck" twin, first coined by Mahony et al. signifies a twin pregnancy in which one fetus is positioned in a severely oligohydramniotic sac causing it to be relatively immobile.[22] It frequently occurs in association with polyhydramnios of the co-twin. This constellation of one "stuck" twin in a severely oligohydramniotic sac and a co-twin in a polyhydramniotic sac has been reported to occur in 42% of diamnionic-monochorionic gestations and in 8% of all twin pregnancies.[53]

In most cases of the "stuck" twin phenomenon, no apparent structural etiology for the severe oligohydramnios or polyhydramnios exists, although in many cases there is disparity of fetal size. Although the constellation of one stuck twin and a polyhydramniotic co-twin undoubtedly represents a manifestation of the twin transfusion syndrome in some cases, 33% of cases reported by Mahony et al. occurred in dichorionic pregnancies and only 33% of cases had other manifestations of the twin transfusion syndrome or of acardiac twinning.[22] Chescheir et al. also reported a similar case in a dichorionic pregnancy with opposite-sex twins, and we have seen other similar cases.[47] In such cases, the etiology for the severe oligohydramnios of one twin and polyhydramnios of the co-twin remains speculative but perhaps relates to discrepancies of compression upon the vessels within the two placentae once the volume of one amniotic cavity differs from the other.

The stuck twin phenomenon signifies a poor prognosis, especially when accompanied by severe polyhydramnios of the co-twin. In the study reported by Mahony et al., all six stuck twins died and all of the polyhydramniotic co-twins also died, but all co-twins with normal amnionic fluid volume survived.[22] Among seven pregnancies with one "stuck" twin and a polyhydramniotic co-twin reported by Chescheir et al., none of ten fetuses who presented prior to 26 weeks gestation survived despite a variety of attempted therapeutic maneuvers, whereas all four fetuses who presented after 26 weeks' gestation survived.[47]

Sonographic Findings

The "stuck" twin appears relatively fixed to the uterine wall, even with changes in maternal position (Figs 15–10 and 15–15). When the "stuck" twin is positioned adjacent to the anterior uterine wall, it appears to defy gravity. However, a fetus is heavier than amnionic fluid and sinks into the dependent portions of the amnionic cavity unless it is prevented from doing so by the amnion. Although the thin separating membrane may or may not be visible, a thorough evaluation of the "stuck" twin usually identifies the membrane as it sweeps off the fetus and approaches the uterine wall (Fig 15–15). The detection of severe oligohydramnios and concomitant polyhydramnios of the co-twin warrants a careful search for associated structural anomalies, although frequently none are evident in this setting.

Twin Transfusion Syndrome

Clinical and Pathologic Findings

The twin transfusion syndrome occurs only in fetuses with monochorionic placentation.[2] Although placental vascular anastomoses are seen in virtually 100% of monochorionic pregnancies, the twin transfusion syndrome occurs in only 5% to 30% of monochorionic twins.[45, 49, 55, 56, 92] It occurs when blood shunts from one twin to the other via placental anastomoses, generally arterial to venous. This classically results in one anemic twin and a fluid-overloaded co-twin, although the clinical picture of the syndrome varies from case to case. Table 15–6 lists the classical signs of the twin transfusion syndrome. The different variations of the clinical syndrome include: Hydrops in the donor, normal amniotic fluid in both sacs, absence of growth discrepancy between the two twins, absence of hydrops, and arterial to arterial anastomoses with no identification of arterial to venous anastomoses.[48, 54, 55]

The twin transfusion syndrome may occur throughout pregnancy. Many cases identified in the early second trimester result in death of both twins at pre-term delivery. Milder cases do occur, often presenting late in pregnancy with survival of both twins. Although no specific therapy has been identified, De

TABLE 15–6.

Classical Signs of the Twin Transfusion Syndrome*

Recipient	Donor
Polyhydramnios	Oligohydramnios
Plethoric	Anemic
Edema	Not edematous
Large for dates	Small for dates
Enlarged viscera	Small viscera
Arterial hypertension	Arterial hypotension
Hyperbilirubinemia	Bilirubin normal

*From Braat DDM, Exalto N, Bernardus R, et al: Twin pregnancy: Case reports illustrating variations in transfusion syndrome. Eur J Obstet Gynecol Reprod Biol 1985; 19:383–390. Used by permission.

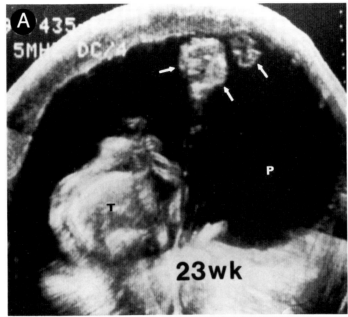

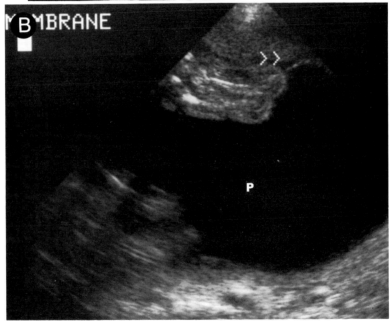

FIG 15–15.
"Stuck" twin. **A,** transverse image through the uterus at 23 weeks shows one twin in a severely polyhydramniotic sac and a "stuck" twin lying adjacent to the anterior uterine wall. The twin in the polyhydramniotic sac sinks into the dependent portion of the amnionic cavity. **B,** scan of a similar case shows a portion of the separating membrane in close proximity to the "stuck" twin. *P* = polyhydramnios; *arrows* = "stuck" twin; *T* = co-twin in polyhydramniotic sac; *arrowheads* = portion of the separating membrane adjacent to the "stuck" twin.

Lia et al. have reported a good outcome in a pregnancy treated with digitalis.[48] Selective termination of the twin with oligohydramnios ("stuck" twin) has also been reported.[58] This case resulted in a good outcome for the surviving, presumably recipient twin. In some cases, the twin with oligohydramnios succumbs during pregnancy and the remaining recipient twin survives without interventional therapy. The polyhydramnios associated with the surviving twin may resolve in less than 2 weeks.[54] However, the surviving twin does have a significant risk of perinatal morbidity and mortality, especially from neurological sequelae presumably related to thromboembolic events from the dead co-twin.

FIG 15–16.
Twin transfusion syndrome. Dual-image sonogram through the abdomen of both twins at 21 weeks shows a large amount of ascites in the twin depicted on the left. Additional scans of this twin demonstrated scalp edema and polyhydramnios indicative of hydrops fetalis. The abdominal circumference of the co-twin depicted on the right is only mean for 18–19 weeks, and this twin is in an oligohydramniotic sac indicative of intrauterine growth retardation. Note that the transverse liver diameter of the hydropic twin is larger than the entire abdominal diameter of the small co-twin. *x graticules* = abdominal circumference of hydropic twin; *+ graticules* = abdominal circumference of growth-retarded twin; *A* = ascites; *L* = liver; *S* = stomach; *P* = polyhydramnios.

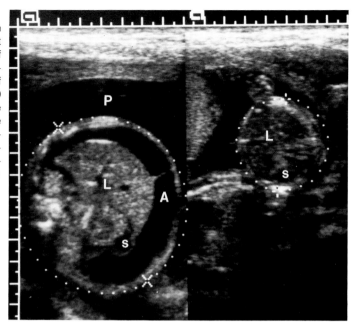

Sonographic Findings

The sonographic criteria suggesting the diagnosis of twin transfusion syndrome include (Fig 15–16) (1) significant disparity in size between fetuses of the same sex with one twin being relatively macrosomic and the other showing evidence for asymmetric growth retardation; (2) disparity in size between the two amniotic sacs; (3) two separate umbilical cords with disparity in size or in number of vessels within the umbilical cords; (4) a single placenta with areas of disparity in echogenicity of the cotyledons supplying the two umbilical cords; and (5) evidence of hydrops in either fetus or findings of congestive cardiac failure in the recipient.[46] Although hydrops is an important part of the twin transfusion syndrome, numerous other causes for hydrops exist and detection of hydrops does not necessarily signify the presence of the twin transfusion syndrome.[52]

Acardiac Twinning

Clinical and Pathologic Findings

Acardiac twinning (chorioangiopagus parasiticus) probably represents the most extreme manifestation of the twin transfusion syndrome in most cases. It has been reported to occur in approximately 1% of monochorionic twin deliveries (i.e., approximately 1 in 25,000 deliveries) and is uniformly fatal to the affected twin.[62] Although the vast majority of acardiac twinning occurs in monochorionic twin pregnancies (especially those which are also monoamnionic), it can occur in dichorionic or even dizygotic pregnancies if the placenta fuses and the umbilical cords originate in close proximity to each other.[64]

The acardiac twin has no direct vascular connections with the placenta. Umbilical arterial-to-arterial anastomoses allow blood to circulate with pulsatile pressure from the normal fetus through the acardiac twin. The acardiac twin, therefore, has reversal of blood circulation (i.e., blood enters via umbilical arteries and exits via the umbilical vein). This pathophysiology, termed twin reversed arterial pressure (TRAP), has been verified with Doppler sonography.[63] If the vascular connection to the acardiac twin is insufficient, early in pregnancy the acardiac embryo will reabsorb, whereas demise later in pregnancy may result in fetus papyraceous.[64] Inclusion of these pregnancies would increase the incidence of TRAP significantly.

The acardiac or "perfused" twin usually has many structural anomalies, probably related to the reversal of circulation rather than to underlying defects (Fig 15–17).[64] Because the acardiac twin receives pulsatile blood into the internal iliac arteries secondarily from the normal or "pump" twin, the structures supplied by the distal abdominal aorta and iliac arteries of the acardiac twin demonstrate the best development. However, even these structures are only relatively well perfused by poorly oxygenated and nutrient-poor blood, whereas the upper trunk and head are not perfused at all. Therefore, various gradations of developmental pathology occur in acardiac twinning (Fig 15–17).[64] Furthermore, approximately 50% of these anomalous fetuses have only one umbilical artery.[64] The co-twin or "pump twin" is usually normal except for cardiomegaly

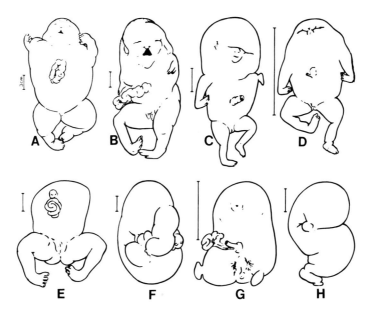

FIG 15–17.
Drawings showing representative examples of acardiac twins with gradation of loss of normal form and relative sparing of the lower body. **A,** anencephaly, midline cleft lip and palate, microophthalmia, radial aplasia, limb reductions, oligodactyly, and syndactyly. **B,** anencephaly, midline cleft lip and palate, microophthalmia, gastroschisis, phocomelia, and oligodactyly. **C,** microophthalmia, radial aplasia, phocomelia, and oligodactyly. **D,** cyclopia, omphalocele, radial aplasia, oligodactyly, absent cranial vault, clubfeet, and marked edema. **E,** absent head, thorax and arms with omphalocele, clubfeet, and oligodactyly. **F,** absent cranial end with partial abdominal cavity, omphalocele, reduced lower limbs, oligodactyly, and syndactyly. **G,** absent cranium, minimal thorax, omphalocele, herniation of the gut from the umbilicus, cloacal exstrophy, and skin tags suggestive of limbs. **H,** hemipelvis, single leg with single toe, omphalocele, and complete absence of thoracic and cranial structures. (From Van Allen MI, Smith DW, Shepard TH: Twin reversed arterial perfusion (TRAP) sequence: A study of 14 twin pregnancies with acardius. Semin Perinatol 1983; 7:285–293. Used by permission.)

and signs of heart failure which usually resolve shortly after birth.[61] However, the pump twin has a 50% mortality, primarily related to prematurity and in utero congestive heart failure.[64]

Sonographic Findings

An acardiac twin pregnancy demonstrates one anomalous twin who moves independently but has no cardiac motion (Fig 15–18). Occasionally, an apparent singleton living pregnancy but with a concomitant amorphous mass of tissue that has recognizable fetal parts represents an acardiac twin upon postnatal examination. Other associated findings include polyhydramnios, two-vessel umbilical cord, structural anomalies in the acardiac twin, and evidence of cardiac failure in the pump twin.[60, 61, 64]

Conjoined Twins

Clinical and Pathologic Findings

Conjoined twins occur in approximately 1 in 50,000 births.[72] All conjoined twins are monoamnionic-monochorionic. Development of conjoined twins is thought to occur after 13 days and before the third week of gestation as a result of arrest of separation in a monozygotic twin.[2, 68] No known predisposing factors result in conjoined twinning. Although the site and extent of fusion varies markedly, conjoined twins are most commonly joined at the chest and/or abdomen and less commonly at the sacrum, ischium, or head and face (Table 15–7).[75, 78–80] Congenital anomalies in conjoined twins may or may not be associated with the site of union.[75] Once the diagnosis of conjoined twins is established, cesarean section is the generally preferred method of delivery in order to avoid dystocia and birth trauma.[71, 79] The morbidity and mortality in conjoined twins relates to the region of fusion and associated anomalies.[70, 75]

Sonographic Findings

All sonographic evaluations of twins must specifically attempt to determine whether the twins are separate or conjoined. Detection of a separating membrane excludes conjoined twinning, but unequivocal documentation of conjoined twinning may be more difficult. The site and extent of fusion of conjoined twins varies, but the sonographic criterion that verifies the presence of conjoined twins in virtually all cases is unequivocal demonstration of continuous external skin contour of

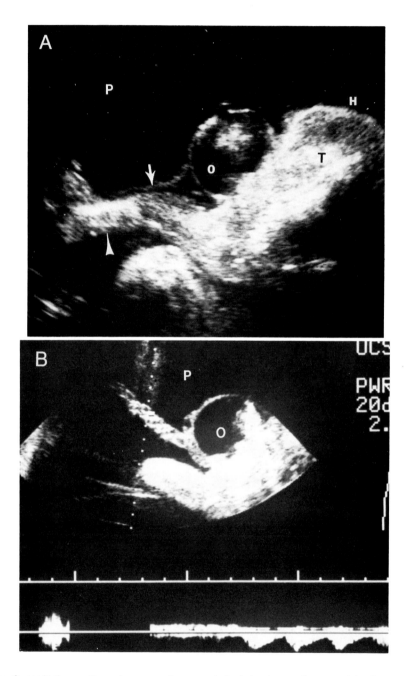

FIG 15–18.
Acardiac twin pregnancy. **A,** sagittal scan through an acardiac, acephalic twin shows absence of fetal structures rostral to the thorax. Although this twin has no cardiac motion, real-time ultrasound demonstrated motion of the lower extremities and subsequent scans showed normal growth of the femora. This twin also has an omphalocele. **B,** Doppler tracing shows blood in the umbilical artery flowing away from the transducer and thus toward the acardiac, acephalic fetus. The ratio between peak systolic and end diastolic velocities is 3 to 2. *T* = thorax; *H* = expected head region; *arrowhead* = lower extremity; *O* = omphalocele; *P* = polyhydramnios in sac of co-twin; *arrow* = membrane separating the acardiac, acephalic twin from the polyhydramniotic co-twin. (From Pretorius DH, Leopold GR, Moore TR, et al: Acardiac twin: Report of Doppler sonography. J Ultrasound Med 1988; 7:413–416. Used by permission.)

TABLE 15–7.

Types, Location of Fusion and Relative Frequency of Conjoined Twins

Type	Relative Frequency (%)	Location of Fusion
Thoracopagus	40	Thorax
Omphalopagus	34	Xiphoid to umbilicus
Pygopagus	18	Sacrum
Ischiopagus	6	Ischium
Craniopagus	2	Head
Diprosopus	<1	Head and body but with two faces
Dicephalus	<1	Body but with two heads
Syncephalus	<1	Face and thorax
Rachipagus	<1	Vertebrae above sacrum
Dipygus (Monocephalus)	<1	Head and thorax with partial or complete duplication of pelvis and lower extremities
Dipygus (Dicephalus)	<1	Trunk with partial or complete duplication of heads, upper extremities, pelvis and lower extremities

both monoamniotic twins (Figs 15–19 to 15–22).[71] This should be suspected whenever a membrane cannot be seen separating the twins, although in most such cases monoamniotic twins are not conjoined or the membrane is not seen because it is immediately adjacent to a "stuck" fetus in an oligohydramniotic sac.[22]

Depending upon the distribution of fusion between conjoined twins, demonstration of shared fetal organs also provides definitive, often obvious evidence for conjoined twinning. Demonstration of a twin pregnancy with a single umbilical cord containing more than three vessels also provides strong, but not definitive evidence for conjoined twinning; the umbilical cord entanglement in monoamnionic, but non–conjoined twins closely resembles a single umbilical cord, and the umbilical cord can have more than three vessels in the absence of conjoined twinning.[19, 23] Other common, but not pathognomonic findings in conjoined twinning include (1) constant relative fetal positioning; and (2) unusual positioning with hyperextension of both cervical spines or unusual extremity posture.[65–67, 69, 71, 73, 74, 76–78, 80–83]

Congenital Anomalies in Twins

Numerous reports indicate that twins have an increased prevalence of congenital anomalies in 6% to 10% of twin births (see Table 15–4).[84, 87, 88, 91] Included among the variety of interesting hypotheses proposed to explain this apparent association between twinning and congenital anomalies are (1) some women may be predisposed to delivering both anomalous fetuses and twins; (2) twinning and certain anomalies may be produced by the same exogenous agents; (3) diagnosis of an anomaly in one twin may lead to a more detailed examination of the apparently normal co-twin; and (4) discordant vascular abnormalities or thromboembolic events may cause many of the anomalies of monozygous twins.[89]

Most authorities now agree that only monozygotic twins have an increased prevalence of anomalies relative to singletons.[39, 91] Thromboembolic insults have been postulated to cause microcephaly, multicystic encephalomalacia, hydrocephaly, hydranencephaly, hemifacial microsomia, limb amputation, intestinal atresia, horseshoe kidney, cardiac malformations, and aplasia cutis in monozygotic twins (Fig 15–23 and Table 15–4).[89, 91] Hence, most twin anomalies probably result from environmental rather than genetic insults.[90] However, monozygotic twins are also at greater risk for congenital anomalies due to abnormal embryologic development. Since monozygous twinning is itself a result of abnormal embryologic development, an association with other anomalies is not surprising.

Twins are probably more likely than singletons to have defects related to crowding and anomalous positioning within the uterus (i.e., talipes, hip dislocation), but this has not been confirmed.[89] Anomalies unique to multiple gestations include conjoined twinning and acardia. Malformations that may be seen in association with monozygotic twins include anencephaly, holoprosencephaly, VACTERL association (vertebral anoma-

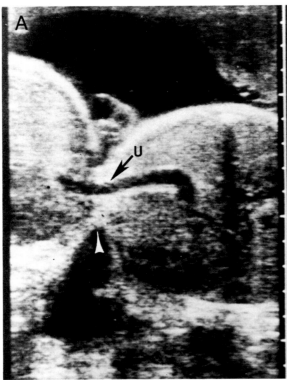

FIG 15–19.
Conjoined twins at abdomen. **A,** transverse sonogram through the conjoined abdomen of both twins shows the shared umbilical vein and continuous external skin. **B and C,** postnatal radiograph and photograph confirm the prenatal findings. U = shared umbilical vein; *arrowhead* = continuous external skin contour. (From Hurren AJ, Sommerville AJ, Warren VF: Antenatal diagnosis of a set of conjoined twins presenting with unusual ultrasound findings. J Clin Ultrasound 1988; 16:672–674. Used by permission.)

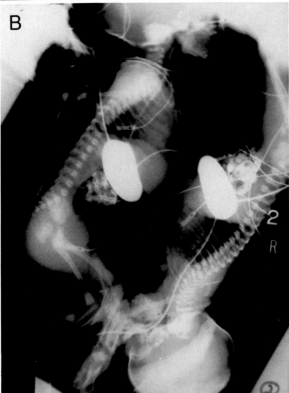

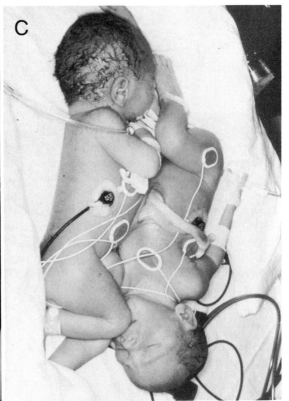

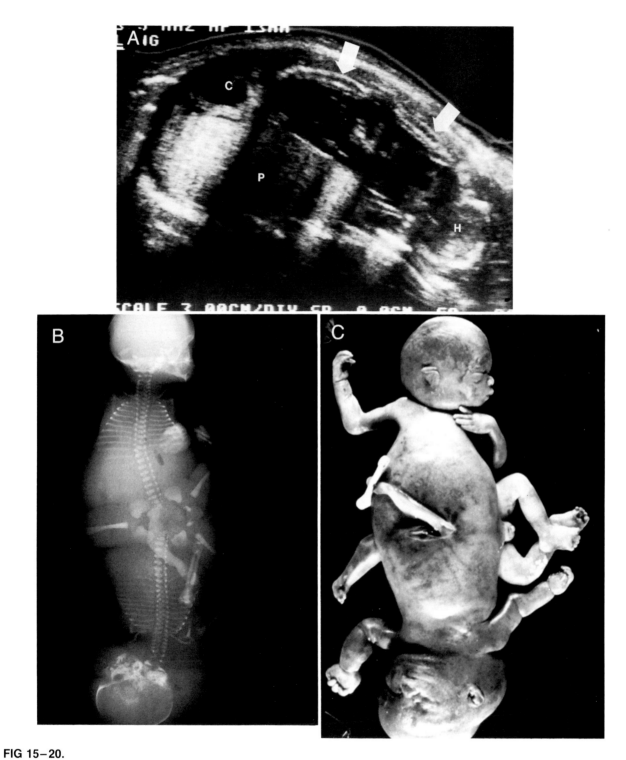

FIG 15–20.
Conjoined twins at ischium. **A,** longitudinal scan through uterus shows a continuous surface between the vertex and breech fetus. The fetal spines are in the same axis. **B and C,** postmortem radiograph and photograph confirm the prenatal findings. *Arrows* = fetal spines; *C* = cyst in neck of breech fetus; *H* = head of vertex fetus; *P* = placenta. (From Wilson DA, Young GZ, Crumley CS: Antepartum ultrasonographic diagnosis of ischiopagus: A rare variety of conjoined twins. J Ultrasound Med 1983; 2:281–282. Used by permission.)

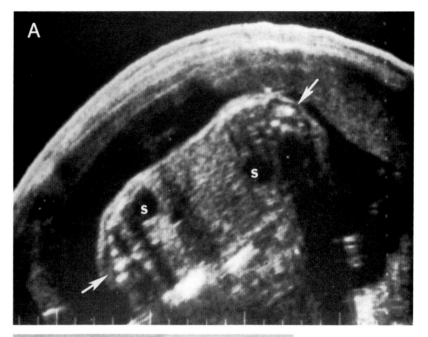

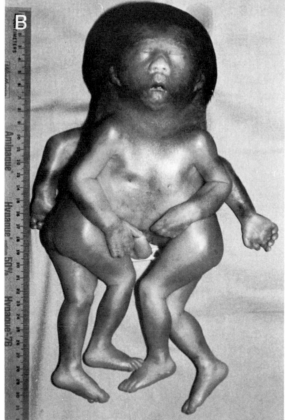

FIG 15–21.
Dipygus. **A,** sonogram shows fusion of the thorax and abdomen with two stomachs and two spines. **B,** postmortem photograph of a similar case illustrates a single head and thorax but duplication of the pelvis and extremities. *S* = stomachs; *arrows* = spines. (Part **B** courtesy of Faye Laing, MD, San Francisco General Hospital, San Francisco, CA.)

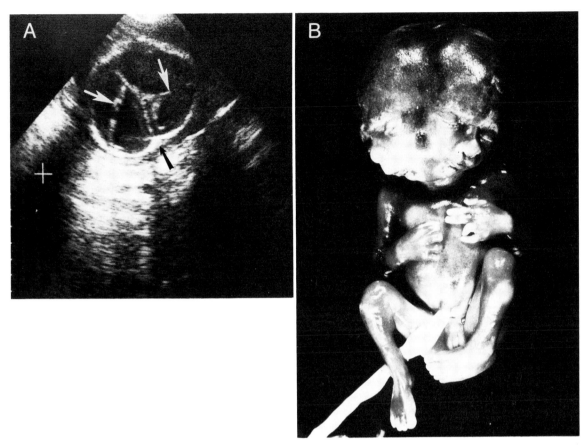

FIG 15–22.
Diprosopus. **A,** sonogram of the head at 20 weeks shows ventricular dilation and two falx cerebri separated by an echogenic membrane. Note the indentation at the junction of the two faces. **B,** postmortem photograph demonstrates the two faces and widened head but single body. *White arrows* = falx cerebri; *black arrow* = indentation at the junction of the two faces. (From Strauss S, Tamarkin M, Engelberg S, et al: Prenatal sonographic appearance of diprosopus. J Ultrasound Med 1987; 6:93–95. Used by permission.)

lies, anal atresia, cardiac anomalies, tracheoesophageal atresia, renal anomalies, and limb deformities), exstrophy of the cloaca, and sirenomelia.[85] Approximately 3.5% of twins, but only 1% of singletons have a single umbilical artery.[86]

DOPPLER SONOGRAPHY IN TWINS

Doppler sonography of the umbilical arteries has been helpful in the evaluation of high-risk pregnancies, particularly those at risk for IUGR. Given the high prevalence of IUGR and fetal anomalies in twins, Doppler sonography probably will also prove to be helpful in the evaluation of twin pregnancies (Fig 15–24).[43]

Several investigators have now reported data from Doppler evaluation of the umbilical arteries in twin pregnancies.[92–96] In an evaluation of 76 twin pregnancies, Giles et al. found that the ratio between peak systolic velocity (A) and end-diastolic velocity (B) in twins agreed closely with the ratio in singletons reported by Trudinger et al.[94, 97] They also found that among 33 twin pregnancies in which one or both infants were small for gestational age (SGA) an abnormal A/B ratio had a positive predictive value of 70% and a specificity of 70% in the diagnosis of the SGA twin. Farmakides et al. found that the difference between A/B ratios between co-twins in 43 twin pregnancies at 30–36 weeks was a helpful indicator of underlying pathology and that a difference of 0.4 or greater of the A/B ratio for twins was predictive of a weight difference of greater than 349 gms.[92] Nimrod et al. studied multiple different Doppler parameters in 30 twin pregnancies and found that a combination of parameters was the most sensitive method of identifying IUGR.[96] Since an abnormal A/B ratio or a difference in ratios can be observed in disease states other than IUGR, however, clinical correlation is necessary.

Doppler sonography has had variable results in the evaluation of fetuses with the twin transfusion syn-

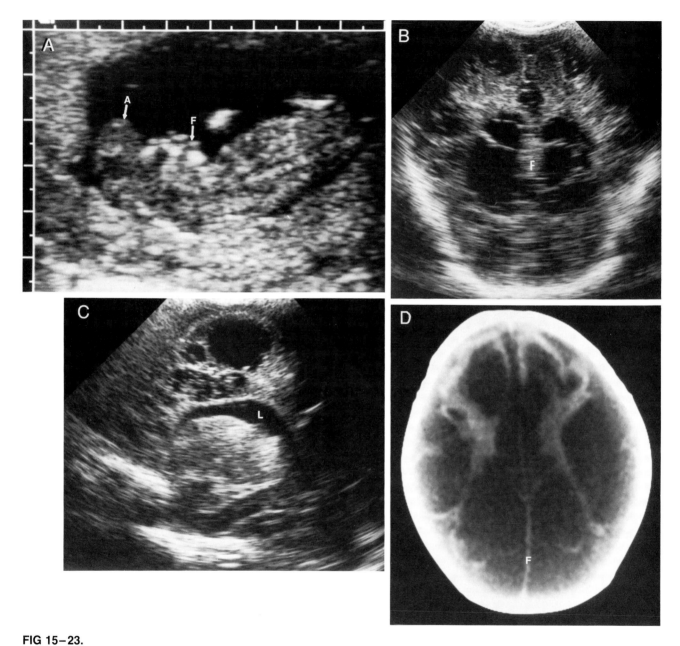

FIG 15–23.
Multicystic encephalomalacea in survivor of a monozygotic co-twin pair. **A,** sonogram at 13 weeks shows anencephaly of one twin. The co-twin appeared normal. The anencephalic twin died several weeks later. **B to D,** postnatal axial **(B)** and parasagittal **(C)** sonograms and axial-computed tomogram **(D)** of the survivor demonstrate extensive multicystic encephalomalacea. *A* = absent calvarium of anencephalic co-twin; *F* = face of anencephalic co-twin; *f* = falx cerebri; *L* = lateral cerebral ventricle.

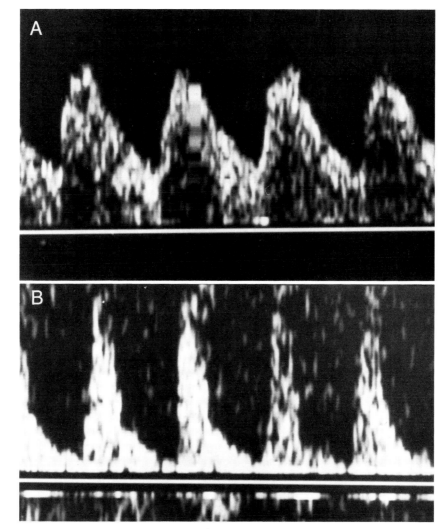

FIG 15–24.
Doppler tracings of a twin pregnancy with one small for gestational age twin at 33 weeks. **A,** normal umbilical artery Doppler tracing in twin A shows an A/B ratio of 2.2. **B,** normal fetal internal carotid artery Doppler tracing in twin A shows minimal diastolic flow. *(Continued.)*

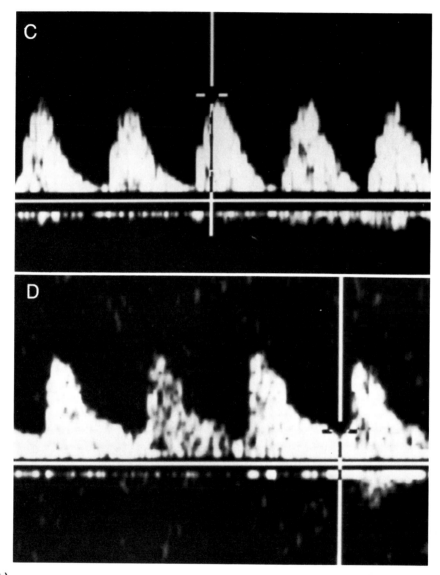

FIG 15–24 (cont.).
C, abnormal umbilical artery Doppler tracing in twin B shows an A/B ratio of 6.3. The biometric measurements for this twin were mean for 2 weeks less than for its co-twin. **D,** abnormal fetal internal carotid artery Doppler tracing in twin B shows significant diastolic flow with an A/B ratio of 3.6. At delivery twin B weighed 25% less than twin A (2,100 gm vs. 2,740 gm).

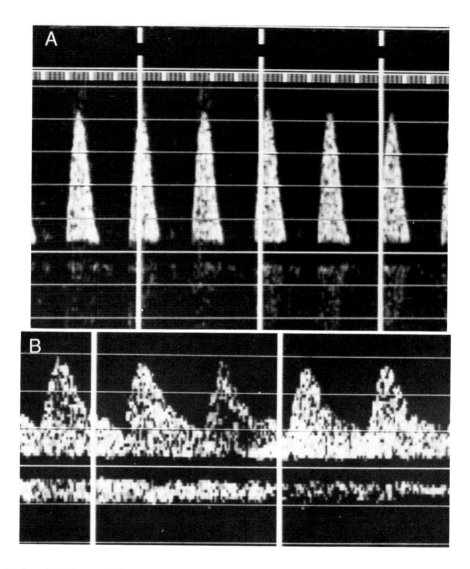

FIG 15–25.
Doppler tracings of twins with twin transfusion syndrome at 28.5 weeks. **A,** abnormal Doppler tracing for twin A shows no diastolic flow in the umbilical artery. **B,** twin B has a normal Doppler tracing in the umbilical artery with an A/B ratio of 3.1. (From Pretorius D, Manchester D, Barkin S, et al: Doppler ultrasound of twin transfusion syndrome. J Ultrasound Med 1988; 7:117–124. Used by permission.)

drome (Fig 15–25). In a review of the literature, Pretorius et al. found that seven of 13 cases with the twin transfusion syndrome had abnormal A/B ratios in at least one twin.[54] Although an abnormal Doppler study suggested a poor outcome, a normal Doppler study was not helpful in predicting outcome. Doppler sonography did not differentiate donor from recipient. Doppler evaluation was helpful when uncertainty existed as to whether the growth discrepancy in a twin pregnancy represented a pathologic state or a normal variation of growth parameters. However, it did not distinguish between the twin transfusion syndrome and IUGR. Clearly, the twin transfusion syndrome may result in complex hemodynamics; Doppler techniques may help to elucidate its pathophysiology in the future.

CONCLUSION

Twin gestations are high-risk pregnancies with relatively high morbidity and mortality. With the goal of improved pregnancy outcome, targeted sonography helps to evaluate these pregnancies for amnionicity and chorionicity, growth retardation, polyhydramnios or oligohydramnios, twin transfusion syndrome, acardiac or conjoined twins, fetal anomalies, and other complications.

REFERENCES

Incidence and Embryology

1. Benirschke K: Accurate recording of twin placentation. A plea to the obstetrician. Obstet Gynecol 1961; 18:334–347.
2. Benirschke K, Kim CK: Multiple pregnancy. I, II. N Engl J Med 1973; 288:1276–1284, 1329–1336.
3. Fox H: *Pathology of the Placenta.* Philadelphia, WB Saunders Co, 1988.
4. Hrubec Z, Robinette D: The study of human twins in medical research. N Engl J Med 1984; 310:435–441.
5. MacGillivray I: Epidemiology of twin pregnancy. Semin Perinatol 1986; 10:4–8.
6. Moore KL: *The Developing Human,* ed 4. Philadelphia, WB Saunders Co, 1988.
7. Nylander PPS: The phenomenon of twinning, in Barron, Thompson (eds): *Obstetrical Epidemiology.* San Francisco, Academic Press, 1983, pp 143–389.
8. Schenker J, Yarkoni S, Granat M: Multiple pregnancies following induction of ovulation. Fertil Steril 1981; 35:105–123.
9. Willson JR, Carrington ER: *Obstetrics and Gynecology,* ed 6. St Louis, CV Mosby Co, 1979.

Perinatal Morbidity and Mortality

10. Benirschke K: Twin placenta in perinatal mortality. NY State J Med 1964; 61:1499.
11. Coleman BG, Grumbach K, Arger PH, et al: Twin gestations: Monitoring of complications and anomalies with US. Radiology 1987; 165:449–453.
12. De Muylder X, Moutquin JM, Desgranges M, et al: Obstetrical profile of twin pregnancies: A retrospective review of 11 years (1969–1979) at Hospital Notre-Dame, Montreal, Canada. Acta Genet Med Gemellol 1982; 31:149–155.
13. Hawrylrshyn P, Barkin M, Bernstein A, et al: Twin pregnancies—A continuing perinatal challenge. Obstet Gynecol 1982; 59:463–466.
14. Naeye R, Tafari N, Judge D, et al: Twins: Causes of perinatal death in 12 United States cities and one African city. Am J Obstet Gynecol 1978; 131:267–272.
15. Newton ER: Antepartum care in multiple gestation. Semin Perinatol 1986; 10:19–29.
16. Persson P-H. Grennert L, Gennser G, et al: On improved outcome of twin pregnancies. Acta Obstet Gynecol Scand 1979; 58:3.
17. Strauss F, Benirschke K, Driscoll SG: Placenta Handuch Der Speziellen Pathologischen Anatome and Histologie Berlin, Springer Verlag, 1967, pp 261.

Sonographic Approach and Assessment of Amnionicity and Chorionicity

18. Barss V, Benacerraf B, Frigoletto F: Ultrasonographic determination of chorion type in twin gestation. Obstet Gynecol 1985; 66:779–783.
19. Beck R, Naulty CM: A human umbilical cord with four arteries. Clin Pediatr 1985; 24:118–119.
20. D'Alton M, Dudley D: Ultrasound in the antenatal management of twin gestation. Semin Perinatol 1986; 10:30–38.
21. Hertzberg B, Kurtz A, Choi H: Significance of membrane thickness in the sonographic evaluation of twin gestations. AJR 1987; 148:151–153.
22. Mahony B, Filly R, Callen P: Amnionicity and chorionicity in twin pregnancies: Prediction using ultrasound. Radiology 1985; 155:205–209.
23. Nyberg D, Filly R, Golbus M, et al: Entangled umbilical cords: A sign of monoamniotic twins. J Ultrasound Med 1984; 3:29–32.
24. Townsend R, Simpson G, Filly R: Membrane thickness in ultrasound prediction of chorionicity of twin gestations. J Ultrasound Med 1988; 7:327–332.
25. Townsend R, Filly RA: Sonography of nonconjoined monoamniotic twin pregnancies. J Ultrasound Med 1988; 7:665–670.

Co-Twin Demise

26. Dudley DKL, D'Alton ME: Single fetal death in twin gestation. Semin Perinatol 1986; 10:65–72.

27. Johnson F, Driscoll SG: Twin placentation and its complications. Semin Perinatol 1986; 10:9–13.
28. Jaunaiux E, Elkazen N, Leroy F, et al: Clinical and morphologic aspects of the vanishing twin phenomenon. Obstet Gynecol 1988; 72:577–581.
29. Landy H, Keith L, Keith D: The vanishing twin. Acta Genet Med Gemellol 1982; 31:179–194.
30. Landy H, Weiner S, Corson S, et al: The "vanishing twin": Ultrasonographic assessment of fetal disappearance in the first trimester. Am J Obstet Gynecol 1986; 155:14–19.
31. Melnick M: Brain damage in survivor after in-utero death of monozygous co-twin. Lancet 1977; ii:1287.
32. Redwine FO, Hays PM: Selective birth. Semin Perinatol 1986; 10:73–81.
33. Sulak L, Dodson M: The vanishing twin: Pathologic confirmation of an ultrasonographic phenomenon. Obstet Gynecol 1986; 68:811–815.
34. Yoshioka H, Kadomoto Y, Mino M, et al: Multicystic encephalomalacia in liveborn twin with a stillborn macerated co-twin. J Pediatr 1979; 95:798–800.

Prematurity, Growth Retardation, and Traumatic Delivery

35. Blickstein I, Shoham-Schwartz Z, Lancet M: Growth discordancy in appropriate for gestational age, term twins. Obstet Gynecol 1988; 72:582–584.
36. Cetrulo CL: The controversy of mode of delivery in twins: The intrapartum management of twin gestation. I. Semin Perinatol 1986; 10:39–43.
37. Chitkara U, Berkowitz G, Levine R, et al: Twin pregnancy: Routine use of ultrasound examinations in the prenatal diagnosis of intrauterine growth retardation and discordant growth. Am J Perinatol 1985; 2:49–54.
38. Grumbach K, Coleman B, Arger P, et al: Twin and singleton growth patterns compared using US. Radiology 1986; 158:237–241.
39. Haney A, Crenshaw M, Dempsey P: Significance of biparietal diameter differences between twins. Obstet Gynecol 1978; 51:609–613.
40. Houlton MC: Divergent biparietal diameter growth rates in twin pregnancies. Obstet Gynecol 1977; 49:542–545.
41. Naeye R, Benirschke K, Hagstrom J, et al: Intrauterine growth of twins as estimated from liveborn birth-weight data. Pediatrics 1966; 37:409–416.
42. Rodis JF, Vintzileos AM, Campbell WA, et al: Antenatal diagnosis and management of monoamniotic twins. Am J Obstet Gynecol 1987; 157:1255–1257.
43. Secher N, Kaern J, Hansen HK. Intrauterine growth in twin pregnancies: Prediction of fetal growth retardation. Obstet Gynecol 1985; 66:63–68.
44. Socol ML, Tamura RK, Sabbagha RE, et al: Diminished biparietal diameter and abdominal circumference growth in twins. Obstet Gynecol 1984; 64:235–238.

Polyhydramnios, Oligohydramnios, and the Twin Transfusion Syndrome

45. Braat D, Exalto N, Bernardus R, et al: Twin pregnancy: Case reports illustrating variations in transfusion syndrome. Eur J Obstet Gynecol Reprod Biol 1985; 19:383–390.
46. Brennan J, Diwan R, Rosen M, et al: Fetofetal transfusion syndrome: Prenatal ultrasonographic diagnosis. Radiology 1982; 143:535–536.
47. Chescheier N, Seeds J: Polyhydramnios and oligohydramnios in twin gestations. Obstet Gynecol 1988; 71:882–884.
48. De Lia J, Emery M, Sheafor S, et al: Twin transfusion syndrome: Successful in utero treatment with digoxin. Int J Gynaecol Obstet 1985; 23:197–201.
49. Falkner F: Implications for growth in human twins, in Falkner F, Tanner LJM (eds): *Human Growth. Principles and Prenatal Growth.* New York, Plenum, 1978.
50. Hashimoto B, Callen P, Filly R, et al: Ultrasound evaluation of polyhydramnios and twin pregnancy. Am J Obstet Gynecol 1986; 154:1069–1072.
51. Jacoby H, Charles D: Clinical conditions associated with hydramnios. Am J Obstet Gynecol 1966; 94:910–919.
52. Machin G: Differential diagnosis of hydrops fetalis. Am J Med Genet 1981; 9:341–350.
53. Mack LA, Patten R, Cyr DR, et al: Disparity of amniotic fluid volume in twin pregnancies: The problem of the stuck twin (abstract). Radiology 1988; 169:209.
54. Pretorius D, Manchester D, Barkin S, et al: Doppler ultrasound of twin transfusion syndrome. J Ultrasound Med 1988; 7:117–124.
55. Rausen A, Seki M, Strauss L: Twin transfusion syndrome: A review of 19 cases studied at one institution. J Pediatr 1965; 66:613–628.
56. Sekiya S, Hafez E: Physiomorphology of twin transfusion syndrome: A study of 86 twin gestations. Obstet Gynecol 1977; 50:288–292.
57. Wallenberg HCS, Wladmiroff JW: The amniotic fluid. II. Polyhydramnios and oligohydramnios. J Perinat Med 1977; 5:233–243.
58. Wittman B, Farquharson D, Thomas W, et al: The role of feticide in the management of severe twin transfusion syndrome. Am J Obstet Gynecol 1986; 155:1023–1026.

Acardiac Twinning

59. Cardwell MS: The acardiac twin: A case report. J Reprod Med 1988; 33:320–322.
60. Lachman R, McNabb M, Furmanski M, et al: The acardiac monster. Eur J Pediatr 1980; 134:195–200.
61. Mack L, Gravett M, Rumack C, et al: Antenatal ultrasonic evaluation of acardiac monsters. J Ultrasound Med 1982; 1:13–18.
62. Napolitani F, Schreiber I: The acardiac monster. Am J Obstet Gynecol 1960; 80:582–589.
63. Pretorius D, Leopold G, Moore T, et al: Acardiac twin

report of Doppler sonography. J Ultrasound Med 1988; 7:413–416.

64. Van Allen M, Smith D, Shepard T: Twin reversed arterial perfusion (TRAP) sequence: A study of 14 twin pregnancies with acardius. Semin Perinatol 1983; 7:285–293.

Conjoined Twins

65. Abrams SL, Callen PW, Anderson RL, et al: Anencephaly with encephalocele in craniopagus twins: Prenatal diagnosis by ultrasonography and computed tomography. J Ultrasound Med 1985; 4:485–488.

66. Appuzio JJ, Ganesh V, Landau J, et al: Prenatal diagnosis of conjoined twins. Am J Obstet Gynecol 1984; 148:343.

67. Chen HY, Hsieh FJ, Huang LH: Prenatal diagnosis of conjoined twins by real-time sonography. J Clin Ultrasound 1983; 11:94–96.

68. Edwards HD, Hagel DR, Thompson J, et al: Conjoined thoracopagus twins. Circulation 1977; 56:491.

69. Fagan CJ: Antepartum diagnosis of conjoined twins by ultrasonography. AJR 1977; 129:921.

70. Filler RM: Conjoined twins and their separation. Semin Perinatol 1986; 10:82–91.

71. Gore R, Filly R, Parer J: Sonographic antepartum diagnosis of conjoined twins. JAMA 1982; 247:3351–3353.

72. Hanson JW: Incidence of conjoined twinning. Lancet 1975; ii:1257.

73. Hartung RW, Yiu-Chin V, Aschenbrener CA: Sonographic diagnosis of cephalo-thoracophagus in a triplet pregnancy. J Ultrasound Med 1984; 3:139–141.

74. Hurren AJ, Sommerville AJ, Warren VF: Antenatal diagnoses of a set of conjoined twins presenting with unusual ultrasound findings. J Clin Ultrasound 1988; 16:672–674.

75. Herbert W, Cefalo R, Koontz W: Perinatal management of conjoined twins. Am J Perinatol 1983; 1:58–62.

76. Okazaki J, Wilson J, Holmes S, et al: Diprosopus: Diagnosis in utero. AJR 1987; 149:147–148.

77. Siegfried MS, Koptik GF: Prenatal sonographic diagnosis of conjoined twins. Postgrad Med 1983; 73:317.

78. Strauss S, Tamarkin M, Engleberg S, et al: Prenatal sonographic appearance of diprosopus. J Ultrasound Med 1987; 6:93–95.

79. Vaugh TC, Powell LC: The obstetrical management of conjoined twins. Obstet Gynecol 1979; 56:491.

80. Weingast GR, Johnson ML, Pretorius DH, et al: Difficulty in sonographic diagnosis of cephalothoracopagus. J Ultrasound Med 1984; 3:421–423.

81. Wilson DA, Young GZ, Crumley CS: Antepartum ultrasonographic diagnosis of ischiopagus: A rare variety of conjoined twins. J Ultrasound Med 1983; 2:281–282.

82. Wilson RL, Shaub MS, Cetrulo CJ: The antepartum findings of conjoined twins. J Clin Ultrasound 1977; 5:35.

83. Wood MJ, Thompson HE, Robertson FM: Real-time ultrasound diagnosis of conjoined twins. J Clin Ultrasound 1981; 9:195.

Congenital Anomalies in Twins

84. Baker ME, Rosenberg ER, Troffater KF, et al: The in utero findings in twin pentalogy of Cantrell. J Ultrasound Med 1984; 3:525–527.

85. Jones KL, Benirschke K: The developmental pathogenesis of structural defects: The contribution of monozygotic twins. Semin Perinatol 1983; 7:239–243.

86. Benirschke K, Sullivan M, Marin-Padilla M: Size and number of umbilical vessels: A study of multiple pregnancy in man and the armadillo. Obstet Gynecol 1964; 24:819–834.

87. Hay S, Wehrung D: Congenital malformations in twins. Am J Hum Genet 1980; 22:662–678.

88. Hendricks C: Twinning in relation to birth weight, mortality and congenital anomalies. Obstet Gynecol 1966; 27:47–53.

89. Little J, Bryan E: Congenital anomalies in twins. Semin Perinatol 1986; 10:50–64.

90. Pysher T: Discordant congenital malformations in monozygous twins. Diagn Gynecol Obstet 1980; 2:221–225.

91. Schinzel A, Smith D, Miller J: Monozygotic twinning and structural defects. J Pediatr 1979; 95:921–930.

Doppler Assessment of Twins

92. Farmakides G, Schulman H, Saldana L, et al: Surveillance of twin pregnancy with umbilical arterial velocimetry. Obstet Gynecol 1985; 153:789–792.

93. Gerson A, Johnson A, Wallace, et al: Umbilical arterial systolic/diastolic values in normal twin gestation. Obstet Gynecol 1988; 72:205–208.

94. Giles W, Trudinger B, Cook C: Fetal umbilical artery flow velocity-time waveforms in twin pregnancies. Br J Obstet Gynaecol 1985; 92:490–497.

95. Giles WB: Doppler assessment in multiple pregnancy. Semin Perinatol 1987; 11:369–374.

96. Nimrod C, Davies D, Harder J, et al: Doppler ultrasound prediction of fetal outcome in twin pregnancies. Am J Obstet Gynecol 1987; 156:402–406.

97. Trudinger BJ, Giles WB, Cook CM, et al: Fetal umbilical artery flow velocity waveforms and placental resistance: Clinical significance. Br J Obstet Gynecol 1985; 92:23.

The Placenta, Placental Membranes, and Umbilical Cord

David A. Nyberg, M.D.

Harris J. Finberg, M.D.

The placenta, placental membranes, and umbilical cord are essentially fetal structures that are derived from the zygote. Abnormalities affecting these structures can affect fetal mortality and morbidity and may also provide important clues to underlying fetal malformations. When compared to what we know about the fetus, however, our knowledge of both normal and pathological conditions affecting the placenta, placental membranes, and umbilical cord is lacking. This lack of information can be attributed, in large part, to the inaccessibility of the placenta and placental membranes within the confines of the uterus. Placental membranes and vascular connections are normally disrupted as part of all deliveries, and pathologic examination of the placenta may not adequately describe its condition in vivo. Correlation with animal models is also limited, because the human placenta differs markedly from those of commonly available laboratory animals, such as rats, rabbits, guinea pigs, and sheep.[9]

In recent years, observations made from antenatal sonography have greatly added to our understanding of the placenta and the fetal-placental unit. Unlike pathologic examination, sonography can evaluate the intact placenta throughout gestation. Serial sonograms have helped to show the natural history of certain placental disorders, such as periplacental hemorrhage. More recently, use of umbilical artery and uterine artery Doppler can also provide physiologic information regarding umbilical and placental flow.

This chapter will deal with common abnormalities of the placenta and associated structures. Emphasis will be placed on those abnormalities which may be associated with fetal anomalies and fetal mortality.

THE PLACENTA

Embryogenesis

Ovulation occurs approximately 14 days following the last menstrual cycle, and fertilization occurs 1–2 days later in the distal fallopian tube.[8] By menstrual day 20, the zygote has formed the blastocyst, a fluid-filled cystic cavity composed of an inner cell mass and an outer trophoblastic layer.[8] The inner cell mass eventually will form the fetus, yolk sac, and allantois; the trophoblasts will form the placenta, chorion, and amnion.

Implantation of the blastocyst in the endometrium begins about 1 week after ovulation and is completed by menstrual day 23.[8] During implantation, trophoblasts erode adjacent maternal capillaries so that maternal blood comes into direct contact with the conceptus. This establishes an intercommunicating lacunar network which will become the intervillous space of the placenta.[10] The endometrium also undergoes a decidual reaction that helps support and control trophoblastic invasion. Frond-like chorionic villi arise from the trophoblast. After menstrual day 29, blood vessels enter primary villi to form true or tertiary villi.

Chorionic villi initially cover the entire surface of the chorionic sac. After 8 weeks, those villi aligned to-

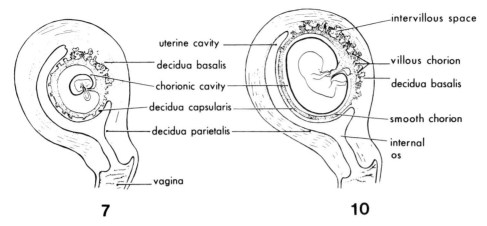

7 **10**

FIG 16–1.
Development of chorionic villi and fetal membranes at 7 menstrual weeks (5 fetal weeks) and 10 menstrual weeks. (From Moore KL: *The Developing Human,* ed 4. Philadelphia, WB Saunders Co, 1988. Used by permission.)

ward the uterine cavity become compressed and their blood supply becomes restricted (Fig 16–1). Degeneration of these villi forms the chorion laevae (smooth chorion). Simultaneously, chorionic villi associated with the decidua basalis rapidly proliferate to form the chorion frondosum which will become the definitive placenta (see Fig 16–1). As pregnancy progresses, the chorionic villi branch and gradually develop into a complex system of 50 to 60 subunits or cotyledons, each of which arises from a primary stem villus and is supplied by primary branches of the umbilical vessels.[10] Each cotyledon is further subdivided into one to five lobules.[10]

The mature placenta weighs 450 to 550 gms and has a diameter of 16 to 20 cm. The fetal surface, which is continuous with the surrounding chorion, is termed the chorionic plate. The maternal surface of the placenta, which lies contiguous with the decidua basalis, is termed the basilar plate.

Fetal-Placental-Uterine Circulation

The fetal-umbilical circulation originates with deoxygenated blood pumped by the fetal heart through the ductus arteriosus and into the descending aorta. Fetal blood continues through the hypogastric arteries to the umbilical arteries and into the umbilical cord. By term, approximately 40% of the fetal cardiac output (300–350 cc/min) is directed through the umbilical circulation. Within the placenta, the umbilical arteries freely divide into multiple capillary branches that course through the tertiary villi. As a result of changes in the trophoblast, only a thin layer normally separates fetal blood from maternal blood. This layer is composed of the capillary wall, the trophoblastic basement membrane, and a thin rim of cytoplasm of the syncytiotrophoblast.

Oxygenated maternal blood is delivered to the placenta through 80 to 100 end branches of the uterine arteries, called spiral arteries.[4, 8, 10] Maternal blood enters the intervillous space near the central part of each placental lobule where it flows around and over the surface of the villi (Fig 16–2).[10] This process permits exchange of oxygen and nutrients with fetal blood flowing in villous capillaries. Maternal blood then returns through a network of basilar, subchorial, interlobular, and marginal veins. The rate of uteroplacental flow increases from about 50 cc/min at 10 weeks to 500–600 cc/min at term. By term, the intervillous space of 150 cc is replaced three to four times per minute.[8]

Normal Sonographic Findings

The placenta (chorionic frondosum) can be identified on sonography as early as 8 menstrual weeks. Between 8 and 20 weeks, the placenta normally appears uniform in echotexture and thickness, measuring less than 2–3 cm (Fig 16–3). After 20 weeks, intraplacental sonolucencies (venous lakes or intervillous thrombi) and placental calcification may begin to appear, and the placenta can measure 4–5 cm in thickness (Fig 16–4).[3, 5]

The placental location is usually in the mid to fundal portion of the uterus, reflecting the site of implantation. However, the apparent location of the placenta can change markedly with distention of the urinary bladder and development of focal uterine contractions. These factors can also produce a false-positive impression of a placenta previa by compressing the lower uterine walls together.[10]

Disproportionately greater growth of the uterus compared to the placenta results in a progressively smaller surface area of placental attachment with ad-

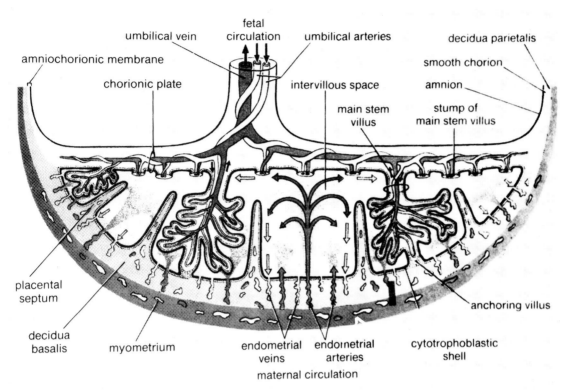

FIG 16–2.
Schematic drawing of term placenta showing the fetal-placental and maternal-placental circulation. Maternal blood supplied by the spiral arteries (endometrial arteries) circulates in the intervillous space, around the placental villi, and out the periplacental veins. (From Moore KL: *The Developing Human,* ed 4. Philadelphia, WB Saunders Co, 1988. Used by permission.)

vancing gestational age. At 20 weeks, the placenta covers approximately one fourth of the myometrium surface area, but near term the placenta covers one eighth the myometrial surface.[6] Differential growth of the lower uterine segment is responsible for the impression of placental ascension during pregnancy ("placental migration"). This process explains the apparent improvement in many low-lying placentas or suspected partial previas after the second trimester.[10]

The placenta is separated from the myometrium by

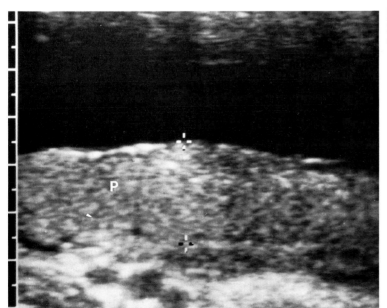

FIG 16–3.
Normal placenta. The normal placenta *(P)* before 20 weeks appears uniform in thickness and echo texture.

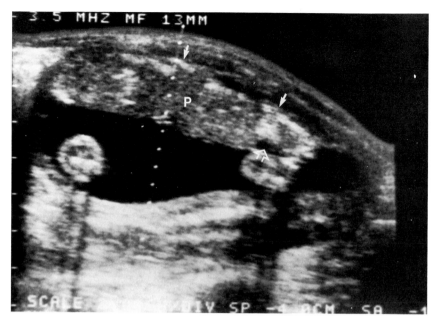

FIG 16–4.
Mature placenta. Sonogram at 35 weeks shows basilar calcification *(straight arrows)* and intraplacental calcification (grade II placenta). Intraplacental sonolucencies *(open arrow)* representing maternal lakes or intervillous thrombosi also are identified.

a subplacental venous complex (basilar and marginal veins).[2] These veins can become quite prominent, particularly for lateral and posterior placentas, and should not be mistaken for retroplacental or marginal hemorrhage. The myometrium can usually be identified as a thin, hypoechoic layer beneath the basilar veins. Together, the basilar veins and myometrium (subplacental complex) measure 9–10 mm in average thickness;[2] this is better appreciated for posterior placentas than anterior placentas.[7]

The cervical canal can be recognized on sagittal scans as an echogenic line, representing the mucosal interface and mucous plug, surrounded by a hypoechoic zone of variable thickness representing submucosal glands. The internal cervical os itself can be identified at the point of a slight "V" configuration or funneling of the amniotic fluid leading to the cervical canal. Scanning with an empty bladder produces a more vertical orientation of the cervix which may be difficult for the inexperienced observer to recognize.[1] Traction or a Trendelenburg position may be necessary for elevating fetal parts out of the pelvis and visualizing the internal cervical os.[26]

Placental Calcification

An association between placental calcification and gestational age has been widely observed since early studies of the placenta. Grannum et al. first proposed a systematic classification for grading placental maturation based on the pattern of calcification: grade 0 is a homogeneous placenta, grade I shows small intraplacental calcifications, grade II shows calcification of the basilar plate (see Fig 16–4), and grade III shows compartmentalization of the placenta from the chorionic plate to the basal layer.[12] Using this classification, Petrusha and Platt found that grade 0 is most common in the first trimester, grade I may appear as early as 14 menstrual weeks and is most common until 34 weeks, and grade II does not usually appear until after 30 weeks and peaks at 36 weeks.[16] Grade III is not usually seen until after 35 weeks and even then is found in only 30% of term placentas.

Despite early enthusiasm, placental grading has been found to be too imprecise for fetal dating or estimation of fetal lung maturity. More relevant is a possible association between premature calcification (grade II before 32 weeks or grade III before 34 weeks) and fetal growth retardation.[14] However, this association may be significant only when the fetus is already known to be small. For example, Kazzi et al. found that a small fetus (<2,700 gm) who demonstrated a grade III placenta had a fourfold greater risk of intrauterine growth retardation (IUGR) than a small fetus without a grade III placenta.[15]

A correlation between premature placental calcification, hypertension, and IUGR was noted by Hills et al. in a study of 128 high-risk pregnancies.[13] In another study of 100 non–diabetic hypertensive patients and 100 controls scanned between 28 and 43 weeks, Kazzi et al. found that accelerated placental calcification was significantly associated with hypertension, out of proportion to any possible effect on fetal size (biparietal diameter).[15] Another report found that premature placental calcification was strongly associated with cigarette smoking but not with decreased fetal weight.[11]

Delayed placental calcification has been linked to certain conditions, notably diabetes mellitus and Rh sensitization. Identification of delayed placental calcification is less helpful than accelerated calcification, however, because of the normal variability in placental calcification at term.

Abnormalities of Placental Size

Placentomegaly is most commonly identified as an abnormally thickened placenta. Hoddick et al. found that placental thickness does not usually exceed 3 cm in thickness before 20 weeks or 4 to 5 cm before 40

TABLE 16–1.

Disorders Associated With Placentomegaly

Maternal diabetes
Maternal anemia
Hydrops
Placental hemorrhage
Intrauterine infection
Congenital neoplasms
Beckwith-Wiedemann syndrome
Sacrococcygeal teratoma
Hydatidiform mole
Chromosomal abnormalities

---

weeks (Fig 16–5).[5] However, thick placentae occasionally may be observed when the surface area of myometrial attachment is unusually small. Estimation of placental volume would be desirable in this situation, although such calculations would be time-consuming and imprecise.

Placentomegaly (Fig 16–6) may be associated with a variety of conditions (Table 16–1) including maternal diabetes, maternal anemia, α-thalassemia, rhesus sensitization or other fetal-maternal blood group incompatibility, feto-maternal hemorrhage, chronic intrauterine infections, the twin transfusion syndrome, and congenital neoplasms. Fetal malformations that have been associated with placentomegaly include the Beckwith-Wiedemann syndrome, sacrococcygeal teratoma, chromosomal abnormalities, and fetal hydrops. Placental enlargement from hydrops is thought to result from retrograde transmission of portal venous pressure induced by fetal hepatomegaly.

An abnormally small placenta may be associated with IUGR, intrauterine infection, and chromosomal abnormalities. However, since there are no established criteria for an abnormally small placenta, this condition has not been described prenatally.

Placenta Previa

Clinical and Pathologic Findings

Placenta previa is found in 1 in 200 pregnancies at the time of delivery.[6, 19, 23–25] Approximately 20% are complete (total) previas, defined as placental tissue completely covering the internal cervical os, and 80% are partial (marginal) previas (Fig 16–7). Factors that have been associated with placenta previa include advanced maternal age, multiparity, and prior cesarean section or uterine surgery.[6]

Painless vaginal bleeding is the clinical hallmark of placenta previa and eventually occurs in nearly all clinically significant cases.[23] Conversely, 3%–5% of all

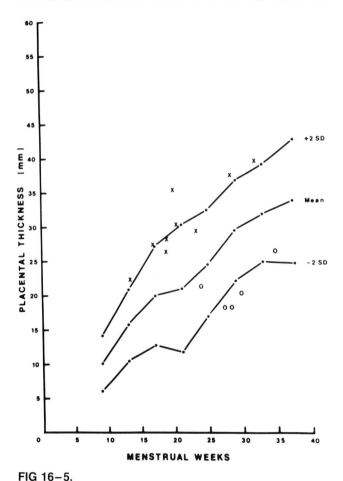

FIG 16–5.
Graph showing that placental thickness progressively increases with menstrual age but rarely exceeds 4–5 cm at any age. Note that placentas with smaller surface area of attachment of the uterus *(x)* tend to be thicker than placentas with a larger area of attachment *(o)*. (From Hoddick WK, Mahony BS, Callen PW, et al. Placental thickness. J Ultrasound Med 1985; 4:479–482. Used by permission.)

FIG 16–6.
Placentomegaly. The placenta *(P)* is markedly thickened (9 cm) in association with fetal hydrops and a large amount of ascites *(As)*. *AF* = amniotic fluid; *Sp* = spine.

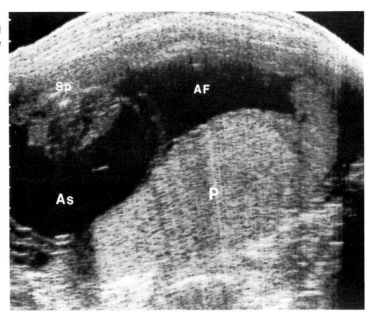

pregnancies are complicated by third-trimester bleeding, and of these, 7%–11% are due to placenta previa. Bleeding usually occurs during the third trimester because uterine thinning and cervical effacement lead to placental detachment and tears in the basilar and marginal veins; in 30% of cases, however, vaginal bleeding initially presents before the third trimester.[23] Vaginal bleeding also apparently can occur from partial previa or a low-lying placenta secondary to tears of marginal veins.

FIG 16–7.
Classification of placental location. **A,** complete placenta previa. **B,** partial (marginal) previa. **C,** low-lying placenta. (From Goplerud CP: Bleeding in later pregnancy, in Danforth DN (ed): *Obstetrics and Gynecology,* ed 5. New York, Harper & Row, 1986. Used by permission.)

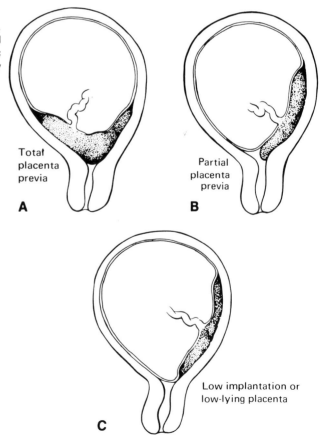

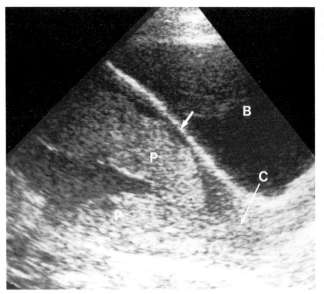

FIG 16–8.
Complete placenta previa. Longitudinal sonogram demonstrates the placenta *(P)* positioned centrally over the cervix *(C)*. Note the normally hypoechoic boundary *(arrow)* representing the myometrium and subplacental veins between the placenta and urinary bladder *(B)*.

Perinatal mortality from placenta previa is less than 5% currently, although it was as high as 40% in the 1950s.[19] Other potential complications of placenta previa include premature delivery and intrauterine growth retardation (IUGR).[23, 29] These complications occur more frequently from complete previas than marginal previas, and are thought to be secondary to premature detachment of the placenta from the lower uterine segment.

Sonographic Findings

Complete placenta previa is diagnosed on sonography when the placenta covers the entire cervical os (Fig 16–8), and a partial previa is suggested when the lower placental margin appears to extend to, but not across, the internal cervical os.[6, 18, 31, 36] Identification of a complete placenta previa is easiest when the pla-

centa is directly implanted over the os, forming a central or symmetric previa (see Fig 16–8). Abnormal fetal lie (transverse or breech) may be an associated finding, because the placenta prevents the fetal head from entering the pelvis. In some cases, periplacental hemorrhage can also be identified.

Complete previa is often not symmetrically located over the cervical os but rather lies predominantly on the anterior, posterior, or lateral uterine wall (Fig 16–9).[30] In this situation, distinguishing an asymmetric complete previa from a partial previa or a very low-lying placenta can be difficult, even when scanning in multiple planes and with variations in urinary bladder filling.[22] To aid in this distinction, transvaginal and transperineal sonography have been proposed.[20] Transperineal sonography can be readily performed with standard transducers and does not carry the theoretic

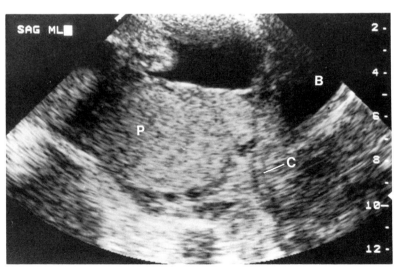

FIG 16–9.
Asymmetric complete placenta previa. Longitudinal scan demonstrates a placenta *(P)* that is predominantly posterior in location but which completely covers the cervix *(C)*. *B* = urinary bladder.

hazard of transvaginal sonography in women with placenta previa.

The reported accuracy of US for diagnosing placenta previa varies widely. While false-negative diagnoses are rare, false-positive diagnoses are common depending on the gestational age, the sonographic technique employed, the type of previa (complete vs. partial), and the indications for sonography.[17, 21, 28, 32] Recent ultrasound studies during the second trimester have reported a placenta previa in 2.5% to 7.5% of all pregnancies.[17, 32] This compares to an actual frequency of only 0.5% at the time of delivery. Earlier US stud-

ies reported an even higher rate of false-positive diagnoses (up to half of all second-trimester pregnancies) although many of these were due to technical factors.[33, 34]

An overly distended urinary bladder and focal uterine contractions are the two most common technical factors responsible for false-positive diagnoses of placenta previa or transabdominal sonography (Figs 16–10 and 16–11).[9, 17, 32, 35] Townsend et al. found that 93% of suspected marginal placenta previas seen before 20 weeks ultimately were found not to have a previa at the time of delivery, and two thirds of false-

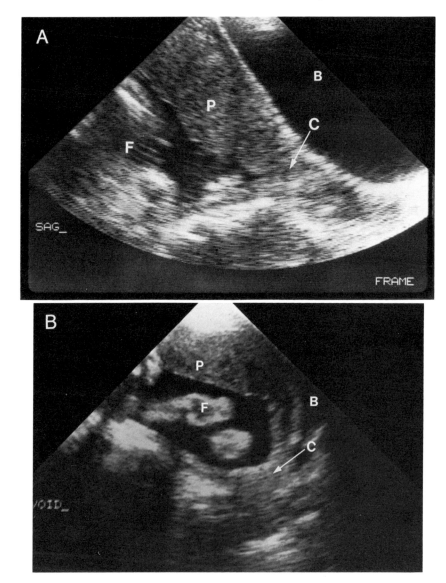

FIG 16–10.
False-positive placenta previa. **A,** longitudinal scan with a distended urinary bladder suggests that the placenta *(P)* is partially covering the cervix *(C). B* = urinary bladder; *F* = fetus. **B,** repeat sonogram with an empty bladder *(B)* shows that the placenta *(P)* is remote from the cervix *(C). F* = fetus.

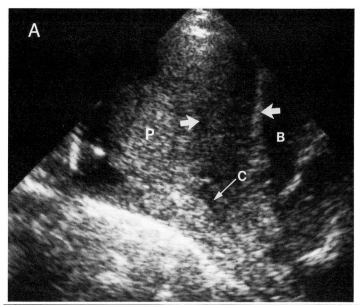

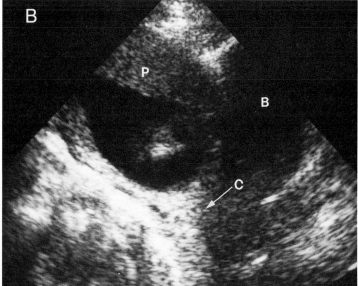

FIG 16–11.
False-positive previa due to uterine contraction. **A,** longitudinal scan suggests that the placenta *(P)* overlies the cervix *(C)* to form a previa. However, note the thickened myometrium *(arrows)* suggesting the presence of a focal uterine contraction. **B,** repeat scan 30 minutes later shows normal relation of placenta *(P)* with cervix *(C)* and resolution of focal contraction. *B* = urinary bladder.

positive diagnoses could be attributed to technical artifacts.[32] Importantly, no false-positive diagnoses were made of complete previas. These authors suggested that an overly distended bladder can be recognized as an abnormally long cervix (>3–4.0 cm). Focal uterine contractions are more difficult to recognize but can be suspected when the myometrial wall is abnormally thick (>1.5 cm). Rescanning after partial voiding in the case of a distended bladder or following a 30- to 60-minute delay in the case of focal uterine contractions usually will resolve normal anatomic relationships.

The risks of overdiagnosing placenta previas should be weighed against the rare, but potentially disastrous error of missing a true previa.[21, 30] False-positive diagnoses can lead to unnecessary additional sonograms, greater expense, emotional stress, hospitalization, and even needless cesarean section. Because of the frequency of false-positive diagnoses, the term "potential placenta previa" has been proposed to describe this appearance during the second trimester.[21] One could argue whether a diagnosis of a low-lying placenta or a partial placenta previa should be made at all in asymptomatic women scanned before 20 weeks. On the other hand, previas probably should continue to be overinterpreted in women with vaginal bleeding or when a complete placenta previa is suspected at any time in gestation.

FIG 16–12.
Classification of placenta accreta, increta, and percreta. *a* = myometrium; *b* = decidua basalis; *c* = decidua spongiosa; *d* = placenta. (From Newton M: Other complications of labor, in Danforth DN (ed): *Obstetrics and Gynecology*, ed 5. New York, Harper & Row, 1986. Used by permission.)

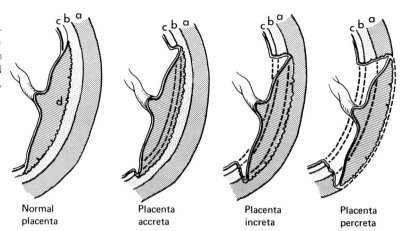

Normal placenta   Placenta accreta   Placenta increta   Placenta percreta

Placenta Accreta, Increta, Percreta

Clinical and Pathologic Findings

Placenta accreta is an abnormally adherent placenta in which the chorionic villi grow directly into the myometrium without intervening decidua.[23] Extension through the myometrium is termed placenta increta, and penetration of the uterine serosa is termed placenta percreta (Fig 16–12). However, this is a theoretical classification since all three conditions may be present in a single pregnancy; the term placenta accreta will be used here to refer to all three conditions.

Placenta accreta results from underdeveloped decidualization of the endometrium.[6] The most common predisposing factor is a uterine scar from previous cesarean section. About 20% of cases are associated with placenta previa secondary to inadequate decidua formation in the lower uterine segment. Potential clinical problems include retention of placental tissue and persistent postpartum bleeding. In severe cases, unsuccessful manual extraction of the placenta may require hysterectomy.

Sonographic Findings

Placenta accreta/increta/percreta occasionally can be suspected on prenatal sonography by demonstrating absence of the usual hypoechoic subplacenta venous complex and myometrium beneath the placenta (Figs 16–13 and 16–14).[109, 110] This can be best demon-

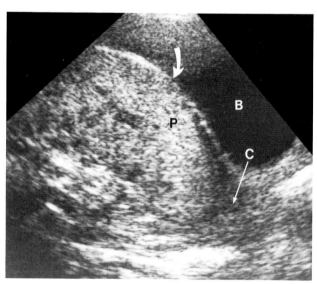

FIG 16–13.
Placenta increta. Longitudinal sonogram demonstrates a placenta previa with the placenta *(P)* covering the cervix *(C)*. Also note the loss of the normal hypoechoic boundary *(curved arrow)* between the placenta and urinary bladder *(B)*. This patient required emergency hysterectomy following cesarean delivery for continued vaginal bleeding.

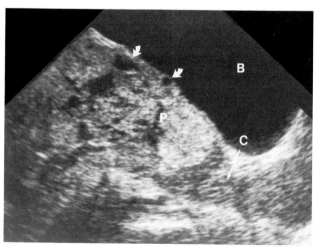

FIG 16–14.
Placenta percreta. Longitudinal sonogram shows placenta previa with placenta *(P)* covering the cervix *(C)*. Note both the loss of the normal boundary between the placenta and urinary bladder *(B)* and the presence of subplacental vessels extending into the bladder wall *(arrows)*. This patient had four prior cesarean deliveries and required hysterectomy at 22.5 weeks for uncontrolled vaginal bleeding.

strated when the placenta is located anteriorly, adjacent to the urinary bladder. A specific diagnosis of placenta percreta can be suggested when placental vessels are seen to extend within the urinary bladder wall (see Fig 16–14). All six cases of placenta accreta reported by de Mendonca were associated with placenta previa.[110] She recommends that when placenta previa is diagnosed, placenta accreta should be specifically considered.

Succenturiate Placenta

Clinical and Pathologic Findings

Succenturiate placenta is defined as the presence of one or more accessory lobes connected to the body of the placenta by blood vessels. These are relatively common, reported in 3%–6% of pregnancies in the series reported by Fox.[4] Retention of a succenturiate lobe at delivery may result in postpartum hemorrhage and infection. Rarely, rupture of the connecting vessels may occur during delivery, resulting in fetal hemorrhage and demise. This potential complication is more likely when the succenturiate lobe is on the opposite myometrial surface, since the body of the placenta and connecting vessels cross over or near the cervical os.

Sonographic Findings

Succenturiate placenta can be suspected prenatally when US demonstrates a discrete lobe separate from the body of the placenta (Fig 16–15).[108] A similar appearance may be seen from a subchorionic hemorrhage, or less likely, from a myometrial contraction or uterine myoma. Occasionally, a vascular band connecting the lobes can be seen within the amniotic fluid.

Extrachorial Placentation

Clinical and Pathologic Findings

Extrachorial placenta (circummarginate placenta and circumvallate placenta) is defined as attachment of the placental membranes to the fetal surface of the placenta rather than to the placental margin.[23] Circumvallate placenta is diagnosed when the placental margin also is folded, thickened, or elevated with underlying fibrin and often hemorrhage; circummarginate placenta is diagnosed when the placental margin is not deformed.[4]

Circummarginate placenta can be found to some degree in up to 20% of placentas, but these are not usually of clinical significance.[4] By contrast, circumvallate placenta occurs in 1%–2% of pregnancies and can be associated with symptoms of bleeding and placental abruption. Prematurity is another potential complication of circumvallate placenta when marginal placental abruption occurs.

Sonographic Findings

Circummarginate placenta probably is not recognizable, since it does not distort the placental shape. On the other hand, circumvallate placenta is potentially detectable by its elevated placental margin or by associated marginal hemorrhage (Fig 16–16).[107] Janniaux et al. propose that demonstration of diffuse subamniotic sonolucent areas may be suggestive of circumvallate placenta.[107]

Placental Abruption and Periplacental Hemorrhage

Clinical and Pathologic Findings

Placental abruption, defined as premature placental detachment, is clinically recognized in 1% of pregnancies.[23, 24] It carries a perinatal mortality rate of

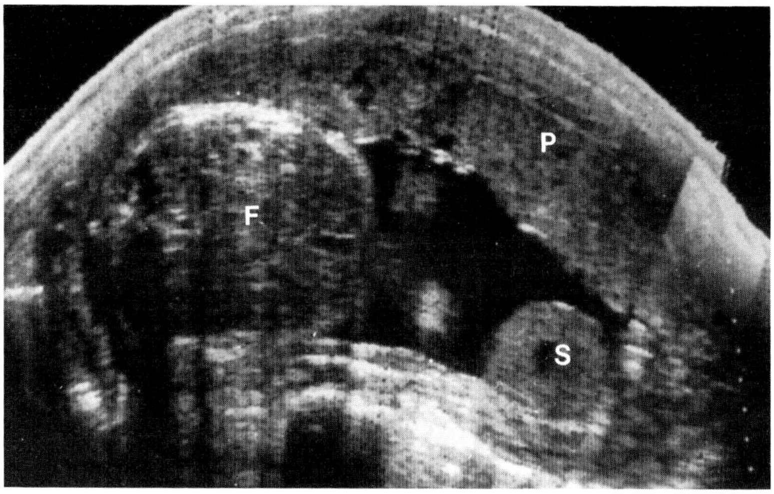

FIG 16–15.
Succenturiate placenta. Transverse sonogram demonstrates a succenturiate lobe *(S)* separate from the anterior placenta *(P)*. F = fetus.

FIG 16–16.
Circumvallate placenta and marginal abruption. Scan at 24 weeks in a woman with vaginal bleeding and uterine contractions shows a hemorrhage (*H,* outlined by arrows) at the margin of the placenta *(P).* Tocolytic therapy was ineffective, and a 740-gm infant was delivered at 25 weeks. A circumvallate placenta with a 7 cm adherent clot was identified at delivery. *F* = fetus.

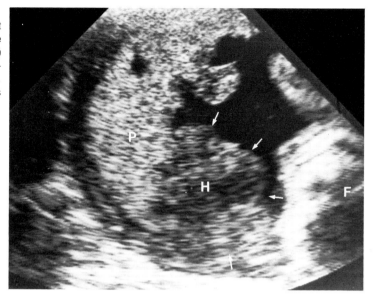

20%–60%, depending on its severity, and accounts for up to 15%–25% of all perinatal deaths.[47] Placental abruption can be categorized into two major groups by the primary area of placental detachment: retroplacental and marginal (Fig 16–17). This distinction is important because of each group's distinctive etiology, clinical symptoms, sonographic findings, and prognosis.

Evidence suggests that retroplacental abruptions usually result from rupture of spiral arteries, producing "high-pressure" bleeds, whereas marginal abruptions appear to result from tears of marginal veins, producing "low-pressure" bleeds.[24, 41–44, 51, 56] Retroplacental abruption has been most strongly associated with hypertension and vascular disease, whereas marginal abruption has been most strongly associated with cigarette smoking.[50, 51] Naeye suggests that cigarette smoking reduces uterine perfusion, especially at the less well-perfused placental margin, causing decidual ne-

crosis and subsequent hemorrhage.[51] One of the strongest risk factors for placental abruption is a previous history of abruption, perinatal death, or premature delivery.[50] Other risk factors for placental abruption include fibroids, trauma, placenta previas or low-lying placentas, and drugs such as cocaine.[24, 62]

Hemorrhage produced by marginal abruption tends to dissect beneath the placental membranes, presumably because it is more easily detached from the myometrium than the placenta itself.[52] Hence, marginal abruptions are associated with little placental detachment, and the resulting subchorionic hematoma often accumulates at a site separate from the placenta. The clinical symptoms of marginal placental abruption are also mild and require a high index of clinical suspicion.[43] Up to 15%–20% of third-trimester vaginal bleeding is attributed to placental abruption, although many of the "idiopathic" causes of vaginal bleeding are probably also due to small marginal detachments.[42, 43]

It is well known that the pathological diagnosis of placental abruption, when defined as a hematoma adherent to the maternal surface of the placenta, is often discordant with the clinical diagnosis. Retroplacental hematomas are found at pathology in up to 4.5% of placentas, even though most are small and are not associated with clinical symptoms.[4] Conversely, pathological findings may be absent following clinical evidence of acute abruption if the hematoma has not had sufficient time to organize. Also, old hematomas may have completely resolved by the time of delivery, leaving only associated findings of fibrin deposition, decidual necrosis, placental infarction, and/or thrombosis of marginal veins.[43]

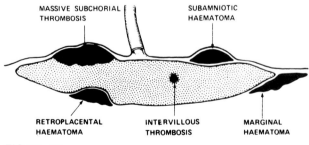

FIG 16–17.
Sites of hemorrhage in and around the placenta that have been described pathologically. Retroplacental hematoma and marginal hematoma correspond to retroplacental and marginal abruptions, respectively. (From Fox H: *Pathology of the Placenta.* Philadelphia, WB Saunders Co, 1978, pp 107–157. Used by permission.)

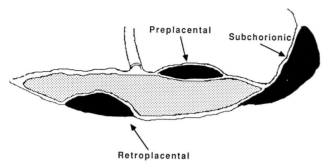

FIG 16–18.
Sites of periplacental hemorrhage that have been described sonographically. Subchorionic hemorrhage may be remote from the placenta but is thought to arise from marginal abruptions. The term "preplacental" hemorrhage has been chosen to describe both subamniotic hematoma and massive subchorial thrombosis. Intraplacental hemorrhage (intervillous thrombi) also may be identified but are difficult to distinguish from placental lakes or other intraplacental sonolucencies.

Sonographic Findings

The primary sonographic evidence for placental abruption is demonstration of a hemorrhage produced by the placental detachment.[60, 61] Sonographic examination has been reported to be negative in most cases of clinically suspected abruption, presumably as a result of free passage of blood through the cervical os.[60] Indeed, some studies have suggested that the primary role of sonography in suspected abruption is only in ex-

cluding placenta previa.[45] Others, however, have found sonography to be useful when the spectrum of sonographic findings that may be seen with placental hemorrhage are recognized.[37, 53] Also, abruptions which form a sonographically detectable hematoma appear to have a worse prognosis than those that do not.[37, 53] It is suggested that sonographers should be highly suspicious of placental abruption in women who are scanned with symptoms of vaginal bleeding and/or uterine irritability.[42, 45]

Categories of periplacental hemorrhage that have been described on sonography include retroplacental, subchorionic, and "preplacental", based on their location relative to the placenta (Fig 16–18).[52] The first two categories (retroplacental and subchorionic) correspond to retroplacental and marginal placental abruptions, respectively. Preplacental hemorrhage is an unusual site that will be discussed separately.

When evaluating women with suspected placental abruption, it is important to realize that the sonographic appearance of periplacental hemorrhage depends on the time the ultrasound examination is performed relative to the onset of hemorrhage.[52] Acute hemorrhage is hyperechoic to isoechoic relative to the placenta, whereas older hemorrhage (>2 weeks) is nearly sonolucent (Fig 16–19). Correlation with the clinical history may be useful in recognizing suspected hemorrhage.

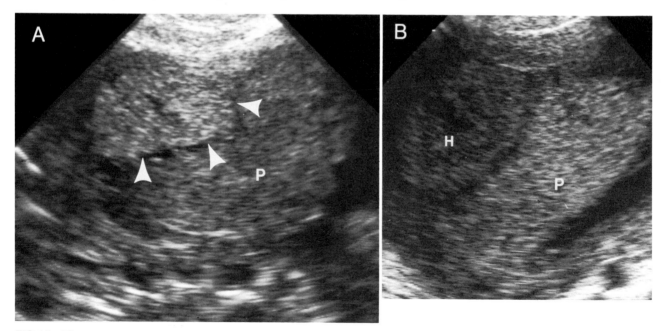

FIG 16–19.
Retroplacental abruption. **A,** sonogram at 25 weeks shows a hyperechoic hematoma *(arrowheads)* in a retroplacental location beneath the placenta *(P)*. **B,** repeat sonogram 1 week later shows the hematoma *(H)* is now hypoechoic compared with adjacent placenta *(P)*. Fetal demise followed repeat vaginal bleeding and contractions consistent with extension of the abruption. (From Nyberg DA, Cyr DR, Mack LA, et al: Sonographic spectrum of placental abruption. AJR 1987; 148:161–164. Used by permission.)

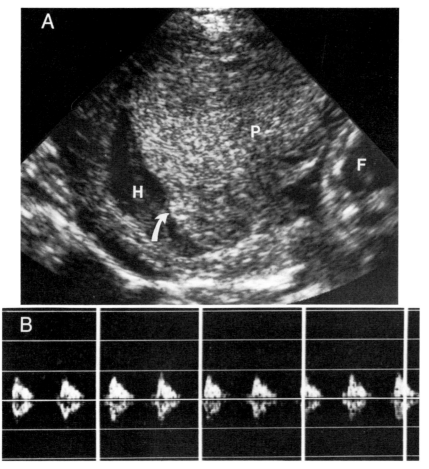

FIG 16–20.
Retroplacental abruption. **A,** sonogram at 34 weeks shows a thickened placenta *(P)* and a retroplacental hematoma *(H)* elevating the placenta. *F* = fetus. **B,** umbilical artery Doppler demonstrates absence of diastolic flow.

A retroplacental abruption occasionally is seen as a well-defined hematoma located between the placenta and uterus (Figs 16–19 and 16–20). However, acute retroplacental hematomas can be difficult to recognize because they dissect into the placenta and/or myometrium and are similar in echogenicity to the adjacent placenta. In these cases, sonography may demonstrate only a thickened, heterogeneous-appearing placenta (Fig 16–21),[46, 48, 49, 52] as well as non–specific findings of rounded placental margins and intraplacental sonolucencies. Jaffe et al. found that the placenta may measure up to 9 cm thick from acute retroplacental abruption, compared to a normal maximum thickness of 4 to 5 cm.[46]

Subchorionic (marginal) hemorrhage is by far the most common site of placental abruption seen on sonography (Figs 16–22 to 16–24).[52, 55] Of 57 periplacental hemorrhages detected on prenatal sonography, Nyberg et al. reported that subchorionic hemorrhage comprised 91% of cases before 20 weeks and 67% of

cases after 20 weeks.[52] While it is thought that nearly all subchorionic hematomas arise from marginal abruptions, in only about half the cases is placental detachment actually demonstrated.[52, 55] The resulting hematoma can mimic other mass lesions including a myoma, succenturiate lobe, chorioangioma, placenta previa, or coexisting molar pregnancy (see Fig 16–24).[49, 52, 60, 63]

As the hematoma resolves, the detached placental membrane (consisting of the fused chorion and amnion) may be the only evidence of prior subchorionic hemorrhage (see Figs 16–23 and 16–24).[5] This membrane can be followed to the placental margin where the chorion is firmly adherent to the chorionic plate. This appearance should be distinguished from chorioamniotic separation, where the membrane (amnion) can be followed over the fetal surface of the placenta to the umbilical cord insertion. However, chorioamniotic separation may also occur from placental hemorrhage. Prominent marginal veins should also be distin-

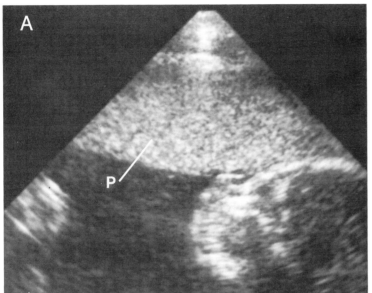

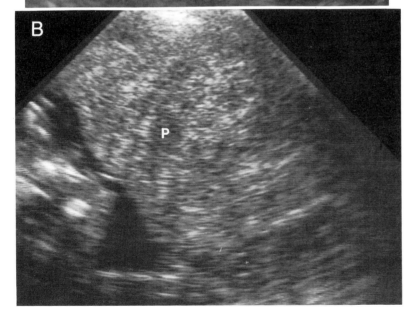

FIG 16–21.
Acute retroplacental abruption. **A,** sonogram at 20 weeks shows a normal-appearing anterior placenta *(P).* **B,** repeat sonogram 5 days later shows a markedly thick and heterogeneous placenta *(P).* A large retroplacental hematoma was found after spontaneous abortion. (From Nyberg DA, Cyr DR, Mack LA, et al: Sonographic spectrum of placental abruption. AJR 1987; 148:161–164. Used by permission.)

FIG 16–22.
Marginal abruption. Sonogram at 28 weeks shows a hematoma elevating the margin of the placenta *(curved arrow)* and extending beneath the chorionic membranes *(straight arrow)* on the opposite uterine surface. *P* = placenta; *H* = hematoma; *F* = fetus.

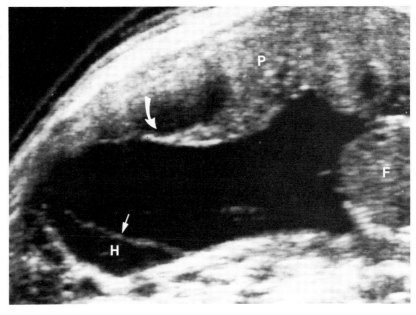

guished from marginal hemorrhage by the lack of mass effect. Detection of flowing blood on real-time sonography may not necessarily be a distinguishing feature, since we also have observed flow at sites of resolving hemorrhage.

In addition to retroplacental and subchorionic hemorrhages, periplacental hemorrhage may occur in a "preplacental" location between the placenta and the amniotic fluid (Fig 16–25). Pathologically, such a hem-

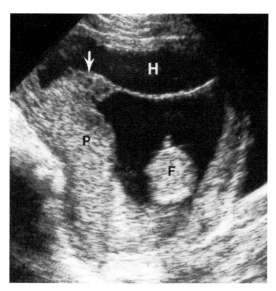

FIG 16–23.
Marginal abruption. Sonogram at 13 weeks shows a large sonolucent hematoma *(H)* that is predominantly subchorionic in location. Hematoma extends beneath the margin of the placenta. *(P),* detaching it from the adjacent myometrium *(arrow). F* = fetus. (From Nyberg DA, Cyr DR, Mack LA, et al: Sonographic spectrum of placental abruption. AJR 1987; 148:161–164. Used by permission.)

orrhage may be located beneath the chorionic plate (subchorial) or between the amnion and chorion (subamniotic), although sonography usually cannot make this distinction.[4] While the etiology of preplacental hemorrhages is uncertain, some authors believe that they may result from rupture of vessels on the placental surface secondary to temporary occlusion of the umbilical vein.[38] Large preplacental hematomas probably correspond to the "massive subchorial" hematomas (Breus mole) which have been well described in the pathological literature.[4, 57]

Anechoic or hypoechoic placental "lakes" beneath the chorionic plate, which may become very large, are more commonly seen than preplacental hemorrhage. Blood flow is often visible within these lakes, indicating they communicate with the intervillous space. These vascular spaces decompress at delivery so that pathologic examination usually shows only areas of fibrin deposition.[4, 10]

Prognosis

Periplacental hemorrhage is frequently associated with premature labor and delivery, probably because the irritating effect of intrauterine blood stimulates uterine contractions.[43, 47] This notion is supported by ultrasound studies showing that nearly all intrauterine hematomas large enough to visualize after 20 weeks are associated with uterine contractions, even in the absence of pain or uterine tenderness.[53] Sustained uterine contractions induced by intrauterine hemorrhage may further worsen hypoxia produced by the placental detachment,[54] thereby explaining the improved fetal outcome for cesarean section compared to vaginal de-

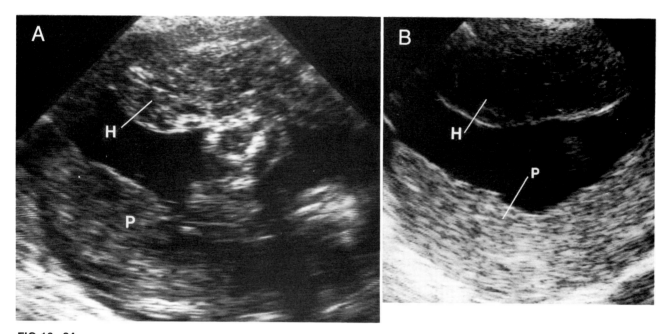

FIG 16–24.
Subchorionic hemorrhage. **A,** sonogram at 31 weeks shows a large subchorionic hematoma *(H)* located on the myometrial surface opposite the placenta *(P)*. This hemorrhage, which is similar in echogenicity to that of the placenta, was initially confused for a succenturiate lobe. **B,** repeat sonogram 2 weeks later shows that the hematoma has become nearly sonolucent in appearance. (From Nyberg DA, Cyr DR, Mack LA, et al: Sonographic spectrum of placental abruption. AJR 1987; 148:161–164. Used by permission.)

livery in some studies.[47, 58] Others have found that mild cases of placental abruption often can be managed expectantly.[59]

It is well established that the clinical significance of placental abruption is directly related to the degree of placental separation.[4] Fetal death, which results from acute hypoxia, does not usually occur from detach-

ments involving less than 30% of the placenta.[4, 39, 45, 58] High-pressure, retroplacental hematomas tend to produce significant placental detachment and are more likely to produce fetal demise as well as other "classic" clinical symptoms of a tense and painful uterus, precipitous delivery, and coagulopathy.[41, 44]

Most prenatal sonographic series suggest that ap-

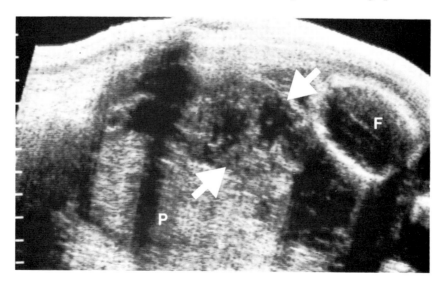

FIG 16–25.
Preplacental hemorrhage. Longitudinal sonogram at 18 weeks shows a large *(arrows)* preplacental hematoma *(H)* located between the placenta *(P)* and the fetus *(F)*. The pregnancy resulted in spontaneous abortion. (From Nyberg DA, Cyr DR, Mack LA, et al: Sonographic spectrum of placental abruption. AJR 1987; 148:161–164. Used by permission.)

proximately 80% of subchorionic hematomas seen before 20 menstrual weeks result in a normal term delivery.[40, 53] Some authors have found that the size of subchorionic hematomas (>60 ml) has prognostic significance,[55] while others have found that even large hematomas may have a normal outcome when only the placental margin is detached.[53] In reporting 59 cases of periplacental hemorrhage seen throughout pregnancy, Nyberg et al. found that perinatal mortality was most strongly associated with the estimated percentage of placental detachment.[53] The location (retroplacental) and size (>60 ml) of the hemorrhage and the menstrual age (>20 weeks) at the time of the examination also were found to be significant risk factors. It is expected that abnormal umbilical artery Doppler patterns would also be associated with a worse outcome (see Fig 16–20).

Large preplacental hematomas may produce clinical symptoms similar to those observed for placental abruption (vaginal bleeding, spontaneous abortion, and premature delivery). Although placental detachment does not occur from preplacental hemorrhage, fetal demise can result when the hematoma is large and compresses the umbilical cord.[53]

Intervillous Thrombosis

Clinical and Pathologic Findings

Intervillous thrombosis is a frequently encountered pathological finding, seen in 36% of term placentas (see Fig 16–17).[4] Intervillous thrombi apparently result from intraplacental hemorrhage caused by breaks in villous capillaries. Pathologically, these lesions are composed of coagulated blood originating from both the maternal and fetal system.[4, 94] As the lesions age, blood is replaced by fibrin, resulting in a white, laminated lesion. Adjacent villi are compressed and may show coagulation necrosis.

While intervillous thrombi are considered to be of little risk to the fetus itself, they have been associated with Rh sensitization and elevated maternal alpha-fetoprotein (AFP) levels from fetal-maternal hemorrhage (discussed further below).[91, 93, 98, 106] Devi found that women with intervillous thrombi were more likely to have circulating fetal red blood cells in the maternal circulation than other women.[89] Intervillous thrombi may also be associated with periplacental hemorrhage.

Sonographic Findings

Sonographic-pathologic correlation has shown that intervillous thrombi may be seen as intraplacental sonolucencies (Fig 16–26).[105, 106] The increasing number of intraplacental sonolucencies observed in normal

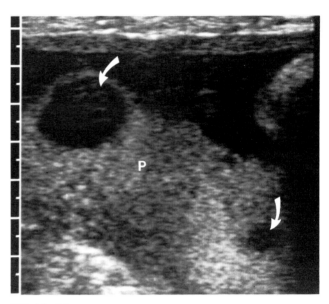

FIG 16–26.
Intervillous thrombi. Sonogram at 18 menstrual weeks in a woman referred for elevated maternal serum alpha-fetoprotein (MS-AFP) shows several intraplacental sonolucencies *(arrows)* consistent with intervillous thrombi. Placental "lakes" may demonstrate a similar appearance but show blood flow on real-time sonography. *P* = placenta.

placentas with advancing gestational age also is consistent with the frequency of intervillous thrombi seen pathologically. The association of maternal lakes with other intraplacental sonolucencies suggests that some may represent sites of prior hemorrhage which have resolved and now communicate with the intervillous space.

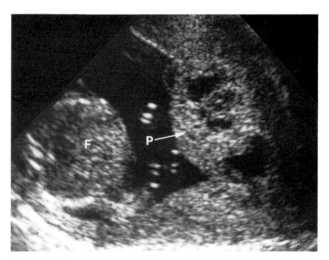

FIG 16–27.
Placental infarcts. Sonogram in a woman with systemic lupus erythematosis demonstrates confluent sonolucencies throughout the placenta *(P)*. Intrauterine fetal demise occurred three weeks after this sonogram with extensive placental infarcts found on pathologic examination. *F* = fetus.

Placental Infarcts

Placental infarcts are found at pathology in up to 25% of normal placentas at term. However, these usually are small and are of no clinical significance.[4] Large infarcts or infarcts that occur during early pregnancy usually reflect underlying maternal vascular disease (Fig 16–27). In some cases, an underlying myoma can contribute to placental infarction.

Sonographically, small infarcts appear similar in echogenicity to the adjacent placenta. Occasionally, large placental infarcts can appear as intraplacental sonolucencies (Fig 16–27) which may be indistinguishable from intervillous thrombi.[61]

Gestational Trophoblastic Disease

Clinical and Pathologic Findings

The prevalence of gestational trophoblastic diseases is approximately 1 in 1,200 pregnancies in the United States; a much greater frequency is observed in other parts of the world (e.g., the Far East).

Gestational trophoblastic disease can be categorized into three major groups: 1) classical or complete mole, 2) partial or incomplete mole, or 3) coexistent mole and fetus.[68] Invasive mole and metastatic trophoblastic disease can be considered as subgroups of a complete mole. Simple hydropic degeneration seen with first-trimester pregnancy losses should be distinguished from trophoblastic disease.

Complete moles are unique in that they contain only paternal chromosomes.[73–75] Histologic features of the classic mole include trophoblastic hyperplasia, hydropic villi, and absence of fetal tissue. Theca lutein cysts secondary to elevated levels of human chorionic gonadotropin are present in up to 50% of cases. Symptoms of molar pregnancies include vaginal bleeding, preeclampsia, and signs of hormonal hyperstimulation (nausea, vomiting, and even hyperthyroidism).[65] Approximately 15%–25% of women with complete mole will develop malignant gestational trophoblastic disease.

Partial hydatidiform moles usually are associated with a fetus or fetal tissue and, unlike complete moles, carry little malignant potential.[76] Histologic features include focal trophoblastic hyperplasia. Partial moles are frequently associated with fetal anomalies and chromosome abnormalities, usually triploidy (see Chapter 17).[73–75] Hydatidiform degeneration or hydropic change is present in nearly all cases in which the extrahaploid set of chromosomes is paternal in origin, but is much less common with a maternal origin.[67]

Coexistent true trophoblastic disease and a living fetus is exceedingly rare.[65, 76] Many of the reported cases appear to represent a partial mole or hydropic degeneration. However, instances of a classic mole and coexisting fetus have been reported, and such moles carry malignant potential.[64, 72] The presumed mechanism for this situation is hydatidiform degeneration arising from a co-twin.[73]

Sonographic Findings

The sonographic appearance of a classic molar pregnancy varies with the gestational age at which the examination is performed.[65] In the first trimester, a hydatidiform mole may be mistaken for an incomplete or missed abortion.[65, 69] After the first trimester, characteristic vesicular changes representing hydropic villi can be demonstrated throughout the placenta.[69]

Sonographic findings of partial hydatidiform mole may include reduced amniotic fluid and a thickened placenta with intraplacental cystic areas (Fig 16–28). However, the sonographic appearance varies widely. A living fetus may or may not be present, and fetal anomalies associated with a triploid fetus may or may not be evident.[66–70]

Sonographic findings of a coexisting mole include an enlarged, hyperechoic placenta with multiple small cysts and a coexisting living embryo (Fig 16–29). This appearance may be difficult to distinguish from a partial mole. A coexisting mole is more likely when more than one placenta is identified, whereas a partial mole is more likely when fetal demise, abnormal fetal tissue, or fetal anomalies are demonstrated.[64] When a live fetus is demonstrated and the correct diagnosis is uncertain, karyotyping the fetus or placenta may help to distinguish a partial mole from a coexistent mole.

Other placental abnormalities that should be considered when molar pregnancy is suspected include intraplacental or periplacental hemorrhage, degenerating uterine leiomyomas, demise of a co-twin, or prominent maternal venous lakes.[64, 70]

Chorioangioma

Clinical and Pathologic Findings

Excluding trophoblastic disease, chorioangioma (hemangioma) is by far the most common "tumor" of the placenta. Other tumors, primarily teratomas and metastatic neoplasms, are exceedingly rare.

Chorioangioma is a benign vascular malformation that probably should be regarded as a hamartoma rather than a true neoplasm because it is composed of tissue normally present in the placenta and does not metastasize. The majority are typical capillary hemangiomas that arise from just beneath the chorionic plate.[79] An association has been noted between chorioangio-

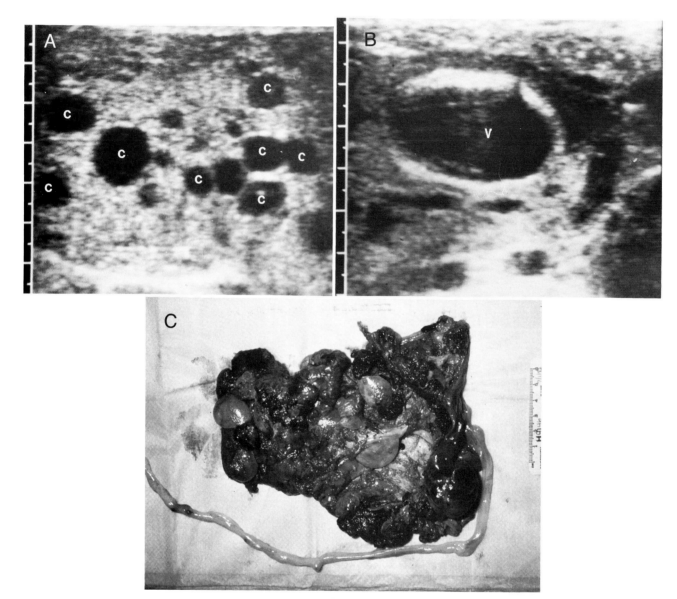

FIG 16–28.
Partial mole and triploidy. **A,** scan shows innumerable cystic areas *(C)* throughout the placenta. **B,** transverse scan of the fetal cranium shows a monventricle *(V),* indicating alobar holoprosencephaly. Other abnormalities identified on sonography included marked oligohydramnios, cystic kidneys, and a myelomeningocele. **C,** photograph at postmortem examination shows multiple cysts of the placenta representing hydatidiform degeneration.

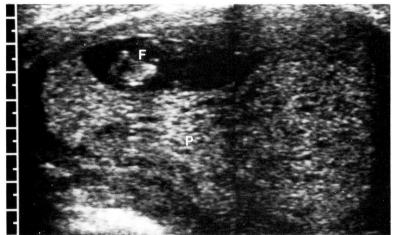

FIG 16–29.
Coexistent mole and fetus. Sonogram at 14 weeks shows a living fetus *(F)* and vesicular changes throughout much of the placenta *(P)*. No fetal anomalies were identified sonographically or at autopsy, and trophoblastic proliferation of the placenta was present.

mas and fetal hemangiomata, twinning, a single umbilical artery, and velamentous insertion.[79] This cluster of anomalies shares anomalies of blood vessels. A female predominance also has been widely observed among such anomalies.[77, 79]

Small chorioangiomas can be identified in 1% of placentas, but these are usually microscopic in size.[4] Tumors that are large enough to produce clinical symptoms and that can be visualized on sonography are uncommon, occurring in 1 in 3,500 to 20,000 births. Potential complications include polyhydramnios, premature labor, fetal hydrops, IUGR, and fetal demise. An increased risk of preeclampsia has been noted by some authors but not by others.[77] Maternal serum AFP levels may be elevated.[86]

Sonographic Findings

Sonographically, chorioangiomas usually are seen as circumscribed solid (hyperechoic or hypoechoic) masses or complex masses that often protrude from the fetal surface of the placenta (Fig 16–30).[81–85] Most reported tumors have been located near the umbilical cord insertion site; intraplacental tumors are more difficult to recognize (Fig 16–31). Polyhydramnios is present in one third of the cases.[85] Fetal hydrops is a poor prognostic finding that may be seen in association with large tumors involving the placenta or umbilical cord.

The mechanism of hydramnios and hydrops in chorioangioma has been disputed. Possible etiologic factors of hydrops include leakage of protein, vascular shunting, and umbilical vessel obstruction. Some authors believe that tumor size is most important,[78] whereas others have emphasized the obstruction resulting from the proximity of the tumor to the cord.[80]

The primary differential diagnosis for a mass within the placenta or arising from the fetal surface of the placenta is hemorrhage. This distinction can occasionally be difficult, since both lesions may be associated with vaginal bleeding and elevated maternal serum alpha-fetoprotein (MS-AFP). Doppler ultrasound may help in this distinction because chorioangiomas should show an arterial signal, whereas placental hemorrhage should not (Fig 16–32).

Relationship of Placental Abnormalities and Oligohydramnios with Elevated MS-AFP

Clinical and Pathologic Findings

Placental abnormalities have long been suspected as a common cause of elevated maternal serum-alpha fetoprotein (MS-AFP).[87–92, 97–100] Because fetal serum AFP is 100,000 times greater than that found in the maternal serum, even a small fetal-maternal hemorrhage can result in significant elevation of MS-AFP. Placental dysfunction and placental hemorrhage can also help explain the association of elevated MS-AFP with placental abruption, premature delivery, and IUGR. Placental dysfunction also may be the underlying cause for oligohydramnios, which has been associated with elevated MS-AFP. Chorioangioma may also be associated with elevated MS-AFP.[86]

Sonographic Findings

Placental hemorrhage associated with elevated MS-AFP theoretically could be either intraplacental (intervillous thrombi) or periplacental in location. Perkes et al. reported intraplacental sonolucencies consistent with intervillous thrombi in 18% of 121 patients with elevated MS-AFP compared to only 3% of 260 controls.[101] Similarly, Kelly et al. observed intraplacental sonolucencies >1.5 cm in diameter in 14 of 76 women (18.4%) referred with elevated MS-AFP, compared to only three women (3.4%) in a control group (p <

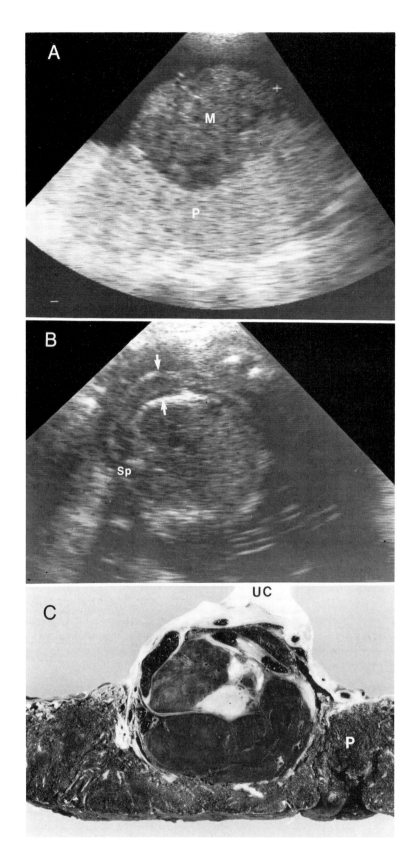

FIG 16–30.
Chorioangioma. **A,** scan at 28 weeks shows a large solid mass *(M)* arising from the fetal surface of the placenta *(P)* near the umbilical cord insertion. **B,** transverse scan of the fetus shows hydrops with skin thickening *(arrows)*. This case resulted in fetal demise. **C,** pathologic section from a similar case shows chorioangioma located near umbilical cord *(UC)* insertion site. *P* = placenta. (Part C from Spirt BA, Gordon L, Cohen WN, et al: Antenatal diagnosis of chorioangioma of the placenta. AJR 1980; 135:1273–1275.)

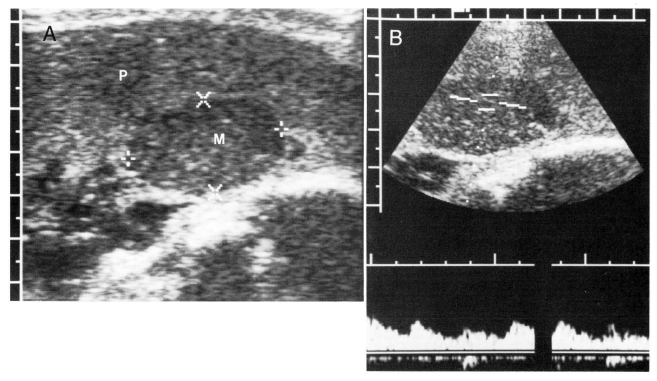

FIG 16–31.
Chorioangioma. **A,** scan at 28 weeks shows a mass *(M)* that is nearly isoechoic to the remainder of the placenta *(P).* **B,** Doppler demonstrates arterial flow signal. Chorioangioma was found at delivery.

0.01).[95] Salafia et al. also noted an increased frequency of intervillous thrombosis in patients with elevated midtrimester MS-AFP levels.[103]

Sonographic evidence of periplacental hemorrhage has also been observed in association with elevated MS-AFP, although pathologic correlation has been lacking (see Fig 16–32). Kelly et al. reported sonographic evidence of periplacental hemorrhage, usually subchorionic, in seven of 76 patients (9%) who were referred with elevated MS-AFP and a normal fetus, compared with no control patients.[95] By comparison, Fleischer noted periplacental hematomas in 16 of 25 patients (64%) referred with elevated AFP.[91] The reason for the larger number of periplacental hemorrhage in this series is unexplained.

An association between elevated MS-AFP and oligohydramnios has been noted in 1%–2% of patients with elevated MS-AFP.[90, 96, 102, 104] Oligohydramnios has been secondary to major urinary tract anomalies in 10% to 37% of series.[102] In reviewing 39 cases of oligohydramnios associated with elevated MS-AFP, Dyer et al. reported that 4 had renal agenesis, 3 had urinary tract obstruction, 2 had extrauterine pregnancies, and 1 had chronic leakage of amniotic fluid.[90] The cause for oligohydramnios for the remaining 29 cases (74%) was unclear. Possible etiologies include utero-

placental dysfunction which could result in fetal hypoxemia and shunting of blood away from the fetal kidneys.

Regardless of the etiology, pregnancies complicated by severe mid-trimester oligohydramnios have a poor prognosis. In the study by Kelly et al., only five of 13 pregnancies with oligohydramnios and elevated MS-AFP (excluding fetal anomalies) resulted in a live term birth, and two of these suffered from growth retardation.[95] Richards et al. reported only four survivors among 19 pregnancies (21%) with elevated MS-AFP and moderate to severe oligohydramnios.[102] Non–survivors included all seven fetuses with major urinary tract anomalies.

MEMBRANES

Various intrauterine membranes, septations, and bands have been described in and about the amniotic cavity (Table 16–2). These include chorioamniotic separation, chorioamniotic elevation, membranes of twins and blighted ova, amniotic bands, and synechiae. Recognition of common, "benign" types of membranes is important so that they are not confused with the amniotic band syndrome.

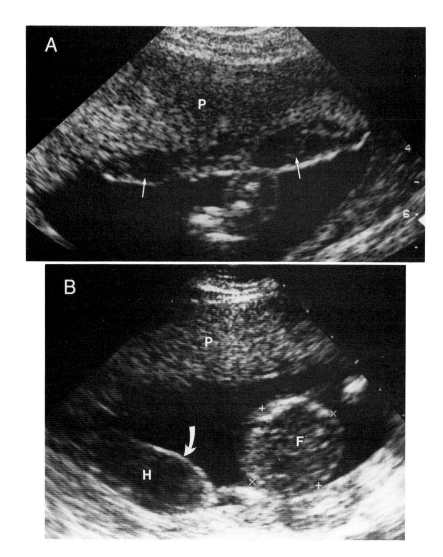

FIG 16–32.
Placental abnormalities and elevated MS-AFP. **A,** scan at 18 menstrual weeks in a woman referred for elevated MS-AFP demonstrates confluent sonolucent areas *(arrows)* beneath the chorionic plate of the placenta *(P).* **B,** different plane shows hematoma *(H)* beneath the chorionic membranes *(arrow).* Both intraplacental sonolucencies and periplacental hemorrhage have been associated with elevated MS-AFP. *P* = placenta; *F* = fetus.

Types of Intrauterine Membranes

Chorioamniotic separation
Chorioamniotic elevation
Multiple gestations
Intrauterine synechiae
Amniotic bands

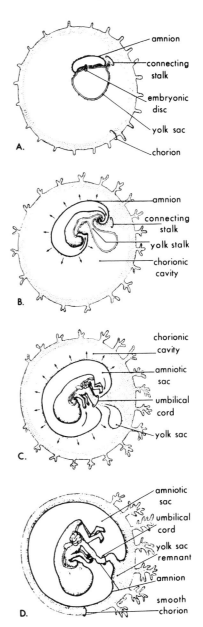

Embryogenesis

The fetal membranes are composed of the chorion, amnion, allantois, and yolk sac.[8] The chorion originates from trophoblastic cells and remains intimately in contact with trophoblasts throughout pregnancy. Reticular fibers extend into the trophoblastic layer to bind it to the underlying uterus.[121] The amnion develops at about the 28th menstrual day (fetal day 14) from cytotrophoblasts immediately adjacent to the dorsal aspect of the bilaminar embryonic disk. Initially, the amnion is attached to the margins of the embryonic disk (Fig 16–33).[8] As the embryo grows and folds ventrally, the junction of the amnion is reduced to a small area on the ventral surface of the embryo (the umbilicus). At the same time, rapid expansion of the amniotic cavity occurs (Fig 16–33). By 16 menstrual weeks the amnion fuses with the chorion, thereby obliterating the space between them (extraembryonic coelom).

The secondary yolk sac forms after regression of the primary yolk sac at 28 menstrual days on the ventral surface of the embryonic disk. Before 5 menstrual weeks, the amniotic sac and secondary yolk sac have been likened to two balloons pressed together with the embryonic disk between them (see Fig 16–33).[8] The whole structure is suspended within another balloon (the chorionic cavity) by the connecting stalk. With subsequent expansion of the amnion, the yolk sac becomes displaced from the embryo and comes to lie between the amnion and chorion.

Chorioamniotic Separation

Clinical and Pathologic Findings

Chorioamniotic separation is a normal finding until 16 menstrual weeks, when the amnion normally should fuse with the chorion (Fig 16–34).[115, 116] The chorioamniotic separation beyond 16 weeks can be associated with polyhydramnios or prior amniocentesis. A similar appearance occasionally can result from periplacental hemorrhage that extends between the amnion and chorion (subamniotic).

Regardless of the cause, chorioamniotic separation is of little clinical significance in itself. Concern that the amnion will subsequently rupture and cause fetal

FIG 16–33.
Formation of placental membranes, yolk sac, and fetus at **A,** 5 menstrual weeks (3 fetal weeks); **B,** 6 menstrual weeks; **C,** 12 menstrual weeks; and **D,** 22 menstrual weeks. (From Moore KL: *The Developing Human,* ed 4. Philadelphia, WB Saunders Co, 1988. Used by permission.)

entrapment and the amniotic band syndrome is not wholly justified. Ring constrictions and amputations from amniotic bands rarely have been observed following mid-trimester amniocentesis, presumably from amniotic rupture.[112, 124, 126] However, major fetal deformities and fetal entrapment caused by the amniotic band syndrome probably occur significantly earlier in pregnancy before amniocentesis and visualization of chorioamniotic separation.[119, 128]

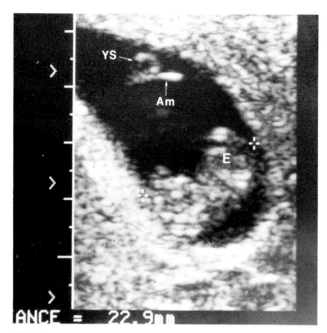

FIG 16-34.
Physiologic chorioamniotic separation. Scan at 9 menstrual weeks shows the thin amnion *(Am)* as it courses perpendicular to the ultrasound beam. Note that the yolk sac *(YS)* is on the opposite surface of the amnion from the embryo *(Em)*.

Sonographic Findings

The sonographic diagnosis of chorioamniotic separation is possible when the amnion is visible as a membrane discrete from the chorion (Fig 16–35).[116] Because the amnion is a very thin, pliable membrane, it usually is seen only when it lies orthogonal to the ultrasound beam. Careful examination will occasionally show that the space between the amnion and chorion (extraembryonic coelom) demonstrates a different echo pattern than amniotic fluid. Unlike chorioamniotic elevation, the membrane does not end at the placental margin but continues to the base of the umbilical cord (see Fig 16–35).

Chorioamniotic Elevation

Clinical and Pathologic Findings

Chorioamniotic elevation is diagnosed when both the chorion and amnion separate from the decidua but remain fused together. Because the chorion normally is adherent to the decidua and the chorionic plate of the placenta, demonstration of chorioamniotic elevation implies the presence of underlying hemorrhage or other mass lesion.

Sonographic Findings

The sonographic appearance of chorioamniotic elevation is distinctive.[116] The detached membrane is thickened and slightly irregular in appearance and can be followed to the placental margin, where it firmly adheres to the chorionic plate (see Figs 16–22 to 16–24). Elevation of the placental margin, consistent with a marginal abruption, also is occasionally demonstrated. A "blighted twin" may appear similar to chorio-

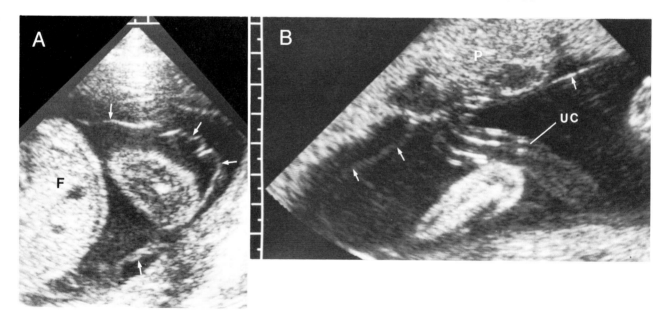

FIG 16-35.
Chorioamniotic separation. **A,** scan at 23 weeks shows detachment of the amnion *(arrows)* from the chorion. *F* = fetus. **B,** different plane shows the detached amnion *(arrows)* coursing over the placental surface to the insertion of the umbilical cord *(UC)*. *P* = placenta.

amniotic elevation, but in this situation the adjacent fluid collection is completely surrounded by echogenic chorionic villi.

Amniotic Band Syndrome

Clinical and Pathologic Findings

The amniotic band syndrome is a rare condition caused by rupture of the amnion during early pregnancy, thereby exposing fetal parts to the injurious chorionic cavity.[119, 128] Common anomalies include craniofacial defects, asymmetric facial clefts, amputation defects of the extremities, abdominal wall defects, and various secondary abnormalities.[113, 119, 120] The estimated date of insult ranges from 6 menstrual weeks to 18 weeks, with the severity of defects related to the age of injury.[119]

The limb-body wall complex is a complex malformation that is closely related to the amniotic band syndrome but is considered distinctive by some authorities.[130, 131] Characteristic features of the limb-body wall complex include marked fetal scoliosis, evisceration of abdominal contents into the extraembryonic coelom, and a shortened umbilical cord.[131]

Sonographic Findings

Sonographic identification of the amniotic band syndrome and limb-body wall complex is possible when characteristic fetal defects are identified. The abnormal membranes may also be demonstrated, but this is usually overshadowed by the severity of fetal defects (Fig 16–36).[117, 122, 127] Identification of one or more membranes alone is unlikely to represent the amniotic band syndrome; rather, this is more likely to indicate chorioamniotic separation, chorioamniotic elevation,

or intrauterine synechiae. Sonographic progression of chorioamniotic separation to the amniotic band syndrome has not yet been observed on prenatal sonography.

Synechiae

Clinical and Pathologic Findings

Intrauterine "synechiae", amniotic "sheets", or "pillars" are frequently observed as an incidental finding during obstetric sonography; however, there have been relatively few published reports regarding them. Mahony et al. first described the sonographic appearance of such membranes in a series of seven patients.[122] They suggested that these structures represent intrauterine synechiae covered by a layer of amnion and chorion (Fig 16–37). This notion was supported by Randel et al., who found that 12 of 17 (71%) patients had a prior history of uterine curettage from therapeutic abortion or following spontaneous abortion.[125] All but three patients delivered healthy babies. Of the remaining patients, one delivered prematurely at 29 weeks, another delivered at 35 weeks with fetal demise and normal autopsy, and the third gave birth to an Rh-immunized infant who required blood transfusions. An intrauterine septum may also be seen from partial uterine duplication (bicornuate uterus or uterine didelphis), in which case the septum represents myometrium coursing in a sagittal plane.

Sonographic Findings

Sonographically, intrauterine synechiae appear as membranes or pillars within the amniotic fluid (Figs 16–38 and 16–39).[125] Characteristically, the membrane demonstrates a broad base that probably repre-

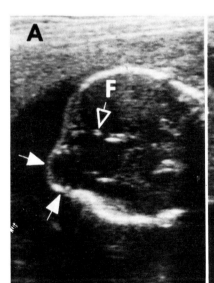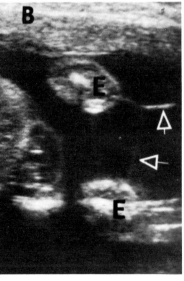

FIG 16–36.
Amniotic band syndrome. **A,** scan through the fetal cranium shows an asymmetrical encephalocele *(solid arrows)*. *F* = falx cerebri. **B,** numerous amniotic bands *(arrows)* attached to the extremities *(E)* were seen to restrict fetal motion. Other scans showed an asymmetric facial cleft. (From Mahony BS, Filly RA, Callen PW, et al: The amniotic band syndrome: Antenatal sonographic diagnosis and potential pitfalls. Am J Obstet Gynecol 1985; 152:63–68. Used by permission.)

FIG 16–37.
Schematic drawing of intrauterine synechia. A layer of amnion and chorion is draped over an intrauterine synechia or septum. There is no restriction of fetal motion. (From Mahony BS, Filly RA, Callen PW, et al: The amniotic band syndrome: Antenatal sonographic diagnosis and potential pitfalls. Am J Obstet Gynecol 1985; 152:63–68. Used by permission.)

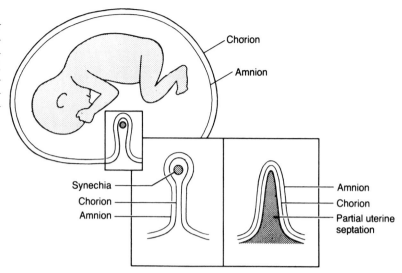

sents the synechia itself; the placental margin occasionally may attach to this base (see Fig 16–39). The sheet-like membrane is similar in thickness to that seen in dichorionic twins and probably represents a double layer of amnion and chorion draped over the synechia or adhesion (see Fig 16–38, A). Although the synechiae appear to be within the amniotic fluid, they are anatomically external to the amniotic sac.[125] The membrane causes no fetal entrapment and does not adhere to the fetus. There are no associated fetal deformities, and fetal parts move freely around the membrane.

In the late third trimester, the membrane no longer may be visualized as it becomes obliterated or compressed.[125] This sonographic appearance should be clearly distinguished from the amniotic band syndrome.

Randel et al. suggest that intrauterine synechiae have no clinical significance in and of themselves.[125] However, we have noted that they can occasionally compartmentalize a large component of the amniotic fluid, thereby limiting fetal mobility (see Fig 16–39). For this reason, there may be an association between

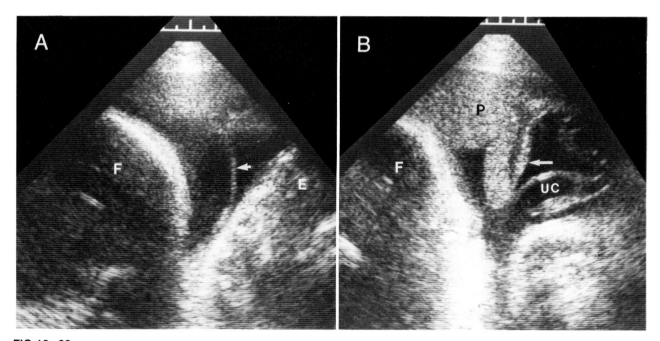

FIG 16–38.
Synechia. **A,** transverse scan shows intrauterine membrane *(arrow)* representing double layer of amnion at lower edge of synechia. The fetus *(F)* is freely mobile around membrane and the extremity *(E)* is found on the opposite side of membrane. **B,** scan at a slightly higher level shows broader base of synechia *(arrow)* with margin of placenta *(P)* attached to it. F = fetus; UC = umbilical cord.

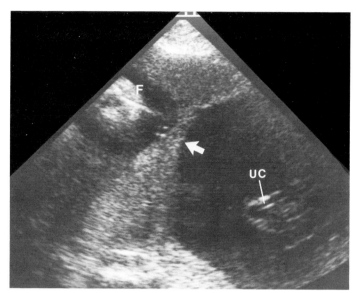

FIG 16–39.
Synechia. Longitudinal sonogram at 32 weeks demonstrates an intrauterine synechia *(arrow)* that obstructed the fetal head from entering the pelvis and resulted in cord presentation. The patient underwent cesarean delivery at term for persistent transverse lie. *F* = fetus; *UC* = umbilical cord.

intrauterine synechiae, abnormal fetal presentation (breech or transverse), and umbilical cord presentation.

Membranes Associated With Twins

Clinical and Pathologic Findings

One third of twin gestations arise from a single fertilized ovum (monozygotic twins) and two thirds arise from separate fertilized ova (dizygotic twins).[8] All dizygotic twins are dichorionic, referring to the presence of separate placental sites, and all dichorionic gestations also are diamniotic. By contrast, monozygotic twins may be dichorionic (30%); monochorionic, diamniotic (60%); or monochorionic, monoamniotic (10%), depending on the time of division. Viewed in another way, all monochorionic gestations result from monozygotic twinning, and 90% of dichorionic gestations result from dizygotic twinning.

Sonographic Findings

All twin gestations except monochorionic, monoamniotic twins contain a separating membrane between the fetuses. The membrane of dichorionic, diamniotic twins is composed of four layers (a double layer of amnion and chorion), whereas the membrane of monochorionic, diamniotic twins is composed of only two layers of amnion.[4, 8] As suggested by the histology, sonographic identification of a thick intervening membrane has been reported to be highly predictive of a dichorionic gestation (see Chapter 15). Identification of a thin membrane is predictive of a monochorionic, diamniotic gestation during early pregnancy but is less helpful during the third trimester, because dichorionic membranes also may become attenuated.[125]

Based on the number of placentae and membrane thickness, Barss et al. correctly classified 100% of dichorionic pregnancies and 91% of monochorionic diamniotic gestations.[114] Similarly, Townsend et al. found that a thick membrane had a predictive value of 83% for dichorionicity, but in the third trimester a thick membrane was seen in only 52% of dichorionic twins.[129] As shown by other studies, the lack of membrane visualization is not sufficient evidence of a monoamniotic gestation.[123]

THE UMBILICAL CORD

The umbilical cord is the fetal lifeline that connects the fetus with the placenta. Although anomalies of the umbilical cord are relatively uncommon, they are potentially serious and may provide important clues to the health of the fetal-placental unit.

Normal Development and Sonographic Findings

Embryogenesis of the umbilical cord and related structures is complex. Briefly, the umbilical cord is formed by the fetal week 5–6 (menstrual week 7–8) when the body stalk coalesces with the yolk stalk.[8] The body stalk connects the embryo with the placenta and contains the umbilical arteries, vein, and allantois. The yolk stalk connects the yolk sac with the embryo and contains the omphalomesenteric duct and associated vitelline vessels. Fusion of the body stalk and yolk stalk coincides with establishment of the placenta as the sole nutritive source for the embryo. Subsequently, both the omphalomesenteric duct and allantois obliterate.

FETO-PLACENTAL CIRCULATION

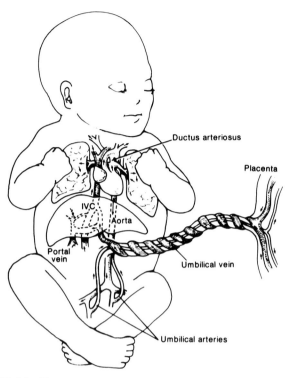

FIG 16–40.
Schematic drawing showing the fetal-placental circulation. Blood pumped by the fetal heart courses through the ductus arteriosus, into the descending aorta, and through two umbilical arteries to the placenta, and then returns via the single umbilical vein. (From Hill MC, Lande IM, Grossman JH III: Obstetric Doppler, in Grant EG, White EM (eds): *Duplex Sonography.* New York, Springer-Verlag, 1987. Used by permission.)

The umbilical cord contains two umbilical arteries that carry deoxygenated blood from the fetus to the placenta and a single umbilical vein that returns oxygenated blood to the fetus (Fig 16–40). The umbilical arteries first appear in the third fetal week (fifth menstrual week) as ventral branches of the paired dorsal aortas. By the time of fusion of the dorsal aortas, the definitive umbilical arteries have arisen as two lateral branches from the caudal end of the descending aorta. Within the fetal abdomen, the two umbilical arteries can be identified as they converge from a location just lateral to the urinary bladder (Fig 16–41). After birth, obliteration of the intracorporeal umbilical arteries forms the medial umbilical ligaments.

At 4 weeks fetal age (6 weeks menstrual age), paired umbilical veins carry blood from the developing placenta to the primitive heart. At 5 weeks (7 menstrual weeks), they join an anastomotic venous network formed by the omphalomesenteric veins in the developing liver, thereby establishing the umbilical-

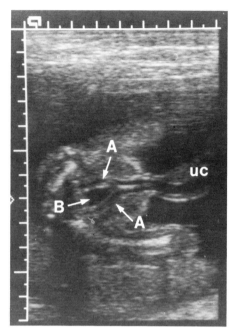

FIG 16–41.
Normal umbilical arteries. Transverse scan of the pelvis demonstrates both umbilical arteries *(A)* coursing around the urinary bladder *(B)* before entering the umbilical cord *(UC).*

portal venous connection. By 6 weeks, the right umbilical vein regresses and the left umbilical vein enlarges to accommodate the increasing flow. The umbilical vein now enters the left portal vein directly. The vast majority of blood flows through branches of the left and right portal veins, through the liver sinusoids, and eventually to the inferior vena cava via the hepatic veins. However, development of the ductus venosus permits a portion of returning blood to flow directly from the left portal vein to the systemic venous system (Fig 16–42). After birth, the intracorporeal umbilical vein obliterates to form the ligamentum teres within the falciform ligament, and the ductus venosus obliterates as part of the fissure for the ligamentum venosum.

On sonography, the intracorporeal umbilical vein can be seen to deviate abruptly from the umbilical arteries after entry through the umbilicus (Fig 16–43). The umbilical vein courses cephalically in the free, inferior margin of the falciform ligament (see Fig 16–43). On entering the liver, the umbilical vein becomes the umbilical portion of the left portal vein, which turns posteriorly and is continuous with the main portal vein and anterior and posterior divisions of the right portal vein. The ductus venosus courses superiorly from the transverse portion of the left portal vein to end in the inferior vena cava near the confluence of the hepatic veins (see Figs 16–42 and 16–43).[132] Be-

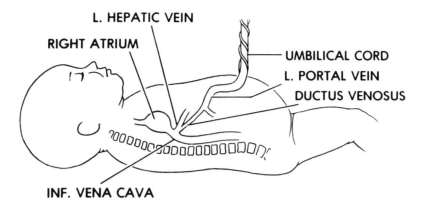

FIG 16–42.
Normal umbilical circulation. Drawing shows normal return of blood to the fetus from the placenta through the umbilical vein. The majority of blood flows through branches of the left and right portal veins, through the liver, and then drains via hepatic veins to the inferior vena cava. A relatively small proportion of blood flows through the ductus venosus and directly to the inferior vena cava or to the left hepatic vein near its confluence with the inferior vena cava. (From Chinn DH, Filly RA, Callen PW: Ultrasonic evaluation of fetal umbilical and hepatic vascular anatomy. Radiology 1982; 144:153–157. Used by permission.)

cause of its cranial-caudal course, the ductus venosus can be visualized in its entirety only on longitudinal scans. However, many textbooks have erroneously mislabeled the ductus venosus as other vascular structures on tranvserse scans of the abdomen.

Because it is bathed by amniotic fluid, the umbilical cord can be readily visualized as early as 8 menstrual weeks (Figs 16–44 and 16–45).[133] Initially, the umbilical cord is small but it grows in both diameter and length during pregnancy (see Fig 16–45). Growth of the umbilical cord parallels growth of the embryo until 28 weeks, when the umbilical cord has attained its final length of 50 to 60 cm (range, 22 to 130 cm).[137, 138] The eventual length of the umbilical cord is related to fetal mobility, with longer cords associated with increased mobility and shorter cords found when fetal movement is inhibited, for example, by oligohydramnios.[135] Short cords also are found in association with certain fetal malformations, such as abdominal wall defects.[135] Unusually long cords may prolapse and are associated with nuchal cords and true knots.

Coiling is an obvious characteristic of the umbilical cord that is established by 9 menstrual weeks.[134] The number of twists is usually between 0 and 40, with more twists present near the fetal insertion site. For unknown reasons, a predominance of left-sided twists (sinistral) have been observed compared to right-sided twists (dextral). In a representative series of 271 cords, Nakari observed that the spiral was left-handed in 87.5%, right-handed in 11.9%, and neither in 0.6%.[136] Lacro et al. suggest that an increased incidence of right twists and absent twists are found in fetuses with a single umbilical artery and that absence of cord twist may be associated with an adverse prognosis.[134]

Single Umbilical Artery

Clinical and Pathologic Findings

The most commonly encountered abnormality of the umbilical cord is a single umbilical artery (SUA), found in 0.2%–1.0% of pregnancies.[139–144] The reported frequency is higher among autopsy series than newborns. Whites have a higher frequency of SUA than blacks or Japanese.[144, 155] An increased frequency of SUA also has been noted in multiple gestations and in association with marginal and velamentous insertion of the umbilical cord. Monozygotic twins are usually discordant for SUA, suggesting that environmental factors are important.

Three possible mechanisms have been proposed to explain the embryogenesis of a single umbilical artery: (1) primary agenesis of one of the umbilical arteries; (2) secondary atrophy or atresia of a previously normal artery; or (3) persistence of the original single allantoic artery of the body stalk.[153] Most cases are likely to result from secondary atrophy or atresia of a previously formed umbilical artery. However, not all cases of SUA necessarily share the same embryogenesis. For example, a single umbilical artery associated with sirenomelia arises from the abdominal aorta directly and probably represents persistence of the vitelline artery.

A single umbilical artery has long been of interest because of its association with major congenital anomalies, perinatal death, premature delivery, IUGR, and chromosomal abnormalities.[140–144, 149] Congenital anomalies are found in 20%–50% of newborns with a SUA, and of these 20% are multiple. The most frequently affected organ systems include the musculoskeletal (23%), genitourinary (20%), cardiovascular

FIG 16-43.

Normal umbilical and fetal circulation. **A,** longitudinal scan shows that the umbilical arteries and umbilical vein abruptly deviate after the umbilical vessels enter the fetal abdomen. *UA* = umbilical artery; *UV* = umbilical vein; *H* = heart; *B* = urinary bladder; *S* = spine; *P* = penis. **B,** slightly different scan shows that the umbilical vein courses in a cephalic direction, then enters the liver to become the umbilical portion of the left portal vein. A portion of blood flow continues in the ductus venosus *(DV)* before entering the heart *(H)*. *UC* = umbilical cord; *S* = spine. **C,** slightly different angle in another fetus shows continuation of flow through the right atrium *(RA)*, right ventricle *(RV)*, pulmonary artery *(PA)*, and then out the ductus arteriosus *(DA)* and down the descending aorta *(Ao)*. *UC* = umbilical cord; *UV* = umbilical vein; *LPV* = umbilical portion of left portal vein; *DV* = ductus venosus; *S* = spine.

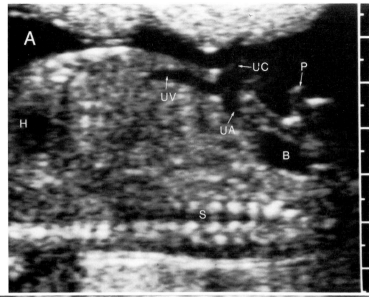

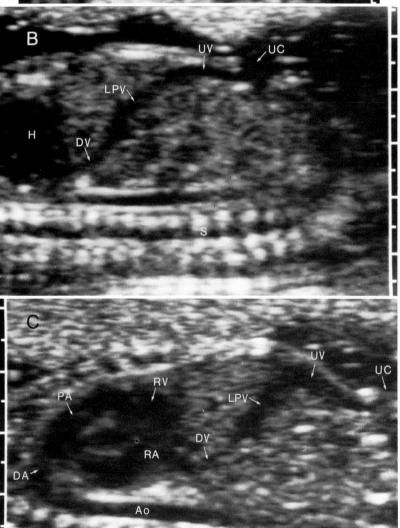

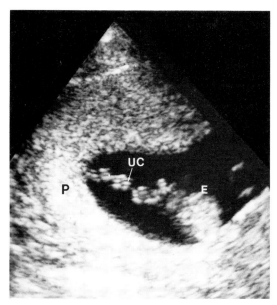

FIG 16–44.
Normal umbilical cord. Scan at 9 menstrual weeks shows the umbilical cord *(UC)* attaching the embryo *(E)* with the developing placenta *(P)* or chorionic frondosum.

(19%), gastrointestinal (10%), and central nervous systems (8%). However, no consistent pattern of anomalies has been recognized, and virtually any malformation may be present. Some types of anomalies, such as sirenomelia and acardiac twins, virtually always have a single umbilical artery. Infants born with a SUA but no other malformation can expect a normal outcome, with only an increased frequency of inguinal hernia observed in comparison to controls.[145]

An increased incidence of chromosome abnormalities has been observed among infants with a SUA.[142, 151, 152] Trisomy 18 has been most commonly reported but other karyotypes include trisomy 13, Turner's syndrome (45,X), and triploidy.[148] The risk of a chromosomal abnormality has been found to depend on the presence of associated anomalies. Vlietinck et al. encountered no chromosomal abnormalities in 19 consecutive live born infants who had a SUA but no congenital malformations.[157] By contrast, Byrne and Blane reported that all nine aborted fetuses with a SUA had other anomalies, and three (33%) of these had a chromosomal abnormality.[142] Similarly, Lenoski noted that three of seven fetuses (43%) with a SUA had aneuploidy.[151] Based on this and our own experience, we do not recommend karyotyping when an isolated SUA is identified (see Chapter 17).

Perinatal mortality is increased in infants with a SUA, primarily due to associated congenital anomalies. The increased frequency of premature delivery also occurs predominantly in the group with anomalies. IUGR, found in 35% of infants with a SUA, may be unrelated to other fetal anomalies but rather related to disturbances in normal placental growth.

Sonographic Findings

Prenatal sonographic detection of a single umbilical artery has been reported by various authors.[147, 150, 154, 156] The two-vessel umbilical cord is best demonstrated on cross-sectional scans, but also can be seen on longitudinal scans (Figs 16–46 and 16–47). Typically, the single umbilical artery is larger than normal and may be nearly as large as the umbilical vein. Atrophy of the accompanying umbilical artery occasionally may be demonstrated.

The accuracy of sonography for identifying a SUA

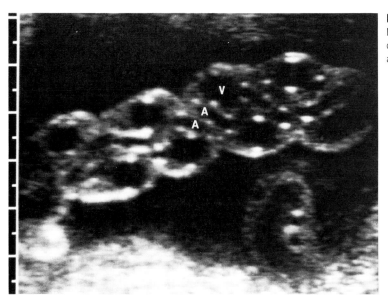

FIG 16–45.
Normal umbilical cord. Longitudinal scan of the umbilical cord at 35 weeks shows two umbilical arteries *(A)* and one umbilical vein *(V)* coiling around each other.

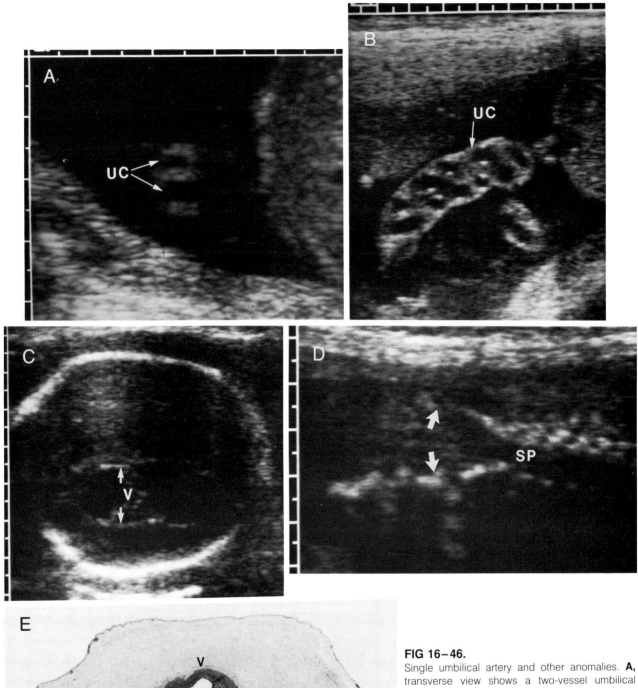

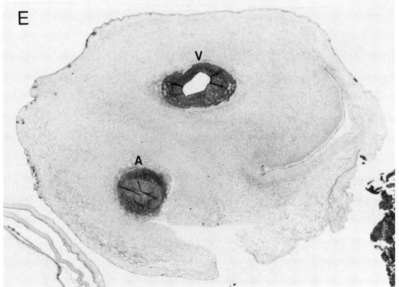

FIG 16–46.
Single umbilical artery and other anomalies. **A,** transverse view shows a two-vessel umbilical cord *(UC)*. **B,** longitudinal view of the umbilical cord *(UC)* shows a vein and artery *(A)* coiled around each other. **C,** axial scan of the cranium shows mild dilatation *(arrows)* of the lateral ventricles *(V)*. **D,** longitudinal view of the spine *(Sp)* shows a large dysraphic defect *(arrows)*. **E,** cross-sectional view of umbilical cord at postmortem examination shows single umbilical artery *(A)* and vein *(V)*. Unilateral absent kidney was also identified.

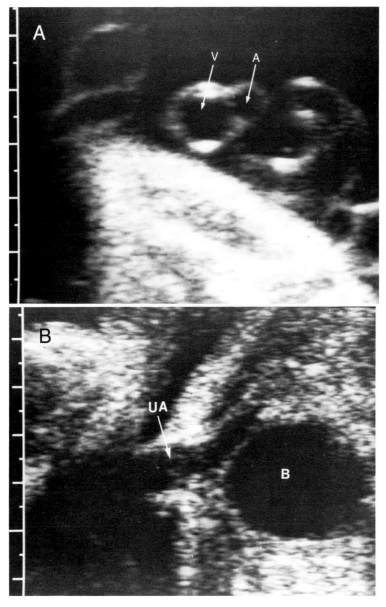

FIG 16–47.
Isolated single umbilical artery. **A,** transverse view of the umbilical cord shows a vein *(V)* and a single artery *(A)*. **B,** angled view through the pelvis shows a single umbilical artery *(UA)* coursing around the urinary bladder *(B)*. No additional abnormalities were identified on sonography or at delivery.

is unknown. In a series of nine cases of SUA reported by Herrman and Sidropoulos, four cases were correctly diagnosed, two cases were suspected, and three were missed.[147] The earliest sonographic diagnosis was made at 23 menstrual weeks. In a series of 20 fetuses with a SUA and a known CNS anomaly reported by Nyberg et al., 6 were identified prospectively, 6 additional cases were identified on retrospective review of the sonograms, and the remaining 8 cases could not be adequately evaluated due to severe oligohydramnios or other technical factors.[154] Identification of a SUA can be difficult before the third trimester because of the small size of the umbilical cord.

A potential false-positive diagnosis of a SUA is possible when the umbilical cord is examined near the placental end since the two umbilical arteries may normally fuse at a variable distance from the placenta. Also, it may be difficult to obtain a true cross-sectional view of the cord due to its tortuosity. A more reliable and earlier diagnoses of SUA should be possible with availability of color Doppler technology.

The majority of reported cases of SUA have been overshadowed by growth disturbances or other anomalies (see Fig 16–46). In the nine cases reported by Herrman and Sidropoulos, eight had IUGR and six had significant other anomalies.[147] In a series of seven cases of SUA reported between 28 to 36 weeks by Tortora et al., five demonstrated major fetal anomalies, polyhydramnios, oligohydramnios, and/or IUGR, and only two were isolated.[156] All cases reported by Nyberg et al.

were known to have a CNS malformation.[154] These data suggest that sonographic identification of a two-vessel cord should initiate a thorough anatomic survey of the fetus for additional anomalies.

Detection of at least one major malformation in addition to a SUA usually predicts the presence of additional, non-detectable anomalies and carries a significant risk of a chromosomal abnormality.[154] However, the sensitivity of sonography for detecting significant anomalies coexisting with a SUA is uncertain. No additional malformations were identified in two fetuses with a SUA reported by Tortora et al., and the absence of anomalies was confirmed at birth.[156] Similarly, a SUA was the only sonographic abnormality (see Fig 16–47) in a series of six cases at Swedish Medical Center, Seattle, Washington, and in none of these cases were additional anomalies detected after birth (unpublished data). The most subtle malformation we have seen in association with a single umbilical artery is unilateral absence of a kidney. Based on this limited experience, we believe that identification of a SUA alone should not alter obstetric management of affected pregnancies.

Multiple Umbilical Vessels

Clinical and Pathologic Findings

Umbilical cords that contain more than the normal complement of three vessels are extremely rare.[158–160] Painter and Russel reported an infant with four vessels (two arteries and two veins) within the umbilical cord who had multiple anomalies including ectopia cordis.[160] By contrast, Murdoch described an apparently normal infant with a four-vessel cord (three arteries and one vein).[159]

Sonographic Findings

Hill et al. reported prenatal sonographic detection of a four-vessel cord in a fetus with holoprosencephaly and polyhydramnios.[158] We have observed an umbilical cord that artifactually appeared to contain six vessels (Fig 16–48), apparently secondary to looping of the cord on itself as a "false knot".

Cord Presentation and Prolapse Cord

Clinical and Pathologic Findings

Umbilical cord presentation, cord prolapse, and nuchal cord are potential causes of umbilical cord compression and fetal distress. Although the first clue to these cord complications usually is made by abnormal fetal heart rate tracings (variable decelerations or mixed acceleration-deceleration),[164] prenatal sonography can play a useful role in diagnosing them.

Prolapse of the umbilical cord through the cervical os at the time of delivery is reported to occur in 1 in 200 deliveries. The high perinatal mortality rate (25% to 60%) is attributed to cord compression during vaginal delivery.[165] The most common contributing factor is abnormal fetal presentation (breech, transverse, or oblique), reported in the majority of cases.[163] Other possible etiologic factors include immaturity, excessive cord length, and polyhydramnios.

Sonographic Findings

Cord presentation with its potential for prolapse frequently has been observed on antenatal sonography (Fig 16–49).[161–163] In the largest series to date, Lange et al. reported nine cases of cord prolapse among 1,471 patients (0.61%) scanned at term.[163] All nine cases of cord prolapse were associated with abnormal fetal lie. Of seven fetuses who were delivered by cesarean section, cord presentation was confirmed in four cases and suspected in three. Two patients had vaginal deliveries, one following spontaneous version and the other resulting in stillbirth. None of the 1,462 patients with sonographically normally positioned cords developed cord prolapse at delivery. Based on this experience, these authors suggest that sonographic evaluation of cord position should be performed whenever abnormal fetal presentation is present at term and vaginal delivery is anticipated.

Nuchal Cord

Clinical and Pathologic Findings

In 4,237 pregnancies, Spellacy et al. found one nuchal loop in 21.3% and two or more nuchal loops in 3.4%.[168] Similarly, in 1,007 consecutive infants, Shui and Eastman noted one loop around the neck in 20.6% of cases, two loops in 2.5%, and three loops in 0.2%.[167] The incidence of nuchal cord has been associated with increased cord length, polyhydramnios, small fetuses, and vertex presentation.[168]

Nuchal cord can produce signs of fetal distress, shown as bradycardia and depressed 1-minute Apgar score.[168, 169] However, no significant difference has been noted in Apgar scores by 5 minutes, and neither Spellacy nor Shui found an increased infant mortality with nuchal cords.[167, 168] Nevertheless, it is our belief that two or more tight nuchal loops may be associated with increased fetal mortality.

Sonographic Findings

Nuchal cord occasionally has been diagnosed by prenatal sonography by demonstration of one or more loops of cord encircling the fetal neck (Fig 16–50).[166]

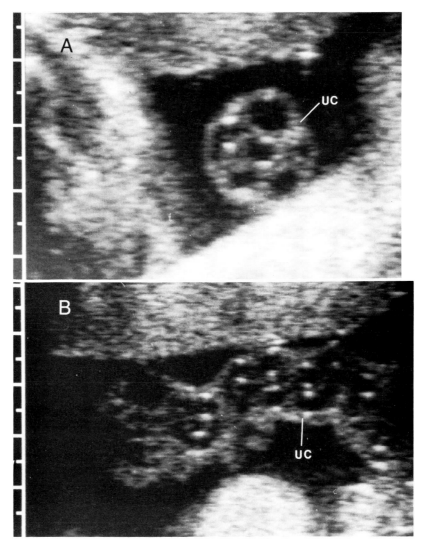

FIG 16–48.
False-positive multiple umbilical vessels. Transverse **(A)** and longitudinal **(B)** views appear to show six vessels within the umbilical cord *(UC)*. At delivery, this proved to be looping of a segment of umbilical cord on itself. Umbilical cords that contain more than three vessels are extremely rare.

This is best evaluated in longitudinal plane to the fetus by visualizing one or more loops of cord in cross-section. This evaluation may be difficult, however, when the head is positioned low in the pelvis, when there is relatively little amniotic fluid, or when the cord loop is particularly tight. In this situation, examination of the area around the neck with Doppler ultrasound may be useful.[166]

Cord Knot

Clinical and Pathologic Findings

True knots occur in the cord in less than 1% of cases.[10] Factors predisposing to cord knots include long umbilical cords, polyhydramnios, small fetuses, and monoamniotic twins.[168] Cord knots are usually loose and have no clinical significance. When tight, however, cord knots can obstruct fetal circulation and cause fetal demise. Secondary thromboses may develop within the cord vessels.

Sonographic Findings

Prenatal sonographic demonstration of a true cord knot (Fig 16–51) has not heretofore been reported to our knowledge. A true cord knot should be distinguished from a "false knot," a term that has been used to describe exaggerated loops of umbilical vessels.[170] A false knot has been given an additional meaning pathologically as focal dilatation of the umbilical vessels or a focal accumulation of Wharton's jelly.[4]

FIG 16–49.
Cord presentation. Longitudinal scan shows a dilated lower uterine segment and cervix with multiple loops of umbilical cord *(arrows)* presenting. *C* = fetal cranium; *B* = bladder.

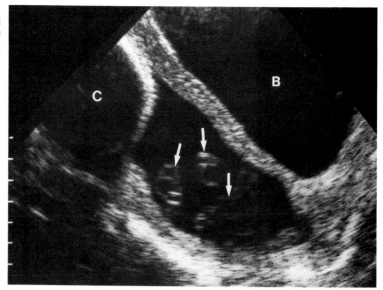

An entangled umbilical cords is a type of cord knot characterized by intertwining of both umbilical cords from two co-twins (Fig 16–52). Since this complication can develop only in the absence of a separating membrane, demonstration of entangled umbilical cords is one of the few diagnostic features of monoamniotic twins.[171]

Velamentous Insertion

Clinical and Pathologic Findings

Velamentous insertion, defined as insertion of the umbilical cord into the membranes before entering the placental tissue, has been reported in 1% of deliveries.[4] By comparison, marginal insertion of the umbilical cord into the periphery of the placenta (battledore placenta) has been reported in 2%–10% of pregnancies. Risk factors for velamentous insertion include abnormalities that may affect alignment of the embryonic body stalk at implantation. Such factors include uterine enlargement, multiple gestations, uterine anomalies, and pregnancies with an intrauterine device.

Velamentous insertion carries the risk of cord rupture during traction of the cord, requiring manual extraction of the placenta. A rare but particularly dangerous type of velamentous insertion is vasa previa, which

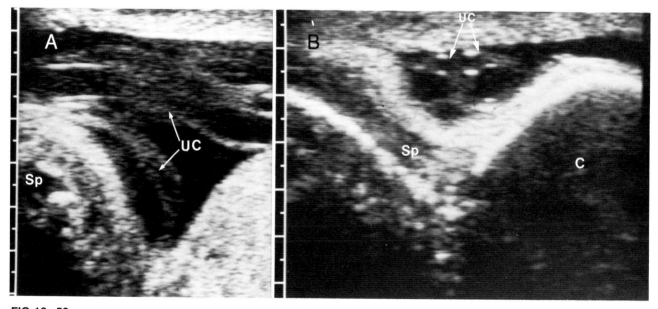

FIG 16–50.
Nuchal cord. Longitudinal **(A)** and transverse **(B)** views of the fetus show two loops of umbilical cord *(UC)* around the fetal neck. *C* = cranium; *Sp* = cervical spine.

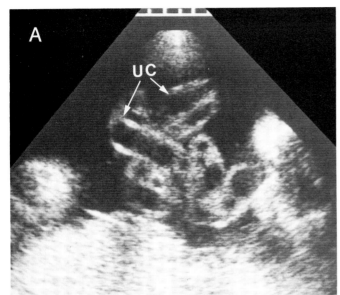

FIG 16–51.
Cord knot. **A,** scan shows loops of umbilical cord *(UC)* intertwined. **B,** photograph of infant at delivery confirms the presence of a cord knot *(arrow)*. The infant did well and showed no evidence of vascular compromise.

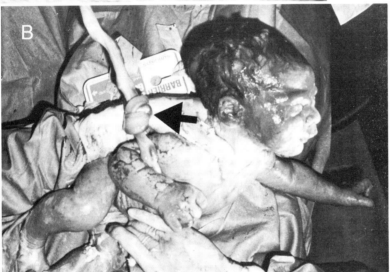

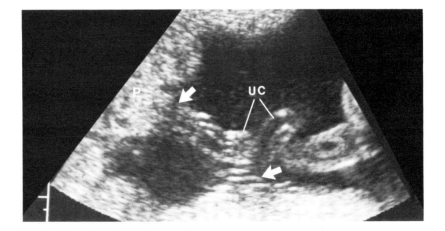

FIG 16–52.
Entangled umbilical cords in monoamniotic twins. Scan shows placental insertion sites of both umbilical cords *(arrows)* in monoamniotic twin gestation. The umbilical cords *(UC)* loop around each other, thereby confirming the absence of an intervening membrane.

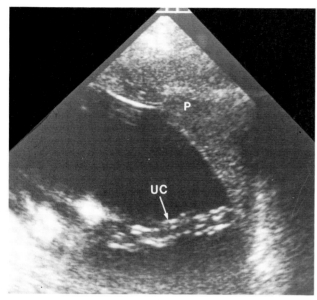

FIG 16–53.
Marginal umbilical insertion. Scan at 17 weeks shows the umbilical cord *(UC)* inserting into the far margin of the placenta *(P)*.

is defined as the umbilical vessels crossing the cervical os. This condition carries a perinatal mortality rate of 60%–70% during vaginal delivery from fetal exsanguination.

Sonographic Findings

No case of velamentous insertion has been reported by prenatal sonography, to our knowledge. However, marginal insertion has been demonstrated (Fig 16–53).

Umbilical Cord Enlargement

Clinical and Pathologic Findings

The normal umbilical cord usually measures 1–2 cm in diameter. However, wide individual variation is noted, depending primarily on the amount of Wharton's jelly present and less often on variations in the size of umbilical vessels.[172] An association between diabetes mellitus and large cords has been noted. Umbilical cord edema can occur in association with hydrops, rhesus sensitization, and stillbirths. Other causes of umbilical cord enlargement include hematoma, umbilical cord tumor (hemangioma), urachal abnormalities, and small bowel-containing omphaloceles[174, 175] (Table 16–3).

DeVore et al. suggest that dilatation of the umbilical vein also may occur prior to development of fetal hydrops or amniotic fluid bilirubin in fetuses with rhesus hemolytic anemia.[174] They propose that liver enlargement compresses intrahepatic venous drainage

TABLE 16–3.
Causes of Umbilical or Paraumbilical Cord Mass

Edema
Mucoid degeneration of Wharton's jelly
Allantoic duct cyst
Omphalomesenteric duct cyst
Urachal cyst
Hemangioma
Hematoma
Varix of umbilical vein
Omphalocele
Gastroschisis
Umbilical hernia

and secondarily enlarges the umbilical vein. However, these observations have not been confirmed by other investigators.[180]

Sonographic Findings

Most commonly, a large umbilical cord is visualized in otherwise normal fetuses due to prominence of Wharton's jelly (Fig 16–54).[172, 179] Umbilical cord edema may also be observed.[178] Periumbilical masses such as bowel-containing omphaloceles, urachal cysts, and omphalomesenteric cysts, may also appear as a thickened umbilical cord at the fetal insertion site.[173, 177, 186, 188] A case of giant dilatation of the intra-abdominal umbilical vein was reported by Fuster et al.[176]

Umbilical Cord Cysts

Clinical and Pathologic Findings

Umbilical cord cysts can originate from remnants of either the omphalomesenteric or allantoic ductal systems. Omphalomesenteric cysts are lined with columnar mucin-secreting cells, and allantoic cysts are lined by a single layer of flattened epithelium. Omphalomesenteric duct cysts are usually small but may be as large as 6 cm in diameter. They usually are observed near the fetal insertion end of the umbilical cord.

In addition to cysts and polyps of the umbilical cord, omphalomesenteric duct remnants may give rise to Meckel's diverticula, intra-abdominal mesenteric cysts, and anomalies of the umbilicus (fistulas, polyps, cysts).[184] Other anomalies that have been associated with a patent omphalomesenteric duct include omphalocele, hernias, cardiac defects, trisomy 21, spina bifida, and cleft lip.[182]

Umbilical cord cysts are usually asymptomatic. Blanc and Allen described an unusual case of sponta-

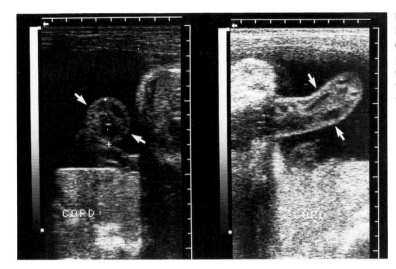

FIG 16–54.
Large umbilical cord. Transverse **(A)** and longitudinal **(B)** views at 33 weeks in association with idiopathic polyhydramnios demonstrate an enlarged umbilical cord that measures 3 cm in diameter *(arrows)*. (From Casola G, Scheible W, Leopold G: Large umbilical cord: A normal finding in some fetuses. Radiology 1985; 156:181–182. Used by permission.)

neous rupture of an omphalomesenteric duct cyst that was lined by gastric mucosa; fetal death resulted from erosion of the gastric mucosa into the umbilical vessels.[181]

Sonographic Findings

Cysts of both the omphalomesenteric duct (Fig 16–55) and allantoic duct (Fig 16–56) have been reported on prenatal sonography (also see Chapter 11).[183, 186–189] Fink and Filly reported an association between allantoic cysts and omphalocele (see Fig 16–56).[183]

Other umbilical abnormalities that can appear cystic on sonography include focal accumulation of Wharton's jelly with mucoid degeneration, resolving hematoma, focal dilatation of umbilical vessels, and umbilical cord hemangiomas. Based on available information, demonstration of an umbilical cord cyst should

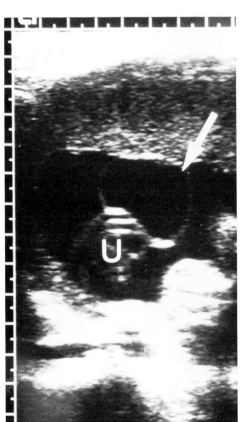

FIG 16–55.
Omphalomesenteric duct cyst. Scan at 20 weeks shows a cyst *(arrow)* arising from the umbilical cord *(U)*. No other abnormalities were identified on sonography or at the time of delivery. (From Rosenberg JC, Chervenak FA, Walker BA, et al: Antenatal sonographic appearance of omphalomesenteric duct cyst. J Ultrasound Med 1986; 5:719–720. Used by permission.)

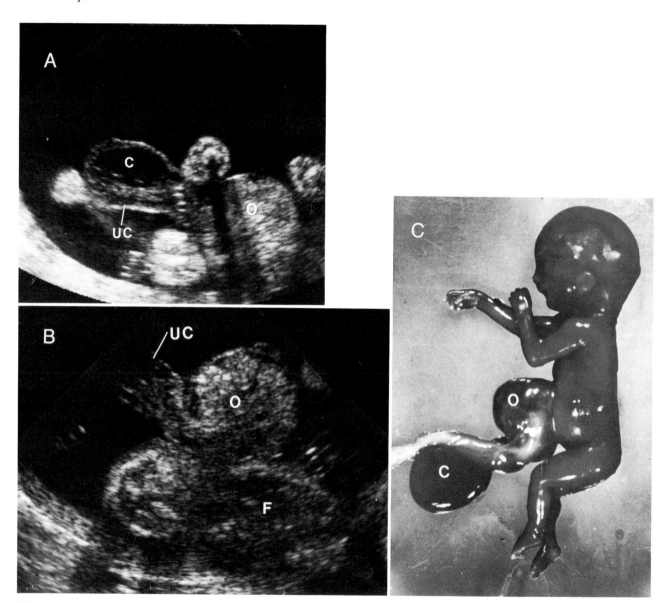

FIG 16–56.
Allantoic cyst. **A,** scan demonstrates a cyst *(C)* arising from the umbilical cord *(UC)* in association with an omphalocele *(O)* and polyhydramnios. **B,** longitudinal scan demonstrates the omphalocele *(O)* arising from the fetal abdomen. *F* = fetus; *UC* = umbilical cord. **C,** photograph of a similar case shows an allantoic cyst *(C)* arising from the umbilical cord in association with an omphalocele *(O).* (Part C from Fink IJ, Filly RA: Omphalocele associated with umbilical cord allantoic cyst: Sonographic evaluation in utero. Radiology 1983; 149:473–476. Used by permission.)

initiate a search for associated anomalies related to the umbilicus or umbilical vessels such as omphalocele, urachal cyst, and hemangioma.

Umbilical Cord Hematoma and Thrombosis

Clinical and Pathologic Findings

Umbilical cord hematomas most commonly result from needle puncture during amniocentesis or other interventional procedures. Spontaneous umbilical cord hematoma is rare, with an estimated prevalence ranging from 1 in 5,000 to 1 in 12,700 deliveries.[4] The hematoma usually is located near the fetal end of the umbilical cord and arises from rupture of the umbilical vein or, less commonly, from an abnormal umbilical artery. Etiologic factors that have been suggested include torsion, trauma during delivery, insufficiency of Wharton's jelly, and fetal hemorrhagic disease. However, no

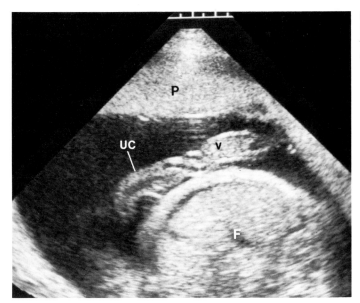

apparent cause is usually evident.[4, 191, 193] The high fetal mortality rate (approaching 50%) may be secondary to either fetal exsanguination or compression of the umbilical vessels by the hematoma.[192, 194, 195]

Sonographic Findings

Prenatal detection of umbilical cord hematomas has been infrequently reported. Ruvinsky et al. reported a case that appeared as a large (6 cm) septated mass adjacent to the anterior abdominal wall at 32 weeks.[194] Fetal demise was also present. Sutro et al. re-

ported another case of umbilical cord hematoma in a fetus with hydrocephalus and trisomy 18 following genetic amniocentesis.[196] In this case, the hematoma appeared as a large echogenic mass conforming to the umbilical cord.

Thrombosis of the umbilical vein has also been infrequently reported. Abrams and Filly reported prenatal detection of such a finding as a sign of fetal death.[190] Umbilical vein thrombosis may occur from umbilical cord needle puncture during fetal blood sampling or intrauterine transfusions (Fig 16–57).[193]

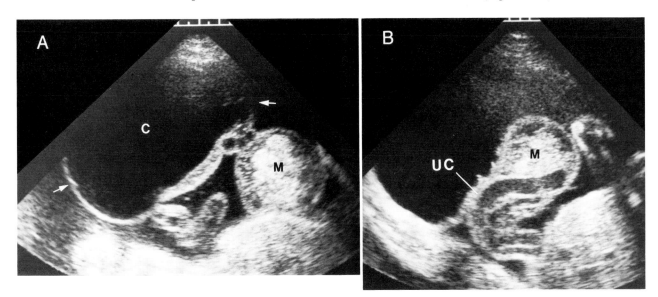

FIG 16–58.
Cord hemangioma and umbilical cord cyst. **A,** scan demonstrates an echogenic mass *(M)* representing a hemangioma within the umbilical cord *(UC)*. **B,** a large cyst *(C)* is demonstrated in association with the mass *(M)*. Cystic areas are commonly demonstrated in association with umbilical cord hemangiomas and probably develop from transudation of fluid.

Umbilical Cord Hemangioma

Hemangiomas of the umbilical cord are similar to hemangiomas of the placenta (chorioangiomas) in origin and significance (see section on chorioangiomas above).[197] Benirschke and Dodds have called these angiomyxomas because of the prominence of myxoid material.[199] Like placental chorioangiomas, umbilical cord hemangiomas may be associated with fetal hydrops and elevated MS-AFP.[201] Fetal demise occasionally has been reported from umbilical cord hemangioma, possibly secondary to umbilical cord compression.[200]

Sonographic Findings

Sonographic detection of umbilical cord hemangiomas has been rarely reported.[198, 201, 202] Most of the reported cases have demonstrated a solid or echogenic mass, often in association with a cystic component (Figs 16–58 and 16–59). The cystic component is thought to result from transudation of fluid from the hemangioma. Like chorioangiomas, umbilical cord hemangiomas may cause fetal hydrops and death. They have also been associated with elevated levels of MS-AFP (see Fig 16–59).[201] Elevated AFP is thought to result from transudation of fetal serum across the thin walled vessels.

UMBILICAL DOPPLER

Doppler analysis has been found to be a useful, non–invasive method of evaluating placental circulation and placental resistance.[204–208, 213–216] This usually involves evaluation of the umbilical vessels, with the umbilical arteries more frequently examined than the umbilical vein. Maternal uterine arteries can also be examined by Doppler, but this appears to be less sensitive than sampling the umbilical circulation.

Umbilical Doppler can be performed by either continuous wave or pulsed technology.[209] Continuous wave ultrasound is emitted from the transducer as a constant beam, and the returning signal originates from any vessel or structure within the line of the Doppler beam.[204] Pulsed Doppler is usually combined with real-time ultrasound as duplex Doppler. The vessel is imaged at the same time a range gate is placed over the vessel of interest. The returning signal originates only from this predetermined depth. Advantages of continuous wave Doppler include lower cost and use of lower power levels; advantages of duplex Doppler include the ability to image and interrogate the vessel of interest simultaneously. However, both continuous wave and pulsed Doppler provide similar information.[203]

Estimation of absolute flow raises a number of potential errors when applied to the umbilical vessels. Due to the normal tortuosity of the umbilical cord, the Doppler angle between the ultrasound beam and the direction of the umbilical artery usually is not known. Also, small errors in measurement of the umbilical arteries can lead to large variations in the estimated cross-sectional area. Estimation of umbilical venous flow is somewhat easier because the vein is larger and single.

Despite the potential errors, estimation of umbilical flow may have clinical value for certain conditions. Gill et al. have calculated that normal umbilical vein flow is 110 to 120 ml/min/kg throughout pregnancy.[206] For an average term infant, this would correspond to approximately 350 ml/min. This is in agreement with Van Lierde et al., who found that the calculated blood

FIG 16–59.
Umbilical cord hemangioma. Composite sonogram shows an echogenic mass *(M)* representing hemangioma near the placental insertion site of the umbilical cord. A cystic area *(C)* is also associated with the mass. The maternal serum alpha-fetoprotein was markedly elevated. *P* = placenta. (From Resta RG, Luthy DA, Mahony BS, et al: Umbilical cord hemangioma associated with extremely high alpha-fetoprotein levels. Obstet Gynecol 1988; 72:488–491. Used by permission.)

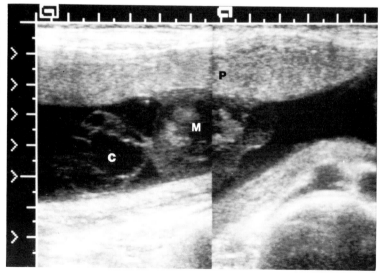

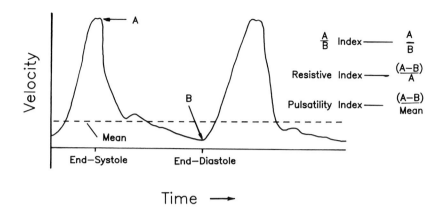

FIG 16–60.

Three commonly used clinical indices of the Doppler wave form: (1) peak systolic velocity *(A)*/end-diastolic peak velocity *(B)* ratio; (2) Pourcelot (resistive) index; and (3) pulsatility index. (From Nelson TR, Pretorius DH: The Doppler signal: Where does it come from and what does it mean? AJR 1988; 151:439–447. Used by permission.)

flow is 366 ± 65 ml/minute at term.[218] They also found that the average umbilical flow aortic flow ratio was 0.54 ± 0.07.

Because of the difficulties in estimating umbilical flow, waveform analysis is the most commonly used method for evaluating placental and umbilical flow.[215, 216] Unlike flow calculations, waveform analysis does not require knowledge of the Doppler angle or vessel dimensions. The umbilical waveform is most commonly expressed as the systolic-to-diastolic ratio (A/B ratio). Other parameters that have been used to describe the waveform are the pulsatility index (PI) and the Pourcelot ratio (Fig 16–60).[209]

Normal values of the systolic-to-diastolic ratio vary with gestational age with increasing end-diastolic flow observed with advancing gestation. However, in general, this ratio is less than 3 to 1 during the third trimester (Fig 16–61). Compromised fetuses may show reduced diastolic flow with various clinical conditions, including maternal hypertension, diabetes mellitus, IUGR, rhesus sensitization, systemic lupus erythematosus, other vascular disease, twin gestations, and fetal anomalies (Figs 16–62 and 16–63).[208, 210–215]

An association between decreased or absent diastolic flow and congenital anomalies is of particular interest. Trudinger and Cook reported that 13 of 26 fetuses (50%) with a major congenital malformation showed decreased diastolic flow.[214] Similarly, Meizner et al. reported decreased diastolic flow in 17 of 32 (53%) pregnancies complicated by a major fetal anomaly (Fig 16–64), whereas only 2 of 32 patients showed abnormal uterine artery flow.[208] Major anomalies in this series included malformations of the central nervous system (n=13), gastrointestinal tract (n=8), urinary tract (n=7), musculoskeletal system (n=2), and one case each of chylothorax and non–immune hydrops. In another study of 15 fetuses with absence of reversal of umbilical artery diastolic flow, Rochelson et al. reported that 11 occurred in association with maternal hypertension and 4 had lethal congenital anomalies (three had trisomy 18 and one had non–immune hydrops).[212] Eight fetuses died, including all four fetuses with congenital anomalies.

Possible mechanisms for decreased diastolic flow in fetuses with congenital anomalies include decreased cardiac output from cardiac anomalies (see Fig 16–62)

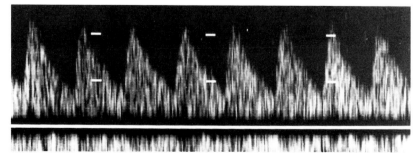

FIG 16–61.

Normal umbilical artery Doppler waveform. Doppler at 30 weeks shows a systolic-to-diastolic ratio of 2.7.

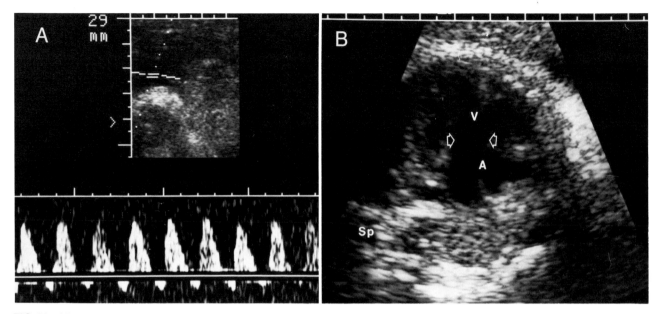

FIG 16-62.
Abnormal umbilical artery Doppler waveform. **A,** simultaneous real-time and duplex Doppler demonstrates reversal of diastolic flow. **B,** scan of the heart demonstrates a large atrioventricular septal defect *(open arrows).* Other anomalies included IUGR, cerebellar hypoplasia, single umbilical artery, and trisomy 18 karyotype. *A* = atria; *V* = ventricles; *Sp* = spine.

or increased placental resistance. Some authors have suggested that the anomalous fetus somehow initiates obliteration of the small arteries in the placenta.[214]

A possible relationship between abnormal umbilical artery waveforms and chromosome abnormalities is unclear. Wladimiroff et al. suggest that fetuses with chromosome abnormalities and IUGR demonstrate normal Doppler patterns.[219] However, we have noted abnormal flow patterns in some of these fetuses (see Fig 16–62 and 16–63). Also, Rochelson et al. suggest that chromosome analysis should be considered when absent diastolic flow is demonstrated in the absence of maternal hypertension or oligohydramnios.[212]

In interpreting umbilical artery waveforms, sonographers should be aware of pitfalls that may contribute to an artifactually large systolic-to-diastolic ratio. These include an unusually steep Doppler angle between the ultrasound beam and the direction of the vessel and setting the wall filter too high. The umbilical artery ratio may also vary with the location along the cord, with higher systolic flows observed near the fetal end of the umbilical cord. Although the waveforms of the two umbilical arteries usually are the same, two different waveforms occasionally can occur when one of the umbilical arteries supplies an area of infarcted placenta.[217]

FIG 16-63.
Trisomy 21. Umbilical artery Doppler at 26 weeks demonstrates decreased diastolic flow. Oligohydramnios, IUGR, and borderline lateral cerebral ventricular dilatation were also demonstrated. Chromosome analysis yielded trisomy 21.

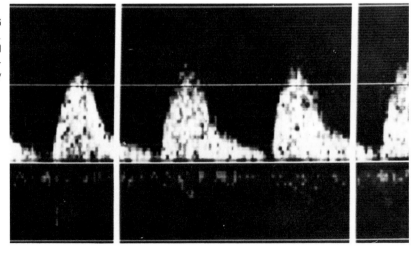

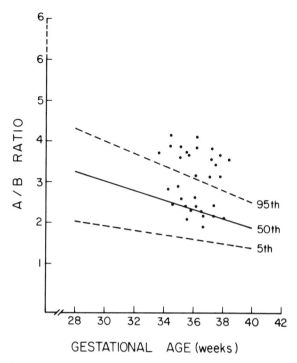

FIG 16–64.
Graph showing A/B (systolic/diastolic) ratios for 32 fetuses with major anomalies. Normal values are demonstrated within the dotted lines. (From Meizner I, Katz M, Lunenfeld E, et al: Umbilical and uterine flow velocity waveforms in pregnancies complicated by major fetal anomalies. Prenat Diagn 1987; 7:491–496. Used by permission.)

SUMMARY

A wide variety of abnormalities affecting the placenta, placental membranes, and umbilical cord can be detected by prenatal sonography. Careful evaluation of the location and appearance of the suspected abnormality should lead to the correct diagnosis and aid in obstetric management of these cases. Increasing use of umbilical and fetal Doppler should further help in identifying compromised or anomalous fetuses.

REFERENCES

The Placenta

Overview and Normal Development

1. Bowie JD, Andreotti RF, Rosenberg ER: Sonographic appearance of the uterine cervix in pregnancy: The vertical cervix. AJR 1983; 140:737–740.
2. Callen P, Filly R: The placental subplacental complex: A specific indicator of placental position on ultrasound. J Clin Ultrasound 1980; 8:21–26.
3. Cooperberg PL, Wright VJ, Carpenter CW: Ultrasonographic demonstration of a placental maternal lake. JCU 1979; 7:62–64.
4. Fox H: *Pathology of the Placenta.* Philadelphia, WB Saunders Co, 1978.
5. Hoddick WK, Mahony BS, Callen PW, et al: Placental thickness. J Ultrasound Med 1985; 4:479–482.
6. Laing FC: Ultrasound evaluation of obstetric problems relating to the lower uterine segment and cervix, in Sanders RC, James AE Jr (eds): *The Principles and Practice of Ultrasonography in Obstetrics and Gynecology,* ed 3. Norwalk, CT, Apple-Century-Crofts 1985, pp 355–367.
7. Marx M, Casola G, Scheible W, et al: The subplacental complex: Further sonographic observations. J Ultrasound Med 1985; 4:459–461.
8. Moore KL: *The Developing Human,* ed 4. Philadelphia, WB Saunders Co, 1988, pp 104–130.
9. Wigglesworth JS: *Perinatal Pathology.* Philadelphia, WB Saunders Co, 1984, pp 48–83.
10. Zemlyn S: The placenta, in Sarti (ed): *Diagnostic Ultrasound,* ed 2. Chicago, Year Book Medical Publishers, 1987, pp 839–856.

Placental Calcification

11. Brown HL, Miller JM Jr, Khawli O, et al: Premature placental calcification in maternal cigarette smokers. Obstet Gynecol 1988; 71:914–917.
12. Grannum RA, Berkowitz RL, Hobbins JC: The ultrasonic changes in the maturing placenta and their relationship to fetal pulmonic maturity. Am J Obstet Gynecol 1979; 133:915.
13. Hills D, Irwin GAL, Tuck S, et al: Distribution of placental grade in high-risk gravidas. AJR 1984; 143:1011–1013.
14. Hopper KD, Komppa GH, Williams BP, et al: A reevaluation of placental grading and its clinical significance. J Ultrasound Med 1984; 3:261–266.
15. Kazzi GM, Gross TL, Solol RJ, et al: Detection of intrauterine growth retardation: A new use for sonographic placental grading. Am J Obstet Gynecol 1983; 145:733–737.
16. Petrucha RA, Platt LD: Relationship of placental grade to gestational age. Am J Obstet Gynecol 1982; 144:733.

Placenta Previa and Vaginal Bleeding

17. Artis AA III, Bowie JD, Rosenberg ER, et al: The fallacy of placental migration: Effect of sonographic techniques. AJR 1985; 144:79–81.
18. Bowie JD, Rochester D, Cadkin AV, et al: Accuracy of placental localization by ultrasound. Radiology 1978; 128:177–180.
19. Crenshaw CJ, Jones DED, Parker RT: Placenta praevia: A survey of twenty years experience with improved

perinatal survival by expected therapy and cesarean delivery. Obstet Gynecol Surv 1975; 28:461–470.

20. Farine D, Fox HE, Jakobson S, et al: Vaginal ultrasound for diagnosis of placenta previa. Obstet Gynecol 1988; 159:566–569.

21. Gallagher P, Fagan CJ, Bedi DG, et al: Potential placenta previa: Definition, frequency, and significance. AJR 1987; 149:1013–1015.

22. Gillieson MS, Winer-Muran HT, Muran D: Low-lying placenta. Radiology 1982; 144:577–580.

23. Goplerud CP: Bleeding in late pregnancy, in Danforth DN (ed): *Obstetrics and Gynecology,* ed 3. Hagerstown, MD, Harper & Row, 1977, pp 378–384.

24. Green-Thompson RW: Antepartum hemorrhage. Clin Obstet Gynecol 1982; 9:479–515.

25. Hibbard LT: Placenta praevia. Am J Obstet Gynecol 1969; 104:172–176.

26. Jeffrey RB, Laing FC: Sonography of the low-lying placenta: Value of Trendelenburg and traction scans. AJR 1981; 137:547–549.

27. King DL: Placental migration demonstrated by ultrasonography. Radiology 1973; 109:167–170.

28. Mittelstaedt CA, Partain CL, Boyce IL Jr, et al: Placenta previa: significance in the second trimester. Radiology 1979; 131:465–468.

29. Naeye RL: Placenta previa: Predisposing factors and effects on the fetus and surviving infants. Obstet Gynecol 1978; 52:521–525.

30. Newton ER, Barss V, Cetrulo CL: The epidemiology and clinical history of asymptomatic midtrimester placenta previa. Am J Obstet Gynecol 1984; 148:743–748.

31. Scheer K: Ultrasonic diagnosis of placenta previa. Obstet Gynecol 1973; 42:707–710.

32. Townsend RT, Laing FC, Nyberg DA, et al: Technical factors responsible for "placental migration:" Sonographic assessment. Radiology 1986; 160:105–108.

33. Wexler P, Gottesfeld KR: Second trimester placenta previa: An apparently normal placentation. Obstet Gynecol 1977; 50:706–709.

34. Wexler P, Gottesfeld KR: Early diagnosis of placenta previa. Obstet Gynecol 1979; 54:231–234.

35. Zemlyn S: The effect of the urinary bladder in obstetrical sonography. Radiology 1978; 128:169–175.

36. Zemlyn S. The placenta, in Sarti D (ed): *Diagnostic Ultrasound,* ed 2. Chicago, Year Book Medical Publishers, Inc, 1987, pp 839–856.

Abruption and Periplacental Hemorrhage

37. Combs CA: Personal communication.

38. Desa DJ: Rupture of fetal vessels on placental surface. Arch Dis Child 1971; 46:495–501.

39. Douglas RG, Buchman MI, MacDonald FA: Premature separation of the normally implanted placenta. J Obstet Gynecol 1955; 72:710–736.

40. Goldstein SR, Subramanyan BR, Raghavendra BN, et al: Subchorionic bleeding in threatened abortion: Sonographic findings and significance. AJR 1983; 141:975–978.

41. Gruenwald P, Levin H, Yousem H: Abruption and premature separation of the placenta. Am J Obstet Gynecol 1968; 102:604–610.

42. Harris BA: Marginal placental bleeding. Am J Obstet Gynecol 1952; 61:53–61.

43. Harris BA, Gore H, Flowers CE: Peripheral placental separation: A possible relationship to premature labor. Obstet Gynecol 1985; 66:774–778.

44. Hibbard BM, Jeffcoate TNA: Abruptio placentae. Obstet Gynecol 1966; 27:155–167.

45. Hurd WW, Miodovnik M, Hertzberg V, et al: Selective management of abruptio placenta: A prospective study. Obstet Gynecol 1983; 61:467–483.

46. Jaffe MH, Schoen WC, Silver TM, et al: Sonography of abruptio placentae. AJR 1981; 137:1049–1054.

47. Knab DR: Abruptio placentae. An assessment of the time and method of delivery. Obstet Gynecol 1978; 52:625–629.

48. McGahan JP, Phillips HE, Reid MH, et al: Sonographic spectrum of retroplacental hemorrhage. Radiology 1982; 142:481–485.

49. Mintz MC, Kurtz AB, Arenson R, et al: Abruptio placentae: Apparent thickening of the placenta caused by hyperechoic retroplacental clot. J Ultrasound Med 1986; 5:411–413.

50. Naeye RL, Harkness WL, Utts J: Abruptio placentae and perinatal death: A prospective study. Am J Obstet Gynecol 1977; 128:740–746.

51. Naeye RL: Abrupto placentae and placenta previa: Frequency, perinatal mortality, and cigarette smoking. Obstet Gynecol 1980; 55:701–704.

52. Nyberg DA, Cyr DR, Mack LA, et al: Sonographic spectrum of placental abruption. AJR 1987; 148:161–164.

53. Nyberg DA, Mack LA, Benedetti TJ, et al: Placental abruption and placental hemorrhage: Correlation of sonographic findings with fetal outcome. Radiology, 1987; 164;357–361.

54. Odendaal HJ: The frequency of uterine contractions in abruptio placentae. S Africa Med J 1976; 50:2129–2131.

55. Sauerbrei EE, Pham DH: Placental abruption and subchorionic hemorrhage in the first half of pregnancy: Ultrasound appearance and clinical outcome. Radiolog 1986; 160:109–112.

56. Sexton LI, Hertig AT, Reid DE, et al: Premature separation of the normally implanted placenta. Am J Obstet Gynecol 1950; 59:13–24.

57. Shanklin DR, Scott JS: Massive subchorial thrombohaematoma (Breus' mole). Br J Obstet Gynaecol 1975; 82:476–487.

58. Sher G: A rational basis for the management of abruptio placentae. J Reprod Med 1978; 31:123–129.

59. Sholl JS: Abruptio placentae: Clinical management in nonacute cases. Am J Obstet Gynecol 1987; 156:40–51.

60. Spirt BA, Kagan EH, Rozanski RM: Abruptio placenta: Sonographic and pathologic correlation. AJR 1979; 133:877–881.
61. Spirt BA, Gordon LP, Kagan EH: The placenta: Sonographic-pathologic correlations. Semin Roentgen 1982; 17:219–230.
62. Townsend RR, Laing FC, Jeffrey RB Jr: Placental abruption associated with cocaine abuse. AJR 1988; 150:1339–1340.
63. Williams CH, VanBergen WS, Prentice RL: Extra-amniotic blood clot simulating placenta previa on ultrasound scan. J Clin Ultrasound 1976; 5:45–47.

Gestational Trophoblastic Disease

64. Bree RL, Silver TM, Wicks JD, et al: Trophoblastic disease with coexistent fetus: A sonographic and clinical spectrum. J Clin Ultrasound 1978; 6:310–314.
65. Callen PW: Ultrasonography in evaluation of gestational trophoblastic disease, in Callen PW (ed): *Ultrasonography in Obstetrics and Gynecology,* Philadelphia, WB Saunders Co, 1983; pp 259–270.
66. Chatterjee MS, Tejani NA, Verma UL, et al: Prenatal diagnosis of triploidy. Int J Gynaecol Obstet 1982; 21:155–157.
67. Jacobs PA, Szulman AE, Funkhauser J, et al: Human triploidy: Relationship between parenteral origin of the additional haploid complement and development of partial hydatidiform mole. Ann Hum Genet 1982; 46:223–231.
68. Lockwood C, Scioscia A, Stiller R, et al: Sonographic features of the triploid fetus. Am J Obstet Gynecol 1987; 157:285–287.
69. Munyer TP, Callen PW, Filly RA, et al: Further observations on the sonographic spectrum of gestational trophoblastic disease. J Clin Ultrasound 1981; 9:349–358.
70. Reid MH, McGahan JP, Oi R: Sonographic evaluation of partial hydatidiform mole and its look-alikes. AJR 1981; 140:307–311.
71. Rubenstein JB, Swayne LC, Dise CA, et al: Placental changes in fetal triploidy syndrome. J Ultrasound Med 1986; 5:545–560.
72. Sauerbrei EE, Salem S, Fayle B: Coexistent hydatiform mole and live fetus in the second trimester. Radiology 1980; 135:415–417.
73. Szulman AE, Surti U: The syndromes of hydatiform mole. I. Cytogenetic and morphologic correlations. Am J Obstet Gynecol 1978; 131:665–671.
74. Szulman AE, Philippe E, Boue JG, et al: Human triploidy: Association with partial hydatidiform moles and nonmolar conceptuses. Hum Pathol 1981; 12:1016–1021.
75. Uchida JA, Freeman VCP: Triploidy and chromosomes. Am J Obstet Gynecol 1985; 151:65–69.
76. Watson EJ, Hernandez E, Miyazawa K: Partial hydatidiform moles: A review. Obstet Gynecol Surv 1987; 42:540–544.

Placental Chorioangioma

77. Asadourian LA, Taylor HB: Clinical significance of placental hemangiomas. Obstet Gynecol 1968; 31:551–555.
78. De Costa EJ, Gerbie AB, Andresen RH, et al: Placental tumors: Hemangiomas. Obstet Gynecol 1956; 7:249.
79. Froehlich LA, Fujikura T, Fisher P: Chorioangiomas and their clinical implications. Obstet Gynecol 1971; 37:51–59.
80. Kuhnel P: Placental chorioangioma. Acta Obstet Gynecol Scand 1933; 13:143.
81. O'Malley BP, Toi A, deSa DJ, et al: Ultrasound appearances of placental chorioangioma. Radiology 1981; 138:159–160.
82. Reiner L, Fries E: Chorioangioma associated with arteriovenous aneurysm. Am J Obstet Gynecol 1965; 93:58–64.
83. Rodan BA, Bean WJ: Chorioangioma of the placenta causing intrauterine fetal demise. J Ultrasound Med 1983; 2:95–97.
84. Spirt BA, Gordon L, Cohen WN, et al: Antenatal diagnosis of chorioangioma of the placenta. AJR 1980; 135:1273–1275.
85. van Wering JH, van der Slikke JW: Prenatal diagnosis of chorioangioma associated with polyhydramnios using ultrasound. Eur J Obstet Gynecol Reprod Biol 1985; 19:255–259.
86. Willard DA, Moeschler JB: Placental chorioangioma: A rare cause of elevated amniotic fluid alpha-fetoprotein. J Ultrasound Med 1986; 5:221–222.

Placental Abnormalities and AFP Levels

87. Brock DJH, Barron L, Duncan P, et al: Significance of elevated mid-trimester maternal plasma-alpha-fetoprotein values. Lancet 1979; i:1281–1282.
88. Brock DJH: Mechanisms by which amniotic-fluid alpha-fetoprotein may be increased in fetal abnormalities. Lancet 1976; ii:345–346.
89. Devi B, Jennison RF, Langley FA: Significance of placental pathology in transplacental haemorrhage. J Clin Path 1968; 21:322–331.
90. Dyer SN, Burton BK, Nelson LH: Elevated maternal serum alpha-fetoprotein levels and oligohydramnios: Poor prognosis for pregnancy outcome. Am J Obstet Gynecol 1987; 157:336–339.
91. Fleischer AC, Kurtz AB, Wapner RJ, et al: Elevated alpha-fetoprotein and a normal fetal sonogram: Association with placental abnormalities. AJR 1988; 150:881–883.
92. Hamilton MPR, Abdalla HI, Whitfield CR: Significance of raised maternal serum alpha-fetoprotein in singleton pregnancies with normally formed fetuses. Obstet Gynecol 1985; 64:465–470.
93. Hoogland HJ, de Haan J, Vooys GP: Ultrasonographic diagnosis of intervillous thrombosis related to Rh

isoimmunization. Gynecol Obstet Invest 1979; 10:237–245.

94. Javert CT, Reiss C: The origin and significance of macroscopic coagulation hematomas (red infarcts) of the human placenta. Surg Gynecol Obstet 1952; 94:257–269.

95. Kelly RB, Nyberg DA, Mack LA, et al: Sonography of placental abnormalities and oligohydramnios in women with elevated alpha-fetoprotein levels: Comparison with control subjects. AJR, in press.

96. Koontz WL, Seeds JH, Adama NJ, et al: Elevated maternal serum alpha-fetoprotein, second-trimester oligohydramnios, and pregnancy outcome. Obstet Gynecol 1983; 62:301–304.

97. Lachman E, Hingley SM, Bates G, et al: Detection and measurement of fetomaternal haemorrhage: Serum alpha-fetoprotein and the Kleihauer technique. Br Med J 1977; 1:1377–1379.

98. Los FJ, de Wolf BTHM, Huisjes HJ: Raised maternal serum-alpha-fetoprotein levels and spontaneous fetomaternal transfusion. Lancet 1979; ii:1210–1212.

99. Main DM, Mennut MT: Neural tube defects: Issues in prenatal diagnosis and counseling. Obstet Gynecol 1986; 67:1–15.

100. Milunsky A, Alpert E: Results and benefits of a maternal serum alpha-fetoprotein screening program. JAMA 1984; 252:1438–1442.

101. Perkes EA, Baim RS, Goodman KJ, et al: Second-trimester placental changes associated with elevated maternal serum alpha-fetoprotein. Am J Obstet Gynecol 1982; 144:935–938.

102. Richards DS, Seeds JW, Katz VL, et al: Elevated maternal serum alpha-fetoprotein with oligohydramnios: Ultrasound evaluation and outcome. Obstet Gynecol 1988; 72:337–341.

103. Salafia CM, Silberman L, Herrera NE, et al: Placental pathology at term associated with elevated midtrimester maternal serum alpha-fetoprotein concentration. Am J Obstet Gynecol 1988; 158:1064–1066.

104. Seller MJ, Child AH: Raised maternal serum alpha-fetoprotein, oligohydramnios, and the fetus. Lancet 1980; i:317–318.

105. Spirt BA, Gordon LP, Kagan EH: Intervillous thrombosis: Sonographic and pathologic correlation. Radiology 1983; 147:197–200.

106. Wentworth P: A placental lesion to account for foetal haemorrhage into the maternal circulation. Br J Obstet Gynecol 1964; 71:379–387.

Other Placental Abnormalities

107. Janniaux E, Auni FE, Conner C, et al: Ultrasonographic diagnosis and morphologic study of placenta circumvallate. J Clin Ultrasound 1989; 17:126–131.

108. Jeanty P, Kirkpatrick C, Verhoogen C, et al: The succenturiate placenta. J Ultrasound Med 1983; 2:9–12.

109. de Mendonca LK: Sonographic diagnosis of placenta accreta: Presentation of six cases. J Ultrasound Med 1988; 7:211–215.

110. Pasto ME, Kurtz AB, Rijkin MD, et al: Ultrasonographic findings of placenta increta. J Ultrasound Med 1983; 2:155–159.

111. Shapiro LR, Duncan PA, Daudian MM, et al: The placenta in familial Beckwith-Wiedemann syndrome. Birth Defects 1982; 18:203–206.

Membranes

Amniotic Band Syndrome

112. Ashkanazu M, Borenstein R, Kate Z, et al: Constriction of the umbilical cord by an amniotic band after midtrimester amniocentesis. Acta Obstet Gynecol Scand 1982; 61:89–91.

113. Baker CJ, Rudolph AJ: Congenital ring constrictions and intrauterine amputations. Am J Dis Child 1971; 121:393–400.

114. Barss VA, Benacerraf BR, Frigoletto FD: Ultrasonographic determination of chorion type in twin gestation. Obstet Gynecol 1985; 66:779–783.

115. Bourne GL: The microscopic anatomy of the human amnion and chorion. Am J Obstet Gynecol 1960; 79:1070–1073.

116. Burrows PE, Lyons EA, Phillips HJ, et al: Intrauterine membranes: Sonographic findings and clinical significance. J Clin Ultrasound 1982; 10:1–8.

117. Fiske CE, Filly RA, Golbus MS: Prenatal ultrasound diagnosis of amniotic band syndrome. J Ultrasound Med. 1982; 1:45–47.

118. Hertzberg BS, Kurtz AB, Choi HY, et al: Significance of membrane thickness in the sonographic evaluation of twin gestations. AJR 1987; 148:151–153.

119. Higgenbottom MC, Jones KL, Hall BD, et al: The amniotic band disruption complex: Timing of amniotic rupture and variable spectra of consequent defects. J Pediatr 1979; 95:544–549.

120. Hunter AGW, Carpenter BF: Implications of malformations not due to amniotic bands in the amniotic band sequence. Am J Med Genet 1986; 24:691–700.

121. Lavery JP: Appendages of the placenta, in Lavery JP (ed): *The Human Placenta-Clinical Perspectives*. Rockville, Maryland, Aspen Publishers, 1987, pp 257–279.

122. Mahony BS, Filly RA, Callen PW, et al: The amniotic band syndrome: Antenatal diagnosis and potential pitfalls. Am J Obstet Gynecol 1985; 152:63–68.

123. Mahony BS, Filly RA, Callen PW: Amnionicity and chorionicity in twin pregnancies: Prediction using ultrasound. Radiology 1985; 155:205–209.

124. Moessinger AC, Blan WA, Byrne J, et al: Amniotic band syndrome associated with amniocentesis. Am J Obstet Gynecol 1981; 141:588–591.

125. Randel SB, Filly RA, Callen PW, et al: Amniotic sheets. Radiology 1988; 166:633–636.

126. Rehder H, Weitzell H: Intrauterine caputation after amniocentesis. Lancet 1978; 1:382.

127. Seeds JW, Cefalo RC, Herbert WNP: Amniotic band syndrome. Am J Obstet Gynecol 1982; 144:243–248.

128. Torpin R: Amniochorionic mesoblastic fibrous strings and amniotic bands. Am J Obstet Gynecol 1965; 91:65–75.
129. Townsend RR, Simpson GF, Filly RA: Membrane thickness in ultrasound prediction of chorionicity of twin gestations. J Ultrasound Med 1988; 7:327–332.
130. Van Allen MI, Curry C, Gallagher: Limb-body wall complex. I: Pathogenesis. Am J Med Genet 1987; 28:529–548.
131. Van Allen MI, Curry C, Walden L, et al: Limb-body wall complex. II: Limb and spine defects. Am J Med Genet 1987; 28:549–565.

The Umbilical Cord

Overview and Umbilical Circulation

132. Chinn DH, Filly RA, Callen PW: Ultrasonic evaluation of fetal umbilical and hepatic vascular anatomy. Radiology 1982; 144:153–157.
133. Hill LM, Kislak S, Runco C: An ultrasonic view of the umbilical cord. Obstet Gynecol Survey 1987; 42:82–88.
134. Lacro RV, Jones KL, Benirschke K: The umbilical cord twist: Origin, direction, and relevance. Am J Obstet Gynecol 1987; 157:833–838.
135. Miller ME, Higginbottom M, Smith DW: Short umbilical cord: Its origin and relevance. Pediatrics 1981; 67:618–621.
136. Nakari BG: Congenital anomalies of the human umbilical cord and their clinical significance: A light and microscopic study. Ind J Med Res 1969; 57:1018–1025.
137. Purola E: The length and insertion of the umbilical cord. Ann Chir Gynaecol 1968; 57:621–622.
138. Walker CW, Pye BG: The length of the human umbilical cord: A statistical report. Br Med J 1960; 1:546–548.

Single Umbilical Artery

139. Benirschke K, Brown WH: A vascular anomaly of the umbilical cord. Obstet Gynecol 1955; 6:399–404.
140. Benirschke K, Bourne GL: The incidence and prognostic implication of congenital absence of one umbilical artery. Am J Obstet Gynecol 1960; 79:251–254.
141. Bryan EM, Kohler HG: The missing umbilical artery: Prospective study based on a maternity unit. Arch Dis Child 1974; 49:844–852.
142. Byrne J, Blane WA: Malformations and chromosome anomalies in spontaneously aborted fetuses with single umbilical artery. Am J Obstet Gynecol 1985; 1:340–342.
143. Faierman E: The significance of one umbilical artery. Arch Dis Child 1960; 35:285–288.
144. Froehlich LA, Fukikura T: Significance of a single umbilical artery. Report from the collaborative study of cerebral palsy. Am J Obstet Gynecol 1966; 94:274–279.
145. Froehlich LA, Fujikura T: Follow-up of infants with single umbilical artery. Pediatrics 1973; 52:6–13.

146. Heifetz SA: Single umbilical artery. Perspect Pediatr Pathol 1984; 8:345–378.
147. Herrman UJ Jr, Sidropoulos D: Single umbilical artery: Prenatal findings. Prenat Diagn 1988; 8:275–280.
148. Hodes ME, Cole J, Palmer CG, et al: Clinical experience with trisomies 18 and 13. J Med Genetics 1978; 15:48–60.
149. Janosko EO, Zona JZ, Belin RP: Congenital anomalies of the umbilicus. Amer Surgeon 1977; 177–185.
150. Jassani MN, Brennan JN, Meshatz IR: Prenatal diagnosis of single umbilical artery by ultrasound. J Clin Ultrasound 1980; 8:447–448.
151. Lenoski EF, Medovy H: Single umbilical artery: Incidence, clinical significance and relation to autosomal trisomy. Can Med Assoc J 1962; 87:1229–1231.
152. Lewis AJ: Autosomal trisomy. Lancet 1962; i:866.
153. Monie IW: Genesis of single umbilical artery. Am J Obstet Gynecol 1970; 108:400–405.
154. Nyberg DA, Shepard T, Mack LA, et al: Significance of a single umbilical artery in fetuses with CNS malformations. J Ultrasound Med 1988; 7:265–273.
155. Peckham CH, Yerushalmy J: Aplasia of one umbilical artery: Incidence by race and certain obstetric factors. Obstet Gynecol 1965; 26:359–366.
156. Tortora M, Chervenak FA, Mayden K, et al: Antenatal sonographic diagnosis of single umbilical artery. Obstet Gynecol 1984; 63:693–696.
157. Vlietinck RF, Thiery M, Orye E, et al: Significance of the single umbilical artery. Arch Dis Child 1972; 47:639–642.

Multiple Vessel Cord

158. Beck R, Naulty CM: A human umbilical cord with four arteries. Clin Pediatr 1985; 24:118–119.
159. Murdock DE: Umbilical cord doubling: Report of a case. Obstet Gynecol 1966; 27:555–557.
160. Painter D, Russel P: Four-vessel umbilical cord associated with multiple congenital anomalies. Obstet Gynecol 1977; 50:505–507.

Cord Presentation and Prolapse

161. Donnelly PB, Rosenberg MA, Kay CJ, et al: Sonographic demonstration of occult umbilical cord prolapse. AJR 1980; 134:1060–1061.
162. Hales ED, Westney LS: Sonography of occult cord prolapse. J Clin Ultrasound 1984; 12:283–285.
163. Lange IR, Manning FA, Morrison I, et al: Cord prolapse: Is antenatal diagnosis possible? Am J Obstet Gynecol 1985; 151:1083–1085.
164. Mendez-Bauer C, Ruiz Canseco A, Ruiz MA, et al: Early decelerations of the fetal heart rate from occlusion of the umbilical cord. J Perinat Med 1978; 6:69–79.
165. Myles TJM: Prolapse of the umbilical cord. Br J Obstet Gynaecol 1959; 66:301–310.

Nuchal Cord

166. Jouppila P, Kirkenen P: Ultrasonic diagnosis of nuchal encirclement by the umbilical cord: A case and methodological report. J Clin Ultrasound 1982; 10:59–62.

167. Shui KP, Eastman NJ: Coiling of the umbilical cord around the fetal neck. Br J Obstet Gynaecol 1957; 64:227–228.

168. Spellacy WN, Gravem H, Fisch RO: The umbilical cord complications of true knots, nuchal coils and cord around the body. Am J Obstet Gynecol 1966; 94:1136.

169. Stembera ZK, Horska S: The influence of coiling of the umbilical cord around the neck of the fetus on its gas metabolism and acid-base balance. Biol Neonate 1972; 20:214.

Cord Knot

170. Hertzberg BJ, Bowie JD, Bradford WD, et al: False knot of the umbilical cord: Sonographic appearance and differential diagnosis. J Clin Ultrasound 1988; 16:599–602.

171. Nyberg DA, Filly RA, Golbus MS, et al: Entangled umbilical cords: A sign of monoamniotic twins. J Ultrasound Med 1984; 3:29–32.

Umbilical Cord Enlargement

172. Casola G, Scheible W, Leopold GR: Large umbilical cord: A normal finding in some fetuses. Radiology 1985; 156:181–182.

173. Chantler C, Baum JD, Wigglesworth JS, et al: Giant umbilical cord associated with patent urachus and fused umbilical arteries. J Obstet Gynecol 1969; 76:273–274.

174. DeVore GR, Mayden K, Tortora M, et al: Dilatation of the fetal umbilical vein in rhesus hemolytic anemia: A predictor of severe disease. Am J Obstet Gynecol 1981; 141:464–467.

175. Ente G, Penzer PH, Keningsberg K: Giant umbilical cord associated with patent urachus. Amer J Dis Child 1970; 120:82–83.

176. Fuster JS, Benasco C, Saad I: Giant dilatation of the umbilical vein. J Clin Ultrasound 1985; 13:363–365.

177. Nyberg DA, Fitzsimmons J, Mack LA, et al: Chromosomal abnormalities in fetuses with omphalocele: The significance of omphalocele contents. J Ultrasound Med 1989; 8:299–308.

178. Quartero HWP, van de Berg W, Kolkman PH: A prenatal diagnosis of umbilical cord oedema made by ultrasound; a case report. Eur J Obstet Gynecol Reprod Biol 1984; 17:409–412.

179. Ramanathan K, Epstein S, Yaghooben J: Localized deposition of Wharton's jelly: Sonographic findings. J Ultrasound Med 1986; 5:339–340.

180. Witter FR, Graham D: The utility of ultrasonically measured umbilical vein diameters in isoimmunized pregnancies. Am J Obstet Gynecol 1983; 146:225–226.

Umbilical Cord Cysts

181. Blanc WA, Allan GW: Intrafunicular ulceration of persistent omphalomesenteric duct with intra-amniotic hemorrhage and fetal death. Am J Obstet Gynecol 1961; 82:1392–1396.

182. Doscher C: The patent omphalomesenteric duct. Illinois Medical Journal 1971; 493–496.

183. Fink IJ, Filly RA: Omphalocele associated with umbilical cord allantoic cyst: Sonographic evaluation in utero. Radiology 1983; 149:473–476.

184. Heifetz SA, Rueda-Pedraza ME: Omphalomesenteric duct cysts of the umbilical cord. Am J Pediatr Pathol 1983; 1:325.

185. Iaccarino M, Baldi I, Persico O, et al: Ultrasonographic and pathologic study of mucoid degeneration of umbilical cord. J Clin Ultrasound 1986; 14:127–129.

186. Petrikovsky BM, Nochimson DJ, Campbell WA, et al: Fetal jejunoileal atresia with persistent omphalomesenteric duct. Am J Obstet Gynecol 1988; 158:173–175.

187. Radade RV, Niphadkar KB, Mysorekar VR: Extraumbilical allantoic cyst: A case report. Indian J Pathol Microbiol 1966; 9:87–89.

188. Sachs L, Fourcroy JL, Wenzel DJ, et al: Prenatal detection of umbilical cord allantoic cyst. Radiology 1982; 145:445–446.

189. Rosenberg JC, Chervenak FA, Walker BA, et al: Antenatal sonographic appearance of omphalomesenteric duct cyst. J Ultrasound Med 1986; 5:719–720.

Umbilical Cord Hematoma, Thrombosis

190. Abrams SL, Callen PW, Filly RA: Umbilical vein thrombosis: Sonographic detection in utero. J Ultrasound Med 1985; 4:283–285.

191. Clare NM, Hayashi R, Khodr G: Intrauterine death from umbilical cord hematoma. Arch Pathol Lab Med 1979; 103:46–47.

192. Dipple AL: Hematoma of the umbilical cord. Surg Gynecol Obstet 1940; 70:51.

193. Gassner CB, Paul RH: Laceration of umbilical cord vessels secondary to amniocentesis. Obstet Gynecol 1976; 48:627–630.

194. Ruvinsky ED, Wiley TL, Morrison JC, et al: In utero diagnosis of umbilical cord hematoma. Am J Obstet Gynecol 1981; 140:833–834.

195. Schreier R: Hematoma of the umbilical cord. Obstet Gynecol 1962; 20:798–800.

196. Sutro WH, Tuck SM, Loesevitz A, et al: Prenatal observation of umbilical cord hematoma. AJR 1984; 142:801–802.

Umbilical Cord Hemangioma

197. Barry FE, McCoy CP, Callahan WP: Hemangioma of the umbilical cord. Am J Obstet Gynecol 1951; 62:675–680.

198. Baylis MS, Jones RY, Hughes M: Angiomyoma of the

umbilical cord detected antenatally by ultrasound. J Obstet Gynecol 1984; 4:243.

199. Benirschke K, Dodds JP: Angiomyxoma of the umbilical cord with atrophy of an umbilical artery. Obstet Gynecol 1967; 30:99–102.

200. Fortune DW, Ostor AG: Angiomyxomas of the umbilical cord. Obstet Gynecol 1980; 55:375–381.

201. Resta RG, Luthy DA, Mahony BS: Umbilical cord hemangioma associated with extremely high alpha-fetoprotein levels. Obstet Gynecol 1988; 72:488–491.

202. Seifer DB, Ferguson JE II, Behrens CM, et al: Nonimmune hydrops fetalis in association with hemangioma of the umbilical cord. Obstet Gynecol 1985; 66:283–286.

Umbilical Doppler

203. Brar HS, Medearis AL, De Vore GR, et al: Fetal umbilical velocimetry using continuous-wave and pulsed-wave Doppler ultrasound in high-risk pregnancies: A comparison of systolic to diastolic ratios. Obstet Gynecol 1988; 72:607–610.

204. Fitzgerald DE, Stuart B, Drumm E, et al: The assessment of the fetoplacental circulation with continuous-wave Doppler ultrasound. Ultrasound Med Biol 1984; 10:371–376.

205. Giles WB, Trudinger BJ, Baird PPJ: Fetal umbilical artery flow velocity waveforms and placental resistance: Pathologic correlation. Br J Obstet Gynaecol 1985; 92:31–38.

206. Gill RW, Kossof G, Warren PS, et al: Umbilical venous flow in normal and complicated pregnancy. Ultrasound Med Biol 1984; 10:349–363.

207. McCowan LM, Erskine LA, Ritchie K: Umbilical artery Doppler blood flow studies in the preterm, small for gestational age fetus. Am J Obstet Gynecol 1987; 156:655–659.

208. Meizner I, Katz M, Lunenfeld E, et al: Umbilical and uterine flow velocity waveforms in pregnancies complicated by major fetal anomalies. Prenat Diagn 1987; 7:491–496.

209. Nelson TR, Pretorius DH: The Doppler signal: Where does it come from and what does it mean? AJR 1988; 151:439–447.

210. Nimrod C, Davies D, Harder J, et al: Doppler ultrasound prediction of fetal outcome in twin pregnancies. Am J Obstet Gynecol 1987; 156:402–406.

211. Pretorius DH, Manchester D, Barkin S, et al: Doppler ultrasound of twin transfusion syndrome. J Ultrasound Med 1988; 7:117–124.

212. Rochelson B, Schulman H, Farmakides G, et al: The significance of absent end-diastolic velocity in umbilical artery velocity waveforms. Am J Obstet Gynecol 1987; 156:1213–1218.

213. Schulman H: The clinical implication of Doppler ultrasound analysis of the uterine and umbilical arteries. Am J Obstet Gynecol 1987; 156:889–893.

214. Trudinger BJ, Cook CM: Umbilical and uterine artery waveforms in pregnancy associated with major fetal abnormality. Br J Obstet Gynaecol 1985; 92:666–670.

215. Trudinger BJ, Cook CM, Jones et al: A comparison of fetal heart rate monitoring and umbilical artery waveforms in the recognition of fetal compromise. Br J Obstet Gynaecol 1986; 93:171–175.

216. Trudinger BJ: The umbilical circulation. Semin Perinat 1987; 11:311–321.

217. Trudinger BJ, Cook CM: Different umbilical artery flow velocity waveforms in one patient. Obstet Gynecol 1988; 71:1019–1021.

218. Van Lierde M, Oberweis D, Thomas K: Ultrasonic measurement of aortic and umbilical blood flow in the human fetus. Obstet Gynecol 1984; 63:801–805.

219. Wladimiroff JW, Touge JM, Stewart PA, et al: Severe intrauterine growth retardation: Assessment of its origin from fetal arterial flow velocity waveforms. Eur J Obstet Gynecol Reprod Biol 1986; 22:23–28.

Chromosome Abnormalities

David A. Nyberg, M.D.

James P. Crane, M.D.

Simply stated, chromosome abnormalities can be considered as genetic mutations large enough to visualize under the microscope.[8] Because large segments of the genome are affected, chromosome abnormalities are associated with multiple congenital anomalies, a high mortality and morbidity rate, and a poor long-term prognosis. For these reasons, detection of major chromosome abnormalities has been a subject of intense interest and research in the last two decades.

This chapter is arranged in three parts. As a basis for understanding chromosome abnormalities, a clinical perspective is discussed in the first part of the chapter. Sonographic risk factors that have been associated with major chromosome abnormalities, primarily autosomal disorders, are discussed in the second part. Due to their frequency and importance, pathologic features of trisomies 21, 18, and 13; 45, X; and triploidy are discussed separately in the third part of the chapter.

CLINICAL PERSPECTIVE

Scope of the Problem

Chromosome abnormalities are present in approximately 1 of every 180 live born infants (0.56%), and, of these, approximately one third are autosomal disorders, one third are sex chromosome abnormalities, and one third are translocations or other rearrangements.[21] However, a much higher prevalence of chromosome abnormalities is found in women undergoing mid-trimester amniocentesis. In a collaborative European study of women undergoing amniocentesis

because of a maternal age $\geq$ 35 years, some type of chromosome abnormality was found in 2.26% of women and, of these, 51% were trisomy 21, 13% were trisomies 18 or 13, 11% were translocations, 17% were sex chromosome abnormalities, and 8% were other types.[9]

The differences between prenatal and neonatal series of chromosome disorders can be attributed both to the higher risk of older women undergoing amniocentesis, and to the high spontaneous loss rate of fetuses with major chromosome abnormalities.

Fetuses with chromosome abnormalities have a high mortality throughout pregnancy, with the greatest loss during the first trimester. Aneuploidy is found in 60% of early spontaneous abortuses and 6% of stillborns compared to only 0.5% of live borns. Approximately one third of fetuses with trisomy 21 and 70% of fetuses with trisomy 18 found at the time of second-trimester amniocentesis will die before birth.[11, 12] The mortality rate continues to be high after birth, since only 50% of infants born with trisomy 21 and few infants with trisomies 18 or 13 will survive to 5 years of age.

Survivors with a major chromosome abnormality can be expected to have significant intellectual impairment. It is estimated that 25% of all individuals with an IQ (intelligence quotient) less than 50 have a chromosome disorder, primarily trisomy 21.[13] The cost of hospitalization and institutionalization of these patients has been emphasized.[13] The psychological and emotional impact on the parents and family unit is even more devastating but more difficult to measure; birth of a child with a major chromosome abnormality or congenital malformation frequently leads to guilt, alterations in lifestyle, and family disruption.

Because of the uniformly dismal outcome associated with a major chromosome abnormality, cesarean delivery generally is considered an unnecessary risk to the mother of an affected fetus.[20] If the underlying fetal abnormality is not recognized, however, intrapartum fetal distress may lead to a higher rate of cesarean deliveries. Schneider et al. reported that during the period 1974 to 1979, 15 of 28 fetuses (56%) with trisomy 18 were delivered by primary cesarean section, and 11 (39%) of these were performed for "fetal distress;" this rate was significantly higher than that of a control group.[20] Other authors have reported a similar experience of fetal distress and cesarean delivery for fetuses with major chromosome abnormalities.

Prenatal detection of fetuses with a major chromosome abnormality before the time of viability provides the option of terminating the pregnancy. Knowledge of the karyotype also is desirable in fetuses with known major malformations before in utero surgery or other aggressive treatment is considered. Even when discovered later in pregnancy, knowledge of an abnormal karyotype will usually influence other obstetric considerations including the place, time, and/or mode of delivery.

Who Is at Risk?

Due to the inherent risks and costs of prenatal chromosome analysis, unselected chromosome testing of all pregnant women who request it is not currently feasible. Therefore, chromosome analysis generally is reserved for pregnancies considered to be at a greater risk for carrying a chromosome abnormality than the general population (Table 17–1). Advanced maternal

TABLE 17–1.

Risk of Chromosome Abnormality*

Older mothers (≥35 years)	2% (see Table 17–2)
Previous aneuploidy	1%–2%
Familial chromosome rearrangement	
Robertsonian translocation	5.5%
Reciprocal translocations	11.6%
Inversions	5.9%
Fragile X carrier	25%
Low maternal serum AFP†	1%–2%
High maternal serum AFP	1%
Sonographically detectable abnormality	See text

*Modified from Ferguson-Smith MA: Prenatal diagnosis of chromosome anomalies: Who is at risk? Rodeck CH, Nicolaides KH (eds): *Prenatal Diagnosis*, New York, John Wiley & Sons, 1984, pp 53–64.
†AFP = alpha-fetoprotein.

TABLE 17–2.

Risks of Chromosome Abnormalities for Live Births Compared With Maternal Age

Maternal Age	Trisomy 21 at Delivery*	All Chromosome Abnormalities‡ at Delivery†
20	1/1734	1/526
21	1/1612	1/526
22	1/1500	1/500
23	1/1408	1/500
24	1/1327	1/476
25	1/1250	1/476
26	1/1186	1/476
27	1/1124	1/455
28	1/1064	1/435
29	1/1014	1/417
30	1/965	1/385
31	1/915	1/385
32	1/794	1/322
33	1/637	1/286
34	1/496	1/238
35	1/386	1/192
36	1/300	1/156
37	1/234	1/127
38	1/182	1/102
39	1/141	1/83
40	1/110	1/66
41	1/86	1/53
42	1/66	1/42
43	1/52	1/33
44	1/40	1/26
45	1/31	1/21
46	1/24	1/16
47	1/19	1/13
48	1/15	1/10
49	1/11	1/8

*Mean of three large studies. From Palomaki GE, Haddow JE: Am J Obstet Gynecol 1987; 156:460–463.
†Adapted from Hook EB: Obstetrics and Gynecology 1981; 58:282.
‡Excluding 47, XXX at ages 20–32.

age (age 35 or older at the time of delivery) is by far the most common clinical indication leading to chromosome analysis (Table 17–2). Other accepted clinical indications for chromosome analysis include a previous child or fetus with aneuploidy and a known balanced translocation or other structural rearrangements in one of the parents.[8] Chromosome analysis also is usually offered to women who undergo mid-trimester amniocentesis for any other reason, such as elevated maternal serum alpha-fetoprotein (MS-AFP) levels. Low MS-AFP levels (discussed below) are a rapidly growing clinical indication for chromosome analysis at many centers, although this has not been universally accepted (see Chapter 4).[2, 4–7, 15–19, 23] Other maternal serum markers, such as human chorionic gonadotropin (HCG), also have been proposed as a method for identifying chromosomally anomalous fetuses.[3, 22]

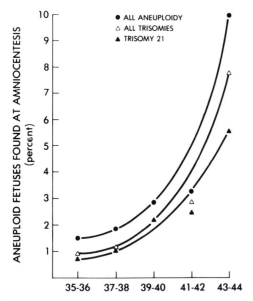

FIG 17–1.
Risk of aneuploid fetus at the time of second-trimester amniocentesis vs. maternal age. Maternal age shows an exponential relationship, with most chromosome abnormalities including trisomes 18, 13, and 21. (From Simpson JL, Golbus MS, Martin AO, et al: *Genetics in Obstetrics and Gynecology,* Philadelphia, Grune & Stratton, 1982. Used by permission.)

Maternal age is positively correlated with various chromosome abnormalities including trisomies 18, 13 and 21, XXX, and XXY, but not 45,X (Fig 17–1).[9] As previously noted, the specific risk of a chromosome abnormality also varies inversely with the menstrual age at the time of chromosome analysis. The specific risk of trisomy 21 at the time of second-trimester amniocentesis varies from 1 in 274 for women 35 years old to 1 in 10 for women 48 years old (Table 17–3). The prevalence of any chromosome abnormality at the time of amniocentesis has been observed to plateau at the older age ranges (> 46 years; see Table 17–3), and this plateau is thought to reflect the inability of these women to maintain anomalous pregnancies until the time of amniocentesis.[9]

The association between low MS-AFP and certain chromosome abnormalities, notably trisomy 21 and trisomy 18, was first reported in 1984 and has been confirmed by several large studies.[17] For example, DiMaio et al. found one fetus with trisomy 21 for each 161 women with low MS-AFP tested.[5] The association between low MS-AFP and chromosomal abnormalities cannot be explained by other factors such as maternal weight, birth weight, fetal sex, or diabetes mellitus. Wald et al. suggest that the hormonal pattern of chromosomally anomalous fetuses (low AFP, low estriol, and high HCG levels) indicates placental immaturity.[22]

Since advanced maternal age and low MS-AFP are independent risk factors for trisomy 21, using both determinants together can detect more fetuses with trisomy 21 than can either alone (Table 17–4).[18] Combining age and AFP can also provide a more precise estimate of risk for individual patients. For example, data reported by Palomaki and Haddow show that a woman aged 35 with an AFP level of 1.0 multiples of the median (MoM) has a lower risk (1 in 381) of carrying a fetus with trisomy 21 than a 25-year-old with an AFP level of 0.4 MoM (risk, 1 in 233).[18]

It is important to recognize the limitations as well as the benefits of current clinical indications when screening for chromosome abnormalities. Because there are many more younger women than older women who conceive, screening all women 35 years or older in the United States would identify only 20% of infants currently born with Down's syndrome.[1, 10] Similarly, screening all women with low MS-AFP levels (< 0.5 MoM) would identify 20% to 30% of fetuses with Down's syndrome but also would require testing 4%–8% of normal pregnancies.[6] Screening all women with either indication potentially could identify nearly half of all fetuses with trisomy 21. However, because less than half the women in known risk groups currently undergo chromosome analysis, the actual number of chromosome abnormalities that are detected is substantially less.

Methods of Diagnosis

Genetic amniocentesis is the time-honored and most common method of chromosome analysis.[33] Approximately 200,000 genetic amniocenteses were performed during 1988 in the United States alone. The major advantages of this method over alternative techniques of chromosome analysis are its simplicity and safety. The rate of spontaneous abortion attributed to amniocentesis is 0.2% to 0.5%.[33, 35] Another potential advantage of amniocentesis is the opportunity for detecting elevated levels of amniotic fluid alpha-fetoprotein (AFP), which may indicate the presence of an underlying malformation. The major disadvantages of amniocentesis are the relatively late date at which the procedure is usually performed (15 to 18 menstrual weeks) and the further delay required for culture of sloughed fetal cells (10 to 14 days).

In recent years, chorionic villous sampling (CVS) has developed as an alternative to genetic amniocentesis for chromosome analysis.[25, 27, 30] The primary advantage of this method is its opportunity for early karyotyping between 8 to 12 weeks and the shorter time

TABLE 17–3.

Comparison of Chromosome Abnormalities With Maternal Age for Live Births
and at the Time of Second-Trimester Amniocentesis

Maternal Age	Trisomy 21		All Chromosome Abnormalities‡	
	Live birth	Amniocentesis*	Live birth	Amniocentesis†
20	1/1734	1/1231	1/526	
21	1/1612	1/1145	1/526	
22	1/1500	1/1065	1/500	
23	1/1408	1/1000	1/500	
24	1/1327	1/942	1/476	
25	1/1250	1/887	1/476	
26	1/1186	1/842	1/476	
27	1/1124	1/798	1/455	
28	1/1064	1/755	1/435	
29	1/1014	1/721	1/417	
30	1/965	1/685	1/385	
31	1/915	1/650	1/385	
32	1/794	1/563	1/322	
33	1/637	1/452	1/286	
34	1/496	1/352	1/238	
35	1/386	1/274	1/192	1/83
36	1/300	1/213	1/156	1/76
37	1/234	1/166	1/127	1/67
38	1/182	1/129	1/102	1/58
39	1/141	1/100	1/83	1/49
40	1/100	1/78	1/66	1/40
41	1/86	1/61	1/53	1/32
42	1/66	1/47	1/42	1/26
43	1/52	1/37	1/33	1/21
44	1/40	1/29	1/26	1/19
45	1/31	1/22	1/21	1/15
46	1/24	1/17	1/16	1/12
47	1/19	1/13	1/13	1/20
48	1/15	1/10	1/10	1/18
49	1/11	1/8	1/8	1/16

*Adapted from Palomaki GE, Haddow JE: Am J Obstet Gynecol 1987; 156:460–463, assuming 29% loss rate between the second trimester and term. These data are also very similar to following reference.

†Data based on values predicted by logistic regression model (Table 17–10). From Ferguson-Smith MA, Yates JRW: Prenat Diagn 1984; 4:5–44.

‡For the autosomal trisomies, an exponential rise in incidence is noted with advancing maternal age over the first part of the age range followed by a plateau at the upper end of the age range. This plateau is thought to reflect the inability to maintain anomalous pregnancies until the time of amniocentesis in these women.

usually required for cell analysis.[32] Disadvantages of CVS include its greater technical failure rate (10%) and occasional placental mosaicism, both of which require subsequent amniocentesis.[27, 36] Also, CVS may carry a slightly greater risk of subsequent abortion than amniocentesis. Although the precise risk is difficult to determine because of the higher rate of spontaneous abortions during the first trimester, some authorities suggest that the abortion rate resulting from CVS is 1%–2% above the baseline rate,[27] while others suggest that this rate is similar to that resulting from amniocentesis.[25]

Chorionic villous sampling is most commonly performed during the first trimester via a transcervical route. However, transabdominal CVS also has been successfully employed in the first trimester. More recently, transabdominal placental aspiration also has been successfully performed in the second and third trimesters.[24, 29, 31, 34] These methods may permit rapid karyotyping within 1–2 days of the procedure.[32]

Direct sampling of fetal blood via percutaneous umbilical vein sampling is an alternative method for rapid karyotyping during the second and third trimesters.[26, 28, 39] Placental aspiration may be technically eas-

TABLE 17–4.

Risk of Down's Syndrome, Reported as Number of Pregnancies per Case of Down's Syndrome, Based on Maternal Age and MS-AFP Level at the Time of Second-Trimester Amniocentesis*

Maternal Age (years)	Maternal Serum AFP Level (Multiples of the Median)								
	Any	0.35	0.4	0.5	0.6	0.7	0.8	0.9	1.00
20	1231	237	323	519	742	977	1219	1465	1710
21	1145	221	301	483	690	909	1134	1363	1590
22	1065	205	280	449	642	845	1054	1268	1479
23	1000	193	262	422	602	794	990	1190	1389
24	942	182	247	397	567	748	933	1121	1308
25	887	171	233	374	534	704	878	1056	1232
26	842	162	221	355	507	668	834	1002	1169
27	798	154	209	337	481	633	790	950	1108
28	755	145	198	319	455	599	748	899	1049
29	721	139	189	304	434	572	714	858	1001
30	685	132	180	289	413	544	678	815	951
31	650	125	171	274	392	516	644	744	903
32	563	108	148	238	339	447	557	670	782
33	452	87	119	191	272	359	448	538	628
34	352	68	92	149	212	279	349	419	489
35	274	53	72	116	165	217	271	326	381
36	213	41	56	90	128	169	211	254	296
37	166	32	44	70	100	132	164	198	231
38	129	25	34	54	78	102	128	154	179
39	100	19	26	42	60	79	99	119	139
40	78	15	20	33	47	62	77	93	108
41	61	12	16	26	37	48	60	73	85
42	47	9	12	20	28	37	47	56	65
43	37	7	10	16	22	29	37	44	51
44	29	6	8	12	17	23	29	35	40
45	22	4	6	9	13	17	22	26	31
46	17	3	4	7	10	13	17	20	24
47	13	3	3	5	8	10	13	15	18
48	10	2	3	4	6	8	10	12	14
49	8	2	2	3	5	6	8	10	11

*Compiled from data of Palomaki GE, Haddow JE: Am J Obstet Gynecol 1987; 156:460–463.

ier to perform,[24] but umbilical vein sampling can provide other important information regarding the fetus. In addition to chromosome analysis, the fetal hematocrit, protein and antibody levels, and viral cultures all can be determined at the time of umbilical vein sampling. Successful karyotyping is also possible by culture of fetal cells obtained from aspiration of available fetal fluid collections such as cystic hygromata, the urinary bladder, and renal cysts.

The Role of Ultrasound

Ultrasound is routinely used before, during, and after chromosome analysis. Accurate fetal dating is necessary to determine the optimal time and method of chromosome testing. Since MS-AFP levels vary with menstrual age, fetal dating also is important for determining whether chromosome analysis is indicated in women who are referred for low AFP levels. Selecting the optimal sampling site for CVS requires sonographic guidance. Although similar benefits have not been proven for amniocentesis, there is general agreement that sonographic guidance is probably a safer method than "blind" amniocentesis.[33]

In addition to fetal dating and guiding procedures, ultrasound plays a potentially important role in identifying malformations that are not detected by chromosome analysis and/or AFP testing, even for women who are already scheduled for these procedures.[37] The additional benefit of ultrasound evaluation over amniocentesis and amniotic fluid AFP determination is that ultrasound is predictably most useful for "internal" malformations, such as hydrocephalus or diaphragmatic hernia. Such defects can be detected during an anatomic survey of the fetus performed at the time of amniocentesis or, alternatively, on repeat examination at 18 to

22 weeks when sonographic accuracy is improved.[37] A detailed sonographic examination is potentially more important following CVS than amniocentesis, because very few anomalies can be detected by ultrasound during the first trimester and because MS-AFP is less sensitive (80%) for detecting spina bifida and other open defects than is amniotic fluid AFP analysis (99%).

Detection of unsuspected malformations in women referred for "routine" obstetric indications currently is one of the most important contributions of ultrasound to prenatal genetic diagnoses. Remember that the majority of fetuses with major chromosome abnormalities are found among such "low risk" patients. In these women, sonographic detection of fetal anomalies is often the sole indication for chromosome analysis. In deciding whether chromosome analysis is indicated for these women, it is important to know the expected frequency of chromosomal abnormalities. The following section will discuss the known risks of chromosome abnormalities for specific anomalies, emphasizing the data from prenatal sonographic studies when available.

THE RISK OF CHROMOSOME ABNORMALITY BASED ON SONOGRAPHIC FINDINGS

Sonographers should be aware that chromosome abnormalities are often associated with multiple structural anomalies. By contrast, single structural abnormalities are most commonly transmitted as multifactorial traits. Therefore, identification of more than one anomaly significantly increases the probability of an underlying chromosome disorder.

The frequency of chromosome abnormalities reported from prenatal sonographic identification of fetal anomalies varies from 11% to 35%, depending primarily on the type of malformations detected.[38, 40–44] These data are substantially greater than the 6% to 7% prevalence of chromosome abnormalities reported among live borns with major malformations. This difference can be attributed to three possible factors: (1) inclusion of more severely anomalous fetuses who often die before birth in prenatal studies, (2) possible ascertainment bias by selecting patients in higher risk groups (for example, older women) for prenatal studies, and (3) the relative insensitivity of ultrasound for diagnosing many minor malformations which are less likely to be associated with chromosome abnormalities.

The reported frequency of chromosome abnormalities among prenatal studies also varies with the method of patient selection. Calculations based on the total number of fetuses with a given malformation may underestimate the true frequency of abnormal karyotypes since not all fetuses undergo chromosome analysis. On the other hand, calculations based only on the number of fetuses who undergo chromosome analysis may overestimate the true frequency of abnormal karyotypes since chromosome analysis is more likely to be requested for severely anomalous fetuses than for fetuses with isolated anomalies.

Although it would be useful to know the risk of a chromosome abnormality for isolated malformations, this information is not available for many anomalies. Even when known, published results may not apply to all institutions because the ability to detect both the primary malformation and concurrent anomalies varies with the skill and experience of the sonographer and the quality of the ultrasound equipment. Other factors contributing to the accuracy of sonography for detecting anomalies include the clinical indication of the sonogram and the gestational age at the time of examination.

With these caveats in mind, an approximate risk of chromosome abnormalities for many major congenital malformations can now be estimated and compared with other types of congenital malformations. In the following section, we review specific sonographic findings that have been associated with chromosome abnormalities and, therefore, might be indications for chromosome analysis. An attempt has been made to distinguish malformations that are strongly associated with chromosome abnormalities (for example, cystic hygroma) from anomalies that are less strongly associated with chromosome abnormalities or that may be significant only when other malformations are present (for example, a single umbilical artery).

CENTRAL NERVOUS SYSTEM MALFORMATIONS

Central nervous system (CNS) disorders have been associated with a variety of chromosome abnormalities, particularly trisomies 13, 18, and triploidy. By contrast, trisomy 21 and 45,X uncommonly demonstrate intracranial abnormalities.

Because the risk of a chromosome disorder varies with the specific malformation, it is important to establish the correct diagnosis when an intracranial abnormality is demonstrated. For example, chromosome abnormalities are frequently associated with holoprosencephaly (Fig 17–2), yet are not associated with hydranencephaly, an anomaly that may closely resemble holoprosencephaly (Fig 17–3). These differences reflect the belief that holoprosencephaly results from a

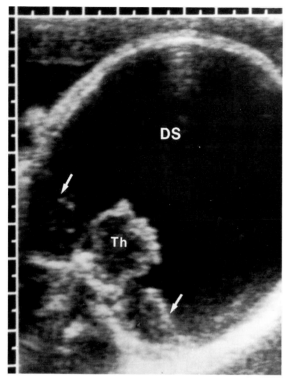

FIG 17–2.
Alobar holoprosencephaly, "pancake" type. Semicoronal scan of the cranium shows fused central thalami *(Th)*, small amount of brain tissue at the base of the cranium *(arrows),* and a large fluid collection representing the dorsal sac *(DS).* Chromosome analysis yielded trisomy 13.

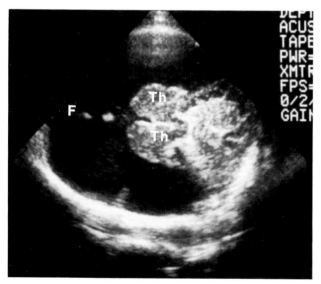

FIG 17–3.
Hydranencephaly. Axial scan demonstrates absence of brain mantle, although the thalami *(Th)* and cerebellum *(C)* remain intact. A falx *(F)* also is demonstrated. Hydranencephaly is not associated with chromosome abnormalities. (From Greene MF, Benacerraf B, Crawford JM: Hydranencephaly: US appearance during in utero evolution. Radiology 1985; 156:779–780. Used by permission.)

primary disorder of early embryogenesis, whereas hydranencephaly is an "acquired" defect secondary to vascular disruption.

In addition to holoprosencephaly, CNS malformations that have been associated with chromosome abnormalities include the Dandy-Walker malformation, hydrocephaly, spina bifida, and agenesis of the corpus callosum. These anomalies are discussed separately below.

Holoprosencephaly

Prenatal studies suggest that an underlying chromosome abnormality may be identified in as many as 40%–60% of fetuses with alobar or semilobar holoprosencephaly (see Fig 17–2). The largest prenatal series to date reported chromosome abnormalities in 43% (10 of 23 fetuses) of the entire series or 59% (10 of 17) of those fetuses who underwent chromosome analysis. Trisomy 13 or a variant of trisomy 13 is the most common chromosome abnormality associated with holoprosencephaly. Other chromosome disorders that have been associated with holoprosencephaly include trisomy 18, triploidy, 5p+, 13q−, 18p−, and various other karyotypes.[49, 50, 55, 59] An underlying chromosome abnormality carries little recurrence risk, whereas a normal karyotype is more likely to be associated with various inheritable syndromes that may also be expressed as holoprosencephaly.

The presence of facial malformations appears to increase the risk of an underlying chromosome abnormality in fetuses with holoprosencephaly.[55] Other extra-facial anomalies, notably omphalocele or renal cystic dysplasia, are strongly predictive of a chromosome abnormality in our experience.

Dandy-Walker Malformation/Cerebellar Hypoplasia

The Dandy-Walker malformation is recognized as a non-specific anomaly with a diversity of causes.[52, 58] Inheritable syndromes that may express the Dandy-Walker malformation include the Ellis-Van Creveld syndrome and the Meckel-Gruber syndrome. Cerebellar abnormalities, including cerebellar hypoplasia or the Dandy-Walker malformation, have also been associated with various chromosome abnormalities, primarily trisomies 18 and 13.[53, 57, 60, 61]

Cerebellar hypoplasia or the Dandy-Walker variant may appear similar to the Dandy-Walker syndrome although, unlike the latter, ventricular dilatation is usually absent.[54] This distinction may be important because cerebellar hypoplasia has been more strongly associated with chromosome abnormalities (Fig 17–4).[53, 57, 60, 61] In a series of seven fetuses with cerebel-

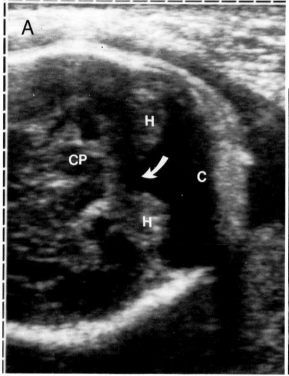

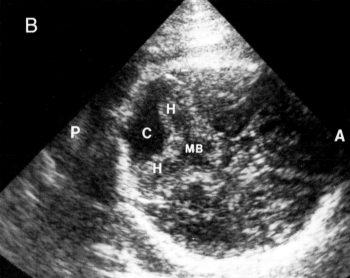

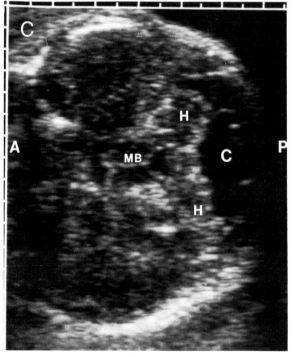

FIG 17–4.

Three examples of the Dandy-Walker variant or cerebellar hypoplasia associated with chromosome abnormalities. Each demonstrates a midline cyst or enlarged cisterna magna in the posterior fossa that was not associated with ventricular dilatation. **A,** mosaic trisomy 13. Posterior fossa cyst is associated with agenesis of the cerebellar vermis *(curved arrow)*. No other abnormalities were demonstrated on sonography, although other anomalies (polydactyly and cardiac anomaly) were identified on postmortem examination. *CP* = cerebral peduncles; *H* = cerebellar hemisphere. **B,** trisomy 18. Posterior fossa cyst *(C)* is identified only as an enlarged cisterna magna. Other abnormalities identified on sonography included atrioventricular septal defect of the heart, intrauterine growth retardation, and reversal of diastolic flow on Doppler examination. *A* = anterior; *P* = posterior; *H* = cerebellar hemispheres; *MB* = midbrain. **C,** trisomy 18. Posterior fossa cyst *(C)* is identified, seen only as an enlarged cisterna magna (15mm). Other abnormalities identified on sonography included large ventricular septal defect and a single umbilical artery. *A* = anterior; *P* = posterior; *H* = cerebellar hemispheres; *MB* = midbrain. (Part **B** courtesy of Fred Hegge, MD, Emanuel Hospital, Portland, OR. Part **C** From Nyberg DA, Shepard T, Mack LA, et al: Significance of a single umbilical artery in fetuses with central nervous system malformations. J Ultrasound Med 1988; 7:265–273. Used by permission.)

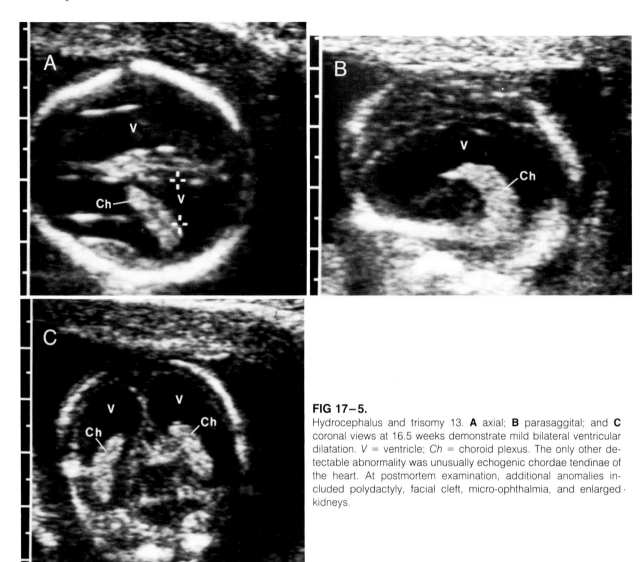

FIG 17–5.
Hydrocephalus and trisomy 13. **A** axial; **B** parasaggital; and **C** coronal views at 16.5 weeks demonstrate mild bilateral ventricular dilatation. *V* = ventricle; *Ch* = choroid plexus. The only other detectable abnormality was unusually echogenic chordae tendinae of the heart. At postmortem examination, additional anomalies included polydactyly, facial cleft, micro-ophthalmia, and enlarged · kidneys.

lar hypoplasia or the Dandy-Walker malformation identified prenatally, chromosome abnormalities were reported in two of four fetuses tested (trisomy 18 and mosaic trisomy 13), and neither demonstrated ventricular dilatation.[54] Based on the available literature as well as our own experience, we believe that demonstration of cerebellar hypoplasia or the Dandy-Walker syndrome is an indication for chromosome analysis.

Hydrocephalus and/or Spina Bifida

Hydrocephalus and/or spina bifida have been associated with various chromosome abnormalities, primarily trisomies 18, 13, and triploidy (Fig 17–5).[47, 48, 56, 62, 160] Occasionally, trisomy 21 can also demonstrate mild ventricular dilatation (Fig 17–6).

Data regarding the prevalence of chromosome abnormalities among fetuses with hydrocephalus or spina bifida are incomplete. Chervenak et al. reported five chromosome abnormalities among 53 cases (9%) of fetal "hydrocephalus" detected in utero.[47] Although it is unclear how many cases may have had additional CNS malformations, such as holoprosencephaly,[47] other authors have reported a similar frequency of chromosome abnormalities in association with hydrocephalus.[56]

The precise risk of a chromosome abnormality undoubtedly varies with the specific malformation present. In an analysis of 107 fetuses with CNS anomalies, Nyberg et al. found chromosome abnormalities in 3% (1 of 30) of fetuses with hydrocephalus, 8% (3 of

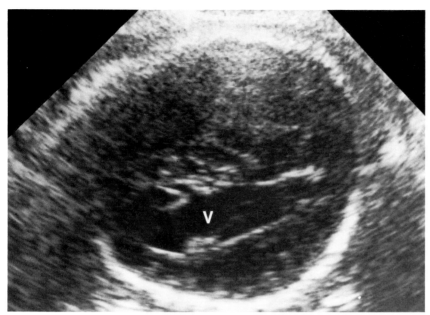

FIG 17-6.
Hydrocephalus and trisomy 21. Axial scan 31 weeks shows mild dilatation of the far lateral ventricle (V). The near ventricle is obscured by acoustic noise. A small amount of fluid was also identified in the duodenum, which proved to represent duodenal stenosis.

38) of fetuses with hydrocephalus and spina bifida, and 33% (3 of 9) of fetuses with spina bifida alone (Table 17-5 and Fig 17-7).[160] Considering only fetuses who underwent chromosome analysis, these figures are 8%, 15%, and 50%, respectively.[160] It is unclear whether the relatively high rate of chromosome abnormalities for fetuses with spina bifida but no ventricular dilatation is representative of the true risk or if it simply reflects a sampling error due to the small number of fetuses studied.

Agenesis of the Corpus Callosum

Agenesis of the corpus callosum has been associated with a variety of chromosome abnormalities including trisomies 13, 18, and 8, triploidy, and translocations. However, the frequency of chromosome ab-

normalities remains uncertain due to the small number of cases reported in utero.[45, 46, 51] In the largest prenatal series of fetuses with agenesis of the corpus callosum, Bertino et al. reported a chromosome abnormality (trisomy 8) in one of seven fetuses (14%), including one of five (20%) fetuses who underwent chromosome analysis.[46]

In summary, CNS malformations frequently are associated with chromosome abnormalities, with the highest risk reported for midline malformations of holoprosencephaly, the Dandy-Walker malformation, and, perhaps, agenesis of the corpus callosum. Demonstration of hydrocephalus or spina bifida probably also justifies chromosome analysis, since the risk of an underlying chromosome abnormality is much higher

TABLE 17-5.

Comparison of Chromosome Abnormalities With the Type of Central Nervous System Malformation*

	No. Cases	Chromosomes Tested	Abnormal	Percent† Abnormal
Hydrocephalus	30	13	1	3%-8%
Hydrocephalus and MM‡	38	20	3	8%-15%
MM	9	6	3	33%-50%
Dandy-Walker malformation	7	4	2	29%-50%
Holoprosencephaly	23	17	10	43%-59%

*Adapted from Nyberg DA, Shepard T, Mack LA, et al: Significance of a single umbilical artery in fetuses with CNS malformations. J Ultrasound Med 1988; 7:265-273.
†Minimum is the number of abnormal chromosomes as a percent of total number of cases; maximum is the number of abnormal chromosomes as a percent of fetuses who underwent chromosome analysis.
‡MM = meningomyelocele.

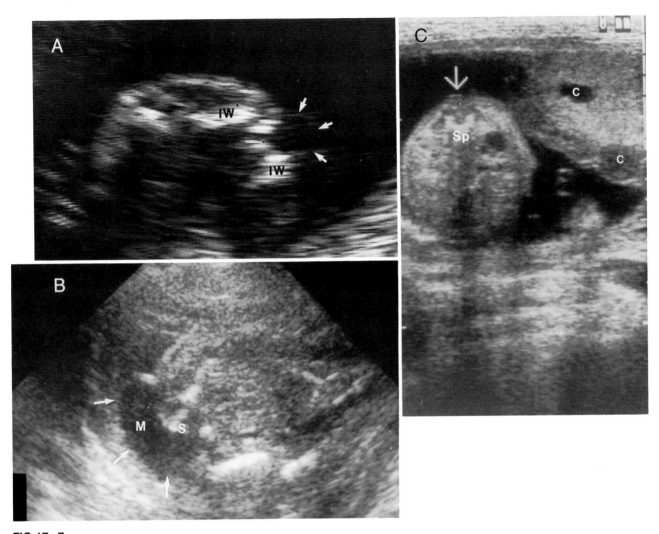

FIG 17−7.
Myelomeningocele and chromosome abnormalities. **A,** trisomy 18. Transverse scan at 18 weeks demonstrates a dysraphic defect with a myelomeningocele sac *(arrows)* involving the lower lumbar spine. A single umbilical artery was also noted. Additional other anomalies found at autopsy included horseshoe kidney, clubfeet, and facial cleft. *IW* = iliac wing. **B,** trisomy 13. Transverse scan of the lower spine *(S)* demonstrates a large *(arrows)* myelomeningocele sac *(M)*. A cystic kidney and marked oligohydramnios also were identified. Other abnormalities found at postmortem examination included a large ventricular septal defect, absent left kidney, single umbilical artery, and abnormalities of the extremities. **C,** triploidy. Transverse view of the lumbar spine *(Sp)* demonstrates splaying of the dorsal vertebral arch. Cystic dysplasia of the kidneys and small cystic areas *(C)* within the placenta were also identified. (Part **A** from Nyberg DA, Shepard T, Mack LA, et al: Significance of a single umbilical artery in fetuses with central nervous system malformations. J Ultrasound Med 1988; 7:265−273. Used by permission.)

than observed in the baseline population, and knowledge of the karyotype may influence obstetric management.[48]

Choroid Plexus Cysts

Recent attention has been directed to the possible association between sonographically detectable choroid plexus cysts and chromosome abnormalities, particularly trisomy 18. Chudleigh et al. first reported detection of choroid plexus cysts on prenatal sonography as benign, transient findings in five fetuses who were

examined between 17 to 19 weeks and in whom the cysts resolved by 20 to 23 weeks (Fig 17−8).[66] Bundy et al. noted bilateral large choroid plexus cysts in a fetus with trisomy 18, but this was thought to be an incidental finding.[63] Nicolaides et al. subsequently reported trisomy 18 in three of four fetuses with bilateral choroid plexus cysts; all fetuses also were noted to have mild dilatation of the occipital horns, suggesting that the cysts were unusually large.[39] One of these fetuses also demonstrated an omphalocele and a ventricular septal defect, and another had obstructive uropathy.

Other authors also have noted a possible associa-

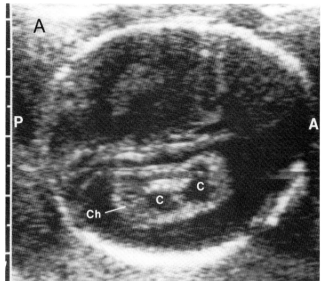

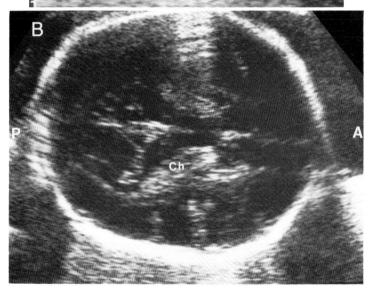

FIG 17–8.
Isolated choroid plexus cysts. **A,** axial scan of the cranium at 18 weeks shows several cysts *(C)* within the choroid plexus *(Ch)* of the far cerebral ventricle. A = anterior; P = posterior. **B,** follow-up scan at 30 weeks shows normal choroid plexus *(Ch)* with resolution of the cysts. A = anterior; P = posterior.

tion between sonographically detectable choroid plexus cysts and chromosome abnormalities; the chromosome abnormalities reported to date are shown in Table 17–6.[65, 67, 70, 70a, 72] All but one case has been associated with trisomy 18. Descriptions of the cyst, when provided, suggest that the majority of chromosome abnormalities are associated with large, bilateral cysts (Fig 17–9). However, it appears that smaller cysts may also be associated with trisomy 18 (Fig 17–10).[70a]

The reported prevalence of choroid plexus cysts among normal fetuses ranges from 0.3% to 2.5% (Table 17–7).[64, 65, 67a, 68, 70a, 71, 71a, 73] The highest prevalence reported by Chan et al. included only women who were scanned between 16 to 24 weeks prior to genetic amniocentesis.[64] By comparison, Chitkara et al. reported detection of one or more choroid plexus cysts in only 0.65% (41 of 6,288) fetuses exam-

ined between 16–42 weeks' gestation.[65] However, all but one fetus with choroid plexus cysts were initially seen before 22 weeks, suggesting that the actual prevalence would have been significantly higher if only second-trimester pregnancies had been considered.

The prevalence of choroid plexus cysts among fetuses with trisomy 18 is uncertain, since this association had not been studied prior to their prenatal detection. In a retrospective, postmortem study of 14 fetuses with trisomy 18, Fitzsimmons and associates found choroid plexus cysts in five cases, including five of seven (71%) fetuses less than 26 weeks of age.[69] By comparison, Chitkara et al. identified choroid plexus cysts on prenatal sonography in only one of five fetuses (20%) with trisomy 18 who were studied prospectively.[65] However, these authors also indicated that since the completion of their studies, bilateral choroid

TABLE 17–6.

Literature Review of Choroid Plexus Cysts Associated With Chromosomal Abnormalities*

Author	Description of Cysts	Other US Findings	Karyotype	Pathology
Bundy et al. (1986)	Large bilateral	NA	Tri 18	
Nicolaides et al. (1986)	Bilateral	Omphalocele, VSD	Tri 18	Omphalocele, VSD
	Bilateral	Obstructive uropathy	Tri 18	Obstructive uropathy
	Bilateral	Mild dilatation of posterior horns of lateral cerebral ventricles	Tri 18	None
Ricketts et al. (1987)	NA	NA	Tri 21	ASD
Farhood et al.[1] (1987)	5 mm	None	Tri 18	Low-set ears, micrognathia, membranous VSD
Furness (1987)	Large bilateral	None	Tri 18	Small VSD, choanal atresia
Chitkara et al. (1988)	Large 20 mm bilateral	Absent stomach	Tri 18	NA (Presumed esophageal atresia)
	Bilateral	None	Tri 18[2]	NA
	Bilateral	None	Tri 18[2]	NA
Ostlere et al.[3] (1989)	Bilateral 10 mm	IUGR	Tri 18	VSD
	Large 15 mm bilateral	Hydronephrosis Polyhydramnios IUGR	Tri 18	
Gabriell et al.[4] (1989)	2 > 10 mm	VSD, rocker-bottom feet	Tri 18	Same plus horseshoe kidney (?)
	2 > 10 mm	VSD, short arms, rocker-bottom feet	Tri 18	Same plus esophageal atresia (?)
		VSD, rocker-bottom feet	Tri 18	Same (?)
		VSD, AGCC, upper mesomelia	Tri 18	Same (?)

*NA = information not available; VSD = ventricular septal defect; ASD = atrial septal defect; AGCC = agenesis of the corpus callosum.
1. Two additional trisomies were mentioned but details were not given. The case reported was also associated with low maternal serum alpha-fetoprotein.
2. Not included in the authors' prospective series.
3. Description of these two cases leaves it unclear which ultrasound findings were associated with the larger (15 mm) choroid plexus cysts.
4. Description is unclear as to pathologic findings seen on sonography and additional pathologic findings present.

plexus cysts were the only detectable abnormality in two additional fetuses with trisomy 18.

The specific risk of trisomy 18 when choroid plexus cysts are identified before 26 weeks is uncertain but can be estimated with available information. Allow-ing for crude assumptions regarding the prevalence of trisomy 18 (1 in 6,000), choroid plexus cysts in nor-mal fetuses (1%–3%), and the prevalence of sono-graphically detectable cysts in second-trimester fetuses with trisomy 18 (20%–71%), the risk of trisomy 18 in

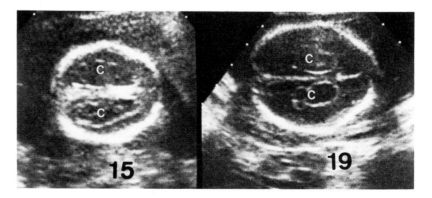

FIG 17–9.
Choroid plexus cysts and trisomy 18. Axial sonograms performed at 15 and 19 weeks' gestation demonstrate large, bilateral choroid plexus cysts *(C)* filling the lateral ventricles. By 36 weeks, the cysts resolved, but polyhydramnios was evident. After birth, trisomy 18, choanal atresia, and small ventricular septal defects were found. (From Furness ME: Choroid plexus cysts and trisomy 18. Lancet 1987; i:693. Used by permission.)

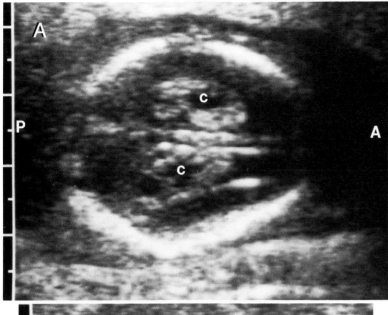

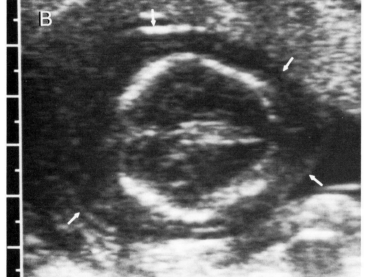

FIG 17–10.
Choroid plexus cysts and trisomy 18. **A,** axial scan of the cranium at 14 weeks demonstrates bilateral choroid plexus cysts *(C)*. A = anterior; *P* posterior. **B,** scan at a lower level shows diffuse lymphangiectasia with marked skin edema *(arrows)*. Trisomy 18 was found on amniocentesis.

a fetus with choroid plexus cysts can be estimated as about 1%. This crude estimate is consistent with available prospective studies which have reported only three chromosome abnormalities among 191 fetuses (1.6%) identified with choroid plexus cysts (see Table 17–7). All three of these fetuses demonstrated unusually large cysts or other sonographic abnormalities. These data suggest that the risk of trisomy 18 in a fetus with isolated choroid plexus cysts is probably much less than 1%.

In summary, available evidence suggests that demonstration of choroid plexus cysts should initiate a careful search for additional abnormalities. In the absence of other risk factors or additional abnormalities, detection of isolated choroid plexus cysts that are typ-

ical in appearance is not considered an indication for amniocentesis by the present authors. However, the risk of trisomy 18 in association with large, bilateral choroid plexus cysts, atypical-appearing cysts, or cysts associated with additional abnormalities would appear to justify chromosome analysis.

FACIAL ABNORMALITIES

Facial Clefts

Facial clefts (cleft lip and palate) have been associated with chromosome abnormalities (trisomies 13 and 18), particularly when central nervous system disorders or other malformations also are present (Fig

TABLE 17–7.

Literature Review of Choroid Plexus Cysts Identified on Sonography
(Prospective Series)

Author	No. Patients	No. Cysts	Prevalence	No. Chromosome Abnormalities
Ostlere et al. (1987)	3627	11	0.3%	0
Chan et al. (1989)	513	13	2.5%	0
Clark et al. (1988)	2820	5	0.2%	0
Chitkara et al. (1988)	6288	41	0.7%	1 (trisomy 18)
Toi et al. (1988)	5800	62	1.1%	0
DeRoo et al. (1988)	2084	17	0.8%	0
Ostlere et al. (1989)	7000	42	0.6%	2 (both trisomy 18)
Total	28,132	191	0.3–2.5%	3 (1.6%)

17–11). In a series of 12 fetuses identified with facial clefts on prenatal sonography, Saltzman et al. reported that four of ten fetuses (40%) who underwent chromosome analysis had an abnormal karyotype, and all four fetuses had other detectable anomalies (two cases of holoprosencephaly and one case each of hydrocephalus and a ventricular septal defect).[79] Another prenatal series reported eight facial clefts in association with alobar or semilobar holoprosencephaly, and six of these had an underlying chromosome abnormality.[78] Identification of an isolated facial cleft has not yet been associated with chromosome abnormalities.[72] Based on current evidence, therefore, identification of a facial cleft should initiate a search for other abnormalities but as an isolated finding may not necessarily be an indication for chromosome analysis.

Ocular Abnormalities

A variety of ocular abnormalities, including cyclopia, hypotelorism, and hypertelorism, may be associated with chromosome abnormalities. When seen in association with other malformations, particularly holoprosencephaly, ocular abnormalities carry a high risk of aneuploidy (Fig 17–12).[78] In this regard, sonographers should recognize that cyclopia may appear as extreme hypotelorism with nearly fused orbits but only a single external opening (Fig 17–12).

An unusual ocular abnormality that possibly is implicated with chromosome abnormalities is persistence of the choroidal artery.[75] The choroidal artery is a normal structure that forms during embryologic development of the orbit and regresses by the third trimester. Birnholz and Farrell reported that the choroidal artery

can be demonstrated during the second trimester, and its persistence into the third trimester is associated with chromosome abnormalities.[75] However, due to the difficulty experienced by most sonographers in eliciting this structure, evaluation of the choroidal artery currently should be considered investigational.

Other Craniofacial Abnormalities

A variety of other facial abnormalities observed on clinical examination have been associated with chromosome abnormalities. For example, micrognathia is present in the majority of fetuses with triploidy or trisomy 18 (Fig 17–13).[74] A facial profile may demonstrate other cranial abnormalities such as a prominent occiput, which is frequently found in fetuses with trisomy 18 (Fig 17–14).

Small, deformed ears have also been associated with chromosome disorders including trisomies 13, 18, and 21.[76] However, ear abnormalities may be difficult to detect, and more obvious findings usually are apparent in fetuses with chromosome abnormalities. For these reasons, the value of examining the fetal ear is questioned.

Cystic Hygroma

Cystic hygromata are cystic fluid collections, typically located in the posterior and lateral neck, which are caused by obstruction of the lymphatic system.[82] Although they may be isolated (Fig 17–15), cystic hygromata are often associated with generalized hydrops, also referred to as lymphangiectasia (Fig 17–16). Obtaining amniotic fluid for chromosome analysis may be

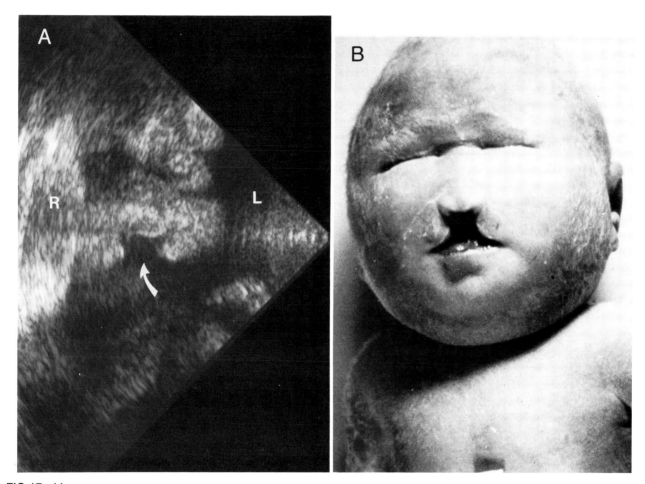

FIG 17–11.
Facial cleft and trisomy 13. **A,** coronal scan demonstrates a large midline facial cleft *(arrow)*. Other abnormalities that were identified included omphalocele and alobar holoprosencephaly. *R* = right; *L* = left. **B,** corresponding postmortem photograph of a similar case shows large facial cleft.

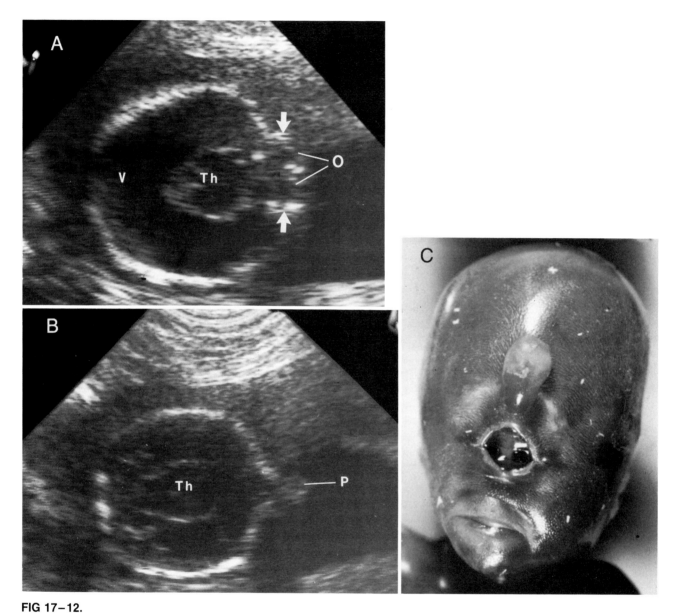

FIG 17–12.
Cyclopia and trisomy 13. **A,** axial scan of the cranium shows marked hypotelorism *(arrows)* of orbits *(O)*. Also noted are fused midline thalami *(Th)* and a large monoventricle *(V)*, consistent with alobar holoprosencephaly. **B,** scan at a slightly more cephalic level shows proboscis *(P)* protruding from the forehead. *Th* = Thalami. **C,** photograph after delivery shows cyclopia and nearly fused orbits with supraorbital proboscis. (From Nyberg DA, Mack LA, Bronstein A, et al: Holoprosencephaly: Prenatal sonographic diagnosis. AJR 1987; 149:1050–1058. Used by permission.)

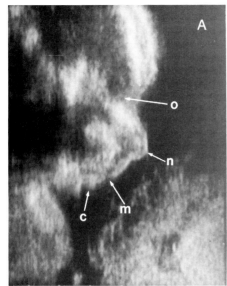

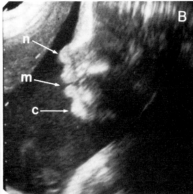

FIG 17–13.
Micrognathia and trisomy 18. **A,** facial profile demonstrates a relatively small chin *(c)* and mouth *(m)*. O = orbit; *n* = nose. **B,** by comparison, facial profile of normal fetus demonstrates normally proportioned chin *(c)* and mouth *(m)*. N = nose. The majority of fetuses with trisomy 18 demonstrate micrognathia.

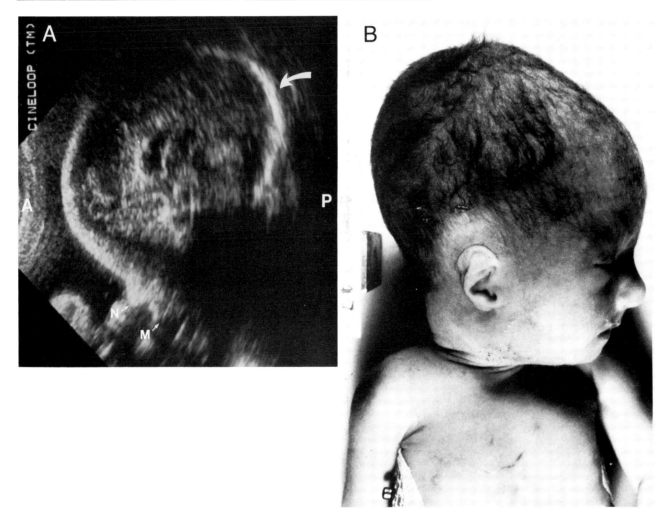

FIG 17–14.
Prominent occiput and trisomy 18. **A,** sagittal view of the face and cranium demonstrates prominent occiput *(curved arrow)*. Chromosome analysis yielded trisomy 18. *N* = nose; M = mouth; *A* = anterior; P = posterior. **B,** postmortem photograph of another fetus with trisomy 18 shows prominent occiput.

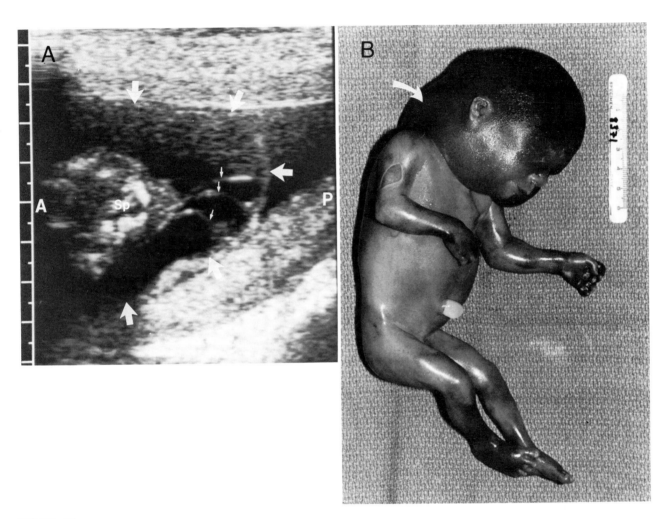

FIG 17–15.
Cystic hygroma **A,** transverse view of the neck demonstrates characteristic cystic hygroma *(outlined by large arrows)* with internal septations *(small arrows). A* = anterior; *P* = posterior; *Sp* = spine. **B,** postmortem photograph of another fetus with trisomy 21 demonstrates
cervical cystic hygroma *(arrow).*

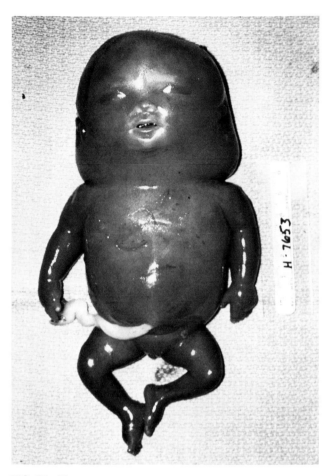

FIG 17–16.
Cystic hygroma with lymphangiectasia. Postmortem photograph demonstrates large cystic hygromata and diffuse hydrops (lymphangiectasia). There have been no reported survivors in fetuses who demonstrated cystic hygroma and lymphangiectasia.

difficult in these pregnancies, since large cystic hygromata may completely fill the available amniotic space. In this situation, successful cell culture has resulted from aspiration of the cystic hygroma itself.

Turner's syndrome (45,X) has been found most frequently with cystic hygroma, although a variety of other karyotypes are possible. A summary of selected prenatally diagnosed cases of cystic hygroma (Table 17–8) shows that when fetal cells are successfully cultured, approximately 75% are associated with a chromosome abnormality, and Turner's syndrome (45,X) accounts for 80% of these.[80–89] Trisomy 18 or trisomy 21 is the most common of other abnormal karyotypes. Of fetuses with normal karyotypes, 46,XX is about twice as common as 46,XY.

Chromosome analysis is recommended whenever a cervical cystic hygroma is identified prenatally. However, the prognosis is poor regardless of the underlying cause. Occasionally, the cystic hygroma resolves or an isolated cystic hygroma can be surgically resected after birth. However, there have been no reported survivors when cystic hygroma was associated with generalized lymphangiectasia. On the other hand, isolated cystic hygromata in an atypical location (non-cervical) do not appear to carry a significant risk of a chromosome abnormality.

Non-immune Hydrops

Non-immune hydrops fetalis, characterized by generalized skin edema, ascites, and pericardial and pleural effusions, is a non-specific endpoint resulting from a variety of fetal and maternal disorders.[92] Fetuses with non-immune hydrops should be distinguished from those who also demonstrate cystic hygromata, since the latter group has a higher frequency of chromosome abnormalities.[83]

The prognosis of fetuses with non-immune hydrops is extremely poor, and intrauterine death may intervene before chromosome analysis is performed. In a series of 22 singletons with non-cardiac related non-immune hydrops, Allan et al. identified chromosome abnormalities in 3 (14%).[90] In another series of 28 fetuses with non-immune hydrops and no cystic hygromata reported by Nicolaides et al., five (18%) had chromosome abnormalities (three cases of trisomy 21, one case of 46XY/92XXYY, and one case of unbalanced partial trisomies of chromosomes 11 and 22).[39]

Percutaneous umbilical vein sampling has proven to be a useful method for evaluating non-immune hydrops. This permits direct evaluation of fetal blood including the hematocrit, serum protein, immunoglobulin titers, and viral cultures and also permits rapid chromosome analysis.[26, 28]

Cardiovascular Malformations

Cardiovascular malformations are found in over 90% of fetuses with trisomy 18 and 13, 40%–50% of fetuses with trisomy 21, and 15%–20% of those with Turner's syndrome (Table 17–9). Hence, the presence of a cardiac malformation significantly increases the risk of an underlying chromosome abnormality (Figs 17–17 and 17–18).[98–101] In an ongoing population-based case-control study, Ferencz et al. reported chromosome disorders in 13% of 2,103 live borns with a cardiovascular malformation compared to only 0.1% of infants without a cardiovascular malformation.[99]

A much greater frequency of chromosome abnormalities has been observed in fetuses with a sonographically detectable cardiac defect compared to postnatal studies.[93, 95–97, 102] In two of the largest prenatal series,

TABLE 17–8.

Literature Review (Not Inclusive) of Prenatally Diagnosed Cases of Cystic Hygroma.

Reference	N	Abnormal Chromosomes					Normal Chromosomes		Unsuccessful Culture or Not Available
		45,X	T18	T13	T21	Other	46,XX	46,XY	
Chervenak et al. (1983)	16	10		1			3	1	1
Pearce et al. (1984)	25	17	1		2		---2----		3
Redford et al. (1984)	5	2	1		1			1	
Marchese et al. (1985)	6	4	1				1		
Garden et al. (1985)	22	11	1			1	2	1	6
Carr et al. (1986)	5	2			1		2		
Nicolaides et al. (1986)	9	6			1			2	
Pijpers et al. (1988)	17	8	1				3	3	2
Total	105	60			12		21		12
% Total		(57% 45, X)			(11% other)		(20%)		(11%)

Crawford et al. reported chromosome abnormalities in 16 of 74 (22%) fetuses with a sonographically detectable cardiac defect,[97] and Copel et al. reported chromosome abnormalities in 11 of 34 fetuses (32%) correctly identified with a cardiac defect (three cases trisomy 18, two cases trisomy 21, two cases trisomy 13, two cases trisomy 9, and one case each of triploidy 1p and

47,XXY).[95] The type of chromosome abnormalities identified in prenatal studies also differs from postnatal studies. Trisomy 21 accounted for nearly 78% of chromosome abnormalities reported by Ferencz et al., while a greater proportion of other major chromosome abnormalities (trisomies 18 and 13) has been reported from prenatal studies.[98]

TABLE 17–9.

Congenital Heart Disease and Chromosome Syndromes Among Live Births*

Chromosomal Abnormality	Prevalence in Live Births	Frequency of Congenital Heart Disease (%)	Typical Defect†
Trisomy 21	1:800	50	VSD, ECD
Trisomy 18	1:5,000	99	VSD, ECD, DORV
Trisomy 13	1:20,000	90	VSD
45X	1:5,000	35	Coarct, Bic AOV
Triploidy	rare	?	VSD
Trisomy 8	rare	50	VSD
Trisomy 22	rare	67	ASD
Trisomy 9	rare	50	VSD
5p−	1:20,000	20	VSD
4p−	rare	40	ASD
13q−	rare	25	VSD
18q−	rare	<50	VSD

*Adapted from Copel JA, Pilu G, Kleinman CS: Congenital heart disease and extracardiac anomalies: Associations and indications for fetal echocardiography. Am J Obstet Gynecol 1986; 154:1121–1132.

†VSD = ventricular septal defect; ASD = atrial septal defect; ECD = endocardial cushion defect (atrioventricular communis); DORV = double-outlet right ventricle; Coarct = coarctation of the aorta; Bic AOV = bicuspid aortic valve.

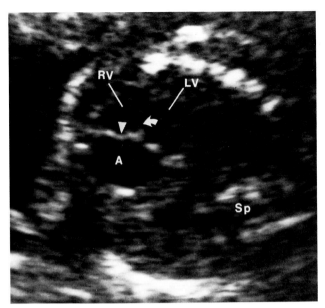

FIG 17–17.
Cardiac malformation and trisomy 21. Transverse scan of the heart demonstrates a large atrioventricular septal defect *(curved arrow)* with a single atrium *(A)* and a pair of atrioventricular valves *(arrowhead)*. *RV* = right ventricle; *LV* = left ventricle; *Sp* = spine.

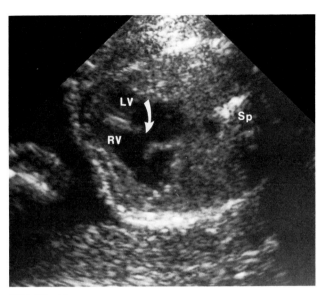

FIG 17–18.
Cardiac malformation and trisomy 18. Four-chamber view demonstrates large ventricular septal defect *(curved arrow)*. Tricuspid dysplasia and transposition of the great vessels were also present. Extracardiac anomalies included cerebellar hypoplasia and a single umbilical artery. *LV* = left ventricle; *RV* = right ventricle; *Sp* = spine.

The differences between prenatal and postnatal studies can be explained by both the natural attrition rate of chromosomally anomalous fetuses during pregnancy[94] and by the insensitivity of prenatal sonography for detecting small defects. Other factors contributing to the frequency of chromosome abnormalities include the clinical indication for the sonogram and the presence of extracardiac anomalies.[93]

Both prenatal and postnatal studies indicate that the risk of a chromosome abnormality varies with the specific type of cardiac anomaly. In their prenatal series, Copel et al. reported that chromosome abnormalities were found in five of seven fetuses with atrioventricular septal defect (endocardial cushion defect), two of three fetuses with double-outlet right ventricle, and two of three fetuses with hypoplastic left heart syndrome.[95] By comparison, no fetus diagnosed with an isolated ventricular septal defect (n = 3) or pulmonic stenosis (n = 4) had a chromosome abnormality.[95] Similarly, Crawford et al. reported chromosome abnormalities in seven of 18 (39%) fetuses with an atrioventricular septal defect (six cases of trisomy 21 and one case of trisomy 18), three of 19 (16%) fetuses with a ventricular septal defect (all trisomy 18), and five of 18 (28%) fetuses with left-sided defects (three cases of 45,X and two cases of trisomy 18) compared to only one of 19 (5%) fetuses with other cardiac defects.[97]

In summary, the strong association between car-

diac malformations and chromosome abnormalities warrants chromosome analysis whenever a structural cardiac defect is detected prenatally. This is particularly important if continuation of the pregnancy is considered.

Duodenal Atresia

Trisomy 21 (Down's syndrome) is present in 20% to 30% of cases of duodenal atresia (Fig 17–19).[103, 105] Unfortunately, characteristic sonographic findings of duodenal atresia ("double bubble" and polyhydramnios) are frequently not apparent until the third trimester, at which time termination of pregnancy usually is not considered a therapeutic option. Occasionally, however, duodenal atresia may be seen before 24 weeks as a mildly dilated duodenum (Fig 17–20).[104] Even when duodenal atresia is not detected until the third trimester, however, knowledge of the fetal karyotype is essential for patient counseling and optimal obstetric management of affected pregnancies. Therefore, chromosome analysis is recommended whenever duodenal atresia is identified prenatally.

Omphalocele

Unlike gastroschisis, omphalocele is frequently associated with concurrent malformations and chromo-

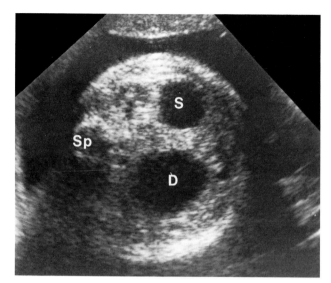

FIG 17–19.
Duodenal atresia and trisomy 21. Transverse scan at 31 weeks demonstrates characteristic "double bubble" with fluid-filled stomach *(S)* and dilated duodenum *(D)*. Also note presence of polyhydramnios. *Sp* = spine.

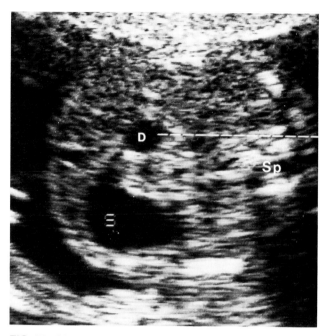

FIG 17–20.
Duodenal atresia at 18 weeks. Transverse scan at 18 weeks demonstrates a fluid-filled duodenum *(D)*. No other abnormalities were identified. Chromosome analysis yielded trisomy 21. Demonstration of duodenal atresia before 24 weeks is unusual. *S* = stomach; *Sp* = spine.

some abnormalities.[109, 112, 115, 116] Trisomies 18 and 13 have been reported most often, followed by trisomy 21, 45,X (Turner's syndrome), and triploidy. A higher frequency of chromosome abnormalities has been observed in most prenatal studies (30%–40%) than in neonatal studies (combined rate of 12%), probably due to the inclusion of more severely anomalous fetuses who die in utero or during the immediate neonatal period.[106, 107, 110, 114]

In a prenatal study, Crawford et al. identified abnormal karyotypes in six of 17 fetuses (35%) identified with omphalocele, including five of eight fetuses with a cardiac malformation (all trisomy 18).[106] Only one fetus with trisomy 18 (14%) had a normal heart. Gilbert and Nicolaides found chromosome abnormalities in 54% of 35 fetuses identified with an omphalocele, and nearly all of these (90%) were trisomy 18.[107] They also reported that chromosome abnormalities were significantly associated with advanced maternal age (>33 years) and male fetuses. The association of trisomy 18 with male fetuses with an omphalocele has also been noted by others.[111]

A more recent prenatal study reported that chromosome abnormalities (trisomies 18, 13, and 21, and 45,X) were most strongly associated with the contents of the omphalocele (liver vs. no liver).[114] Chromosome abnormalities were found in only two of 18 fetuses in whom the liver was in the omphalocele sac (see Fig 17–18) compared to all eight fetuses in whom only bowel was contained within the omphalocele sac (p<.001) (Figs 17–21 and 17–22). Other risk factors

found to be associated with chromosome abnormalities in this series included concurrent anomalies identified by sonography (p = .05) and advanced maternal age (p = .03).[114] Further studies are necessary to confirm these observations.

Currently, chromosome analysis is recommended whenever omphalocele is diagnosed prenatally. Sonographers should be aware that bowel-containing omphaloceles tend to be small and can be missed or mistaken for gastroschisis.[108, 113, 114]

Hydrothorax

Fetal hydrothorax occasionally has been associated with chromosome abnormalities, particularly 45,X (Turner's syndrome) or trisomy 21 (Fig 17–23).[117–120] Nicolaides reported that one of three fetuses with massive unilateral pleural effusions had trisomy 21; this fetus also had evidence of an atrioventricular septal defect.[39] Blott et al. reported prenatal pleuro-amniotic shunting of 11 fetuses identified with pleural effusions and, of these, one had trisomy 21.[117] Similarly, Rodeck et al. reported trisomy 21 in one of eight fetuses with hydrothorax who were managed with pleuro-amniotic shunts.[119] Based on this limited available data, fetal hydrothorax appears to carry a significant risk of an underlying chromosome abnormality. Hence, chromo-

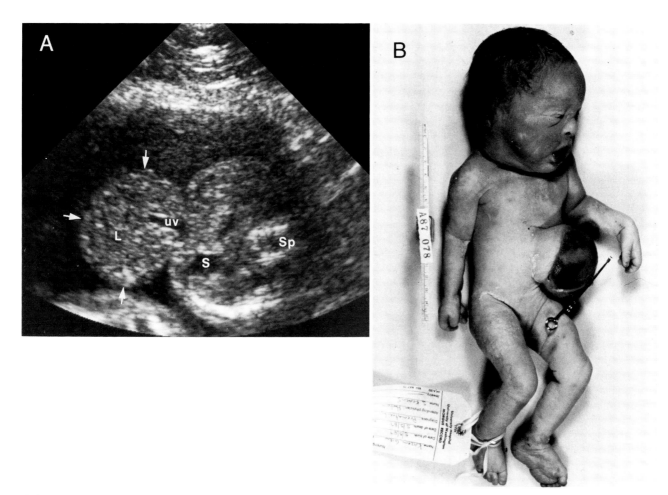

FIG 17–21.
Omphalocele and normal karyotype. **A,** transverse scan demonstrates an omphalocele *(arrows)* containing liver *(L)*. Note the umbilical vein *(UV)* coursing through the abdominal defect. *S* = stomach; *Sp* = spine. **B,** postmortem photograph, following respiratory death at 32 weeks, shows the liver within the omphalocele sac. Other anomalies identified at autopsy included hypoplastic lungs, ventricular septal defect, atrial septal defect, agenesis of the gallbladder, and imperforate vagina. The karyotype was a normal female. (From Nyberg DA, Fitzsimmons J, Mack LA, et al: Chromosomal abnormalities in fetuses with omphalocele: The significance of omphalocele contents. J Ultrasound Med, in press. Used by permission.)

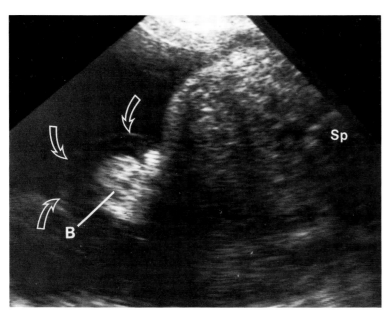

FIG 17–22.
Omphalocele and trisomy 13. Scan of the abdomen at 31 weeks shows omphalocele limited by membrane *(arrows)* and containing bowel *(B)* and ascites but no liver. Alobar holoprosencephaly and renal cystic dysplasia were also identified. Postmortem photograph is shown in Figure 17–35. *Sp* = spine. (From Nyberg DA, Mack LA, Bronstein A, et al: Holoprosencephaly: Prenatal sonographic diagnosis. AJR 1987; 149:1050–1058. Used by permission.)

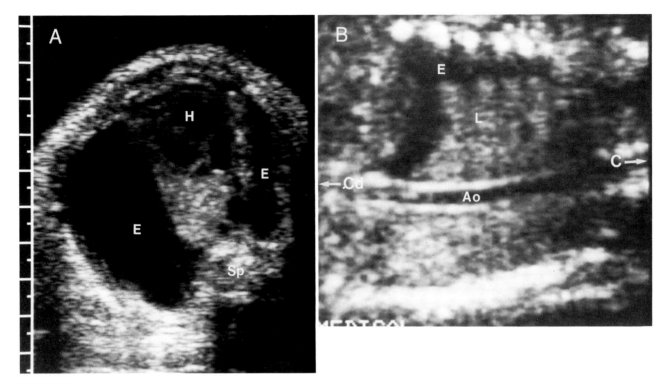

FIG 17–23.
Hydrothorax and trisomy 21. **A,** transverse scan of the thorax demonstrates bilateral pleural effusions *(E)* and polyhydramnios without other evidence of hydrops. The heart *(H)* is displaced to the right. In utero aspiration of the larger pleural effusion was performed. Chromosome analysis yielded trisomy 21. *Sp* = spine. **B,** coronal view of another fetus with trisomy 21 demonstrates a right-sided pleural effusion *(E)* surrounding the lung *(L)*. *Ao* = aorta; *C* = cephalad; *Cd* = caudal.

some analysis is encouraged whenever hydrothorax is identified prenatally, particularly when intrauterine drainage of the hydrothorax or other surgical procedure is considered.

Diaphragmatic Hernia

Diaphragmatic hernia has been associated with various chromosome abnormalities including trisomies 18, 13, and 21, Turner's syndrome, and 13q−.[123] However, the reported frequency of chromosome abnormalities varies markedly between neonatal and prenatal series. In a neonatal series, Puri reported two chromosome abnormalities (trisomy 18 and trisomy 13) among 36 infants (6%) born with a diaphragmatic hernia.[125] By contrast, Comstock reported chromosome abnormalities in two of eight fetuses (25%) who were diagnosed with a diaphragmatic hernia prenatally (both with trisomy 18).[124] Similarly, Benacerraf and Adzick reported 4 chromosome abnormalities among 19 cases (21%) of diaphragmatic hernia diagnosed in utero (two cases of trisomy 18, one case of tetraploidy, and one case of trisomy 21).[122] In 94 cases of diaphragmatic hernia collated from a multi-institutional survey, Adzick et al. reported that only four (4.2%) had chromosome abnormalities. However, the number of fetuses who actually underwent chromosome analysis was not reported in this study.[121] Also, the results may have reflected underreporting from other centers, since the frequency of additional anomalies also was lower (16%) than suggested by other prenatal studies (50%).

The frequency of chromosome abnormalities suggests that chromosome analysis is indicated whenever diaphragmatic hernia is diagnosed prenatally. Knowledge of the karyotype is even more important when in utero surgical correction or other aggressive therapy is considered.

Genitourinary Anomalies

Anomalies of the genitourinary tract are among the most commonly detected by prenatal sonography. As in other organ systems, the risk of a chromosome abnormality in the genitourinary tract appears to vary with the specific malformation present. The highest frequency of chromosome abnormalities has been reported in fetuses with bladder outlet obstruction (urethrovesical obstruction), most commonly from trisomy 18 or trisomy 13 (Figs 17–24 and 17–25). In a series of

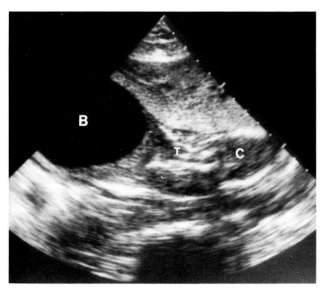

FIG 17–24.
Urethrovesical obstruction and trisomy 18. Longitudinal view demonstrates a markedly enlarged urinary bladder (B) and marked oligohydramnios from urethrovesical obstruction. Chromosome analysis yielded trisomy 18. C = cranium; T = thorax. (Part **B** courtesy of Dolores H Pretorius, MD.)

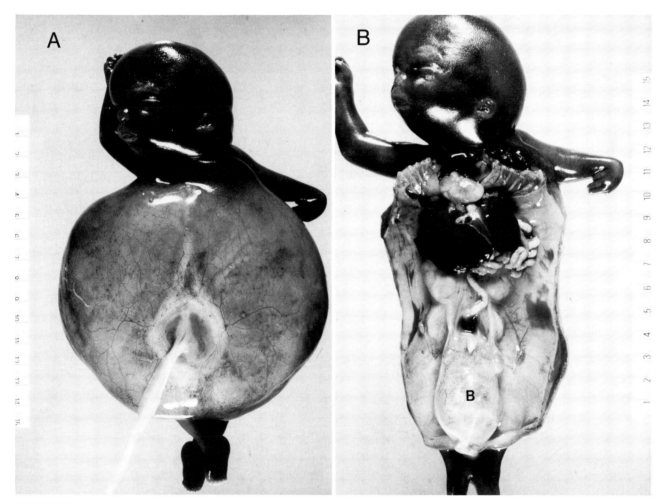

FIG 17–25.
Urethrovesical obstruction and trisomy 18. **A,** postnatal photograph of a case similar to Figure 17–24 shows marked dilatation of the abdomen with a prune-belly deformity. Marked abdominal dilatation was detected on antenatal sonography at 18 weeks, but this was suspected to represent an abdominal wall defect. **B,** internal anomalies include a markedly enlarged urinary bladder (B), absence of the urethra, hydroureters, and urinary ascites. Other anomalies included a complex cardiac defect, micrognathia, low-set ears, and finger flexion deformities. (From Nevin NC, Nevin J, Dunlop JM, et al: Antenatal detection of grossly distended bladder owing to absence of the urethra in a fetus with trisomy 18. J Med Genet 1983; 20:132–133. Used by permission.)

39 fetuses with obstruction at or distal to the urethrovesical junction, Nicolaides et al. reported chromosome abnormalities in nine (23%).[39] Although it is uncertain whether this estimate is representative of the true risk, an association between urethrovesical obstruction and chromosome abnormalities has been noted in many additional case reports.[42, 44, 127, 128, 130, 131]

Chromosome abnormalities have been reported less frequently for more proximal urinary malformations. In a series of 25 fetuses with obstruction at the ureteropelvic junction (UPJ), Kleiner et al. reported that one (4%) had a chromosome abnormality (trisomy 18).[129] In a series of 17 fetuses with multicystic dysplastic kidneys, Rizzo et al. reported that two (12.5%) had chromosome abnormalities (trisomy 13 and 4q+) and five had normal karyotypes (chromosome results were not available in ten cases).[132] Our own experience suggests that the presence of renal cystic dysplasia and concurrent anomalies of other organ systems should suggest a chromosome abnormality (Fig 17–26). If necessary, aspiration of renal cysts can be performed for chromosome analysis.[133]

The frequency of chromosome disorders associated with renal agenesis is uncertain, because chromosome analysis is often not performed in the presence of a lethal malformation. The presence of marked oligohydramnios probably also contributes to infrequent use of chromosome analysis when renal agenesis is suspected.

Based on available evidence, chromosome analysis is recommended for fetuses with bladder outlet obstruction, particularly when in utero surgery or drainage procedures are considered.[126] It is presently uncertain whether chromosome analysis is indicated for other types of genitourinary malformations when no additional anomalies are identified. The present authors do not currently recommend chromosome analysis when unilateral cystic dysplasia or UPJ obstruction is demonstrated.

Clubfoot (Talipes Equinovarus)

Clubfoot has been associated with multiple chromosome abnormalities including trisomy 18, trisomy 13, 4p–, and 18q–.[135–137] Since fetuses with a myelomeningocele frequently have clubfeet on a neuromuscular basis, the risk of a chromosome abnormality for these fetuses probably should be considered separately. Excluding five fetuses with a myelomeningocele who had normal karyotypes, Benacerraf reported 13 fetuses with clubfoot diagnosed on prenatal sonography, including ten (77%) with other major congenital anomalies, and four (31%) with chromosome abnor-

malities (three cases of trisomy 18 and one case of 5p+).[135] All four fetuses with abnormal karyotypes had other sonographic abnormalities including diaphragmatic hernia, intrauterine growth retardation, omphalocele, or short extremities.[135]

In a smaller series, Jeanty et al. reported that two of eight fetuses (25%) with clubfoot detected on sonography had a chromosome abnormality (trisomy 18 and trisomy 20).[137] Each case demonstrated additional sonographic abnormalities including oligohydramnios (trisomy 20) and short limbs (trisomy 18). These data suggest that clubfoot usually is identified only after other abnormalities are detected.

In summary, current evidence suggests that clubfeet are an indication for chromosome analysis when additional malformations are detected. However, there is insufficient information to recommend chromosome analysis when clubfoot is seen in isolation.[136]

Limb Reduction/Other Extremity Malformations

Limb reduction abnormalities have been associated with chromosome abnormalities, particularly trisomy 18.[139–145] For example, it has been suggested that 16% of fetuses with trisomy 18 may demonstrate a limb reduction abnormality (8% in the upper limb and 8% in the lower limb).[140] Bundy et al. reported that 1 of 15 fetuses with trisomy 18 demonstrated micromelia of both forearms, and this was a readily visible finding.[63] Jeanty et al. reported another fetus with trisomy 18 who demonstrated shortened extremities and clubfeet.[137] Radial or thumb aplasia also has been associated with trisomy 18 in 5%–10% of cases.[142]

A wide variety of other extremity abnormalities have been associated with chromosome abnormalities.[143] Polydactyly (Fig 17–27) is found in 80% of fetuses with trisomy 13. Triploidy is often characterized by syndactyly, although this finding is extremely difficult to demonstrate sonographically. Fetuses with trisomy 18 often have flexion deformities of the hands and overlapping fingers, most commonly seen as the second finger overlapping the third finger (Fig 17–28). Trisomy 21 frequently is accompanied by two extremity deformities: hypoplasia of the middle phalanx of the fifth digit resulting in clinodactyly[138] and a widened space between the first and second toes. An association between shortened femurs and trisomy 21 also has been noted, but since this has often been reported in conjunction with nuchal thickening, it is discussed separately below.

In summary, a wide variety of skeletal anomalies have been associated with chromosome abnormalities. Although relatively few such anomalies have been reported on prenatal sonography, shortened extremities

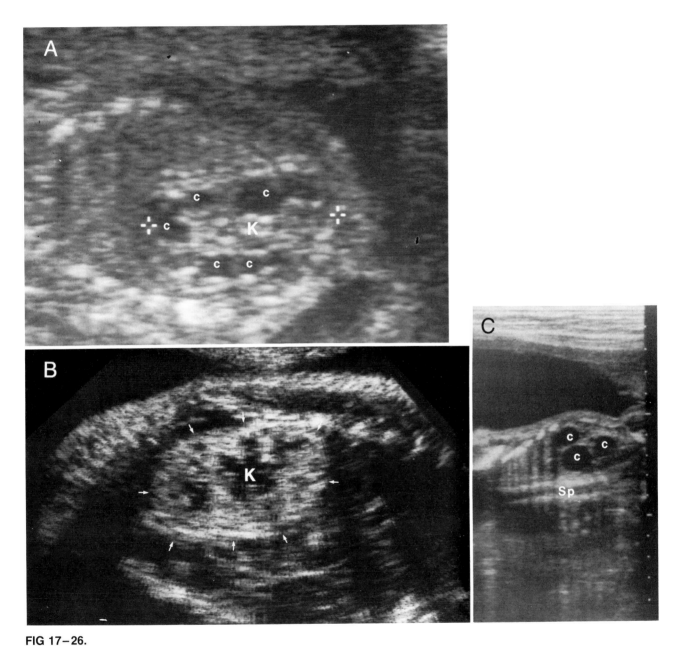

FIG 17–26.
Renal cystic dysplasia and chromosome abnormalities. **A,** trisomy 18. Longitudinal scan of the right kidney *(K)* at 19 weeks demonstrates multiple cysts *(c)* of varying sizes consistent with cystic dysplasia. The left kidney was not visualized, and marked oligohydramnios was present. **B,** trisomy 13. Longitudinal scan shows large echogenic kidney (*K,* outlined by small arrows) secondary to innumerable small cysts. From same case as Figure 17–22. **C,** triploidy. Longitudinal scan shows multiple cysts *(c)* of the fetal kidney. A myelomeningocele was identified on other views (same fetus as Figure 17–7,C. *Sp* = spine. (From Nyberg DA, Mack LA, Bronstein A, et al: Holoprosenceph-aly: Prenatal sonographic diagnosis. AJR 1987; 149:1050–1058. Used by permission.)

FIG 17-27.
Polydactyly and trisomy 13. **A,** transverse scan through hand at 31 weeks shows polydactyly with six digits. Other abnormalities identified included alobar holoprosencephaly and cebocephaly. **B,** another fetus with trisomy 13 shows postaxial polydactyly with the extra digit oriented nearly perpendicular to other digits.

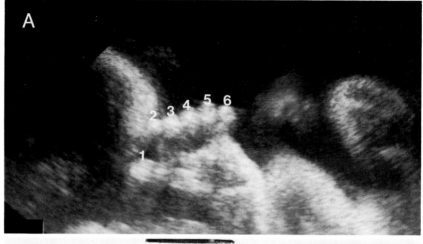

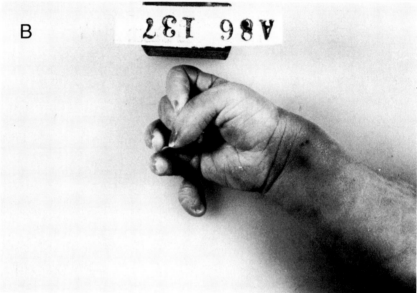

should be readily demonstrated, and this finding shows the strongest association with trisomy 18.

Nuchal Thickening/Short Femur Lengths

Redundant skin in the nuchal region is present in 80% of newborns with trisomy 21,[150] as well as other chromosome abnormalities (trisomies 13, 18, and 45,X). In some cases, nuchal thickening apparently results from cystic hygromata that have resolved.[148, 153]

Identification of an easily reproducible sonographic finding that might be associated with trisomy 21 is a desirable goal. To this end, Benacerraf and her colleagues have proposed that nuchal thickness and/or disproportionately short femur lengths may be useful findings as a method for screening fetuses with trisomy 21.[146, 147] They reported that nuchal thickening (> 5 mm) can be demonstrated in up to 42% of fetuses with trisomy 21 during the mid-trimester, compared to only

0.06% of normal fetuses (Fig 17–29).[146, 147] Using a ratio of actual femur length (FL) measurement to the expected FL (based on the biparietal diameter), these authors reported a ratio of 0.91 or lower had a sensitivity of 68% and a specificity of 98% for detecting fetuses with trisomy 21 between 15 and 21 weeks.[147] Using both nuchal thickening and a low FL/expected FL ratio, trisomy 21 was identified with a sensitivity of 75% and a specificity of 98%, with a positive predictive value of 3.6%.

These observations have stimulated additional studies by a number of other investigators. Toi et al. point out that nuchal fold measurement varies significantly with the plane and angle of the scan.[154] Assuming the sensitivity and specificity reported by Benacerraf, they also note that the positive predictive value of nuchal thickening is relatively low in the general population. However, this frequency compares favorably with commonly accepted clinical indications for chro-

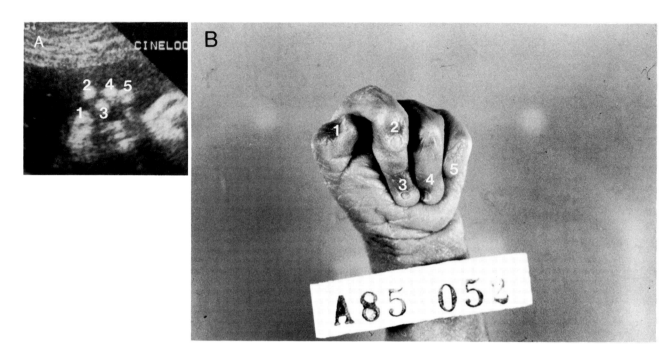

FIG 17-28.
Overlapping fingers with trisomy 18. **A,** transverse view of the hand shows overlapping fingers with the second finger *(2)* overlapping the third *(3)*. **B,** postmortem photograph of another fetus with trisomy 18 shows overlapping fingers with second finger *(2)* over the third *(3)*.

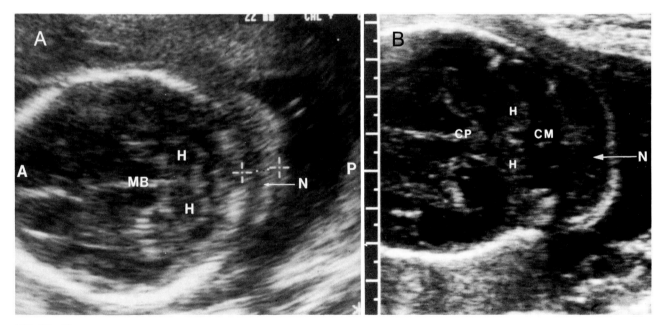

FIG 17-29.
Nuchal thickening and chromosome abnormalities. **A,** trisomy 21. Transverse scan oriented through the posterior fossa at 20 weeks shows abnormal thickening (8 mm) of the nuchal fold *(N,* marked by cursors). *A* = anterior; *P* = posterior; *H* = cerebellar hemispheres; *MB* = midrain. **B,** Turner's syndrome. Similar view in another fetus with Turner's syndrome (45,X) at 26 weeks also shows marked thickening of the nuchal area *(N),* representing a resolving cystic hygroma. Subsequent scans showed resolution of nuchal thickness. *CM* = cisterna magna; *H* = cerebellar hemispheres; *CP* = cerebral penduncles.

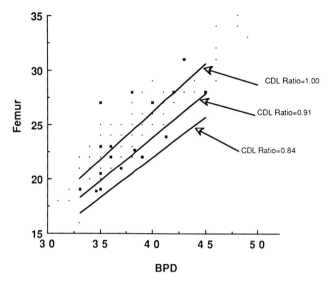

FIG 17–30.
Femur length and trisomy 21. Femur length plotted against biparietal diameter (BPD) for 128 normal control group *(dots)* and 28 fetuses with trisomy 21 *(black squares)*. The three lines correspond to critical decision lines (CDL) for measured-to-expected femur-length ratios of 1.0, 0.91, and 0.84. A measured-to-expected femur length ratio of less than 0.91 would have detected five of 28 fetuses with trisomy 21 and resulted in a positive predictive value of 3%, assuming the prevalence of trisomy 21 is 1 in 250. Regression line for expected femur length = 0.878–BPD–.89594. (From Perrella R, Duerinckx AJ, Grant EG, et al: Second-trimester sonographic diagnosis of Down syndrome: Role of femur-length shortening and nuchal fold thickening. AJR 1988; 151:981–985. Used by permission.)

mosome analysis including advanced maternal age and low MS-AFP levels.

Perrella et al. retrospectively evaluated the usefulness of both nuchal thickening and short femur length in a series of 28 fetuses with trisomy 21.[152] In 14 fetuses, sonograms were considered adequate to determine the nuchal thickness, and three of these (21%) were considered thickened. By comparison, 12 of their 128 control patients (9%) also demonstrated a thickened nuchal fold. These authors did not support a role for routine measurements of nuchal thickness as a screening procedure. While they did find that short femur length had a positive predictive value of 3% for identifying trisomy 21 in women with advanced maternal age (Fig 17–30), the predictive value decreases to 1% in the general population (prevalence of trisomy 21, 1 in 700).[152]

In a retrospective by Dicke et al., a biparietal diameter (BPD)/FL ratio > 1.5 SD identified 18% of Down's syndrome pregnancies with only a 4% false-positive rate and a positive predictive value of 1/169.[149] When trisomies 21, 18, and 13 were considered collectively, a sensitivity of 29% and predictive value of 1 in 78

were achieved with no increase in the false-positive rate (4%). The FL observed/FL expected ratio (using a derived formula) was less valuable in detecting chromosomally abnormal fetuses with a sensitivity of only 15%, a false-positive rate of 10%, and a positive predictive value of only 1 in 455.

Lynch et al. retrospectively studied nine pairs of twins consisting of one fetus with Down's syndrome and one normal co-twin.[151] Actual femur length to expected femur length was concordant (normal or abnormal) in seven of nine pairs of twins, suggesting that shortened femur length was not of value in identifying the anomalous twin. On the other hand, nuchal fold thickening (6 mm or more) was identified in five of nine fetuses with trisomy 21 and was not present in any of the normal co-twins.

Experience from Swedish Medical Center, Seattle, Washington, (unpublished data) suggests that marked nuchal thickening (10 mm) is likely to be associated with trisomy 21, although it is uncommonly encountered, while mild nuchal thickening (5–6 mm) is more likely to be found in normal fetuses. At this institution, femur length shortening has not been found to be useful as a screening procedure. Also, sonographers should recognize that published formulas that derive the expected femur length from the biparietal diameter vary significantly.[146, 152] The reason for these differences is unknown, but is more likely to reflect variations in methods of measurement, particularly for the femur length, rather than actual regional or racial differences in fetal size.

In summary, some studies support the notion that nuchal thickening and/or disproportionately small femur length may be associated with trisomy 21, whereas other studies do not. A stronger case can be made for the value of nuchal thickening, particularly when obviously thickened. Whether a disproportionately short femur length justifies chromosome analysis currently is uncertain, and further investigation is encouraged.

Single Umbilical Artery

A single umbilical artery has long been of interest because of its association with congenital malformations and chromosome abnormalities.[155–160] Over 50% of fetuses with trisomy 18 and 10%–50% of fetuses with trisomy 13 have a single umbilical artery (Fig 17–31). Turner's syndrome (45,X), triploidy, and other chromosome abnormalities also appear to have an increased frequency of a single umbilical artery over the general population (1%).

The risk of a chromosome abnormality from a sin-

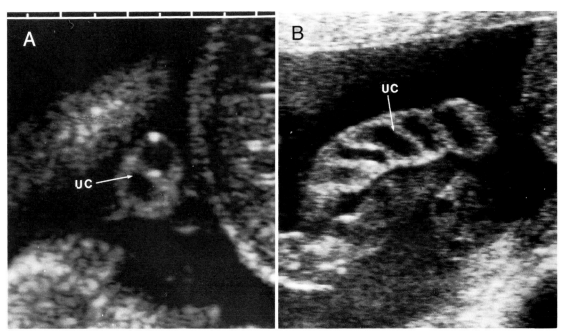

FIG 17–31.
Single umbilical artery and trisomy 18. Transverse **(A)** and longitudinal **(B)** views of the umbilical cord *(UC)* shows a two-vessel umbilical cord (single umbilical artery) rather than the normal three vessels. Other abnormalities identified on sonography included cerebellar hypoplasia and a complex cardiac anomaly (same fetus as Figures 17–4,C and 17–18). (From Nyberg DA, Shepard T, Mack LA, et al: Significance of a single umbilical artery in fetuses with central nervous system malformations. J Ultrasound Med 1988; 7:265–273. Used by permission.)

gle umbilical artery clearly depends on the presence of associated anomalies. Vlietinck et al. found no chromosome abnormalities in 19 consecutive live born infants who had a single umbilical artery but no congenital malformations.[161] By contrast, Byrne and Blane reported that all nine aborted fetuses with a single umbilical artery had other anomalies and three (33%) of these had a chromosome abnormality.[156] Similarly, Lenoski and Medovy noted that three of seven fetuses (43%) with a single umbilical artery had a trisomic karyotype.[157]

In a prenatal ultrasound study the presence of a single umbilical artery significantly increased the risk of concurrent malformations and chromosome abnormalities in fetuses with known central nervous system malformations (holoprosencephaly, Dandy-Walker malformation, hydrocephalus, or spina bifida).[160] Based on available evidence, we believe that identification of a single umbilical artery should initiate a search for additional malformations but is not itself an indication for chromosome analysis.

Placental Abnormalities

Placental abnormalities such as thickening or cystic changes may be a clue to an underlying chromosome abnormality, particularly triploidy (Fig 17–32).[163, 188]

Other chromosome abnormalities may also demonstrate placental changes; Jouppila and associates observed intraplacental cystic areas in five of 11 fetuses with trisomy 18 and one of two fetuses with trisomy 13.[162] Therefore, a chromosome abnormality should be considered when multiple cystic areas are identified in the placenta, especially in association with oligohydramnios and/or early-onset intrauterine growth retardation (IUGR). Placental abnormalities also can result in an abnormal systolic/diastolic ratio with umbilical artery Doppler (see Chapter 16).

Abnormal Amniotic Fluid Volume

Polyhydramnios

Polyhydramnios is often the initial or primary manifestation of an underlying fetal disorder.[168] The greater the degree of polyhydramnios, the greater the likelihood of finding a major malformation and an accompanying chromosome abnormality (Fig 17–33).[164] The presence of both polyhydramnios and IUGR has been said to be characteristic of trisomy 18, although oligohydramnios also may be demonstrated from trisomy 18.[166]

Barkin et al. reviewed 191 singleton pregnancies complicated by polyhydramnios including 138 (71%) with mild polyhydramnios and 57 (29%) with severe

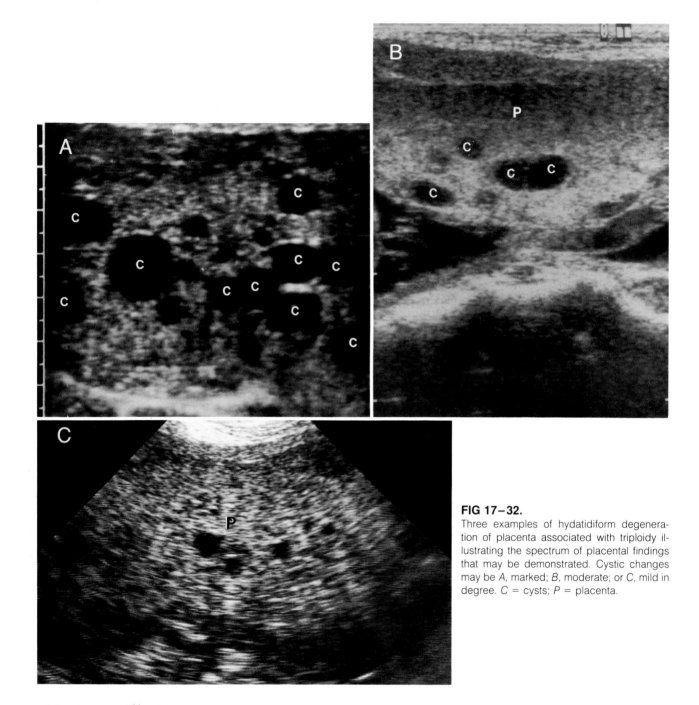

FIG 17–32.
Three examples of hydatidiform degeneration of placenta associated with triploidy illustrating the spectrum of placental findings that may be demonstrated. Cystic changes may be *A,* marked; *B,* moderate; or *C,* mild in degree. *C* = cysts; *P* = placenta.

polyhydramnios.[164] Of the 57 fetuses with severe polyhydramnios, congenital anomalies were found in 75% (43 cases) and chromosome abnormalities were found in six (10.5%). Five of the fetuses with chromosome abnormalities had other detectable anomalies, and one fetus had ascites only. By comparison, 29% of fetuses with mild polyhydramnios had anomalies, and none of these fetuses had chromosome abnormalities.

Similarly, Filly reported malformations in 25 of 28

fetuses (89.3%) with marked polyhydramnios, compared to six of 31 fetuses (19%) with mild polyhydramnios.[167] Three of 28 fetuses (11%) with marked polyhydramnios had chromosome abnormalities (two cases of trisomy 21 and one case of trisomy 13), and fetal abnormalities were demonstrated in two of these three cases. In another study, Landy et al. found one chromosome abnormality (trisomy 18) among 99 fetuses with polyhydramnios, including 59 fetuses with

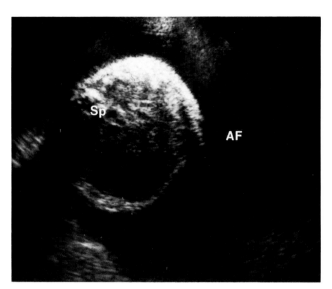

FIG 17–33.
Polyhydramnios and trisomy 18. Transverse scan of the abdomen at 31 weeks shows markedly increased amount of amniotic fluid *(AF)*. The fetal stomach was not visualized, and cerebellar hypoplasia also was identified. Chromosome analysis yielded trisomy 18. Multiple anomalies were found at autopsy including esophageal atresia with tracheoesophageal fistula (same fetus as Figure 17–36). *Sp* = spine.

idiopathic polyhydramnios.[165] Unlike the other series, however, these authors did not distinguish mild from severe polyhydramnios.

Based on available evidence, demonstration of marked polyhydramnios should initiate a careful search for an underlying fetal malformation. Demonstration of an associated anomaly or IUGR carries a significant risk of a chromosome abnormality. Whether "idiopathic" polyhydramnios is an indication for chromosome analysis will undoubtedly depend on other factors including the severity of polyhydramnios.

Oligohydramnios

Oligohydramnios may reflect an underlying chromosome abnormality when seen in association with IUGR or a renal malformation. However, the risk of a chromosome abnormality in this situation remains uncertain due to the paucity of reports.

Intrauterine Growth Retardation

Early "symmetric" IUGR is a common manifestation of major chromosome abnormalities, particularly trisomies 18 and 13, and triploidy.[169–171] Jouppila et al. demonstrated early growth retardation in 9 of 11 fetuses with trisomy 18, 2 of 2 fetuses with trisomy 13, and 2 of 5 fetuses with 45,X, compared to only 2 of 18

fetuses with trisomy 21.[162] Demonstration of early symmetric IUGR in association with oligohydramnios also should suggest a chromosome abnormality (Fig 17–34). Of six cases with early IUGR and oligohydramnios found not to be due to renal agenesis, Nicolaides et al. reported chromosome abnormalities in two, both representing triploidy.[39]

In summary, current evidence suggests that early (second trimester) symmetric IUGR should initiate a careful search for fetal anomalies and, if the pregnancy is continued, stimulate chromosome analysis. When early IUGR is demonstrated, chromosome analysis can be performed from fetal blood obtained by umbilical vein sampling.

Summary

The risk of aneuploidy is increased for a wide range of sonographically detectable abnormalities. Even sonographic abnormalities that may be considered to have a relatively low likelihood of aneuploidy usually carry a greater risk than commonly accepted clinical indications for karyotyping such as advanced maternal age and low MS-AFP levels. Anomalies that appear to carry the greatest risk at an underlying chromosome abnormality are listed in Table 17–10.

It might appear that virtually any congenital anomaly increases the risk of an underlying chromosome abnormality. While this may be true for malformations that occur during embryologic development, "acquired" disorders or anomalies which are thought to result from tissue disruption probably do not carry an increased risk of a chromosome abnormality. Examples of these disorders include hydranencephaly, amniotic band syndrome, limb-body wall complex, tumors, jejunoileal atresia caused by vascular insufficiency, and gastroschisis.

As we have attempted to indicate, the two most important determinants in attempting to define the risk of a chromosome abnormality are the specific type of malformation identified and the presence of associated anomalies. Whether sonographic abnormalities are considered to justify the expense and risk of chromosome analysis will vary from institution to institution. Chromosome analysis is particularly important if expensive and aggressive surgical management is considered as a therapeutic option (for example, urethrovesical obstruction), even if associated chromosome abnormalities are relatively uncommon. Other factors that influence the ultimate decision include the gestational age at detection, skill of the sonographer(s), available options in management, the approach of the

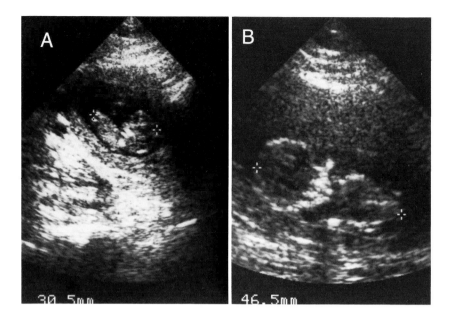

FIG 17–34.
Early intrauterine growth retardation and triploidy. **A,** longitudinal scan in a woman known to be 11.5 menstrual weeks by an earlier US examination shows a crown rump length of 30 mm, corresponding to 10 weeks. **B,** repeat sonogram 2 weeks later (13.5 weeks) shows a crown rump length of 46 mm, corresponding to 11.5 weeks. Chromosome analysis yielded triploidy. (From Benacerraf BR: Intrauterine growth retardation in the first trimester associated with triploidy. J Ultrasound Med 1988; 7:153–154. Used by permission.)

obstetrician and genetic counselor and, of course, the wishes of the patient.

Patients occasionally may choose not to undergo chromosome analysis, regardless of the frequency of chromosome abnormalities. This decision is particu-larly likely if the malformation is perceived as uni-formly fatal or if multiple other malformations are iden-tified. However, patients should be made aware that knowledge of a chromosome disorder is important when counseling about future pregnancies, because

TABLE 17–10.

Partial List of Sonographic Findings That Carry a Significant Risk of a Chromosomal Abnormality

Central nervous system anomalies
  Holoprosencephaly
  Dandy-Walker malformation, cerebellar hypoplasia
  Hydrocephalus
  Spina bifida
  Agenesis of the corpus callosum
Choroid plexus cysts—large or associated with other abnormalities
Facial abnormalities
Cystic hygroma
Nuchal thickening
Cardiac malformations
Duodenal atresia
Omphalocele
Hydrothorax
Genitourinary anomalies
  Obstructive uropathy (obstruction at or distal to the urethrovesical junction)
  Renal cystic dysplasia with other abnormalities
Clubfoot with other abnormalities
Severe IUGR*
Polyhydramnios or oligohydramnios and other abnormalities
Single umbilical artery with other anomalies
Multiple placental cysts

*IUGR = intrauterine growth retardation.

malformations due to an underlying chromosome abnormality carry a lower risk of recurrence (1%–2%) than most inheritable syndromes.

TYPICAL PATHOLOGIC AND SONOGRAPHIC FEATURES OF SPECIFIC CHROMOSOMAL ABNORMALITIES

In addition to knowing the frequency of chromosome abnormalities based on a specific sonographic finding, it is useful to be aware of typical pathologic and clinical features of the major chromosome abnormalities (trisomies 13, 18, and 21; triploidy, and 45X). These are discussed separately below.

Trisomy 13 (Patau's Syndrome)

Clinical and Pathologic Findings (Table 17–11)

Trisomy 13 and its association with certain congenital malformations was first described by Patau in 1960.[189] The prevalence of trisomy 13 is 1 in 6,000 births, but it accounts for about 1% of spontaneous first-trimester abortions. A bimodal distribution of maternal ages has been noted with peaks at 25 and 38 years, consistent with age-independent and age-dependent subgroups.[200]

TABLE 17–11.

Pathologic Features of Trisomy 13

Single umbilical artery (10%–50%)
Craniofacial
  Microcephaly
  Cyclopia
  Anophthalmia
  Microphthalmia
  Cleft lip and palate
  Low-set, deformed ears
  Capillary hemangiomas
  Central nervous system
  Holoprosencephaly
  Agenesis of the corpus callosum
Cardiovascular malformations (VSD, ASD, PDA*)
Gastrointestinal
  Omphalocele, umbilical hernia (40%)
Urogenital malformations
  Cystic renal dysplasia
  Hydronephrosis
  Duplicated kidney
  Ambiguous genitalia
Skeletal
  Polydactyly (70%)
  Rocker bottom feet
  Scalp defects

*VSD = ventricular septal defects; ASD = atrial septal defects; PDA = patent ductus arteriosus.

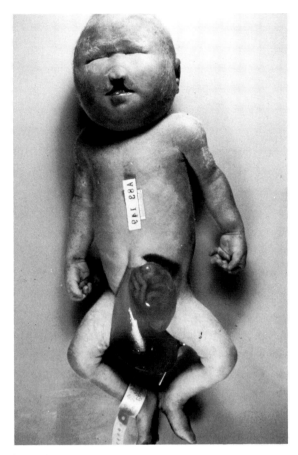

FIG 17–35.
Trisomy 13. Postmortem photograph shows characteristic findings of trisomy 13 including facial cleft, hypotelorism, omphalocele, and polydactyly. Alobar holoprosencephaly and renal cystic dysplasia were also identified on prenatal sonography.

The phenotype of trisomy 13 is so striking that a diagnosis can frequently be made on the basis of clinical observations alone (Fig 17–35).[184, 189, 191, 198, 200] Characteristic physical findings include microcephaly, anophthalmia, or micro-ophthalmia; receding forehead; cleft lip and palate (60% to 70%); flexed and overlapping fingers; and postaxial polydactyly (75%). Of internal anomalies, malformations of the central nervous system are among the most common and severe. These include some form of holoprosencephaly (78%), agenesis of the corpus callosum (22%), cerebellar anomalies (28%), and hydrocephalus (13%).[200] Cardiovascular malformations also are common (>80%) and may include VSD, ASD, patent ductus arteriosus (PDA), mitral or aortic atresia, pulmonary stenosis, and anomalous venous return. Genitourinary anomalies (30%) include renal cystic dysplasia (31%), hydronephrosis, and duplication abnormalities. Omphalocele or umbilical hernia is found in nearly one third of cases. The calcaneus is often prominent and the feet rocker have a bottom shape. Other features of trisomy 13 that would not normally be detected on sonograms include colobomas, capillary hemangioma of the forehead, and localized scalp defects over the parieto-occipital region.

Sonographic Findings

Trisomy 13 may present with early-onset IUGR and third-trimester polyhydramnios. Malformations of the CNS, particularly holoprosencephaly, are the most common specific anomalies reported. Other malformations that have been detected include cyclopia, hypotelorism, facial cleft, renal cystic dysplasia or hydronephrosis, cardiovascular malformations, polydactyly, and clubfoot.

Certain sonographic findings of trisomy 13 are shared by the Meckel-Gruber syndrome, an autosomal recessive disorder that is characterized by cystic kidneys and one or more additional findings of polydactyly and a midline central nervous system malformation (occipital encephalocele, holoprosencephaly, or Dandy-Walker malformation). Distinction between these disorders is important, since the recurrence risk of trisomy 13 is low (1%–2%) compared to Meckel-Gruber syndrome (25%).

Because of the severity of malformations usually present, the sensitivity of sonography for detecting trisomy 13 would be expected to be high. Benacerraf et al. reported sonographic recognition of nine fetuses with trisomy 13 encountered during a 3-year period.[172] All nine fetuses had facial abnormalities, seven fetuses demonstrated holoprosencephaly, and three fetuses demonstrated abnormalities of the hands and feet (polydactyly or clubfoot).

Prognosis

The prognosis for infants with trisomy 13 is extremely poor. About half die within the first month, 75% die by 6 months, and less than 5% survive more than 3 years. The mean survival for live borns is 130 days. Death usually occurs within the first month of life; long-term survivors rarely have been reported.[191] Common neonatal problems include hypotonia or hypertonia, seizures, apnea, feeding difficulties, and failure to thrive.

Trisomy 18

Clinical and Pathologic Findings (Table 17–12).

Trisomy 18 is one of the most common autosomal disorders with a prevalence of 1 in 3,000 to 1 in 6,000. Intrauterine demise or stillbirth is common; it is esti-

mated that 50% to 90% of fetuses alive at 16 weeks will not survive to live birth.[11, 185] Males experience a higher mortality rate both during pregnancy and after birth, leading to a female-male preponderance among newborns. Like other major autosomal disorders, trisomy 18 is positively correlated with maternal age, although there also are a large number of "age-independent" cases.[11]

Characteristic clinical findings of trisomy 18 include IUGR, loose skin, hypoplasia of skeletal muscle, and diminished fetal activity (Fig 17–36).[178, 195, 196] The head is dolichocephalic and frequently microcephalic with a prominent occiput. Facial features include a small mouth, micrognathia, and low, pointed "pixie" ears. Cleft lip and/or palate is much less common (15%) than with trisomy 13. The hands often are clenched with overlapping fingers, most frequently with the index finger overlapping the middle finger and with the fifth finger curved inward (Fig 17–28). Cardiovascular malformations, present in approximately 90% of cases, include VSD, ASD, PDA, double-outlet right ventricle, and bicuspid aortic and pulmonic valves.[100, 187] The placenta is small, and a single umbilical artery is present in over 50% of cases.

In addition to the common malformations noted above, over 100 different abnormalities involving virtually every organ system have been noted in conjunction with trisomy 18.[194] These include diaphragmatic and inguinal hernias, omphalocele (Fig 17–37), umbilical hernia, genitourinary anomalies (hydronephrosis, hydroureter, bladder outlet obstruction, horseshoe kidney, and duplication abnormalities), and anomalies of the gastrointestinal tract (tracheoesophageal fistula, anorectal atresia). Central nervous system anomalies may include hydrocephalus, cerebellar hypoplasia, agenesis of the corpus callosum, and spina bifida.[180, 194–196] Limb reduction abnormalities have been noted in 16% of cases, equally divided between lower and upper extremities.[140] Other skeletal problems include prominent heels, rocker bottom feet, arthrogryposis, and short sternum.

Sonographic Findings

The diversity of prenatal sonographic findings reported with trisomy 18 reflects the pathologic findings. Symmetric IUGR, often in association with polyhydramnios or oligohydramnios, may be the initial clue to the presence of trisomy 18. Specific sonographic malformations that have been reported include cystic hygroma, non-immune hydrops, hydrocephalus, spina bifida, facial cleft, diaphragmatic hernia, tracheoesophageal fistula, genitourinary anomalies, cardiovascular

TABLE 17–12.

Pathologic Features of Trisomy 18

Intrauterine growth retardation
Polyhydramnios or oligohydramnios
Single umbilical artery (>80%)
Cystic hygroma
Non-immune hydrops
Craniofacial abnormalities
    Dolichocephaly, microcephaly
    Low-set "pixie" ears
    Micrognathia
    Cleft lip or palate (10%–20%)
Central nervous system abnormalities
    Hydrocephalus
    Myelomeningocele (10%–20%)
Cardiovascular malformations (VSD, ASD, PDA,* double-outlet right
    ventricle, bicuspid aortic, and pulmonic valves)
Gastrointestinal anomalies
    Esophageal atresia/tracheoesophageal fistula
    Omphalocele
    Diaphragmatic hernia
    Anorectal atresia
Genitourinary anomalies
    Urethrovesical obstruction
    Renal dysplasia
    Horseshoe kidney
    Ambiguous genitalia
Skeletal
    Short extremities
    Overlapping fingers, flexed hands (>80%)
    Rocker bottom feet
    Shortened first toes

*VSD = ventricular septal defects; ASD = atrial septal defects; PDA = patent ductus arteriosus.

malformations, omphalocele, clubfoot, short extremities, overlapping fingers, and single umbilical artery.

Few studies have addressed the sensitivity of ultrasound for detecting fetuses with trisomy 18. Bundy et al. described prenatal sonographic findings in 12 fetuses with trisomy 18.[63] All five fetuses seen after 20 weeks demonstrated IUGR and of these two also demonstrated oligohydramnios and one demonstrated polyhydramnios. Of seven fetuses seen before 20 weeks, three were interpreted as normal, and one each demonstrated lymphangiectasia, micromelia, hydrocephalus, and large choroid plexus cysts. Benacerraf et al. reported that 12 of 15 fetuses (80%) with trisomy 18 demonstrated sonographic abnormalities of polyhydramnios, diaphragmatic hernia, omphalocele, cardiovascular malformation, and/or neural tube defect.[172] Eleven fetuses also had abnormalities of the hands or feet.

Prognosis

The prognosis of fetuses with trisomy 18 is uniformly poor. Many undiagnosed cases are delivered prematurely (secondary to polyhydramnios) and by cesarean section. The median survival for infants born with trisomy 18 is 5 days, with a mean of 48 days.[175] Less than 10% of infants are still alive at 1 year of age. Males with trisomy 18 are overrepresented in deaths at all stages of pregnancy and, if born alive, their life expectancy is less than that of females.[11] Common neonatal problems include feeding difficulties, poor sucking reflex, hypotonia, and failure to thrive.

Trisomy 21 (Down's Syndrome)

Clinical and Pathologic Findings (Table 17–13)

Trisomy 21 is one of the most common chromosome abnormalities, with an overall prevalence of 1 in 660 newborns. Trisomy 21 comprises nearly half of all chromosome abnormalities detected at the time of second-trimester amniocentesis. The precise risk of trisomy 21 varies significantly with maternal age (see Table 17–2). Other risk factors that increase the likelihood of trisomy 21 include a family history of Down's syndrome and low MS-AFP levels.

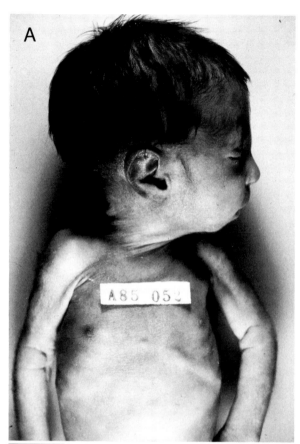

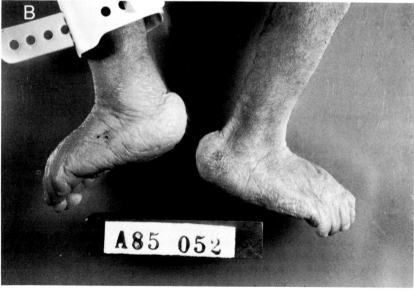

FIG 17–36.
Trisomy 18. **A,** lateral view of fetus with trisomy 18 shows micrognathia, skin laxity, underdeveloped musculature, and prominent occiput. **B,** rocker bottom feet. Other anomalies identified at autopsy included overlapping fingers (see Fig 17–28, A), esophageal atresia with tracheoesophageal fistula, cerebellar hypoplasia, small ventricular septal defect, and bicuspid aortic valve.

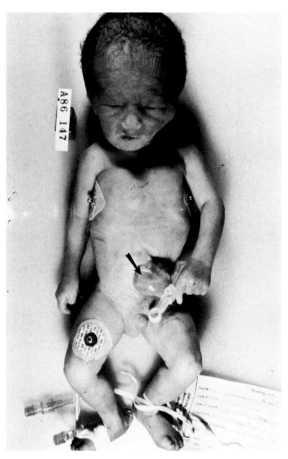

FIG 17–37.
Trisomy 18. Postmortem photograph of an infant with trisomy 18 shows micrognathia, a small bowel-containing omphalocele *(arrow),* and clenched hands. Other anomalies identified at autopsy included rocker bottom feet, esophageal atresia with tracheoesophageal fistula, short sternum, tiny (0.4 cm) ventricular septal defect, bicuspid aortic and pulmonic valves cerebellar hypoplasia, and single umbilical artery.

TABLE 17–13.
Pathologic Features of Trisomy 21

Cystic hygroma
Non-immune hydrops
Hydrothorax
Craniofacial
    Brachycephaly
    Epicanthic folds
    Short nose
    Round, low ears
    Broad neck
    Protruding tongue
Cardiovascular malformations (VSD, ASD, PDA*)
Gastrointestinal
    Duodenal atresia
    Esophageal atresia (tracheoesophageal fistula)
    Anorectal atresia
    Omphalocele
Genitourinary
    Undescended testis
Skeletal
    Flattening of acetabular angles
    Widening of iliac wings
    Short, broad hands
    Clinodactyly
    Short lower extremities
    Increased space between first and second toes

*VSD = ventricular septal defects; ASD = atrial septal defects; PDA = patent ductus arteriosus.

The characteristic clinical features of trisomy 21 were first described in 1866 by Dr. John Langdon Down, well before the corresponding chromosome abnormality was discovered in 1959.[190] However, clinical features during the neonatal period are often absent or poorly developed compared to the adult. Hall identified 10 major clinical features of Down's syndrome from a group of 48 newborns.[150] Characteristic craniofacial features include brachycephaly; a relatively flat occiput and mild microcephaly; flat, small nose; low nasal bridge; protruding tongue; epicanthal folds; and small, low-set ears that show overfolding of the upper helix.[190, 192] There may be excess skin on the back of a rather short neck (Fig 17–38). The hands are short and broad. The mid-phalanx of the fifth finger is hypoplastic and curved inward (clinodactyly) in 60% of cases. A single palmar crease is present in 30% of cases. There may be a wide gap between the first and second toes. The pelvis is hypoplastic with an outward flaring of the iliac wings and shallow acetabular angle. Cardiac anomalies, primarily ventricular septal defects and endocardial cushion defects, are present in approximately 25% of infants with trisomy 21. A similar frequency has been found in fetal specimens.[187] Gastrointestinal anomalies include duodenal atresia or stenosis (8%) and tracheoesophageal fistula.

Morphologic features of trisomy 21 in fetuses are even less developed than in neonates and have been studied infrequently. Stephens and Shepard examined 13 fetuses with trisomy 21 who were aborted during the second trimester and found very few consistent features.[197] The most consistent findings were a simian crease, hypoplasia of deformed middle phalanx of the fifth finger (91%), and a cleft between the first and second toes.[197] In another group of 26 fetuses with trisomy 21 who underwent autopsy, Keeling reported the following anomalies: transverse palmar crease (65%), low-set ears (54%), ventricular septal defect or atrioventricular septal defect (19%), short digits (8%), hydrops fetalis (8%), duodenal atresia (8%), and hydrocephalus (4%).[187]

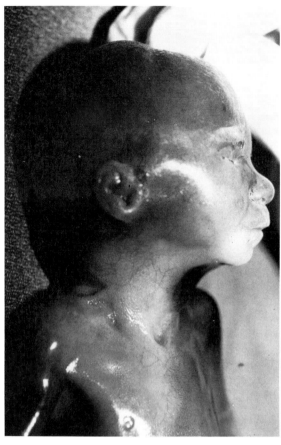

FIG 17–38.
Down's syndrome. Postmortem photograph of fetus with trisomy 21 shows low-set ears and mild nuchal thickening.

Sonographic Findings

Prenatal sonography is predictably less sensitive for detecting trisomy 21 than it is for detecting trisomies 18 and 13. The most characteristic findings of trisomy 21 on sonography are duodenal atresia and endocardial cushion defect. Other sonographic findings that have been reported with trisomy 21 include cystic hygroma, non–immune hydrops, hydrothorax, omphalocele, nuchal thickening, disproportionately short femurs, and clinodactyly.[39, 90, 117, 138, 139]

Prognosis

In previous years, approximately 20%–30% of infants with trisomy 21 died during the first year of life, and 50% died by age 5. Currently, the mean survival age is now nearly 20 years. Mental retardation is invariably present in adults, with a mean IQ of 50–60. There is a 20-fold increased association with acute leukemia.[193] Other medical problems include congestive heart failure, frequent respiratory infections, strabismus (20%), cataract formation, and premature aging.

TABLE 17–14.
Pathologic Markers of Triploidy

Intrauterine growth retardation
Oligohydramnios
Hydatidiform degeneration of
　placenta
Craniofacial
　Low, malformed ears
　Micro-ophthalmia, colobomata
　Cleft lip or palate
　Micrognathia
Central nervous system
　Holoprosencephaly
　Agenesis of the corpus callosum
　Hydrocephalus
　Myelomeningocele
Cardiovascular (VSD, ASD, PDA*)
Gastrointestinal
　Omphalocele
Genitourinary
　Ambiguous genitalia
Skeletal
　Syndactyly, third and fourth fingers

*VSD = ventricular septal defects; ASD = atrial septal defects; PDA = patent ductus arteriosus.

Triploidy

Clinical and Pathologic Findings (Table 17–14)

Triploidy is found in 12% of all early abortuses. This frequency is greatly reduced by the time of delivery, when it is present in only 1 in 2,500 births. A paternal origin of the extra-haploid set of chromosomes accounts for 73% of cases.[199] However, because fetuses with triploidy of paternal origin are more likely to abort during early pregnancy, a maternal origin of triploidy may be more common by the time of sonographic diagnosis.[188] Among abortuses, about 60% are 69,XXY; 37% are 69,XXX; and only 3% are XYY.[186] Those with 69 XYY manifest the least embryonic development.

Clinical features of triploidy include hypotonia and low birth weight, with head-abdomen discordance (Fig 17–39). Common facial features include micro-ophthalmia; hypertelorism; colobomas; facial asymmetry; low-set, malformed ears (50%); cleft palate (25%); and micrognathia (30%). Syndactyly of the third and fourth fingers is found in over 50% of cases (see Fig 17–38), and talipes equinovarus frequently is present. Central nervous system malformations are common and include holoprosencephaly, hydrocephalus (50%), agenesis of the corpus callosum, and myelomeningocele (25%). Less common anomalies include cardiovascular malformations (60%), omphalocele or umbili-

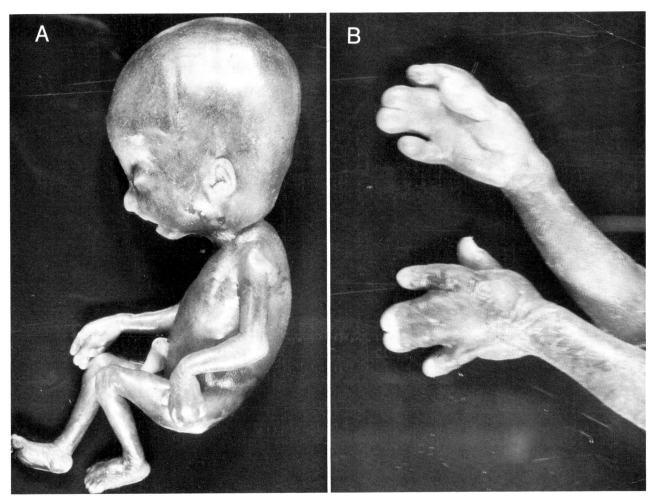

FIG 17–39.
Triploidy. **A,** postmortem photograph shows disproportionate size of head to trunk, and micrognathia. **B,** photograph of hands shows characteristic syndactyly of third and fourth digits. (From Crane NP, Beaver HA, Cheung SW: Antenatal ultrasound findings in fetal triploidy syndrome. J Ultrasound Med 1985; 4:519–524. Used by permission.)

cal hernia (23%), adrenal hypoplasia, and genitourinary anomalies (cystic renal dysplasia, hydronephrosis, hypospadius, cryptorchidism).[173]

Sonographic Findings

Intrauterine growth retardation is universally present in prenatally reported cases of triploidy. Marked oligohydramnios also is nearly always demonstrated, although polyhydramnios occasionally has been reported.[176] Lockwood et al. reported six cases of triploidy, all of which demonstrated severe IUGR and oligohydramnios.[188] The head/abdominal circumference ratio was greater than the 95th percentile for gestational age in all cases. Similar findings were reported by Crane et al., who reported three cases and reviewed six additional cases detected in utero.[177] Intrauterine growth retardation from triploidy has been diagnosed as early as 12 weeks by Benacerraf (see Fig 17–34).[169]

Placental abnormalities of hydatidiform degeneration or hydropic changes are present in nearly all cases in which the extra-haploid set of chromosomes is paternal in origin, but are much less common with a maternal origin.[186] The placenta may appear thickened or demonstrate cystic changes on sonography. However, these findings are highly variable and are not specific for triploidy (see Fig 17–32). In six cases of triploidy seen prenatally (only two with a live fetus), Rubenstein et al. observed hydropic degeneration in all cases ranging from an 11 cm cystic mass to small (less than 1 cm) scattered cysts in the first trimester.[163] By comparison, Lockwood et al. reported that only one of six (17%) fetuses with triploidy showed histologic evidence of hydropic changes in the placenta, and none showed ultrasound abnormalities.[188] It is the opinion of the present authors that placental abnormalities may help suggest the diagnosis of triploidy, especially in combination with early-onset IUGR and oligohydramnios.

Sonographic identification of specific anomalies is often difficult in the presence of marked oligohydramnios. Central nervous system malformations are the most frequent specific malformations identified and are present in most fetuses with triploidy who survive to term. Other anomalies that may be detected include spina bifida, omphalocele, and cardiovascular malformations.

Prognosis

True triploidy is uniformly lethal, with most fetuses spontaneously aborted during early pregnancy. Mosaic individuals may live a normal life span.

Turner's Syndrome (45,X)

Clinical and Pathologic Findings

Turner's syndrome (45,X) occurs in 1 in 2,500 to 5,000 live female births but as many as 9% of first-trimester abortuses.

The most characteristic congenital malformation associated with Turner's syndrome is cystic hygroma. However, this anomaly is not specific for Turner's syndrome and also can be associated with other chromosome abnormalities, as well as a normal karyotype. Other common problems include non-immune hydrops and cardiovascular malformations (25%), including coarctation of the aorta. Genitourinary anomalies include ovarian dysgenesis, present in all affected females; horseshoe kidney; hydronephrosis; renal agenesis; or renal hypoplasia.

Sonographic Findings

The most common sonographic malformation associated with Turner's syndrome is cystic hygroma. Four of six fetuses (66%) with Turner's syndrome reviewed by Brown and Thompson showed cystic hygroma.[174] Conversely, 75% of fetuses with cystic hygroma and successful karyotypes prove to have Turner's syndrome. Other sonographic findings that have been reported with Turner's syndrome include hydrothorax and nonimmune hydrops.

Prognosis

If a fetus with Turner's syndrome survives to a live birth, the long-term survival rate is good. Turner's syndrome in adults is characterized by sexual infantilism, primary amenorrhea, webbed neck, and cubitus valgus. Breast development is poor, and the chest is shield-shaped with wide-spaced nipples. Adults are uniformly short. The verbal IQ usually is normal, but the motor IQ is lower than average due to difficulty with spatial relationships. Hearing loss is present in about 50% of cases.

REFERENCES

Clinical Risk Factors

1. Adams MM, Erickson JD, Layde PM, et al: Down's syndrome: Recent trends in the United States. JAMA 1981; 246; 758–760.
2. Baumgarten A, Schoenfeld M, Mahoney MH, et al: Prospective screening for Down syndrome using maternal serum AFP. Lancet 1985; 1:1280–1281.
3. Bogart MH, Pandian MR, Jones OW: Abnormal maternal serum chorionic gonadotropin levels in pregnancies with fetal chromosomal abnormalities. Prenat Diagn 1978; 7:623–670.
4. Cuckle HS, Wald NJ, Lindenbaum RH: Maternal serum alpha-fetoprotein measurement: A screening test for Down's syndrome. Lancet 1984; 1:926–929.
5. DiMaio MS, Baumgarten A, Greenstein RM, et al: Screening for fetal Down's syndrome in pregnancy by measuring maternal serum alpha-fetoprotein levels. N Engl J Med 1987; 317:342–346.
6. Doran T, Cadesky K, Wong P, et al: Maternal serum alpha-fetoprotein and fetal autosomal trisomies. Am J Obstet Gynecol 1986; 154:277–281.
7. Drugan A, Dvorin E, Koppitch FC III, et al: Counseling for low maternal serum alpha-fetoprotein should emphasize all chromosome anomalies, not just Down syndrome! Obstet Gynecol 1989; 73:271–274.
8. Ferguson-Smith MA: Prenatal diagnosis of chromosome anomalies: Who is at risk?, in Rodeck CH, Nicolaides KH (eds): *Prenatal Diagnosis.* New York, John Wiley & Sons, 1984, pp 53–64.
9. Ferguson-Smith MA, Yates JRW: Maternal age specific rates for chromosome aberrations and factors influencing them: Report of a collaborative European study on 52,965 amniocenteses. Prenat Diagn 1984; 4:5–44.
10. Heuther CA: Projection of Down's syndrome births in the United States 1979–2000, and the potential effects of prenatal diagnosis. Am J Public Health 1983; 73:1186–1189.
11. Hook EB: Chromosome abnormalities and spontaneous fetal death following amniocentesis: Further data and associations with maternal age. Am J Hum Genet 1983; 35:110–116.
12. Hook EB: Spontaneous deaths of fetuses with chromosomal abnormalities diagnosed prenatally. N Engl J Med 1978; 299:1036–1038.
13. Kaback MM: The utility of prenatal diagnosis, in Rodeck CH, Nicolaides KH (eds): *Prenatal Diagnosis.* New York, John Wiley & Sons, 1984, pp 53–64.
14. Kalter H, Warkany J: Congenital malformations: Etiologic factors and their role in prevention. N Engl J Med 1983; 308:424–431.

15. Lindenbaum RH, Ryynanen M, Holmes-Siedle M, et al: Trisomy 18 and maternal serum and amniotic fluid alpha-fetoprotein. Prenat Diagn 1987; 7:511–519.

16. Kaffe S, Perlis TE, Hsu LYF: Amniotic fluid alpha-fetoprotein levels and prenatal diagnosis of autosomal trisomies. Prenat Diagn 1988; 8:183–187.

17. Merkatz IR, Nitowsky HM, Macri JN, et al: An association between low maternal serum alpha-fetoprotein and fetal chromosome abnormalities. Am J Obstet Gynecol 1984; 148:886–894.

18. Palomaki GE, Haddow JE: Maternal serum alpha-fetoprotein, age, and Down syndrome risk. Am J Obstet Gynecol 1987; 156:460–463.

19. Pueschel SM: Maternal alpha-fetoprotein screening for Down's syndrome. N Engl J Med 1987; 317:376–378.

20. Schneider AS, Mennuti MT, Zacki EH: High caesarean section rate in trisomy 18 births: A potential indication for late prenatal diagnosis. Am J Obstet Gynecol 1981; 140:367–370.

21. Simpson JL, Golbus MS, Martin AO, et al: *Genetics in Obstetrics and Gynecology.* Philadelphia, Grune & Stratton, 1982.

22. Wald NJ, Cuckle HS, Densem JW, et al. Maternal serum screening for Down's syndrome in early pregnancy. Br Med Journal 1988; 297:883–887.

23. Wu LR: Maternal serum alpha-fetoprotein screening and Down's syndrome [letter]. Am J Obstet Gynecol 1986; 155:1362.

Methods of Diagnosis

24. Basaran S, Miny P, Pawlowitzki I-H, et al: Rapid karyotyping for prenatal diagnosis in the second and third trimesters of pregnancy. Prenat Diagn 1988; 8:315–320.

25. Crane JP, Beaver HA, Cheung SW: First trimester chorionic villus sampling versus mid-trimester genetic amniocentesis—preliminary results of a controlled prospective trial. Prenat Diagn 1988; 8:355–366.

26. Daffos F, Capella-Pavlovsky M, Forestier F: Fetal blood sampling during pregnancy with use of a needle guided by ultrasound: A study of 606 consecutive cases. Am J Obstet Gynecol 1985; 153:665.

27. Elias S, Simpson JL: Chorionic villous sampling, in Sabbagha RE (ed): *Diagnostic Ultrasound Applied to Obstetrics and Gynecology,* 2 ed. Philadelphia, JB Lippincott Co, 1987, pp 83–90.

28. Gosden C, Rodeck CH, Nicolaides KH, et al: Fetal blood chromosome analysis: Some new indications for prenatal karyotyping. Br J Obstet Gynaecol 1985; 92:915–920.

29. Hogdall CK, Doran TA, Shime J, et al: Transabdominal chorionic villus sampling in the second trimester. Am J Obstet Gynecol 1988; 158:345–349.

30. Hogge WA, Schonberg SA, Golbus MS: Chorionic villus sampling: Experience of the first 1,000 cases. Am J Obstet Gynecol 1986; 154:1249–1252.

31. Nicolaides KH, Southill PW, Rodeck CH, et al: Why confine chorionic villus sampling to the first trimester? Lancet 1986; 1:543–544.

32. Simoni G, Brambati B, Danesino C, et al: Efficient direct chromosome analysis and enzyme determinations from chorion villi samples in the first trimester of pregnancy. Hum Genet 1983; 63:349.

33. Simpson JL, Elias S: Genetic amniocentesis, in Sabbagha RE (ed): *Diagnostic Ultrasound Applied to Obstetrics and Gynecology,* 2 ed. Philadelphia, JB Lippincott Co, 1987, pp 64–82.

34. Smidt-Jensen S, Hahnemann N: Transabdominal fine needle biopsy from chorionic villi in the first trimester. Prenat Diagn 1984; 4:163–169.

35. Tabor A, Phillip J, Madsen M, et al: Randomized controlled trial of genetic amniocentesis in 4,606 low-risk women. Lancet 1986; 1:1287–1292.

36. Verjaal M, Leschot J, Wolf H, et al: Karyotypic differences between cells from placenta and other fetal tissues. Prenat Diagn 1987; 7:345–348.

General Ultrasound Studies

37. Hegge FN, Prescott GH, Watson PT: Sonography at the time of genetic amniocentesis to screen for fetal malformations. Obstet Gynecol 1988; 71:522–525.

38. Marchese CA, Carozzi F, Mosso R, et al: Fetal karyotype in malformations detected by ultrasound. Amer J Hum Genet 1985; 37:A223.

39. Nicolaides KH, Rodeck CH, Gosden CM: Rapid karyotyping in nonlethal fetal malformations. Lancet 1986; 1:283–287.

40. Palmer CG, Miles JH, Howard-Peebles PN, et al: Fetal karyotype following ascertainment of fetal anomalies by ultrasound. Prenat Diagn 1987; 7:551–555.

41. Platt LD, DeVore GR, Lopez E, et al: Role of amniocentesis in ultrasound-detected fetal malformations. Obstet Gynecol 1986; 68:153–155.

42. Vandenberghe K, De Wolf F, Fryns JP, et al: Antenatal ultrasound diagnosis of fetal malformations: Possibilities, limitations, and dilemmas. Eur J Obstet Reprod Biol 1984; 18:279–297.

43. Wladimiroff JW, Sachs ES, Reuss A, et al: Prenatal diagnosis of chromosome abnormalities in the presence of fetal structural defects. Am J Med Genet 1988; 29:289–291.

44. Williamson RA, Weiner CP, Patil S, et al: Abnormal pregnancy sonogram: Selective indication for fetal karyotype. Obstet Gynecol 1987; 69:15–20.

CNS Malformations

45. Amato M, Howald H, von Muralt G: Fetal ventriculomegaly, agenesis of the corpus callosum and chromosomal translocation—Case report. J Perinat Med 1986; 14:271–274.

46. Bertino RE, Nyberg DA, Cyr DR, et al: Prenatal diagnosis of agenesis of the corpus callosum. J Ultrasound Med 1987; 7:251–260.

47. Chervenak FA, Duncan C, Ment LR, et al: Outcome of fetal ventriculomegaly. Lancet 1984; ii:179–181.

48. Chervenak FA, Goldberg JD, Chiu T-H, et al: The importance of karyotype determination in a fetus with ventriculomegaly and spina bifida discovered during the third trimester. J Ultrasound Med 1986; 5:405–406.

49. Chervenak FA, Isaacson G, Hobbins JC, et al: Diagnosis and management of fetal holoprosencephaly. Obstet Gynecol 1985; 66:322–326.

50. Cohen MM: An update on the holoprosencephalic disorders. J Pediatr 1982; 101:865–869.

51. Comstock C, Culp D, Gonzalez J, et al: Agenesis of the corpus callosum in the fetus: Its evolution and significance. J Ultrasound Med 1985; 4:613–616.

52. Murray J, Johnson J, Bird T: Dandy-Walker malformation: Etiologic heterogeneity and empiric recurrence risks. Clin Genet 1985; 28:272–283.

53. Norman RM: Neuropathological findings in trisomies 13–15 and 17–18 with special reference to the cerebellum. Dev Med Child Neurol 1966; 8:170–177.

54. Nyberg DA, Cyr DR, Mack LA, et al: The Dandy-Walker malformation: Prenatal sonographic diagnosis and its clinical significance. J Ultrasound Med 1988; 7:65–71.

55. Nyberg DA, Mack LA, Bronstein A, et al: Holoprosencephaly: Prenatal sonographic diagnosis. AJR 1987; 149:1050–1058.

56. Nyberg DA, Mack LA, Hirsch J, et al: Fetal hydrocephalus: Sonographic detection and clinical significance of associated anomalies. Radiology 1987; 163:187–191.

57. Passarge E, True CW, Sueoka WT, et al: Malformations of the central nervous system in trisomy 18 syndrome. J Pediatr 1966; 69:771–778.

58. Pilu G, Romero R, De Palma L, et al: Antenatal diagnosis and obstetric management of Dandy-Walker syndrome. J Reprod Med 1986; 31:1017–1022.

59. Pilu G, Romero R, Rizzo N, et al: Criteria for the prenatal diagnosis of holoprosencephaly. Am J Perinatol 1987; 4:41–49.

60. Sumi SM: Brain malformations in the trisomy 18 syndrome. Brain 1970; 93:821–830.

61. Tamaraz JC, Rethore M-O, Iba-Zizen M-T, et al: Contribution of magnetic resonance imaging to the knowledge of CNS malformations related to chromosomal aberrations. Hum Genet 1987; 76:265–273.

62. Williamson RA, Schauberger CW, Varner MW, et al: Heterogeneity of prenatal onset hydrocephalus: Management and counseling implications. Am J Med Genet 1984; 17:497–508.

(Also see references 40,160.)

Choroid Plexus Cysts

63. Bundy AL, Saltzman DH, Pober B, et al: Antenatal sonographic findings in trisomy 18. J Ultrasound Med 1986; 5:361–364.

64. Chan L, Hixson JL, Laifer SA, et al: A sonographic karyotypic study of second-trimester fetal choroid plexus cysts. Obstet Gynecol 1989; 73:703–706.

65. Chitkara U, Cogswell C, Norton K, et al: Prenatal diagnosis of choroid plexus cysts: A benign anatomical variant or pathological entity? Report of 41 cases and review of the literature. Obstet Gynecol 1988; 72:185–189.

66. Chudleigh P, Pearce JM, Campbell S, et al: The prenatal diagnosis of transient cysts of the fetal choroid plexus. Prenat Diagn 1984; 4:135–137.

67. Clark SL, DeVore GR, Sabey PL: Prenatal diagnosis of cysts of the fetal choroid plexus. Obstet Gynecol 1988; 72:585–587.

67a. DeRoo TR, Harris RD, Sargent SK, et al: Fetal choroid plexus cysts: Prevalence, clinical significance, and sonographic appearance. AJR 1988; 151:1179–1181.

68. Farhood AE, Morris JH, Bieber FR: Transient cysts of the fetal choroid plexus: Morphology and histogenesis. Am J Med Genet 1987; 27:977–982.

69. Fitzsimmons J, Wilson D, Pascoe-Mason J, et al: Choroid plexus cysts in fetuses with trisomy 18. Obstet Gynecol 1989; 73:257–260.

70. Furness ME: Choroid plexus cysts and trisomy 18. Lancet 1987; ii:693.

70a. Gabrielli S, Reece A, Pilu G, et al: The clinical significance of prenatally diagnosed choroid plexus cysts. Am J Obstet Gynecol 1989; 160:1207–1210.

71. Ostlere SJ, Irving HC, Lilford RJ: Choroid plexus cysts in the fetus. Lancet 1987; i:1491.

71a. Ostlere SJ, Irving HC, Lilford RJ: A prospective study of the incidence and significance of fetal choroid plexus cysts. Prenat Diagn 1989; 9:205–211.

72. Ricketts NEM, Lowe EM, Patel NB: Prenatal diagnosis of choroid plexus cysts. Lancet 1987; i:213–214.

73. Toi A, Cullinan J, Blankier J, et al: Choroid plexus cysts in the fetus: Report of 62 cases. Presented to the World Federation for Ultrasound in Medicine and Biology Meeting, Washington, Poster session, Oct. 17–21, 1988.

Facial Abnormalities

74. Benacerraf BR, Frigoletto FD Jr, Green MF: Abnormal facial features and extremities in human trisomy syndromes: Prenatal US appearance. Radiology 1986; 159:243–246.

75. Birnholz JC, Farrell EE: Fetal hyaloid artery: Timing of regression with US. Radiology 1988; 166:781–783.

76. Birnholz JC, Farrell EE: Fetal ear length. Pediatrics 1988; 81:555–558.

77. Hegge FN, Prescott GH, Watson PT: Fetal facial abnormalities identified during obstetric sonography. J Ultrasound Med 1986; 5:679–684.

78. Nyberg DA, McGahan JP, Mack LA, et al: Holoprosencephaly: Correlation of chromosome abnormalities with sonographic and pathologic findings. Presented to the 75th Scientific Assembly and Annual Meeting of the

Radiological Society of North America, Chicago, Nov 26–Dec 1, 1989.

79. Saltzman DH, Benacerraf BR, Frigoletto FD: Diagnosis and management of fetal facial clefts. Am J Obstet Gynecol 1986; 155:377–379.

Cystic Hygroma

80. Byrne J, Blanc WA, Warburton D, et al: The significance of cystic hygroma in the fetus. Hum Pathol 1984; 15:61–67.

81. Carr RF, Ochs R, Ritter DA, et al: Fetal cystic hygroma and Turner's syndrome. Am J Dis Child 1986; 140:580.

82. Chervenak FA, Isaacson G, Blakemore KJ, et al: Fetal cystic hygroma: Cause and natural history. N Engl J Med 1983; 309:822–825.

83. Chodirker BN, Harman CR, Greenberg CR: Spontaneous resolution of a cystic hygroma in a fetus with Turner syndrome. Prenat Diagn 1988; 8:291–296.

84. Garden AS, Benzie RJ, Miskin M, et al: Fetal cystic hygroma colli: Antenatal diagnosis, significance, and management. Am J Obstet Gynecol 1986; 154:221–225.

85. Marchese C, Savin E, Dragone E, et al: Cystic hygroma: Prenatal diagnosis and genetic counseling. Prenat Diagn 1985; 5:221.

86. Pearce JM, Griffin D, Campbell S: Cystic hygromata in trisomy 18 and 21. Prenat Diagn 1984; 4:371–375.

87. Pijpers L, Reuss A, Stewart PA, et al: Fetal cystic hygroma: Prenatal diagnosis and management. Obstet Gynecol 1988; 72:223–224.

88. Redford DHA, McNay MB, Ferguson-Smith ME, et al: Aneuploidy and cystic hygroma detectable by ultrasound. Prenat Diagn 1984; 4:327–328.

89. Weingast GR, Hopper KD, Gottesfeld SA, et al: Congenital lymphangiectasia with fetal cystic hygroma: Report of two cases with coexistent Down's syndrome. J Clin Ultrasound 1988; 16:663–668.

(Also see references 39,174.)

Non-immune Hydrops

90. Allan LD, Crawford DC, Sheridan R, et al: Aetiology of non–immune hydrops: The value of echocardiography. Br J Obstet Gynecol 1986; 93:223–225.

91. Holzgreve W, Curry CJR, Golbus MS, et al: Investigation of nonimmune hydrops fetalis. Am J Obstet Gynecol 1984; 150:805–812.

92. Mahony BS, Filly RA, Callen PW, et al: Severe nonimmune hydrops fetalis: Sonographic evaluation. Radiology 1984; 151:757.

(Also see references 28,39.)

Cardiovascular Malformations

93. Benacerraf BR, Pober BR, Sanders SP: Accuracy of fetal echocardiography. Radiology 1987; 165:847–849.

94. Berg KA, Clark EB, Aslemborski J, et al: Prenatal detection of cardiovascular malformations by echocardiography: An indication for cytogenetic evaluation. Am J Obstet Gynecol 1988; 159:477–481.

95. Copel JA, Cullen M, Green JJ, et al: The frequency of aneuploidy in prenatally diagnosed congenital heart disease: An indication for fetal karyotyping. Am J Obstet Gynecol 1988; 158:409–413.

96. Copel JA, Pilu G, Kleinman CS: Congenital heart disease and extracardiac anomalies: Associations and indications for fetal echocardiography. Am J Obstet Gynecol 1986; 154:1121–1132.

97. Crawford DC, Chita SK, Allan LD: Prenatal detection of congenital heart disease: Factors affecting obstetric management and survival. Am J Obstet Gynecol 1988; 159:352–356.

98. Ferencz C, Rubin JD, McCarter RJ, et al: Cardiac and noncardiac malformations: Observations in a population based study. Teratology 1987; 35:367–378.

99. Greenwood RD, Rosenthal A, Parisi L, et al: Extracardiac abnormalities in infants with congenital heart disease. Pediatrics 1975; 55:485–492.

100. Matsuoka R, Misugi K, Goto A, et al: Congenital heart anomalies in the trisomy 18 syndrome, with reference to congenital polyvalvular disease. Am J Med Genet 1983; 14:657–668.

101. Nora JJ, Nora AH: Congenital heart disease: Chromosomal anomalies, in Nora JJ, Nora AH (eds): *Genetics and Counseling in Cardiovascular Diseases.* Springfield, IL, Charles C Thomas, 1978, pp 9–44.

102. Wladimiroff JW, Stewart PA, Sachs ES, et al: Prenatal diagnosis and management of congenital heart defect: Significance of associated fetal anomalies and prenatal chromosome studies. Am J Med Genet 1985; 21:285–290.

Duodenal Atresia

103. Fonkalsrud EW, DeLorimier AA, Hays DM: Congenital atresia and stenosis of the duodenum. A review compiled from the members of the Surgical Section of the American Academy of Pediatrics. Pediatrics 1969; 43:79–83.

104. Romero R, Ghidini A, Costigan K, et al: Prenatal diagnosis of duodenal atresia: Does it make any difference? Obstet Gynecol 1988; 71:739–741.

105. Touloukian RJ: Intestinal atresia. Clin Perinatol 1978; 5:3–18.

Omphalocele

106. Crawford DC, Chapman MG, Allan LD: Echocardiography in the investigation of anterior abdominal wall defects in the fetus. Br J Obstet Gynecol 1985; 92:1034–1036.

107. Gilbert WM, Nicolaides KH: Fetal omphalocele: Associated malformations and chromosomal defects. Obstet Gynecol 1987; 70:633–635.

108. Griffiths DM, Gough MH: Dilemmas after ultrasound diagnosis of fetal abnormality. Lancet 1985; 1:623.

109. Hauge M, Bugge M, Nielsen J: Early prenatal diagnosis of omphalocele constitutes indication for amniocentesis. Lancet 1983; 2:507.

110. Hughes MD, Nyberg DA, Mack LA, et al: Fetal omphalocele: Prenatal detection of concurrent anomalies and other predictors of outcome. Radiology, in press.

111. Lindenbaum RH, Ryynanen M, Holmes-Siedle M, et al: Trisomy 18 and maternal serum and amniotic fluid alpha-fetoprotein. Prenat Diag 1987; 7:511–519.

112. Mabogunje OOA, Mahour GH: Omphalocele and gastroschisis: Trends in survival across two decades. Am J Surg 1984; 148:679–686.

113. Muller LM, de Jong G: Prenatal ultrasonographic features of the Pena-Shokeir syndrome and the trisomy 18 syndrome. Am J Med Gen 1986; 25:119–129.

114. Nyberg DA, Fitzsimmons J, Mack LA, et al: Chromosomal abnormalities in fetuses with omphalocele: The significance of omphalocele contents. J Ultrasound Med 1989; 8:299–308.

115. Schwaitzenberg SD, Pokorny WJ, McGill CW, et al: Gastroschisis and omphalocele. Am J Surg 1982; 144:650–654.

116. Wladimiroff JW, Molenaar JC, Niermeijer MF, et al: Prenatal diagnosis and management of omphalocele. Eur J Obstet Gynecol Reprod Biol 1983; 16:19–23.

Hydrothorax

117. Blott M, Nicolaides KH, Greenough A: Pleuroamniotic shunting for decompression of fetal pleural effusions. Obstet Gynecol 1988; 71:798–800.

118. Lange IR, Manning FA: Antenatal diagnosis of congenital pleural effusions. Am J Obstet Gynecol 1981; 140:839–840.

119. Rodeck CH, Fisk NM, Fraser DF, et al: Long-term in utero drainage of fetal hydrothorax. N Engl J Med 1988; 310:1135–1138.

120. Yoss BS, Lipsitz PJ: Chylothorax in twin mongoloid infants. Clin Genet 1977; 12:357–360.
(Also see reference 39.)

Diaphragmatic Hernia

121. Adzick NS, Harrison MR, Glick PL, et al: Diaphragmatic hernia in the fetus: Prenatal diagnosis and outcome in 94 cases. J Pediatr Surg 1985; 20:357–361.

122. Benacerraf BR, Adzick NS: Fetal diaphragmatic hernia: Ultrasound diagnosis and clinical outcome in 19 cases. Am J Obstet Gynecol 1987; 156:573–576.

123. Benjamin DR, Juul S, Siebert JR: Congenital posterolateral diaphragmatic hernia: Associated malformations. J Pediatr Surg 1988; 23:899–903.

124. Comstock CH: The antenatal diagnosis of diaphragmatic anomalies. J Ultrasound Med 1986; 5:391–396.

125. Puri P, Gorman F: Lethal non–pulmonary anomalies associated with congenital diaphragmatic hernia: Implications for early intra-uterine surgery. J Pediatr Surg 1984; 19:29–32.

Genitourinary

126. Appleman Z, Golbus MS: The management of fetal urinary tract obstruction. Clin Obstet Gynecol 1986; 29:483–489.

127. Flake AW, Harrison MR, Sauer L, et al: Ureteropelvic junction obstruction in the fetus. J Ped Surg 1986; 21:1058–1063.

128. Frydman M, Magenis RE, Mohandas RK, et al: Chromosome abnormalities in infants with prune belly syndrome: association with trisomy 18. Am J Med Genet 1983; 15:145–148.

129. Kleiner B, Callen PW, Filly RA: Sonographic analysis of the fetus with ureteropelvic junction obstruction. AJR 1987; 148:359–363.

130. McKeown CME, Donnai D: Prune belly in trisomy 13. Prenat Diagn 1986; 6:379–381.

131. Nevin NC, Nevin J, Dunlop JM, et al: Antenatal diagnosis of grossly distended bladder owing to absence of urethra in a fetus with trisomy 18. J Med Genet 1983; 20:132–133.

132. Rizzo N, Gabrielli S, Pilu G, et al: Prenatal diagnosis and obstetrical management of multicystic dysplastic kidney disease. Prenat Diagn 1987; 7:109–118.

133. Temmerman M, Levi S, Verboven M, et al: Puncture of unilateral renal cyst in utero. Eur J Obstet Gynecol Reprod Biol 1986; 13:107–110.

134. Zerres K, Volpel MC, Weiss H: Cystic kidneys. Genetics, pathologic anatomy, clinical pictures and prenatal diagnosis. Hum Genet 1984; 68:104–135.

Clubfoot

135. Benacerraf BR: Antenatal sonographic diagnosis of congenital clubfoot: A possible indication for amniocentesis. J Clin Ultrasound 1986; 14:703–706.

136. Hashimoto BE, Filly RA, Callen PW: Sonographic diagnosis of clubfoot in utero. J Ultrasound Med 1986; 5:81–83.

137. Jeanty P, Romero R, d'Alton M, et al: In utero sonographic detection of hand and foot deformities. J Ultrasound Med 1985; 4:595–601.

Limb Reduction and Other Extremity Malformations

138. Benacerraf BR, Osathanondh R, Frigoletto FD: Sonographic demonstration of hypoplasia of the middle phalanx of the fifth digit: A finding associated with Down syndrome. Am J Obstet Gynecol 1988; 159:181–183.

139. Bofinger MK, Dignan PSJ, Schmidt RE, et al: Reduction malformations and chromosome anomalies. Am J Dis Child 1973; 125:135–143.

140. Christianson AL, Nelson MM: Four cases of trisomy 18

syndrome with limb reduction malformation. J Med Genet 1984; 21:293.

141. Kajii T: Phocomelia in trisomy 18 syndrome. Lancet 1967; 1:385–386.

142. Oikawa K, Kochen JA, Schorr JB, et al: Trisomy 17 syndrome with phocomelia due to complete and partial chromosomal trisomy. J Pediatr 1963; 63:715–717.

143. Pfeiffer RA, Santelmann R: Limb anomalies in chromosomal aberrations. Birth Defects 1977; 13:319–337.

144. Rabinowitz JG, Moseley JE, Mitty HA, et al: Trisomy 18, esophageal atresia, anomalies of the radius and congenital hypoplastic thrombocytopenia. Radiology 1967; 89:488–491.

145. Zellweger H, Huff DS, Abbo G: Phocomelia and trisomy E. Acta Genet Med Gemellol (Roma) 1965; 14:164–173.

Nuchal Thickening

146. Benacerraf BR, Gelman R, Frigoletto FD Jr: Sonographic identification of second-trimester fetuses with Down's syndrome. N Engl J Med 1987; 317:1371–1376.

147. Benacerraf BR, Barss VA, Laboda LA: A sonographic sign for the detection in the second trimester of the fetus with Down's syndrome. Am J Obstet Gynecol 1985; 151:1078–1079.

148. Chodirker BN, Harman CR, Greenberg CR: Spontaneous resolution of a cystic hygroma in a fetus with Turner syndrome. Prenat Diagn 1988; 8:291–292.

149. Dicke JM, Gray DL, Songster GS, Crane JP: The use of sonographically obtained femur length and biparietal diameter-to-femur length ratio for the detection of fetal trisomies. Official Proceedings 1988 World Federation for Ultrasound in Medicine and Biology Meeting. J Ultrasound Med 1988; 7:265.

150. Hall B: Mongolism in newborn infants. Clin Pediatr 1966; 5:4–12.

151. Lynch L, Berkowitz GS, Chitkara U, et al: Ultrasound detection of Down syndrome: Is it really possible? Obstet Gynecol 1988; 73:267–270.

152. Perrella R, Duerinckx AJ, Grant EG, et al: Second-trimester sonographic diagnosis of Down syndrome: Role of femur-length shortening and nuchal-fold thickening. AJR 1988; 151:981–985.

153. Rodis JF, Vintzileos AM, Campbell WA, et al: Spontaneous resolution of fetal cystic hygroma in Down's syndrome. Obstet Gynecol 1988; 71:976–977.

154. Toi A, Simpson GF, Filly RA: Ultrasonically evident fetal nuchal skin thickening: Is it specific for Down syndrome? Am J Obstet Gynecol 1987; 156:150–153.

Single Umbilical Artery

155. Bryan EM, Kohler HG: The missing umbilical artery: Prospective study based on a maternity unit. Arch Dis Child 1974; 49:844–852.

156. Byrne J, Blane WA: Malformations and chromosome anomalies in spontaneously aborted fetuses with single umbilical artery. Am J Obstet Gynecol 1985; 151:340–342.

157. Lenoski EF, Medovy H: Single umbilical artery: Incidence, clinical significance and relation to autosomal trisomy. Can Med Assoc J 1962; 87:1229–1231.

158. Lewis AJ: Autosomal trisomy. Lancet 1962; 1:866.

159. Monies IW: Genesis of single umbilical artery. Am J Obstet Gynecol 1970; 108:400–405.

160. Nyberg DA, Shepard T, Mack LA, et al: Significance of a single umbilical artery in fetuses with central nervous system malformations. J Ultrasound Med 1988; 7:265–273.

161. Vlietinck RF, Thiery M, Orye E, et al: Significance of the single umbilical artery. Arch Dis Child 1972; 47:639–642.

Placental Abnormalities

162. Jouppila P, Kirkinen P, Kahkonen M, et al: Ultrasonic abnormalities associated with the pathology fetal karyotype results during the early second trimester of pregnancy. Official Proceedings 1988 World Federation for Ultrasound in Medicine and Biology Meeting. J Ultrasound Med 1988; 7:218.

163. Rubenstein JB, Swayne LC, Dise CA, et al: Placental changes in fetal triploidy syndrome. J Ultrasound Med 1986; 4:545–550.

(Also see references 186,188.)

Polyhydramnios

164. Barkin SZ, Pretorius DH, Beckett MK, et al: Severe polyhydramnios: Incidence of anomalies. AJR 1987; 148:155–159.

165. Landy HJ, Isada NB, Larsen JW Jr: Genetic implications of idiopathic hydramnios. Am J Obstet Gynecol 1987; 157:114–117.

166. Liang ST, Yam AWC, Tang MHY, et al: Trisomy 18: The value of late prenatal diagnosis. Eur J Obstet Gynecol Reprod Biol 1986; 22:95–97.

167. Filly RA: Polyhydramnios, in Marguilis AR, Gooding CA (eds): *Diagnostic Radiology* 1987, pp 263–270.

168. Moya F, et al: Hydramnios and congenital anomalies. JAMA 1960; 173:1552–1556.

IUGR

169. Benacerraf BR: Intrauterine growth retardation in the first trimester associated with triploidy. J Ultrasound Med 1988; 7:153–154.

170. Golbus MS, Hall BD, Creasy RK: Prenatal diagnosis of congenital anomalies in an intrauterine growth retarded fetus. Hum Genet 1976; 32:349–352.

171. Reisman LE: Chromosomal abnormalities and intrauterine growth retardation. Pediat Clin North Am 1970; 17:101–110.

Pathologic Markers of Specific Chromosome Abnormalities

172. Benacerraf BR, Miller WA, Frigoletto FD Jr: Sonographic detection of fetuses with trisomies 13 and 18: Accuracy and limitations. Am J Obstet Gynecol 1988; 158:404–409.

173. Blackburn WR, Miller WP, Superneau DW, et al: Comparative studies of infants with mosaic and complete triploidy: An analysis of 55 cases. Birth Defects 1982; 18:251–274.

174. Brown BSJ, Thompson DL: Ultrasonographic features of the fetal Turner syndrome. J Can Assoc Radiol 1984; 35:40–46.

175. Carter PE, Pearn JH, Bell J, et al: Survival in trisomy 18. Life tables for use in genetic counselling and clinical paediatrics. Clin Genet 1986; 27:59–61.

176. Chaterjee MS, Tejani N, Verma UL, et al: Prenatal diagnosis of triploidy. Int J Gynaecol Obstet 1983; 21:155–157.

177. Crane JP, Beaver HA, Cheung SW: Antenatal ultrasound findings in fetal triploidy syndrome. J Ultrasound Med 1985; 4:519–524.

178. Edwards JH, Harnden DG, Cameron AH, et al: A new trisomic syndrome. Lancet 1960; 1:787–789.

179. Edwards MT, Smith WL, Hanson J, et al: Prenatal sonographic diagnosis of triploidy. J Ultrasound Med 1986; 5:279–281.

180. Flannery DB, Kahler SG: Neural tube defects in trisomy 18. Prenat Diag 1986; 6:97–99.

181. Fryns JP: Chromosomal anomalies and autosomal syndromes. Birth Defects 1987; 23:7–32.

182. Gilbert EF, Aryas Laxova R, Opitz JM: Pathology of chromosome abnormalities in the fetus—pathologic markers. Birth Defects 1987; 23:293–296.

183. Gorlin RJ: Classical chromosome disorders, in Yunis JJ (ed): *New Chromosomal Syndromes.* London, Academic Press, 1977, pp 59–117.

184. Hodes ME, Cole J, Palmer CG, et al: Clinical experience with trisomies 18 and 13. J Med Genet 1978; 15:48–60.

185. Hook EB, Woodbury DF, Albright SG: Rates of trisomy 18 in livebirths, stillbirths, and at amniocentesis. Birth Defects 1979; XV,5C:81–93.

186. Jacobs PA, Szulman AE, Funkhauser J, et al: Human triploidy: Relationship between parenteral origin of the additional haploid complement and development of partial hydatidiform mole. Ann Hum Genet 1982; 46:223–231.

187. Keeling JW: Examination of the fetus following prenatal suspicion of congenital abnormality, in Keeling JW (ed): *Fetal and Neonatal Pathology,* New York, Springer-Verlag, 1987, pp 99–122.

188. Lockwood C, Scioscia A, Stiller R, et al: Sonographic features of the triploid fetus. Am J Obstet Gynecol 1987; 157:285–287.

189. Patau K, Smith DW, Theman E, et al: Multiple congenital anomaly caused by an extra chromosome. Lancet 1960; 1:790–793.

190. Penrose LS, Smith GF: Down's anomaly. London, Churchill, 1966.

191. Redheendran R, Neu RL, Bannerman RM: Long survival in trisomy-13-syndrome: 21 cases including prolonged survival in two patients 11 and 19 years old. Am J Med Genet 1981; 8:167–172.

192. Rex AP, Preus M: A diagnostic index for Down syndrome. J Pediatr 1982; 100:903–906.

193. Simpson JL, Golbus MS, Martin AO, et al: Autosomal chromosome abnormalities, in Genetics in Obstetrics and Gynecology. Philadelphia, Grune & Stratton, 1982, pp 53–78.

194. Smith DW: Recognizable Patterns of Human Malformations, 3 ed. Philadelphia, WB Saunders Co, 1982, pp 10–19.

195. Smith DW, Patau K, Therman E, et al: A new autosomal trisomy syndrome: Multiple congenital anomalies caused by an extra chromosome. J Pediatr 1960; 57:338–345.

196. Smith DW, Patau K, Therman E, et al: The no. 18 trisomy syndrome. J Pediatr 1962; 57:338–345.

197. Stephens TD, Shepard TH: The Down syndrome in the fetus. Teratology 1980; 22:37–41.

198. Taylor AI: Autosomal trisomy syndromes: A detailed study of 27 cases of Edwards' syndrome and 27 cases of Patau's syndrome. J Med Genet 1968; 5:227–241.

199. Uchida IA, Freeman VCP: Triploidy and chromosomes. Am J Obstet Gynecol 1985; 151:65–69.

200. Warkany J: Syndromes of chromosomal abnormalities, in Congenital Malformations. Chicago, Year Book Medical Publishers, Inc, 1971, pp 296–345.

201. Warkany J, Passarge E, Smith LB: Congenital malformations in autosomal trisomy syndromes. Am J Dis Child 1966; 112:502–517.

Surgical Management of Prenatally Diagnosed Malformations

Jacob C. Langer, M.D.

N. Scott Adzick, M.D.

Routine obstetrical sonography has changed the surgical management of many congenital anomalies. In some cases, it simply permits appropriate guidance and counseling. In others, various forms of in utero therapy may be possible either now or in the future. Prenatal diagnosis may also influence the timing (Table 18–1) or the mode (Table 18–2) of delivery and in some cases may lead to elective termination of the pregnancy (Table 18–3). The perinatal management of these patients involves many different medical disciplines, including obstetricians, sonographers, neonatologists, geneticists, pediatric surgeons, and pediatricians. It is essential that the affected family be managed using a team approach, and that information and experience be exchanged freely.

The present chapter discusses the authors' current approach to the management of congenital diaphragmatic hernia, abdominal wall defects, hydronephrosis, sacrococcygeal teratoma, and gastrointestinal obstruction. Further discussion of these anomalies can be found in Chapters 8, 11, 12, 6, and 10, respectively.

CONGENITAL DIAPHRAGMATIC HERNIA

Congenital diaphragmatic hernia (CDH) is an anatomically simple defect that is easily correctable after birth. Despite this, the mortality associated with CDH has traditionally been approximately 50%. In addition, routine maternal sonography has identified a large group of fetuses with CDH who die in utero or soon after birth, representing a "hidden mortality" which was not previously appreciated.[13] Because of this dismal outlook, there have been a number of innovations developed in recent years for the management of fetuses and neonates with this disease.

Prenatal Management

Correct management of the fetus with prenatally diagnosed CDH is dependent on an understanding of the natural history, pathophysiology, and prognostic factors determining outcome. In a large survey of 94 prenatally diagnosed cases, we found that overall mortality was 80%, despite maximum conventional therapy. Polyhydramnios was common and was associated with an increased mortality.[1] Nonsurvivors also tended to have larger defects. In a subsequent study of 19 cases, recently updated to include a total of 38 cases from a single institution in Boston,[1,3] we confirmed that polyhydramnios was associated with a poor prognosis, but noted that the polyhydramnios did not appear until the third trimester in most cases, presumably after pulmonary hypoplasia was well established. In addition, we found that associated anomalies and diagnosis before 24 weeks' gestation were associated with a poor outcome. Our recent experience with 45 prenatally diagnosed cases of CDH at the University of California in San Francisco has confirmed these findings.

More recently, sonographic demonstration of abnormally low ratios of lung/total thoracic volume[20] and of left-right ventricular volume[10] have been suggested

TABLE 18–1.

Surgical Conditions That May Require Induced
Pre-term Delivery for Early Correction Ex Utero

Obstructive hydronephrosis
Obstructive hydrocephalus
Amniotic band malformation complex
Gastroschisis or ruptured omphalocele
Intestinal ischemia/necrosis secondary to volvulus,
  meconium ileus, and similar conditions
Sacrococcygeal teratoma
Hydrops fetalis
Intrauterine growth retardation

TABLE 18–2.

Conditions Which May Require Caesarean
Delivery

Conjoined twins
Giant omphalocele
Large hydrocephalus
Large sacrococcygeal teratoma
Large cystic hygroma
Large or ruptured meningomyelocele
Malformations requiring pre-term delivery in the
  presence of inadequate labor or fetal
  distress

as indicators of a poor prognosis. In our initial experience with these ratios, we have found them to be difficult to interpret, and their accuracy has been inconsistent.

It has been suggested that prenatal repair of CDH in poor-risk fetuses could prevent compression of the growing lungs and improve neonatal outcome. This concept is supported by a considerable amount of evidence from the fetal lamb model. Compression of the lung with an intrathoracic balloon results in pulmonary hypoplasia and neonatal death.[14] Simulated correction by deflating the balloon partway through gestation permits sufficient lung growth to support respiratory function at birth.[15] Surgical creation of a diaphragmatic hernia in utero also

TABLE 18–3.

Malformations Usually Managed by Elective
Termination

Anencephaly, porencephaly, encephalocele, and
  giant hydrocephalus
Severe anomalies associated with chromosomal
  abnormalities: Trisomy 13, trisomy 18, and similar
  conditions
Renal agenesis or bilateral polycystic kidney
  disease
Inherited chromosomal, metabolic, and hematologic
  abnormalities: Hemoglobinopathies, Tay-Sachs
  disease, and similar conditions

results in fatal pulmonary hypoplasia,[11] and correction using open fetal surgery permits survival at term (Fig 18–1).[16, 25] Morphometric analysis of the lungs in this model has confirmed that in utero repair results in improved lung growth.[2] Techniques for open fetal surgery have been developed in non–human primates.[17] However, despite the fact that in utero repair of CDH makes sense physiologically and has been shown to be technically feasible, it continues to remain a highly experimental prospect.

Prior to making any management decision, the following information should be obtained. Amniocentesis should be done to rule out chromosomal abnormalities, and a detailed ultrasound examination and a determination of alpha-fetoprotein levels should be performed to ascertain whether there are associated lethal anomalies which may influence further management.[23] Some prognostic information may be gained by noting the gestational age at diagnosis, the presence of polyhydramnios, liver in the chest, and perhaps measurements of lung-thoracic and left-right ventricular volumes. If the diagnosis is made in the first or early in the second trimester, elective termination may be offered, especially if there are associated lethal anomalies. In the future, open fetal surgery may be another alternative for poor-risk fetuses without associated anomalies, who are diagnosed before 28 weeks' gestation. If the decision is made not to intervene, or if the diagnosis is made after 28 weeks' gestation, serial ultrasound examinations should be done to look for the development of polyhydramnios, hydrops, or anomalies which may not have been evident before.

Clearly, one of the most important advantages of prenatal diagnosis is the anticipation of a desperately ill newborn. The mother should be transferred to an appropriate perinatal center where neonatal, ventilatory, and surgical expertise are available. This avoids the unnecessary mortality associated with transporting the sick neonate and the delay in appropriate medical and ventilatory care that this entails. The timing or mode of delivery should not be influenced significantly by prenatal diagnosis. Pre-term delivery, although permitting earlier decompression of the thorax, adds the additional insult of lung immaturity to the preexisting pulmonary hypoplasia. There is no advantage to cesarean section in this condition, unless it is done for obstetrical indications.

Postnatal Management

Some newborns with CDH present with minimal to moderate respiratory distress, respond well to ventilation and operative repair, and survive to lead normal

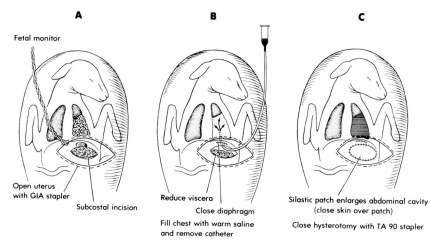

FIG 18–1.
Technique for repair of diaphragmatic hernia in utero, developed in a fetal lamb model.

lives. Others are born in extremis, are never resuscitable, and die within the first few hours or days of life due to persistent hypoxia and hypercarbia. There is a middle group, however, who have a brief "honeymoon period," after which rapid deterioration takes place.[12] Current understanding of the pathophysiology in this group is outlined in Figure 18–2. Management techniques are designed to interrupt the vicious cycle of hypoxia, hypercarbia, and persistent fetal circulation due to pulmonary vascular hypertension. These patients are salvageable, because there is sufficient pulmonary capacity present as long as the deleterious vasoactive events of the first few days can be overcome.

In the late 1970s, the role of increased pulmonary vascular resistance and right-to-left shunting was recognized, and a battery of different pharmacologic agents were tried in an attempt to decrease pulmonary vascular resistance.[7] Although these drugs are used widely, there is no good evidence that they are efficacious. Positive inotropic agents also have been used extensively to improve function in the failing heart, and one

group has recommended prolonged general anesthesia as a means for improving the hemodynamic picture.[28] None of these approaches, however, appears to have had a major impact on survival.

In the past 5 years, there have been several new concepts and techniques suggested to improve survival in CDH, including extracorporeal membrane oxygenation (ECMO), high-frequency oscillation (HFO), and delayed repair of the hernia.

ECMO

Neonatal ECMO has rapidly gained in popularity since the first report in 1976,[4] and is now done in over 50 centers across North America. The most serious ECMO complication is intracranial bleeding, which is much more common in premature infants. As with most new therapeutic modalities, the key issue is appropriate patient selection. Current recommendations suggest ECMO for babies who have had a "honeymoon period," are not premature, have no evidence of intracranial bleeding, and who have no other anomalies.[5]

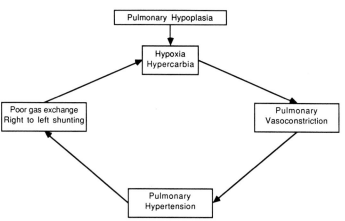

FIG 18–2.
Pathophysiology in infants with CDH who deteriorate after an intitial "honeymoon" period. Medical and pharmacological therapy is aimed at interruption of this vicious cycle.

Stolar et al.[26] reported 14 infants who met the criteria for ECMO, 12 of whom (86%) survived. Others have not done as well, probably because of less stringent exclusion criteria.[19] In the only report of ECMO for prenatally diagnosed CDH, we had only three neonatal survivors out of 12 cases.[3] With more accurate patient selection, ECMO may become an important part of the management of the neonate with CDH who deteriorates after an initial "honeymoon period."

High-frequency Oscillation

This new ventilation technique has been used experimentally in respiratory distress syndrome and meconium aspiration with encouraging preliminary results.[8] There is good evidence that HFO permits ventilation with a lower mean airway pressure and that it is extremely effective in lowering arterial PCO_2 levels.[21] However, further experience is necessary to determine if survival is improved when this technique is applied to babies with CDH.

Timing of Surgery

The standard surgical approach to CDH has always been immediate surgery to decompress the chest. However, ventilatory management is not as good during transport to and from the operating room, infants often deteriorate after surgery, and the pathophysiology of the deterioration is related not to the presence of the bowel in the chest, but to changes in pulmonary vascular resistance superimposed on preexisting pulmonary hypoplasia. In fact, after paralysis and positive pressure ventilation, it is common on chest x-ray to see the lungs expand, the mediastinal shift resolve, and the bowel move down into the abdomen. Sakai et al. have shown that surgical repair of the defect actually worsens thoracic compliance and PCO_2, suggesting that emergency repair may be harmful to the already borderline infant.[24]

For these reasons, several groups have advocated delaying surgical repair until the patient has been stabilized.[9, 18, 22, 27] This may take only a few hours in good-risk patients or up to 7 days in patients who are extremely borderline. During this time, HFO may be used if there is persistent hypercarbia,[27] and ECMO may be attempted if there is a honeymoon period followed by deterioration in oxygenation. In the future, using ECMO as a "bridge," lung transplantation may be the only hope for the severely affected newborn who cannot be resuscitated.

Surgical Repair

Repair of the defect is usually the most straightforward part of the management of CDH. Preoperative considerations include appropriate ventilatory and fluid management, nasogastric drainage to prevent bowel distension, and preoperative antibiotics. Although not usually needed, blood should be available.

Through a left subcostal abdominal incision, the viscera are pulled out of the chest through the defect. The diaphragm is closed using interrupted non–absorbable sutures. In some cases, the defect is too large for primary closure, and prosthetic material or an abdominal muscle flap is used. Prior to closure, the abdominal musculature is manually stretched to make room for the viscera. There is controversy regarding whether a chest tube should be inserted prior to closure, but because of the high incidence of postoperative pneumothorax due to high pressure ventilation, we continue to use one.

ABDOMINAL WALL DEFECTS

Abdominal wall defects, including both gastroschisis and omphalocele, can be diagnosed and differentiated prenatally by routine sonography.[40] The two conditions differ with respect to both prenatal and postnatal management, and a number of controversies exist, particularly surrounding the issues of timing and mode of delivery.

Prenatal Management

When an abdominal wall defect is diagnosed in the first or second trimester, options include elective termination of the pregnancy, early delivery before or at lung maturity, or delivery at term. The decision to terminate the pregnancy usually is made because of the presence of associated anomalies. Omphalocele has a very high incidence of associated anomalies (approximately 50%), whereas gastroschisis does not (<10%);[49] these figures are higher in series which include prenatally diagnosed cases.[50] It is probably wise to perform a detailed ultrasound examination and a karyotype analysis in all cases. It is important to remember, however, that in the absence of associated anomalies, most fetuses with abdominal wall defects will, with appropriate perinatal management, grow up to be normal children.[29] Counseling should reflect this positive outlook, and termination should be advised only in properly selected cases.

Important management considerations should include the timing of delivery, the mode of delivery, and transport of the patient to an appropriate center. Our current approach to these decisions is summarized in Figure 18–3.

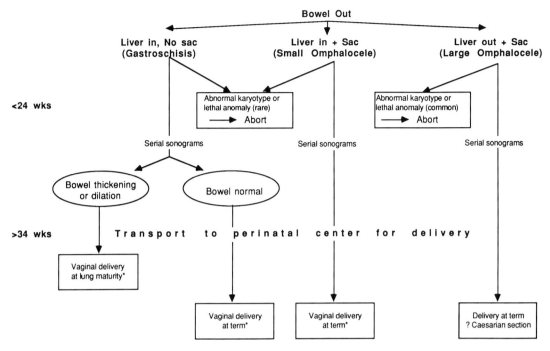

FIG 18–3.
The authors' current management plan for prenatally diagnosed abdominal wall defects.

Timing of Delivery

Postnatal outcome in omphalocele is related to the presence or absence of associated structural and chromosomal anomalies, and, therefore, there is no advantage to early delivery. In gastroschisis, however, postnatal morbidity is due to intestinal damage, resulting in atresia, ischemia, and severe motility and absorption defects.[48] Classic teaching has held that the damage is caused by exposure to amniotic fluid, and we had previously proposed early delivery to minimize this damage.[45] However, recent clinical and experimental evidence has suggested that the bowel damage may be due to constriction at the level of the abdominal wall, rather than to amniotic fluid alone.[42] Using ultrasound, it is possible to predict the condition of the exteriorized bowel in fetal gastroschisis. Fetuses with bowel dilation and thickening tend to have a poor outcome, whereas those with normal caliber bowel tend to do well postnatally.[31] Using these criteria, we now can properly select patients who require early delivery.

Mode of Delivery

It is controversial whether fetuses with an abdominal wall defect should be delivered by cesarean section to prevent visceral damage or whether it is safe to deliver them vaginally. In the case of gastroschisis, some studies strongly support the use of cesarean section and others just as strongly oppose it.[30, 33–35, 41, 50] Most

of these studies suffer from their small numbers and their retrospective nature. In addition, in their analysis few differentiate between those patients who were diagnosed prenatally and those who were not. Most studies also do not take into consideration the timing of delivery or the need for preoperative transportation, both of which may be important factors in neonatal outcome.

We reserve cesarean section for those that require it for purely obstetrical reasons. In the experience at our institution, we have not seen any adverse effects from vaginal delivery.[39] It has become clear, however, that this issue will not be settled definitively until a prospective, randomized, controlled trial is done; a multicenter trial currently is underway.

Maternal Transport

These fetuses should be delivered in a center which is capable of expert, rapid resuscitation and surgical intervention. The child with an omphalocele and a missed cardiac, neural tube, or other anomaly requires appropriate expertise to manage these conditions, as well as an experienced pediatric surgeon to deal with the omphalocele. The child with gastroschisis needs appropriate resuscitation and early surgical management of the abdominal wall defect. Time spent in unnecessary transportation of the infant increases the risk of infection, fluid depletion, temperature instability, and difficulty with closure of the abdomen due to increasing bowel distension.

Postnatal Management

Resuscitation

Infants with an abdominal wall defect require (1) adequate fluid support, with an intravenous line and monitoring of urine output, (2) protection of the herniated viscera with a watertight occlusive dressing, (3) nasogastric drainage to minimize bowel distension, (4) antibiotics, and (5) temperature stabilization in an isolette. Because the viscera are covered with a relatively tough membrane in infants with omphalocele, the issues of fluid loss and visceral protection are less important than in infants with gastroschisis.

Due to the relatively greater risk of fluid loss, temperature instability, and infection, infants with gastroschisis should be taken to the operating room as soon as possible after they have been evaluated and stabilized in the neonatal intensive care unit. Infants with omphalocele can wait longer before surgical intervention, and preoperative investigation for potentially life-threatening associated anomalies is appropriate.

Surgical Repair

Most infants will have the defect closed without difficulty shortly after birth. However, the large size of some defects, the bowel distension and edema sometimes seen in gastroschisis, and the small volume of the peritoneal cavity make primary closure impossible in some cases. Most of these more complicated defects can be closed within a week of birth using a "chimney" technique,[47] which involves placing a sheet of Silastic over the viscera and gradually squeezing them back into the abdomen over a period of 3 to 6 days; at that time, the Silastic is removed and the fascia closed. For a few rare and exceptional lesions that cannot be closed shortly after birth, simple skin coverage without fascial closure[38] or non–operative coverage with Op-site[36] or Mercurochrome[51] are other options. These methods require a subsequent ventral hernia repair, which may be extremely difficult. Non–operative coverage is only appropriate for giant omphaloceles in high-risk neonates or in infants with other lethal anomalies which preclude an aggressive approach.

Because of the acute rise in intra-abdominal pressure generated by closure of the defect, it is important that these newborns be ventilated postoperatively,[32] often with sedation and muscle paralysis. Appropriate fluid management and monitoring are essential, since

there may be changes in venous return due to caval compression as well as alterations in renal, hepatic, and intestinal blood flows resulting from vascular compression.[44] Because of the presence of poor small bowel motility in many children with gastroschisis,[46] many surgeons routinely place a gastrostomy and a central venous line for total parenteral nutrition at the time of the initial closure. This probably is only necessary in patients who require a staged repair or in whom there is evidence of severe intestinal damage.

CONGENITAL HYDRONEPHROSIS

Fetal hydronephrosis frequently is recognized sonographically, because the dilated bladder and renal pelvis are easily visualized and because the associated oligohydramnios is a common obstetrical indication for sonography. Fetal hydronephrosis may be due to obstruction, neuropathy, vesicoureteral reflux, or a combination of these factors. Bilateral hydronephrosis may have devastating consequences, including chronic renal failure and pulmonary hypoplasia from the associated oligohydramnios.[65]

Prenatal Management

Based on our substantial clinical experience with fetal renal anomalies, we have developed an approach to management, which is outlined in Figure 18–4.[57, 58, 62] Detailed sonography and karyotype analysis must be done to rule out associated anomalies. The fetus with unilateral or mild bilateral hydronephrosis and evidence of continuing renal function does not require prenatal intervention but will benefit from early recognition and prompt postnatal repair. On the other hand, the fetus with severe irreversible renal damage evidenced by longstanding oligohydramnios or marked renal dysplasia prior to 20 weeks' gestation usually cannot be salvaged, and elective termination should be advised. The fetus with bilateral hydronephrosis secondary to urethral obstruction who develops oligohydramnios between 18 and 32 weeks may benefit from in utero decompression to halt ongoing damage to developing kidneys and lungs. If oligohydramnios develops later than 32 weeks, the child should be delivered at lung maturity, and the urinary tract decompressed ex utero.

Selection of appropriate management for the fetus with obstructive uropathy requires an accurate assessment of the severity of existing renal damage and the potential for recovery of renal function with decom-

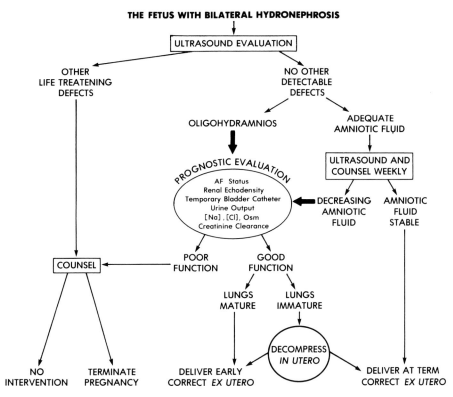

FIG 18–4.
The authors' current management plan for prenatally diagnosed urinary tract obstruction.

pression. Clinical assessment, using such methods as urine reaccumulation after bladder aspiration,[5] Lasix stimulation of urine output,[72] or sonographic appearance of the kidneys,[68] has been unreliable. The amniotic fluid status is useful only in extreme cases; e.g., normal volume late in gestation suggests adequate function, whereas severe oligohydramnios early in gestation suggests poor function.[63] Because fetuses with obstructive uropathy and renal dysplasia produce small amounts of nearly isotonic urine, we have found that fetal urine osmolarity, urine electrolytes, and hourly urine output appear to be predictive for renal damage.[61] In combination with the presence of oligohydramnios and the sonographic appearance of renal dysplasia, fetal urine electrolytes and osmolarity have been closely correlated with outcome in humans (Fig 18–5).[56] Finally, our laboratory studies indicate that fetal creatinine clearance, determined from fetal urine and maternal serum samples, may be a simple, quantitative estimate of fetal renal function.[52]

In experimental models, we have shown that prenatal decompression of fetal urinary tract obstruction arrests the adverse effects on renal development and reverses otherwise lethal pulmonary hypoplasia.[59, 60, 64, 65] Initial clinical application of this information involved placement of percutaneous fetal shunt

catheters. Although we and others have had some success with these catheters (Fig 18–6), they are prone to obstruction and migration, requiring close observation and frequent replacement.[69] These problems, and the fact that an intermittently malfunctioning tube provides suboptimal drainage, led us to develop techniques for surgical exteriorization of the fetal urinary tract (Fig 18–7).

Open fetal surgery for urethral obstruction avoids the problems associated with catheters and provides long-term, reliable decompression. In our preliminary experience with five fetuses operated on for bladder outlet obstruction, all tolerated the procedure well, were completely decompressed for the remainder of gestation, and were born alive;[55] two had severe preexisting renal damage and died of pulmonary hypoplasia. The other three regained normal amniotic fluid volume and were born with normal pulmonary reserve. One died of unrelated causes at 9 months of age, one has an elevated serum creatinine at 2½ years of age and may require renal transplantation in the future, and one is thriving with normal renal function at 16 months of age. Maternal morbidity was minimal, and two of the mothers have had subsequent successful pregnancies. The future role of this modality awaits further experience and improved patient selection.

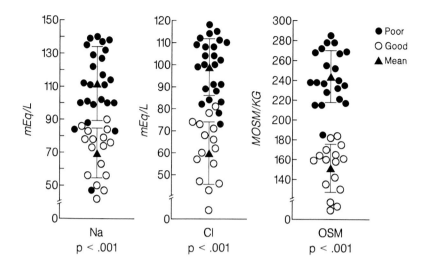

FIG 18–5.
Separation of fetuses with bilateral hydronephrosis into "good prognosis" and "poor prognosis" groups according to urinary electrolyes, osmolarity, and sonographic appearance of renal dysplasia. Fetuses were considered to be in the "good" group if there was no evidence of renal dysplasia on sonogram, if the urine sodium was less than 100 mEq/L urine chloride was less than 90 mEq/L, and urine osmolarity was less than 210 moSm/kg. Fetuses were placed in the "poor" group if any one of these features were abnormal. Overall survival in the "good" group was 13 of 16 fetuses (81.2%), and overall survival in the "poor" group was 3 of 24 fetuses (12.5%). The three survivors in the "poor" group all underwent bladder decompression in utero.

FIG 18–6.
Technique for catheter drainage of the fetal bladder. This technique has been complicated by catheter dislodgement and occlusion and by infection, leading to the development of techniques for open fetal vesicostomy.

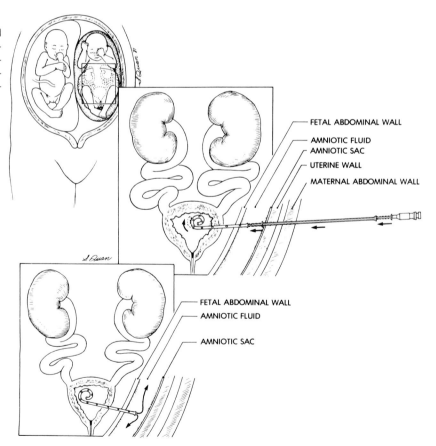

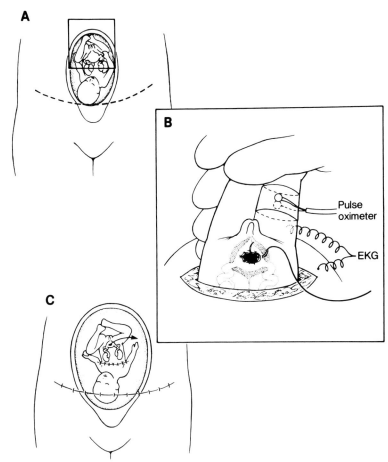

FIG 18–7.
Technique for open fetal vesicostomy. The fetus is monitored electrocardiographically using a pulse oximeter. The caudal half of the fetus is delivered, the vesicostomy is performed, and the fetus is returned to the uterus. Amniotic fluid is restored using physiological saline.

Postnatal Management

Neonatal sonography is the first step in the confirmation and characterization of the anomalies found during the prenatal studies and should be done several days after delivery to avoid demonstrating falsely normal-appearing kidneys in the first 24 to 48 hours postnatally.[67] Voiding cystourethrography is essential to determine the presence or absence of reflux or outlet obstruction. Renal nuclear medicine studies are helpful in assessing overall and differential renal function.

Early relief of urinary tract obstruction, either unilateral[57, 66] or bilateral,[70] is necessary to optimize functional recovery, because impaired growth and maturation of cortical nephrons result from unrelieved obstruction during the first year of life.[71]

Unilateral obstruction either at the ureteropelvic or ureterovesical level is corrected as soon as the baby's overall condition permits, and we have demonstrated that dismembered pyeloplasty can be successfully performed, even in the premature infant.[57] Some of the neonates with bilateral obstructive uropathy may be delivered early. If primary transurethral valve ablation is not technically feasible in premature infants

with posterior urethral valves, then a temporary cutaneous umbilical vesicostomy can be performed.[53]

How does the antenatal diagnosis of urinary tract obstruction influence clinical management? First, many cases of obstruction requiring surgical decompression would otherwise go undetected in the neonatal period. Second, early detection leads to early repair and, presumably, maximal salvage of renal function. Finally, prenatal diagnosis permits termination of pregnancy, prenatal decompression, or early delivery and repair in selected instances.

SACROCOCCYGEAL TERATOMA

Sacrococcygeal teratoma (SCT) is the most common tumor in newborns. It arises from the sacral region and may contain elements from all three primordial layers.[83] Recently, prenatal sonography has identified a previously unrecognized population of fetuses with large SCTs who die in utero, raising a number of issues with respect to the appropriate management of these fetuses.

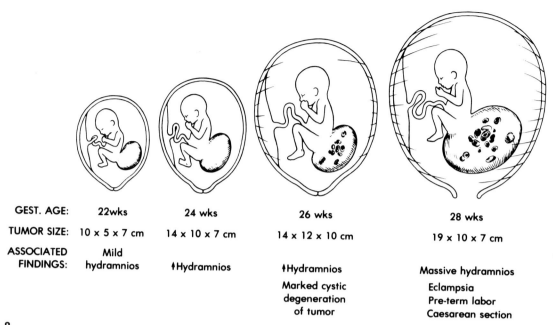

GEST. AGE:	22wks	24 wks	26 wks	28 wks
TUMOR SIZE:	10 x 5 x 7 cm	14 x 10 x 7 cm	14 x 12 x 10 cm	19 x 10 x 7 cm
ASSOCIATED FINDINGS:	Mild hydramnios	↑Hydramnios	↑↑Hydramnios Marked cystic degeneration of tumor	Massive hydramnios Eclampsia Pre-term labor Caesarean section

FIG 18-8.
Progression of large fetal sacrococcygeal teratoma from placentomegaly and polyhydramnios to hydrops, premature labor, and maternal preeclampsia.

Prenatal Management

Appropriate management of the fetus with SCT requires an understanding of the natural history and pathophysiology. These tumors may remain very small and not cause any physiologic disturbance. On the other hand, they may grow to be extremely large and vascular. In these cases, maternal sonography has revealed a previously unrecognized chain of events, which begins with placentomegaly and polyhydramnios and progresses to fetal hydrops. These changes ultimately lead to premature labor, fetal demise, and a preeclampsia-like state in the mother (Fig 18–8).[77] Although there have been a number of theories to explain this syndrome, the most likely is high-output cardiac failure due to arteriovenous shunting through the tumor.[76] Fetal echocardiography with Doppler ultrasound has documented a vastly increased cardiac output in these cases.[75] The cause of the maternal hypertension, hyperdynamic circulation, and pulmonary edema is less clear, but probably is related to release of human chorionic gonadotropin and vasoactive compounds by the hypertrophied placenta.[80, 82]

Currently, prenatal management is limited to careful observation for evidence of placentomegaly or hydrops. Associated anomalies are rare. Other potential prognostic features such as tumor/fetus size ratio[78] and bleeding into the tumor[73] can be assessed and followed. Serial echocardiography with Doppler ultrasound may allow detection of a fetal hyperdynamic circulation, which may precede fulminant hydrops. Early delivery at lung maturity should be done if there is evidence of shunting through the tumor, unequivocal placentomegaly or hydrops, or increased cardiac output on Doppler. In the future, fetal surgery to resect the tumor or interrupt its blood supply may be the only alternative in cases that have begun to deteriorate in the second trimester.

The mode of delivery for SCT also is important. Large tumors may cause dystocia, and prenatal diagnosis permits both transport to a perinatal center and the use of elective cesarean delivery;[79] complications such as bleeding and rupture can be avoided in this way. Needle decompression of SCT prior to delivery has been reported,[81] but rarely is warranted.

Postnatal Management

For fetuses who survive to term, the tumor is rarely life threatening, and resection can be scheduled within the first few days of life. The extent of pelvic involvement is assessed by rectal examination and sonography. Most SCTs in newborns are primarily external, and the vast majority are benign.

The principles of surgical excision involve complete resection of the tumor with removal of the coccyx.[74] This is important, since remaining tumor may undergo malignant degeneration with time if not removed in the newborn period. A posterior approach usually is sufficient, although occasionally a combined abdomino-perineal approach is necessary for intrapelvic extension. The cosmetic result usually is quite acceptable, and long-term survival is to be expected in the vast majority of cases.

GASTROINTESTINAL OBSTRUCTION

There are many causes of gastrointestinal obstruction, including congenital atresia, stenosis, webs, or other mechanical causes (midgut volvulus, internal hernias), intraluminal obstruction (meconium ileus), or disturbed motility (Hirschsprung's disease). Obstruction results in proximal dilation with the potential for necrosis or perforation and inability to absorb swallowed fluids.

Prenatal Management

The diagnosis of gastrointestinal obstruction often is made because of the presence of polyhydramnios. This is particularly true with proximal obstruction, since the swallowed amniotic fluid cannot be absorbed into the fetal circulation and eliminated through the placenta. In esophageal atresia, the typical findings are polyhydramnios associated with lack of fluid in the stomach. A dilated proximal esophageal pouch is only rarely seen in utero. Although these findings are relatively specific, they are often not present, and, therefore, the diagnosis is often missed prenatally.[94] Duodenal obstruction presents with polyhydramnios and a typical "double-bubble," consisting of the dilated stomach and duodenum. In both of these conditions, polyhydramnios typically does not appear until the third trimester.

With distal intestinal obstruction, polyhydramnios is not a constant finding. Dilated bowel loops usually are seen and are particularly significant if there is increased peristalsis. Intra-abdominal calcification often implies a perforation with meconium peritonitis, although it also may be seen with cytomegalovirus infection and urinary tract obstruction. In addition, some fetuses with intra-abdominal calcification do not have any evidence of gastrointestinal obstruction postnatally.[86] Although meconium peritonitis usually is thought to be associated with meconium ileus, most such cases do not in fact have cystic fibrosis.[86] Prenatal diagnosis of Hirschsprung's disease[96] and imperforate anus[89] is rare, presumably because neither typically causes polyhydramnios and colonic dilation usually does not occur until after birth.

Outcome in the prenatally diagnosed fetus with gastrointestinal obstruction is largely related to the presence of associated anomalies. Therefore, careful sonographic screening, amniocentesis, and a family history for cystic fibrosis are very important.[91]

Apart from associated anomalies, the most important determinant of morbidity in esophageal and duodenal obstruction is the speed with which neonatal and surgical management are undertaken at birth. Aspiration pneumonia from repeated vomiting and regurgitation, as well as fluid depletion and electrolyte imbalance, can occur with delayed diagnosis and treatment.[87] It is clear that morbidity is decreased by early recognition of these conditions, and prenatal diagnosis with maternal transport to a perinatal center permits immediate treatment with minimal complications.[95]

The prognosis of distal intestinal obstruction is related to the length of viable intestine remaining at birth. It is difficult to predict prenatally which fetuses will have non–viable bowel and in most cases to know when bowel necrosis occurs. The presence of intra-abdominal calcification and ascites does not necessarily imply a poorer prognosis, but it seems prudent to deliver these babies as soon as lung maturity has occurred. There is no evidence that cesarean delivery offers any advantage over vaginal delivery for these fetuses, unless it is for obstetrical reasons.

Decompression of the fetal abdomen in utero has been reported and advocated for management of intestinal perforation on the grounds that it would prevent neonatal distress.[84] There is no good evidence that this is true, however, and we have found that the ascites tends to resolve spontaneously. Therefore, we would not agree with this approach.[88]

Postnatal Management

The most important aspect of postnatal management is adequate resuscitation (including fluid management), nasoesophageal or nasogastric drainage, and nutritional support.[87] In the absence of associated anomalies, early definitive repair of esophageal and duodenal obstruction can be accomplished within the first few days of life. For premature babies or those with associated anomalies, initial gastrostomy (and ligation of a tracheoesophageal fistula if present) can be done, with definitive repair being delayed until the patient is a better surgical risk.[90] Babies with isolated "long-gap" esophageal atresia usually are treated with gastrostomy followed by definitive repair at approximately 3 months of age.[85]

After resuscitation, infants with distal gastrointestinal obstruction should undergo early laparotomy to assess the amount of viable bowel and resect nonviable bowel. In the case of meconium ileus, the bowel is irrigated with saline, Gastrografin, or N-acetylcysteine solution. If possible, resection should be followed by a primary anastomosis.[92, 93] In utero perforation is managed by peritoneal irrigation and careful hemostasis, since there are often dense adhesions due to chemical peritonitis. In infants suspected of having cystic fibrosis, the diagnosis can be made by stool analysis, liver biopsy, or sweat chlorides; early attention to pulmonary and nutritional care is important.

REFERENCES

Congenital Diaphragmatic Hernia

1. Adzick NS, Harrison MR, Glick PL, et al: Diaphragmatic hernia in the fetus: Prenatal diagnosis and outcome in 94 cases. J Pediatr Surg 1985; 20:357–361.
2. Adzick NS, Outwater KM, Harrison MR, et al: Correction of congenital diaphragmatic hernia in utero. IV: An early gestational fetal lamb model for pulmonary vascular morphometric analysis. J Pediatr Surg 1985; 20:673–680.
3. Adzick NS, Vacanti JP, Lillehei CW, et al: Fetal diaphragmatic hernia: Ultrasound diagnosis and clinical outcome in 38 cases from a single medical center. J Pediatr Surg 1989; 24:654–658.
4. Bartlett RH, Gazzaniga AB, Jefferies R, et al: Extracorporeal membrane oxygenation (ECMO) cardiopulmonary support in infancy. Trans Am Soc Artif Intern Organs 1976; 22:80–88.
5. Bartlett RH, Gazzaniga AB, Toomasian J, et al: Extracorporeal membrane oxygenation (ECMO) in neonatal respiratory failure: 100 cases. Ann Surg 1986; 204:236–245.
6. Benacerraf BR, Adzick NS: Fetal diaphragmatic hernia: Ultrasound diagnosis and clinical outcome in 19 cases. Am J Obstet Gynecol 1987; 156:573.
7. Bloss RS, Arandsa JV, Beardmore HE: Congenital diaphragmatic hernia: Pathophysiology and pharmacologic support. Surgery 1981; 89:518–524.
8. Boros SJ, Mammel MC, Coleman JM, et al: Neonatal high frequency ventilation: Four years experience. Pediatrics 1985; 75:657–663.
9. Cartlidge PHT, Mann NP, Kapila L: Preoperative stabilisation in congenital diaphragmatic hernia. Arch Dis Child 1986; 61:1226–1228.
10. Crawford D, Wright VM, Drake DP, et al: Fetal diaphragmatic hernia: The value of fetal echocardiography. Presented at the meeting of the International Fetal Medicine and Surgery Society, Bonn, Germany, June 1–4, 1988.
11. deLorimier AA, Tierney DF, Parker HR: Hypoplastic lungs in fetal lambs with surgically produced congenital diaphragmatic hernia. Surgery 1967; 62:12–17.
12. Geggel RL, Murphy JD, Langleben D, et al: Congenital diaphragmatic hernia: Arterial structural changes and persistent pulmonary hypertension after surgical repair. J Pediatr 1985; 107:457–464.
13. Harrison MR, Bjordal RI, Langmark F, et al: Congenital diaphragmatic hernia: The hidden mortality. J Pediatr Surg 1978; 13:227–230.
14. Harrison MR, Jester JA, Ross NA: Correction of congenital diaphragmatic hernia in utero. I: The model: Intrathoracic balloon produces fatal pulmonary hypoplasia. Surgery 1980; 88:174–182.
15. Harrison MR, Bressack MA, Churg AM, et al: Correction of congenital diaphragmatic hernia in utero. II: Simulated correction permits fetal lung growth with survival at birth. Surgery 1980; 88:260–268.
16. Harrison MR, Ross NA, deLorimier AA: Correction of congenital diaphragmatic hernia in utero. III: Development of a successful surgical technique using abdominoplasty to avoid compromise of umbilical blood flow. J Pediatr Surg 1981; 16:934.
17. Harrison MR, Anderson J, Rosen M, et al: Fetal surgery in the primate. I: Anesthetic, surgical, and tocolytic management to maximize fetal-neonatal survival. J Pediatr Surg 1982; 17:115.
18. Hazebroek FWJ, Pattenier JW, Tibboel D, et al: Congenital diaphragmatic hernia: The impact of preoperative stabilization. Presented at the meeting of the American Pediatric Surgical Association, Tucson, AZ, May 11–14, 1988.
19. Hendren WH, Lillehei CW: Pediatric surgery. N Engl J Med 1988; 319:86–96.
20. Kamata S, Hasegawa T: Personal communication, 1988.
21. Karl SR, Ballantine TVN, Snider MT: High-frequency ventilation at rates of 375 to 1800 cycles per minute in four neonates with congenital diaphragmatic hernia. J Pediatr Surg 1983; 18:822–828.
22. Langer JC, Filler RM, Bohn DJ, et al: Timing of surgery for congenital diaphragmatic hernia: Is emergency operation necessary? J Pediatr Surg 1988; 23:731–734.
23. Puri P, Gorman F: Lethal nonpulmonary anomalies associated with congenital diaphragmatic hernia: Implications for early intrauterine surgery. J Pediatr Surg 1984; 19:29–32.
24. Sakai H, Tamura M, Hosokawa Y, et al: Effect of surgical repair on respiratory mechanics in congenital diaphragmatic hernia. J Pediatr 1987; 111:432–438.
25. Soper RT, Pringle KC, Scofield JC: Creation and repair of diaphragmatic hernia in the fetal lamb: Techniques and survival. J Pediatr Surg 1984; 19:33–40.
26. Stolar C, Dillon P, Reyes C: Selective use of extracorporeal membrane oxygenation in the management of congenital diaphragmatic hernia. J Pediatr Surg 1988; 23:207–211.
27. Tamura M, Tsuchida Y, Kawano T, et al: Piston-pump-type high frequency oscillatory ventilation for neonates with congenital diaphragmatic hernia: A new protocol. J Pediatr Surg 1988; 23:478–482.
28. Vacanti JP, Crone RK, Murphy JD, et al: The pulmonary hemodynamic response to perioperative anesthesia in

the treatment of high-risk infants with congenital diaphragmatic hernia. J Pediatr Surg 1984; 19:672–679.

Abdominal Wall Defects

29. Berseth CL, Malachowski N, Cohn RB, et al: Longitudinal growth and late morbidity of survivors of gastroschisis and omphalocele. J Pediatr Gastroent Nutr 1982; 1:375–379.
30. Bethel CAI, Seashore JH, Touloukian RJ: Caesarean section does not improve outcome in gastroschisis. Presented at the meeting of the American Pediatric Surgical Association, Tucson, AZ, May 11–14, 1988
31. Bond SJ, Harrison MR, Filly RA, et al: Severity of intestinal damage in gastroschisis: Correlation with prenatal sonographic findings. J Pediatr Surg 1988; 23:520–525.
32. Bower RJ, Bell MJ, Ternberg JL, et al: Ventilatory support and primary closure of gastroschisis. Surgery 1982; 91:52–55
33. Calisti A, Manzoni C, Perrelli L: The fetus with an abdominal wall defect: management and outcome. J Perinat Med 1987; 15:105–111.
34. Carpenter MW, Curci MR, Dibbins AW, et al: Perinatal management of ventral wall defects. Obstet Gynecol 1984; 64:646–651.
35. Davidson JM, Johnson TRB, Rigdon DT, et al: Gastroschisis and omphalocele: Prenatal diagnosis and perinatal management. Prenatal Diagnosis 1984; 4:355–363.
36. Ein SH, Shandling B: A new non-operative treatment of large omphaloceles with a polymer membrane. J Pediatr Surg 1978; 13:255–257.
37. Fitzsimmons J, Nyberg DR, Cyr DR, et al: Perinatal management of gastroschisis. Obstet Gynecol 1988; 71:910–913.
38. Gross RE: A new method for surgical treatment of large omphaloceles. Surgery 1948; 24:277.
39. Grundy H, Anderson RL, Filly RA, et al: Gastroschisis: Prenatal diagnosis and management. Fetal Therapy, in press.
40. Hasan S, Hermansen MC: The prenatal diagnosis of ventral abdominal wall defects. Am J Obstet Gynecol 1986; 155:842–845.
41. Kirk EP, Wah RM: Obstetric management of the fetus with omphalocele or gastroschisis: A review and report of one hundred twelve cases. Am J Obstet Gynecol 1983; 146:512–518.
42. Langer JC, Longaker MT, Crombleholme TM, et al: Etiology of bowel damage in gastroschisis. I: Effects of amniotic fluid exposure and bowel constriction in a fetal lamb model. J Pediatr Surg, in press.
43. Lenke RR, Hatch EJ: Fetal gastroschisis: A preliminary report advocating the use of caesarean section. Obstet Gynecol 1986; 67:395–398.
44. Masey SA, Koehler RC, Buck JR, et al: Effect of abdominal distention on central and regional hemodynamics in neonatal lambs. Pediatr Res 1985; 19:1244–1249.
45. Nakayama D, Harrison MR, Gross BH, et al: Management

of the fetus with an abdominal wall defect. J Pediatr Surg 1984; 19:408–413.
46. Oh KS, Dorst JP, Dominguez R, et al: Abnormal intestinal motility in gastroschisis. Radiology 1978; 127:457–460.
47. Rubin SZ, Ein SH: Experience with 55 Silon pouches. J Pediatr Surg 1976; 11:803–807.
48. Rubin SZ, Martin DJ, Ein SH: A critical look at delayed intestinal motility in gastroschisis. Can J Surg 1978; 21:414–416.
49. Schuster SR: Omphalocele and gastroschisis, in Welch KJ, Randolph JG, Ravitch MM, et al. (eds): *Pediatric Surgery.* Chicago, Year Book Medical Publishers, Inc, 1986, pp 740–762.
50. Sermer M, Benzie RJ, Pitson L, et al: Prenatal diagnosis and management of congenital defects of the anterior abdominal wall. Am J Obstet Gynecol 1987; 156:308–312.
51. Venugopal S, Zachary RB, Spitz L: Exomphalos and gastroschisis: A 10-year review. Br J Surg 1976; 63:523–525.

Congenital Hydronephrosis

52. Adzick NS, Harrison MR, Flake AW, et al: Development of a fetal renal function test using endogenous creatinine clearance. J Pediatr Surg 1985; 20:602.
53. Adzick NS, Harrison MR, Glick PL, et al: Temporary cutaneous umbilical vesicostomy in premature infants with urethral obstruction. J Pediatr Surg 1986; 21:171–172.
54. Bellinger MF, Comstock C, Grosso D, et al: Fetal posterior urethral valves and renal dysplasia at 15 weeks gestational age. J Urol 1983; 129:1238.
55. Crombleholme TM, Harrison MR, Langer JC, et al: Early experience with open fetal surgery for congenital hydronephrosis. J Pediatr Surg 1988; 23:1114–1121.
56. Crombleholme TM, Harrison MR, Anderson RL, et al: Early experience with fetal intervention in bilateral congenital hydronephrosis. Presented to the American Pediatric Surgical Association, Tucson, AZ, May 11–14, 1988.
57. Flake AW, Harrison MR, Sauer L, et al: Ureteropelvic junction obstruction in the fetus. J Pediatr Surg 1986; 21:1058–1063.
58. Flake AW, Adzick NS, Glick PL, et al: Evaluation of the fetus with hydronephrosis, in White RW, Palmer JM, (eds): *New Techniques in Urology,* New York, Futura Publishing, 1987, pp 269–286.
59. Glick PL, Harrison MR, Noall R, et al: Correction of congenital hydronephrosis in utero. III: Early mid-trimester urethral obstruction produces renal dysplasia. J Pediatr Surg 1983; 18:681.
60. Glick PL, Harrison MR, Adzick NS, et al: Correction of congenital hydronephrosis in utero. IV: In utero decompression prevents renal dysplasia. J Pediatr Surg 1984; 19:649.
61. Glick PL, Harrison MR, Golbus MS, et al: Management of

the fetus with congenital hydronephrosis. II: Prognostic criteria and selection for treatment. J Pediatr Surg 1985; 20:376.

62. Harrison MR, Golbus MS, Filly RA: Management of the fetus with a urinary tract malformation. JAMA 1981; 246:635.

63. Harrison MR, Golbus MS, Filly RA, et al: Management of the fetus with congenital hydronephrosis. J Pediatr Surg 1982; 17:728.

64. Harrison MR, Ross NA, Noall R, et al: Correction of congenital hydronephrosis *in utero*. I: The model: Fetal urethral obstruction produces hydronephrosis and pulmonary hypoplasia in fetal lambs. J Pediatr Surg 1983; 18:247.

65. Harrison MR, Nakayama DK, Noall R, et al: Correction of congenital hydronephrosis in utero. II: Decompression reverses the effects of obstruction on the fetal lung and urinary tract. J Pediatr Surg 1982; 17:965.

66. King LR, Coughlen PWF, Bloch EC, et al: The case for immediate pyeloplasty in the neonate with ureteropelvic junction obstruction. J Urol 1984; 132:303–306.

67. Laing FC, Burke VD, Wing VW, et al: Postpartum evaluation of fetal hydronephrosis: Optimal timing for followup sonography. Radiology 1984; 152:423–424.

68. Mahony BS, Filly RA, Callen PW, et al: Sonographic evaluation of fetal renal dysplasia. Radiology 1984; 152:143.

69. Manning FA, Harrison MR, Rodeck C: Catheter shunts for fetal hydronephrosis and hydrocephalus. Report of the international fetal surgery registry. N Engl J Med 1986; 315:336.

70. Mayer G, Genton N, Torrado A, et al: Renal function in obstructive uropathy: Long-term results of reconstructive surgery. Pediatrics 1975; 56:740–745.

71. Spitzer A, Brandis M: Functional and morphologic maturation of superficial nephrons. J Clin Invest 1974; 53:279–283.

72. Wladimiroff JW: Effect of furosemide on fetal urine production. Br J Obstet Gynaecol 1975; 82:221.

Sacrococcygeal Teratoma

73. Alter DN, Reed KL, Marz GR, et al: Prenatal diagnosis of congestive heart failure in a fetus with a sacrococcygeal teratoma. Obstet Gynecol 1988; 71:978–981.

74. Altman RP, Randolph JG, Lilly JR: Sacrococcygeal teratoma: American Academy of Pediatrics Surgical Section Survey, 1973. J Pediatr Surg 1974; 9:389–398.

75. Bond SJ, Harrison MR, Schmidt KG, et al: Death from high output cardiac failure in fetal sacrococcygeal teratoma. J Pediatr Surg, in press.

76. Cousins L, Benirschke K, Porreco R, et al. Placentomegaly due to fetal congestive failure in a pregnancy with a sacrococcygeal teratoma. J Reprod Med 1980; 25:142–144.

77. Flake AW, Harrison MR, Adzick NS, et al: Fetal sacrococcygeal teratoma. J Pediatr Surg 1986; 21:563–566.

78. Grisoni ER, Gauderer MWL, Wolfson RN, et al: Antenatal diagnosis of sacrococcygeal teratomas: Prognostic features. Pediatr Surg Int 1988; 3:173–175.

79. Horger EO, McCarter L: Prenatal diagnosis of sacrococcygeal teratoma. Am J Obstet Gynecol 1979; 134:228–229.

80. Jeffcoate TNA, Scott JS: Some observations on the placental factor in pregnancy toxemia. Am J Obstet Gynecol 1959; 77:475–489.

81. Mintz MC, Mennuti M, Fishman M: Prenatal aspiration of sacrococcygeal teratoma. Am J Roentg 1983; 141:367–368.

82. Nisula BC, Taliadouros GS. Thyroid function in gestational trophoblastic neoplasia: Evidence that the thyrotropic activity of chorionic gonadotropin mediates the thyrotoxicosis of choriocarcinoma. Am J Obstet Gynecol 1980; 138:77–85.

83. Woolley MM: Sacrococcygeal teratomas, in Welch KJ, Randolph JG, Ravitch MM, et al (eds): *Pediatric Surgery*. Chicago, Year Book Medical Publishers, Inc, 1985, pp 267–269.

Gastrointestinal Obstruction

84. Baxi LV, Yeh M-N, Blanc WA, et al: Antepartum diagnosis and management of in utero intestinal volvulus with perforation. N Engl J Med 1983, 308;1519–1521.

85. deLorimier AA, Harrison MR: Long gap esophageal atresia. Primary anastomosis after esophageal elongation by bougienage and esophagomyotomy. J Thorac Cardiovasc Surg 1980; 79:138–141.

86. Foster MA, Nyberg DA, Mahony BS, et al: Meconium peritonitis: Prenatal sonographic findings and their clinical significance. Radiology 1987; 165:661–665.

87. Ghory MJ, Sheldon CA: Newborn surgical emergencies of the gastrointestinal tract. Surg Clin North Am 1985; 65:1083–1098.

88. Glick PL, Harrison MR, Filly RA: Antepartum diagnosis of meconium peritonitis. N Engl J Med 1983; 309:1392.

89. Harris RD, Nyberg DA, Mack LA, et al: Anorectal atresia: Prenatal sonographic diagnosis. AJR 1987; 149:395–400.

90. Ito T, Sugito T, Nagaya M: Delayed primary anastomosis in poor-risk patients with esophageal atresia associated with tracheoesophageal fistula. J Pediatr Surg 1984; 19:243–247.

91. Langer JC, Adzick NS, Filly RA, et al: Gastrointestinal obstruction in the fetus. Presented to the Pacific Coast Surgical Association, Vancouver, BC, Feb. 19–22, 1989.

92. Louw JH: Resection and end-to-end anastomosis in the management of atresia and stenosis of the small bowel. Surgery 1967; 62:940.

93. Mabogunje OA, Wang CI, Mahour GH: Improved sur-

vival of neonates with meconium ileus. Arch Surg 1982; 117:37–40.

94. Pretorius DH, Drose JA, Dennis MA, et al: Tracheoesophageal fistula in utero: Twenty-two cases. J Ultrasound Med 1987; 6:509–513.

95. Romero R, Ghidini A, Costigan K, et al: Prenatal diagno-

sis of duodenal atresia: Does it make any difference? Obstet Gynecol 1988; 71:739–741.

96. Vermish M, Mayden KL, Confino E, et al: Prenatal sonographic diagnosis of Hirschsprung's disease. J Ultrasound Med 1986; 5:37–39.

APPENDIX A

Growth Measurements

TABLE A–1.

Predicted Fetal Measurements at Specific Menstrual Age*

Menstrual Age (wk)	Biparietal Diameter (cm)†	Head Circumference (cm)‡	Abdominal Circumference (cm)§	Femur Length (cm)¶
12.0	1.7	6.8	4.6	0.7
12.5	1.9	7.5	5.3	0.9
13.0	2.1	8.2	6.0	1.1
13.5	2.3	8.9	6.7	1.2
14.0	2.5	9.7	7.3	1.4
14.5	2.7	10.4	8.0	1.6
15.0	2.9	11.0	8.6	1.7
15.5	3.1	11.7	9.3	1.9
16.0	3.2	12.4	9.9	2.0
16.5	3.4	13.1	10.6	2.2
17.0	3.6	13.8	11.2	2.4
17.5	3.8	14.4	11.9	2.5
18.0	3.9	15.1	12.5	2.7
18.5	4.1	15.8	13.1	2.8
19.0	4.3	16.4	13.7	3.0
19.5	4.5	17.0	14.4	3.1
20.0	4.6	17.7	15.0	3.3
20.5	4.8	18.3	15.6	3.4
21.0	5.0	18.9	16.2	3.5
21.5	5.1	19.5	16.8	3.7
22.0	5.3	20.1	17.4	3.8
22.5	5.5	20.7	17.9	4.0
23.0	5.6	21.3	18.5	4.1
23.5	5.8	21.9	19.1	4.2
24.0	5.9	22.4	19.7	4.4
24.5	6.1	23.0	20.2	4.5
25.0	6.2	23.5	20.8	4.6
25.5	6.4	24.1	21.3	4.7
26.0	6.5	24.6	21.9	4.9
26.5	6.7	25.1	22.4	5.0
27.0	6.8	25.6	23.0	5.1

(Continued.)

TABLE A–1 (cont.).

Menstrual Age (wk)	Biparietal Diameter (cm)†	Head Circumference (cm)‡	Abdominal Circumference (cm)§	Femur Length (cm)¶
27.5	6.9	26.1	23.5	5.2
28.0	7.1	26.6	24.0	5.4
28.5	7.2	27.1	24.6	5.5
29.0	7.3	27.5	25.1	5.6
29.5	7.5	28.0	25.6	5.7
30.0	7.6	28.4	26.1	5.8
30.5	7.7	28.8	26.6	5.9
31.0	7.8	29.3	27.1	6.0
31.5	7.9	29.7	27.6	6.1
32.0	8.1	30.1	28.1	6.2
32.5	8.2	30.4	28.6	6.3
33.0	8.3	30.8	29.1	6.4
33.5	8.4	31.2	29.5	6.5
34.0	8.5	31.5	30.0	6.6
34.5	8.6	31.8	30.5	6.7
35.0	8.7	32.2	30.9	6.8
35.5	8.8	32.5	31.4	6.9
36.0	8.9	32.8	31.8	7.0
36.5	8.9	33.0	32.3	7.1
37.0	9.0	33.3	32.7	7.2
37.5	9.1	33.5	33.2	7.3
38.0	9.2	33.8	33.6	7.4
38.5	9.2	34.0	34.0	7.4
39.0	9.3	34.2	34.4	7.5
39.5	9.4	34.4	34.8	7.6
40.0	9.4	34.6	35.3	7.7

*From Hadlock FP, Deter RL, Harrist RB, et al: Estimating fetal age: Computer-assisted analysis of multiple fetal growth parameters. Radiology 1984; 152:497–501. Used by permission.
†BPD = $-3.08 + 0.41$ (MA) $- 0.000061$ MA^3,r^2 = 97.6%; 1 SD = 3 mm.
‡HC = $-11.48 + 1.56$ (MA) $- 0.0002548$ MA^3, r^2 = 98.1%; 1 SD = 1 cm.
§AC = $-13.3 + 1.61$ (MA) $- 0.00998$ MA^2, r^2 = 97.2%; 1 SD = 1.34 cm.
¶FL = $-3.91 + 0.427$ (MA) $- 0.0034$ MA^2, r^2 = 97.5%; 1 SD = 3 mm.

TABLE A–2.

Normal Values for Head Circumference and Abdominal Circumference*

Menstrual Age (MA) (wk)	Head Circumference (HC)			Abdominal Circumference (AC)		
	Lower Limit (cm)††	Predicted Value (cm)†	Upper Limit (cm)††	Lower Limit (cm)††	Predicted Value (cm)†	Upper Limit (cm)††
12	5.8	7.3	8.8	5.4	6.3	7.1
13	7.2	8.7	10.2	6.4	7.4	8.3
14	8.6	10.1	11.6	7.4	8.4	9.5
15	9.9	11.4	12.9	8.3	9.5	10.8
16	11.3	12.8	14.3	9.3	10.6	12.0
17	12.6	14.1	15.6	10.2	11.7	13.3
18	13.9	15.4	16.9	11.2	12.8	14.5
19	15.2	16.7	18.2	12.1	13.9	15.7
20	16.4	17.9	19.4	13.1	15.0	17.0
21	17.7	19.2	20.7	14.0	16.1	18.2
22	18.9	20.4	21.9	15.0	17.2	19.5
23	20.0	21.5	23.0	16.0	18.3	20.7
24	21.2	22.7	24.2	16.9	19.4	22.0
25	22.3	23.8	25.3	17.9	20.5	23.2
26	23.4	24.9	26.4	18.8	21.6	24.4
27	24.4	25.9	27.4	19.8	22.7	25.7
28	24.4	26.9	29.4	20.7	23.8	26.9
29	25.4	27.9	30.4	21.7	24.9	28.2

TABLE A–2 (cont.).

Menstrual Age (MA) (wk)	Head Circumference (HC)			Abdominal Circumference (AC)		
	Lower Limit (cm)††	Predicted Value (cm)†	Upper Limit (cm)††	Lower Limit (cm)††	Predicted Value (cm)†	Upper Limit (cm)††
30	26.3	28.8	31.3	22.6	26.0	29.4
31	27.2	29.7	32.2	23.6	27.1	30.6
32	28.1	30.6	33.1	24.6	28.2	31.9
33	28.9	31.4	33.9	25.5	29.3	33.1
34	29.7	32.2	34.7	26.5	30.4	34.4
35	30.4	32.9	35.4	27.4	31.5	35.6
36	31.1	33.6	36.1	28.4	32.6	36.9
37	31.7	34.2	36.7	29.3	33.7	38.1
38	32.3	34.8	37.3	30.3	34.8	39.3
39	32.9	35.4	37.9	31.2	35.9	40.6
40	33.4	35.9	38.4	32.2	37.0	41.8

*From Deter RL, Harrist RB, Hadlock FP, et al: Fetal head and abdominal circumference. II: Critical reevaluation of the relationship to menstrual age. J Clin Ultrasound 1982; 10:365–372. Used by permission.
†Predicted values
  $HC = -10.3676 + 1.5021 \, (MA) - .0002136 \, (MA)^3$
  $AC = -6.9300 + 1.0985 \, (MA)$
††HC: Lower limit (<28 weeks) = predicted value − 1.5 cm
    Lower limit (>28 weeks) = predicted value − 2.5 cm
    Upper limit (<28 weeks) = predicted value + 1.5 cm
    Upper limit (>28 weeks) = predicted value + 2.5 cm
  AC: Lower limit = predicted value − .13 (predicted value)
    Upper limit = predicted value + .13 (predicted value)

TABLE A–3.

Mean and Standard Deviation of Head Circumference as a Function of Gestational Age.*

Week No	SD Above Mean		Mean	SD Below Mean				
	+2	+1		−1	−2	−3	−4	−5
20	204	189	175	160	145	131	116	101
21	216	201	187	172	157	143	128	113
22	228	213	198	184	169	154	140	125
23	239	223	210	195	180	166	151	136
24	250	235	221	206	191	177	162	147
25	261	246	232	217	202	188	173	158
26	271	257	242	227	213	198	183	169
27	282	267	252	238	223	208	194	179
28	291	277	262	247	233	218	203	189
29	301	286	271	257	242	227	213	198
30	310	295	281	266	251	236	222	207
31	318	304	289	274	260	245	230	216
32	327	313	297	283	268	253	239	224
33	334	320	305	290	276	261	246	232
34	341	327	312	297	283	268	253	239
35	348	333	319	304	289	275	260	245
36	354	339	325	310	295	281	266	251
37	360	345	330	316	301	286	272	257
38	364	350	335	320	306	291	276	262
39	369	354	339	325	310	295	281	266
40	372	358	343	328	314	299	284	270
41	375	360	346	331	316	302	287	272
42	377	363	348	333	319	304	289	275

*From Chervenak FA, Jeanty P, Cantraine F, et al: The diagnosis of fetal microcephaly. Am J Obstet Gynecol 1984; 149:512–517. Used by permission.

TABLE A–4.

Predicted Femur Length at Different Gestational Ages*

| Menstrual Age (wk) | Femur Length† | | |
	Lower Limit (cm)‡	Predicted Value (cm)	Upper Limit§ (cm)
12	0.6	0.7	0.8
13	0.9	1.0	1.1
14	1.1	1.3	1.5
15	1.4	1.6	1.8
16	1.7	2.0	2.3
17	2.0	2.3	2.6
18	2.2	2.6	3.0
19	2.5	2.9	3.3
20	2.7	3.1	3.5
21	2.9	3.4	3.9
22	3.2	3.7	4.4
23	3.4	4.0	4.6
24	3.6	4.2	4.8
25	3.9	4.5	5.1
26	4.0	4.7	5.4
27	4.2	4.9	5.6
28	4.5	5.2	5.9
29	4.6	5.4	6.2
30	4.8	5.6	6.4
31	5.0	5.8	6.6
32	5.2	6.0	6.8
33	5.3	6.2	7.1
34	5.5	6.4	7.3
35	5.7	6.6	7.5
36	5.8	6.8	7.8
37	5.9	6.9	7.9
38	6.1	7.1	8.1
39	6.3	7.3	8.3
40	6.4	7.4	8.4

*From Warda AH, Deter RL, Rossavik IK, et al: Fetal femur length: A critical re-evaluation of the relationship to menstrual age. Obstet Gynecol 1985; 66:69. Used by permission.

†Femur Length = $-3.8929 + 0.42062$ (menstrual age) $- 0.0034513$ (menstrual age)^2.

‡Lower Limit = predicted value $- 0.14$ (predicted value).

§Upper Limit = predicted value $+ 0.14$ (predicted value).

TABLE A–5.

Normal Extremity Long Bone Lengths and Biparietal Diameter at Different Menstrual Ages*†

Menstrual Age (wk)	Biparietal Diameter	Femur	Tibia	Fibula	Humerus	Radius	Ulna
13	2.3(0.3)	1.1(0.2)	0.9(0.2)	0.8(0.2)	1.0(0.2)	0.6(0.2)	0.8(0.3)
14	2.7(0.3)	1.3(0.2)	1.0(0.2)	0.9(0.3)	1.2(0.2)	0.8(0.2)	1.0(0.2)
15	3.0(0.1)	1.5(0.2)	1.3(0.2)	1.2(0.2)	1.4(0.2)	1.1(0.1)	1.2(0.1)
16	3.3(0.2)	1.9(0.3)	1.6(0.3)	1.5(0.3)	1.7(0.2)	1.4(0.3)	1.6(0.3)
17	3.7(0.3)	2.2(0.3)	1.8(0.3)	1.7(0.2)	2.0(0.4)	1.5(0.3)	1.7(0.3)
18	4.2(0.5)	2.5(0.3)	2.2(0.3)	2.1(0.3)	2.3(0.3)	1.9(0.2)	2.2(0.3)
19	4.4(0.4)	2.8(0.3)	2.5(0.3)	2.3(0.3)	2.6(0.3)	2.1(0.3)	2.4(0.3)
20	4.7(0.4)	3.1(0.3)	2.7(0.2)	2.6(0.2)	2.9(0.3)	2.4(0.2)	2.7(0.3)
21	5.0(0.5)	3.5(0.4)	3.0(0.4)	2.9(0.4)	3.2(0.4)	2.7(0.4)	3.0(0.4)
22	5.5(0.5)	3.6(0.3)	3.2(0.3)	3.1(0.3)	3.3(0.3)	2.8(0.5)	3.1(0.4)
23	5.8(0.5)	4.0(0.4)	3.6(0.2)	3.4(0.2)	3.7(0.3)	3.1(0.4)	3.5(0.2)
24	6.1(0.5)	4.2(0.3)	3.7(0.3)	3.6(0.3)	3.8(0.4)	3.3(0.4)	3.6(0.4)
25	6.4(0.5)	4.6(0.3)	4.0(0.3)	3.9(0.4)	4.2(0.4)	3.5(0.3)	3.9(0.4)
26	6.8(0.5)	4.8(0.4)	4.2(0.3)	4.0(0.3)	4.3(0.3)	3.6(0.4)	4.0(0.3)
27	7.0(0.3)	4.9(0.3)	4.4(0.3)	4.2(0.3)	4.5(0.2)	3.7(0.3)	4.1(0.2)
28	7.3(0.5)	5.3(0.5)	4.5(0.4)	4.4(0.3)	4.7(0.4)	3.9(0.4)	4.4(0.5)
29	7.6(0.5)	5.3(0.5)	4.6(0.3)	4.5(0.3)	4.8(0.4)	4.0(0.5)	4.5(0.4)
30	7.7(0.6)	5.6(0.3)	4.8(0.5)	4.7(0.3)	5.0(0.5)	4.1(0.6)	4.7(0.3)
31	8.2(0.7)	6.0(0.6)	5.1(0.3)	4.9(0.5)	5.3(0.4)	4.2(0.3)	4.9(0.4)
32	8.5(0.6)	6.1(0.6)	5.2(0.4)	5.1(0.4)	5.4(0.4)	4.4(0.6)	5.0(0.6)
33	8.6(0.4)	6.4(0.5)	5.4(0.5)	5.3(0.3)	5.6(0.5)	4.5(0.5)	5.2(0.3)
34	8.9(0.5)	6.6(0.6)	5.7(0.5)	5.5(0.4)	5.8(0.5)	4.7(0.5)	5.4(0.5)
35	8.9(0.7)	6.7(0.6)	5.8(0.4)	5.6(0.4)	5.9(0.6)	4.8(0.6)	5.4(0.4)
36	9.1(0.7)	7.0(0.7)	6.0(0.6)	5.6(0.5)	6.0(0.6)	4.9(0.5)	5.5(0.3)
37	9.3(0.9)	7.2(0.4)	6.1(0.4)	6.0(0.4)	6.1(0.4)	5.1(0.3)	5.6(0.4)
38	9.5(0.6)	7.4(0.6)	6.2(0.3)	6.0(0.4)	6.4(0.3)	5.1(0.5)	5.8(0.6)
39	9.5(0.6)	7.6(0.8)	6.4(0.7)	6.1(0.6)	6.5(0.6)	5.3(0.5)	6.0(0.6)
40	9.9(0.8)	7.7(0.4)	6.5(0.3)	6.2(0.1)	6.6(0.4)	5.3(0.3)	6.0(0.5)
41	9.7(0.6)	7.7(0.4)	6.6(0.4)	6.3(0.5)	6.6(0.4)	5.6(0.4)	6.3(0.5)
42	10.0(0.5)	7.8(0.7)	6.8(0.5)	6.7(0.7)	6.8(0.7)	5.7(0.5)	6.5(0.5)

*From Merz E, Mi-Sook KK, Pehl S: Ultrasonic mensuration of fetal limb bones in the second and third trimesters. J Clin Ultrasound 1987; 15:175–183. Used by permission.
†Mean values (cm); value of 2 SD in parentheses.

TABLE A–6.

Estimates of Fetal Weight (in Grams) Based on Abdominal Circumference and Femur Length*

Femur Length (cm)	Abdominal Circumference (cm)																				
	20.0	20.5	21.0	21.5	22.0	22.5	23.0	23.5	24.0	24.5	25.0	25.5	26.0	26.5	27.0	27.5	28.0	28.5	29.0	29.5	30.0
4.0	663	691	720	751	783	816	851	887	925	964	1006	1048	1093	1139	1188	1239	1291	1346	1403	1463	1525
4.1	680	709	738	769	802	836	871	907	946	986	1027	1070	1115	1162	1211	1262	1315	1371	1429	1489	1551
4.2	697	726	757	788	821	855	891	928	967	1007	1049	1093	1138	1186	1235	1287	1340	1396	1454	1515	1578
4.3	715	745	776	808	841	875	912	949	988	1029	1071	1116	1162	1209	1259	1311	1365	1422	1480	1541	1605
4.4	734	764	795	827	861	896	933	971	1010	1051	1094	1139	1185	1234	1284	1336	1391	1448	1507	1568	1632
4.5	753	783	815	847	882	917	954	993	1033	1074	1118	1163	1210	1259	1309	1362	1417	1474	1534	1596	1660
4.6	772	803	835	868	903	939	976	1015	1056	1098	1142	1187	1235	1284	1335	1388	1444	1501	1561	1623	1688
4.7	792	823	856	889	924	961	999	1038	1079	1122	1166	1212	1260	1310	1361	1415	1471	1529	1589	1652	1717
4.8	812	844	877	911	947	984	1022	1062	1103	1146	1191	1237	1286	1336	1388	1442	1498	1557	1618	1681	1746
4.9	833	865	899	933	969	1007	1046	1086	1128	1171	1216	1263	1312	1363	1415	1470	1527	1585	1647	1710	1776
5.0	855	887	921	956	993	1031	1070	1111	1153	1197	1243	1290	1339	1390	1443	1498	1555	1615	1676	1740	1806
5.1	877	910	944	980	1016	1055	1095	1136	1179	1223	1269	1317	1367	1418	1471	1527	1584	1644	1706	1770	1837
5.2	899	933	967	1004	1041	1080	1120	1162	1205	1250	1296	1344	1395	1447	1500	1556	1614	1674	1737	1801	1868
5.3	922	956	992	1028	1066	1105	1146	1188	1232	1277	1324	1373	1423	1476	1530	1586	1645	1705	1768	1833	1900
5.4	946	981	1016	1053	1091	1131	1172	1215	1259	1305	1352	1401	1452	1505	1560	1617	1675	1736	1799	1865	1933
5.5	971	1005	1041	1079	1118	1158	1199	1242	1287	1333	1381	1431	1482	1535	1591	1648	1707	1768	1832	1897	1966
5.6	995	1031	1067	1105	1144	1185	1227	1271	1316	1362	1411	1461	1513	1566	1622	1679	1739	1801	1864	1931	1999
5.7	1021	1057	1094	1132	1172	1213	1255	1299	1345	1392	1441	1491	1544	1598	1654	1712	1772	1834	1898	1964	2033
5.8	1047	1084	1121	1160	1200	1242	1285	1329	1375	1422	1472	1523	1575	1630	1686	1744	1805	1867	1932	1999	2068
5.9	1074	1111	1149	1188	1229	1271	1314	1359	1406	1454	1503	1555	1608	1663	1719	1778	1839	1902	1966	2034	2103
6.0	1102	1139	1178	1217	1258	1301	1345	1390	1437	1485	1535	1587	1641	1696	1753	1812	1873	1936	2002	2069	2139
6.1	1130	1168	1207	1247	1289	1331	1376	1421	1469	1518	1568	1620	1674	1730	1788	1847	1908	1972	2038	2105	2175
6.2	1160	1198	1237	1278	1319	1363	1408	1454	1501	1551	1602	1654	1709	1765	1823	1882	1944	2008	2074	2142	2212
6.3	1189	1228	1268	1309	1351	1395	1440	1487	1535	1585	1636	1689	1744	1800	1858	1919	1981	2045	2111	2180	2250
6.4	1220	1259	1299	1341	1384	1428	1473	1520	1569	1619	1671	1724	1779	1836	1895	1956	2018	2082	2149	2218	2289
6.5	1251	1291	1332	1373	1417	1461	1507	1555	1604	1655	1707	1760	1816	1873	1932	1993	2056	2121	2188	2256	2328
6.6	1284	1324	1365	1407	1451	1496	1542	1590	1640	1691	1743	1797	1853	1911	1970	2031	2094	2160	2227	2296	2367
6.7	1317	1357	1399	1441	1486	1531	1578	1626	1676	1728	1780	1835	1891	1949	2009	2070	2134	2199	2267	2336	2408
6.8	1351	1391	1433	1477	1521	1567	1615	1663	1713	1765	1819	1873	1930	1988	2048	2110	2174	2240	2307	2377	2449
6.9	1385	1427	1469	1513	1558	1604	1652	1701	1752	1804	1857	1913	1970	2028	2089	2151	2215	2281	2348	2418	2490
7.0	1421	1463	1506	1550	1595	1642	1690	1740	1791	1843	1897	1953	2010	2069	2130	2192	2256	2322	2391	2461	2533
7.1	1458	1500	1543	1588	1633	1681	1729	1779	1830	1883	1938	1994	2051	2110	2171	2234	2299	2365	2433	2504	2576
7.2	1495	1538	1581	1626	1673	1720	1769	1819	1871	1924	1979	2035	2093	2153	2214	2277	2342	2408	2477	2547	2620
7.3	1534	1577	1621	1666	1713	1761	1810	1861	1913	1966	2021	2078	2136	2196	2258	2321	2386	2453	2521	2592	2665
7.4	1573	1616	1661	1707	1754	1802	1852	1903	1955	2009	2065	2122	2180	2240	2302	2365	2431	2498	2566	2637	2710
7.5	1614	1657	1702	1749	1796	1845	1895	1946	1999	2053	2109	2166	2225	2285	2347	2411	2476	2543	2612	2683	2756
7.6	1655	1699	1745	1791	1839	1888	1939	1990	2043	2098	2154	2211	2270	2331	2393	2457	2523	2590	2659	2730	2803
7.7	1698	1742	1788	1835	1883	1933	1983	2035	2089	2144	2200	2258	2317	2378	2440	2504	2570	2638	2707	2778	2851
7.8	1741	1786	1833	1880	1928	1978	2029	2082	2135	2191	2247	2305	2365	2426	2488	2553	2618	2686	2755	2827	2899
7.9	1786	1832	1878	1926	1975	2025	2076	2129	2183	2238	2295	2353	2413	2474	2537	2602	2668	2735	2805	2876	2949
8.0	1832	1878	1925	1973	2022	2073	2124	2177	2232	2287	2344	2403	2463	2524	2587	2652	2718	2785	2855	2926	2999
8.1	1879	1926	1973	2021	2071	2121	2173	2227	2281	2337	2394	2453	2513	2575	2638	2702	2769	2837	2906	2977	3050
8.2	1928	1974	2022	2070	2120	2171	2224	2277	2332	2388	2446	2504	2565	2626	2690	2754	2821	2889	2958	3029	3102
8.3	1978	2024	2072	2121	2171	2223	2275	2329	2384	2440	2498	2557	2617	2679	2743	2807	2874	2942	3011	3082	3155

Femur Length (cm)	Abdominal Circumference (cm)																			
	30.5	31.0	31.5	32.0	32.5	33.0	33.5	34.0	34.5	35.0	35.5	36.0	36.5	37.0	37.5	38.0	38.5	39.0	39.5	40.0
4.0	1590	1658	1729	1802	1879	1959	2042	2129	2220	2314	2413	2515	2622	2734	2850	2972	3098	3230	3367	3511
4.1	1617	1685	1756	1830	1907	1987	2071	2158	2249	2344	2442	2545	2652	2764	2880	3002	3128	3260	3397	3540
4.2	1644	1712	1783	1858	1935	2016	2100	2187	2279	2373	2472	2575	2683	2794	2911	3032	3159	3290	3427	3570
4.3	1671	1740	1812	1886	1964	2045	2129	2217	2308	2404	2503	2606	2713	2825	2942	3063	3189	3321	3458	3600
4.4	1699	1768	1840	1915	1993	2075	2159	2247	2339	2434	2533	2637	2744	2856	2973	3094	3220	3352	3488	3630
4.5	1727	1797	1869	1944	2023	2105	2189	2278	2370	2465	2565	2668	2776	2888	3004	3125	3251	3383	3519	3661
4.6	1756	1826	1898	1974	2053	2135	2220	2309	2401	2497	2596	2700	2807	2919	3036	3157	3283	3414	3550	3692
4.7	1785	1855	1928	2004	2084	2166	2251	2340	2432	2528	2628	2732	2840	2952	3068	3189	3315	3446	3582	3723
4.8	1814	1885	1959	2035	2115	2197	2283	2372	2464	2560	2660	2764	2872	2984	3100	3221	3347	3478	3613	3754
4.9	1845	1916	1990	2066	2146	2229	2315	2404	2497	2593	2693	2797	2905	3017	3133	3254	3380	3510	3645	3786
5.0	1875	1947	2021	2098	2178	2261	2347	2437	2530	2626	2726	2830	2938	3050	3166	3287	3412	3542	3677	3818
5.1	1906	1978	2053	2130	2210	2294	2380	2470	2563	2659	2760	2864	2972	3084	3200	3320	3445	3575	3710	3850
5.2	1938	2010	2085	2163	2243	2327	2413	2503	2597	2693	2794	2898	3006	3117	3234	3354	3479	3608	3743	3882
5.3	1970	2043	2118	2196	2277	2360	2447	2537	2631	2728	2828	2932	3040	3152	3268	3388	3513	3642	3776	3915
5.4	2003	2076	2151	2229	2311	2395	2482	2572	2665	2762	2863	2967	3075	3186	3302	3422	3547	3676	3809	3948
5.5	2036	2109	2185	2264	2345	2429	2516	2607	2700	2797	2898	3002	3110	3221	3337	3457	3581	3710	3843	3981
5.6	2070	2143	2220	2298	2380	2464	2552	2642	2736	2833	2933	3038	3145	3257	3372	3492	3616	3744	3877	4015
5.7	2104	2178	2254	2333	2415	2500	2587	2678	2772	2869	2970	3074	3181	3293	3408	3527	3651	3779	3911	4048
5.8	2139	2213	2290	2369	2451	2536	2624	2714	2808	2905	3006	3110	3218	3329	3444	3563	3686	3814	3946	4082
5.9	2175	2249	2326	2405	2488	2573	2660	2751	2845	2942	3043	3147	3254	3366	3480	3599	3722	3849	3981	4117
6.0	2211	2286	2363	2442	2525	2610	2698	2789	2883	2980	3080	3184	3292	3403	3517	3636	3758	3885	4016	4151
6.1	2248	2323	2400	2480	2562	2647	2736	2827	2921	3018	3118	3222	3329	3440	3554	3673	3795	3921	4052	4186
6.2	2285	2360	2438	2518	2600	2686	2774	2865	2959	3056	3157	3260	3367	3478	3592	3710	3832	3957	4087	4222
6.3	2323	2398	2476	2556	2639	2725	2813	2904	2998	3095	3195	3299	3406	3516	3630	3747	3869	3994	4124	4257
6.4	2362	2437	2515	2595	2678	2764	2852	2943	3037	3134	3235	3338	3445	3555	3668	3785	3906	4031	4160	4293
6.5	2401	2477	2555	2635	2718	2804	2892	2983	3077	3174	3274	3378	3484	3594	3707	3824	3944	4069	4197	4329
6.6	2441	2517	2595	2675	2759	2844	2933	3024	3118	3215	3315	3418	3524	3633	3746	3863	3983	4106	4234	4366
6.7	2481	2557	2636	2716	2800	2885	2974	3065	3159	3256	3355	3458	3564	3673	3786	3902	4021	4144	4271	4402
6.8	2523	2599	2677	2758	2841	2927	3016	3107	3200	3297	3397	3499	3605	3714	3826	3941	4060	4183	4309	4439
6.9	2564	2641	2719	2800	2884	2969	3058	3149	3242	3339	3438	3541	3646	3754	3866	3981	4100	4222	4347	4477
7.0	2607	2683	2762	2843	2927	3012	3101	3192	3285	3381	3481	3583	3688	3796	3907	4022	4140	4261	4386	4514
7.1	2650	2727	2806	2887	2970	3056	3144	3235	3328	3424	3523	3625	3730	3838	3948	4062	4180	4300	4425	4552
7.2	2694	2771	2850	2931	3014	3100	3188	3279	3372	3468	3567	3668	3772	3880	3990	4104	4220	4340	4464	4591
7.3	2739	2816	2895	2976	3059	3145	3233	3323	3416	3512	3610	3712	3816	3922	4032	4145	4261	4381	4503	4629
7.4	2785	2861	2940	3021	3105	3190	3278	3369	3461	3557	3655	3756	3859	3966	4075	4187	4303	4421	4543	4668
7.5	2831	2908	2987	3068	3151	3236	3324	3414	3507	3602	3700	3800	3903	4009	4118	4230	4344	4462	4583	4708
7.6	2878	2955	3034	3115	3198	3283	3371	3461	3553	3648	3745	3845	3948	4053	4161	4272	4387	4504	4624	4747
7.7	2926	3003	3081	3162	3245	3331	3418	3508	3600	3694	3789	3891	3993	4098	4205	4316	4429	4545	4665	4787
7.8	2974	3051	3130	3211	3294	3379	3466	3555	3647	3741	3838	3937	4039	4143	4250	4360	4472	4588	4706	4827
7.9	3024	3100	3179	3260	3343	3427	3514	3604	3695	3789	3885	3984	4085	4188	4295	4404	4515	4630	4748	4868
8.0	3074	3151	3229	3310	3392	3477	3564	3653	3744	3837	3933	4031	4131	4234	4340	4448	4559	4673	4790	4909
8.1	3125	3202	3280	3360	3443	3527	3614	3702	3793	3886	3981	4079	4179	4281	4386	4493	4604	4716	4832	4950
8.2	3177	3253	3332	3412	3494	3578	3664	3752	3843	3935	4030	4127	4226	4328	4432	4539	4648	4760	4875	4992
8.3	3230	3306	3384	3464	3546	3630	3716	3803	3893	3985	4080	4176	4275	4376	4479	4585	4693	4804	4918	5034

*From Hadlock FP, Harrist RB, Carpenter RJ, et al: Sonographic estimation of fetal weight. Radiology 1984; 150:535–540. Used by permission.

TABLE A–7.

Clavicle Length as Obtained From Gestational Age*

Gestational Age (wk)	Clavicle Length (mm)† Percentile		
	5th	50th	95th
15	11	16	21
16	12	17	22
17	13	18	23
18	14	19	24
19	15	20	25
20	16	21	26
21	17	22	27
22	18	23	28
23	19	24	29
24	20	25	30
25	21	26	31
26	22	27	32
27	23	28	33
28	24	29	34
29	25	30	35
30	26	31	36
31	27	32	37
32	28	33	38
33	29	34	39
34	30	35	40
35	31	36	41
36	32	37	42
37	33	38	43
38	34	39	44
39	35	40	45
40	36	41	46

*From Yarkoni S, Schmidt W, Jeanty P, et al: Clavicle measurement: A new biometric parameter for fetal evaluation. J Ultrasound Med 1985 4:467–470. Used by permission.

†Clavicle length = 1.118303 + 0.9788639 (gestational age); r^2 = 0.807; standard deviation = 2.92 mm

TABLE A–8.

Calculated Fetal Lengths† Based on Femur Length*

Ultrasound Femur Length (mm)	Mean Fetal Length (cm)	SE (cm)	Fifth Percentile (cm)	95th Percentile (cm)
30	23.880	.636	22.634	25.126
31	24.470	.616	23.262	25.677
32	25.060	.596	23.892	26.228
33	25.650	.576	24.521	26.779
34	26.240	.556	25.150	27.330
35	26.830	.536	25.779	27.881
36	27.420	.517	26.407	28.433
37	28.010	.497	27.035	28.985
38	28.600	.478	27.664	29.536
39	29.190	.458	28.292	30.088
40	29.780	.439	28.919	30.641
41	30.370	.420	29.547	31.193
42	30.960	.401	30.174	31.746
43	31.550	.382	30.801	32.299
44	32.140	.364	31.427	32.853

TABLE A-8 (cont.).

Ultrasound Femur Length (mm)	Mean Fetal Length (cm)	SE (cm)	Fifth Percentile (cm)	95th Percentile (cm)
45	32.730	.345	32.053	33.407
46	33.320	.327	32.679	33.961
47	33.910	.309	33.304	34.516
48	34.500	.292	33.928	35.072
49	35.090	.275	34.551	35.629
50	35.680	.258	35.173	36.187
51	36.270	.243	35.794	36.746
52	36.860	.228	36.414	37.306
53	37.450	.214	37.031	37.869
54	38.040	.201	37.646	38.434
55	38.630	.189	38.259	39.001
56	39.220	.179	38.868	39.572
57	39.810	.171	39.474	40.146
58	40.400	.166	40.075	40.725
59	40.990	.162	40.672	41.308
60	41.580	.162	41.263	41.897
61	42.170	.164	41.849	42.491
62	42.760	.168	42.431	43.089
63	43.350	.175	43.007	43.693
64	43.940	.184	43.580	44.300
65	44.530	.194	44.149	44.911
66	45.120	.207	44.715	45.525
67	45.710	.220	45.279	46.141
68	46.300	.235	45.840	46.760
69	46.890	.250	46.400	47.380
70	47.480	.266	46.959	48.001
71	48.070	.283	47.516	48.624
72	48.660	.300	48.072	49.248
73	49.250	.317	48.628	49.872
74	49.840	.335	49.183	50.497
75	50.430	.354	49.737	51.123
76	51.020	.372	50.291	51.749
77	51.610	.391	50.844	52.376
78	52.200	.410	51.397	53.003
79	52.790	.429	51.950	53.630
80	53.380	.448	52.502	54.258
81	53.970	.467	53.054	54.886
82	54.560	.487	53.606	55.514
83	55.150	.506	54.158	56.142
84	55.740	.526	54.709	56.771
85	56.330	.546	55.261	57.399
86	56.920	.565	55.812	58.028
87	57.510	.585	56.363	58.657
88	58.100	.605	56.914	59.286
89	58.690	.625	57.465	59.915
90	59.280	.645	58.016	60.544

*From Vintzileos AM, Campbell WA, Neckles S, et al: The ultrasound femur length as a predictor of fetal length. Obstet Gynecol 1984; 64:779–782. Used by permission.
†Confidence intervals and SE based on the regression line. SE = standard error of the mean.

TABLE A–9.

Predicted Foot Length at Different Gestational Ages*†

Gestational Age (wk)	−2 SD (mm)	Predicted Value (mm)	+2 SD (mm)
12	7	8	9
13	10	11	12
14	13	15	16
15	16	18	20
16	19	21	23
17	22	24	27
18	24	27	30
19	27	30	34
20	30	33	37
21	32	36	40
22	35	39	43
23	37	42	46
24	40	45	50
25	42	47	53
26	45	50	55
27	47	53	58
28	49	55	61
29	51	58	64
30	54	60	67
31	56	62	68
32	58	65	72
33	60	67	74
34	62	69	77
35	64	71	79
36	66	74	82
37	67	76	84
38	69	78	86
39	71	80	88
40	72	81	90

*From Mercer BM, Sklar S, Shariatmader A, et al: Fetal foot length as a predictor of gestational age. Am J Obstet Gynecol 1987; 156:350–355. Used by permission.
†Predicted foot length based upon polynomial regression ±2 standard deviations.

TABLE A–10.

Normal Length of the Fetal Kidneys at Different Gestational Ages*

Menstrual Age (wk)	−2 SD‡ (mm)	Predicted Value† (mm)	+2 SD‡ (mm)
24	22.0	24.5	27.0
25	22.6	25.1	27.7
26	23.3	25.8	28.3
27	24.0	26.5	29.0
28	24.7	27.2	29.8
29	25.5	28.0	30.5
30	26.3	28.8	31.3
31	27.1	29.6	32.1
32	27.9	30.4	32.9
33	28.8	31.3	33.8
34	29.6	32.2	34.7
35	30.5	33.1	35.6
36	31.5	34.0	36.5
37	32.4	35.0	37.5
38	33.4	36.0	38.5
39	34.5	37.0	39.5
40	35.5	38.0	40.5
41	36.6	39.1	41.6
42	37.7	40.2	42.7

*From Bertagnoli L, Lalatta F, Gallicchio R, et al: Quantitative characterization of growth of the fetal kidney. J Clin Ultrasound 1983; 11:349–356. Used by permission.
†Length = 16.8933 + 0.0132 (menstrual age)^2.
‡Standard deviation = 1.259 mm.

TABLE A–11.

Normal Anterior-Posterior Diameter of the Fetal Kidneys at Different Gestational Ages*

Menstrual Age (wk)	−2 SD‡ (mm)	Predicted Value† (mm)	+2 SD‡ (mm)
22	8.9	11.3	13.7
23	9.3	11.7	14.1
24	9.7	12.1	14.5
25	10.2	12.6	15.0
26	10.7	13.1	15.5
27	11.3	13.7	16.1
28	11.9	14.3	16.7
29	12.5	15.0	17.4
30	13.2	15.6	18.0
31	14.0	16.4	18.8
32	14.8	17.2	19.6
33	15.6	18.0	20.4
34	16.5	18.9	21.3
35	17.5	19.9	22.3
36	18.5	20.9	23.3
37	19.5	21.9	24.4
38	20.7	23.1	25.5
39	21.8	24.3	26.7
40	23.1	25.5	27.9

*From Bertagnoli L, Lalatta F, Gallacio R, et al: Quantitative characterization of growth of the fetal kidney. J Clin Ultrasound 1983; 11:349–356. Used by permission.
†Predicted value = 8.457278951 + .00026630314 (menstrual age)^3.
‡Standard deviation (SD) = 1.209

APPENDIX B

Commonly Recognized Syndromes

Achondrogenesis
Inheritance: autosomal recessive.
Primary features: skeletal dysplasia with severe limb shortening, often with decreased skeletal ossification, especially of the vertebral bodies.

Achondroplasia
Inheritance: 80% spontaneous mutations; autosomal dominant.
Primary features: moderate rhizomelia, relatively large calvarium with small skull base, absent nasal bridge, thoracolumbar kyphosis with lack of caudal increase in interpedicular distance, trident hands, squared iliac ala.

Acrocallosal syndrome
Inheritance: autosomal recessive.
Primary features: macrocephaly, hypertelorism, polydactyly, mental retardation, agenesis of the corpus callosum, postaxial polydactyly of feet, as well as hallucal duplication.

Adrenogenital syndrome
Inheritance: mutant gene; autosomal recessive trait for 21-hydroxylase deficiency.
Primary features: virilization, ambiguous genitalia.

Amniotic band syndrome
Inheritance: sporadic.
Primary features: variable deformities, often including constriction rings, extremity amputations or lymphedema, bizarre facial clefts, large abdominal wall or chest wall defects, and asymmetric encephaloceles.

Apert's syndrome
Inheritance: autosomal dominant, many cases new mutations.
Primary features: coronal craniosynostosis, acrocephaly, beaked nose, hypertelorism, hydrocephalus, syndactyly.

Asphyxiating thoracic dysplasia (Jeune's syndrome)
Inheritance: autosomal recessive.
Primary features: skeletal dysplasia with mild-to-moderate rhizomelic shortening and small thorax; renal dysplasia; polydactyly (14%).

Basal cell nevus syndrome
Inheritance: autosomal dominant.
Primary features: macrocephaly, facial cleft, calcification of falx cerebri, skin changes after birth.

Beckwith-Wiedemann syndrome
Inheritance: probably autosomal dominant with variable expressivity.
Primary features: omphalocele or umbilical hernia, macroglossia, visceromegaly, neonatal hypoglycemia, ear crease, hemihypertrophy, Wilms tumor.

Bloom syndrome
Inheritance: autosomal recessive.
Primary features: immunodeficiency, low birthweight, photosensitive rash after birth, increased rate of sister chromatid exchange.

Campomelic dysplasia
Inheritance: mostly sporadic, occasionally autosomal recessive.
Primary features: ventral bowing of the tibiae and femora, talipes equinovarus, absent or hypoplastic fibulae and scapulae.

Cenani-Lenz syndrome
Inheritance: autosomal recessive.
Primary features: severe mesomelic dwarfism with complete syndactyly, fusion of radius and ulna.

Cerebro-hepato-renal syndrome of Zellweger
(See Zellweger syndrome.)

CHARGE association
Inheritance: unknown, mostly sporadic.
Primary features: **C**olobomatous malformations, **H**eart defects, **A**tresia of the choanae, **R**etarded growth or mental development, **G**enital anomalies, and **E**ar anomalies.

Chondrodysplasia punctata—rhizomelic type
Inheritance: autosomal recessive.
Primary features: severe micromelia, especially of the humeri, and femora with stippled epiphyses.

Chondroectodermal dysplasia (Ellis-van Creveld syndrome)
Inheritance: autosomal recessive.
Primary features: heart defects (especially atrial septal defects), polydactyly, distal limb shortening, narrow chest.

Cleidocranial dysplasia
Inheritance: autosomal dominant or spontaneous mutation.
Primary features: partial or total aplasia of the clavicles, brachycephaly.

Crouzon syndrome (craniofacial dysostosis)
Inheritance: autosomal dominant.
Primary features: brachycephaly, prominent forehead, proptosis, mid-face hypoplasia, beaked nose, short upper lip.

Cystic fibrosis
Inheritance: autosomal recessive.
Primary features: electrolyte and mucous disturbances, meconium ileus, pancreatic insufficiency, recurrent respiratory infections after birth.

De Lange's syndrome
Inheritance: autosomal dominant.
Primary features: microcephaly, low birthweight, characteristic facial features, cleft palate, micrognathia, dysplastic kidneys, cardiac malformations, genital anomalies.

Diastrophic dysplasia
Inheritance: autosomal recessive.
Primary features: skeletal dysplasia with micromelia, "hitchhiker thumb," talipes, micrognathia, cleft palate.

DiGeorge syndrome
Inheritance: mostly sporadic.
Primary features: cellular immunodeficiency, hypoparathyroidism, cardiac defects including defects of aortic arch.

Ectrodactyly-ectodermal dysplasia-clefting syndrome
Inheritance: autosomal dominant.
Primary features: cleft lip +/− cleft palate, maxillary hypoplasia, syndactyly or absence of fingers.

Ehlers-Danlos syndromes
Inheritance: variable.
Primary features: subluxation and dislocation of joints, delayed calvarial ossification, kyphoscoliosis.

Ellis-Van Creveld syndrome
(see chondroectodermal dysplasia)

Fanconi anemia
Inheritance: autosomal recessive.
Primary features: abnormal chromosomal breakage, low birthweight, hypoplasia of thumb or radius, pancytopenia after birth.

Fragile X syndrome
(See Martin-Bell syndrome.)

Fryns syndrome
Inheritance: autosomal recessive.
Primary features: central nervous system anomalies, microphthalmia, facial anomalies, pulmonary hypoplasia/abnormal lobation, diaphragmatic defects, kidney cysts, and distal limb anomalies.

Goldenhar-Gorlin syndrome
Inheritance: mostly sporadic.
Primary features: asymmetric abnormalities common including hypoplasia of maxilla and mandible, microphthalmia or anophthalmia dysplastic ears, epibul-

bar dermoid of eye, coloboma, vertebral defects, cardiac malformations, renal anomalies.

Holt-Oram syndrome
Inheritance: autosomal dominant.
Primary features: cardiac malformations, radial defects of upper extremities.

Hydrolethalus syndrome
Inheritance: autosomal recessive.
Primary features: hydrocephalus, polyhydramnios, micrognathia, polydactyly (postaxial of hands, preaxial of feet), abnormal lobulation of lungs, cleft palate, heart defect in over half, clubfoot in over half. Differential diagnosis includes Meckel syndrome (includes polycystic kidneys), and Smith-Lemli-Opitz syndrome (pancreatic giant cells).

Hypophosphatasia (congenita)
Inheritance: autosomal recessive.
Primary features: moderate-to-severe extremity bone shortening, diffuse hypomineralization.

Infantile polycystic kidney disease
Inheritance: autosomal recessive.
Primary features: enlarged and echogenic kidneys, often with innumerable tiny cysts, oligohydramnios, hepatic fibrosis.

Ivemark syndrome
Inheritance: mostly sporadic.
Primary features: cardiosplenic syndrome resulting in asplenia syndrome (bilateral left sidedness) or polysplenia syndrome (bilateral right sidedness). Asplenia syndrome includes asplenia, situs inversus, complex heart defects, atrial isomerism, heart block, bilateral trilobed lungs; polysplenia syndrome includes polysplenia, heart defects, bilateral bilobed lungs.

Jarcho-Levin syndrome (spondylothoracic dysplasia, spondylocostal dysplasia)
Inheritance: autosomal recessive.
Primary features: bone dysplasia with vertebral and rib anomalies, small thorax.

Jeune's syndrome
(See asphyxiating thoracic dysplasia.)

Kaufman-McKusick syndrome
Inheritance: autosomal recessive.
Primary features: vaginal atresia or duplication, hydrometrocolpos, other genitourinary anomalies, anorectal atresia, cardiac defects, polydactyly.

Klippel-Trenaunay-Weber syndrome
Inheritance: mostly sporadic.
Primary features: hypertrophy of limbs, hemihypertrophy, hemangioma of skin.

Kneist dysplasia
Inheritance: probably autosomal dominant.
Primary features: mild-to-moderate micromelia with metaphyseal and epiphyseal splaying, kyphoscoliosis, platyspondyly.

Larsen's syndrome
Inheritance: sporadic.
Primary features: multiple dislocations of large joints, talipes, abnormal vertebral segmentation with kyphoscoliosis, hypertelorism, depressed nasal bringe, micrognathia, prominent forehead.

Laurence-Moon-Bardett-Biedl syndrome
Inheritance: variable, autosomal recessive.
Primary features: polydactyly, genitourinary anomalies.

Lenz's syndrome
Inheritance: X-linked.
Primary features: microphthalmos or anophthalmos, microcephaly, renal dysgenesis.

Limb-body wall complex
Inheritance: sporadic.
Primary features: severe kyphoscoliosis, thoracoabdominalschisis, neural tube defects, bizarre facial clefts, absent extremities, positional deformities.

Marden-Walker syndrome
Inheritance: probably autosomal recessive.
Primary features: micrognathia, hypertelorism, low-set ears, small mouth, multiple joint contractures, renal cysts.

Marfan syndrome
Inheritance: autosomal dominant.
Primary features: tall stature, high arched palate, aortic and mitral valve insufficiency after birth.

Martin-Bell syndrome (fragile X syndrome)
Inheritance: X linked.
Primary features: second only to Down's syndrome in its contribution to mental retardation in males, it is due to fragile site on X chromosome at Xq28 with a frequency of 1:000 to 1:1500 in males. Since culture of

amniotic fluid leads to uncertain expression or mitotic index, fetal blood remains the only reliable method for diagnosis.

Meckel-Gruber syndrome

Inheritance: autosomal recessive.

Primary features: cystic kidneys a constant feature plus occipital encephalocele and/or polydactyly (postaxial). Other features include microcephaly, microphthalmia, cleft palate, genitourinary anomalies.

Megacystis-microcolon-hypoperistalsis syndrome

Inheritance: autosomal recessive.

Primary features: dilated bladder, hydronephrosis, microcolon, dilated proximal duodenum. Most common in females.

Metatropic dysplasia

Inheritance: autosomal recessive.

Primary features: micromelia with marked metaphyseal flaring, narrow thorax but relatively long trunk, progressive kyphoscoliosis.

Mohr Syndrome

(See oro-facial-digital syndrome II.)

Nager acrofacial dysostosis

Inheritance: usually sporadic.

Primary features: micrognathia, deformed external ears, upper extremity anomalies.

Neu-Laxova syndrome

Inheritance: autosomal recessive.

Primary features: central nervous system anomalies including agenesis of the corpus callosum and lissencephaly, microcephaly, sloped forehead, hypertelorism, micrognathia, flat nose, flexion deformities, overlapping fingers.

Noonan's syndrome

Inheritance: probable autosomal dominant.

Primary features: short stature, webbed neck, lymphedema (including cystic hygromas, hydrops, and pulmonary lymphangiectasis), facial anomalies, congenital heart defects, and mental retardation.

Opitz-G syndrome

Inheritance: probable autosomal dominant, penetrance greater for males.

Primary features: hypertelorism, dolicocephaly, facial abnormalities, micrognathia, cleft lip or palate, esoph-

ageal dysfunction, hydrops, cardiovascular anomalies (VSD, ASD, coarctation of aorta), mild mental retardation in 60%.

Oro-facial-digital syndrome I

Inheritance: X-linked dominant.

Primary features: hydrocephalus, brain malformations including porencephaly, cleft palate, polydactyly of feet, buccal-alveolar webbing and facial milia, mental retardation. Lethal in males.

Oro-facial-digital syndrome II (Mohr syndrome)

Inheritance: autosomal recessive.

Primary features: cleft lip and palate, lobate tongue, dental abnormalities, hypoplasia of mandible, bilateral polydactyly of hands and feet (preaxial), conductive hearing deficit.

Osteopetrosis congenita

Inheritance: autosomal recessive.

Primary features: Hepatosplenomegaly, anemia or pancytopenia, thick and dense bones.

Pallister-Hall syndrome

Inheritance: autosomal recessive.

Primary features: hypothalamic hamartoblastoma.

Pena-Shokeir phenotype (fetal akinesia/hypokinesia sequence)

Inheritance: mostly sporadic, some cases autosomal recessive.

Primary features: phenotype caused by various conditions leading to reduced fetal movement. Features include intrauterine growth retardation, craniofacial anomalies (hypertelorism, micrognathia, cleft palate, short neck), limb anomalies (contractures, hypoplasia, occasional pterygia), pulmonary hypoplasia, short umbilical cord, and polyhydramnios. Differential diagnosis includes cerebro-ocular-facial syndrome, Neu-Laxova syndrome, lethal multiple pterygium syndromes, and trisomy 18.

Pierre-Robin syndrome

Inheritance: sporadic.

Primary features: micrognathia, cleft palate, glossoptosis.

Popliteal pterygium syndrome

Inheritance: mostly sporadic, autosomal dominant.

Primary features: contractures with webbing of popliteal regions, cleft lip and palate, syndactyly, talipes equinovarus.

Radial aplasia-thrombocytopenia (TAR) syndrome
Inheritance: autosomal recessive.
Primary features: radial aplasia, lower extremity defects, thrombocytopenia, and cardiac defects.

Roberts' syndrome
Inheritance: autosomal recessive.
Primary features: severe micromelia with most severe defects appearing as phocomelia (pseudo-thalidomide syndrome). Other features include facial cleft, cardiac defects, and genitourinary anomalies. Karyotyping shows characteristic abnormalities of centromere.

Rubenstein-Taybi syndrome
Inheritance: mostly sporadic.
Primary features: microcephaly, beaked nose, glaucoma, mental retardation, cardiac defects, broad thumb, or big nose.

Short-rib polydactyly syndrome
Inheritance: autosomal recessive.
Primary features: micromelia, narrow thorax with short ribs, polydactyly, renal dysplasia.

Smith-Lemli-Opitz syndrome
Inheritance: autosomal recessive.
Primary features: microcephaly, hydrocephalus, cerebellar hypoplasia, cardiac anomalies, genital anomalies, facial anomalies including incomplete cleft palate, facial capillary hemangioma and micrognathia, polydactyly in severe form. Differential diagnosis includes Meckel-Gruber syndrome, hydrolethalus syndrome, or Pallister-Hall syndrome.

Spondyloepiphyseal dysplasia congenita
Inheritance: autosomal dominant.
Primary features: shortened and mildly bowed femora, short trunk, micrognathia.

Stickler syndrome
Inheritance: autosomal dominant.
Primary features: cataracts, myopia, micrognathia, scoliosis.

Thanatophoric dysplasia
Inheritance: sporadic.
Primary features: skeletal dysplasia with severe micromelia, cloverleaf skull, platyspondyly, narrow spinal canal.

Thrombocytopenia-absent radius syndrome
(See radial aplasia-thrombocytopenia syndrome.)

Treacher-Collins syndrome
Inheritance: mostly autosomal dominant.
Primary features: deafness, malformed ears, malar and mandibular hypoplasia, cleft palate.

Tuberous sclerosis
Inheritance: autosomal dominant.
Primary features: intracranial calcifications, mental retardation, seizures, renal cysts, renal tumors (angiomyolipomas), cardiac tumors (rhabdomyoma), depigmented skin lesions.

Twin transfusion syndrome
Inheritance: sporadic.
Primary features: growth-retarded twin with large, hydropic co-twin.

VACTERL (VATER) association
Inheritance: sporadic.
Primary features: VACTERL is association of **V**ertebral anomalies, **A**norectal atresia, **C**ardiac defects, **T**racheo-**E**sophageal fistula, **R**enal anomalies, and **L**imb anomalies.

Von Hipple-Lindau syndrome
Inheritance: autosomal dominant.
Primary features: ocular and cerebellar hemangiomata, tumors of kidneys, pancreas.

Walker-Warburg syndrome
Inheritance: autosomal recessive.
Primary features: encephalocele, agenesis of midline brain structures, lissencephaly, hydrocephalus, eye abnormalities.

Williams syndrome
Inheritance: autosomal dominant.
Primary features: cardiac defects, especially supravalvular aortic stenosis, elfin like face.

Zellweger syndrome
Inheritance: autosomal recessive.
Primary features: hypotonicity, limb contractures, seizures, calcified epiphyses especially patella. Underlying defect is error in fatty acid metabolism.

Index